AF669450

101 Medical Autopsy Cases
Adult and Pediatric

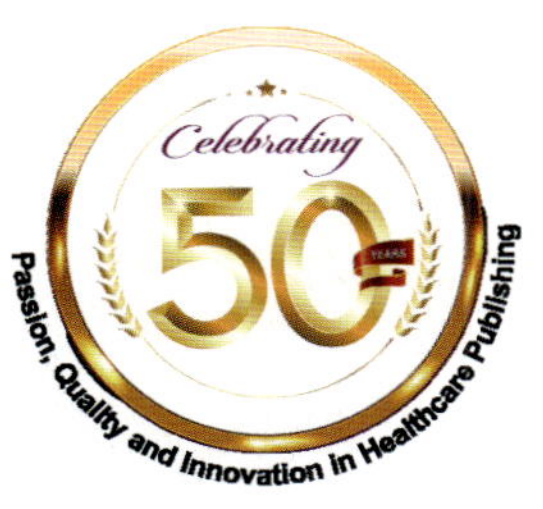

101 Medical Autopsy Cases Adult and Pediatric

(With Complete Pathological/Clinical Details and Review of Literature)

Editor

Nandita Bharadwaj Kakkar MD FICPath
Professor
Department of Histopathology
Post Graduate Institute of Medical Education and Research
Chandigarh, India

Foreword

Vinay Kumar MBBS MD FRCPath

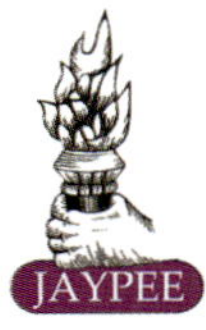

JAYPEE BROTHERS MEDICAL PUBLISHERS
The Health Sciences Publisher
New Delhi | London | Panama

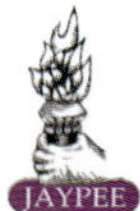

Jaypee Brothers Medical Publishers (P) Ltd

Headquarters

Jaypee Brothers Medical Publishers (P) Ltd
4838/24, Ansari Road, Daryaganj
New Delhi 110 002, India
Phone: +91-11-43574357
Fax: +91-11-43574314
E-mail: jaypee@jaypeebrothers.com

Overseas Offices

J P Medical Ltd
83 Victoria Street, London
SW1H 0HW (UK)
Phone: +44 20 3170 8910
Fax: +44 (0)20 3008 6180
E-mail: info@jpmedpub.com

Jaypee-Highlights Medical Publishers Inc
City of Knowledge, Bld. 235, 2nd Floor, Clayton
Panama City, Panama
Phone: +1 507-301-0496
Fax: +1 507-301-0499
E-mail: cservice@jphmedical.com

Jaypee Brothers Medical Publishers (P) Ltd
Bhotahity, Kathmandu, Nepal
Phone: +977-9741283608
Email: kathmandu@jaypeebrothers.com

Website: www.jaypeebrothers.com
Website: www.jaypeedigital.com

101 Medical Autopsy Cases: Adult and Pediatric

First Edition: **2019**

ISBN: 978-93-5270-612-9

Printed at Replika Press Pvt. Ltd.

OM SAI RAM

Dedicated to

All the 101 Cadavers on whom medical autopsies were performed and who paved the way to this wealth of knowledge
The Almighty
My Angels
Late Pandit Shanti Parkash and Raj Rani Bharadwaj
Late Amolak and Kamla Malhotra
My mother, (Late) Mrs Meena Bharadwaj
My mother-in-law, (Late) Mrs Sneh Kakkar
My father-in-law, Mr BR Kakkar (IAS Retd)
My husband, Dr Niraj Kakkar,
My daughters, Dr Aaina and Dr Apsara
and

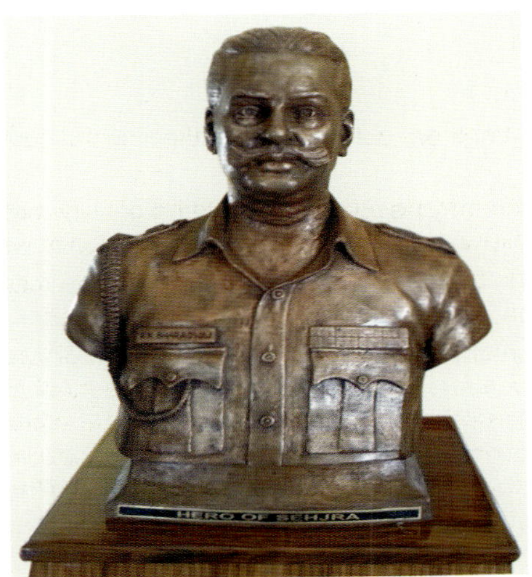

My father, Late Col RK Bharadwaj—'The Hero of Sehjra'

Contributors

AK Banerjee
Ex-Professor and Head
Department of Histopathology
PGIMER, Chandigarh, India

Akshay Kumar
Professor
Department of Radiodiagnosis and Imaging
PGIMER, Chandigarh, India

Anand Bardia
Junior Resident
Department of Pathology
PGIMER, Chandigarh, India

Anil Narang
Ex-Professor and Head
Department of Pediatrics
PGIMER, Chandigarh, India

Anupam Lal
Professor
Department of Radiodiagnosis and Imaging
PGIMER, Chandigarh, India

Aparna Mishra
Junior Resident
Department of Pediatrics
PGIMER, Chandigarh, India

Archana KS
Senior Resident
Department of Pathology
PGIMER, Chandigarh, India

Arun Bansal
Professor
Department of Pediatrics
PGIMER, Chandigarh, India

Arun Baranwal
Professor
Department of Pediatrics
PGIMER, Chandigarh, India

Arun Kumar
Junior Resident
Department of Pathology
PGIMER, Chandigarh, India

Aseem Bassha M
Junior Resident
Department of Pediatrics
PGIMER, Chandigarh, India

Ashim Das
Professor
Department of Histopathology
PGIMER, Chandigarh, India

Ashish Agarwal
Junior Resident
Department of Pediatrics
PGIMER, Chandigarh, India

Ashish Bhalla
Professor
Department of Internal Medicine
PGIMER, Chandigarh, India

Ashish Jain
Associate Professor
Department of Transfusion Medicine
PGIMER, Chandigarh, India

Baijayantimala Mishra
Department of Virology
PGIMER, Chandigarh, India

BD Radotra
Professor
Department of Histopathology
PGIMER, Chandigarh, India

Biman Saikia
Professor
Department of Immunopathology
PGIMER, Chandigarh, India

Bhavneet Bharti
Professor
Department of Pediatrics
PGIMER, Chandigarh, India

BR Thapa
Professor and Head
Department of Gastroenterology
PGIMER, Chandigarh, India

Charan Singh Rayat
Tutor
Department of Histopathology
(Electron Microscopy)
PGIMER, Chandigarh, India

Charan Singh
Technical Assistant
Department of Histopathology
PGIMER, Chandigarh, India

Debasish Sahoo
Junior Resident
Department of Pediatrics
PGIMER, Chandigarh, India

Deepak Bansal
Professor
Department of Pediatrics
PGIMER, Chandigarh, India

Deepak Bhasin
Ex-Professor and Head
Department of Gastroenterology
PGIMER, Chandigarh, India

Devi Dayal
Professor
Department of Pediatrics
PGIMER, Chandigarh, India

Dhananjay Zutshi
Professor
Department of Internal Medicine
PGIMER, Chandigarh, India

*PGIMER: Post Graduate Institute of Medical Education and Research

Dhiraj Khurana
Professor
Department of Neurology
PGIMER, Chandigarh, India

Gaurav Garg
Junior Resident
Department of Pathology
PGIMER, Chandigarh, India

Gaurav Prakash
Additional Professor
Department of Internal Medicine
PGIMER, Chandigarh, India

Gunasekaran Singh
Junior Resident
Department of Internal Medicine
PGIMER, Chandigarh, India

Gurpreet Singh
Laboratory Technician
Immunohistochemistry
Department of Histopathology
PGIMER, Chandigarh, India

Gurpreet Singh
Professor and Head
Department of Surgery
PGIMER, Chandigarh, India

Gurwinder Kaur
Senior Resident
Department of Pathology
PGIMER, Chandigarh, India

Jashan Sandhu
Senior Resident
Department of Pathology
PGIMER, Chandigarh, India

Jasmina Ahluwalia
Professor
Department of Hematology
PGIMER, Chandigarh, India

Jasmine Kaur
Senior Resident
Department of Radiodiagnosis and Imaging
PGIMER, Chandigarh, India

Jawaharlal G
Junior Resident
Department of Internal Medicine
PGIMER, Chandigarh, India

Jayshree M
Professor
Department of Pediatrics
PGIMER, Chandigarh, India

JK Mahajan
Professor
Department of Pediatric Surgery
PGIMER, Chandigarh, India

JL Mathew
Professor
Department of Pediatrics
PGIMER, Chandigarh, India

Kanya Mukhopadhyay
Professor
Department of Pediatrics
(Neonatology Division)
PGIMER, Chandigarh, India

Kartar Singh
Ex-Professor and Head
Department of Gastroenterology
PGIMER, Chandigarh, India

Karthi N
Additional Professor
Department of Pediatrics
PGIMER, Chandigarh, India

Khushboo
Junior Resident
Department of Pathology
PGIMER, Chandigarh, India

KL Gupta
Professor and Head
Department of Nephrology
PGIMER, Chandigarh, India

KS Sodhi
Professor
Department of Radiodiagnosis and Imaging
PGIMER, Chandigarh, India

Kumar Sangam
Junior Resident
Department of Pathology
PGIMER, Chandigarh, India

Kunal Sehgal
Junior Resident
Department of Pathology
PGIMER, Chandigarh, India

Kusum Joshi
Ex-Professor and Head
Department of Histopathology
PGIMER, Chandigarh, India

Kusum Sharma
Professor
Department of Medical Microbiology
PGIMER, Chandigarh, India

Late RK Marwaha
Professor
Department of Pediatrics
PGIMER, Chandigarh, India

Late SD Deodhar
Professor
Department of Internal Medicine
PGIMER, Chandigarh, India

L Dhaliwal
Ex-Professor and Head
Department of Obstetrics and Gynaecology
PGIMER, Chandigarh, India

Madhusudhan
Junior Resident
Department of Pathology
PGIMER, Chandigarh, India

Mandeep Walia
Assistant Professor
Department of Pediatrics
PGIMER, Chandigarh, India

Man Updesh Singh Sachdeva
Additional Professor
Department of Hematology
PGIMER, Chandigarh, India

Manjay Singh
Junior Resident
Department of Pediatrics
PGIMER, Chandigarh, India

Manphool Singhal
Additional Professor
Department of Radiodiagnosis and Imaging
PGIMER, Chandigarh, India

Meenu Singh
Professor
Department of Pediatrics
PGIMER, Chandigarh, India

Mini P Singh
Professor
Department of Virology
PGIMER, Chandigarh, India

Mukin Kumar S
Junior Resident
Department of Pathology
PGIMER, Chandigarh, India

Nandita Bhardwaj Kakkar
Professor
Department of Histopathology
PGIMER, Chandigarh, India

Narender Kumar
Assistant Professor
Department of Hematology
PGIMER, Chandigarh, India

Narendra Dhaka
Assistant Professor
Department of Gastroenterology
PGIMER, Chandigarh, India

Naveen Kalra
Professor
Department of Radiodiagnosis and Imaging
PGIMER, Chandigarh, India

Navneet Sharma
Professor
Department of Internal Medicine
PGIMER, Chandigarh, India

Neelam Chaudhary
Department of Obstetrics and Gynecology
PGIMER, Chandigarh, India

Neelam Varma
Professor and Head
Department of Hematology
PGIMER, Chandigarh, India

Niranjan Khaire
Junior Resident
Department of Internal Medicine
PGIMER, Chandigarh, India

NK Khandelwal
Professor and Head
Department of Radiodiagnosis and Imaging
PGIMER, Chandigarh, India

Pankaj C Vaidya
Professor
Department of Pediatrics
PGIMER, Chandigarh, India

Pankaj Kaul
Tutor
Department of Histopathology
PGIMER, Chandigarh, India

Pankaj Malhotra
Professor
Department of Internal Medicine
PGIMER, Chandigarh, India

Parimal Agrawal
Senior Resident
Department of Pathology
PGIMER, Chandigarh, India

Parminder S Otaal
Assistant Professor
Department of Cardiology
PGIMER, Chandigarh, India

Pavithra HN
Junior Resident
Department of Pathology
PGIMER, Chandigarh, India

Prasanna Kumar
Junior Resident
Department of Internal Medicine
PGIMER, Chandigarh, India

Pranjali Vasisht
Fellow-PDCC (Pediatric Pathology)
Department of Histopathology
PGIMER, Chandigarh, India

Praveen Kumar
Professor and Head
Department of Pediatrics
PGIMER, Chandigarh, India

Pulkit Rastogi
Assistant Professor
Department of Histopathology
PGIMER, Chandigarh, India

R Nithiyanandan
Junior Resident
Department of Internal Medicine
PGIMER, Chandigarh, India

Rajesh Vijayvergiya
Professor
Department of Cardiology
PGIMER, Chandigarh, India

Rajindra Prasad
Ex-Professor and Head
Department of Biochemistry
PGIMER, Chandigarh, India

Rakesh Kumar
Associate Professor
Department of Pediatrics
PGIMER, Chandigarh, India

Ramandeep Singh
Department of Biochemistry
PGIMER, Chandigarh, India

Ranjana Minz
Professor and Head
Department of Immunopathology
PGIMER, Chandigarh, India

Reena Das
Professor
Department of Hematology
PGIMER, Chandigarh, India

Renu Suthar
Assistant Professor
Department of Pediatrics
PGIMER, Chandigarh, India

Richa Jain
Assistant Professor
Department of Pediatrics
(Hematology Oncology Division)
PGIMER, Chandigarh, India

Rimesh Pal
Junior Resident
Department of Internal Medicine
PGIMER, Chandigarh, India

RJ Dash
Ex-Professor and Head
Department of Endocrinology
PGIMER, Chandigarh, India

RK Dhiman
Professor and Head
Department of Hepatology
PGIMER, Chandigarh, India

RK Kochhar
Professor and Head
Department of Gastroenterology
PGIMER, Chandigarh, India

RK Vasishta
Professor and Head
Department of Histopathology
PGIMER, Chandigarh, India

Rohit Bhowmick
Junior Resident
Department of Pediatrics
PGIMER, Chandigarh, India

S Reddy
Additional Professor
Department of Cardiology
PGIMER, Chandigarh, India

S Singhi
Ex-Professor and Head
Department of Pediatrics
PGIMER, Chandigarh, India

Sadhana Lal
Professor
Department of Gastroenterology
PGIMER, Chandigarh, India

Saniya Sharma
Senior Resident
Department of Pathology
PGIMER, Chandigarh, India

Sanjay Bhadada
Additional Professor
Department of Endocrinology
PGIMER, Chandigarh, India

Sarla Gopalan
Ex-Professor and Head
Department of Obstetrics and Gynaecology
PGIMER, Chandigarh, India

Sarla Malhotra
Ex-Professor and Head
Department of Obstetrics and Gynecology
PGIMER, Chandigarh, India

Saumya Gupta
Senior Resident
Department of Pathology
PGIMER, Chandigarh, India

Saurabh Datta
Professor
Department of Pediatrics
(Neonatology Division)
PGIMER, Chandigarh, India

Savita Kumari
Professor and Head
Department of Internal Medicine
PGIMER, Chandigarh, India

SC Varma
Ex-Professor and Head
Department of Internal Medicine
PGIMER, Chandigarh, India

Setu Gupta
Junior Resident
Department of Internal Medicine
PGIMER, Chandigarh, India

Shalini Gainder
Additional Professor
Department of Obstetrics and Gynecology
PGIMER, Chandigarh, India

Shano Naseem
Associate Professor
Department of Hematology
PGIMER, Chandigarh, India

Shilpi Thakur
Junior Resident
Department of Pathology
PGIMER, Chandigarh, India

Shiv Bagga
Additional Professor
Department of Cardiology
PGIMER, Chandigarh, India

Shiv Sajan Saini
Assistant Professor
Department of Pediatrics
(Neonatology Division)
PGIMER, Chandigarh, India

Shivani Chandel
Junior Resident
Department of Internal Medicine
PGIMER, Chandigarh, India

Shobha Sehgal
Ex-Professor and Head
Department of Immunopathology
PGIMER, Chandigarh, India

Shreya Shrivastava
Junior Resident
Department of Pathology
PGIMER, Chandigarh, India

SK Jindal
Ex-Professor and Head
Department of Pulmonary Medicine
PGIMER, Chandigarh, India

SK Mehta
Ex-Professor and Head
Department of Gastroenterology
PGIMER, Chandigarh, India

SK Singh
Professor
Department of Urology
PGIMER, Chandigarh, India

SK Sinha
Professor
Department of Gastroenterology
PGIMER, Chandigarh, India

SN Mathuriya
Ex-Professor and Head
Department of Neurosurgery
PGIMER, Chandigarh, India

Sudha Sharma
Senior Resident
Department of Pathology
PGIMER, Chandigarh, India

Sumita Bhogal
Junior Resident
Department of Internal Medicine
PGIMER, Chandigarh, India

Suraj Khanal
Associate Professor
Department of Cardiology
PGIMER, Chandigarh, India

Suravi Mohanty
Fellow-PDCC (Pediatric Pathology)
PGIMER, Chandigarh, India

Surinder Rana
Additional Professor
Department of Gastroenterology
PGIMER, Chandigarh, India

Surjit Singh
Professor and Head
Department of Pediatrics
PGIMER, Chandigarh, India

Surjit Singh
Ex-Professor
Department of Internal Medicine
PGIMER, Chandigarh, India

TD Yadav
Professor
Department of General Surgery
PGIMER, Chandigarh, India

Tushar Sehgal
Senior Resident
Department of Hematology
PGIMER, Chandigarh, India

Vani Bharani
Senior Resident
Department of Pathology
PGIMER, Chandigarh, India

Vanita Jain
Professor
Department of Obstetrics and Gynecology
PGIMER, Chandigarh, India

Vanita Suri
Professor and Head
Department of Obstetrics and Gynecology
PGIMER, Chandigarh, India

Varun Dhir
Additional Professor
Department of Internal Medicine
PGIMER, Chandigarh, India

Venkataseshan S
Professor
Department of Pediatrics
PGIMER, Chandigarh, India

Vikarn Vishwajeet
Senior Resident
Department of Pathology
PGIMER, Chandigarh, India

Vikram Thakur
PhD Student
Department of Virology
PGIMER, Chandigarh, India

Vikrant
Junior Resident
Department of Pathology
PGIMER, Chandigarh, India

Vinay Sakhuja
Ex-Professor and Head
Department of Nephrology
PGIMER, Chandigarh, India

Vinita Garg
Junior Resident
Department of Pediatrics
PGIMER, Chandigarh, India

Vipul Gupta
Assistant Professor
Department of Pediatrics
PGIMER, Chandigarh, India

Virender Singh
Professor
Department of Gastroenterology
PGIMER, Chandigarh, India

Vishrut
Junior Resident
Department of Pathology
PGIMER, Chandigarh, India

Vivek Kumar
Assistant Professor
Department of Nephrology
PGIMER, Chandigarh, India

Vivek Lal
Professor and Head
Department of Neurology
PGIMER, Chandigarh, India

YK Chawla
Former Director
Ex-Professor and Head
Department of Hepatology
PGIMER, Chandigarh, India

Foreword

It is a great pleasure, indeed, privilege, for me to write about this unique book which represents a scholarly compilation of 101 cases of adult and pediatric autopsies, collected by Dr Nandita Bharadwaj Kakkar over her illustrious career spanning 27 years. For those who prefer to avoid reading long introductions, I will be very brief; this is an outstanding book, skip rest of the foreword and go to Case 1 and do not stop until you reach Case 101! But this short statement, true though it is, does not do justice to this book which is unlike any other that I have seen.

Indeed the word autopsy in the title is often assumed to indicate a long and dull description of morbid anatomy. Far from it, this book is interesting and filled with knowledge. The first thing that struck me was the organization of each case. It is often said that when teaching something, start with what you are going to tell, then tell them what you wish to tell and finally, tell them what you told them. Following this time-honored sequence, each chapter starts with the case highlights, followed by clinical and pathological details ending with take home message. The section between the highlights of the case and take home message is further subdivided into clinical details, autopsy findings, final diagnosis, a discussion of the disease and commentary on the index case. While clinical details and autopsy findings are factual recordings, the section on the primary diagnosis is a scholarly and scientifically up-to-date discussion of the disease. As an example, in Case 1, the diagnosis is Mantle cell lymphoma. The write-up includes not only the definition and histologic description, but also includes cytogenetic features, surface antigens (flow cytometry) and molecular pathogenesis. All these attributes are then compared with other entities that constitute the differential diagnosis. Each case is beautifully illustrated with 8–12 figures, including clinical appearance of the patient (where relevant), gross and microscopic pathology. Cases that come to autopsy are by definition complex with multiple complications. It is to the credit of the author that each case has been carefully "dissected" to ensure that the big picture is not lost in the details. Autopsies, unfortunately, are going "out of fashion" as they say. It is assumed that with modern imaging techniques and invasive investigations, the diagnosis can be made clinically and hence autopsies are of little value. Nothing could be farther from the truth—as this book clearly indicates. Autopsies have always been and will remain a powerful educational tool, provided one is willing to put in the kind of effort that Dr Nandita Bharadwaj Kakkar has. Reading this book reminded me of my days as a resident at All India Institute of Medical Sciences. Under the enlightened leadership of the department at that time, each autopsy was expected to be written up as if it was a case report to be submitted for publication. The author has gone one step further and produced a book. I hope it will inspire the residents and faculty alike to treat each autopsy write-up as a chapter in a book. I hope that there will be many more volumes in this series and others will follow where this has left.

I could write more, but rather than consume more time of those who have read so far, I will end by congratulating Dr Nandita Bharadwaj Kakkar and thanking her for service to our discipline. It truly is a labor of love.

Vinay Kumar MBBS MD FRCPath
Alice Hogge and Arthur A Baer Distinguished Service Professor
Chairman Emeritus
Department of Pathology
Biological Sciences Division and
The Pritzker School of Medicine
University of Chicago
Chicago, Illinois, USA
Editor-in-Chief
Robbins and Cotran Pathologic Basis of Disease and
Robbins Basic Pathology

Preface

Medical Autopsy is the strongest teaching tool in medicine and has no substitute. It is the most scientific method to learn pathology and medicine, by correlating the clinical details and pathology of a patient via the "Clinicopathologic Correlation Conferences". Unfortunately, the practice of medical autopsy has declined worldwide. In the prestigious Post Graduate Institute of Medical Education and Research (PGIMER), Chandigarh, India, the Department of Histopathology still performs 500–600 medical autopsies per year, round the clock, i.e. 24 × 7 hours, which include adults, children, infants, neonates, stillbirths and the previable terminated fetuses. Three clinicopathological correlation conferences are held every week in the main lecture theater, which is attended by the entire medical fraternity. These conferences are also relayed "LIVE" by our "Telemedicine Department" to 14 postgraduate medical institutes and medical schools, across India and are a "**Pride of PGIMER**". Apart from this, we have neonatal and stillbirth mortality rounds where the obstetricians, neonatologists and the pathologists meet once in a month and discuss all the autopsied cases.

The Salient Features of the Book

- Comprehensive compilation of 101 Medical Autopsy Cases (48 Adults and 53 Pediatrics—children, infants, neonates, stillbirths and terminated fetuses) in a case-based manner.
- First book in the world literature to have compiled medical autopsy cases with complete clinical/pathological details/gallery of gross and microscopic pictures with review of literature.
- The cases have been grouped in the following order:
    - Hematologic Disorders, Malignancies, Infections, Hepatobiliary and Pancreatic Disorders, Cardiovascular System, Systemic Vasculitides, Primary Renal Mucormycosis, Histiocytosis, Primary Immunodeficiency, Infantile Nephrotic Syndromes, Congenital Heart Disease, Storage Disorder and Pediatric Renal Cystic Disease (developmental/genetic/syndromes).
- Introductory text chapters—Introduction to Medical Autopsy, Systemic Vasculitides, Tubercular Meningitis and Pediatric Renal Cystic Diseases are added for better understanding.
- Each AUTOPSY CASE is a complete journey of the patient/deceased and has been concisely discussed under the following headings—title, highlights of the case, clinical details, investigations, clinical diagnosis, complete histopathological or autopsy findings with a gallery of gross and microscopic photographs (>3000), final autopsy diagnosis, review of literature, commentary index case, take home message and suggested reading or references.
- This book will be a great teaching material for the pathologists, medical physicians, pediatricians, neonatologists, obstetricians, radiologists along with undergraduates/postgraduates students of medicine. It will give what the existing books and other experiences cannot teach.

The pathology of all these medical autopsy cases were worked up and presented in the institutes, Clinicopathologic Correlation Conferences (CPCC)/neonatal and stillbirth mortality meets and is a collection of my 27 years of service in this institute. To present the "Pathology" of a case in the **"Clinicopathologic Correlation Conference"** is a cumbersome task for a histopathologist as he/she has to make the **"FINAL AUTOPSY DIAGNOSIS"**. Remember "A Pathologist can never go wrong" as his/her is the final say. So toiling for hours with the slides, reading, looking at references (the cumbersome Index Medicus in the 90s), correlating clinical details, investigations and radiology, getting special stains, immunohistochemistry and looking at electron microscopy where needed, taking gross and microscopic pictures and finally making the power point presentation (to begin with, it was the 3 × 2 projection slides). Each case is an infinite "Wealth of Knowledge" and I think it is rightly said that **"Medical autopsy is the strongest teaching tool in medicine"**.

The idea for the compilation of this academic wealth goes to my father "Late Col RK Bharadwaj". So I thought why not share this wealth of knowledge with the world and this was a **"Call beyond my duty"** to compile this immensely valuable learning material, which would have got deleted from my computer, once I would retire.

For Information

For this book, I have inserted my maiden name as my middle name, which goes as 'Dr Nandita Bharadwaj Kakkar'. All my publications before this and my profile in PGIMER carry my name as 'Dr Nandita Kakkar'.

Nandita Bharadwaj Kakkar

Acknowledgments

It was a great pleasure and learning experience to work on, present and write-up these 101 Medical Autopsy Cases, which have featured in the Clinicopathologic Correlation Conferences, over the last 27 years of my working in Postgraduate Institute of Medical Education and Research (PGIMER), Chandigarh, India.

It is with folded hands and deep gratitude that I embark on this duty of thanking all those who have contributed to the successful completion of this book.

At the onset I thank the "Almighty" for helping me complete this book and making a dream come true. The onus for each case in this book goes to many, the clinicians in-charge who treated the patients, the diagnosticians who performed the investigations, the clinical residents who motivated the relatives of the deceased for getting a medical autopsy done, the relatives of the deceased and parents of the little "angels" who gave the consent for the medical autopsy, the pathology residents who toiled for many hours (even at night) in the mortuary, performing the autopsies, the histopathology technical staff for processing the tissues, doing a volley of special stains, immunohistochemistry, electron microscopy and my senior colleagues, who gave valuable inputs in helping me make the ***"Final Autopsy Diagnosis".*** I thank each one of them from the core of my heart.

My heartfelt gratitude to all my teachers, who have shaped me and brought me till here. I thank Professor BD Sabharwal, Professor Vineeta Malhotra and Professor Kuldeep Chander who guided me during my MD training in Dayanand Medical College and Hospital, Ludhiana, Punjab, India, Professor BN Datta and Professor AK Banerjee, my mentors who gave me a break in PGIMER and from whom I imbibed a lot, Professor RK Vasishta, my present Head of Department, who with his inspirational clarity of vision always guided and encouraged me to be an astute morphologist, Professor Kusum Joshi, my Ex-Head of Deptartment, who taught me to toil despite all circumstances, my senior colleagues Professor BD Radotra and Professor Ashim Das who were always there when I wanted help, Professor Neelam Marwaha with whom I worked as a Senior Resident and Professor KK Talwar, Former Director PGI, who were both a deep source of inspiration for me.

We are grateful for the constant support and encouragement of Shri Jitendar P Vij (Group Chairman) and Mr Ankit Vij (Managing Director) of M/s Jaypee Brothers Medical Publishers (P) Ltd, New Delhi, India, in publishing this book and also their associates, particularly Ms Chetna Malhotra Vohra (Associate Director—Content Strategy) and Ms Madhuri Aggarwal (Development Editor) who have been prompt, efficient and most helpful.

I thank my three Angels, my father Col RK Bharadwaj, my mothers, Mrs Meena Bharadwaj and Mrs Sneh Kakkar, who left for their heavenly abode recently, but are still with me, holding my hand. It was in fact my father who gave me the idea of compiling this academic wealth. Special thanks to my father-in-law Mr BR Kakkar (IAS retd), who has himself authored 15 spiritual books, for his constant encouragement. Dr Niraj, my amazing husband and my two princesses, my loving daughters, Aaina and Apsara, the trio being the best thing that happened to me in my life, for their immense love and care, without which I could not have completed this marathon task. My sisters, Namrata and Rohini, who were always by my side. My pug Sherry, who follows me everywhere like a lamb and is a bundle of love. I sincerely thank Ms Nila and Ms Padma who meticulously took care of my house and my kitchen in the years that I was busy with the book.

Contents

Section 3: Infections—Adult Cases

Section 4: Hepatobiliary and Pancreatic Disorders—Adult Cases

Section 5: Cardiovascular System—Adult Cases

Section 6: Systemic Vasculitides—Adult and Pediatric Cases

Introduction

Medical Autopsy: The Strongest Teaching Tool in Medicine

Nandita Bharadwaj Kakkar

Autopsy is the dissection of a dead human body and is performed to find the cause of death. The Greek word "autopsy" means "to see with one's own eyes". Autopsy pathology is the best method of learning pathology and medicine. "Pathology" was actually born at the autopsy table. The history of autopsy dates back to 3000 BC when the ancient Egyptians used to practice the removal and examination of the internal organs of dead humans in their religious practice of "mummification". The word autopsy comes from the Greek, meaning "to see with one's own eyes." Synonymous terms are *"necropsy/postmortem"* but the term *"autopsy"* is more popular and hence widely used.

Autopsies are of two kinds:

- ***Forensic/Medicolegal/Coroner's autopsy:*** This is ordered by law, when death occurs under suspicious circumstances, sudden death or accidental death.
- ***Medical/Clinical/Pathological autopsy*:** They are performed to find the cause of death and for research purposes. In this book, I have used the term "Medical Autopsy". For a medical autopsy, mandatory prerequisite is to get the consent from the "next of kin", after explaining the procedure in clear words along with the benefits. No force should be applied. The job of the clinician is to only recommend but "cannot order" a medical autopsy. The next of kin are generally recognized in the following order—spouse, children of legal age, parents, siblings of legal age and legal guardians/custodians.

MEDICAL AUTOPSY TECHNIQUES

- ***Rudolf Virchow***, in the 19th century, established and published specific autopsy protocols which till date bear his name. It is known as the "Technique of R Virchow" wherein the organs are removed one by one.
- ***C Rokitansky*** established a technique characterized by in situ dissection combined with en-block removal of the organ blocks.
- ***Ghon's technique*** is characterized by "en bloc" removal of thoracic/cervical organs, abdominal organs and urogenital system. Thus, in this technique there are multiple organ blocks.
- ***M Letulle*** established the technique of "en masse" removal where in the thoracic, cervical, abdominal and pelvic organs are removed as one organ block and then subsequently dissected into individual organ blocks. This technique is cumbersome and needs more experience. This is a quick method and the body can be returned to the relatives in a shorter time. The dissection can then be done subsequently with ease.

TYPES OF MEDICAL AUTOPSIES

- Abdominal with/without brain
- Abdominothoracic with/without brain
- Brain only
- Brain with spinal cord
- Any special instruction
- Multiple biopsy autopsies (In PGIMER, this if done is done by the clinicians)

We generally use the term partial autopsy for abdominothoracic without removal of the brain and complete autopsy for abdominothoracic with brain.

BENEFITS OF MEDICAL AUTOPSY

- ***To Find the "Cause of Death"***
    - In the adult medical autopsies, the relatives get to know the exact cause of death and this satisfies their mind. Any infectious disease like tuberculosis (which is rampant in India) can be diagnosed and the relatives can be given adequate treatment.
    - In the pediatric age group, the benefits are many. Death of a child, infant, neonate and still births (early and late) is the most devastating event for parents. Due to advancements in radiology, a new group has come up for medical autopsies, i.e. the fetuses (Previable fetuses <20 weeks gestation) who undergo medical termination for various malformations.
        - Medical autopsy establishes the exact cause of death and this satisfies the parents to some extent in bearing with the loss of their child.
        - Valuable information about congenital malformations, genetic or inherited diseases is obtained and this helps in planning the next pregnancy.
- ***Audit***
  Autopsy gives you the complete pathology of the disease process occurring in every organ of the body and hence it teaches the clinicians, where they went wrong in their diagnosis and treatment and how to rectify it. This is the best audit available in the field of medicine.
- ***Final Autopsy Diagnosis***
  Pathologist gives the final answer. This helps in bringing revolution in treatments, better techniques and makes a remarkable difference in patient care.
- ***Unraveling New Entities in a Particular Part of the World***
  New pathological entities are diagnosed, which had never been seen in the area. This changes the mindset of the clinicians and if they see such a case again, it helps them in making an early and correct diagnosis. Examples from PGIMER—(1) Familial hemophagocytic lymphohistiocytosis with severe involvement of the central nervous system was first diagnosed at autopsy in 1996. This awareness led the clinicians to diagnose and treat subsequent patients. (2) Hepatosplenic γδ T cell lymphoma was first diagnosed at autopsy when it was a provisional entity in the WHO classification and this awareness was very fruitful. (3) The presence of "Leptospirosis" was first proven at autopsy in PGIMER, for which the serological confirmation was done on the postmortem sample from Lal Path Laboratory, New Delhi. Thereafter a strong laboratory support was established in our institute for leptospirosis and more such cases are being diagnosed and treated ever since.
- ***Pediatric Autopsies—Special Benefits***
    - Medical autopsy is the best audit for neonatal deaths, stillbirths (early and late) and terminated fetuses. All autopsied cases are discussed in the neonatal/stillbirth mortality rounds held once in a month in our institute.
    - The "Final Autopsy Diagnosis" of all terminated fetuses (with various congenital malformations) is correlated with the radiological diagnosis for which the pregnancy was terminated. This gives immense relief to the parents that their decision for MTP was correct. They are then sent to the "Genetic clinic" for further management and planning a subsequent pregnancy.

PROCEDURE FOR MEDICAL AUTOPSY AT PGIMER, CHANDIGARH, INDIA

We are more or less following the Letulle's technique as most of our incision permissions are abdominothoracic and we remove the entire organs "en masse" and later dissect them out meticulously.

- The organs are dissected and kept flat in a tray as follows for 7–10 days in 10% formalin.
    - ***As complexes***—(1) Organ complex comprising of both the lungs (adequately sliced) and the tracheobronchial tree. (2) Organ complex comprising of slice of liver, c loop of duodenum, pancreas, gallbladder with the dissected biliary tract and slice of spleen. (3) Organ complex comprising of both kidneys, ureters, urinary bladder, abdominal aorta, para-aortic lymph nodes and part of inferior vena cava. (4) Testes with their respective spermatic cords. (5) Uterus with cervix, fallopian tubes and both ovaries. (6) Heart with its arch and part of descending aorta, dissected along the flow of blood from right to the left side.
    - ***As individual organs***—Remaining slices of liver and spleen, adrenals, thymus, lymph nodes, stomach with esophagus, small and large intestine, mesentery, bone piece from the vertebrae, skin, psoas muscle, thyroid/parathyroids.
- *The brain* is kept intact with the brain stem floating in a bucket of 20% formalin hanging from a thread passing

via the Circle of Villus, the thread tied on either side to the handles of the bucket. The meninges and the pituitary gland are also kept. After fixing for 10–12 days, the brain is cut.

- *Postmortem samples*: Blood sample is kept and fresh tissues if needed (i.e. kidney etc.) are kept at –80° (for immunofluorescence and molecular techniques if needed later on) and in glutaraldehyde for electron microscopy.
- *Organ review conference*: This is done after 7–10 days of fixing the organs. Gross autopsy diagnosis is made and adequate sections (minimum 30–35 in an adult autopsy) are taken and sent for processing. Gross photographs are taken.
- *Brain review conference*: The brain cutting is done 10–12 days after fixation. Five standard sections and additional sections if needed are taken and sent for processing.
- *Pediatric autopsies*: Anthropometric measurements, weight of the body and external gross photographs are taken at the time of autopsy. External congenital malformations are meticulously enumerated and photographed. Infantogram is taken if needed. The heart–lung complex is kept together. For Arnold Chiari malformation, the incision is given on the nape of the neck and the displacement of the brainstem into the foramen magnum is documented.
- *Review of slides*: Hematoxylin and eosin stained slides are examined. Special stains, electron microscopy, immunohistochemistry and other special tests, i.e. PCR confirmation of infections etc. are done if needed. Clinical details are sought for, correlations are done and a "Final Autopsy Diagnosis" is made. Gross and photomicrographs are taken and a 20-minute PowerPoint presentation is made.

CLINICOPATHOLOGIC CORRELATION CONFERENCE—CPCC

Three CPCCs are done every week in the main lecture theater of the institute and this is attended by the entire medical fraternity of PGIMER and doctors/students from the local Medical college and other hospitals of Chandigarh. This CPCC is relayed "live" by the Telemedicine department to 14 medical institutes and medical schools across India. In the one hour session, the clinician presents the case along with the relevant investigating team, i.e. the radiologists, hematopathologists, cytologists, microbiologists, etc. The clinician thus gives his clinical diagnosis which is followed by open house discussion for 5–8 minutes. The pathologist then takes 20 minutes to explain the entire case organ wise, to reach to the "Final Autopsy Diagnosis" which is then followed by open house discussion. CPCC is the strongest teaching tool in medicine and this is the pride of PGIMER, Chandigarh, India.

SUGGESTED READING

1. Connolly AJ, Finkbeiner WI, Ursell PC, et al. Autopsy Pathology: A Manual and Atlas, 3rd edition. US: Elseviers; 2016.
2. Enid GB, Spicer DE, et al. Handbook of Pediatric Autopsy Pathology, 2nd edition. New York: Springer; 2014.
3. Lanjerwar D, Vaideeswar P. Autopsy Practices, 1st edition. New Delhi: Jaypee Brothers Medical Publishers (P) Ltd; 2017.
4. Ludwig J. Handbook of Autopsy Practice, 3rd edition. Totowa New Jersey: Humana Press; 2002.

SECTION 1

Hematological Disorders Adult Cases

CASE 1

Mantle Cell Lymphoma, Presenting with Florid Cutaneous Lesions, with Common Variant Morphology in the Nodal/ Extranodal Sites and Blastoid Morphology in the Peripheral Blood: PM 25983

Nandita Bharadwaj Kakkar

HIGHLIGHTS OF THE CASE

A 42-year-old male presented with erythematous maculopapular rashes on the entire body with multiple skin nodules on the face causing considerable disfiguration of his face. There was fever, shortness of breath, left pleural effusion, generalized lymphadenopathy, hepatosplenomegaly, anemia, thrombocytopenia and total leukocyte count of 4,00,000/ UL with 85% blast-like cells in the peripheral blood. A diagnosis of chronic lymphocytic leukemia (CLL) with massive cutaneous involvement was made. Autopsy revealed a mantle cell lymphoma (MCL) (common variant) involving the lymph nodes with florid infiltration into the bone marrow, peripheral blood (blastoid variant), skin, spleen, liver, GIT, lungs, pancreas and muscle. Worth stressing points are first time presentation with florid cutaneous lesions, heavy tumor load, blastoid morphology in the peripheral blood and common variant morphology in the nodal and other extranodal sites and discrepancy in CD5 results [immunohistochemistry (IHC) on paraffin embedded sections negative and positive on peripheral blood flow cytometry].

Keywords: Mantle cell lymphoma, first presentation, cutaneous involvement, autopsy.

CLINICAL DETAILS

Date of Admission: 20.03.2014, Date of Death: 21.03.2014, and Duration of Hospital Stay: 40 Hours

A 42-year-old male was referred to PGIMER, Chandigarh with the chief complaints of multiple skin nodules/ erythematous maculopapular rashes since 4 months, left upper abdominal lump, fever since 3 months and shortness of breath since 2 weeks. This patient was apparently well, till 4 months ago, when he started developing erythematous maculopapular/nodular skin lesions over both lower limbs. These lesions were painless, erythematous, slowly increasing in size, number, extent and soon involved the entire body, including the face (Fig 1), causing significant disfiguration. This was soon accompanied by feeling of a lump in the left upper abdomen and development of masses in the axilla and groin. There was associated fever, weight loss and night sweats. Two weeks prior to admission to our institute, he started having shortness of breath with minimal cough. He was first evaluated in December 2013 (4 months back) in a private hospital, found to have raised total leukocyte count and due to worsening general condition, he was referred to the local medical college. There, he was documented to have generalized lymphadenopathy, hepatosplenomegaly, anemia, thrombocytopenia, lymphocytosis and hypercellular marrow with markedly raised lymphocytes along with neoplastic lymphocytes in the skin biopsy specimen. A provisional

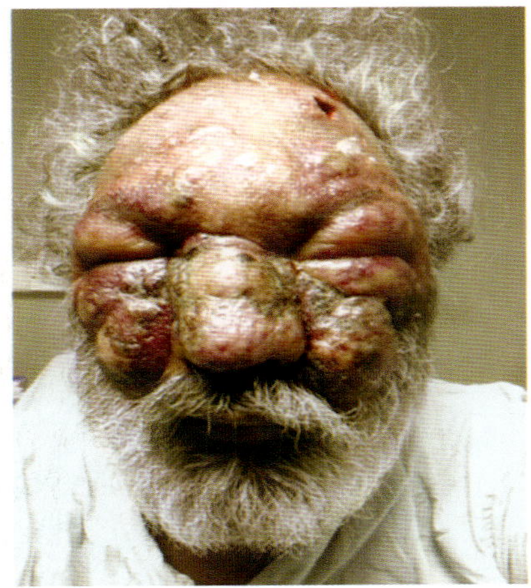

Fig 1: Erythematous maculopapular/nodular skin lesions over face and marked periorbital edema.
(*Courtesy*: Dr Gaurav Prakash)

diagnosis of CLL with cutaneous involvement was made and he was started on chlorambucil 4 mg/day. There was some improvement in symptoms after start of therapy. He was discharged, but he discontinued the medications after 2 months, on his own. This was followed by rapid progression of the skin lesions to involve the upper body and face with development of cervical lymphadenopathy. He was readmitted and restarted on chlorambucil at the same dose, along with prednisolone. He developed shortness of breath and was then referred to our institute, where he succumbed after 12 hours of hospital stay. *On examination* he was found to have pallor, multiple skin nodules involving the face—forehead, nose, cheeks and ears. Cervical, axillary, epitrochlear and inguinal lymph nodes were enlarged. They were multiple, firm, nontender and discrete measuring up to 5 cm in size. He had a disfigured (due to the multiple nodules) edematous face with periorbital puffiness and difficulty in opening his eyes (Fig. 1). There was bilateral pitting pedal edema with diffuse nodular skin infiltration. Liver and spleen were palpable, 10 cm and 12 cm below their respective costal margins. Chest examination revealed decreased breath sounds in left hemithorax. Rest of the systemic examination was normal.

Investigations

Investigations at admission revealed a hemoglobin (Hb) of 6.7 g/dL, total leukocyte count (TLC) 3,93000/μL, platelets 77 × 10^3/uL, PBF showed mild anisocytosis, macrocytes, macroovalocytes, blast-like cells (85%) (Fig 2), nucleated red blood cells (nRBCs)—5/100 and numerous smudge cells. Blood biochemistry revealed deranged renal function tests (urea—86 mg/dL, creatinine—2.2 mg/dL). The chest X-ray showed a left-sided pleural effusion. Bone marrow aspiration done in the local medical college was particulate, hypercellular and revealed 80% lymphoid cells, was suggestive of CLL. The skin biopsy done at that time showed dermal deposits of lymphoid cells, forming nodules at places—suggestive of cutaneous infiltration by CLL.

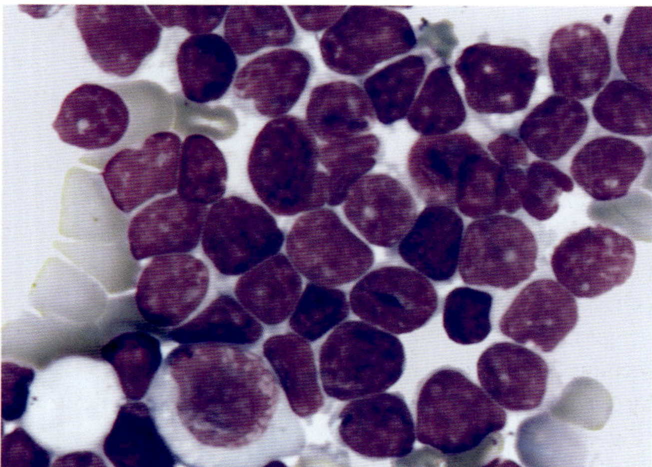

Fig 2: Atypical lymphoid cell with large nuclei, few cleaved with prominent nucleoli and blastic morphology in the peripheral blood. (*Courtesy*: Dr Tushar Sehgal)

Patient was found to have tachycardia, tachypnea, with falling saturation, requiring high flow oxygen therapy with Ventimask. Due to progressive deterioration of respiratory status, he had to be intubated. He subsequently sustained a cardiac arrest and could not be revived. Unit's final diagnosis: CLL with left-sided pleural effusion and renal dysfunction ? transformation to prolymphocytic leukemia ? Richter's transformation. Sample for peripheral blood flow cytometry was taken before the demise of the patient, but was processed after death. Acute leukemia panel revealed positivity for the following markers—HLA-DR, CD20, CD19, CD38, and CD79a; negativity for CD13, CD33, CD117, myeloperoxidase (MPO), CD14, CD64, CD11c, CD34, Tdt, CD10, CD22, CD1a, CD2, CD3, CD4, CD5, CD7, and CD8. Chronic lymphoproliferative disorder (CLPD) panel showed positivity for CD5, CD19, CD20, CD22, CD79b, CD38, and antilambda and negativity for CD23, CD10, antikappa, CD2, CD1a, CD3, CD4, CD8, FMC-7, CD200, and CD43. This labeled this case as a B lymphoproliferative disorder. The Matutes scoring for CLL was 2/5, which should be 4 or 5 for a diagnosis of CLL. Thus, a diagnosis of B-cell lymphoproliferative disorder (CD5+, CD23–, CD10–, B-cell markers positive, and immaturity markers negative) with a possibility of Mantle cell lymphoma (MCL) with leukemic conversion was suggested.

AUTOPSY FINDINGS: PM 25983

This 42-year-old male underwent a partial autopsy. The prosector noted multiple lesions on the face and the entire body, which were both nodular and blister like. The pleural cavity contained 2 liters of hemorrhagic fluid and the pericardial and peritoneal cavity were within normal limits. The ***lymph nodes*** (Figs 3A–C)—supraclavicular, hilar, carinal, paratracheal, epitrochlear, axillary, peripancreatic, splenic, nodes along the GIT, mesenteric, paraaortic, inguinal were enlarged and ranged in size from 1 cm to 5 cm in diameter. Cut section was fleshy. Sections examined from the lymph nodes revealed an effaced nodal architecture, due to a predominantly diffuse (Fig 3D) monomorphic infiltrate with formation of vague nodules (Fig 4A) in areas. There was a diffuse replacement by atypical lymphoid cells, which were small to medium sized, with slightly irregular nuclear

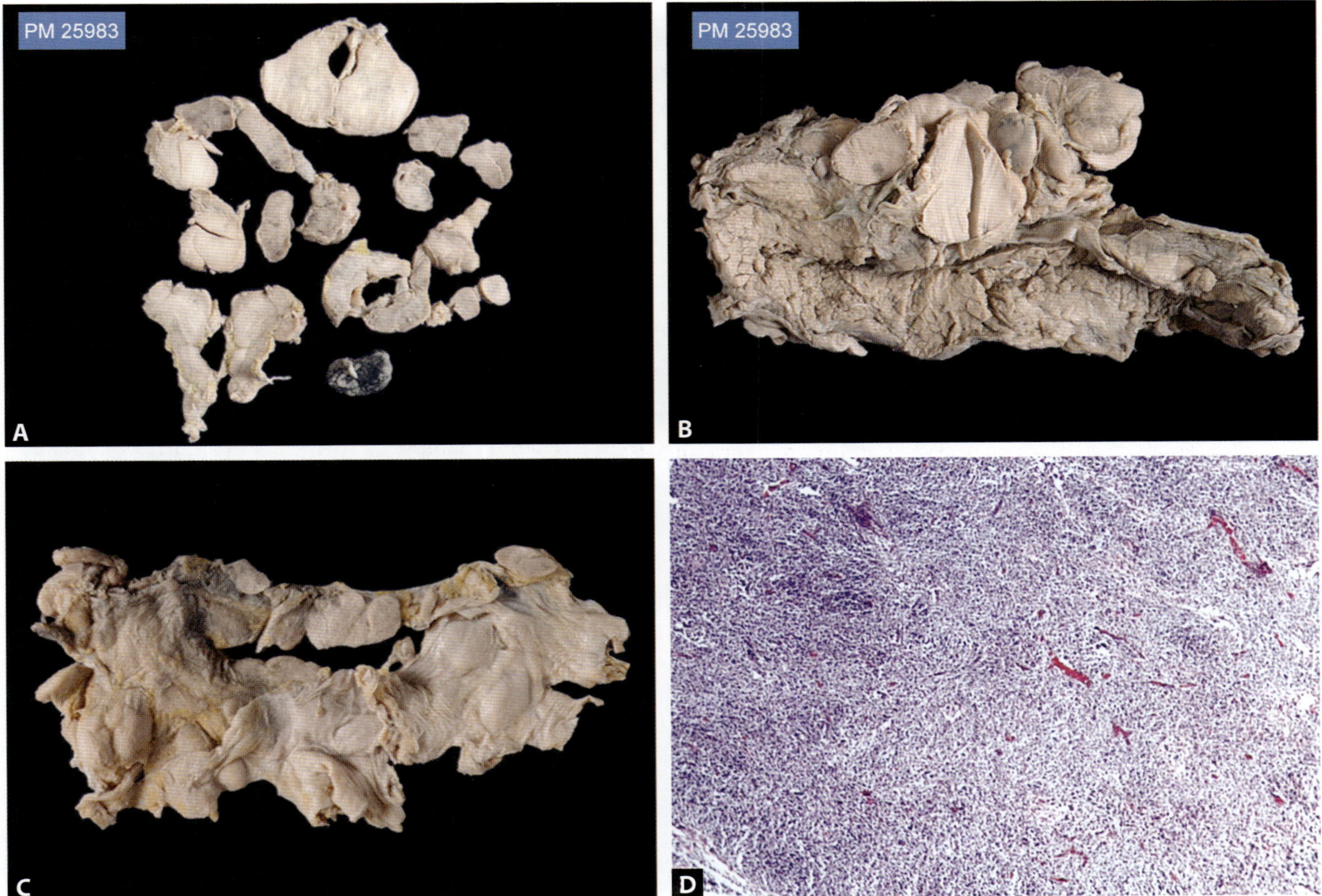

Figs 3A–D: (A) Various groups of enlarged lymph nodes; (B) Enlarged peripancreatic lymph nodes; (C) Enlarged mesenteric lymph nodes; (D) Lymph node showing a diffuse monomorphic infiltrate.

contours, resembling centrocytes (Figs 4B–C). The nuclei had a dispersed chromatin and inconspicuous nucleolus. IHC revealed positivity with CD20 (Fig 4D), cyclin D1 (Fig 4E), Bcl-2 (Fig 4F) and CD43. IHC with CD5, CD3, CD23 and CD10 were negative. The morphology and IHC were consistent with a diagnosis of MCL. The section from the ***skin*** (Figs 5A–C) revealed extensive infiltration by the lymphoma cells, forming large nodules in the deeper dermis, around adnexal structures and also in the subcutis. ***Spleen*** (Fig 5D) was markedly enlarged and weighed 1,600 g. It was adherent to the left lobe of the liver and the diaphragm. Cut section showed diffusely scattered, tiny white nodules, ranging in size from 0.2 cm to 0.8 cm (Fig 5E). Few peripheral infarcts were noted. Microscopy revealed marked expansion of the white pulp forming large nodules (Fig 5F), composed of atypical lymphoid cells with morphology of the cells, similar to that seen in the lymph nodes. Areas of diffuse infiltration were also seen (Fig 6A). The ***liver*** (Fig 6B) was also enlarged and weighed 1,850 g. Cut section was unremarkable. On microscopic examination the portal tracts (Figs 6C–D) were expanded and revealed extensive infiltration by the lymphoma cells. These cells were also seen prominently infiltrating into the sinusoids (Fig 6E). The porta hepatis showed extensive infiltration by the lymphoma cells. The ***kidneys*** (Fig 7A) were enlarged, showing blotchy congestion on the capsular aspect as well as on the cut section. Microscopy revealed massive infiltration (Fig 7B) by lymphoma cells in the cortex and the medulla. The ***lungs*** (Fig 7C) weighed 650 g. The left lung was collapsed and its pleura was dull and corrugated. Microscopy from both the lungs (Fig 7D) revealed alveolar spaces packed with lymphoma cells along with intra-alveolar hemorrhage.

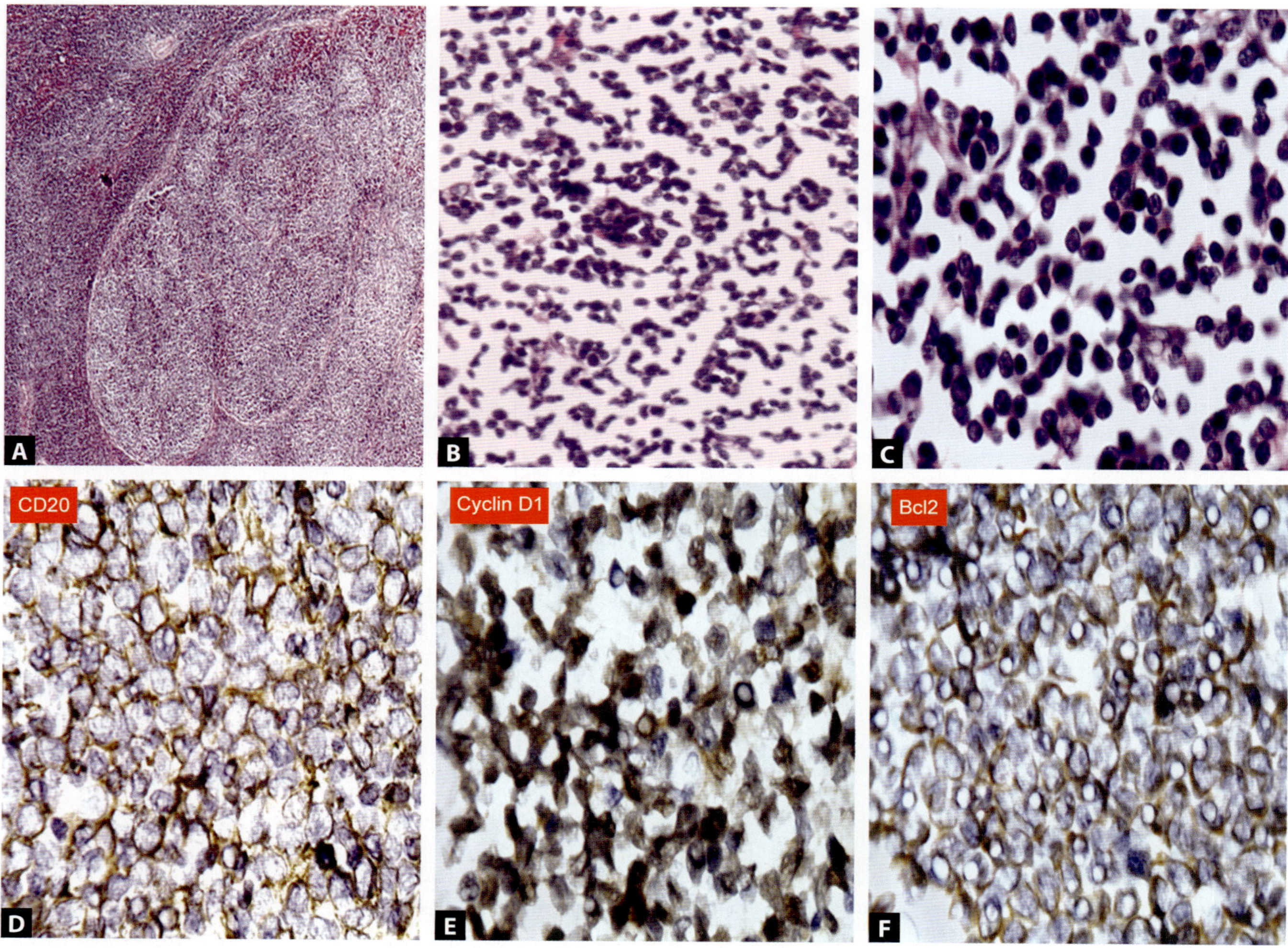

Figs 4A–F: (A) Lymph node showing a vague nodular pattern; (B–C) Atypical lymphoid cells are small to medium sized, with slightly irregular nuclear contours with dispersed chromatin and inconspicuous nucleolus, resembling centrocytes; (D) CD20 shows diffuse strong membranous positivity; (E) Cyclin D1 showing strong nuclear positivity; and (F) Bcl-2 positivity.

The subpleural space was also seen to be infiltrated by the lymphoma cells. The mucosa of the ***stomach*** (Fig 8A) was thickened, rugae were prominent, and an occasional nodule was seen along the greater curvature. The ***duodenal*** mucosa was also thickened. Rest of the GIT showed patchy mucosal thickening. Microscopic examination from all sites of the GIT (Figs 8B–D) showed infiltration by lymphoma cells in the mucosa, in areas extending into the submucosa and the muscularis propria. ***Bone marrow*** (Figs 8E–F) was totally replaced by lymphoma cells and no hematopoietic elements were discernable. Pancreas showed areas of infiltration (Fig 9A). Section from the ***muscle*** (Fig 9B) showed infiltration and destruction of muscle fibers. The ***heart*** was within normal limits. Right ***testis*** was undescended, was present in the inguinal canal and showed florid atrophic changes with no evidence of intratubular germ cell neoplasia or infiltration.

FINAL AUTOPSY DIAGNOSIS: PM 25983

42 Years Male

- Mantle cell lymphoma (common variant) involving the lymph nodes (hilar, carinal, paratracheal, epitrochlear, peripancreatic, splenic, along GIT, paraaortic and mesenteric) with florid infiltration into the bone marrow, peripheral blood (blastoid variant), skin, spleen, liver, GIT, lungs, pancreas and muscle.
- Hemorrhagic pleural effusion (left), pulmonary hemorrhage.
- Right atrophic undescended testis.

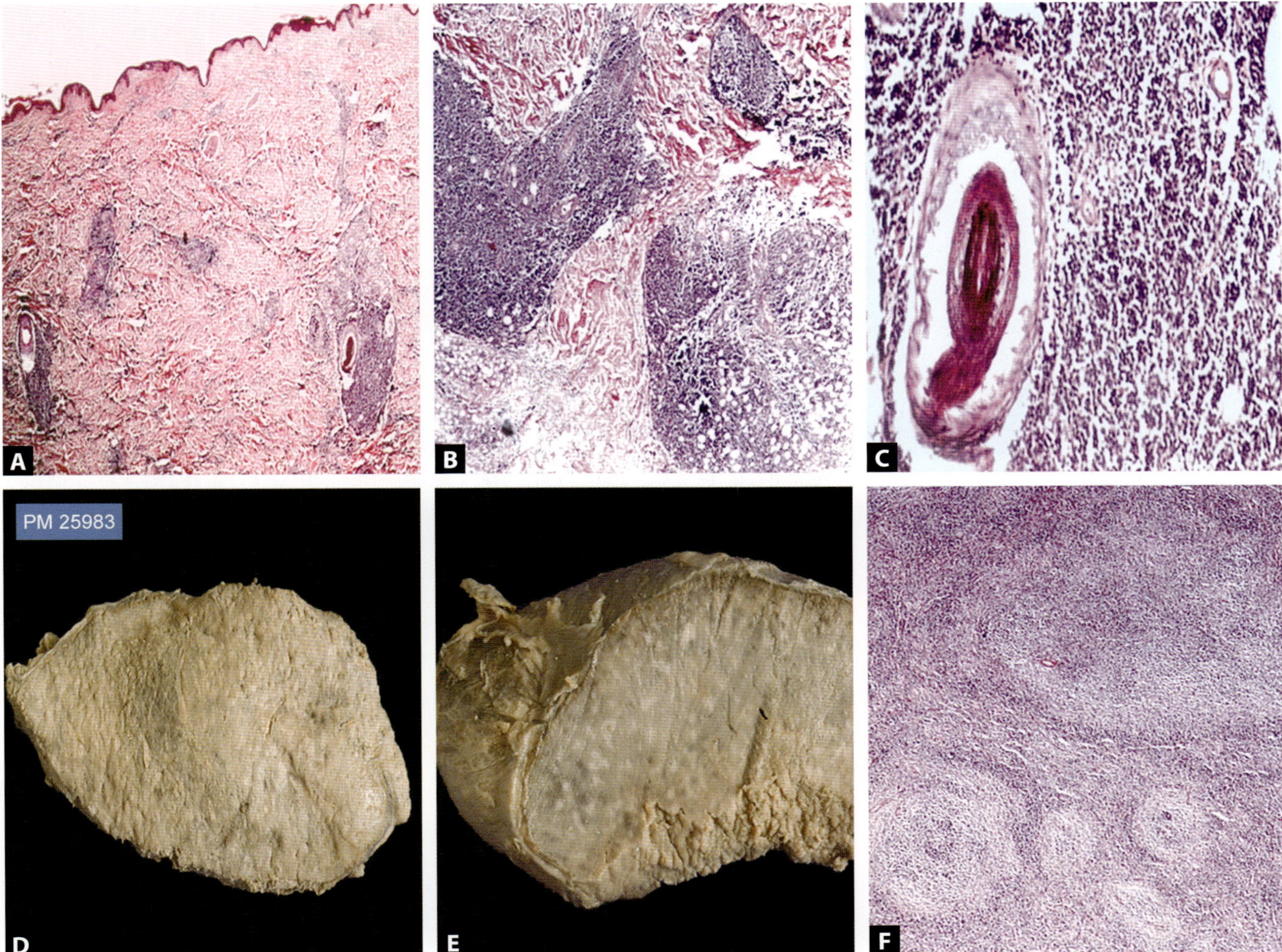

Figs 5A–F: (A) Section of the skin shows nodular infiltrate in the deep dermis; (B) Large nodular deposits in the subcutis; (C) Deposits around adnexal structures; (D) Coronal slice of the enlarged spleen; (E) Spleen shows tiny whitish nodules; and (F) Photomicrograph of the spleen showing nodules.

MANTLE CELL LYMPHOMA

Mantle cell lymphoma is an aggressive B-cell neoplasm which responds poorly to treatment. Its defining characteristic is mutation and overexpression of cyclin D1, a cell cycle gene that contributes to the abnormal proliferation of the malignant cells. Expression of cyclin D1 is pathognomonic for MCL and is an indirect evidence of translocation t(11;14). It is characterized by cyclin D1+, CD5+, CD23–, and CCND1 translocation t(11;14)(q13;q32). MCL is positive for pan B-cell markers (CD79a, CD19, CD20, and CD22), as well as T-cell marker CD5 and CD43, Bcl-2 and is usually negative for CD10 and CD23. It originates from the pregerminal center B lymphocyte which resides in the primary lymphoid follicles and mantle zones. It was initially known as centrocytic lymphoma due to the resemblance to centrocytes. They constitutes 3–10% of non-Hodgkin lymphomas, generally occur in elderly men with a median age of 65 years, with stage III/IV disease. Extranodal involvement is very frequent. Patients present with lymphadenopathy, bone marrow involvement (>80%), hepatosplenomegaly, lymphomatoid polyposis of small bowel and other extranodal involvements like that of the Waldeyer's ring, however, the skin is rarely affected. Central nervous system (CNS) is involved in 10% of cases. In approximately 50% cases, it presents in the leukemic phase with less than 20,000 absolute lymphocytes and this is associated with a worse outcome. Fever, night sweats and weight loss occurs in 30%.

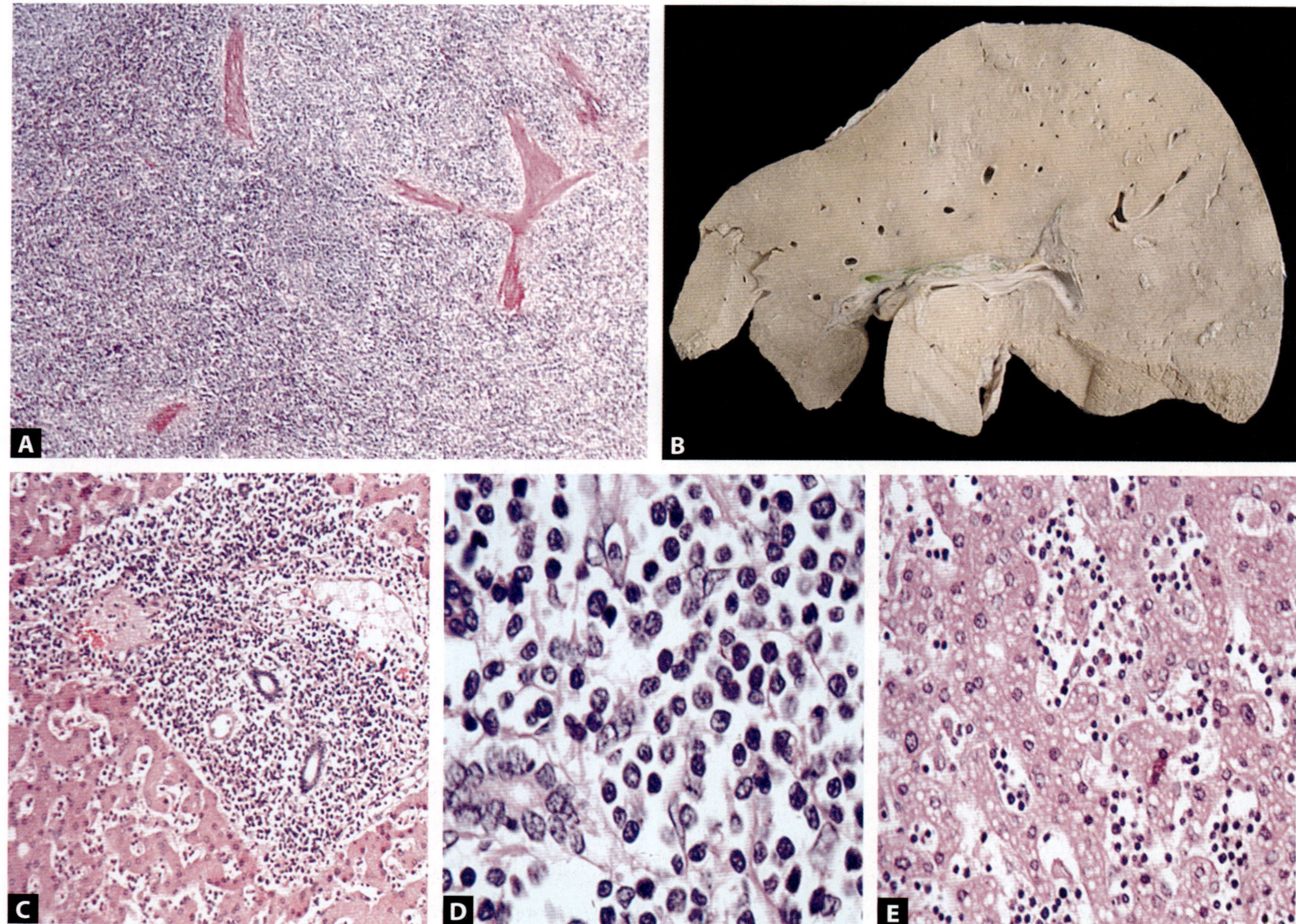

Figs 6A–E: (A) Spleen showing diffuse infiltration; (B) Coronal slice of the enlarged liver. No nodules are seen; (C–D) Lymphoma infiltrate in the portal tracts; and (E) Infiltrate in the sinusoids.

Mantle cell lymphoma is composed of monomorphic, small to medium-sized lymphoid cells with indented nuclear contours, clumped chromatin and scanty cytoplasm. Nucleoli are not seen. These cells most closely resemble centrocytes. Large cells and proliferation centers are seen. Three patterns of tumor infiltration can be seen, i.e. diffuse replacement of the lymph node, expanded mantle zone showing infiltration, or a vague nodular pattern. Scattered epithelioid histiocytes (occasionally impart a starry sky appearance) and prominent hyalinized vessels are seen. More aggressive variants of MCL include: (1) Blastoid variant wherein the cells show a dispersed chromatin, high mitosis (20–30/10 HPF) and resemblance to lymphoblasts, (2) Pleomorphic variant wherein the cells are large with irregular nuclear contours, prominent nucleoli in some, and a pale cytoplasm, (3) Small cell variant resembling a small lymphocytic lymphoma, and (4) Marginal zone-like variant containing cells with abundant pale cytoplasm. IHC panel specific for MCL is CD5+, CD20+ (strong), CD23- and cyclin D1/Bcl-1+. Rare cases have all morphologic features of MCL but are negative for cyclin D1 and these cases may be positive for cyclin D2/D3. The main genetic event is t(11;14)(q13;q32) between IGH and cyclin D1 (CCND1) genes which is present in almost all cases. This results in a deregulated overexpression of CCND1 messenger ribonucleic acid (mRNA) and protein which overcomes the cell cycle suppressive effect of RB1 and p27kip1, leading to the development of MCL. Fluorescent in situ hybridization for cyclin D1/Bcl-1 is more sensitive/specific than the IHC, but has cost considerations.

Differential diagnosis of MCL include small B-cell lymphomas—SLL/CLL, marginal zone lymphomas, follicular lymphomas and lymphoplasmacytic lymphomas.

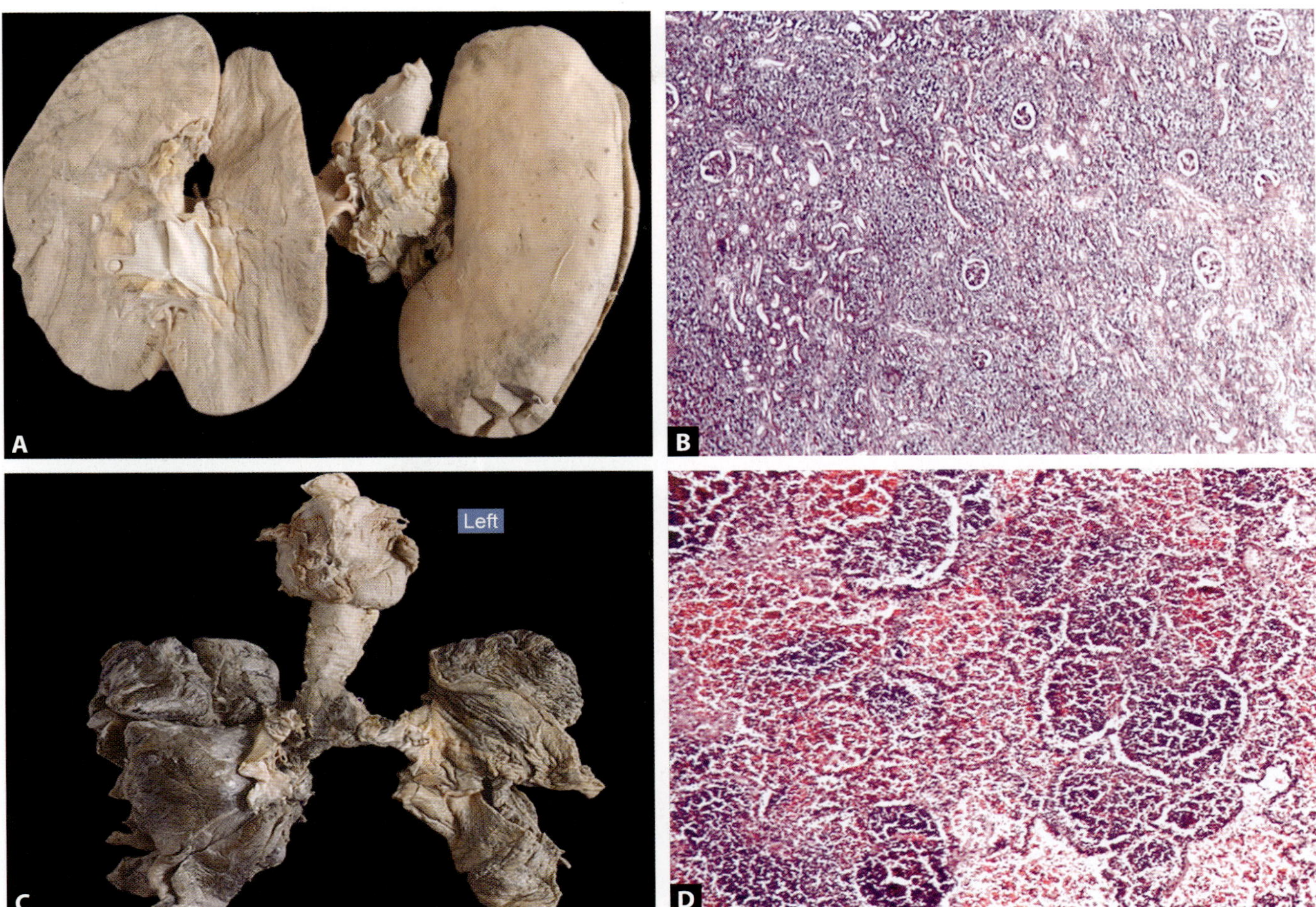

Figs 7A–D: (A) Enlarged kidneys showing blotchy congestion; (B) Kidney showing diffuse infiltration by mantle cell lymphoma (MCL); (C) Both lungs, wherein the left lung shows puckered pleura along with collapse; and (D) Alveolar spaces packed with lymphoma cells and hemorrhage.

(1) ***MCL***—Uniform cells, have irregular cleaved nuclei, residual germinal centers may be prominent imparting a vague nodular pattern, expanded mantle zones around germinal centers may be seen, scattered histiocytes seen at times giving a starry sky appearance, cells are positive for cyclin D1 (85%), CD20, CD5 (80%), CD43 (85%), Bcl-1 (95%), and negative for CD23 and CD10 in 98% cases, (2) ***SLL/ CLL***—Cells have a round nuclei, proliferation centers are present, no mantle zone, no vague nodular pattern, histiocytes are not prominent, they are positive for CD5 (80%), CD23 (85%), CD43 (80%), Bcl-2 (95%), weak CD19 and CD20 positive, and negative for CD10 and cyclin D1, (3) ***Follicular lymphoma***—Show distinct follicles composed of cleaved cells, mantle pattern rare, positive for Bcl-2 (95%) and CD10 (85%), negative for CD5, cyclin D1, 7% show positivity for CD43, 25% show positivity for CD23, (4) ***Marginal zone lymphoma***—Show enlarged marginal and mantle zones, polymorphous population of cells, negative for cyclin D1, CD5, CD10, CD43 (+ in 35%, 2% in splenic MZL), CD23 (+ in 8%) and Bcl-2 (+ in 65–90%), (5) ***Lymphoplasmacytic lymphomas***—Round nuclear membrane, lymphoplasmacytoid appearance, cyclin D1 negative, CD20/ CD19 negative, CD5 (+ 10%), CD10 (+ in 3%), CD43 (+ in 10–30%) and Bcl-2 (+ in > 50%), (6) ***Hairy cell leukemia***—CD25, CD103 expression by flow cytometry.

Cyclin D1 or Bcl-1 expression is very important in the diagnosis of MCL, as it is negative in all small B-cell proliferations, except for an occasional case of atypical SLL/CLL, some cases of splenic MZL, and in approximately 40% of hairy cell leukemias. Distinguishing MCL from other low-grade B-cell lymphomas is of utmost importance due to the differences in the treatment modality and clinical outcome.

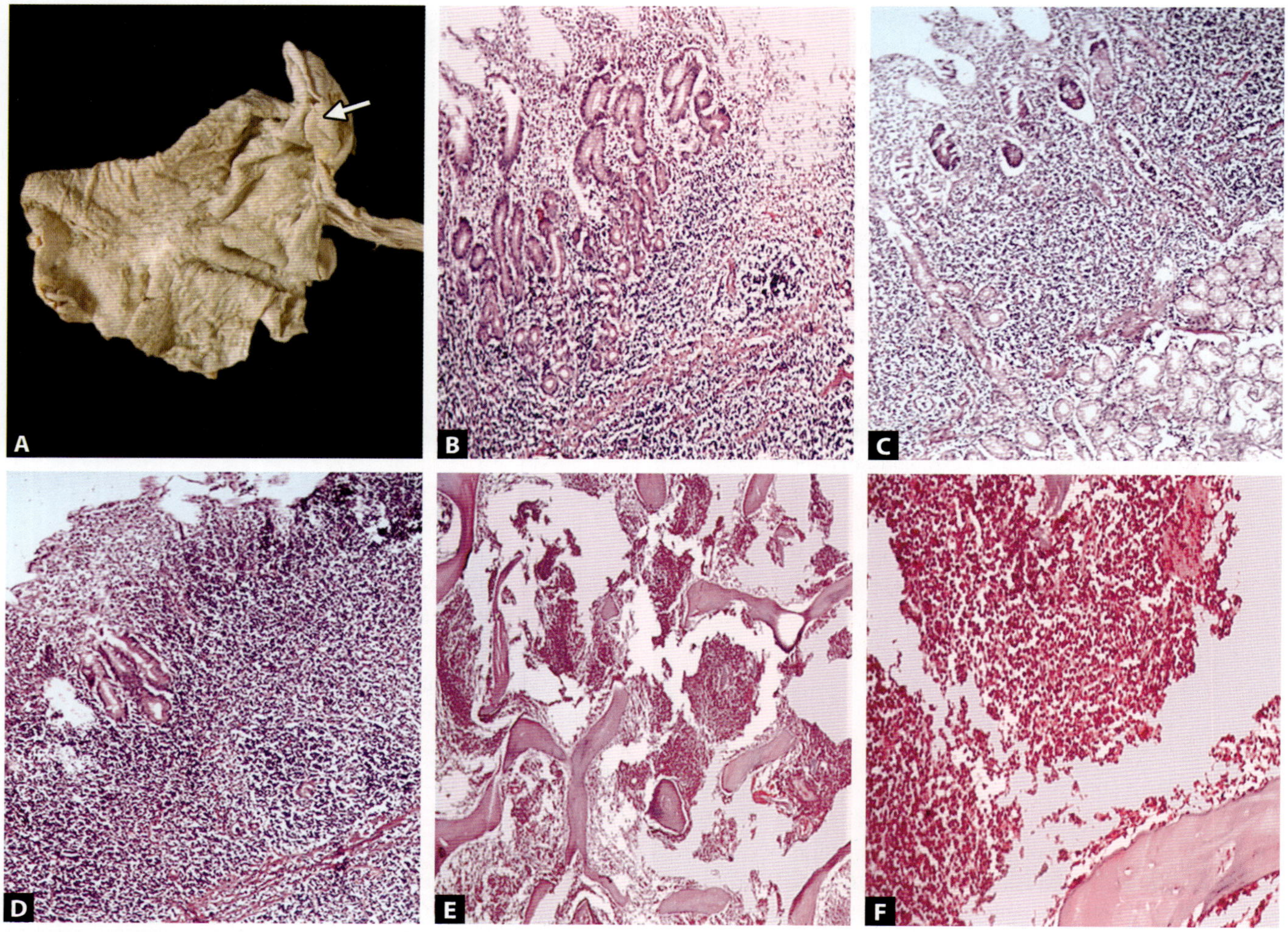

Figs 8A–F: (A) Stomach shows a thickened wall along with a nodule (arrow); GIT shows infiltration by MCL in the (B) Stomach; (C) Duodenum; (D) Small intestine; and (E and F) Postmortem bone marrow shows extensive infiltration by MCL cells.

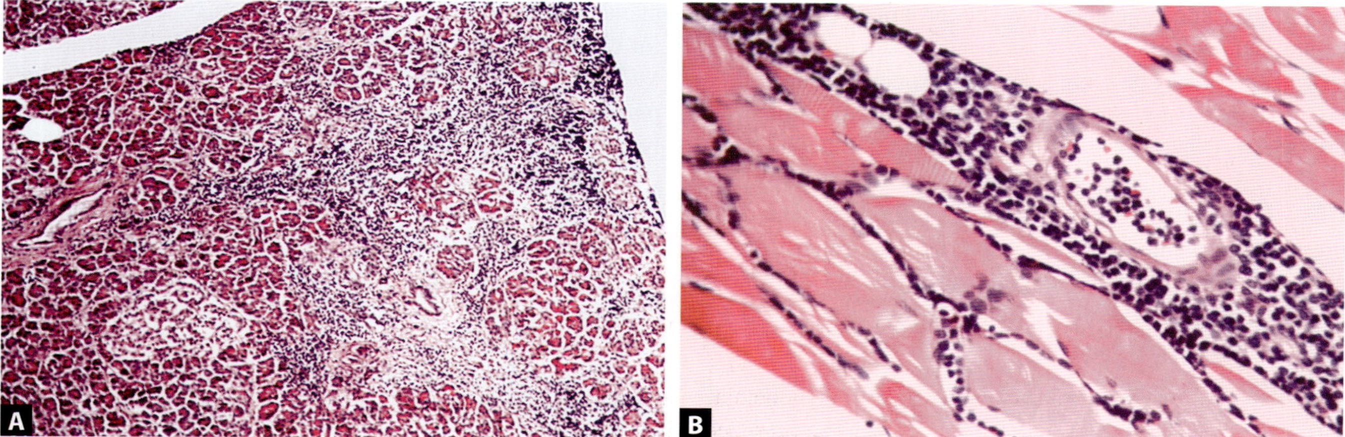

Figs 9A–B: Mantle cell lymphoma (MCL) infiltrating the (A) Pancreas; and (B) Skeletal muscle.

The prototypic MCL is CD5+, cyclin D1+, CD10– and CD23–. If CD5 is negative, and for some reason the cyclin D1 does not work, a diagnosis of low-grade B-cell lymphoma of the non-MCL type will be made, with dangerous repercussions. Liu et al reported 25 cases of CD5 negative (on IHC and flow cytometry) B-cell NHL with positive cyclin D1 expression and morphologic features consistent with MCL. They believed that these cases represent an antigenic variant of MCL and turn out to be a diagnostic pitfall. Recently SOX11 expression has been studied by various workers and is considered very useful in the diagnosis of MCL, including the cyclin D1-negative MCL. Kern et al detected SOX11 in 93% of conventional MCLs and also in their 12 cyclin D1 negative cases and concluded that it is a highly specific marker for both cyclin D1 positive and negative MCL.

Primary skin involvement in MCL is rare. However, skin can get secondarily involved in about 18% of stage IV MCL and in the blastoid variants. Skin involvement indicates a poor prognosis and may be the first manifestation of the disease. Skin lesions are generally nodular or macular/maculopapular. However, tumoral or infiltrated plaques and subcutaneous nodules may be present.

COMMENTARY INDEX CASE: PM 25983

This 42-year-old male, presented with erythematous maculopapular rashes on the entire body with multiple skin nodules on the face, causing considerable disfiguration of his face. There was fever, shortness of breath, left pleural effusion, generalized lymphadenopathy, hepatosplenomegaly, anemia, thrombocytopenia, TLC of 3,93,000/uL with 85% atypical lymphocytes in the peripheral blood and 80% atypical lymphoid cells in the bone marrow. Skin biopsy revealed nodular deposits in the deep dermis and subcutis. A diagnosis of CLL with massive cutaneous involvement was made. He was put on chlorambucil, to which he initially responded and later discontinued the medicine on his own. He deteriorated and was referred to our institute where he died within 10 hours. Flow cytometry (reported after the death of the patient), however, was suggestive of a MCL. Autopsy revealed a disseminated MCL involving the lymph nodes with florid infiltration into the extranodal sites like the bone marrow, peripheral blood, skin, spleen, liver, GIT, lungs, pancreas and muscle. The cell morphology in the nodal and all extranodal sites (except the bone marrow and peripheral blood) was of the classic MCL, with a monomorphic population of small cells with slightly irregular nuclei, scanty cytoplasm, inconspicuous nucleoli and low mitosis. The cells in the peripheral blood conformed to the morphology of blastoid variant. IHC done on the lymph node and skin were positive for cyclin D1, CD20, CD43, Bcl-2 and negative for CD5 (done twice, internal control positive), CD3, CD23 and CD10. CD5 was, however, positive on the flow cytometry. Worth stressing points in this case are—first time presentation with florid cutaneous lesions, heavy tumor load, blastoid morphology in the peripheral blood and common variant morphology in the nodal and other extranodal sites and discrepancy in CD5 results (IHC on paraffin embedded sections negative but CD5 positive on peripheral blood flow cytometry).

TAKE HOME MESSAGE

- Mantle cell lymphoma is a distinct clinicopathologic entity, occurring in elderly men with a median age of 65 years. It is an aggressive B-cell lymphoma and commonly presents with extranodal involvement.
- Expression of cyclin D1 is pathognomonic for MCL and is an indirect evidence of translocation t(11;14).
- Skin involvement in MCL is uncommon, occurs in the blastoid variant of MCL with disseminated disease and is associated with a poor prognosis. It may be the first manifestation of the disease, as in the index case.
- Recently SOX11 expression has been studied by various workers and is considered very useful in the diagnosis of MCL, including the cyclin D1-negative MCL.

SUGGESTED READING

1. Argatoff LH, Connors JM, Klasa RJ, et al. Mantle cell lymphoma: a clinicopathologic study of 80 cases. Blood. 1997;89:2067.
2. Canpolat F, Taş E, Albayrak-Sönmez A, et al. Cutaneous presentation of mantle cell lymphoma. Acta Dermatol Venereol. 2010;90:548-50.
3. Dorfman DM, Pinkus GS. Distinction between small lymphocytic and mantle cell lymphoma by immunoreactivity for CD23. Mod Pathol. 1994;7:326.
4. Ferrer A, Salaverria I, Bosch F, et al. Leukemic involvement is a common feature in mantle cell lymphoma. Cancer. 2007;109:2473.
5. Ishibashi M, Yamamoto K, Kudo S, et al. Mantle cell lymphoma with skin invasion characterized by the common variant in the subcutis and blastoid transformation in the overlying dermis. Am J Dermatopathol. 2010;32:180-2.
6. Liu Z, Dong HY, Gorczyca W, et al. CD5- Mantle cell lymphoma. Am J Clin Pathol. 2002;118:216.
7. Motegi S, Okada E, Nagai Y, et al. Skin manifestation of mantle cell lymphoma. Eur J Dermatol. 2006;16:435-8.
8. Mozos A, Royo C, Hartmann E, et al. SOX11 expression is highly specific for mantle cell lymphoma and identifies the cyclin D1-negative subtype. Hematologica. 2009;94:1555-62.

9. Phelps A, Elaba Z, Murphy MJ. Blastoid mantle cell lymphoma with cutaneous involvement and aberrant immunophenotype. Am J Dermatopathol. 2014;36:526-7.
10. Salaverria I, Royo C, Carvajal-Cuenca A, et al. CCND2 rearrangements are the most frequent genetic events in cyclin D1(-) mantle cell lymphoma. Blood. 2013;121:1394.
11. Samaha H, Dumontet C, Ketterer N, et al. Mantle cell lymphoma: a retrospective study of 121 cases. Leukemia. 1998;12:1281-7.
12. Sen F, Medeiros LJ, Lu D, et al. Mantle cell lymphoma involving skin: cutaneous lesions may be the first manifestation of disease and tumors often have blastoid cytologic features. Am J Surg Pathol. 2002;26:1312-8.
13. Yatabe Y, Suzuki R, Tobinai K, et al. Significance of cyclin D1 overexpression for the diagnosis of mantle cell lymphoma: A clinicopathologic comparison of cyclin D1-positive MCL and cyclin D1-negative MCL-like B-cell lymphoma. Blood. 2000;95:2253.

CONTRIBUTIONS BY:

1. Dr RK Vasishta, Professor and Head, Department of Histopathology (Consultation)
2. Dr Pankaj Kaul, Tutor, Department of Histopathology (Immunohistochemistry)
3. Dr Gaurav Prakash, Additional Professor, Department of Internal Medicine (Clinician In-Charge)
4. Dr Tushar Sehgal, Senior Resident, Department of Hematology (Providing Fig 2)
5. Dr Neelam Varma, Professor and Head, Department of Hematology
6. Dr SC Varma, ex Professor and Head, Department of Internal Medicine (Clinician In-Charge)

Post Graduate Institute of Medical Education and Research, Chandigarh, India.

CASE 2

Primary Myelofibrosis, Cellular Phase with Formation of Sclerosing Extramedullary Hematopoietic Tumors: PM 27873

Nandita Bharadwaj Kakkar

HIGHLIGHTS OF THE CASE

A 50-year-old-male came with pallor, jaundice, abdominal distension, hepatosplenomegaly, high SAAG ascites, bilateral pedal edema, loss of weight and appetite. Investigations revealed pancytopenia, deranged coagulogram, hyperbilirubinemia, raised alkaline phosphatase, CECT showed presence of multiple hypodense lesions in liver, spleen, a pancreatic mass lesion, nodular lesions in the lung parenchyma, cervical and retroperitoneal lymphadenopathy and ascites. PET scan revealed FDG avid lymph nodes on both side of diaphragm, hepatosplenomegaly with multiple coalescing lesions in liver, spleen and pancreas, multiple lung nodules and bone marrow lesions. Clinical diagnosis was Pancytopenia, High grade lymphoma ? DLBCL ? Carcinoma of unknown primary with bone marrow infiltration, metastasis to liver, spleen, lung, bone with ? Portal hypertension. Autopsy diagnosis was Primary Myelofibrosis, cellular phase with extensive extramedullary hematopoiesis and formation of sclerosing extramedullary hematopoietic tumors in the pancreas and lungs.

Keywords: Massive splenomegaly, pancytopenia, primary myelofibrosis, cellular phase, myeloid metaplasia, extramedullary hematopoiesis, sclerosing extramedullary hematopoietic tumor, pancreas, lungs.

CLINICAL DETAILS

Date of Admission and Death: 20.12.2016, Duration of Hospital Stay: 1 Hour

A 50-year-old male, a two wheeler mechanic by occupation was brought to the emergency in an unresponsive state. On examination he was E1V1M1 with unrecordable blood pressure and pulse rate, so was intubated and cardiopulmonary resuscitation was started. Patient revived but then he again suffered a cardiac arrest and was declared dead. As per history from patient's relatives and his old records, in March 2016 he had left supraclavicular lymphadenopathy, a fine-needle aspiration was done, diagnosis was suggestive of granulomatous inflammation [acid-fast bacilli (AFB) status not mentioned] and he was given antitubercular therapy for 6 months. In November 2016, he developed abdominal distension which was insidious in onset, progressive in nature associated with jaundice, high colored urine, swelling of both feet, loss of weight/appetite and was admitted at an outside facility. He underwent *CECT* of the chest, abdomen, and pelvis which showed presence of multiple hypodense lesions in liver, spleen with a pancreatic mass lesion along with cervical and retroperitoneal lymphadenopathy. He was then referred to PGIMER out patient department (OPD). There was history of fever, cough, pruritis, vomiting, loose stools, clay colored stools, melena and hematemesis. There was no history of oliguria, shortness of breath, chest pain, or facial puffiness. There was no history of diabetes mellitus, hypertension, pulmonary tuberculosis, bronchial asthma, or any malignancy/tuberculosis in the family. Patient was an occasional alcohol consumer for 30 years with alcohol intake of 150–250 g/week. He was not a smoker and there were no addictions. On ***examination*** (in PGIMER OPD) he was conscious, oriented with stable vitals. He had pallor, jaundice, left supraclavicular lymphadenopathy (3 × 3 cm, firm, nontender) and bilateral pitting edema. The abdomen was distended, soft, nontender, liver was just palpable with sharp margins, spleen was palpable 3 cm below costal margin and there was presence of free fluid, fluid thrill and bowel sounds were present. Cardiovascular/respiratory/central nervous systems were within normal limits.

Investigations

Hemogram—30.11.2016: Pancytopenia—Hb: 6.6 g/dL (2 unit PRBC transfused), TLC: 2600/μL, Platelet count: 92000/μL. **08.12.16**—Hb: 10.2 g/dL, TLC: 3600/μL, DLC—N/L/M/E/B: 77/10/01/10/02, platelet count: 35000/μL, Peripheral smear: platelets reduced. Coagulogram was deranged- PT/PTI/INR/aPTT: 15'/73%/1.4/39.7'.

Biochemistry—30.11.16: Na^+: 124 mEq/L, K^+: 4.0 mEq/L, serum urea/creatinine: 48/0.6 mg%, serum bilirubin: 3.2 mg%, SGOT/SGPT/ALP: 197/143/1115 U/L, serum total protein/albumin: 5.9/2.2 gm, serum Ca: 7.7 mg%, random blood sugar: 84 mg%. Urine routine microscopy: WNL, HIV/HBsAg/Anti-HCV: Non-reactive. ***Ascitic fluid*** (08/12/16): Total cells: 220, Neutrophils: 30%, Lymphocytes: 70%, protein low: 0.8 g/dL, sugar: 105 mg/dL, bilirubin: 1.0, amylase: 175 IU/L, ADA: 22 IU/L, SAAG high: 1.7 g/dL, malignant cytology: Negative. ***FNAC*** of SOL liver showed few clusters of hepatocytes with reactive changes. ***Upper GI endoscopy*** within normal limits. ***Colonoscopy***: multiple ulcers in ascending colon and internal piles at 6 O'clock position. ***Biopsy ascending colon***: Mild lymphocytic infiltration in lamina propria, no evidence of malignancy, cryptitis or crypt abscess. ***CECT***: (Figs 1A–B) A well-defined mass lesion seen in the tail of the pancreas, multiple variable sized hypodense lesions seen in liver and spleen, gross ascites present, few nodular lesions seen in the lungs with lymphadenopathy (cervical and retroperitoneal). ***PET scan***: FDG avid lymph nodes seen on both side of diaphragm, hepatosplenomegaly with multiple coalescing lesions in liver, spleen and pancreas, multiple lung nodules and marrow lesions—suggestive of ? Lymphomatous etiology ? Granulomatous inflammation ? IgG4 related disease ? Mitotic etiology.

Clinical diagnosis was Pancytopenia, High grade lymphoma-DLBCL ? Carcinoma of unknown primary with bone marrow infiltration, metastasis to liver, spleen, lung, bone with ? portal hypertension.

AUTOPSY FINDINGS: PM 27873

A complete autopsy was performed. The deceased was thin built, icteric, with pedal edema and petechiae on right lower abdomen. The peritoneal cavity yielded 1.5 L of yellowish fluid. Microscopically the postmortem ***bone marrow*** was hypercellular (Fig 2A) with an increase in number of megakaryocytes and marked preponderance of granulocytic series (Fig 2B). Erythropoiesis was depressed and few erythroid series of cells were discernable. Reticulin stain showed 1+ fibrosis (Fig 2C). Masson's trichrome stain did not show any fibrosis. The megakaryocytes (Figs 2D–H) showed varied morphology with hyperlobated/hypolobated/doughnut-shaped/macro/micromegakaryocytes. These atypical megakaryocytes had hyperchromatic, cloudy appearing nuclei on H&E stain. The prominent granulocytic hyperplasia was better appreciated by the myeloperoxidase (MPO) immunohistochemistry (Fig 2I). Considering the clinical picture, i.e. massive splenomegaly, hepatomegaly, and pancytopenia, overall features were consistent with a diagnosis of ***cellular phase of primary myelofibrosis***. The ***spleen*** (Fig 3A) was massively enlarged and weighed 1,180 g. Cut surface of spleen shows multiple firm white areas which looked like infarcts (Fig 3B). Microscopically

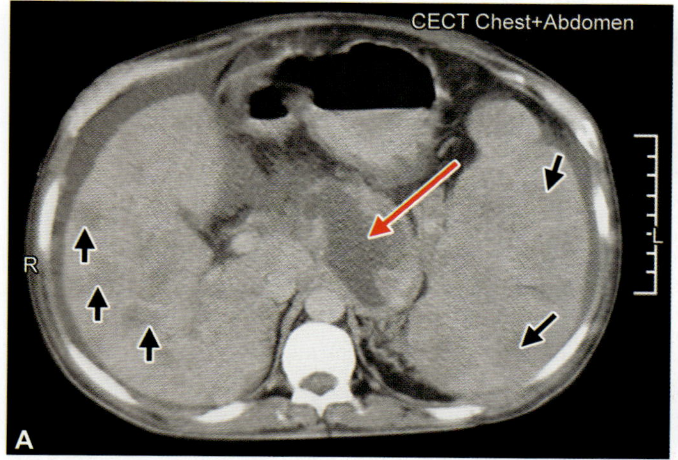

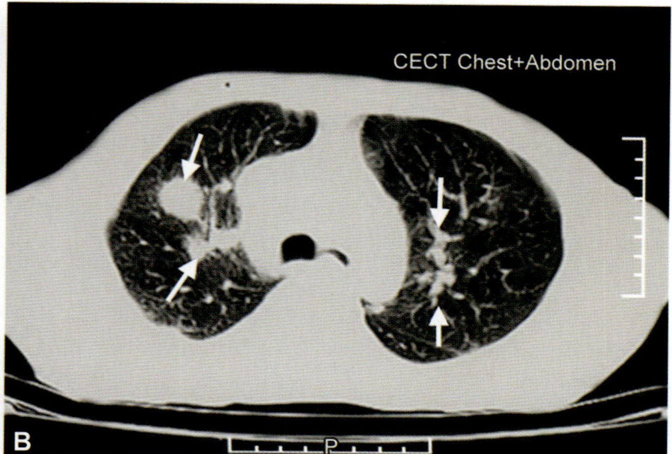

Figs 1A–B: (A) Contrast-enhanced computed tomography (CECT) shows heterogeneous lesion with central nonenhancing component seen abutting the tail of the pancreas (red arrow). Also seen are multiple hypodense lesions in the liver and spleen (black arrows); and (B) Multiple variable-sized nodules seen in both lung parenchyma (arrows).

the spleen showed marked congestion with extensive extramedullary hematopoiesis (EMH), i.e. myeloid metaplasia (Fig 3C), showing presence of marked granulocytic preponderance with MPO positivity (Figs 3D–E), admixed with atypical megakaryocytes (Figs 3F–H) and barely discernable erythroid series of cells. There were areas showing sparse EMH admixed with spindle-shaped fibroblasts and sclerosis of varying degrees (Fig 3I). Further there were areas where only sclerosis was noted and which corresponded to the firm, white and infarct-like areas noted on gross examination (Fig 3J). The ***liver*** (Fig 4A) was enlarged and weighed 1,700 g. Cut section was firm and showed multiple areas of congestion admixed with whitish areas, giving it a nutmeg appearance. On microscopic examination (Figs 4B–C) there were areas of congestion and diffusely present EMH in the parenchyma, which corresponded to the whitish areas seen on gross examination. The EMH was also present in the perivenular areas (Fig 4D) and in the portal tracts. These hematopoietic foci (Figs 4E–G) showed preponderance of granulocytic series (MPO strongly positive) of cells admixed with atypical megakaryocytes and few erythroid cells in a highly sclerotic/collagenized background. The ***lymph nodes*** (hilar, peripancreatic, para-aortic, and splenic) were mild to moderately enlarged, cut section was firm with areas of hemorrhage. On microscopy (Figs 5A–C), the lymph node architecture was totally effaced, no follicles were appreciated, areas of hemorrhage were noted, sparse lymphoid cells were identified, mostly at the periphery in the subcapsular sinuses and there was extensive sclerosis. At a high power

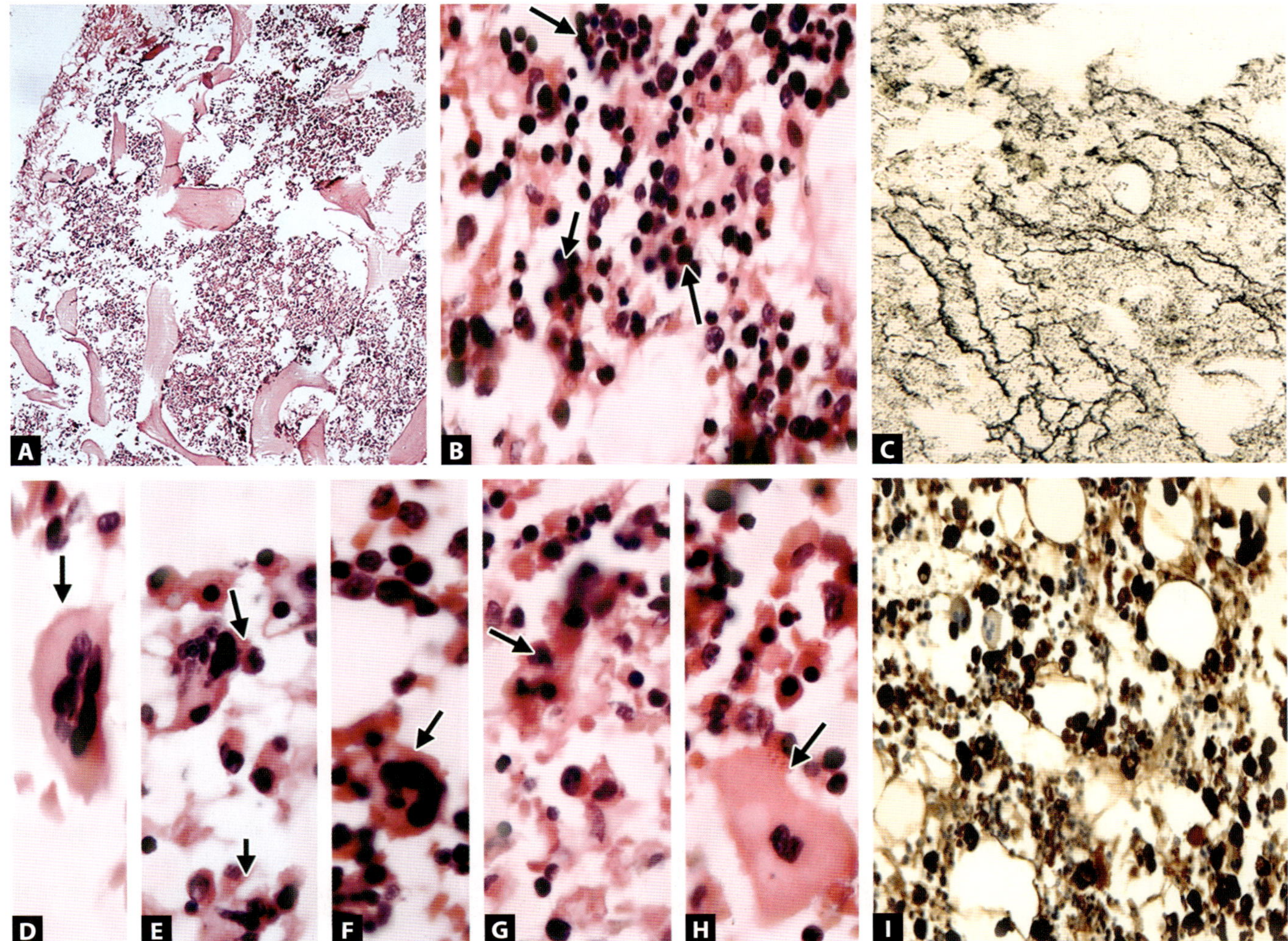

Figs 2A–I: Photomicrographs of the postmortem bone marrow shows (A) Hypercellularity; (B) Granulocytic preponderance (arrows); (C) Reticulin fibrosis 1+; (D–H) Atypical megakaryocytes (arrows); and (I) Myeloperoxidase (MPO) stain shows a granulocytic preponderance.

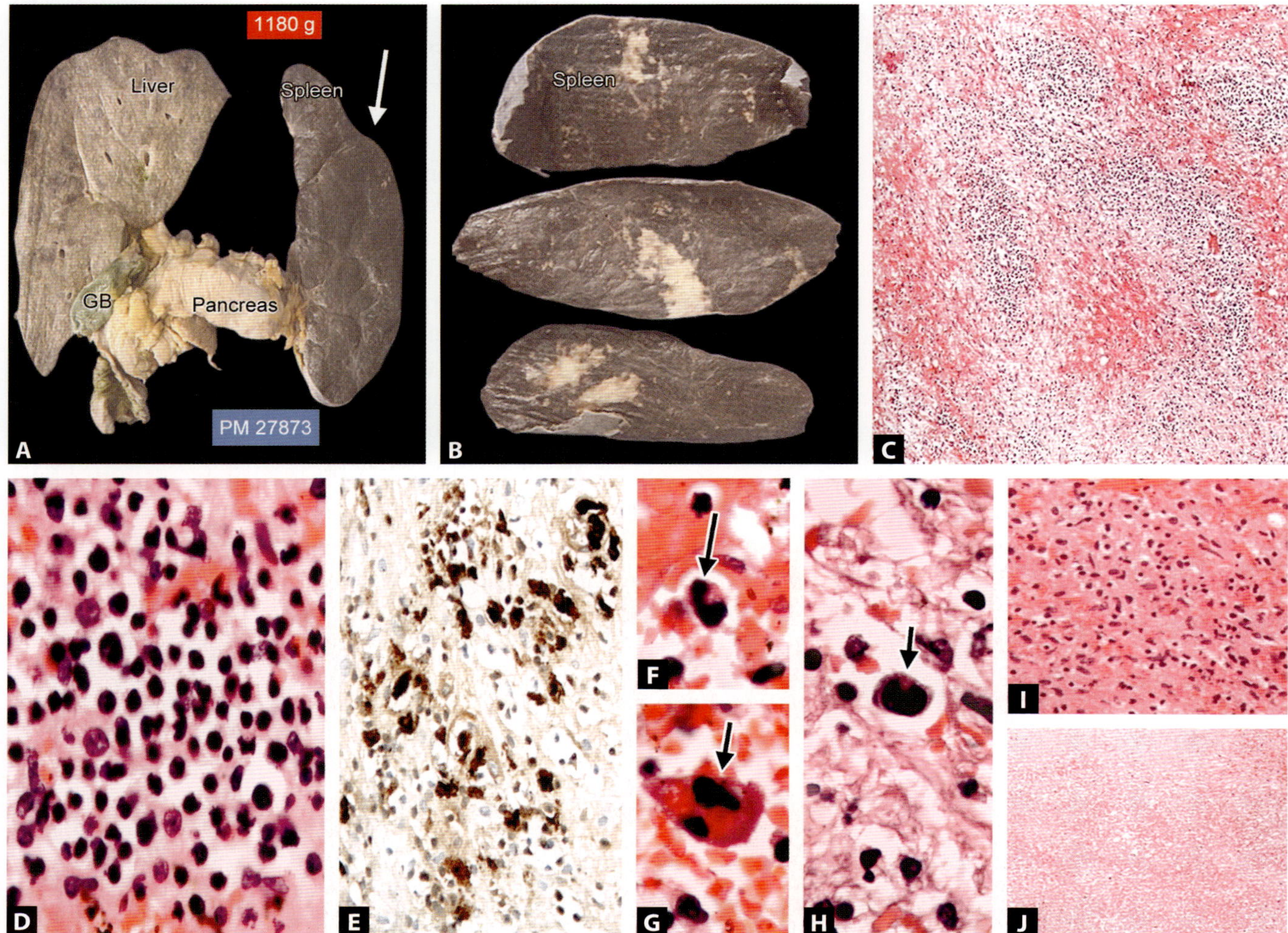

Figs 3A–J: (A) Organ complex of the slice of liver, gallbladder, pancreas and slice of spleen. The spleen shows massive enlargement and its slice is as big as that of the liver; (B) Slices of the enlarged spleen showing areas of sclerosis mimicking infarcts; Photomicrographs of the spleen showing (C) Foci of EMH along with congestion; (D–E) Foci of EMH showing granulocytic preponderance with MPO strongly positive (in E); (F–H) Atypical megakaryocytes (arrows); (I) Areas showing spindle-shaped cells with fibrosis and sparse EMH; (J) Extensive sclerosis.

(Figs 5D–F) cells present in the sclerotic background were foci of EMH showing granulocytic preponderance (MPO strongly positive) admixed with atypical megakaryocytes and barely discernable erythroid cells. The tail and part of the body of the ***pancreas*** was bulky and contained a well-circumscribed, homogeneous firm white, mass measuring 5 × 4 × 3 cm (Fig 6A). The texture of the mass was firm, sclerotic and appreciably different from the adjacent normal pancreas (Fig 6B). Microscopically (Figs 6C–G) sections from the mass revealed EMH with granulocytic preponderance (MPO strongly positive) admixed with atypical megakaryocytes, few erythroid cells, in a densely sclerotic background. Sections from the pancreas (Figs 7A–B) immediately adjacent to the mass showed similar infiltrates of EMH, destroying the acini along with beginning of sclerosis and inspissated secretions in pancreatic ducts. The peripancreatic area (Fig 7C), especially around the mass also showed similar EMH and sclerosis, entrapping the nerves. The ***lungs*** (Figs 7D–E) on cut section showed areas of hemorrhage and firm, white, solid nodules measuring 0.5–2 cm in diameter, more in the left lung than right lung. Microscopic sections from the lung (Figs 7F and 8A–E) nodules showed similar findings as seen in the pancreatic mass, i.e. EMH with granulocytic preponderance, atypical megakaryocytes, and fibrosis. Along with this there were foci of necrosis. However, special stains with PAS, AFB, and Grams were

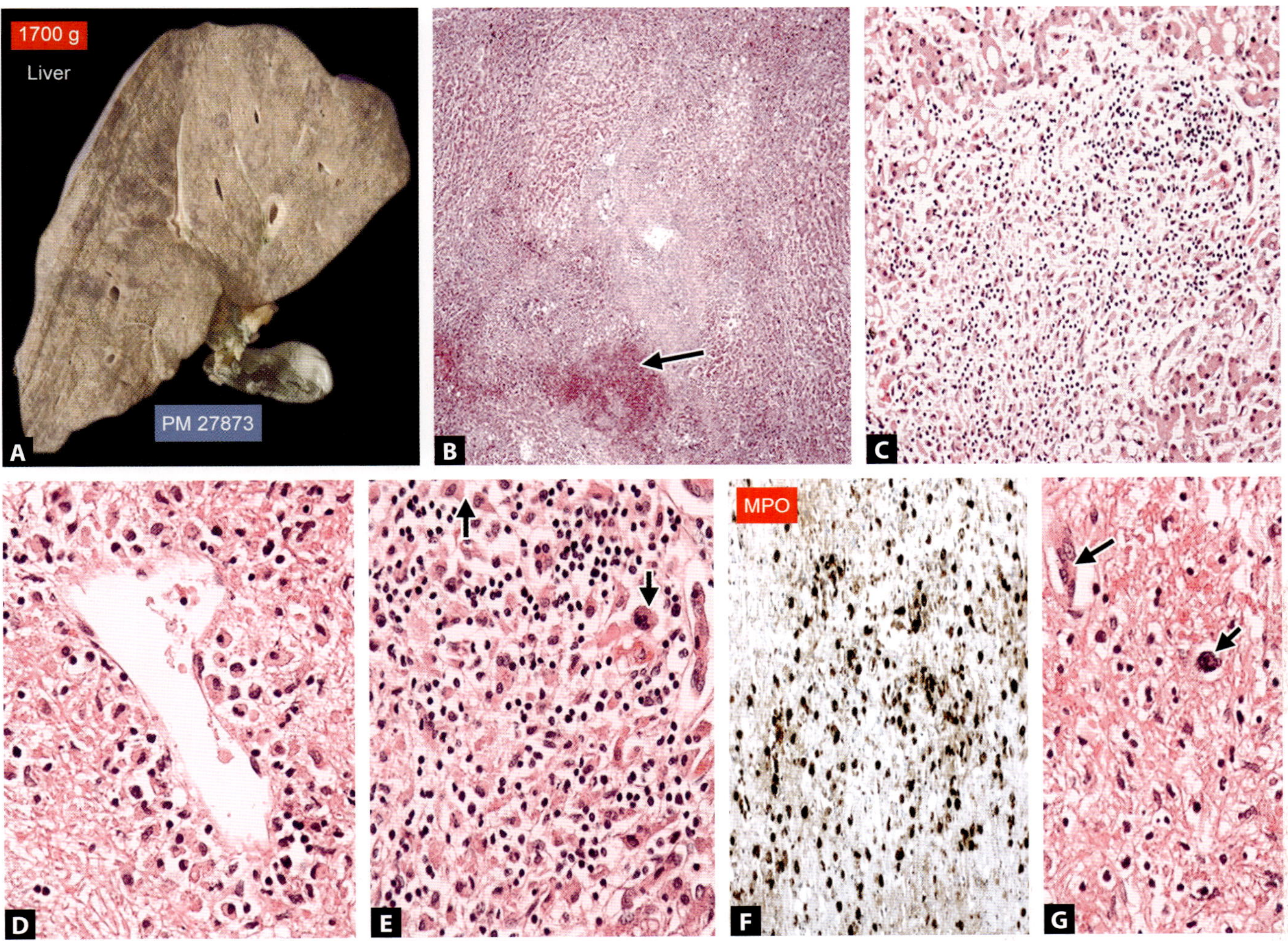

Figs 4A–G: (A) Slice of the liver showing multiple areas of congestion admixed with whitish areas, giving it a nutmeg appearance; Photomicrographs of the liver (B) Showing areas of congestion (arrow) and diffuse EMH; (C) Foci of EMH; (D) Perivenular EMH; (E) Cellular foci of EMH with atypical megakaryocyte (arrows) and granulocytic precursors; (F) Granulocyte precursors strongly positive for MPO immunostain; and (G) Sclerotic areas with sparse cells and few atypical megakaryocytes (arrows).

negative for any infective pathology. Other areas of the lungs showed extensive alveolar hemorrhage. The EMH in all the organs was accompanied with extensive sclerosis (Figs 8F–G) which was highlighted by Masson's trichrome stain. In some areas, only sclerotic tissue could be seen which was devoid of EMH cells. In the pancreas and the lung, it formed well-circumscribed nodules, but had the patient lived for some more time, well-circumscribed tumors would have been seen in liver and spleen as well. The presence of large atypical cells and sclerosis made us think of Hodgkin's lymphoma (lymphocyte depleted/nodular sclerosis type) but the morphology of the large cells was not consistent with the Hodgkin's cells, as they lacked prominent eosinophilic nucleoli and were negative for CD15/CD30. Immunostain for megakaryocytic marker CD61 did not work well but the morphology of the cells and PAS positivity was enough to label them as megakaryocytes.

FINAL AUTOPSY DIAGNOSIS: PM 27873

50 Years Male with Pancytopenia and Massive Splenomegaly

- *Primary myelofibrosis*—Cellular phase
    - With extensive extramedullary hematopoiesis (EMH) with preponderance of granulocytic series and presence of atypical megakaryocytes in spleen, liver, lymph nodes, pancreas, lungs and peripancreatic areas.

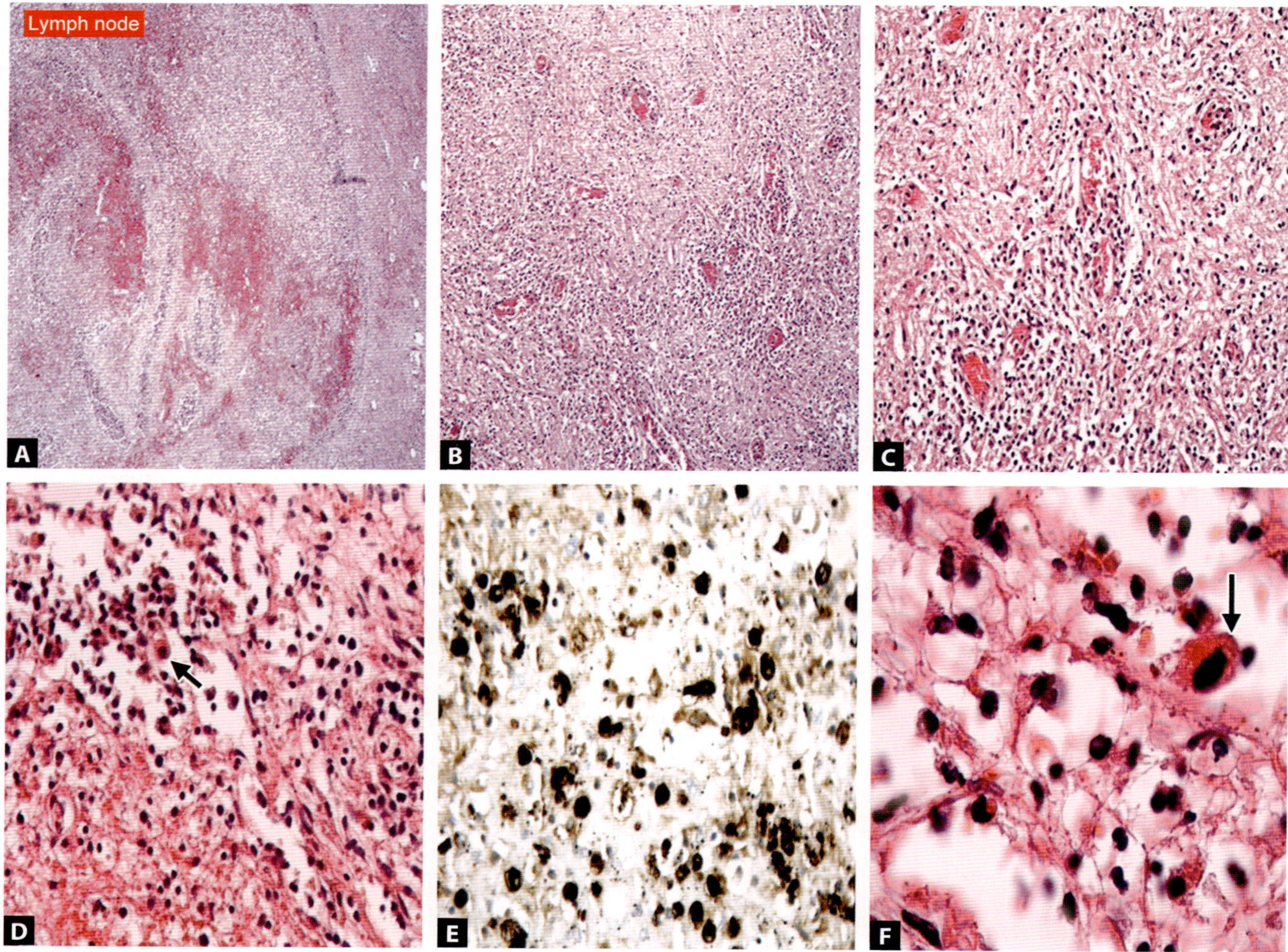

Figs 5A–F: Photomicrographs of the lymph nodes. (A) Total loss of architecture with areas of hemorrhage; (B) Extensive sclerosis with prominent vessels; (C–D) EMH with few large cells (arrow) in the background of sclerosis; (E) MPO stain shows granulocytic preponderance; and (F) Atypical megakaryocyte (arrow).

- *Sclerosing extramedullary hematopoietic tumors (SEMHT)*—Pancreas and lungs
- Pulmonary hemorrhage
- Ascites.

Primary Myelofibrosis

Refer to Case 3 PM 23618.

SCLEROSING EXTRAMEDULLARY HEMATOPOIETIC TUMORS

Chronic myeloproliferative disorders at times give rise to SEMHTs which occur in organs where EMH is going on. EMH is morphologically more cellular and with increasing fibrosis, leads to the formation of well-defined masses which are labeled as SEMHT. They were first described by Beckman and Oehrle in 1982. These tumors are a real diagnostic dilemma in an undiagnosed case of a myeloproliferative disorder. Its correct diagnosis is of utmost importance as it brings into light the basic underlying disease, for the initiation of the proper treatment. Morphologically they are composed of proliferating atypical megakaryocytes, a large number of granulocytic precursors and few erythroid series of cells in a highly sclerotic/fibrotic background. They have been reported in the liver, lungs, retroperitoneum, serosa, mesentery, lymph nodes, breast, lacrimal gland, skin, adrenal gland and kidneys. Awareness is the key to the

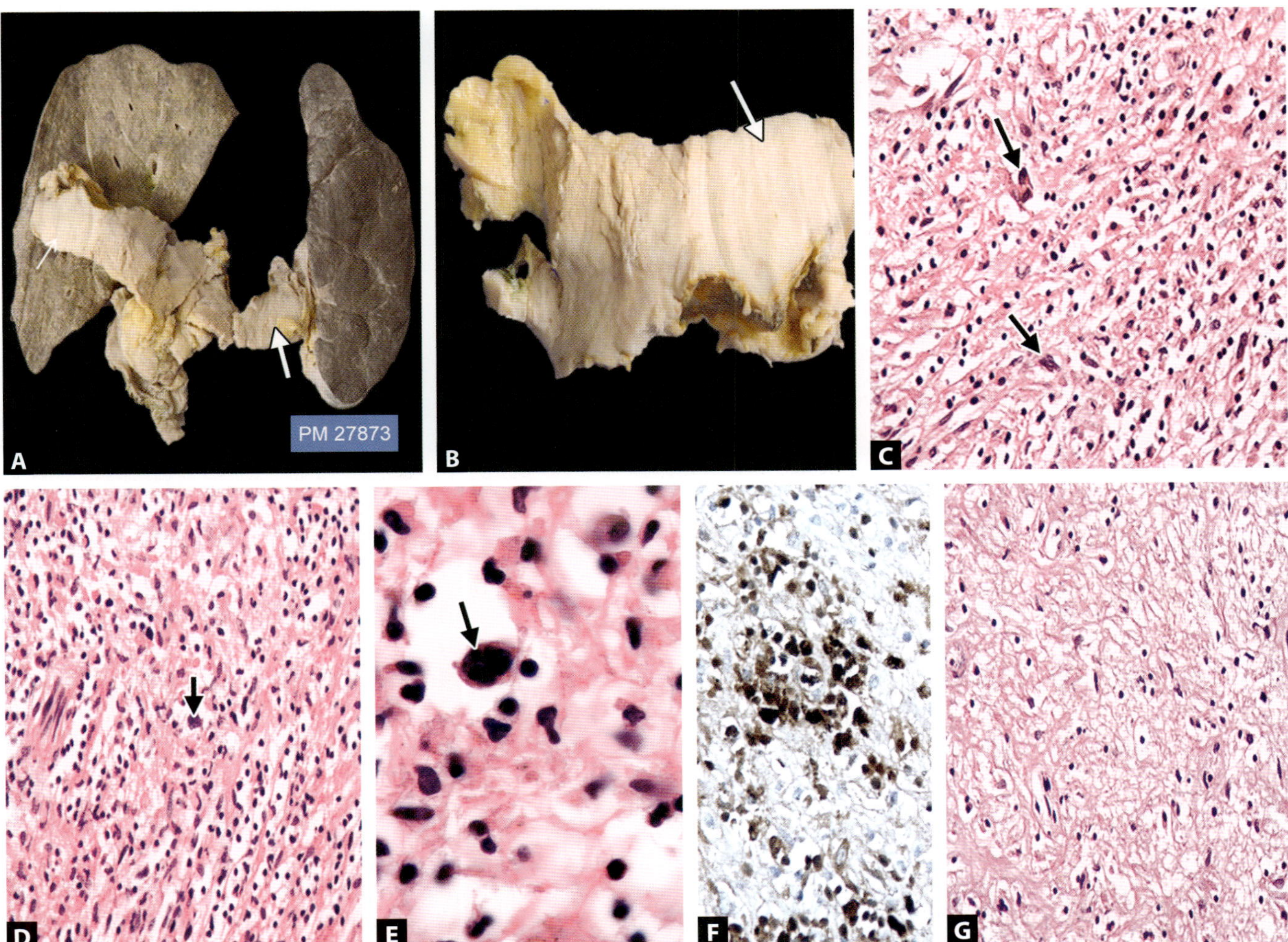

Figs 6A–G: (A and B) Pancreas showing a well-circumscribed firm white tumor in the tail extending into the body (arrows); (C–E) Photomicrographs from the pancreatic tumor shows EMH with atypical megakaryocytes (arrows) in a sclerotic background; (F) MPO immunostain positive in the granulocytic precursors; and (G) Areas of extensive sclerosis.

diagnosis as the eyes will not see what the mind does not know. As a result of the extensive fibrosis, the morphology of the cells is often distorted as also seen in the index case. The bulbous/cloud-shaped megakaryocytes usually seen in primary myelofibrosis, due to the distortion appear like some pleomorphic giant cells, leading to varied erroneous diagnosis. Thus, the differential diagnosis of SEMHT is wide and includes fibrohistiocytic tumors, mesenchymal tumors, Hodgkin's lymphoma (lymphocyte depleted/nodular sclerosis), sarcomas, poorly differentiated/spindle cell/sclerotic carcinomas, melanoma, sclerosing inflammatory diseases like IgG4 disease and leukemia cutis. Immunohistochemistry with CD61/Factor VIII for highlighting the megakaryocytic lineage, MPO for granulocytic series and glycophorin for erythroid series of cells, helps in making a diagnosis. EMH as the name suggests is the presence and proliferation of hematopoietic tissue outside of the bone marrow and is seen in various hematological conditions like thalassemia, spherocytosis, sickle cell anemia, Gaucher's disease, osteopetrosis and myeloproliferative disorders especially primary myelofibrosis. Most commonly, EMH occurs in the spleen, liver and lymph nodes, but can be seen in the lung, kidneys, skin, breast, thyroid gland and GI tract. In primary myelofibrosis, the hallmark is the increase in megakaryocytes which are dysplastic. They liberate platelet-derived growth

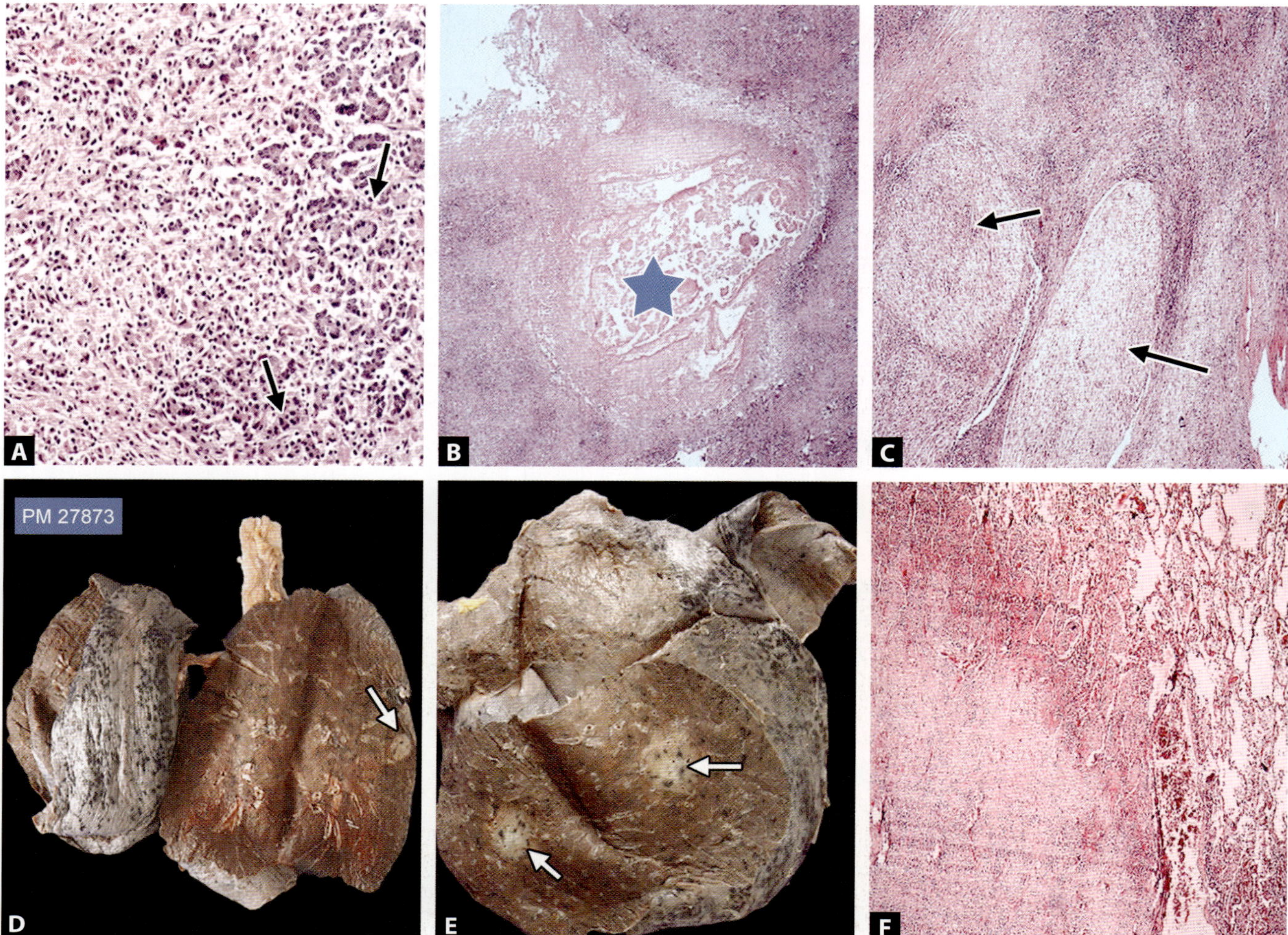

Figs 7A–F: Photomicrographs of the pancreas adjacent to the mass shows (A) Extramedullary hematopoiesis extending into and destroying the acini (arrows); (B) Dilated ducts with inspissated secretions (star); (C) Extensive EMH surrounding the nerves (arrows) in the peripancreatic areas; (D–E) Gross photograph of the lungs showing well-circumscribed firm, white nodules (arrows); and (F) Lung nodule at low power.

factor, transforming growth factor, and endothelial/epidermal growth factors which stimulate fibroplasias.

COMMENTARY—INDEX CASE: PM 27873

A 50-year-old male came with pallor, jaundice, abdominal distension, hepatosplenomegaly, high SAAG ascites, bilateral pedal edema, loss of weight and appetite. Investigations revealed pancytopenia, deranged coagulogram, hyperbilirubinemia, raised alkaline phosphatase, CECT showed presence of multiple hypodense lesions in the liver, spleen, a pancreatic mass lesion, nodular lesions in the lung parenchyma, cervical and retroperitoneal lymphadenopathy, and ascites. PET scan revealed FDG avid lymph nodes on both sides of diaphragm, hepatosplenomegaly with multiple coalescing lesions in liver, spleen and pancreas, multiple lung nodules and marrow lesions. Clinical diagnosis was pancytopenia, high-grade lymphoma, ? DLBCL ? Carcinoma of unknown primary with bone marrow infiltration and metastasis to liver, spleen, lung and bone with portal hypertension.

Autopsy diagnosis in this 50-year-old male with pancytopenia and massive splenomegaly (1,180 g) was primary myelofibrosis (cellular phase) with extensive EMH and formation of well-circumscribed tumors labeled as SEMHTs in the pancreas and lungs. This diagnosis was not considered during

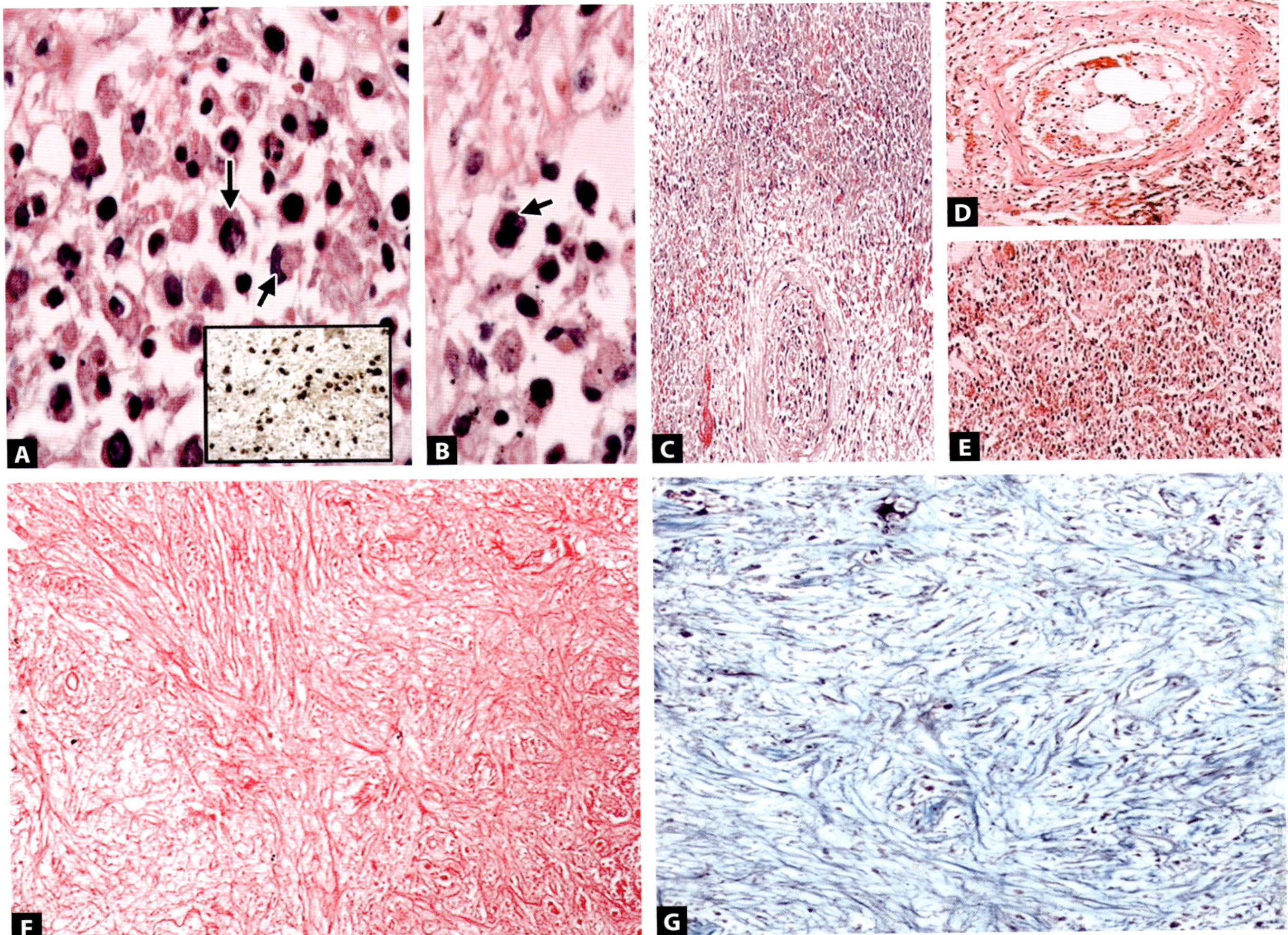

Figs 8A–G: Photomicrographs of the lung nodule shows (A–B) EMH with atypical large cells (arrows) and sclerosis. Inset shows MPO positivity; (C) Areas of necrosis; (D) Bone marrow emboli; (E) Adjacent lung shows alveolar hemorrhage; and (F–G) Areas of extensive sclerosis seen in all organs (H&E and Masson's trichrome).

the life of this patient. To make this diagnosis at postmortem was a herculean task as the extensive sclerosis accompanying the EMH, was actually distorting the morphology of the hematopoietic cells. The well-circumscribed SEMHTs in the pancreas and lungs looked like fibrohistiocytic tumors. Antemortem peripheral blood examination was not available in the file and we were unaware of the leukoerythroblastic picture, presence of anisopoikilocytosis or tear drop cells. Antemortem bone marrow examination and molecular workup were not done. What led us toward the final autopsy diagnosis was: (a) Massive splenomegaly, (b) Peripheral pancytopenia, (c) Cellular bone marrow with preponderance of granulocyte precursors along with increased number and atypical forms of megakaryocytes. The reticulin was only 1+ in the marrow, hence this was a cellular phase of myelofibrosis, and (d) The EMH accompanied by extensive sclerosis distorted the morphology of the cells. Large atypical cells when seen in a reactive background with sclerosis suggest a Hodgkin's lymphoma—nodular sclerosis/lymphocyte depleted. But in the index case, the large atypical looking cells were not so large like the Hodgkin's cells, did not have an eosinophilic nucleoli and were negative for CD30 and CD15. They looked like megakaryocytes with atypicality and thus this took us toward a diagnosis of EMH with extensive sclerosis and SEMHTs in the pancreas and lungs. With time, the liver and spleen would also have developed similar mass lesions.

TAKE HOME MESSAGE

- Peripheral pancytopenia, massive splenomegaly, cellular bone marrow with increased number of atypical megakaryocytes and a marked granulocytic preponderance should take us toward a diagnosis of cellular phase of primary myelofibrosis.
- Sclerosing extramedullary hematopoietic tumors are rare manifestation of chronic myeloproliferative disorders, especially primary myelofibrosis.
- Sclerosing extramedullary hematopoietic tumors are a diagnostic pitfall, especially in an undiagnosed case of myelofibrosis and awareness of this entity is the key to the diagnosis.

SUGGESTED READING

1. Gu MJ. Sclerosing extramedullary hematopoietic tumor presenting as an inguinal mass in a patient with primary myelofibrosis: a diagnostic pitfall. Int J Clin Exp Pathol. 2015;8:3381-3.
2. Karaarslan S, Nese N, Oncel G, et al. Sclerosing extramedullary hematopoietic tumor mimicking intra-abdominal sarcoma. J Pathol Transl Med. 2015;49:335-8.
3. LeBlanc RE, Lester L, Kwong B, et al. JAK2-positive cutaneous myelofibrosis presenting as sclerosing extramedullary hematopoietic tumors on the scalp: case presentation and review of the literature. J Cutan Pathol. 2015;42:858-62.
4. Yang X, Bhuiya T, Esposito M. Sclerosing extramedullary hematopoietic tumor. Ann Diagn Pathol. 2002;6:183-7.

CONTRIBUTIONS BY:

1. Dr Shivani Chandel, Junior Resident, Department of Internal Medicine (Compilation of Clinical Details)
2. Dr Gaurav Garg, Junior Resident, Department of Pathology (Helping with Gross Photographs)
3. Dr Jasmine Kaur, Senior Resident, Department of Radiodiagnosis and Imaging (Figs 1A and B)
4. Dr Ashish Bhalla, Professor, Department of Internal Medicine (Clinician In-Charge)

Post Graduate Institute of Medical Education and Research, Chandigarh, India.

CASE 3

Primary Myelofibrosis, Cellular Phase with Extensive Extramedullary Hematopoiesis and Transformation into Acute Leukemia: PM 23618

Nandita Bharadwaj Kakkar

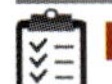

HIGHLIGHTS OF THE CASE

This was a 55-year-old male who was diagnosed as a case of primary myelofibrosis (PMF) (prefibrotic cellular phase) one year before his demise. He first presented with pancytopenia and a leukoerythroblastic picture. Bone marrow revealed a cellular phase of myelofibrosis with 4% blasts. BCR-ABL fusion gene and JAK2 mutation on peripheral blood cells was negative. He was on treatment, but became transfusion dependent. During his last admission, he had exertional dyspnea, easy fatigability, joint pains and fever. There was pancytopenia with 30% blasts in the peripheral blood. Autopsy revealed a prefibrotic cellular phase of PMF progressing into acute leukemia (30% blasts in peripheral blood), extensive extramedullary hematopoiesis (EMH)/myeloid metaplasia, secondary hemosiderosis, coronary artery disease and features of heart failure.

Keywords: Myelofibrosis, primary, cellular phase, prefibrotic phase, myeloid metaplasia, extramedullary hematopoiesis, acute leukemia, transformation, autopsy.

CLINICAL DETAILS

Date of Admission: 11.03.2010, Date of Death: 30.03.2010, and Hospital Stay: 19 Days

This was a 55-year-old-male who was diagnosed as a case of Primary Myelofibrosis (Prefibrotic cellular phase) in February 2009, one year before his demise. He first presented in 2009 with pancytopenia and a leucoerythroblastic picture. Bone marrow revealed a cellular phase of myelofibrosis with 4% blasts. BCR-ABL fusion gene and JAK 2 mutation on peripheral blood cells was negative. He was treated with oral thallidomide, danazole and medrol. He was transfusion dependent and received approximately 70-80 units of blood transfusions from Feb 2009 till Feb 2010. There was thrombocytopenia with history of bleeding from the gums and epistaxis, for which platelet transfusions were administered. He was an occasional alcohol consumer and a smoker (one packet per day). He had worked in a paint factory, where he had been exposed to nitrobenzene. In the year preceding his demise, he had had multiple admissions for fever, bleeding per rectum and palpitations. In Nov 2009, the serum ferritin levels were 6691 ng/mL (N<200 ng/mL). In March 2010, he was admitted with complaints of exertional dyspnea and easy fatigability since few months, pain in the joints since one month and fever. The fever was acute in onset, high grade, intermittent and was followed by yellow discoloration of sclera and urine. No pruritis or clay colored stools were noted. Pain was present both in the large/small joints i.e. bilateral knees, ankles, shoulder and small joints of the hands. There was no accompanying swelling, redness, warmth or stiffness. There was no paroxysmal nocturnal dyspnea, orthopnea or chest pain. There was right abdominal pain since one month, dull, worsening on deep inspiration and coughing, but not related to food intake. Swelling on feet and petechial spots on feet and legs were noted for the last 3 days. On ***examination*** there was pallor, icterus, platonychia, enlarged lymph nodes in the axilla and left cervical region, raised jugular venous pressure, positive Kausmaul's sign, pedal edema, no cyanosis, no clubbing, petechial spots and purpura present on dorsum of feet and legs, bronze pigmentation of face, Café au lait spots present on the hand, normal genitalia, pulse rate 74/mt and BP-100/70 mmHg. Per abdomen there was tenderness in the right hypochondrium, liver and spleen were palpable 4 cm and 3 cm below their respective costal margins. No free fluid was noted and bowel sounds were normal. Cardiovascular system- S_1/S_2-normal, fourth heart sound heard and presysytolic murmur heard in the tricuspid area. The chest and CNS were within normal limits.

Investigations and Course of Management

Hematological: Hemogram revealed pancytopenia with Hb-4.6-5.9 g/dL, TLC 2300-3200/uL, DLC - N10,L8,M,E1,-Blasts 30, Absolute neutrophil count - 320, platelets - 2000 -6000/uL, peripheral blood film showed marked anisopoikilocytosis, macrocytes, microcytes, tear drop cells, retic count - 0.5-1.7%. Coagulogram deranged - PTI-60%, PTTK- 35 secs. Flow cytometry for PNH negative, G6PD-normal, ANA-1+(speckled), urine and plasma Hb negative.

Blood biochemistry/others: S. bilirubin 0.9-1.4 mg%, SGOT/SGPT -40/90 U/L, total proteins / albumin -6.8/3.5 gm, S. alkaline phosphatase 57 U/L, Ca^{2+}/P -8.3/5.1 mg%, S.urea/creatinine- 37/1 mg%, Na^+/K^+ -138/2.7 mEq/L, Blood culture sterile, Serology for HBsAg / HIV / HCV negative, Urine for hemosiderin negative, Thyroid function tests normal. ***X ray chest*** – bilateral ground glass opacities.

Course and Management: Patient was diagnosed as Primary Myelofibrosis and was on therapy. He continued to have features of bicytopenia and later on pancytopenia, requiring considerable amounts of blood and platelet support. After 70 transfusions he was evaluated for iron overload and was found to have markedly raised serum ferritin. He had fever which resolved with antibiotics and congestive cardiac failure for which diuretics were given. But the bone marrow failure persisted. The peripheral blood showed 30% blasts and transformation into acute leukaemia was considered. The patient soon deteriorated, cyanosis was observed and he suffered a cardiac arrest from which he could not be revived. ***Units clinical diagnosis*** was (1) Primary Myelofibrosis progressing to acute leukemia. (2) Secondary haemosiderosis-Chronic transfusion therapy.

AUTOPSY FINDINGS: PM 23618

A complete autopsy was performed on this 55-year-old male. All serous cavities were within normal limits. The ***bone marrow*** was hypercellular (Fig 1A) with depression of the erythroid component and marked granulocytic hyperplasia (Fig 1B) documented by strong positivity with myeloperoxidase (MPO) immunostain (Fig 1C). It was not possible to comment on the number of blasts on the bone marrow section. There was prominent megakaryocytic hyperplasia with marked dysplasia in the form of micro/macromegakaryocytes, abnormal nuclear–cytoplasmic ratio, hyperchromatic nuclei, irregularly folded, balloon like or bulbous with abnormal chromatin clumping and presence of bare forms (Figs 1D–E). The periodic acid-Schiff (PAS) stain stained the cytoplasm of these megakaryocytes deep magenta (Figs 1F–H). These dysplastic megakaryocytes were seen in clusters adjacent to the bone marrow trabeculae (Fig 2A) and vascular sinuses. CD61, a megakaryocyte marker, highlighted these megakaryocytes (Fig 2B). CD34 positive stem cells were increased in the bone marrow (Fig 2C). Reticulin stain showed 1+ fibrosis (Fig 2D). Masson's trichrome stain did not reveal any increase in collagen fibers (Fig 2E). The Prussian blue stain revealed 1+ iron stores (Fig 2F). Taking into account the whole picture in totality, i.e. peripheral pancytopenia with a leukoerythroblastic picture and 30% blasts, a hypercellular marrow with marked granulocytic hyperplasia, erythroid depression, abundant dysplastic megakaryocytes (hallmark and key to the recognition of MF), a reticulin of 1 + with no collagen fibers, and a BCR-ABL fusion gene and JAK2 mutation on peripheral blood cells being negative, a diagnosis of cellular phase of myelofibrosis with transformation into acute leukemia was made. The ***spleen*** weighed 520 g, was markedly enlarged but did not show any focal lesion (Fig 3A). Microscopy (Figs 3B–F) revealed florid EMH, i.e. myeloid metaplasia with granulocytic series of cells (MPO positive) and abundant dysplastic megakaryocytes (CD61, PAS+) in the red pulp. CD34 immunostain showed a large number of positive cells, thereby indicating their sequestration in the spleen. The Prussian blue stain showed 2+ positivity. The ***lymph nodes***, mesenteric (Fig 4A), para-aortic, peripancreatic and hilar were moderately enlarged. Microscopy (Figs 4B–F) showed sinuses packed with florid EMH with abundant dysplastic megakaryocytes (CD61, PAS+). The MPO immunohistochemistry showed positivity in the granulocytic series of cells. The ***liver*** (Fig 5A) was enlarged, weighed 2,220 g and was brown in color. The portal tract and sinuses showed EMH with many dysplastic megakaryocytes (Fig 5B). MPO immunostain showed positivity in the cells present in the sinuses and portal tracts, indicating them to be granulocytic precursors. Hepatocytes and Kupffer cells were loaded with iron which showed 4+ positivity with Prussian blue stain (Fig 5C). Microscopic sections of the ***kidneys*** revealed EMH. The ***lungs*** were heavy and weighed 1,950 g. Cut section revealed hemorrhagic consolidation (Fig 5D). On microscopy (Figs 5E–F) extensive pulmonary hemorrhage, edema and plenty of hemosiderin laden macrophages indicating chronic passive venous congestion was noted. The ***heart*** weighed 430 g. The valves were normal. There was left ventricular hypertrophy, wall thickness 2.2 cm (Fig 5G) and right ventricular dilatation. The coronaries revealed coronary artery disease with 70% occlusion of the left anterior descending artery (Fig 5G—inset), 50% occlusion of the left circumflex artery and 30% occlusion of the right coronary artery. Other organs including the brain were within normal limits.

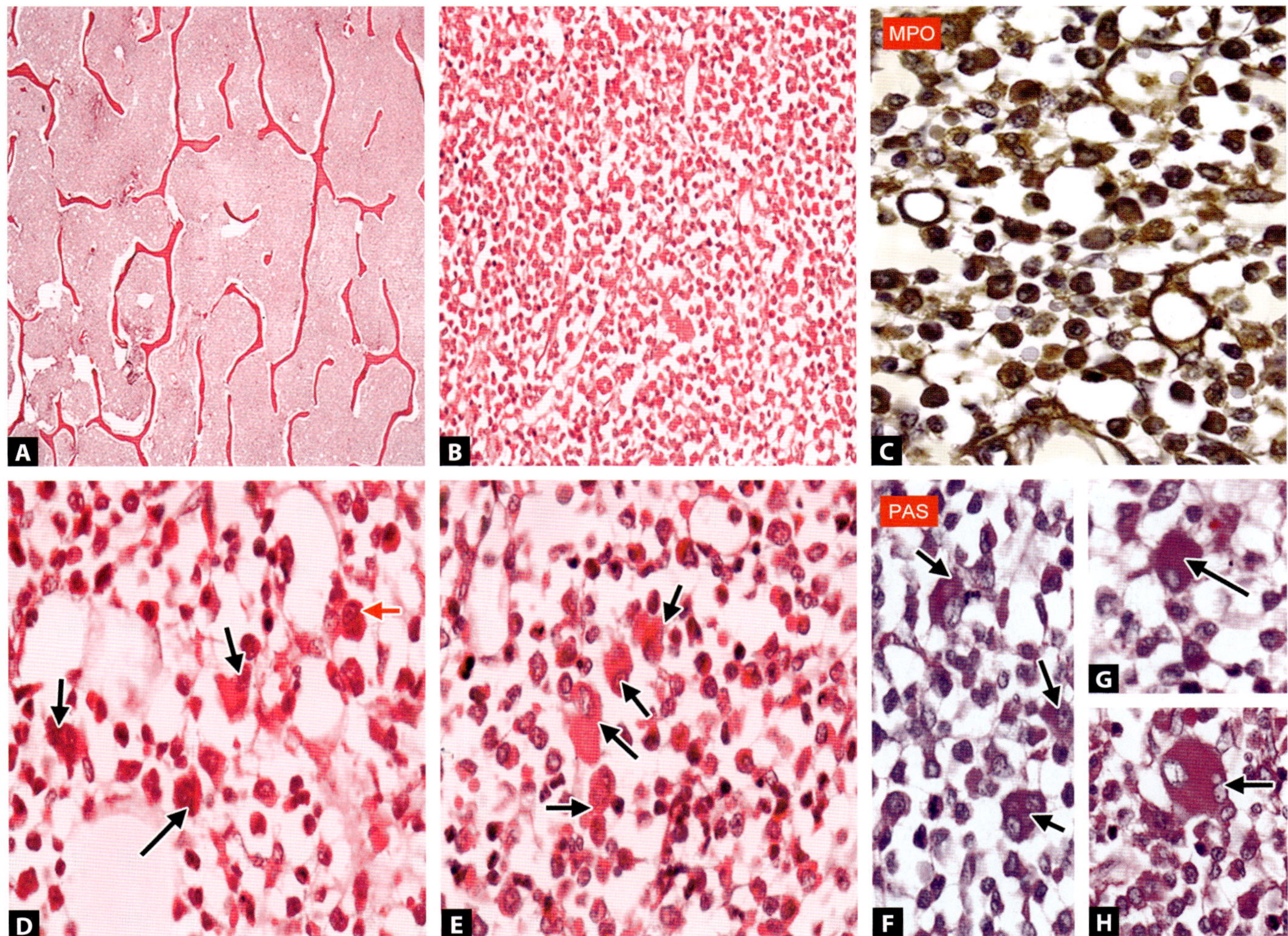

Figs 1A–H: Photomicrographs of the postmortem bone marrow showing (A) Hypercellular marrow spaces; (B) Marked granulocytic hyperplasia; (C) Myeloperoxidase immunostain substantiates the granulocytic hyperplasia; (D–E) Clusters of dysplastic megakaryocytes (arrows); and (F–H) Periodic acid-Schiff (PAS) stain, stains the cytoplasm of the atypical megakaryocytes magenta (arrows).

FINAL AUTOPSY DIAGNOSIS: PM 23618

55 Years Male

- Primary myelofibrosis, cellular phase, progressing into acute leukemia (30% blasts in peripheral blood).
- Extensive extra medullary hematopoiesis, i.e. myeloid metaplasia in the spleen, lymph nodes, liver and kidneys.
- *Secondary hemosiderosis*—Liver, spleen.
- Left ventricular hypertrophy with dilated right ventricle.
- *Coronary artery disease*—Left anterior descending—70%, left circumflex—50% and right coronary—30% occlusion.
- Extensive pulmonary hemorrhage, edema with chronic passive venous congestion.

PRIMARY MYELOFIBROSIS

Primary myelofibrosis along with polycythemia vera and essential thrombocythemia come under the umbrella of myeloproliferative disorders. PMF is a clonal myeloproliferative neoplasm, wherein the bone marrow shows an evolution from a prefibrotic cellular phase with minimal or absent reticulin fibrosis to a frankly fibrotic stage with marked reticulin/collagen fibrosis along with EMH/myeloid metaplasia. One-third of the patients with PMF are incidentally detected on a routine checkup, by the presence of splenomegaly, anemia, leukocytosis, thrombocytosis, leukoerythroblastic picture, and raised lactate dehydrogenase. PMF may come to light by the presence of dyspnea, fatigue, night sweats, weight

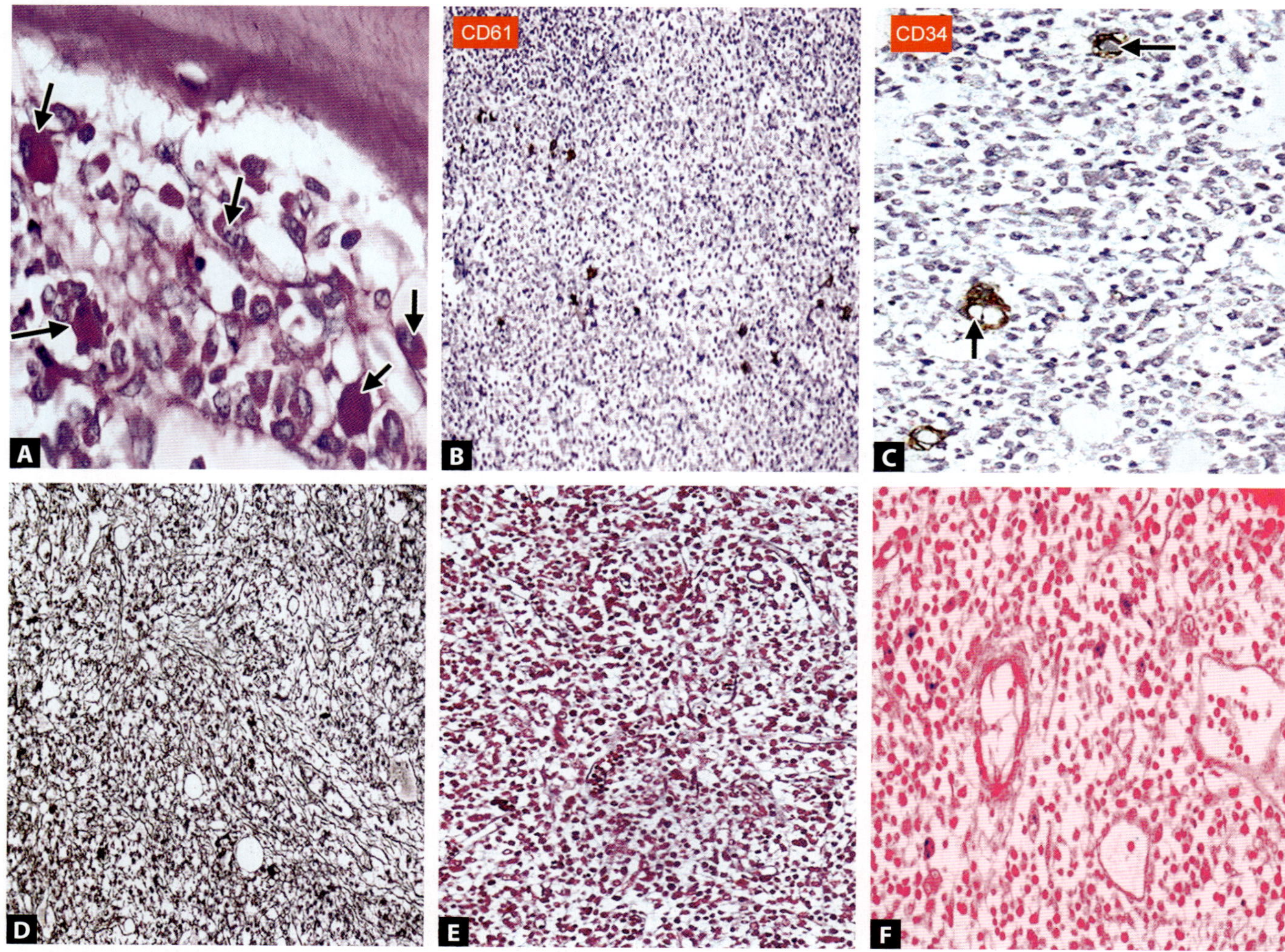

Figs 2A–F: Photomicrographs of the bone marrow. (A) Periodic acid-Schiff (PAS) stain highlights the clusters of atypical megakaryocytes adjacent to the bone marrow trabeculae; (B) CD61 immunostain highlights the increased number of megakaryocytes; (C) CD34 shows increase in the number of CD34 positive stem cells (arrows); (D) Reticulin stain shows 1+ fibrosis; (E) Masson's trichrome stain shows no increase in collagen fibers; and (F) Prussian blue stain does not show any increase in iron.

loss, low-grade fever, bleeding tendencies, gouty arthritis and renal stones. About 90% of patients have splenomegaly which may be massive and about 40–50% have hepatomegaly. Blood and bone marrow (prefibrotic to fibrotic phase) are always involved and EMH becomes prominent with evolution of the disease. In the early stages, CD34 positive progenitors are increased in the bone marrow and in later stage in the peripheral blood as well. This increase is seen in PMF and not in polycythemia vera or essential thrombocythemia. Initially there is a trilineage hyperplasia with progressive laying down of fibrous tissue, leading to hypoplasia and cytopenias. The hallmark is the increase in megakaryocytes which are dysplastic. They liberate platelet-derived growth factor, transforming growth factor, and endothelial/epidermal growth factors which stimulate fibroplasia. Diagnostic criteria for PMF need to meet all three major and two minor criteria. ***Major criteria***: (1) Megakaryocytic proliferation and atypia (micro/macromegakaryocytes with aberrant nuclear/cytoplasmic ratio, nuclei hyperchromatic, irregularly folded, or bulbous) usually accompanied by reticulin/collagen fibrosis or in the cellular prefibrotic phase the megakaryocytes must be accompanied by an increased bone marrow cellularity due to granulocytic hyperplasia and decreased erythropoiesis, (2) World Health Organization (WHO) criteria for polycythemia, chronic myeloid leukemia (presence of BCR-ABL1), myelodysplastic syndrome (presence of

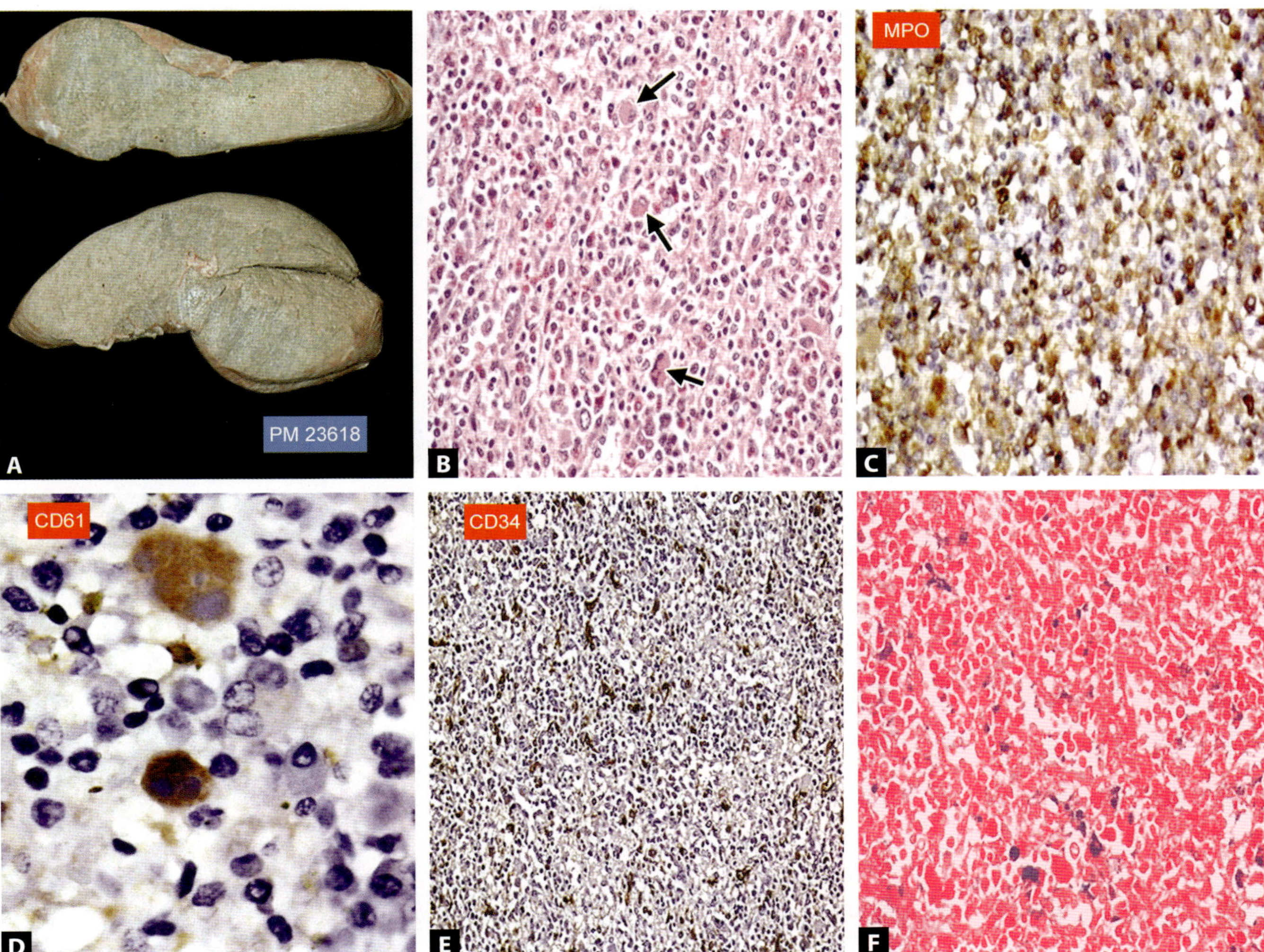

Figs 3A–F: (A) Coronal slices of the diffusely enlarged spleen. Photomicrographs of the spleen (B) Red pulp shows extensive myeloid metaplasia with prominent granulocytic series and atypical megakaryocytes (arrows); (C) Myeloperoxidase immunostain strongly positive in the granulocytic precursors; (D) CD61 immunostain, stains the macro/micromegakaryocyte; (E) Red pulp replete with CD34 positive stem cells; and (F) Prussian blue stain shows hemosiderin deposits in the red pulp.

dyserythropoiesis and dysgranulopoiesis) and other myeloid neoplasms not met, and (3) Demonstration of JAK2 V617F or other clonal marker like MPL W515K/L or in the absence of clonal marker, all secondary causes of bone marrow fibrosis should be ruled out (infections, autoimmune disorders, hairy cell leukemia, metastasis, etc.). ***Minor criteria*** include leukoerythroblastosis, increased serum lactate dehydrogenase levels, anemia and splenomegaly. About 50% of the patients with PMF show the JAK2 V617F mutation, which can also be seen in polycythemia vera and essential thrombocythemia. Philadelphia chromosome is negative in PMF. The presence of either del 13q12-22 or der (6)t(1;6)(q21-23;p21.3) is strongly suggestive of PMF. Patients diagnosed with cellular phase survive for 10–15 years and those diagnosed in the fibrotic stage survive for 3–7 years. Bad prognostic factors are, age more than 70 years, Hb less than 10 g/dL, platelet count less than 100 $\times$ 10^3/uL, and an abnormal karyotype. Causes of mortality are bone marrow failure, infection, hemorrhage, thromboembolic events, cardiac failure and acute leukemia. Accelerated phase of PMF is defined as the presence of 10–19% blasts in the peripheral blood and/or bone marrow and detection of increased number of CD34+ cells by immunohistochemistry. Acute phase is defined as more than 20% blasts in the peripheral blood and/or bone marrow.

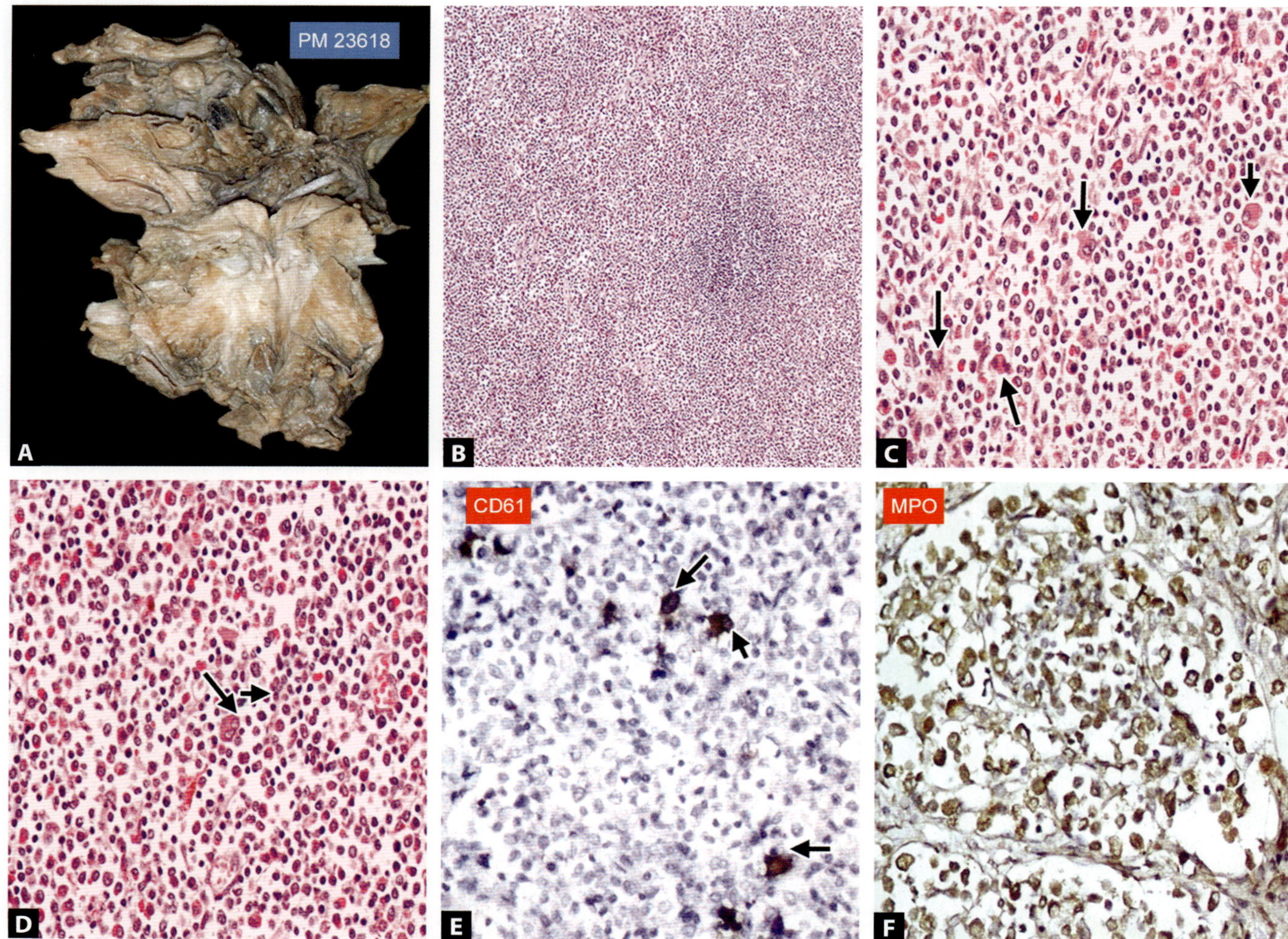

Figs 4A–F: (A) Mesentery showing enlarged lymph nodes. Photomicrographs of the lymph nodes showing (B) Paracortical expansion and compressed follicle; (C–D) Extensive myeloid metaplasia with prominent granulocytic series and atypical megakaryocytes (arrows); (E) Paracortex replete with CD61 positive megakaryocytes (arrows); and (F) Myeloperoxidase (MPO) stain strongly stains the granulocytic component.

Morphology of Primary Myelofibrosis

Peripheral blood shows a leukoerythroblastic picture wherein there is a shift to left with myelocytes/metamyelocytes/promyelocytes, nucleated red blood cells (RBCs) and marked erythropoikilocytosis with tear drop-shaped RBCs (typical finding of PMF). Hemogram shows low hemoglobin, mild leukocytosis with shift to left and normal to high platelets to begin with, followed by a decrease in later stages. The neutrophil alkaline phosphatase score is elevated, i.e. it is between 200 and 300 (N 40–100).

Prefibrotic Cellular Stage of Primary Myelofibrosis

Less than 50% cases are detected in the prefibrotic stage of PMF. Here the bone marrow is hypercellular with increase in the granulocytic series showing a mild shift to left, increased number of megakaryocytes which are atypical and reduced erythropoiesis. The abnormal and increased number of megakaryocytes is the key morphologic feature for the diagnosis. The dysplastic megakaryocytes are seen in clusters of variable sizes adjacent to the bone marrow trabeculae and vascular sinuses. The megakaryocytic abnormalities include—micro/macromegakaryocytes, abnormal nuclear-cytoplasmic ratio, hyperchromatic nuclei which are irregularly folded, balloon like or bulbous with abnormal chromatin clumping and presence of bare forms. CD61 immunohistochemistry and PAS stain highlight the abnormal megakaryocytes, at times not discernable on hematoxylin and eosin (H&E) stain. Megakaryocytes are most atypical in PMF than in any other type of myeloproliferative neoplasm. Reticulin fibrosis is absent

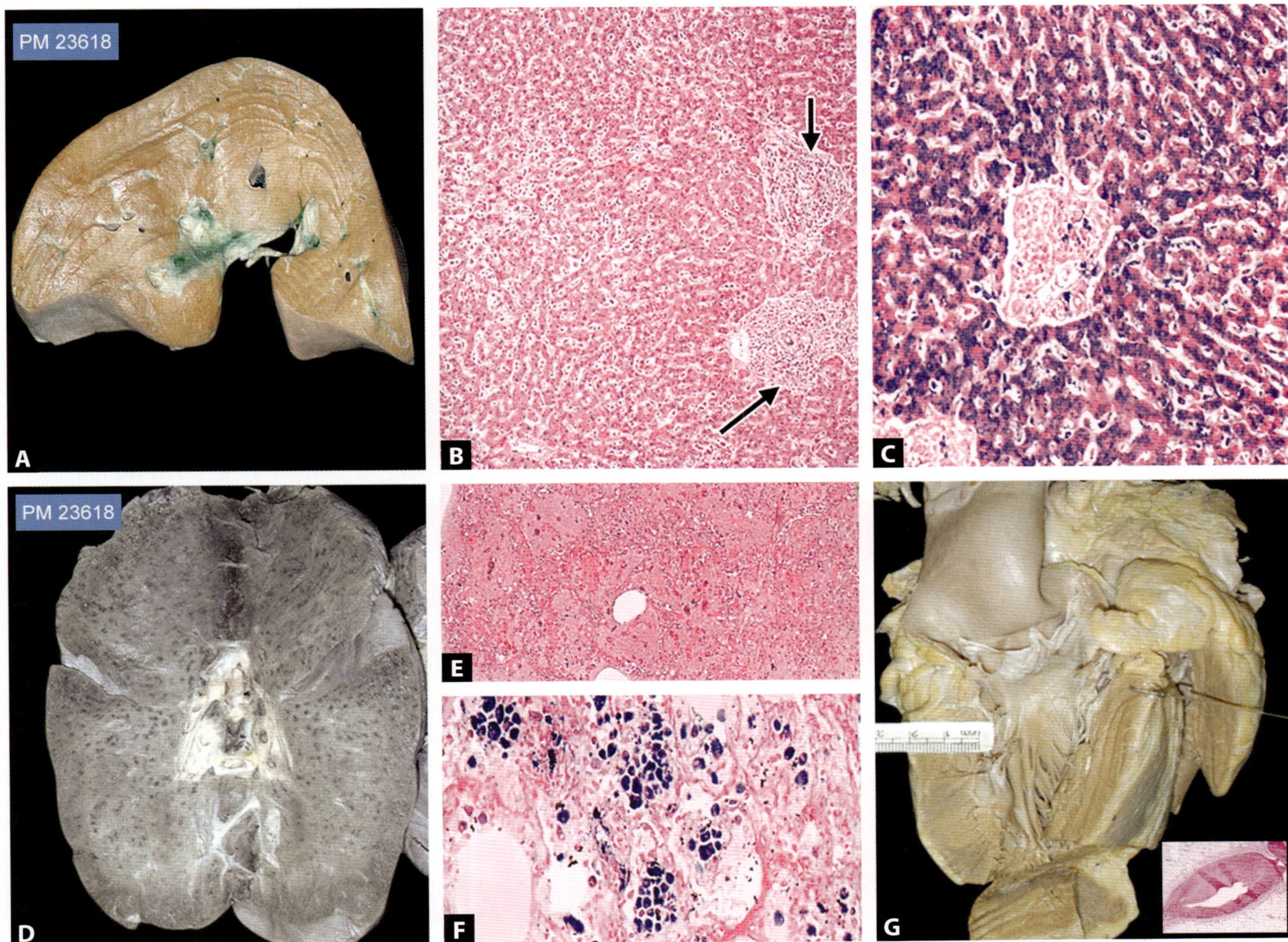

Figs 5A–G: (A) Coronal slice of the enlarged liver which is brown in color; (B) Portal tracts (arrows) and sinusoids showing myeloid metaplasia; (C) Prussian blue stain shows extensive hemosiderin deposition in the hepatocytes and Kupffer cells; (D) Cut section of the lung showing hemorrhagic consolidation; (E) Lung showing hemorrhagic necrosis; (F) Alveolar spaces packed with hemosiderin laden macrophages, i.e. heart failure cells; and (G) Gross picture of the heart showing the left outflow tract with left ventricular wall hypertrophy (2 cm). *Inset*: Left anterior descending artery showing 70% occlusion by a plaque.

or minimal (around vessels only). The early cellular stage progresses to the fibrotic stage.

Fibrotic Stage of Primary Myelofibrosis

Most patients of PMF are diagnosed in this stage. Bone marrow in most cases show hypocellularity, alternating with areas of normocellularity or hypercellularity with frank grade 2 or 3 reticulin or collagen fibrosis. Atypical megakaryocytes in sheets or clusters are the most conspicuous finding. Foci of immature cells may be seen but myeloblasts are less than 10%. Along with the fibrosis, there is a proliferation of tortuous, distended vessels showing intrasinusoidal hematopoiesis. Osteosclerotic phase shows broad irregular trabeculae which can eventually occupy more than 50% of the bone marrow space. Accelerated phase of disease shows 10–19% blasts and increased number of CD34+ cells with cluster formation. Acute transformation shows more than 20% blasts.

EXTRAMEDULLARY HEMATOPOIESIS

Also known as myeloid metaplasia, especially when seen in the lymph nodes, liver and other organs. It can be seen in any phase of PMF in the spleen, liver and lymph nodes. Other sites include kidneys, adrenal glands, gastrointestinal tract, duramater, lung, pleura, breast, skin and soft tissues. Atypical megakaryocytes are the most conspicuous component and EMH is picked up by seeing them (PAS and CD61 positive) admixed with granulocytic (proven by using MPO immunostain) and a minor erythroid component.

COMMENTARY INDEX CASE: PM 23618

This was a 55-year-old male who was diagnosed as a case of PMF (prefibrotic cellular phase) one year before his demise. He first presented in 2009 with pancytopenia and a leukoerythroblastic picture. Bone marrow revealed a cellular phase of myelofibrosis with 4% blasts. Report of BCR-ABL fusion gene and JAK2 mutation on peripheral blood cells was negative. He was on treatment, but became transfusion dependent and was given 70 units of blood transfusions in 1 year. He had multiple admissions during this time. During his last admission in March 2010, he had exertional dyspnea, easy fatigability, joint pains and fever. There was pancytopenia with 30% blasts in the peripheral blood. Autopsy revealed a prefibrotic cellular phase of PMF with acute transformation, i.e. progressing into acute leukemia (30% blasts in peripheral blood), extensive EMH, secondary hemosiderosis, coronary artery disease and features of heart failure. Patients diagnosed with cellular phase normally survive for 10–15 years. The index case did not respond to the treatment. He was transfusion dependent from the start, i.e. had bone marrow failure. He had other bad prognostic factors like Hb less than 10 g/dL, platelet count less than 100 × 10^3/uL, cardiac failure, and terminally, transformation to acute leukemia.

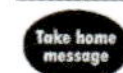

TAKE HOME MESSAGE

- Primary myelofibrosis is a clonal myeloproliferative neoplasm, wherein the bone marrow shows an evolution from a prefibrotic cellular phase to a frankly fibrotic stage, along with extensive EMH/myeloid metaplasia.
- Hallmark is the presence of increased number of megakaryocytes in the bone marrow, which are dysplastic along with fibrosis. But in the cellular phase there is minimal fibrosis with granulocytic hyperplasia and decreased erythropoiesis.
- In PMF, CD34 positive progenitors are increased in the bone marrow and in later stage in the peripheral blood as well.
- In PMF, 50% patients exhibit JAK2 V617F mutation. BCR-ABL1 fusion gene, i.e. Philadelphia chromosome is absent.

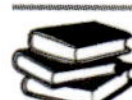

SUGGESTED READING

1. Kakkar N, Bharani V, Srinivasan VK, et al. Myeloproliferative neoplasm with extensive myeloid metaplasia: a diagnostic dilemma. JPMER. 2015;49:148-54.
2. Kakkar N, Vasishta RK, Banerjee AK, et al. Primary pulmonary malignant teratoma with yolk sac element associated with hematologic neoplasia. Respiration. 1996;63:52-4.
3. Thiele J, Kvasnicka HM, Tefferi A, et al. Primary myelofibrosis. In: Swerdlow SH, Campo E, Harris NL (Eds). WHO Classification of Tumors of Hematopoietic and Lymphoid Tissues, 4th edition. Lyon: IARC; 2008. pp. 44-7.

CONTRIBUTIONS BY:

1. Dr Jasmina Ahluwalia, Professor, Department of Hematology (Hematologist In-Charge)
2. Dr Navneet Sharma, Professor, Department of Internal Medicine (Compilation of Clinical Details)
3. Dr SC Varma, Ex Professor and Head, Department of Internal Medicine (Clinician In-Charge)

Post Graduate Institute of Medical Education and Research (PGIMER), Chandigarh, India.

CASE 4

Hepatosplenic T-cell Lymphoma: PM 23096

Nandita Bharadwaj Kakkar

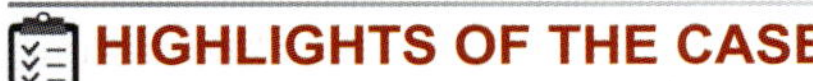

HIGHLIGHTS OF THE CASE

A young 25-year-old female presented with fever, jaundice, and weight loss. There was massive hepatosplenomegaly, no lymphadenopathy and bicytopenia with 10% blasts. The bone marrow, however, showed 60% blasts. The patient had a stormy course and died. Autopsy revealed a hepatosplenic T-cell lymphoma with sinusoidal localization of malignant T cells in the spleen, liver and bone marrow. Admixture with erythrophagocytizing benign histiocytes was seen.

Keywords: Hepatosplenic lymphoma, T cell, γδ T cell, sinusoidal localization of malignant cells, autopsy.

CLINICAL DETAILS

Date of Admission: 26.03.2009, Date of Death: 08.04.2009, and Duration of Hospital Stay: 16 Days

A 25-years female had three admissions in our hospital.

1st admission Dec 2008: She was admitted with fever since 45 days, jaundice since 20 days, weight loss and headache since 2 days. The liver (4 cms) and spleen (6 cms) were enlarged. On investigations, she had bicytopenia with 10% blasts in the peripheral blood (Hb 6.5 g/dl, TLC 11,700/ul, Platelet 24000/ul) and markedly deranged liver function tests. The bone marrow examination revealed 60% blasts, which were MPO negative and T-lineage markers (CD3, CD2, HLA-DR) positive on flow cytometry. A diagnosis of T-cell acute lymphoblastic leukemia (ALL)/leukemic conversion of T-cell lymphoma was given. She was put on a 7 week regime of chemotherapy with prophylactic antibiotics and she improved symptomatically. Bone marrow done after 4 weeks of induction phase showed 8-10% atypical cells and 3% blasts.

2nd Admission 7th March 2009: She was readmitted with pancytopenia (Hb 3g/dl, TLC 2700/ul with 70-80% blasts and platelets 27000/ul). Blood culture grew pseudomonas aeruginosa which was treated and she improved. Subsequently, she developed breakthrough fever for which amphotericin B was added. She also received 4 units of blood transfusion and platelet rich plasmas (PRP). She soon became afebrile and therefore the next cycle of chemotherapy was given on 17th March 2009. She was discharged but within a few days, developed high grade fever and cough.

***3rd admission 26th March 2009*:** She was again readmitted. On examination she was febrile. Hepatosplenomegaly was present. There were crepts and bronchial breathing in the right axillary, mammary and interscapular areas. CVS and CNS were within normal limits. Investigations revealed pancytopenia: Hb-5.4 g/dl, TLC- 1300/µl with an occasional blast and low platelets 52000/µl. Serum bilirubin was 0.9 mg%, SGOT/SGPT -236/37 U/L, alkaline phosphatase 226 U/L and uric acid 9.3mg%. The HRCT chest showed B/L ground glass appearance and few nodular shadows. She was put on cefoperazone, selbactum and ciplox. Subsequently amphotericin B and vancomycin were added in view of persistent fever and clindamycin was added to cover Pneumocystic carinii infection. The Units clinical diagnosis was - T Cell ALL/Hepatosplenic lymphoma with leukemic conversion, febrile neutropenia and b/l bronchopneumonia ? PCP ? fungal. She developed a cardiorespiratory arrest from which she could not be revived.

AUTOPSY FINDINGS: PM 23096

A partial autopsy was performed on this young female. All serous cavities were within normal limits. The ***liver*** was enlarged and weighed 2,200 g. There was no focal lesion seen (Figs 1A–B). On microscopic examination large atypical malignant cells were seen to pack the sinusoids, known as sinusoidal localization of malignant cells (Figs 1C–D). These cells showed open nuclear chromatin, irregular nuclear contours (Figs 1D and 2A), nuclear indentations and ample cytoplasm. Admixture with benign erythrophagocytizing histiocytes (Figs 2B–C) was noted. The malignant cells were strongly positive for T-cell marker, CD3 (Fig 2D), and negative for the B-cell marker CD20. The ***spleen*** was markedly enlarged and weighed 1,200 g (Figs 1A and 3A). No focal lesion or any infarct was seen. Microscopy revealed markedly congested red pulp. The sinuses were packed with atypical lymphoid cells (Figs 3B–C) which were CD3 positive (Fig 3D). Admixture with erythrophagocytizing benign histiocytes was seen. The postmortem ***bone marrow*** also showed infiltration by atypical cells in the sinuses (Figs 4A–B). The ***lymph nodes*** were not enlarged and on microscopic examination did not show any infiltration by lymphoma, but showed sinus histiocytosis with hemophagocytosis (Figs 4C–D). The hilar node showed an old healed focus of tuberculosis. The ***lungs*** weighed 880 g and the pleural surface was dull with hemorrhages (Fig 5A). On serial slicing extensive hemorrhagic consolidation (Fig 5A) was noted. Microscopy, however, revealed extensive bilateral pulmonary hemorrhages

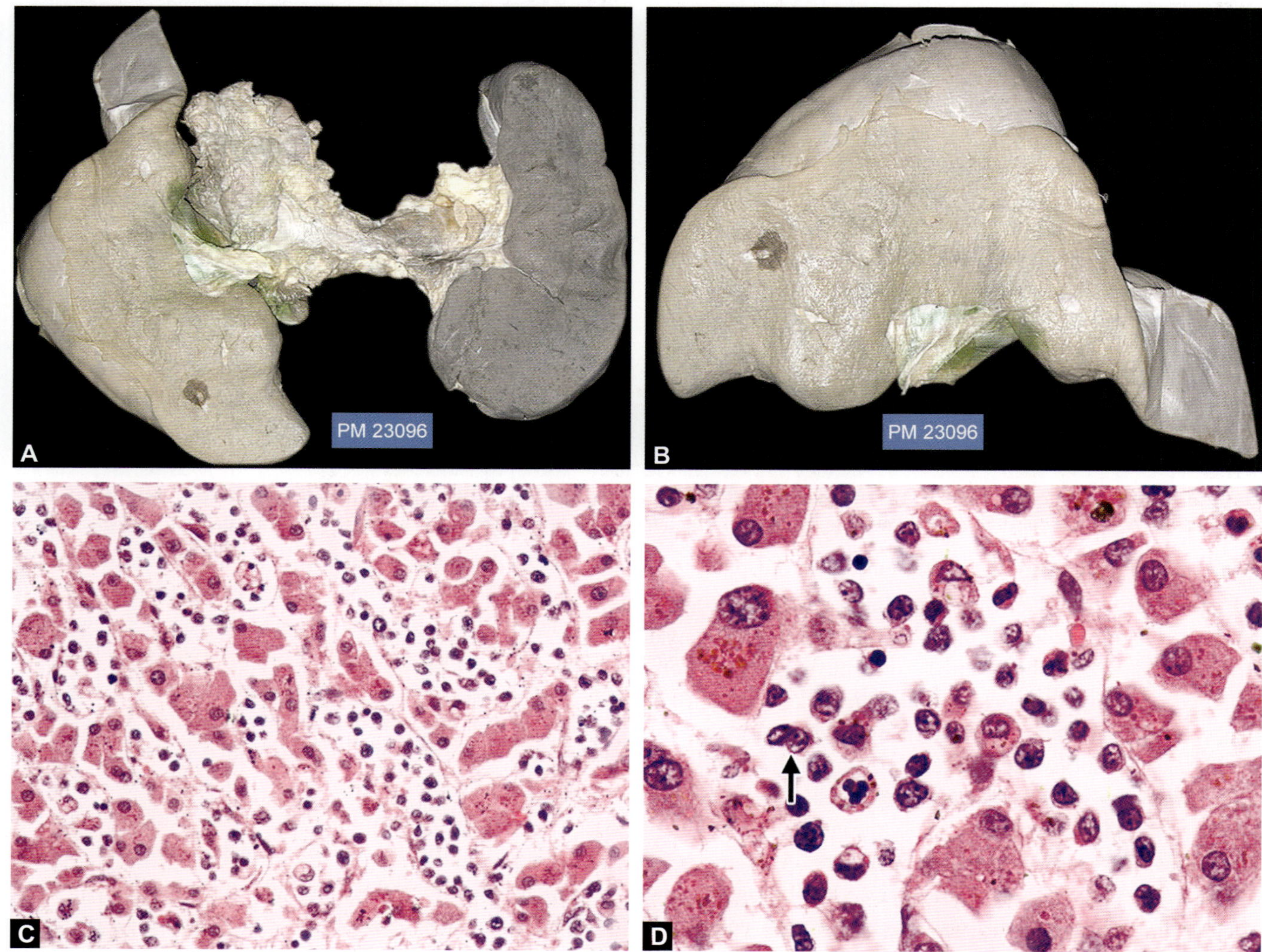

Figs 1A–D: (A) Organ complex comprising of a slice of liver, spleen, loop of duodenum, and pancreas. Spleen (1,200 g) and liver (2,200 g) show diffuse enlargement. No focal lesions or infarcts seen; (B) Slice of liver showing diffuse enlargement. No focal lesion seen; and (C and D) Photomicrographs of the liver at different magnifications showing dense sinusoidal localization of the malignant cells. Many of the cells show nuclear indentations (arrow).

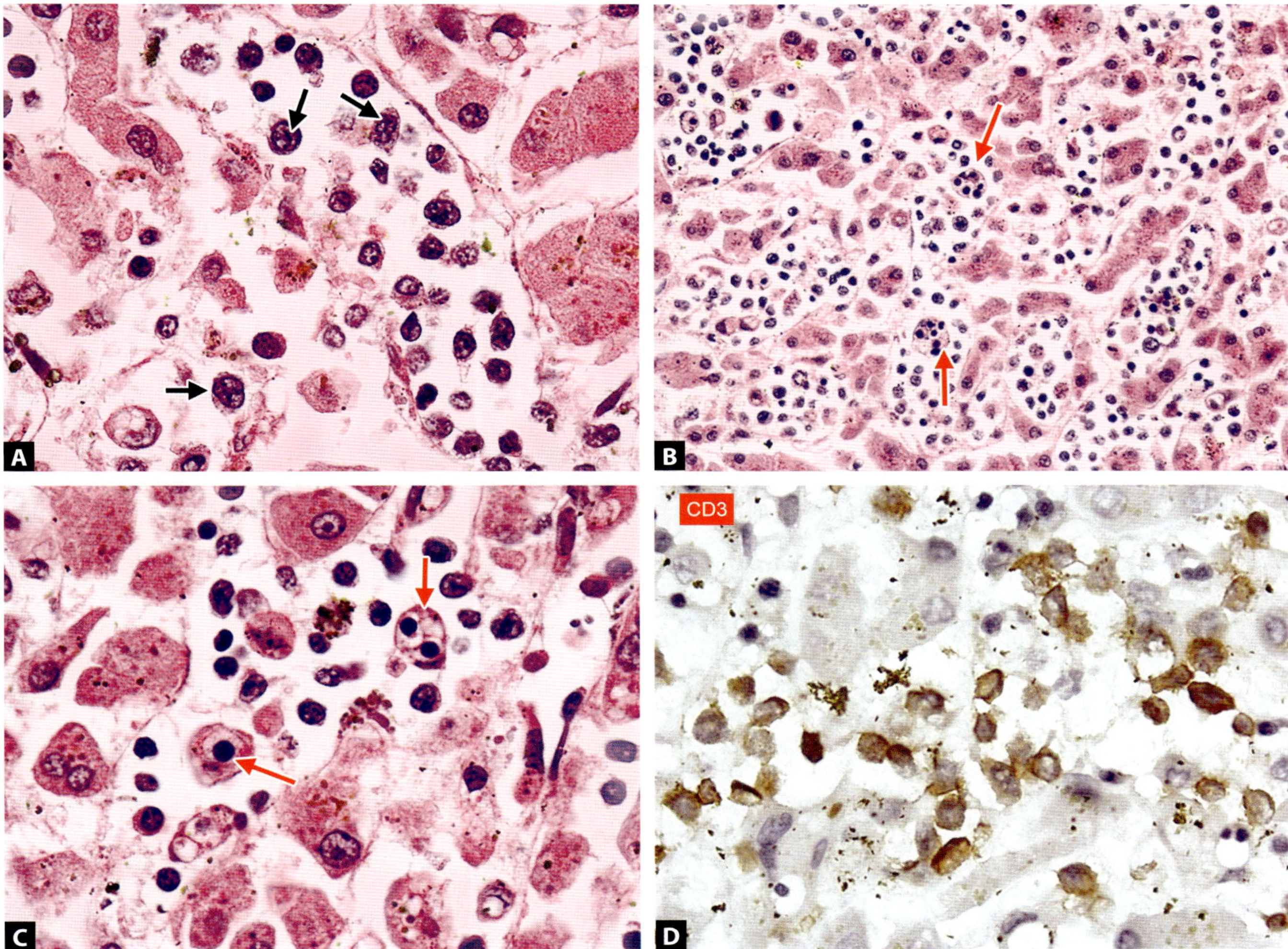

Figs 2A–D: Photomicrographs of the liver. (A) Malignant cells in the sinusoids showing nuclear indentations (arrows); (B and C) Malignant infiltrate showing admixture with erythrophagocytizing benign histiocytes (arrows); and (D) Malignant cells are positive for T-cell marker CD3.

(Fig 5B), diffuse alveolar damage with prominent hyaline membrane formation (Fig 5C) and organizing pneumonia (Fig 5D). The blood vessels were packed with atypical cells (Fig 5E). Rest of the organs were within normal limits.

FINAL AUTOPSY DIAGNOSIS: PM 23096

25 Years Female

- Hepatosplenic T-cell Non-Hodgkin lymphoma (NHL) with infiltration of bone marrow and peripheral blood.
- Extensive B/L pulmonary hemorrhages, diffuse alveolar damage and organizing pneumonia.
- Secondary hemophagocytosis in the liver, spleen, lymph nodes and occasionally in the bone marrow.

HEPATOSPLENIC T-CELL LYMPHOMAS

Hepatosplenic T-cell lymphoma[1-6] is a variety of aggressive peripheral T-cell lymphoma (constituting 5%) which occurs in younger individuals, more in the males and has a very poor prognosis. It is an extranodal systemic Non Hodgkins lymphoma (comprising $< 1\%$ of all NHLs) originating from $\gamma\delta$ T cells. Now it has also been reported to express the $\alpha\beta$ T-cell receptor.[7] Patients present with marked splenohepatomegaly without any lymph node enlargement, clinically significant cytopenias particularly anemia and thrombocytopenia, pronounced constitutional symptoms and an aggressive clinical course. The malignant T cells preferentially localize in the sinusoids of the liver

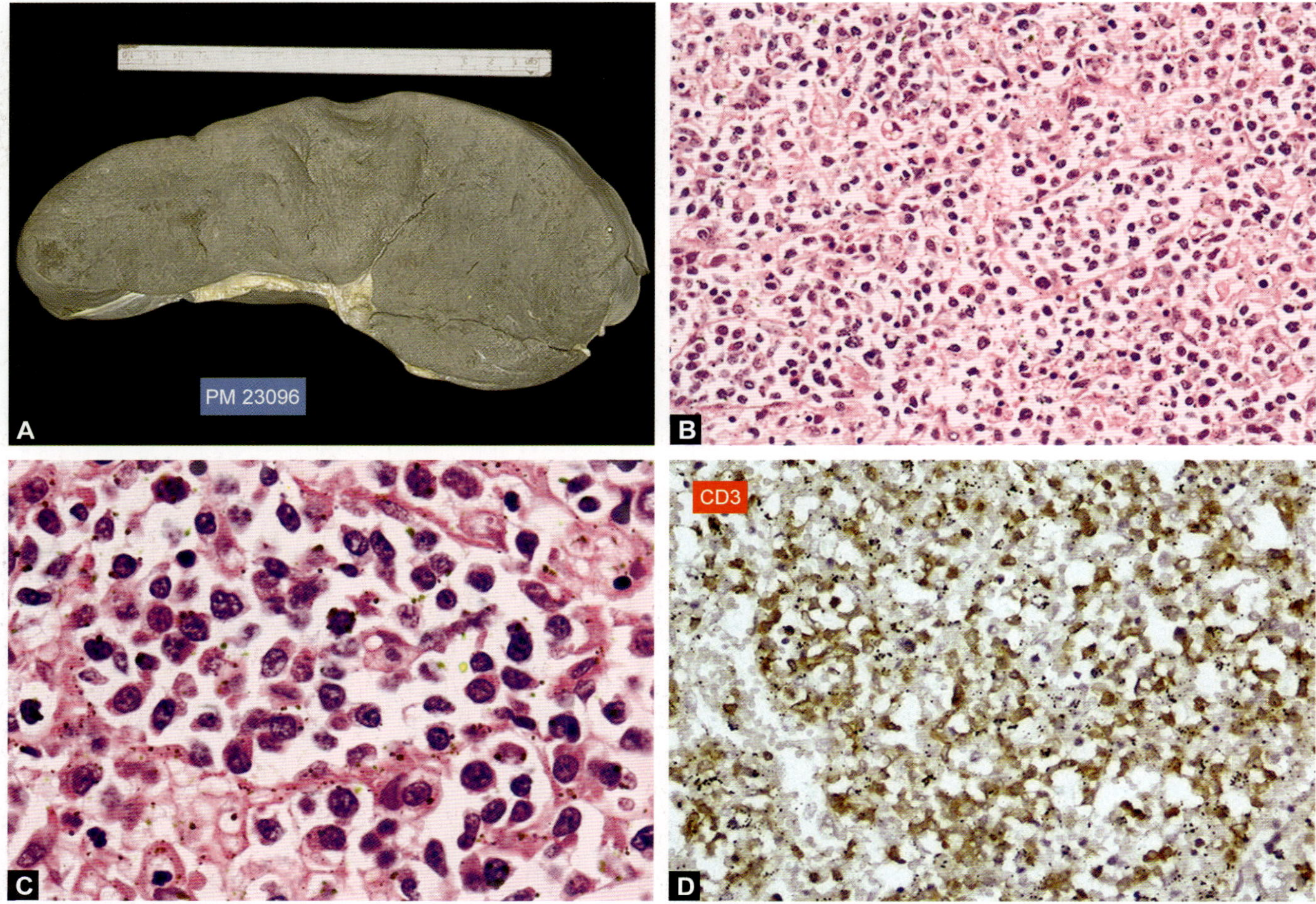

Figs 3A–D: (A) Slice of spleen showing diffuse enlargement; (B and C) Sinusoids of the spleen packed with atypical lymphoid cells; and (D) Atypical lymphoid cells show strong positivity with T-cell marker CD3.

and spleen. Bone marrow (sinuses) and peripheral blood are involved later in the evolution of the disease. Patients usually present in stage IV with bone marrow involvement. Secondary hemophagocytic lymphohistiocytosis (HLH) is a critical complication and leads to a cytokine storm which evokes a fulminant clinical course. The malignant cells have indented nuclei, opened up chromatin and moderate amount of granular cytoplasm. The clinical course is aggressive and despite multiagent chemotherapy, the median survival is less than one year. Hepatosplenic T-cell lymphoma was first enlisted as a provisional entity in the 1994 Revised European-American Lymphoma (REAL) classification of lymphoid neoplasms and later as a distinct entity in the World Health Organization (WHO) classification.

Most peripheral T-cell lymphomas (PTCLs) express αβ T-cell receptors, but the hepatosplenic T-cell lymphomas generally express the γδ T cell receptors. The latter show a unique 'double negative' T cell phenotype (CD4-, CD8-, CD5-, CD3+, CD2+,CD7+) with a co-expression of one or more NK cell associated antigen (generally CD16 or CD56). A consistent expression of Vδ1 containing δ chain is an indication that hepatosplenic γδ T-cell lymphoma is derived from normal Vδ1 + γδ T cells which normally populate the spleen and thymus. The largest percentage of γδ T cells is found in the splenic (Vδ1) red pulp in the Cords of Billroth and this explains the origin and homing of "hepatosplenic γδ T-cell lymphoma" at this site. Chromosomal aberrations[8,9] seen in hepatosplenic T-cell lymphoma are mostly isochromosome 7 and less frequently trisomy 8 and loss of a Y chromosome. Twenty percent of the hepatosplenic T-cell lymphomas arise in a setting of prolonged immunosuppression which leads to an expansion of the γδ T-cell population. Risk factors associated with worse outcome include male gender, failure to achieve a remission,

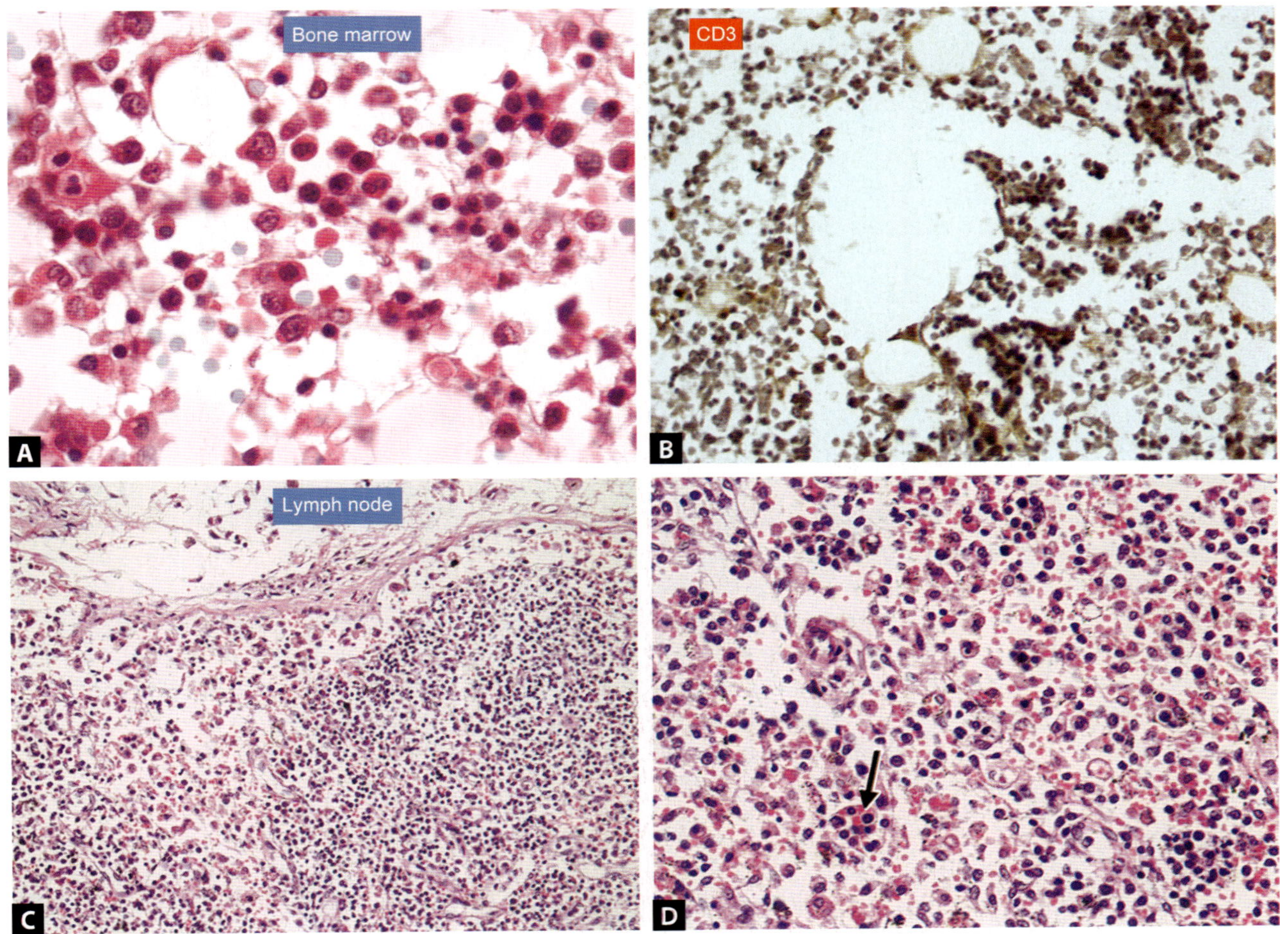

Figs 4A–D: Photomicrographs from the bone marrow showing (A) Infiltration by atypical cells; (B) Atypical cells positive for T-cell marker CD3; (C) Photomicrographs from the lymph node shows dilated sinuses packed with benign histiocytes; and (D) Benign histiocytes showing hemophagocytosis (arrow).

history of immunocompromise, absence of a T-cell receptor gene rearrangement in the gamma chain and bone marrow involvement at presentation.

COMMENTARY—INDEX CASE: PM 23096

The index case was a classical case of hepatosplenic T-cell lymphoma with a fulminant downhill course. The patient was a young female who presented with fever and jaundice. There was massive splenohepatomegaly, no lymphadenopathy, cytopenias, blasts in the peripheral blood and characteristic sinusoidal localization of malignant T cells in the spleen, liver and bone marrow admixed with benign erythrophagocytizing histiocytes. The lymph nodes, however, did not show any infiltration.

ARCHIVAL CASES

So far in our autopsy archives, there are three autopsy cases (including the index case) of hepatosplenic T-cell lymphomas. All were young adults, two females and one male and had an aggressive clinical course. All presented with fever, weight loss, jaundice, cytopenias (bi/pan), deranged liver function tests, atypical cells in the peripheral blood and bone marrow (two cases) and marked splenohepatomegaly with absence of lymphadenopathy. In the first case[6] (published) a clinical diagnosis of hepatosplenomegaly ? cause was given (1995) and in the second case a clinical diagnosis of megaloblastic anemia and lymphoreticular malignancy was suggested (1997). But in the third case (2009) a clinical diagnosis of T-cell ALL/hepatosplenic lymphoma with

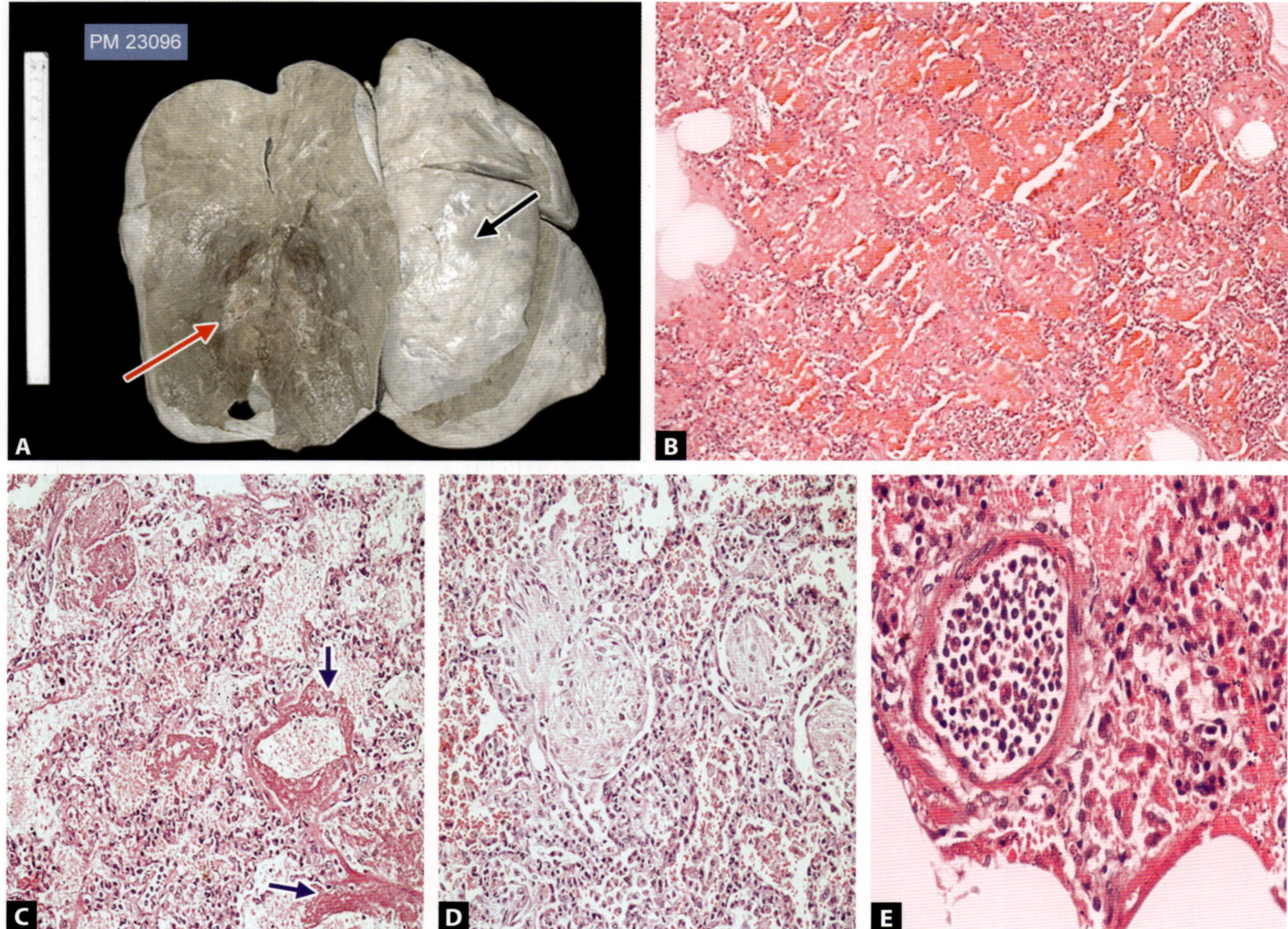

Figs 5A–E: (A) Gross photograph of the lungs showing hemorrhages on the pleura (black arrow) and extensive hemorrhagic consolidation in the right lower lobe (red arrow); Photomicrographs from the lung showing (B) Extensive alveolar hemorrhage; (C) Diffuse alveolar damage with prominent hyaline membrane formation (arrows); (D) Organizing pneumonia; and (E) Vessels packed with atypical cells.

leukemic conversion was given, highlighting the fact that autopsy makes us much wiser. Autopsy (in all three cases) revealed massive enlargement of the liver (3.1, 3.2, and 2.2 kg) and spleen (2.6, 0.6, and 1.2 kg), no lymphadenopathy, sinusoidal localization of malignant T cells in the liver, spleen, bone marrow and presence of erythrophagocytizing benign histiocytes in liver, spleen, bone marrow and lymph nodes. No atypical cell was seen in the lymph nodes. Focal infiltration was seen in other organs in lungs/kidney in case 1 and in kidney, pancreas, adrenals and heart in case 2.

TAKE HOME MESSAGE

- Hepatosplenic T-cell lymphoma is a subset of extranodal, peripheral T-cell lymphoma, with an aggressive clinical course.
- Affects young adults, seen more in the males.
- Patients present with marked splenohepatomegaly, cytopenias, but with absence of lymphadenopathy.
- Diagnostic feature is the sinusoidal localization of malignant T cells in the liver, spleen and bone marrow.
- Secondary HLH is a critical complication and leads to a cytokine storm.

REFERENCES

1. Cooke CB, Krenacs L, Stetler-Stevenson M, et al. Hepatosplenic T-cell lymphoma: a distinct clinicopathologic entity of cytotoxic gamma delta T-cell origin. Blood. 1996;88: 4265-74.
2. de Wolf-Peeters C, Achten R. Yδ T cell lymphomas-A homogeneous entity? Histopathology. 2000;36:294-305.

3. Gaulard P, Belhadj K, Reyes F. Gamma-delta T-cell lymphomas. Semin Hematol. 2003;40:233-43.
4. Weidmann E. Hepatosplenic T cell lymphoma. A review on 45 cases since the first report describing the disease as a distinct lymphoma entity in 1990. Leukemia. 2000;14:991-7.
5. Belhadj K, Reyes F, Farcet JP, et al. Hepatosplenic gamma-delta T-cell lymphoma is a rare clinicopathologic entity with poor outcome: report on a series of 21 patients. Blood. 2003;102:4261-9.
6. Kakkar N, Marwaha N, Banerjee AK, et al. Hepatosplenic Yδ T cell lymphoma-sinusoidal localization of malignant T cells. Am J Hematol. 1996;53:278-9.
7. Macon WR, Levy NB, Kurtin PJ, et al. Hepatosplenic alpha-beta T-cell lymphomas: A report of 14 cases and comparison with hepatosplenic gamma-delta T-cell lymphomas. Am J Surg Pathol. 2001;25:285-96.
8. Wang CC, Tien HF, Lin MT, et al. Consistent presence of isochromosome 7q in hepatosplenic T gamma/delta lymphoma: a new cytogenetic-clinicopathologic entity. Genes Chromosomes Cancer. 1995;12:161-4.
9. Francois A, Lesesve JF, Stamatoullas A, et al. Hepatosplenic gamma/delta T-cell lymphoma: a report of two cases in immunocompromised patients, associated with isochromosome 7q. Am J Surg Pathol. 1997;21:781-90.

CONTRIBUTIONS BY:

1. Dr SC Varma, ex Prof and Head, Dept of Internal Medicine (Clinician In-Charge)
2. Dr Pankaj Malhotra, Professor, Dept of Internal Medicine, (Clinician In-Charge)
3. Dr Savita Kumari, Professor and Head, Dept of Internal Medicine (Compilation of Clinical Details)

Post Graduate Institute of Medical Education and Research, Chandigarh, India.

CASE 5

Acute Promyelocytic Leukemia with Early Death due to Disseminated Intravascular Coagulation and Right Temporal Lobe Hemorrhage: PM 26880

Nandita Bharadwaj Kakkar

HIGHLIGHTS OF THE CASE

A young male came with a short history of 2 weeks with fever, bleeding gums, ecchymotic patches, black tarry stools, shortness of breath and pancytopenia. A diagnosis of acute promyelocytic leukemia (APML), t(15;17) positive with disseminated intravascular coagulation (DIC) was made and he was given one dose of all trans-retinoic acid (ATRA) and arsenic trioxide (ATO). He deteriorated within few hours and a possibility of differentiation syndrome (DS) was kept. Autopsy revealed leukemic infiltration in various organs, right temporal lobe parenchymal hemorrhage with subarachnoid extension and tonsillar herniation along with DIC. No DS was present.

***Keywords*:** Acute promyelocytic leukemia, t(15;17), leukemic infiltration, differentiation syndrome, temporal lobe hemorrhage, disseminated intravascular coagulation, autopsy.

CLINICAL DETAILS

Date of Admission: 26.8.2015 at 4 PM, Date of Death: 27.8.15 at 9 PM and Duration of Hospital Stay: 29 Hours

A 27-year-old-male came with fever, bleeding gums/ecchymotic patches since 15 days and black tarry stools along with shortness of breath since 7 days. The fever was high grade, intermittent, not associated with rigors and chills or any diurnal variation. There was no cough, jaundice or any localizing sign. He was treated at an outside facility with antibiotics and antimalarials. Bleeding manifestations were seen in the form of painless ecchymotic patches on the limbs, gum bleeding, black tarry semi-solid stools, 4–5 times a day and hemorrhagic spots in the eyes. There was shortness of breath which progressed from NYHA class II to class IV. Easy fatiguability was present. There was no paroxysmal nocturnal dyspnea, chest pain, cough, hemoptysis, hematemesis, hematuria, headache, seizures or altered sensorium. On *examination* the splenic tip was palpable. The liver was not palpable, bowel sounds were present and there was no abdominal tenderness or any free fluid. There was tachypnea, bilateral scattered crepitations, rhonchi and harsh breathing sounds. He was irritable, was moving all four limbs and there were no focal neurological deficits.

Investigations and Course of Management

Hematological: Hemoglobin (Hb) 5.1 g/dL, total leukocyte count 2,300/μL, differential count in 50 counted cells—N03 L12 E02 promyelocytes 33, platelets 9,000/μL, absolute neutrophil count—138, peripheral blood film showed pancytopenia, 87% promyelocytes (Figs 1A–B) many showing Auer rods, normocytic normochromic red blood cells (RBCs) and schistocytes. Antemortem bone marrow aspirate (Figs 1C–D) was hypercellular with 87% promyelocytes which were strongly positive for myeloperoxidase (MPO) immunohistochemistry. Many promyelocytes showed faggots (Fig 1E) of Auer rods highly characteristic of APML. Flow cytometry: HLA-DR and CD34—negative; CD13, CD33, CD45, CD38, CD117 and MPO—positive. PML retinoic acid receptor alpha (RARα) (t15-17) was positive. Coagulogram: PT—39 s, PTI—34%, INR—2.92, aPTT—39 s, fibrinogen—2.74 g/L and D-dimers positive.

Biochemistry: Na^+/K^+—139/3.88 mEq/L, urea/creatinine—52/1.45 mg%, total bilirubin/conjugated fraction—2.5/1.02 mg%, SGOT—5778 U/L, SGPT—2872 U/L, ALP -185 U/L, uric acid-7.7 mg%, total proteins/albumin—7.1/3.22 gms, HIV negative and blood cultures—sterile.

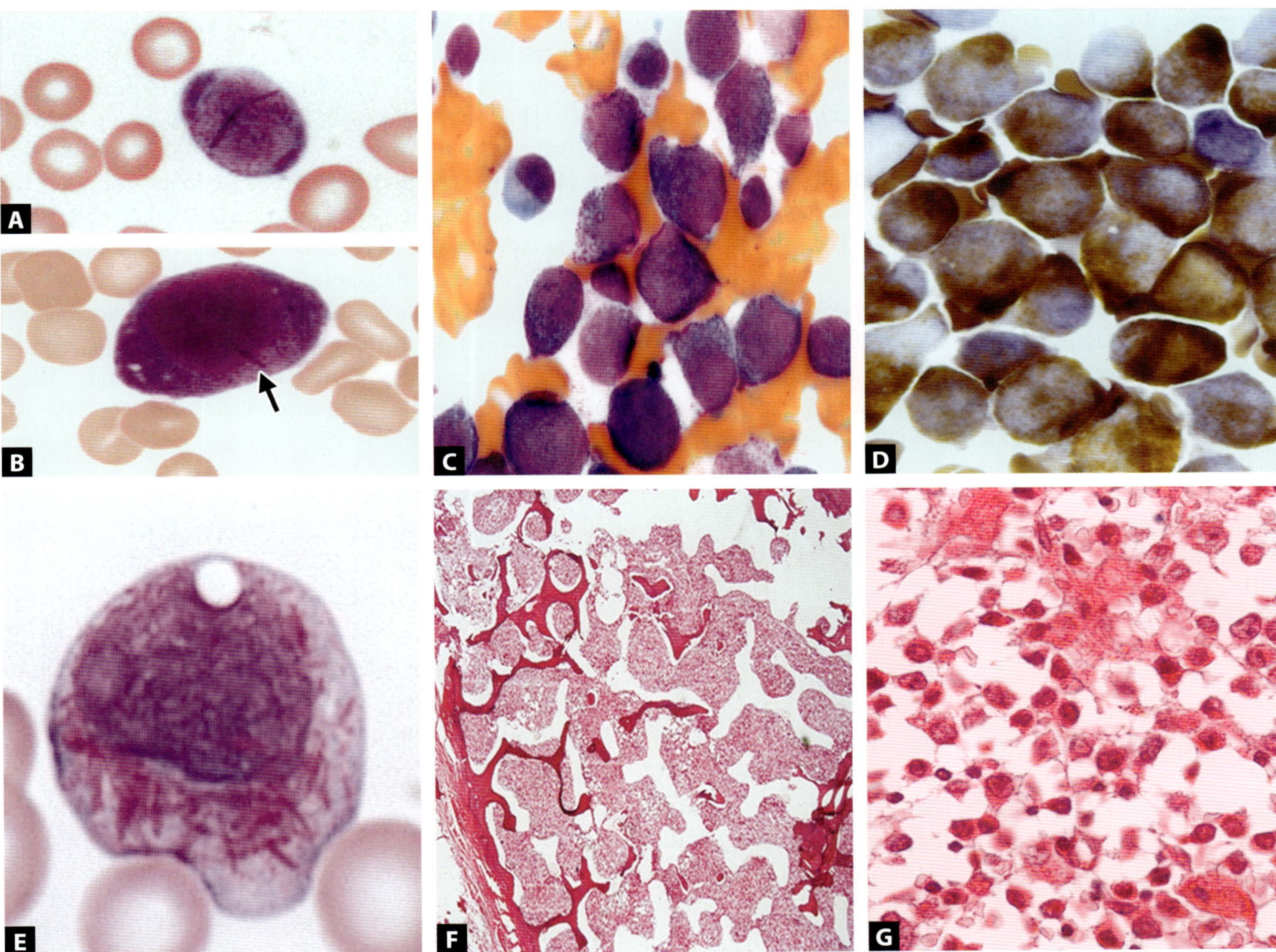

Figs 1A–G: (A and B) Peripheral blood showing promyelocytes containing abundant granules in the cytoplasm and Auer rod (arrow); (C) Antemortem bone marrow aspirate showing sheets of promyelocytes with abundant cytoplasmic granules; (D) Promyelocytes show strong cytoplasmic positivity with myeloperoxidase (MPO) immunostain; (E) Promyelocyte showing Faggots of Auer rods; (F) Postmortem bone marrow shows marked hypercellularity; and (G) Postmortem bone marrow shows sheets of promyelocytes.

ECG: Sinus tachycardia, X-ray chest—bilateral infiltrates, no cardiomegaly, *USG*: Hepatosplenomegaly, no free fluid present.

This 27-year-old male presented with fever, bleeding manifestations, respiratory distress, splenomegaly and pancytopenia. He was diagnosed as a case of APML and was started on cefoperazone, sulbactum, ATRA and ATO at 7 PM on the 26.08.2015. He was put on oxygen by ventimask, transfused one unit packed red blood cells (PRBC) and four units of fresh frozen plasma. At 2 AM on 27.08.2015, there was worsening of respiratory distress with weight gain and fever. Oxygen was now given by Hudson mask. Antibiotics were hiked to imipenem and dexamethasone and lasix was administered. At 9 AM there was worsening of anemia, increasing respiratory distress and decreased urine output. Lasix was given along with packed RBC and fresh frozen plasma. By 7 PM the SpO_2 became low, ABG showed mixed acidosis and he was intubated. Endotracheal aspirate was blood stained. At 9 PM he developed a cardiac arrest from which he could not be revived. Clinical diagnosis was APML, DIC and DS.

AUTOPSY FINDINGS: PM 26880

A complete autopsy was performed. The peritoneal cavity yielded 3 L, pleural cavities 300 mL and pericardial cavity 100 mL of hemorrhagic fluid. The postmortem ***bone marrow*** (Figs 1F–G) was hypercellular and replaced by sheets of promyelocytes. The ***liver*** (Fig 2A) was enlarged and weighed 2,000 g. Leukemic infiltrate was present in the portal tracts and sinusoids (Figs 2B–C). The infiltrate was strongly positive with MPO immunostain (Fig 2D). There was extensive centrizonal hemorrhagic necrosis, indicating shock (Fig 2E). In these foci, reticulin collapse without any fibrosis was seen. The ***spleen*** (Figs 2A and F) weighed 220 g and showed leukemic infiltrate in red and white pulp. The ***small intestine*** showed multiple ulcers ranging in size from 0.5 cm to 1.5 cm in diameter. Microscopy (Figs 3A–D) revealed ulcerated epithelium with submucosal dense leukemic infiltrate, strongly positive for MPO immunostain. Some of the ulcers (Figs 3E–F), however showed mucosal necrosis replete with gram-positive cocci and fungal profiles of Candida. The stomach and large intestine were unremarkable. The ***lymph nodes*** (mesenteric, pre- and para-aortic and peripancreatic) were enlarged and showed diffuse leukemic infiltration (Figs 4A–C). The ***kidneys*** (Figs 4D–F) showed small areas of hemorrhages on the capsular aspect (0.5–1 cm). Microscopy revealed congested glomerular capillary loops and arterioles (afferent and efferent). Martius scarlet blue (MSB) stain showed the presence of red colored fibrin thrombi as a part of the DIC. The tubules showed acute tubular necrosis. The ***lungs*** (Figs 5A–C) were subcrepitant to feel and tracheal mucosa showed hemorrhages. Microscopy revealed diffuse pulmonary edema and focal alveolar hemorrhage. There were thrombi in large pulmonary vessels on right side. No leukemic infiltrate or any differentiating cells clogging the

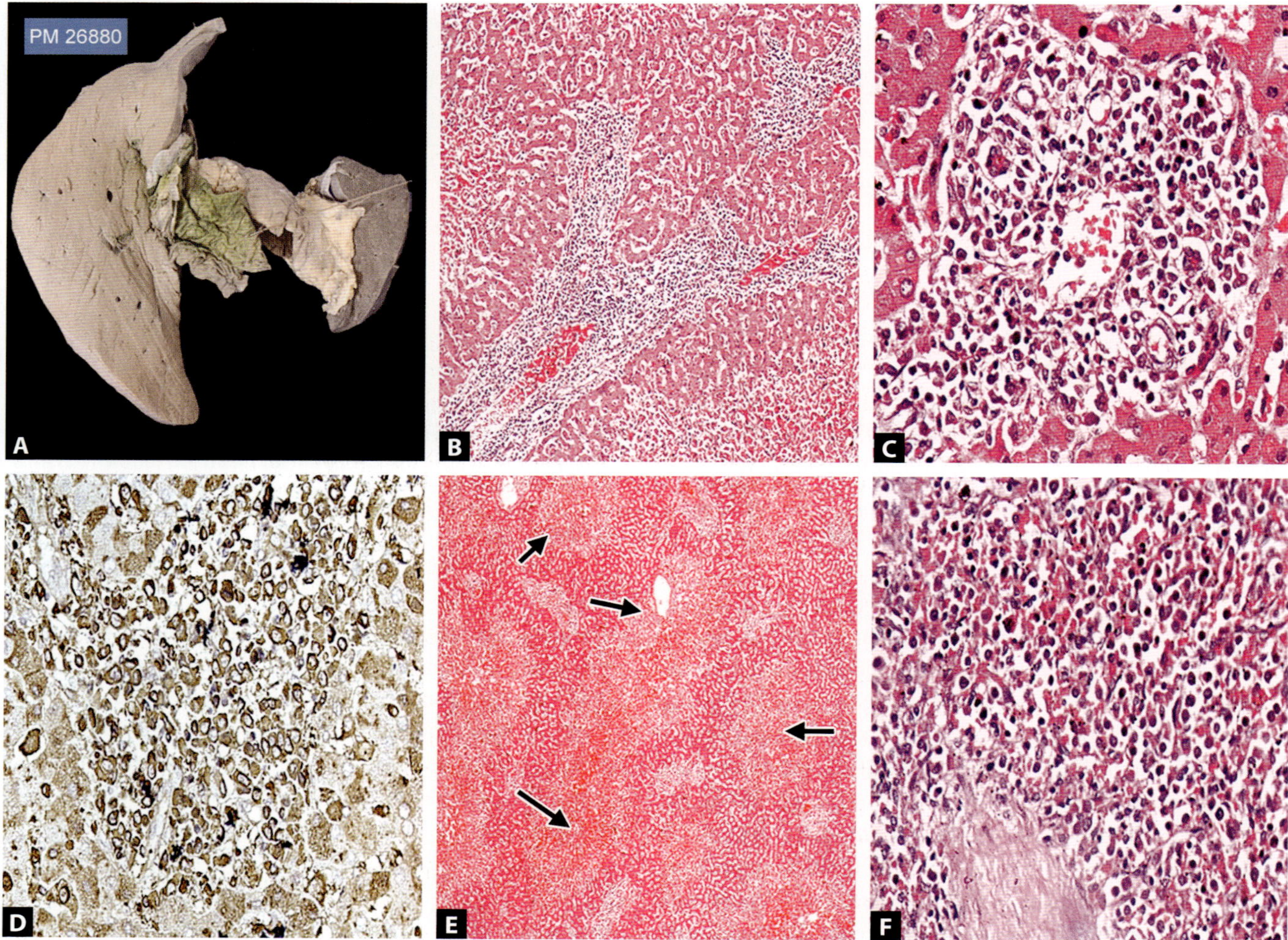

Figs 2A–F: (A) Organ complex of the slice of enlarged liver/spleen, pancreas and c loop of duodenum; (B and C) Photomicrograph of the liver showing expanded portal tract with extensive leukemic infiltrate; (D) Leukemic infiltrate strongly positive with myeloperoxidase (MPO) immunostain; (E) Photomicrograph of the liver showing florid centrizonal hemorrhagic necrosis (arrows); and (F) Photomicrograph of the spleen showing leukemic infiltrate in the red pulp.

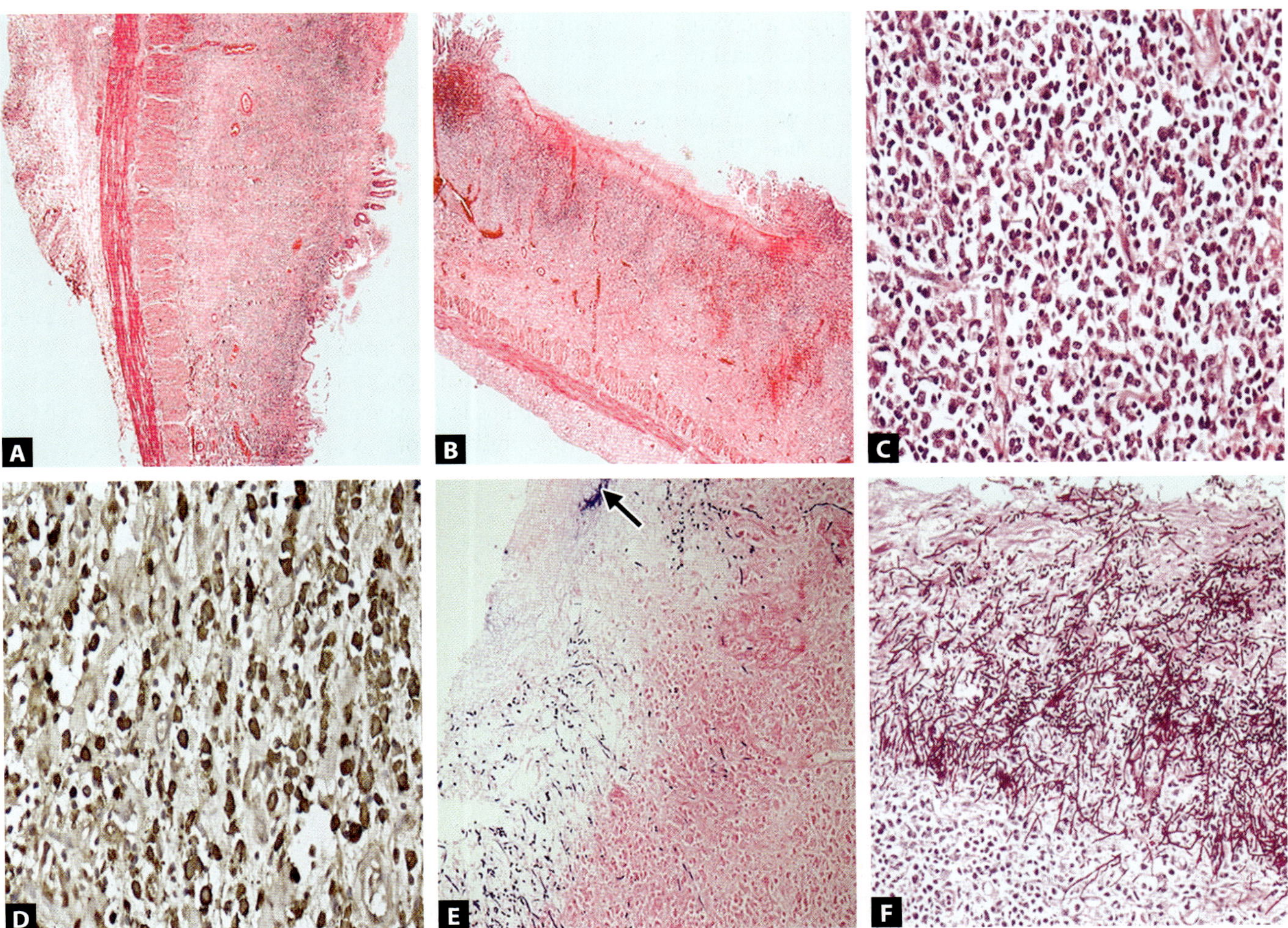

Figs 3A–F: Photomicrographs from the small intestine showing: (A and B) Ulcers with dense submucosal leukemic infiltrate; (C and D) Submucosal infiltrate composed of sheets of promyelocytes, positive with myeloperoxidase (MPO) immunostain; (E) Small intestine ulcer showing necrosis along with cluster of gram-positive cocci (Gram stain–arrow); and (F) Small intestine ulcer replete with fungal profiles of Candida (PAS stain).

microvasculature was seen. Vessels in the section from the testis showed fibrin thrombi (Fig 5D). The ***brain*** (Figs 5E–F) weighed 1,474 g. Subarachnoid hemorrhage was seen in the frontal, temporal and occipital lobes. The gyri were flattened and the sulci were narrowed, indicating edema. There was bilateral tonsillar herniation. Coronal slicing revealed a well-circumscribed area of parenchymal hemorrhage in the right temporal lobe measuring 3 × 2.5 × 2 cm. On microscopic examination (Figs 6A–C) the area surrounding the hemorrhage showed rarefaction, edema, reactive astrocytosis, hemosiderin laden macrophages, perivascular clearing and lymphocyte cuffing. Extension of the intracranial hemorrhage led to subarachnoid hemorrhage. Periadrenal hemorrhage was also noted.

FINAL AUTOPSY DIAGNOSIS: PM 26880

A 27-year-old male with clinical diagnosis of APML, DIC with DS:

- Acute promyelocytic leukemia, RT-PCR (polymerase chain reaction) for t(15;17): Positive
- Leukemic infiltration in liver, spleen, lymph nodes and small intestine.
- Right temporal lobe hemorrhage with subarachnoid extension and ischemic changes.
- Disseminated intravascular coagulation with fibrin thrombi in kidneys, testis and small intestine.
- Pulmonary thromboembolism (Rt lung) and diffuse pulmonary edema.

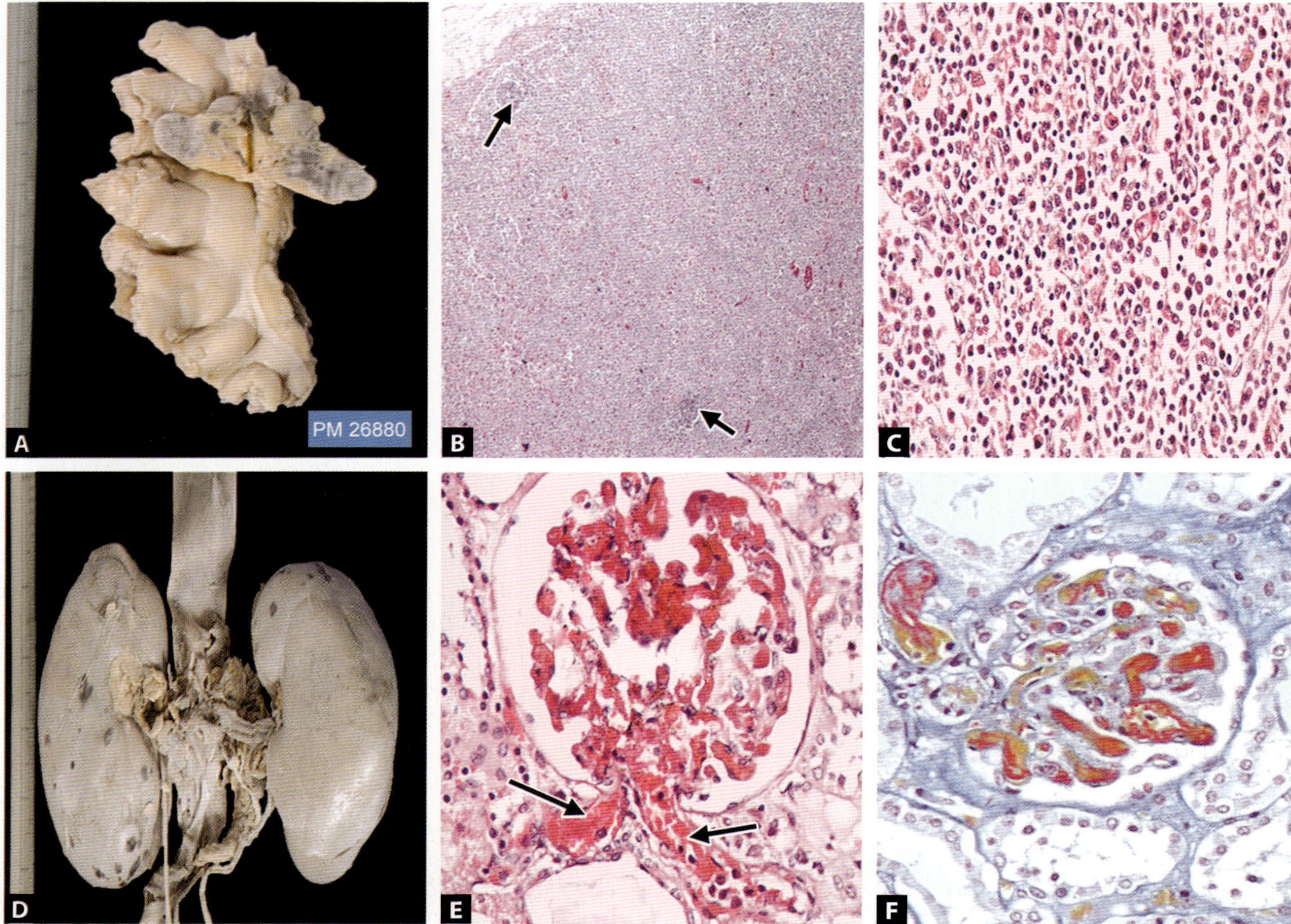

Figs 4A–F: (A) Mesentery showing enlarged lymph nodes; (B and C) Photomicrograph of the lymph node showing small compressed follicles (arrows) and diffuse replacement by sheets of promyelocytes; (D) Gross picture of the kidneys showing capsular hemorrhages; (E) Photomicrograph of the kidney showing fibrin thrombi in the glomerular capillary loops and in the afferent and efferent arterioles (arrows); (F) Martius scarlet blue stain, stains the fibrin thrombi red in color.

- Small intestine ulceration with candidiasis and superadded gram-positive bacterial infection.
- *Shock*: Centrizonal hemorrhagic necrosis (liver) and acute tubular necrosis (kidneys).

ACUTE PROMYELOCYTIC LEUKEMIA

Acute promyelocytic leukemia[1] is a subtype of acute myeloid leukemia (AML-M3) which accounts for 7–8% of adult AML and is characterized by distinct clinical, morphological and cytogenetic abnormality. Unique feature of APML is that it can cause coagulopathy and death due to hemorrhagic manifestations, if not treated early. In the pre-ATRA era, approximately one-fifth of the patient died due to cerebral hemorrhage. The median age of occurrence is 47 years, but can occur at any age and has a higher incidence in males. APML is characterized by balanced reciprocal translocation between chromosome 15 and 17, resulting in expression of promyelocytic leukemia (PML) and RARα fusion protein. About 1–2% of APML cases can have variant translocations usually involving RARα. APML frequently present with leukopenia and patients have weakness, fatigue, infection and bleeding. The less common hypogranular or microgranular variant will have leukocytosis. The classic or hypergranular variant shows increase in abnormal promyelocytes with bilobed nuclei, abundant cytoplasm containing heavy, red to purple cytoplasmic granules, that may obscure the nuclear-cytoplasmic margin. These granules are typically larger than the normal neutrophil granules. Auer rods are

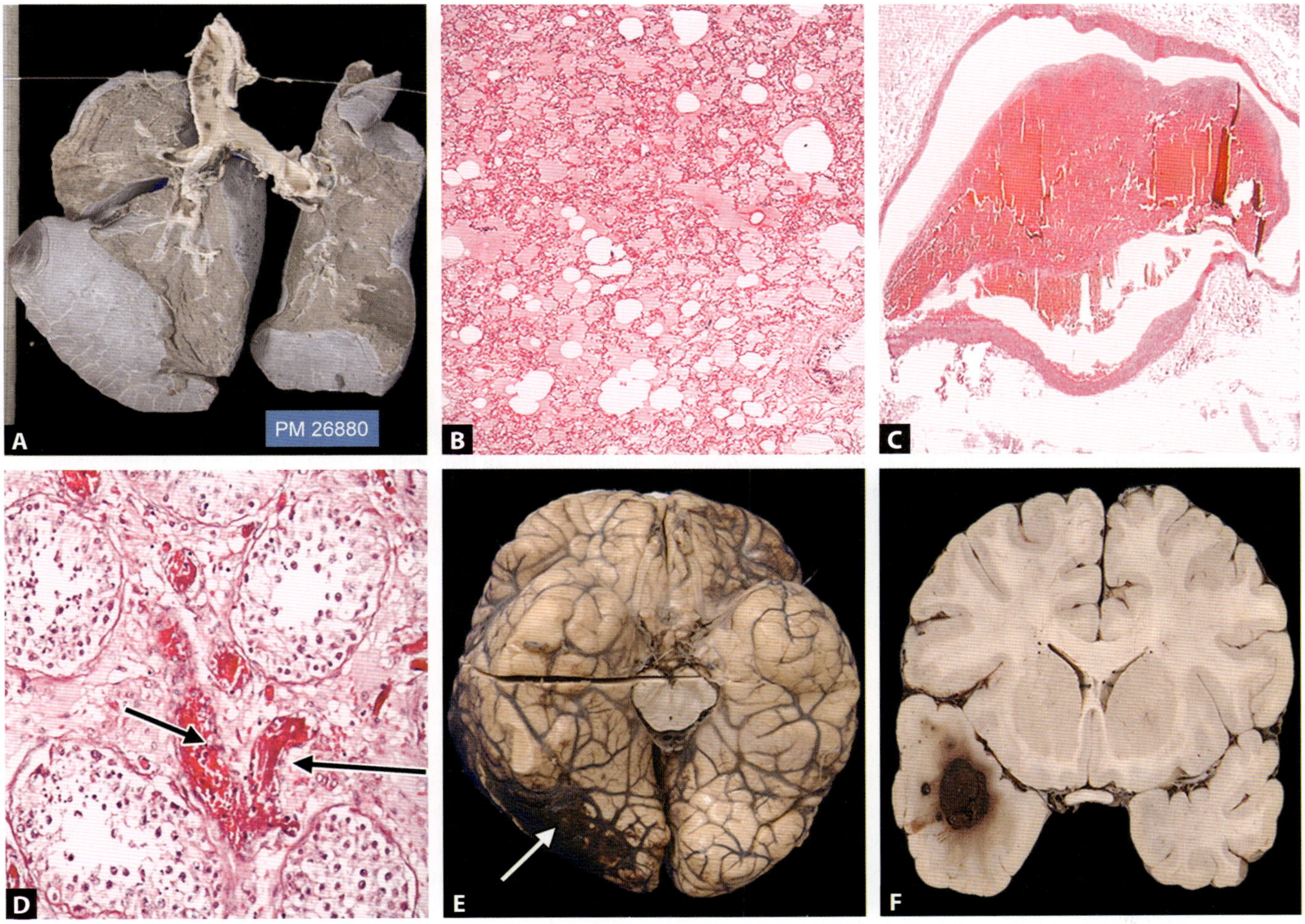

Figs 5A–F: (A) Gross photograph of the subcrepitant lungs. Trachea shows hemorrhages. (B) Photomicrograph of the lung showing diffuse pulmonary edema. No leukemic infiltrate was seen. (C) Lobar artery of the right lung showing thrombus. (D) Fibrin thrombi in the vessels of the testis (arrows). (E) Basilar aspect of the brain showing tonsillar herniation and subarachnoid hemorrhage over the right temporo-occipital lobe (arrow). (F) Coronal slice of the brain showing a well-circumscribed area of parenchymal hemorrhage.

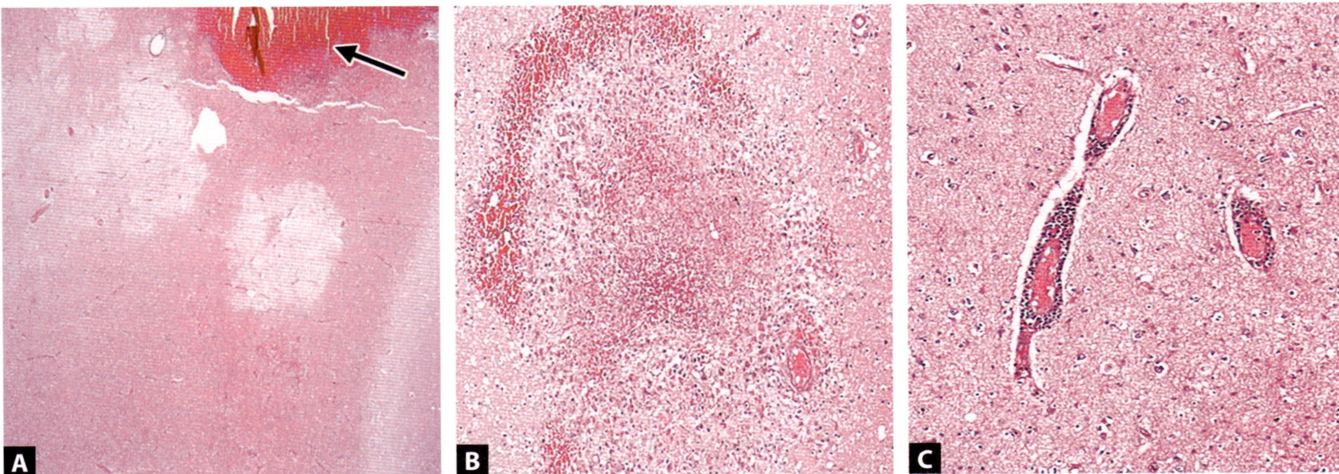

Figs 6A–C: (A) Photomicrograph of the brain showing hemorrhage (arrow) and the surrounding area shows areas of rarefaction and edema; (B) Smaller foci of hemorrhage seen around the main hemorrhage; and (C) Blood vessels in the surround show perivascular lymphocytic cuffing.

present in 90% cases. Pathognomonic cell is the Faggot cell, which contains clusters of Auer rods. The hypogranular/ microgranular variant shows abnormal promyelocytes with markedly irregular nucleus and sparser/finer granules, as compared with the hypergranular variant. Faggot cells are rare. Cases of APML with variant translocations usually present with morphology similar to that of the hypergranular variant, exception being ZBTB16-RARA t(11;17) variant. Promyelocytes are positive for MPO and Sudan black B stains. The hypergranular variant has increased side scatter with bright CD33 positivity, bright MPO positivity and variable CD13 expression. They are negative for human leukocyte antigen DR (HLA-DR) and CD34. The microgranular variant is similar with regard to the expression of CD13, CD33 and MPO, but can aberrantly express CD2. It can also exhibit dim HLA-DR and CD34 expression. About 15–20% cases have positivity for CD56 and this expression is associated with shorter complete remission and poorer survival. ZBTB16/RARA APML variant is more commonly associated with CD56 expression. The major cause of early death (<30 days) in APML is thrombo-hemorrhagic syndrome followed by sepsis and DS. Early death due to hemorrhage, before and during induction therapy, currently remains the main cause for treatment failure in APML. Intracranial hemorrhage is associated with 67% mortality, occurs in 65% cases of APML, 75% of which are intraparenchymal, 31% subarachnoid and 20% subdural. Pulmonary hemorrhage occurs in 32% of cases. Prognosis is favorable in children less than 10 years and in adults, if DIC and hemorrhage are adequately controlled.

Treatment of Acute Promyelocytic Leukemia and Differentiation Syndrome

Treatment of APML has been revolutionized by the use of two drugs, i.e. ATRA with anthracycline-containing drug or arsenic trioxide (ATO). This drug has improved the complete remission rates as well as the overall survival of APML patients by combating the severe coagulopathy that is present in this subset of AML. This has led to cure rates of 80% and remission rates of more than 90%. ATRA is related to vitamin A compounds known as retinoids and it triggers the promyelocytes to mature into granulocytes. This differentiation process leads to degradation of the PML-RARα complex, which further unwinds the mechanisms needed for terminal maturation, which eventually leads to cell death. Arsenic trioxide is the other agent used in the treatment of APML. It is known as a carcinogenic agent, but is usually well tolerated and is known to degrade PML-RARα by attacking its PML moiety.

Both ATRA and ATO, alone or in combination, can trigger DS,[2-8] an unpredictable, but well-known complication of APML treatment, which was first described by Frankel et al,[7] previously known as ATRA syndrome and now designated as "differentiation syndrome". It occurs within 2–47 days of initiating treatment and is heralded by increasing leukocyte counts in most patients, but a few patients develop signs and symptoms at normal leukocyte counts. Some say it occurs within the first 21 days of treatment. It is uncommon during maintenance treatment. Differentiation syndrome is a fatal complication and hence early diagnosis and treatment is crucial. It is characterized clinically by respiratory distress due to pulmonary infiltrates/pleural effusion, weight gain, fever not attributable to infection, pericardial effusion, chest pain typical of coronary obstruction, hypotension, hepatic dysfunction and acute renal failure. Leukocytosis is common in DS, but leukocyte counts may be normal. Literature states that DS occurs in 25% cases of APML. There is no diagnostic clinical sign or laboratory test to diagnose DS. Hence, DS is often misdiagnosed and mostly overdiagnosed. Most clinicians however consider DS in the presence of a minimum of three of the following, i.e. fever in the absence of infection, weight gain, respiratory distress, pulmonary infiltrates, pleural or pericardial effusions, hypotension and renal failure. According to Frankel et al,[7] the diagnosis of DS is established by the presence of at least three of the following signs: weight gain, respiratory distress, unexplained fever, interstitial pulmonary infiltrates, pleural or pericardial effusions. Thus, the diagnosis of DS which is essentially based on clinical and radiological features, requires the exclusion of alternative causes that could explain the signs and symptoms of the syndrome. Histopathology of the lung in DS reveals extensive interstitial and intra-alveolar pulmonary infiltration by maturing myeloid cells, presence of precursors clogging the microvasculature, pulmonary edema/hemorrhage, small vessel inflammation and fibrinous exudates. Postmortem examinations in APML patients who have died with progressive hypoxemia and multiorgan failure show extensive infiltration of maturing myeloid cells in the lung, skin, kidney, liver and lymph nodes. The presence of precursors clogging the microvasculature is also noted.

Pathophysiology of hyperleukocytosis and the ATRA syndrome is not completely understood, but research suggests changes in the adhesive properties of APML cells by the action of ATRA. Clinical signs of DS are similar to those seen in endotoxic shock and in the adult respiratory distress syndrome. Hyperleukocytosis occurs due to production of interleukin-Ib (IL-Ib) and granulocyte colony-stimulating factor (G-CSF) by the APML cells under ATRA. Leukocyte activation and adhesion occurs due to production of interleukins—IL-Ib, IL 6, IL-8 and tumor necrosis factor (TNF) alpha by the APML cells.[9] Cathepsin G, a serine protease is produced which enhances the capillary permeability. Cell adhesion molecule on the APML cells such as CD15s and integrin CD11a and CD11b interact with the endothelial cell receptor ICAM (intercellular adhesion molecule) and this is a possible cause of endothelial damage. Increased expression of IL-I in APML cells may induce endothelial cell expression of ICAM-I and vascular cell adhesion molecule (VCAM-I) which allows for increased binding of APML cells to the endothelium.[10] Also the exposure of the promyelocyte leukemic cell line NB4 to ATRA promotes formation of leukoaggregates via LFA-1/ICAM-2 interaction providing a potential mechanism contributing to the syndrome.[11] These mechanisms lead to endothelial damage and extravasation of APML cells causing heavy infiltration into the tissues. Thus prevention or early treatment of DS is required to improve its outcome.

A combination of ATRA and ATO is associated with fewer complications than ATRA or ATO alone. Differentiation syndrome can clinically mimic adult respiratory distress syndrome, engraftment syndrome after stem cell transplantation and leukostasis which occurs in AML. Differentiation syndrome occurs as a result of a hightened inflammatory response, i.e. a "cytokine storm" which is invoked by the leukemic cells in the process of their maturation, leading on to increased production of chemokines by the APML cells. As a result of this hyperinflammatory response, various organs, especially the lungs show infiltration by blasts and extravasation of fluids (capillary leak syndrome) into alveolar spaces leading to pulmonary edema. Thus, chest X-ray showing diffuse opacification of lungs, i.e. suggestive of edema in a patient on ATRA/ATO treatment, should alert the clinician of an impending DS. Ventilatory support, intravenous steroids and in severe cases discontinuation of the treatment for a short while is the mainstay of treatment. Diagnosis of DS is a challenge.

COMMENTARY INDEX CASE: PM 26880

This young male presented to our institute with fever, anemia, bleeding manifestations, gum hypertrophy, tachycardia, tachypnea and hypoxia. Investigations revealed pancytopenia, blood film showed predominant promyelocytes, the bone marrow aspirate was consistent with a diagnosis of APML, PCR was positive for t(15;17) and the coagulogram was markedly deranged. Apart from this, the renal function tests were deranged along with raised LDH and transaminases. The patient received one dose of ATRA and ATO at 7 PM and within a few hours started to have worsening of respiratory distress and anemia with weight gain, fever and decreased urine output. Differentiation syndrome was thought of and he was given adequate support with intravenous steroids, but succumbed to his illness after 26 hours of receiving the first dose of ATRA and ATO. Autopsy revealed extensive leukemic infiltration in the liver, spleen, lymph nodes and small intestine, right temporal lobe parenchymal hemorrhage with subarachnoid extension and tonsillar herniation along with DIC. There was diffuse pulmonary edema with right pulmonary thromboembolism. Clinically, DS was strongly considered, as within hours the patient had worsening of respiratory distress, anemia with weight gain, fever and decreased urine output. But these symptoms were there at first presentation. DS generally develops within 2–47 days of starting the treatment and DS developing within few hours of the treatment has not been documented. The lungs did not show any leukemic infiltrate or any differentiating cells clogging the microvasculature. Kidneys revealed florid changes of DIC, which was the cause of renal failure. The leukemic infiltrate found in the liver, spleen, lymph nodes and small intestine seemed to be a part of the disease per se and was not due to DS. This infiltrate did not show any differentiation and the microvasculature in these organs were not clogged by differentiating cells. The large temporal lobe parenchymal hemorrhage and the DIC, actually took away the patient. Thus, DS is ruled out in this case at autopsy.

TAKE HOME MESSAGE

- Acute promyelocytic leukemia is a subtype of acute myeloid leukemia, accounts for 7–8% of adult AML and is characterized by distinct clinical, morphological and cytogenetic abnormality.
- Acute promyelocytic leukemia still has a very high incidence of coagulopathy, DIC and subsequent hemorrhagic complications.
- In the pre-ATRA period 80–90% of patients at diagnosis presented with severe hemorrhagic syndrome, out of proportion to the degree of thrombocytopenia and this was the major cause of death.
- ATRA therapy has revolutionized the treatment of APML M3. It has improved the cure rate and overall survival of patients by ameliorating the severe coagulopathy present in APML, although it has not reduced the rate of fatal hemorrhage seen in the first 10 days of induction therapy.

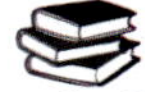

REFERENCES

1. Wang ZY, Chen Z. Acute promyelocytic leukemia: from highly fatal to highly curable. Blood. 2008;111:2505-15.

2. Rego EM, De Santis GC. Differentiation Syndrome in Promyelocytic Leukemia: Clinical Presentation, Pathogenesis and Treatment. Mediterr J Hematol Infect Dis. 2011; 3(1):e2011048.
3. Grimwade D, Mistry AR, Solomon E, et al. Acute promyelocytic leukemia: a paradigm for differentiation therapy. Cancer Treat Res. 2010;145:219-35.
4. Tallman MS, Andersen JW, Schiffer CA, et al. Clinical description of 44 patients with acute promyelocytic leukemia who developed the retinoic acid syndrome. Blood. 2000;95:90-5.
5. Larson RS, Tallman MS. Retinoic acid syndrome: manifestations, pathogenesis and treatment. Best Pract Res Clin Haematol. 2003;16:453-61.
6. Luesink M, Jansen JH. Advances in understanding the pulmonary infiltration in acute promyelocytic leukaemia. Br J Haematol. 2010;151:209-20.
7. Frankel SR, Eardley A, Lauwers G, et al. The "retinoic acid syndrome" in acute promyelocytic leukemia. Ann Intern Med. 1992;117:292.
8. Kakkar N, Dhameja, N, Jasmina, et al. ATRA syndrome with extensive organ infiltration. Am J Hematol. 2002;71:62-4.
9. Dubois C, Schlageter MH, de Gentile A, et al: Modulation of IL-8, IL-1 beta and G-CSF secretion by all-trans retinoic acid in acute promyelocytic leukemia. Leukemia. 1994;8:1750-7.
10. Marchetti M, Falanga A, Giovanelli S, et al. All-trans-retinoic acid increases adhesion to endothelium of the human APML cell line NB 4. Br J Haematol. 1996;93:360-6.
11. Larson RS, Brown DC, Sklar LA. Retinoic acid induces aggregation of the acute promyelocytic leukaemia cell line NB 4 by utilization of LFA-1 and ICAM-2. Blood. 1997;90: 2747-56.

CONTRIBUTIONS BY:

1. Dr Arun Kumar, Junior Resident, Department of Pathology (In Taking Photographs)
2. Dr Jashan Sandhu, Senior Resident, Department of Pathology (In Taking Photographs)
3. Dr Gunasekaran Singh, Junior Resident, Department of Internal Medicine (Compilation of Clinical Details)
4. Dr Narender Kumar, Assistant Professor, Department of Hematology (Contributing Fig 1A–E)
5. Dr SC Varma, Ex Professor and Head Department of Internal Medicine (Clinician In-Charge)

Post Graduate Institute of Medical Education and Research, Chandigarh, India

CASE 6

Acute Promyelocytic Leukemia with Differentiation Syndrome: PM 17959

Nandita Bharadwaj Kakkar

 HIGHLIGHTS OF THE CASE

This is a case of acute promyelocytic leukemia—APML who received all-trans-retinoic acid (ATRA) therapy for 3 weeks, a drug that has revolutionized the treatment of acute promyelocytic leukemia. The patient developed a well-known complication of this therapy called "differentiation syndrome" and succumbed to his illness.

***Keywords*:** Differentiation syndrome, ATRA syndrome, acute promyelocytic leukemia, AML M3, heavy infiltration, all organs.

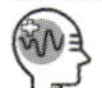 CLINICAL DETAILS

First Admission (August 2001)

A 35-year-male came with weakness, cervical lymphadenopathy and gum swelling of 5 months duration. On examination the liver and spleen were enlarged, 5 cm and 1 cm below the respective costal margins. Generalized lymphadenopathy was present.

Investigations

Hemogram: Hb—12 g/dL, TLC—8,500/μL, platelet count 73,000/μL, DLC—88% blasts, 2% polymorphs, 8% lymphocytes and 2% monocytes.

Bone marrow aspiration: Myeloid:erythroid ratio of 100:1 with 40% blasts, 56% promyelocytes, 2% metamyelocytes, 1% lymphocytes and 1% polymorphs; erythropoiesis was markedly depressed but normoblastic; megakaryocytes were decreased; myeloperoxidase (MPO) was strongly positive in the blasts and promyelocytes. A diagnosis of acute promyelocytic leukemia (APL-AML M3) was made and the patient was started on ATRA therapy (on 29th August 2001). Liver and renal function tests were within normal limits.

Second Admission

Date of second admission: 21/09/2001, Date of Death: 23/09/2001, Duration of Hospital Stay: 2 Days

All-trans-retinoic acid was given for 21 days and thereafter the patient came back with fever and respiratory distress (respiratory rate—36/min). There was jaundice, gingival hyperplasia and sternal tenderness. Liver (8 cm) and spleen (3 cm) were now further enlarged. Cardiovascular system and nervous system were normal.

Investigations: Hb—8.9 g/dL (was 12 g/dL at start of therapy), total leukocyte count of 158,900/μL (was 8,500/μL at start of therapy) with peripheral blood showing 80% blasts/promyelocytes and a platelet count of 76,000/μL. Serum bilirubin (9.8 mg%), transaminases (SGOT-51U/L and SGPT-21 U/L) and alkaline phosphatase (49 U/L) were raised. Blood urea was 140 mg% and serum creatinine was 4.2 mg%. X-ray chest revealed confluent opacities on both sides. A diagnosis of *differentiation (ATRA) syndrome* was made and the patient was immediately put on steroids, but he succumbed to his illness within 24 hours. A partial necropsy was performed after due consent.

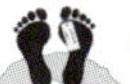 AUTOPSY FINDINGS: PM 17959

A partial necropsy was performed. Both pleural cavities and the pericardial cavity yielded 100 mL each of straw colored fluid.

The ***lungs*** (Fig 1A) were heavy, firm and weighed 1980 g. The pleura was thickened and at places small nodules could be palpated. Cut section (Fig 1B) was firm. On microscopic examination (Fig 1C) there was heavy infiltration by maturing leukemic cells in the subpleural location and the nodules palpated at gross examination also showed similar atypical

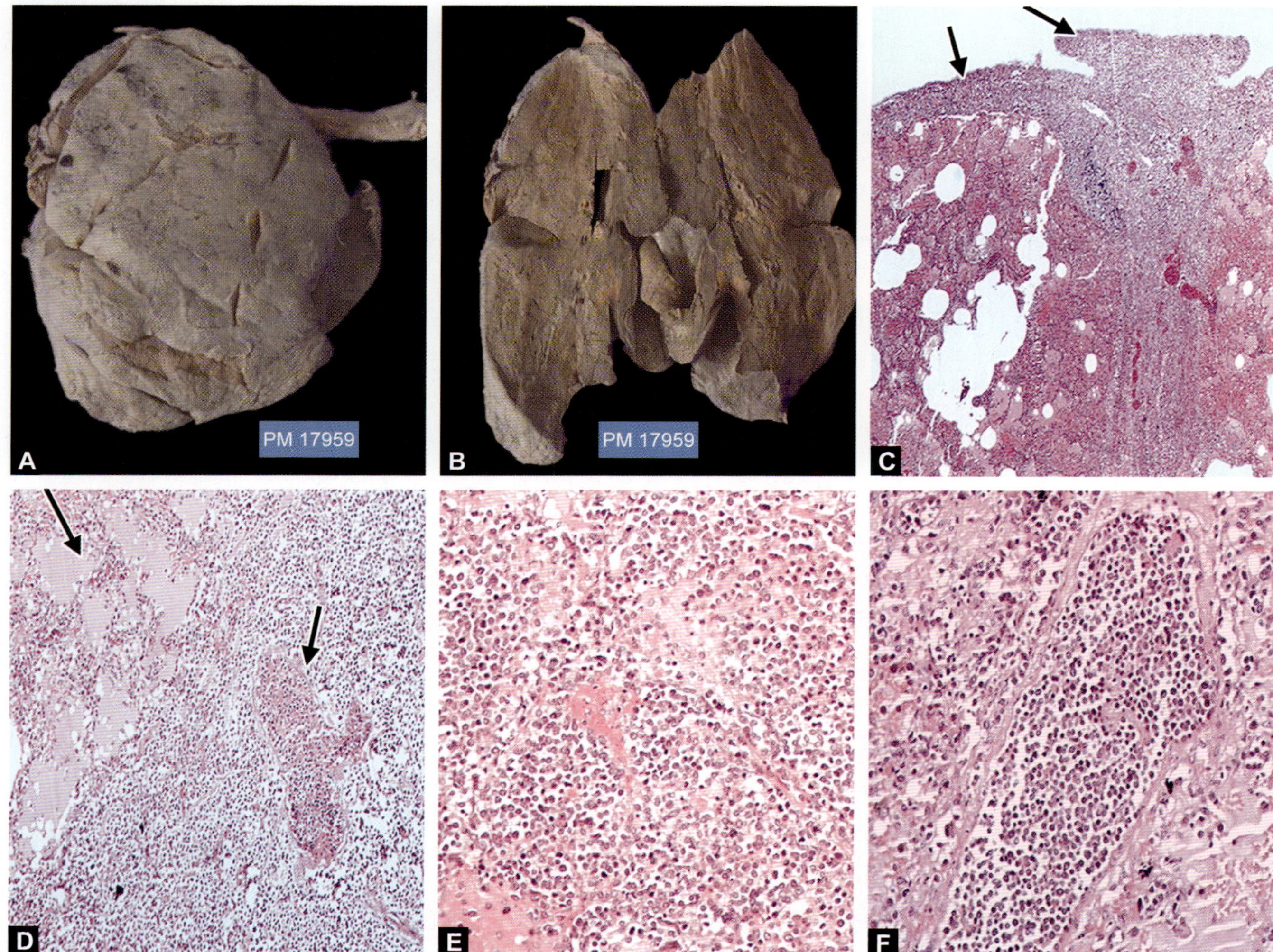

Figs 1A–F: (A) Right lung is enlarged and the pleura is opaque; (B) Cut section of the lung showing a firm parenchyma. Photomicrographs of the lung showing; (C) Pleural infiltrates (arrows); (D) Edema (upper arrow), dense alveolar infiltrates and a blood vessel clogged with atypical cells (lower arrow); (E) Alveoli packed with atypical cells; and (F) A blood vessel clogged with atypical cells.

cells. The alveolar spaces (Figs 1D and E) exhibited a heavy infiltration by atypical cells along with edema, as a result of which the lungs appeared solid. There was florid leukostasis (Figs 1D and F). Apart from this, there was infiltration by atypical cells into the alveolar septae which appeared thick and into the walls of the bronchi/bronchioles (Figs 2A–B). Hyaline membranes, indicating an acute adult respiratory syndrome like picture were also seen (Fig 2C). Alveolar hemorrhage was noted, but there was no evidence of any infection. The ***bone marrow*** (Figs 2D–F) was hypercellular and revealed total replacement by leukemic cells, showing maturation.

The ***liver*** (Figs 3A–C) weighed 1868 g, coronal slicing did not reveal any focal lesion. There was a florid infiltration by the atypical cells in the portal tracts and sinusoids. The ***spleen*** (Figs 3D–F) weighed 510 g and on microscopic examination revealed extensive infiltration by the atypical malignant cells. **Other organs** (Figs 4–5), i.e. lymph nodes (para-aortic, mesenteric and mediastinal), pancreas, kidneys, periadrenal/adrenals, heart (myocardium and pericardium), prostate, testis and mucosa of stomach showed a very heavy infiltration by the malignant cells. Immunohistochemistry with anti-MPO antibodies was done on sections of the lung and liver and were found to be strongly positive (Figs 6A–B).

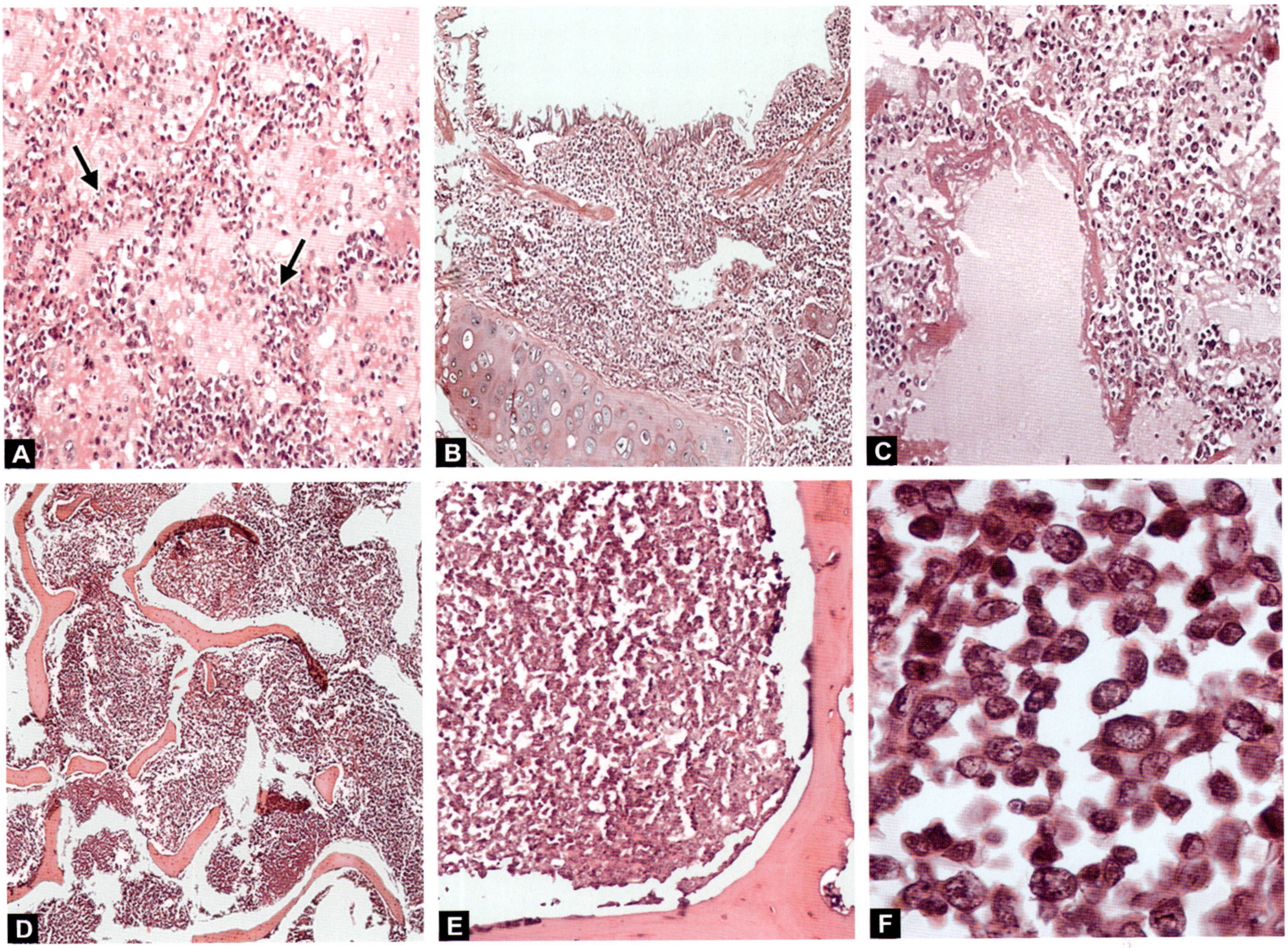

Figs 2A–F: Photomicrographs of the lung showing: (A) Alveolar septae infiltrated by atypical cells (arrows) along with edema; (B) Wall of the bronchi showing presence of atypical cells; (C) Hyaline membrane formation. Photomicrographs of the postmortem bone marrow shows. (D) Hypercellular marrow spaces; and (E and F) Sheets of blasts.

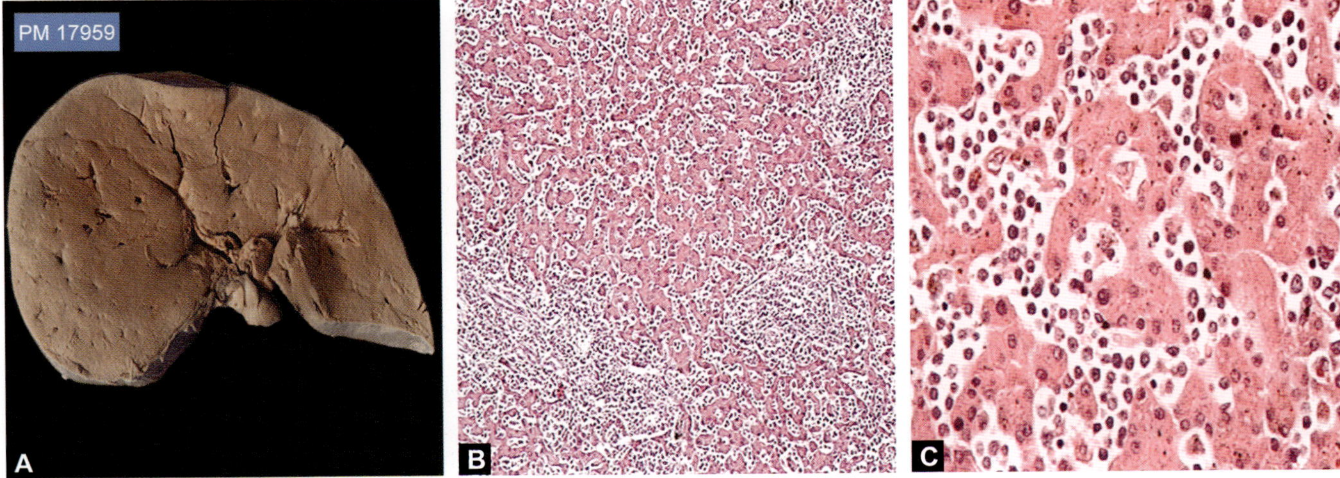

Figs 3A–C:

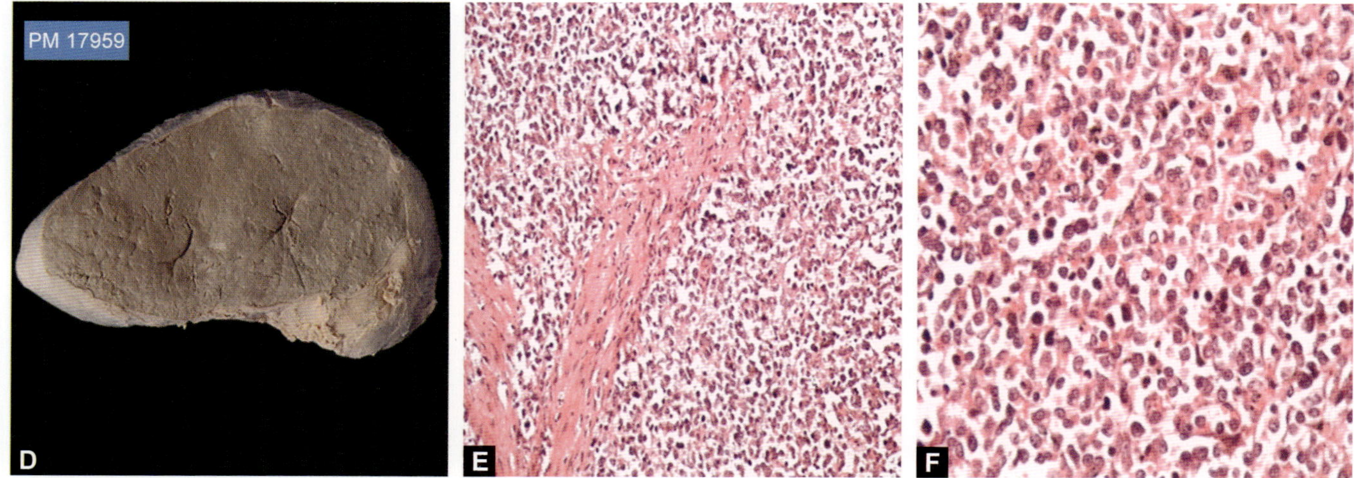

Figs 3A–F: (A) Coronal slice of the liver showing diffuse enlargement; (B–C) Portal tracts and sinusoids show heavy infiltration by atypical cells; (D) Coronal slice of the enlarged spleen; and (E–F) Spleen shows heavy infiltration by atypical cells.

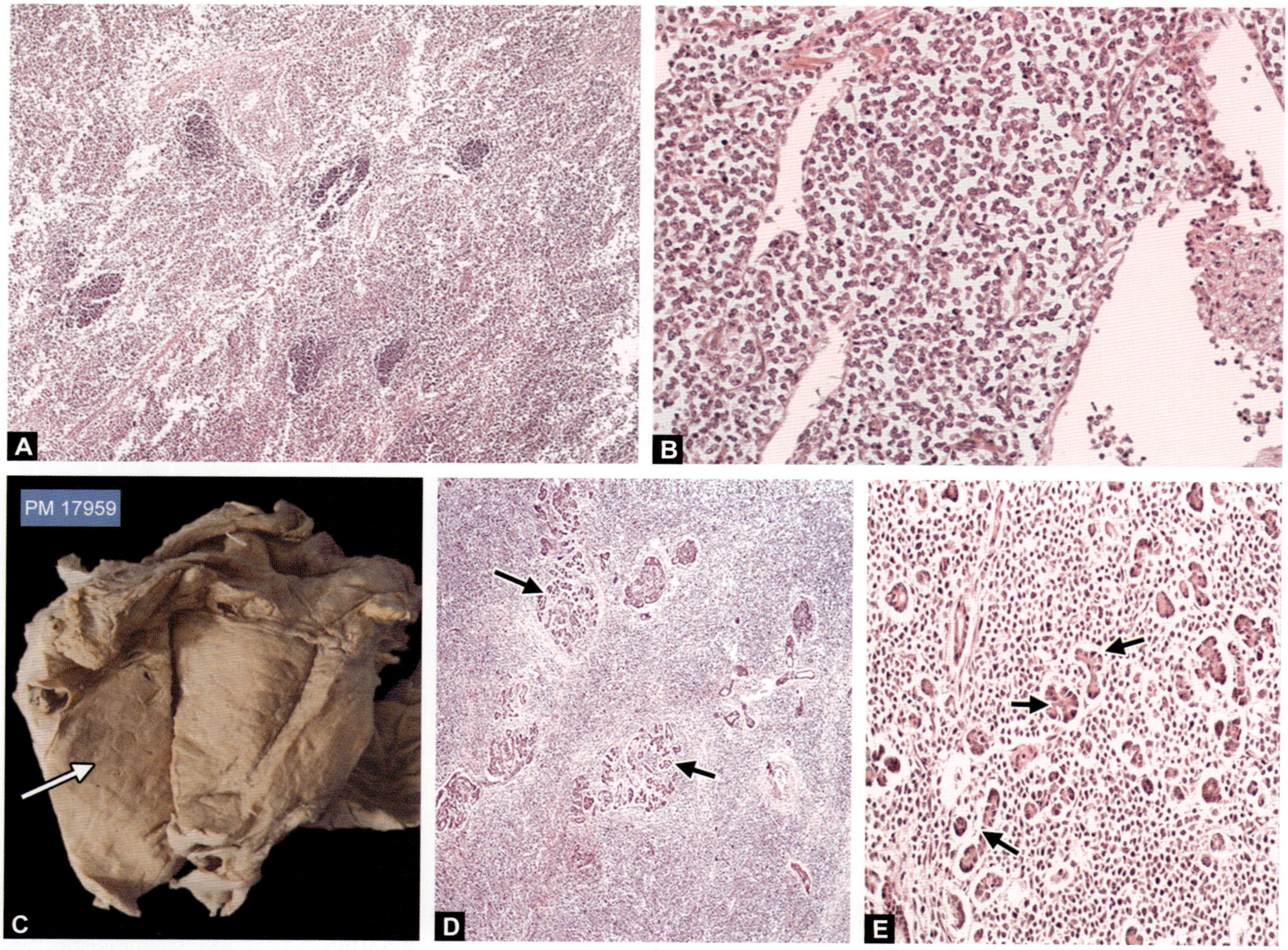

Figs 4A–E: (A–B) Lymph nodes showing loss of architecture and infiltration by atypical cells. (C) Gross photograph of the enlarged pancreas showing nodules (arrow); (D–E) Photomicrographs of the pancreas showing a heavy infiltration by atypical cells. The islets (arrows in "D") and acini (arrows in "E") can be seen amidst the heavy infiltrate.

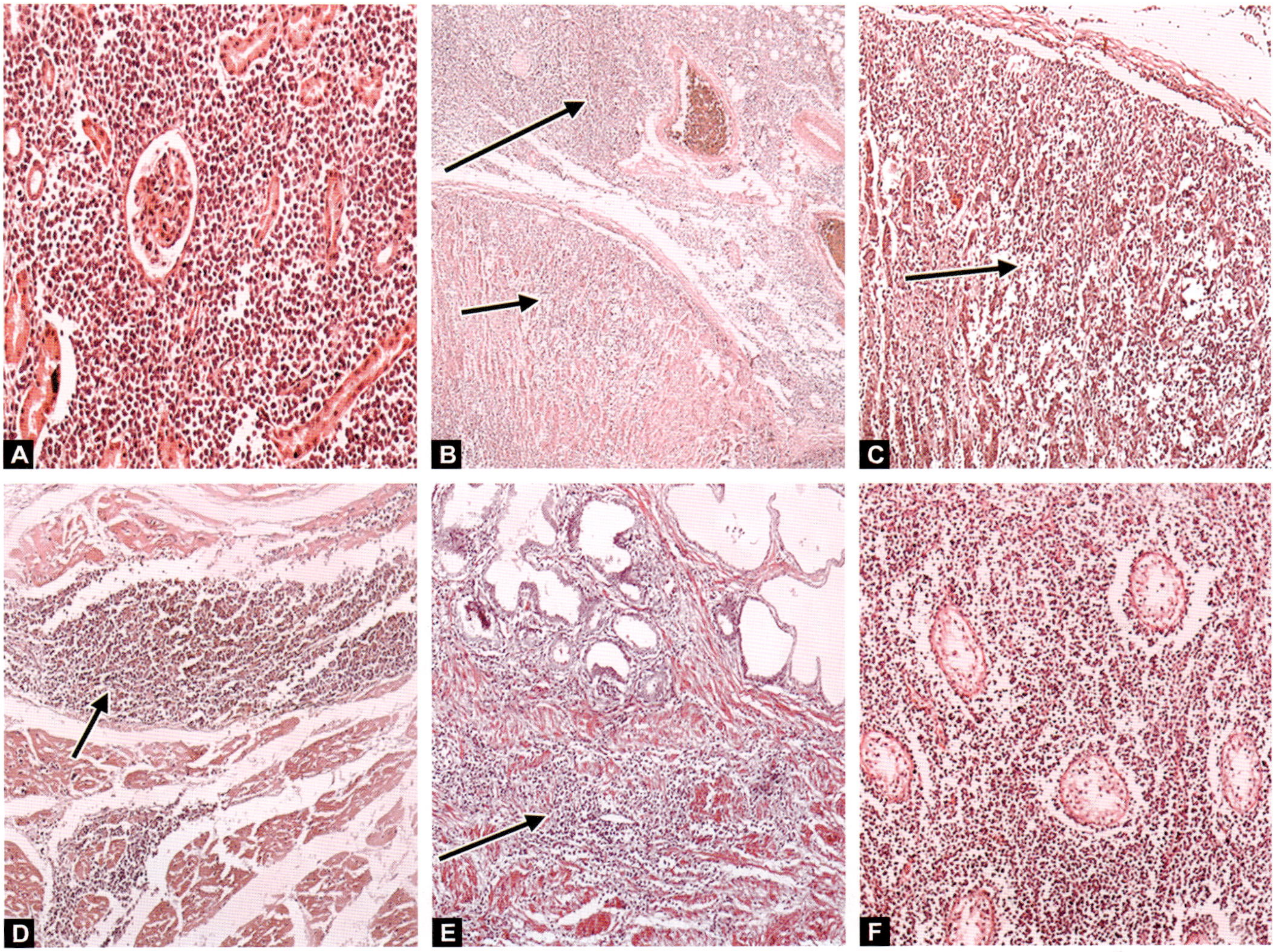

Figs 5A–F: Photomicrographs showing atypical cells infiltrating the (A) Kidney; (B) Adrenal gland (lower arrow) and periadrenal tissue (upper arrow); (C) Adrenal gland (arrow); (D) Myocardium; (E) Prostate (arrow); and (F) Testis, where the seminiferous tubules can be seen amidst the infiltrate.

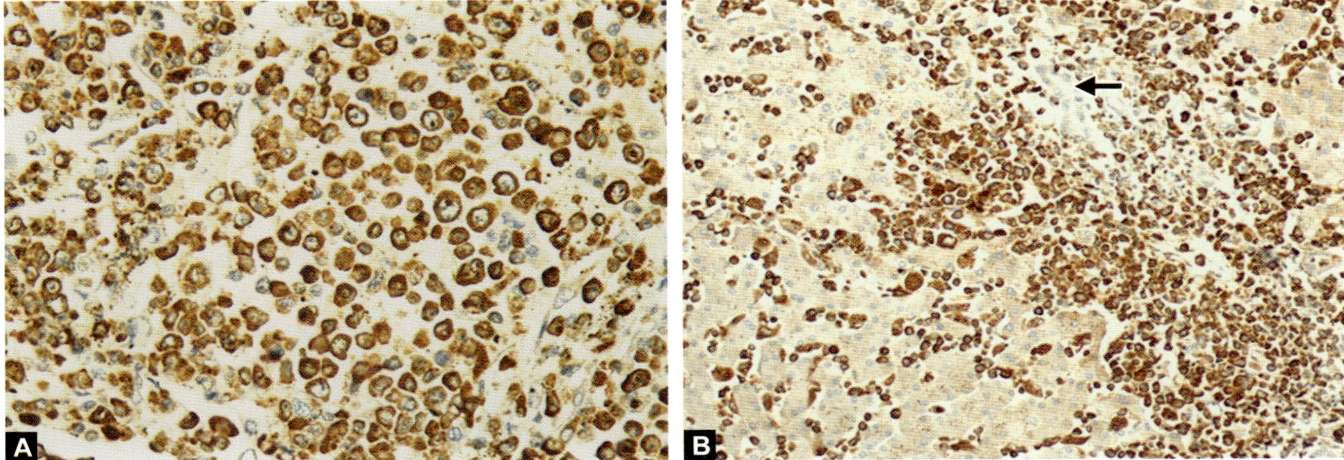

Figs 6A–B: Anti-myeloperoxidase (MPO) antibody showing strong cytoplasmic positivity. (A) In the cells infiltrating the alveolar spaces; and (B) In the cells infiltrating the portal tract and sinusoids. A bile duct (arrow) can be seen in the portal tract (immunoperoxidase stain).

FINAL AUTOPSY DIAGNOSIS: PM 17959

C/O AML M3 on All-Trans-Retinoic Acid Treatment for 3 Weeks

Differentiation/ATRA syndrome-heavy infiltration by the maturing leukemic cells in the lungs, liver, spleen, lymph nodes, bone marrow, kidneys, pancreas, adrenals, testes, myocardium, pericardium and mucosa of stomach.

About Acute Promyelocytic Leukemia and Differentiation Syndrome—Refer to Case 5 "PM 26880"

COMMENTARY INDEX CASE

This is a classical case of AML M3—hypergranular variant. Patient was put on ATRA therapy and within 3 weeks he developed its worst complication—the differentiation syndrome. The patient came back with fever and severe breathlessness. His hematologic profile showed a fall in hemoglobin and marked hyperleukocytosis. The liver and spleen had increased in size. The liver and renal function tests were deranged. The patient succumbed to his illness and necropsy revealed effusions (pleural and pericardial), extensive pulmonary edema, clogging of microvasculature and heavy infiltration of all organs of the body by the maturing atypical leukemic cells. Patient succumbed to his illness, despite the treatment.

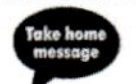

TAKE HOME MESSAGE

- Treatment of APML has been revolutionized by the use of a combination of ATRA with anthracycline-containing chemotherapy or arsenic trioxide (ATO).
- Differentiation syndrome is a life-threatening complication, occurs in 6–27% of patients on ATRA. It develops within 2–47 days of starting therapy and is preceded by increasing white blood cell counts in most patients.
- Autopsy studies in DS show extensive infiltration by maturing myeloid cells into lung, skin, kidney, liver and lymph nodes. The presence of precursors clogging the microvasculature is also noted.

Acknowledgement

This case was published as a "Letter to the Editor" ATRA syndrome with extensive organ infiltration. Am J Hematol. 2002;71:62-4.

CONTRIBUTIONS BY:

1. Gurpreet Singh, Laboratory Technician, Department of Histopathology
2. Dr Jasmina Ahluwalia, Professor, Department of Hematology. (Hematologist In-Charge)
3. Dr SC Varma, ex-Prof and Head, Department of Internal Medicine. (Clinician In-Charge)

Post Graduate Institute of Medical Education and Research, Chandigarh, India.

CASE 7

Chronic Lymphatic Leukemia, Post-Bone Marrow Transplantation with Recurrence, Massive Lymphadenopathy and Hemophagocytosis: PM 21710

Nandita Bharadwaj Kakkar

 HIGHLIGHTS OF THE CASE

This was a 39-year-old male, diagnosed with chronic lymphocytic leukemia (CLL) in September, 2000. He responded well to the treatment initially and after 18 months, developed recurrence for which the chemotherapeutic agents were changed. Being a young patient, he underwent nonmyeloablative allogeneic bone marrow transplantation [human leukocyte antigen (HLA) full house matched] in March, 2006. Post-transplant, he recurred within 7 months and developed anemia, thrombocytopenia, marked leukocytosis (TLC > 1.5 lacs with 96% lymphocytes), massive lymphadenopathy, hepatosplenomegaly, myositis and high-resolution computed tomography (HRCT) revealed bilateral consolidation with left midzone ground glass opacity. Cytomegalovirus-polymerase chain reaction (CMV-PCR) was positive. The patient was appropriately treated and remained in hospital for 34 days, but succumbed to his illness. Autopsy revealed—CLL with recurrence, massive lymphadenopathy with leukemic infiltration, secondary hemophagocytic lymphohistiocytosis (HLH) and invasive pulmonary aspergillosis.

Keywords: Chronic lymphatic leukemia, young, bulky lymphadenopathy, nonmyeloablative allogeneic bone marrow transplantation, hemophagocytosis and autopsy.

 CLINICAL DETAILS

Date of Admission: 27.10.2006, Date of Death: 30.11.2006, Duration of Hospital Stay: 34 Days

A 39-year-old male was diagnosed as a case of CLL in September, 2000. The peripheral blood revealed Hb—9.1 g/dL, TLC—59,900/μL (90% lymphocytes) and platelets—144,000/μL. The bone marrow aspirate [A—698/2,000 (Fig 1A)] showed scanty particles, a cellular aspirate, few megakaryocytes, M:E ratio—16:1 and 88% lymphoid cells. The trephine biopsy (Fig. 1B) revealed interstitial and focal nodular excess of lymphoid cells with suppression of all the other normal hematopoietic elements. On flow cytometry, lymphoma cells were positive for CD3 and CD23. A diagnosis of chronic lymphoid leukemia was given. He received chlorambucil, fludarabine and cyclophosphamide as initial therapy and was apparently asymptomatic for 18 months. Thereafter, he developed recurrence of disease and his chemotherapeutic drugs were changed to chlorambucil, fludarabine, mitoxantrone, vincristine, prednisolone and rituximab was also included. The patient underwent nonmyeloablative allogeneic bone marrow transplantation (HLA full house matched) on 8th March, 2006 (after 5.5 years of diagnosis) at AIIMS, New Delhi. Post-transplant, he was followed up in PGIMER, Chandigarh, was on maintenance intravenous immunoglobulins and tapering doses of cyclosporine and appropriate prophylaxis (Bactrim DS, fluconazole and acyclovir). He recurred within 7 months of the transplant and was admitted to PGIMER, Chandigarh in October, 2006. His present age was 46 years. At this point of time he presented with history of intermittent high-grade fever along with painful, progressively increasing swelling of right thigh. On examination the patient was conscious, oriented and had a poor nutritional status. The pulse was 100/min and BP 130/80 mm Hg. There was severe pallor and generalized lymphadenopathy. There was no icterus, cyanosis, clubbing, rash and the jugular venous pressure was normal. The liver (3 cm below costal margin) and spleen (5 cm below costal margin) were palpable. Bilateral crepitations were present.

Investigations and Course of Management

Investigations revealed anemia (Hb—5.2 g/dL), thrombocytopenia (5,000/μL) and leukocytosis (TLC 1,785,200/μL with 96% lymphocytes, no prolymphocytes seen). Autoimmune hemolytic anemia was ruled out by a negative Coombs

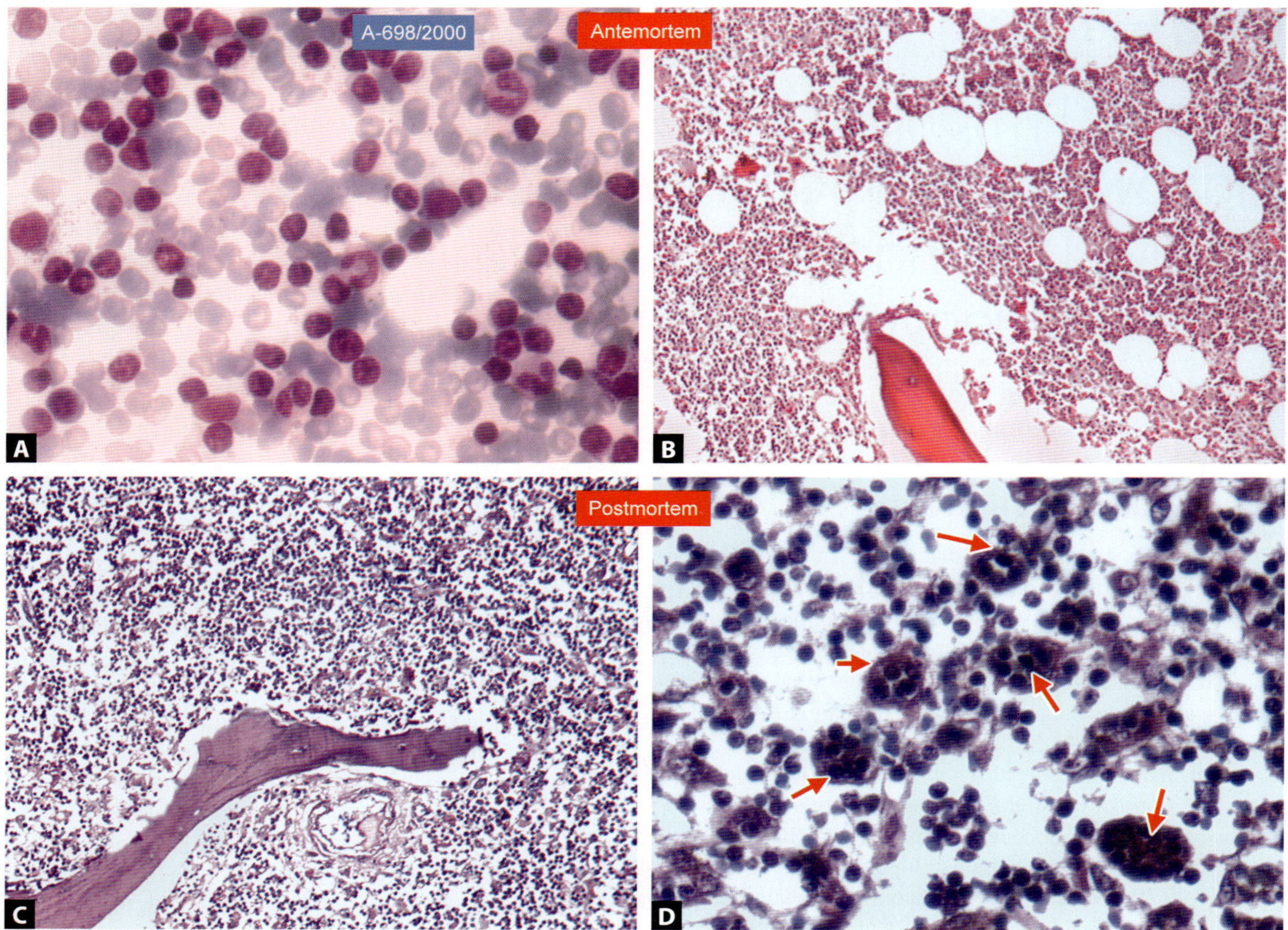

Figs 1A–D: (A) Antemortem bone marrow aspirate showing increased number of lymphoid cells; (B) Antemortem trephine biopsy shows hypercellular marrow spaces with increase in the number of lymphoid cells; (C) Postmortem bone marrow showing hypercellular marrow spaces with more than 90% lymphoid cells; and (D) Bone marrow showing extensive hemophagocytosis (arrows).

test. Liver and renal function tests were within normal limits. There was hyponatremia and hypokalemia. MRI performed on right thigh was suggestive of myositis. Chest X-ray showed shadows in both lungs and HRCT showed bilateral consolidation and left midzone ground glass opacity. CMV-PCR was positive (30,000 copies/mL) and he was treated with ganciclovir. Itraconazole was also added. Repeat CMV-PCR after treatment for 1 month was negative. He was put on antibiotics (Magnex and vancomycin) and initially the fever showed a downward trend, but recurred again. CT scan of right thigh after a week showed small pockets of pus collections. US-guided drainage yielded pus, which was sterile. The right thigh swelling decreased in size (from 42 cm to 38 cm). In view of recurrence of fever, antibiotics were changed to meropenem and vancomycin. Patient received multiple units of PRBC and single-donor apheresis platelets, i.e. SDAP (irradiated) and was transfusion dependent. Repeat chest X-rays showed an increase in chest infiltrates and patient was started on liposomal amphotericin-B, 3 mg/kg/day. Possibility of graft versus host disease (GVHD) was considered and he was put on thalidomide. Respiratory distress further worsened and he required intubation and mechanical ventilation. He soon developed cardiac arrest and could not be revived. ***Units final clinical diagnosis*** was—refractory CLL (Rai stage IV), postallogeneic bone marrow transplantation (nonmyeloablative), right thigh pyomyositis, B/L bronchopneumonia, CMV infection, fungal sepsis with septic shock.

AUTOPSY FINDINGS: PM 21710

A complete autopsy was performed on this 45-years-male. Pericardial cavity yielded 250 mL of straw-colored fluid.

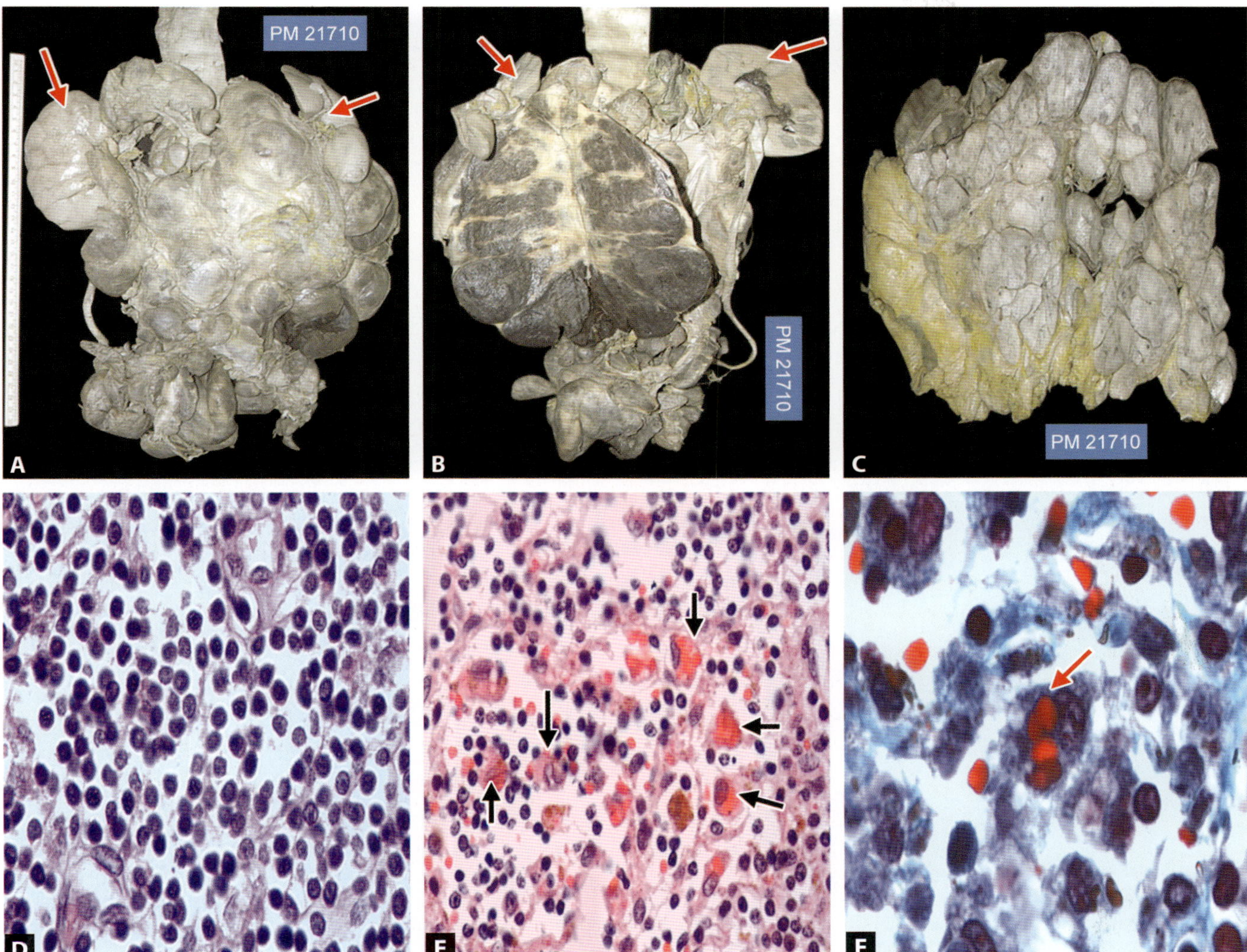

Figs 2A–F: (A) A large conglomerate of para-aortic lymph nodes, measuring 25 × 10 cm. The kidneys can be seen (red arrows in Figs A and B) (B) Cut section of the mass which is hemorrhagic; (C) Enlarged mesenteric lymph nodes, fish flesh in appearance; (D) Photomicrograph of the lymph nodes showing effaced architecture and replacement by sheets of small lymphocytes; (E) Lymph node showing in addition hemophagocytosis (arrows); and (F) Masson's trichrome stain showing red blood cells engulfed by the histiocytes (red arrow).

Pleural and peritoneal cavity showed the presence of blood clots. Petechiae were seen over the trunk and lower limbs. Bone marrow (Fig 1C) showed hypercellular marrow spaces with diffuse infiltration by CLL cells. In addition, numerous histiocytes were seen which showed extensive hemophagocytosis (Fig 1D—arrows). The patient had generalized massive lymphadenopathy and a large conglomerate of para-aortic lymph nodes, measuring 25 × 10 cm was present, encasing the aorta and inferior vena cava (Fig 2A). The cut surface (Fig 2B) of the lymph nodes varied from hemorrhagic to fish flesh like. The mesenteric lymph nodes (Fig 2C) were also enlarged, ranging in size from 1–4.5 cm in diameter. Apart from these, the peripancreatic, portal, hilar, carinal, mediastinal, gastric and nodes all along the small and large intestines were significantly enlarged and fish flesh like. Microscopically, the lymph nodes showed total effacement of architecture and diffuse infiltration by CLL cells (Fig 2D). The leukemic cells were small, monomorphic with round to slightly irregular nuclei. No larger cells and no evidence of Richter transformation was noted in the multiple sections studied from the lymph nodes. Foci of necrosis and prominent hemophagocytosis were noted (Figs 2E to F). Liver (Fig 3A) was markedly enlarged, weighing 2,300 g and was grossly bronze colored. Nodular aggregates (Figs 3B and C) of leukemic infiltrates were seen in the portal tracts and in the parenchyma. In addition, there was extensive

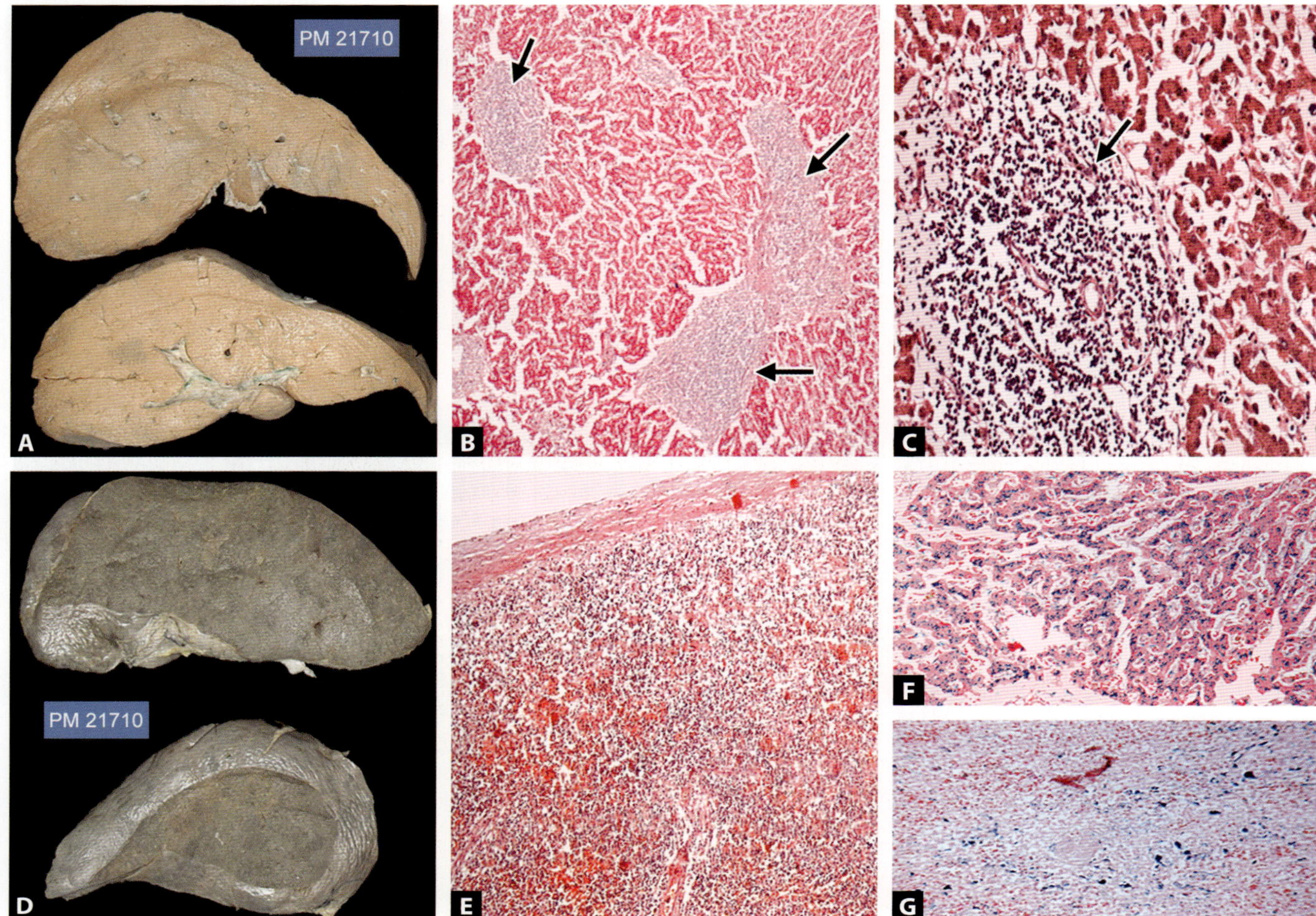

Figs 3A–G: (A) Coronal slices of the liver showing diffuse enlargement; (B and C) Photomicrographs of the liver showing infiltration by the leukemic cells in the portal tracts (arrows); (D) Coronal slices of the enlarged spleen; (E) Spleen showing infiltration by leukemic cells; and (F and G) Photomicrographs of the liver and spleen showing increased deposition of hemosiderin (Prussian blue stain).

hemosiderin pigment deposition in both the hepatocytes and Kupffer cells, which was confirmed on Perls stain (Fig 3F). The spleen (Fig 3D) was also massively enlarged and weighed 770 g. Microscopically, it showed prominent leukemic infiltrate in the red pulp (Fig 3E) and extensive hemosiderin deposition, which was confirmed on Perls stain (Fig 3G). Both the lungs were solid and together weighed 1,365 g. The pleura was thickened. Cut surface showed areas of extensive hemorrhagic consolidation (Figs. 4A—arrows). A whitish coin-shaped lesion, measuring 1 cm diameter was noted in the right upper lobe (Fig 4B—arrow). No thromboemboli were seen. Hilar and carinal lymph nodes were enlarged. Microscopically, the alveolar spaces (Figs. 4C and D) were expanded and packed with leukemic infiltrate and edema fluid. Peribronchiolar leukemic infiltrate (Fig 4E—arrow) was also seen along with bronchopneumonia. Sections from the lung also showed prominent hemophagocytosis (Fig 4F). Sections from the necrotic areas showed coagulative necrosis (Fig 5A) and were replete with septate fungal profiles with acute angle branching, conforming with the morphology of aspergillus (Fig 5B). Periodic Acid-Schiff (Fig 5C) and Grocott's stain (Fig 5D) better highlighted the fungal profiles. Vessels were clogged with thrombi (Fig 5E), replete with fungal profiles (Fig 5F). Both the ***kidneys*** were mildly enlarged, weighed 400 g and microscopically (Fig 6A) showed extensive leukemic infiltration in the interstitium. Glomeruli were unremarkable and tubules showed a few hyaline casts. The ***adrenals*** also showed leukemic infiltrate (Fig 6B). Grossly the brain weighed 1,250 g and the left ventricular cavity was enlarged and dilated, the cause of which could not be pin-pointed. Sections studied showed edematous meninges

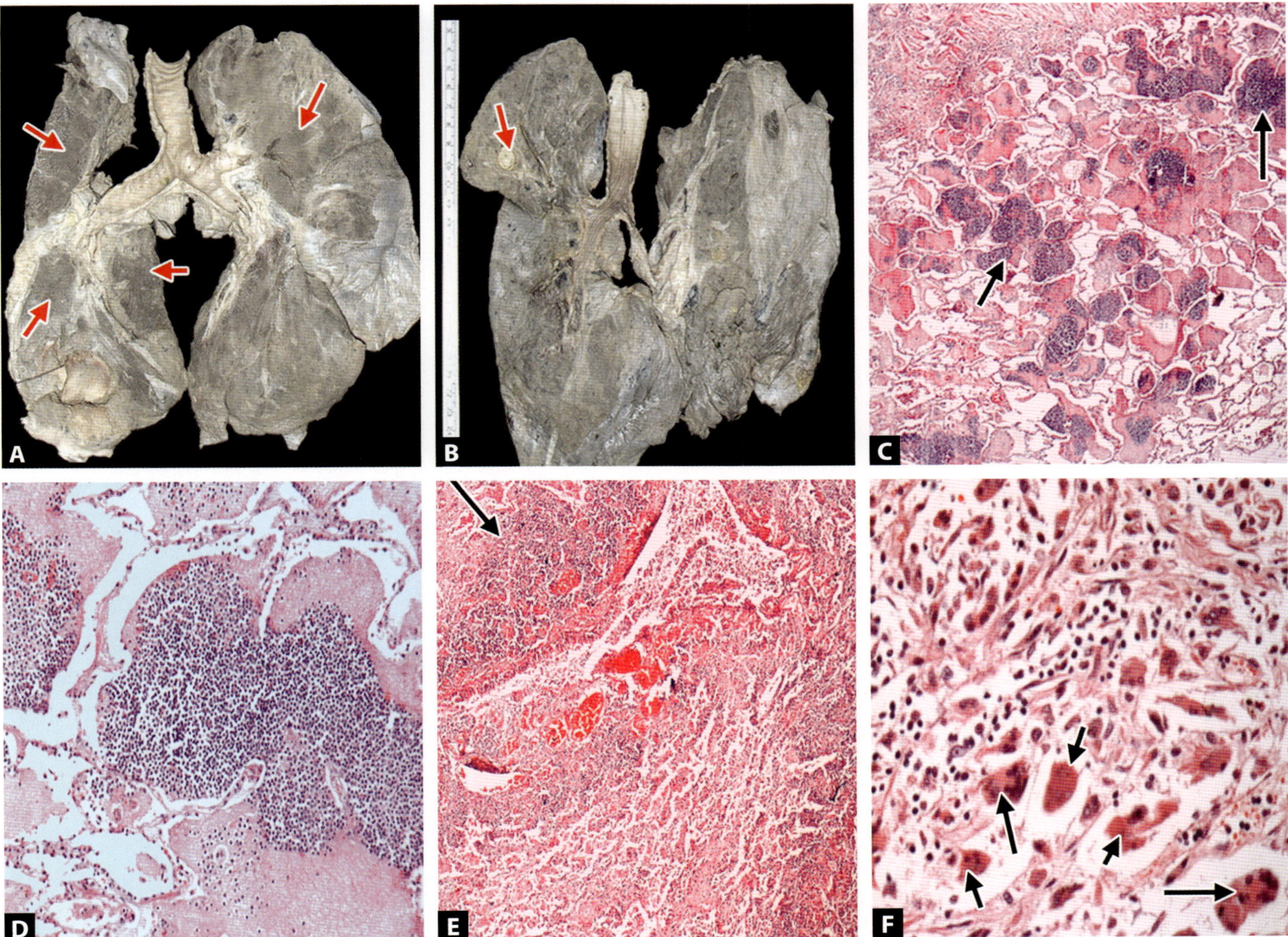

Figs 4A–F: (A) Cut section of the lungs showing areas of hemorrhagic consolidation (red arrows); (B) Small whitish well-circumscribed lesion in the right upper lobe (red arrow); (C and D) Lung showing extensive leukemic infiltrate (arrows) in the alveolar spaces along with edema; (E) Lung showing necrosis and leukemic infiltrate (arrow) destroying the bronchiole; and (F) Lung showing macrophages exhibiting hemophagocytosis (arrows).

and leukemic infiltrates were seen in the Virchow–Robins spaces (Fig 6C). No parenchymal infiltrates were however seen.

FINAL AUTOPSY DIAGNOSIS: PM 21710

45 Years Male, A Case of CLL, Post-bone Marrow Transplantation

- Chronic lymphocytic leukemia (recurrence in peripheral blood and bone marrow) with extensive leukemic infiltration involving:
  - Lymph nodes (massively enlarged): Para-aortic, mesenteric, peripancreatic, portal, paracolic, gastric, hilar, carinal and mediastinal.
  - Liver, spleen, lungs, kidneys, adrenals and brain.
- Extensive secondary Hemophagocytic Lymphohistocytosis (HLH) in bone marrow, lymph nodes and lungs.
- Invasive pulmonary aspergillosis, pulmonary edema and alveolar hemorrhage.
- Secondary hemosiderosis in the liver and spleen.

CHRONIC LYMPHOCYTIC LEUKEMIA/SMALL LYMPHOCYTIC LYMPHOMA

Chronic lymphocytic leukemia/small lymphocytic lymphoma (CLL/SLL) is the most common leukemia in adults. For its diagnosis, presence of equal to or more than 5×10^9/L, clonal B lymphocytes (5,000/μL) in the peripheral blood

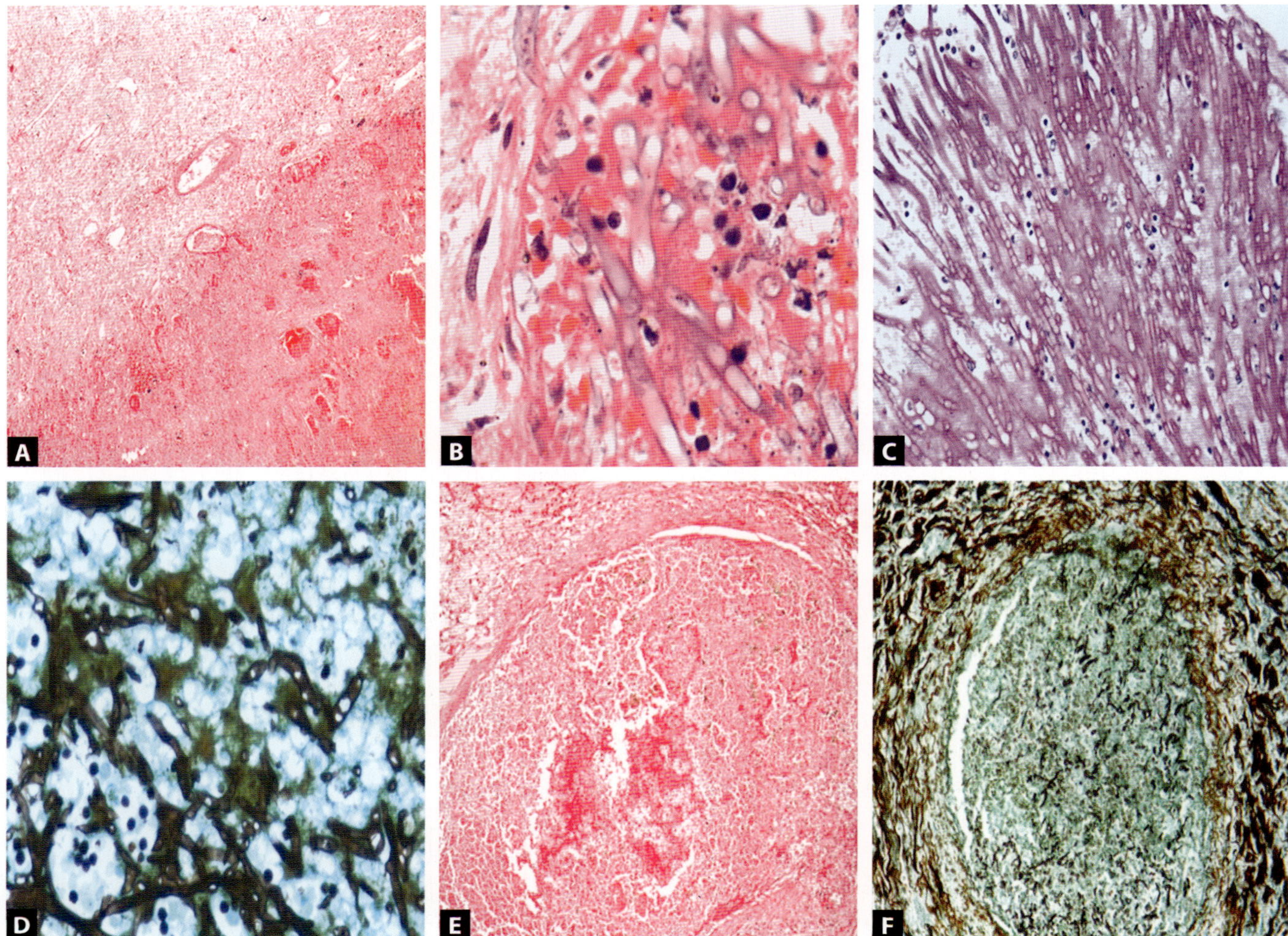

Figs 5A to F: Photomicrograph of the lung showing: (A) Areas of hemorrhagic necrosis; (B) Areas of necrosis replete with septate fungal profiles of *Aspergillus*; (C) Periodic acid-Schiff (PAS) stain, stain the fungal profiles deep pink; (D) Grocott's stain, stain the fungal profiles black; (E) Blood vessel showing a thrombus replete with fugal hyphae; and (F) Grocott's stain showing fungal profiles of *Aspergillus* within the lumen of the vessel.

for a duration of a minimum of at least 90 days is needed. Clonality is established by flow cytometry, by the detection of a single type of antibody light chains, kappa (κ) or lambda (λ), on the abnormal B-cells. The leukemic cells are characteristically small, monomorphic, slightly irregular mature B lymphocytes with a scanty cytoplasm and a nucleus showing chromatin which is predominantly dense with indiscernible nucleoli. Prolymphocytes, which are larger cells with cleaved nuclei can be seen along with and if their population is more than 55%, a diagnosis of prolymphocytic leukemia (B-cell PLL) is considered. The leukemic cells are very fragile and when smeared onto a glass slide, give rise to many broken cells, known as "smudge" cells, which are characteristic morphologic features found in CLL. CLL cells co-express both B-cell surface antigens CD19, CD20, CD23 and the T-cell antigen CD5. It has a male predilection and majority, i.e. 75% of the newly diagnosed cases of CLL are above the age of 50 years. The disease in some, to begin with is symptomless and comes to light in a routine blood test. Others present with fatigue, anemia, autoimmune hemolytic anemia, lymphadenopathy, hepatosplenomegaly and infections. The term SLL is used for the nonleukemic cases with B lymphocytes in the peripheral blood less than 5×10^9/L, showing lymphadenopathy with morphology and immunophenotype of CLL, but with absent marrow involvement. CLL/SLL accounts for 6.7% of non-Hodgkin lymphomas in biopsies. CLL has the highest genetic predisposition of all hematologic neoplasias.

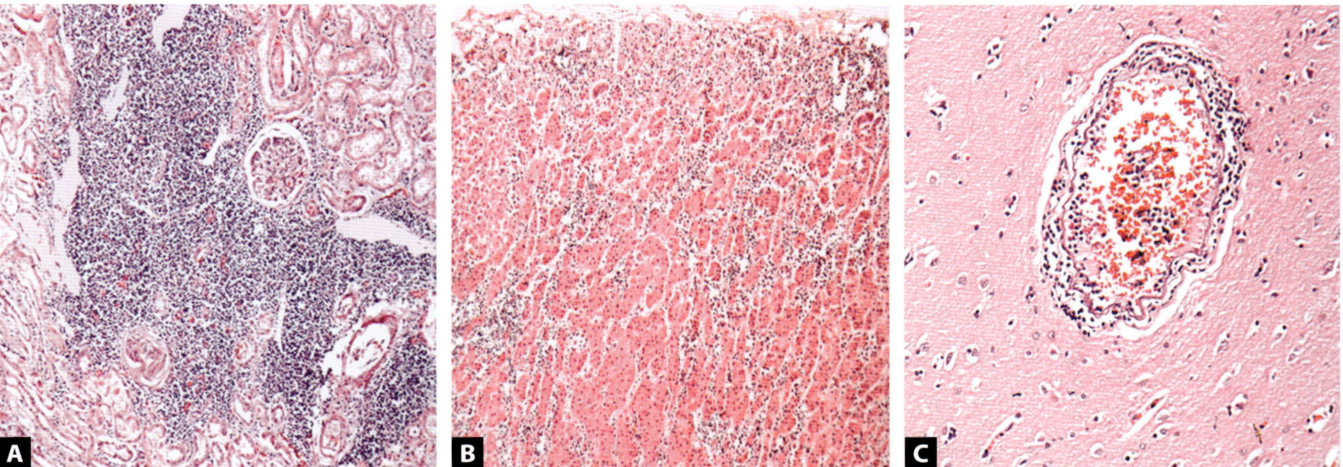

Figs 6A–C: Leukemic cells infiltrating the (A) Kidney; (B) Adrenal gland; and (C) Perivascular spaces in the brain.

Fluorescence in situ hybridization (FISH) detects cytogenetic abnormalities in 80% cases of CLL. About 50% show del 13q14.3 (targets being miR-16-1 and miR-15a), 20% show trisomy 12 and less commonly seen deletions are 11q22-23 (target being ATM), 17p13 (target being *TP53*) and 6q21. The distribution of these abnormalities varies depending on the mutational status. Unmutated CLL has a poorer prognosis and shows a higher percentage of trisomy 12, 11q del and 17p del. Expression of ZAP-70 and CD38 are both associated with an adverse prognosis. Deletion 11q22-23, del 17p13 and del 6q are associated with a worse outcome and isolated del 13q14.3 has a favorable clinical course. Döhner et al found 13q14 (*RB1* and/or *D13S25*) deletions in 45% of their cases followed by 11q deletions (20%), trisomy 12 (15%) and deletion of 17p, i.e. *TP53* gene (10%).

The patients with 11q22.3 (ATM) deletion group are younger, have more advanced and progressive clinical disease, shorter treatment-free interval, indicating thereby that the deletions occurred early in the course of the disease or even represented the primary event and are associated with bulky and extensive lymphadenopathy (extensive peripheral, abdominal and mediastinal). 11q deletions are predictive of poor survival and the negative prognostic effect of 11q deletion is seen only in the younger patients, i.e. in patients younger than 55 years of age. These patients suffer from B symptoms more frequently. About 90% of the patients of CLL, who are younger than 50 years and have 11q deletion, present in Rai stage 0–2 at diagnosis, but their disease progression is much faster. Thus, 11q deletion is a very important predictor of early disease progression and survival that is independent of stage. It has become a biologic prognostic factor for younger patients with B-CLL.

COMMENTARY—INDEX CASE: PM 21710

This was a 39-year-old male, diagnosed with CLL in September, 2000. He responded well to the treatment initially and after 18 months, developed recurrence for which the chemotherapeutic agents were changed. Being a young patient, he underwent nonmyeloablative allogeneic bone marrow transplantation (HLA full house matched) in March, 2006. Post-transplant, he was followed up, was on maintenance intravenous immunoglobulins and tapering doses of cyclosporine and appropriate prophylaxis. He recurred within 7 months (October, 2006) of the transplant and developed anemia, thrombocytopenia, marked leukocytosis (TLC > 1.5 lacs with 96% lymphocytes), massive lymphadenopathy, hepatosplenomegaly, myositis, bilateral crepitations and HRCT revealed bilateral consolidation with left midzone ground glass opacity. CMV-PCR was positive. The patient was appropriately treated and remained in hospital for 34 days, but succumbed to his illness. ***Autopsy revealed*** (1) Recurrence of CLL in peripheral blood and bone marrow with extensive leukemic infiltration involving the lymph nodes (massively enlarged), liver, spleen, lungs, kidneys, adrenals and brain (focal). Patients with bulky lymphadenopathy, inferior clinical outcome and aggressive disease as seen in the index case, generally show 11q22.3 deletion. This deletion was however not confirmed in the index case. (2) Extensive secondary HLH was noted in the bone marrow, lymph nodes and lungs. HLH can be associated with malignancies, is a known fact. But HLH is also a rare complication of nonmyeloablative allogeneic bone marrow transplantation which results from an alloimmune response. Since, 6 months after the transplant, the patient deteriorated and developed anemia, points toward the nonmyeloablative allogeneic bone marrow transplantation as the trigger for HLH. Patient had become transfusion dependent. (3) There was invasive pulmonary aspergillosis in the lungs which was acquired due to the immunosuppressive state of the patient. (4) There was secondary hemosiderosis in the liver and spleen. The cause was multiple blood transfusions in the index case as autoimmune hemolytic anemia was ruled out.

TAKE HOME MESSAGE

- Chronic lymphocytic leukemia is the most common leukemia in adults, diagnosis needs the presence of more than or equal to 5×10^9/L monclonal B lymphocytes (5,000/μL) in the peripheral blood, present for a duration of at least 3 months.
- The patients with 11q22.3 deletion group are younger, have more advanced and progressive clinical disease, shorter treatment-free interval and are associated with bulky and extensive lymphadenopathy.
- Hemophagocytic lymphohistiocytosis is a rare complication of nonmyeloablative allogeneic bone marrow transplantation, which results from an alloimmune response.

SUGGESTED READING

1. Abe Y, Choi I, Hara K, et al. Hemophagocytic syndrome: a rare complication of allogeneic nonmyeloablative hematopoietic stem cell transplantation. Bone Marrow Transplant. 2002;29:799-801.
2. Dickinson JD, Gilmore J, Iqbal J, et al. 11q22.3 deletion in B-chronic lymphocytic leukemia is specifically associated with bulky lymphadenopathy and ZAP-70 expression but not reduced expression of adhesion/cell surface receptor molecules. Leuk Lymphoma. 2006;47:231-44.
3. Döhner H, Stilgenbauer S, James MR, et al. 11q deletions identify a new subset of B-cell chronic lymphocytic leukemia characterized by extensive nodal involvement and inferior prognosis. Blood. 1997;89:2516-22.
4. Hallek M, Cheson BD, Catovsky D, et al. Guidelines for the diagnosis and treatment of chronic lymphocytic leukemia: a report from the International Workshop on Chronic Lymphocytic Leukemia updating the National Cancer Institute-Working Group 1996 guidelines. Blood. 2008;111: 5446-56.
5. Ishikawa J, Maeda T, Miyazaki T, et al. Early onset of hemophagocytic syndrome following allogeneic bone marrow transplantation. Int J Hematol. 2000;72:243-6.
6. Joshi AD, Dickinson JD, Hegde GV, et al. Bulky lymphadenopathy with poor clinical outcome is associated with ATM downregulation in B-cell chronic lymphocytic leukemia patients irrespective of 11q23 deletion. Cancer Genet Cytogenet.2007;172:120-6.

CONTRIBUTIONS BY:

1. Dr Kunal Sehgal, Junior Resident, Department of Pathology (In taking photographs)
2. Dr Reena Das, Professor, Department of Hematology (Figs 1A and B)
3. Dr SC Varma, Ex-Professor and Head, Department of Internal Medicine (Clinician In-Charge)

Post Graduate Institute of Medical Education and Research, Chandigarh, India.

CASE 8

Symptomatic Plasma Cell Myeloma with Primary Systemic Amyloidosis Showing a Predominant Involvement of the Heart and Gastrointestinal Tract: PM 19667

Nandita Bharadwaj Kakkar

HIGHLIGHTS OF THE CASE

A 40-year-male was diagnosed as a case of symptomatic plasma cell myeloma as he fulfilled all criteria. The bone marrow revealed more than 90% plasma cells, serum electrophoresis revealed a normal pattern with no M band, urine for Bence Jones proteins was positive, urine electrophoresis showed M band and immunodiffusion revealed lambda light chains. There was anemia, hypercalcemia, compression of lumbar vertebrae L4–L5, lytic lesions of ribs and renal insufficiency. He was given two cycles of chemotherapy, but he soon went into renal failure. Autopsy revealed primary systemic amyloidosis [(AL) amyloid light chain type] with extensive involvement of the heart, gastrointestinal tract, spleen, mesentery and bone marrow, along with cast nephropathy.

***Keywords*:** Plasma cell myeloma, lambda light chain, primary systemic amyloidosis, extensive, involvement, heart, gastrointestinal tract (GIT), spleen, autopsy.

CLINICAL DETAILS

Date of Admission: 08.12.2013, Date of Death: 18.12.2013, Duration of Hospital Stay: 11 Days

A 40-year-old male came with complaints of progressively increasing low back pain and generalized weakness since 3 months. On investigating (in PGIMER), he was found to have compression of lumbar vertebrae (L4–L5) and X-rays revealed lytic lesions of the ribs. The antemortem bone marrow revealed more than 90% plasma cells, serum electrophoresis revealed a normal pattern and no M band, urine for Bence Jones proteins was positive (2+), urine electrophoresis showed M band and immunodiffusion revealed lambda light chains. He was diagnosed as a case of plasma cell myeloma (lambda light chain type) and started on melphalan and prednisolone. After receiving 2 cycles, he developed lower lobe pneumonia, which improved with antibiotics. A month later, i.e. the present admission, he presented with complaints of nausea and vomiting since 4 days and oliguria since 2 days. There was no history of abdominal pain, diarrhea, constipation, abdominal distension, GI bleed or any swelling of the body. The patient was having hypothyroidism for the last 12 years and was on treatment with a good compliance. There was no history of diabetes, hypertension or tuberculosis. On *examination* he was conscious, oriented, BP 110/70 mm Hg subsequently 86/50 mm Hg, PR: 80/min–100/min, afebrile, pallor +, no cyanosis, clubbing, edema or jaundice. Respiratory system revealed a dull note and coarse crepitations in bilateral infrascapular and infra-axillary areas. The liver and spleen were palpable 3 cm and 4 cm, below their respective costal margins. No free fluid was noted and bowel sounds were present. The cardiovascular and central nervous systems were within normal limits.

Investigations

Hemogram: Hb—8.2 g/dL, TLC—12,400/μL, DLC—N75, L20, M02, E03, platelets—195,000/μL, ESR—70 in the first hour, serum urea 151 mg%, serum creatinine—7.6 mg%, random blood sugar—103 mg%, Ca^{2+}/PO_4—14/12 mg%, Na^+/K^+—127/3.5 mEq/L, total serum proteins/albumin/globulins—4.1/2.5/2.2 g and thyroid function tests revealed low T3 and T4. He was put on peritoneal dialysis and subsequently developed hypotension, for which he was put on inotropes. But he continued to have oliguria and hypotension (creatinine gradually rose to 10.2 mg/dL) and sustained a cardiac arrest from which he could not be revived. ***Units clinical diagnosis*** was Plasma cell myeloma, hypothyroidism, acute renal failure, sepsis and acute tubular necrosis.

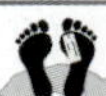 AUTOPSY FINDINGS: PM 19667

A partial autopsy was performed on this 40 years male, a known case of plasma cell myeloma on treatment. All serous cavities were within normal limits. The postmortem ***bone marrow*** (Figs 1A–B) showed an increase in plasma cells along with deposition of amorphous, eosinophilic, hyaline extracellular material, i.e. amyloid. This was positive with Congo red stain and showed a green birefringence with polarized light. Megakaryocytes, erythroid series and myeloid series were well represented. The ***heart*** (Figs 2A–D) weighed 460 g was enlarged and firm. All four chambers showed dilatation. The mitral valve was irregularly thickened (Figs 2C–D). Other valves appeared normal. The coronaries were within normal limits. The endocardium of both atria and left ventricle was firm and puckered. On microscopic examination extensive nodular deposits of an amorphous, eosinophilic, hyaline extracellular substance, i.e. amyloid was seen in the endocardium (Figs 2E–F), mitral valve leaflets (Figs 3A–C), myocardium (Figs 3D–F) and around the vessels in the pericardium. The amyloid showed a positive staining with Congo red stain and revealed an apple green birefringence with polarized light. The amyloid was not sensitive (did not loose its color) to $KMnO_4$ pretreatment, thus negating the possibility of secondary amyloid. Immunohistochemistry revealed a negative staining with AA and a positive for lambda light chain, thus indicating it to be AL amyloid. Overall features in the heart were those of cardiac amyloidosis. The ***spleen*** (Figs 4A–C) was enlarged and weighed 280 g. Cut section was firm to feel. Microscopy revealed extensive amyloid deposition in the white and red pulp. The ***liver*** weighed 1700 g and minimal amyloid deposition was seen around the blood vessels only (Fig 5A). Pancreas revealed amyloid deposition (Fig 5B). The ***kidneys*** (Fig 5C) weighed 510 g and on microscopy, minimal amyloid deposition was seen in a few glomeruli and around the blood vessels (Figs 5D–E). The tubules were clogged by casts, some of which were fractured, but no giant cell reaction was seen (Figs 5F–G). This was indicative of a myeloma kidney. Section from the ***stomach, duodenum, small/large intestine and mesentery*** showed extensive amyloid deposition in the lamina propria and in the wall of the blood vessels (Figs 6A–F). The ***lungs*** (Figs 7A–C) revealed pulmonary hemorrhage, grade 1 pulmonary arterial hypertension, minimal amyloid deposition in the alveolar septae and in the wall of few blood vessels.

FINAL AUTOPSY DIAGNOSIS: PM 19667

A known case of plasma cell myeloma (lambda light chain type) on treatment with:

- Primary systemic amyloidosis (AL type) with extensive involvement of the heart, GIT, spleen, pancreas, mesentery and bone marrow. Focal involvement of liver, kidneys and lungs.
- Cast nephropathy—Myeloma kidney.
- Pulmonary hemorrhage, grade 1 pulmonary arterial hypertension.

PLASMA CELL MYELOMA AND AMYLOIDOSIS

Plasma cell myeloma is a plasma cell neoplasm which is multifocal, generally shows disseminated bone marrow involvement and M-protein in serum/urine. The clinical spectrum is variable with asymptomatic to aggressive forms

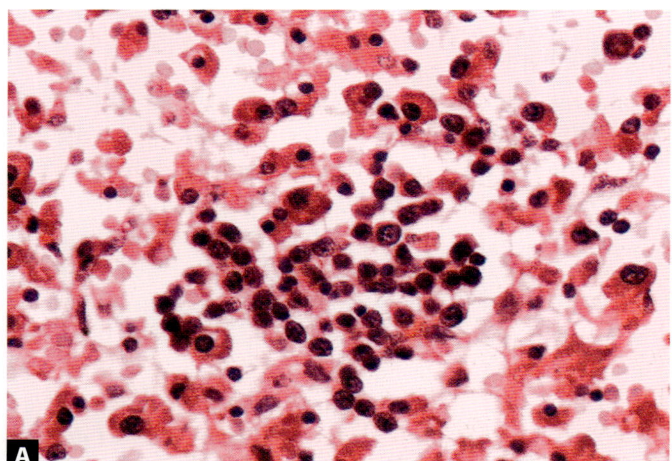

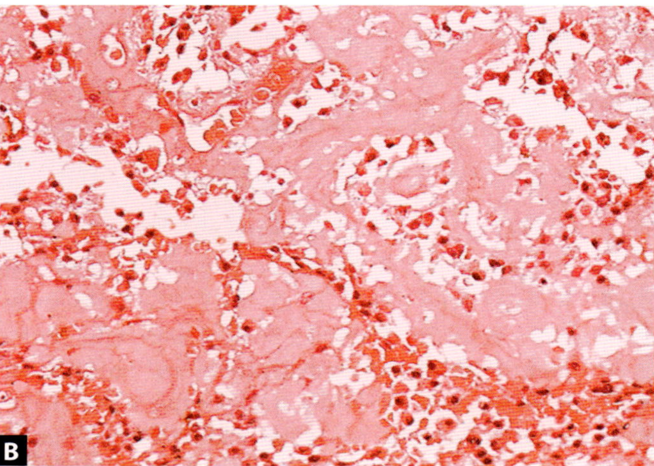

Figs 1A–B: Postmortem bone marrow showing: (A) Cluster of plasma cells; and (B) Extensive amyloid deposition (H & E).

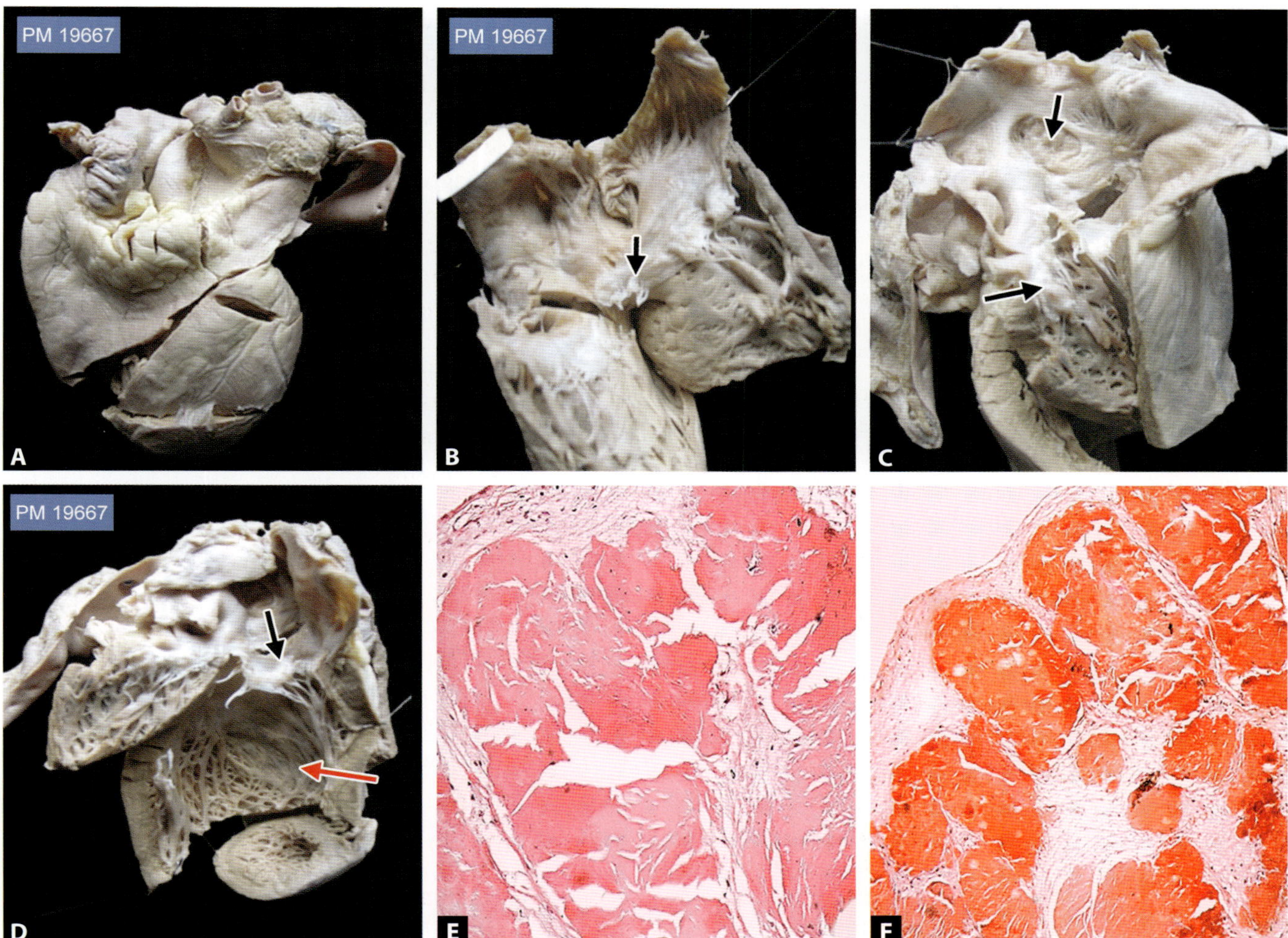

Figs 2A–F: (A) Gross picture of the flabby heart; (B) Right side of the heart showing dilatation (arrow points on the tricuspid valve); (C) Dilated left atrium (upper arrow) and the irregularly thickened mitral valve (lower arrow); (D) Dilated left ventricular cavity (red arrow) and the thickened mitral valve (black arrow); (E) Nodular deposition of amyloid in the endocardium (H & E stain); and (F) Amyloid stains bright orange with Congo red stain.

and includes various conditions associated with deposition of abnormal immunoglobulin chains in tissues. The diagnosis is achieved with a combination of pathological, radiological and clinical features. Symptomatic plasma cell myeloma should show all the following three criteria: (1) Clonal bone marrow plasma cells more than or equal to 10%, (2) Presence of serum and/or urinary monoclonal protein (except in patients with non-secretory myeloma), (3) Evidence of end-organ damage attributed to the underlying plasma cell proliferative disorder leading to CRAB which consists of (i) **C**-hypercalcemia, serum calcium more than or equal to 11.5 mg%, (ii) **R**-renal insufficiency serum creatinine more than 2 mg/dL, (iii) **A**-anemia with hemoglobin levels 2 g/dL below the lower limit of normal or Hb less than 10 g/dL, (iv) **B**-bone lesions—lytic lesions, severe osteopenia or pathological fracture. The revised[1] updated criteria of the international myeloma working group for the diagnosis of multiple myeloma allows in addition to the classic CRAB features, the following three markers as "myeloma defining events" (MDEs). (1) Bone marrow shows more than or equal to 60% plasma cells (clonal); (2) Ratio of serum light chains (involved/uninvolved) more than or equal to 100, wherein the level of the involved free light chain is at least 100 mg/L; (3) MRI shows greater than one lesion (>5 mm). Regardless of the presence or absence of symptoms/CRAB features, presence of at least one of these markers is sufficient for a diagnosis of multiple myeloma.

Amyloidosis associated with plasma cell disorders is usually systemic and of AL type.[2] This occurs due to a clonal

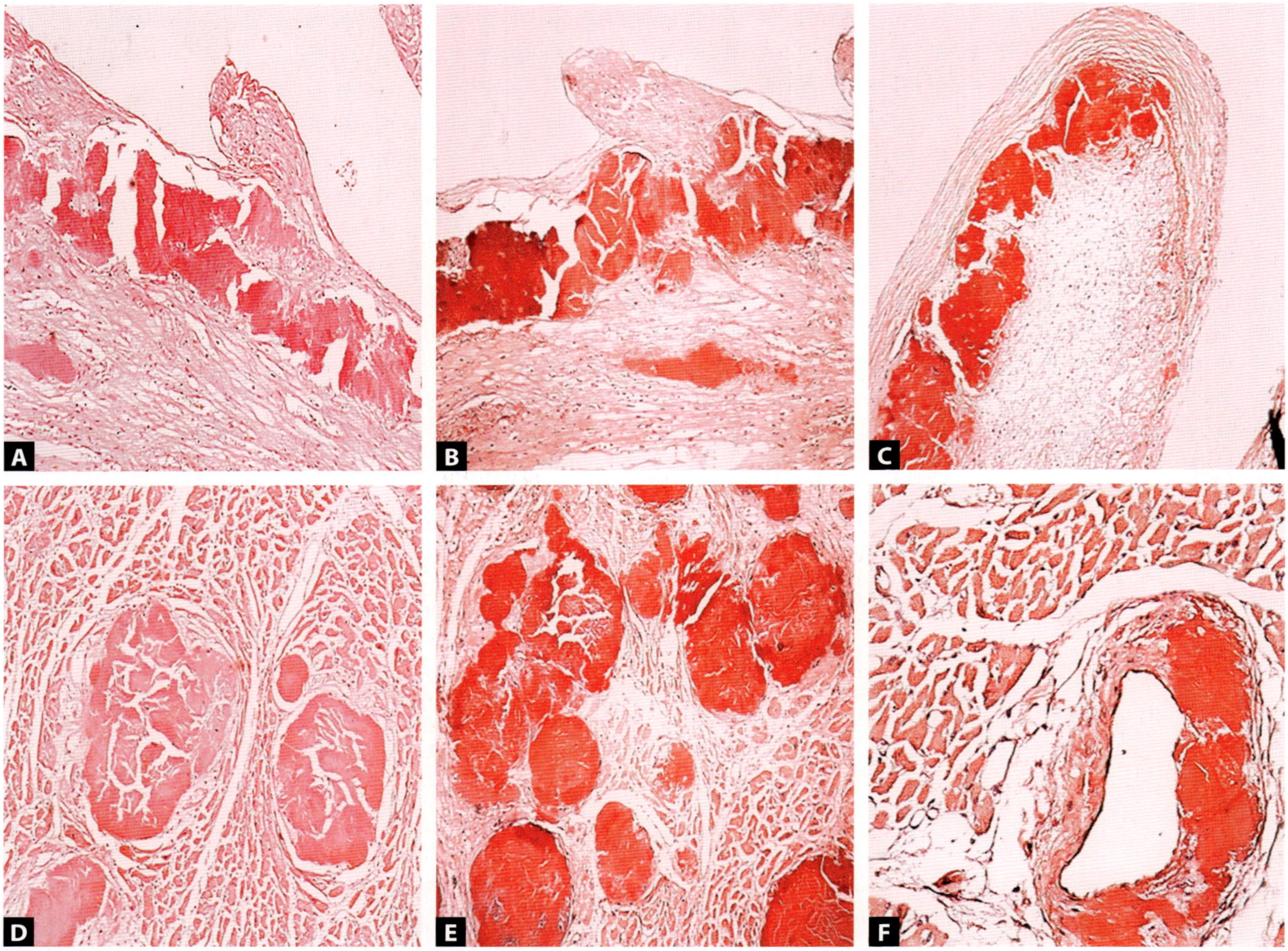

Figs 3A–F: Sections of the mitral valve leaflet showing: (A) Extensive deposition of amyloid (H & E); (B–C) Amyloid stains bright orange with Congo red stain; (D–E) Extensive nodular deposits of amyloid in the myocardium—H & E and Congo red stain; and (F) Amyloid in the perivascular location in the myocardium (Congo red stain).

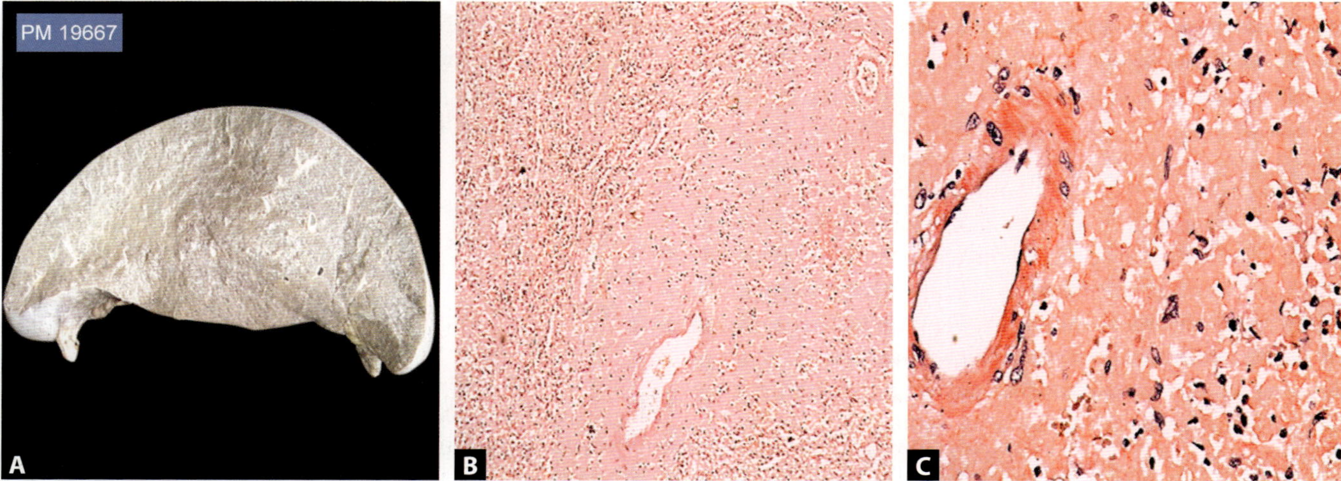

Figs 4A–C: (A) Coronal slice of the diffusely enlarged, firm spleen. Photomicrographs of the spleen showing; (B) Extensive deposition of amyloid (H & E); and (C) Amyloid stains brightly with Congo red stain.

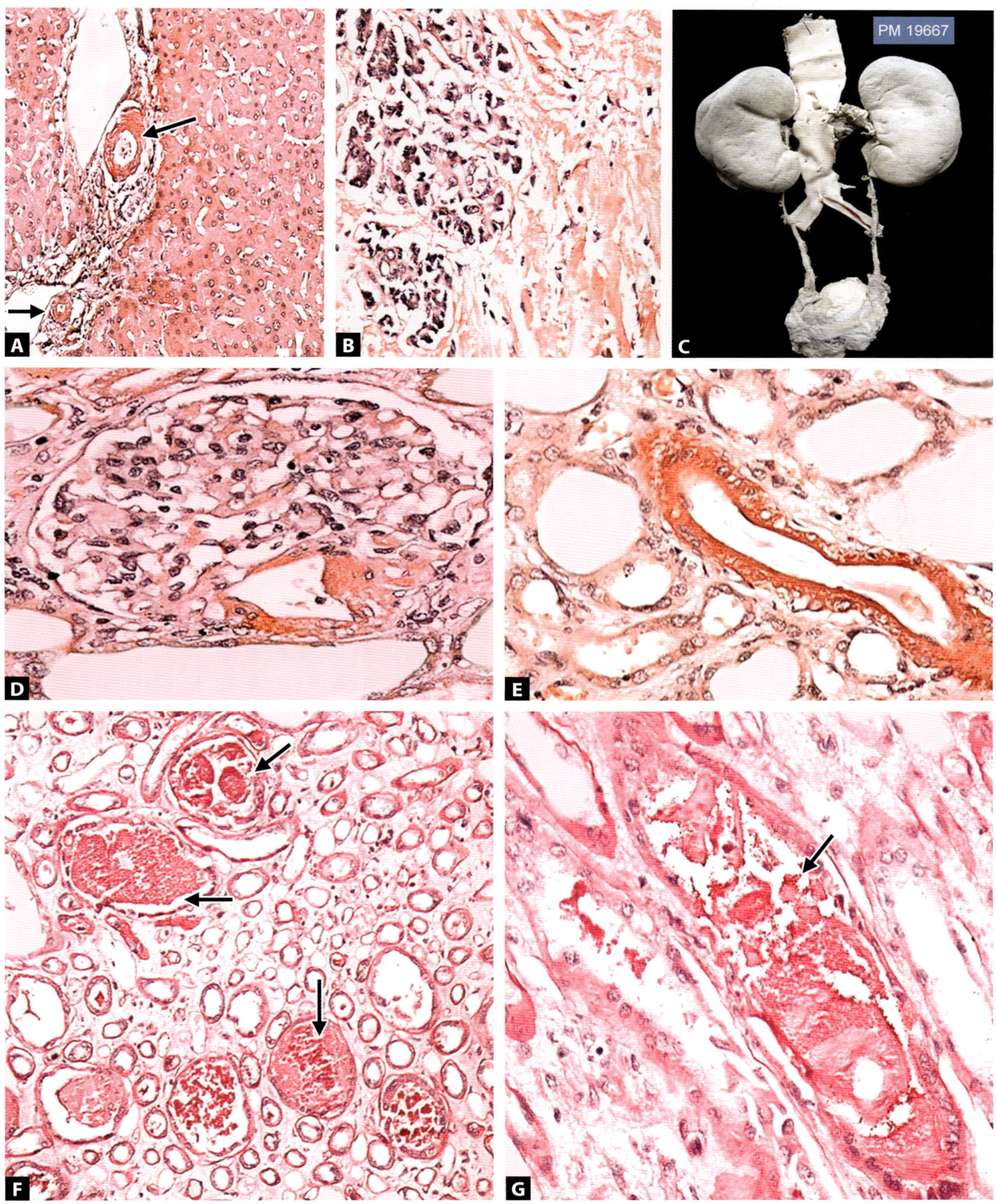

Figs 5A–G: (A) Photomicrograph of the liver showing perivascular deposition of amyloid (arrow); (B) Congo red stain showing deposition of amyloid in the pancreas; (C) Gross photograph of the normal looking kidneys, ureters, urinary bladder and abdominal aorta; (D–E) Photomicrograph of the kidneys showing amyloid deposition (Congo red stain) in the afferent arteriole and interlobular artery; and (F–G) Photomicrograph of the kidneys showing fractured casts (arrows).

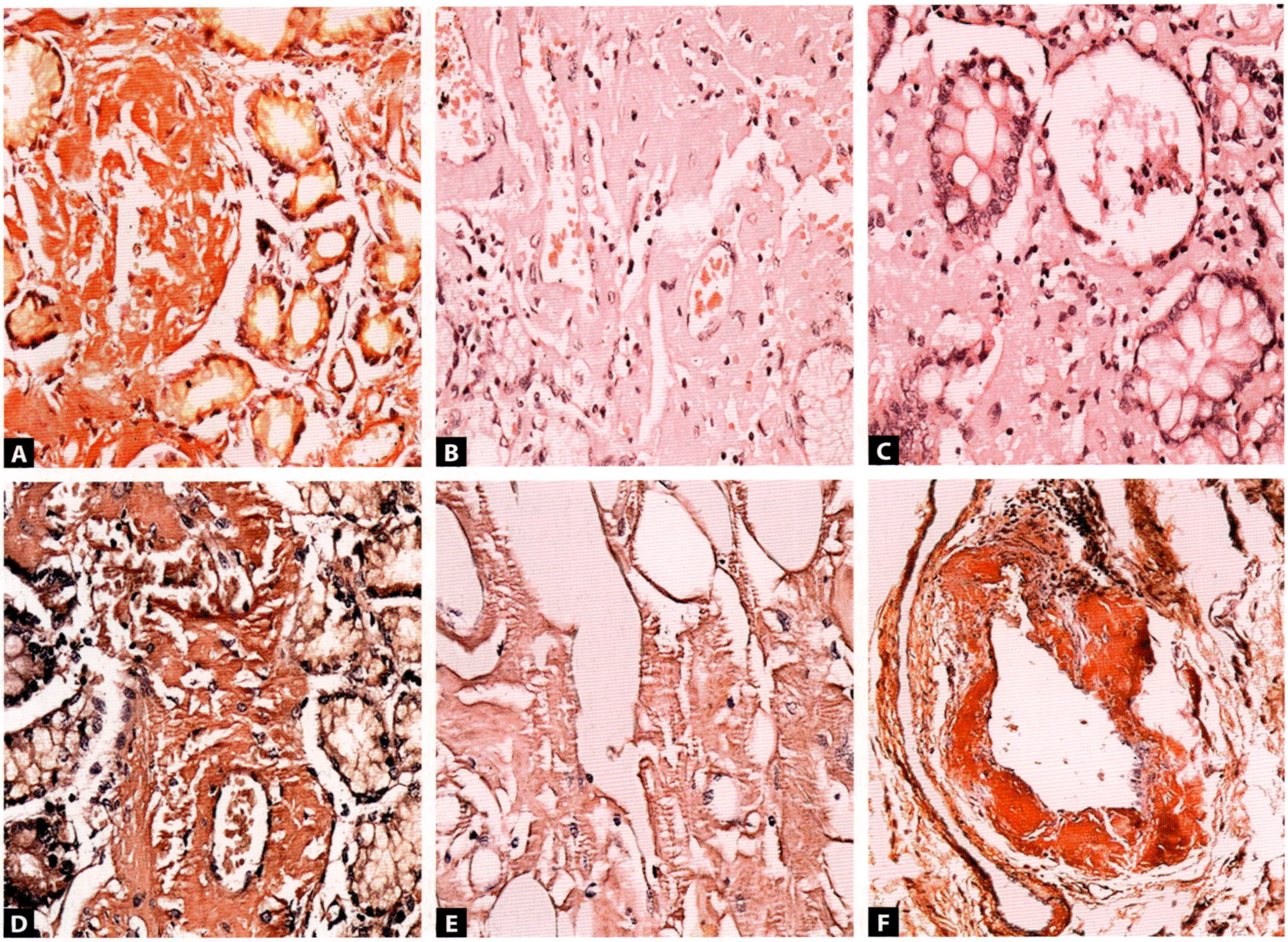

Figs 6A–F: Photomicrographs of the GIT showing amyloid deposits in the (A) Lamina propria of the stomach (Congo red stain); (B) In the lamina propria of the ileum; (C and D) Lamina propria of the colon (H & E and Congo red stains); (E) Mesentery; and (F) Wall of a mesenteric artery (Congo red stain).

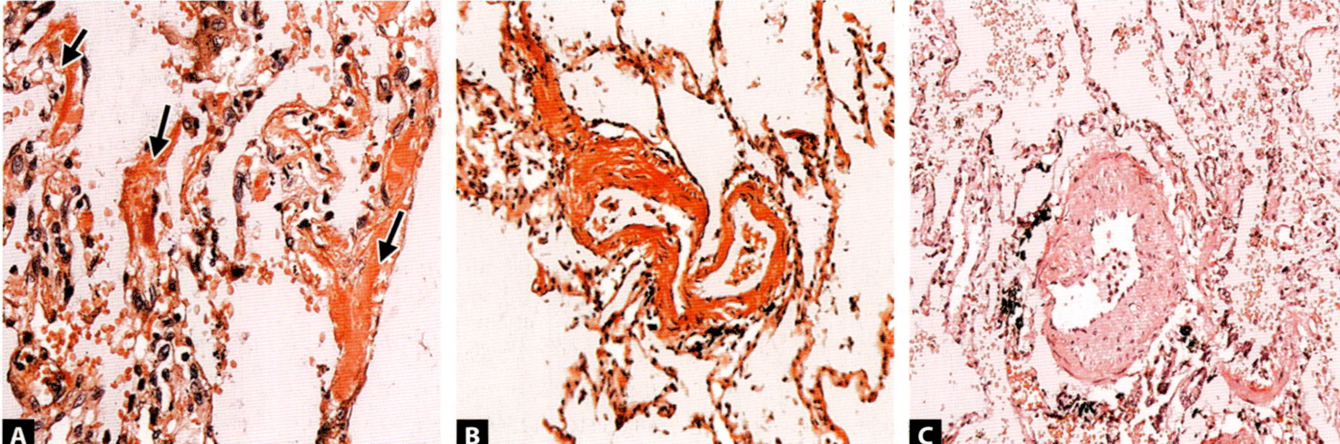

Figs 7A–C: Photomicrographs of the lung showing amyloid deposition in the (A) Alveolar septa (arrows); (B) Vessel wall (Congo red stain); and (C) Photomicrograph of the lung showing arteriopathy.

proliferation of plasma cells that synthesizes an immunoglobulin, which due to its intrinsic physicochemical properties leads to the formation of amyloid. In plasma cell myeloma, systemic amyloidosis occurs in 5–15% of cases. The malignant plasma cells may synthesize whole Ig molecules or free unpaired kappa or lambda light chains referred to as Bence Jones proteins or both. Bence Jones proteins may be found in the serum, but due to their small molecular weight, are excreted in the urine. These light chains can get deposited in the tissues as amyloid. The amyloidogenic potential of a light chain is determined by its specific amino acid sequences. In plasma cell myeloma and other monoclonal plasma cell proliferations which develop amyloidosis, the major fibril protein is AL and the chemically related precursor protein is the immunoglobulin light chains, chiefly the lambda chains or their fragments. Kappa chains are seen in a minority of cases. Amyloid deposition in the tissues causes oxidant stress, disruption of the architecture leading to organ dysfunction. Cardiac involvement is seen most commonly in the AL variety, but can be seen in secondary, hereditary and in senile amyloidosis. The deposition is seen mostly in the myocardium, but can be seen in the endocardium, pericardium, vessels and the atria. Cardiac amyloidosis leads to ischemia, infarction, myocardial dysfunction, heart failure, conduction system abnormalities and arrhythmias.

COMMENTARY—INDEX CASE: PM 19667

A 40-year-old male, was diagnosed as a case of symptomatic plasma cell myeloma as he fulfilled all criteria. He had compression of lumbar vertebrae L4–L5, lytic lesions of ribs, bone marrow revealed more than 90% plasma cells, serum electrophoresis revealed a normal pattern and no M band, urine for Bence Jones proteins was positive, urine electrophoresis showed M band and immunodiffusion revealed lambda light chains. There was anemia (Hb <10 g/dL), hypercalcemia (Ca—14 mg%), lytic bone lesions and renal insufficiency (serum creatinine 7.6–10.2 mg%). He was given two cycles of chemotherapy, but he went into renal failure. Autopsy revealed primary systemic amyloidosis (AL type) with an extensive deposition of amyloid in the heart, GIT and spleen along with cast nephropathy. The unique feature of this case was the extensive nodular deposits of amyloid in the endocardium, mitral valve and myocardium as seen in the photomicrographs. The chambers were dilated with some degree of stiffness of the ventricles, indicating a contractile failure, as what would happen in restrictive cardiomyopathy. The lamina propria of the stomach, duodenum, small and large gut also showed diffuse amyloid deposition. The lambda light chains are more amyloidogenic and this explains the occurrence of primary systemic amyloidosis in the index case. Renal failure in cases of multiple myeloma can be due to cast nephropathy, light chain deposition disease, primary amyloidosis, hypercalcemia, renal tubular dysfunction, volume depletion, intravenous contrast dye and nephrotoxic medicines. In the index case, there was cast nephropathy and hypercalcemia which contributed to the renal failure. Amyloid deposition was very minimal in the kidney.

TAKE HOME MESSAGE

- Plasma cell myeloma is a multifocal, plasma cell neoplasm, the diagnosis of which is a combination of pathology, radiology and clinical features.
- Systemic amyloidosis occurs in 5–15% of cases of plasma cell myeloma.
- The lambda light chains are more amyloidogenic as compared to the others.

REFERENCES

1. Rajkumar SV, Dimopoulos MA, Palumbo A. International Myeloma Working Group updated criteria for the diagnosis of multiple myeloma. Lancet Oncol. 2014;15:e538-48.
2. Ramirez-Alvarado M. Amyloid formation in light chain amyloidosis. Curr Top Med Chem. 2012;12:2523-33.

CONTRIBUTIONS BY:

1. Dr SC Varma, Ex-Professor and Head, Department of Internal Medicine (Clinician In-Charge)
2. Dr KL Gupta, Professor and Head, Department of Nephrology (Compilation of Clinical Details)
3. Dr Reena Das, Professor, Department of Hematology (Hematologist In-Charge)

Post Graduate Institute of Medical Education and Research, Chandigarh, India.

SECTION 2

Malignancy Adult Cases

CASE 9

Microscopic/Occult Testicular Seminoma with Germ Cell Neoplasia in situ and Widespread Nonseminomatous Metastasis in a Young Male: PM 14170

Nandita Bharadwaj Kakkar

 HIGHLIGHTS OF THE CASE

This is a case of a histologically proven (antemortem) metastatic (supraclavicular lymph node), occult testicular germ cell neoplasm, where the testes was found to be normal on examination. X-ray chest revealed bilateral cannonball shadows. On ultrasonography a 6 mm focal hypoechoic area and an ill-defined 5 mm heterogeneous area was found in left testis. The right testis was normal on ultrasonography. Ultrasound guided fine-needle aspiration cytology (FNAC) of left testis revealed a benign cystic lesion. Autopsy revealed an occult/microscopic/regressed seminoma, with germ cell neoplasia in situ (GCNIS) and atrophy in the left testis. There was widespread nonseminomatous metastasis of yolk sac/endodermal sinus type in the lung and embryonal type in the lymph nodes. This case highlights the diagnostic problems of occult germ cell tumors of the testis and the nonseminomatous metastasis from a pure seminoma.

***Keywords*:** Seminoma, occult, microscopic, regressed, germ cell neoplasia in situ, nonseminomatous metastasis, autopsy.

 CLINICAL HISTORY

Date of Admission: 27.07.1994, Date of Death: 08.08.1994, Duration of Hospital Stay: 12 Days

A 30-year-old male presented with low-grade intermittent fever of 5 months duration associated with a nonproductive cough and 2–3 episodes of hemoptysis. He had swelling over the left lower limb extending up to the groin and affecting the genitalia. He complained of a dull backache on both sides (Rt > Lt), with radiation of pain toward the testes. There was significant loss of weight and appetite. On ***examination***, bilateral supraclavicular lymph nodes were enlarged, hard, nontender and mobile. No organomegaly or free fluid was noted and physical examination of the testes was normal. Chest examination revealed bilateral equal movements, tenderness in right inframammary areas and diminished breath sounds.

Investigations

Investigations revealed a normal hemogram and blood biochemistry. X-ray chest brought out "cannonball" shadows in both lung fields. Fine-needle aspiration cytology of supraclavicular lymph node revealed a poorly differentiated metastatic carcinoma ? embryonal carcinoma. Later, a biopsy of this lymph node exhibited a poorly discernable tumor with extensive necrosis and a diagnosis of a metastatic carcinoma was given. On ultrasonography, there was a 6 mm focal hypoechoic lesion and another ill-defined 5 mm heterogeneous area in the left testis, which was normal in size and outline. The right testis was normal on ultrasonography. Ultrasound guided FNAC of left testis revealed a benign cystic lesion. Pregnancy color test for human chorionic gonadotropin (hCG) in urine was strongly positive. A diagnosis of disseminated malignancy with primary in left testis ? embryonal carcinoma ? choriocarcinoma ?? undifferentiated teratoma was made. Patient had sudden onset of dyspnea and died after a hospital stay of 11 days.

AUTOPSY FINDINGS: PM 14170

A complete autopsy was performed. All serous cavities were within normal limits. Left testis (Fig 1A) felt firm and measured 3 × 1.5 × 1 cm. Cut surface revealed an area of fresh hemorrhage related to FNA procedure. Because of a strong suspicion of a primary in the left testis and no obvious tumor on gross examination, it was blocked in toto. Microscopically, a wide range of changes were seen in the left testis. There was a well-defined microscopic focus of tumor with histology of a typical seminoma, composed of cells with clear cytoplasm, centrally placed nucleus and prominent nucleoli (Figs 1B–D). Few seminiferous tubules with GCNIS were discernable in-between the seminoma cells [Figs 1B–C (arrows)]. The solitary focus of seminoma along with the entrapped/surrounding seminiferous tubules harboring GCNIS, showed strong nuclear positivity with OCT4 (Figs 2A–C) and strong membranous positivity with CD117 (Figs 2D–F). The adjacent testis showed features of GCNIS (Figs 3A–C), wherein tubules lacking spermatogenesis, contained clear seminoma like cells with enlarged hyperchromatic nuclei and prominent nucleoli, aligned along the basement membrane. Distinctly, normal tubules with spermatogenesis could be seen adjacent to the tubules with GCNIS [Fig 3A (star)]. The left testes further showed areas showing atrophic seminiferous tubules (Fig 3D) with basement membrane thickening and Leydig cell hyperplasia. Foci of GCNIS showed strong nuclear positivity with OCT4 (Figs 4A–B) and strong membranous positivity with CD117 (Figs 4C–E). Adjacent normal seminiferous tubules were distinctly negative for these stains [Figs 4A,C,D (arrows)]. Sections studied from the tunica albuginea, epididymis and spermatic cord were normal. ***Right testis*** was normal both grossly and microscopically (blocked in toto). ***Lungs*** (Figs 5A–B) weighed 1,800 g and were studded with multiple well-circumscribed nodules, 1–5 cm in diameter. Hilar/carinal/paratracheal lymph nodes were enlarged and matted, forming

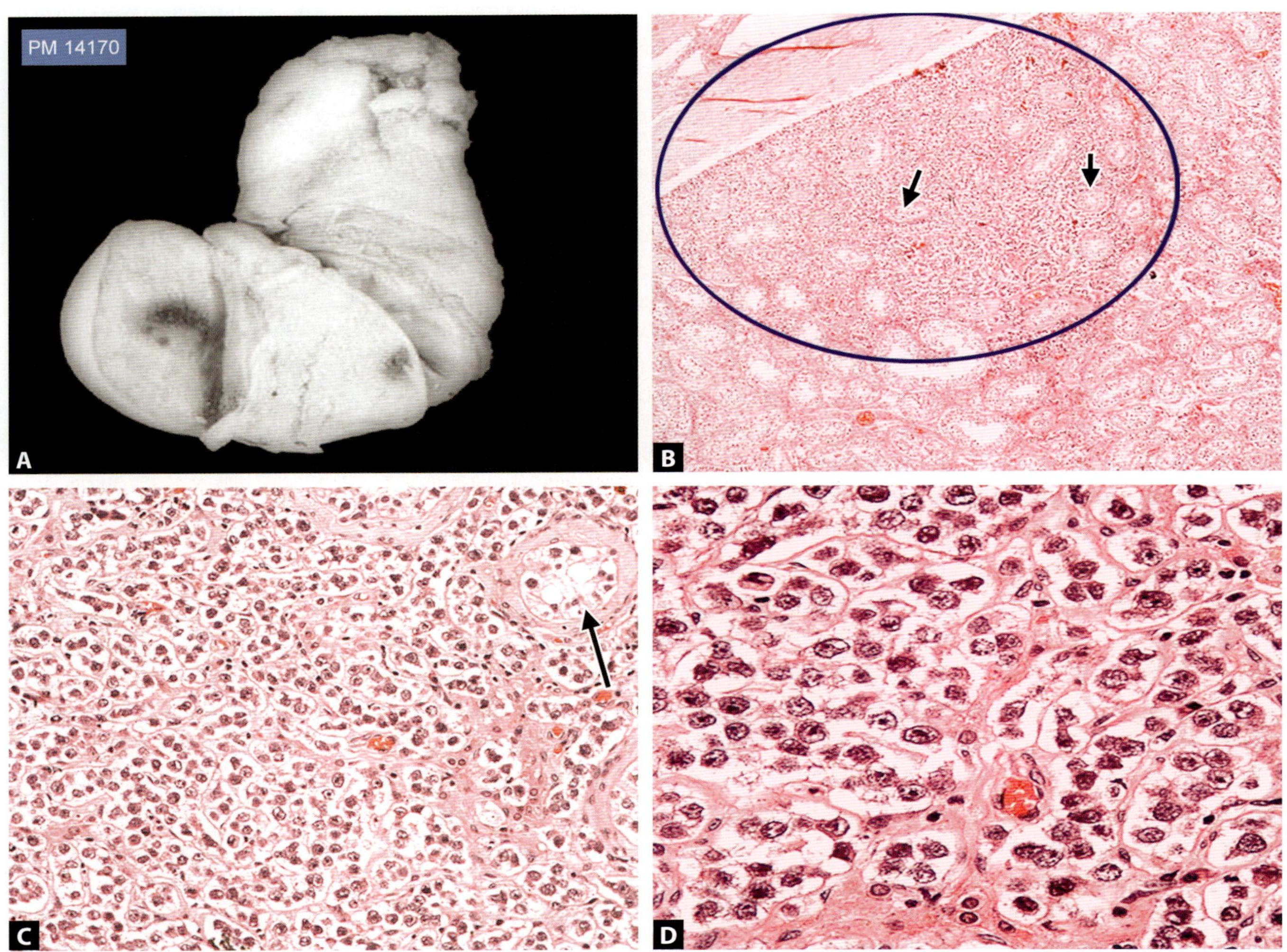

Figs 1A–D: (A) Gross picture of the left testis showing an area of hemorrhage [fine-needle aspiration cytology (FNAC) induced]. The testis is normal in size, consistency and there is no evidence of any tumor. (B) Photomicrograph from the left testis shows the solitary microscopic focus of seminoma wherein interspersed seminiferous tubules are discernable (arrows). (C–D) The seminoma cells show abundant clear cytoplasm, centrally placed nucleus with a prominent nucleolus.

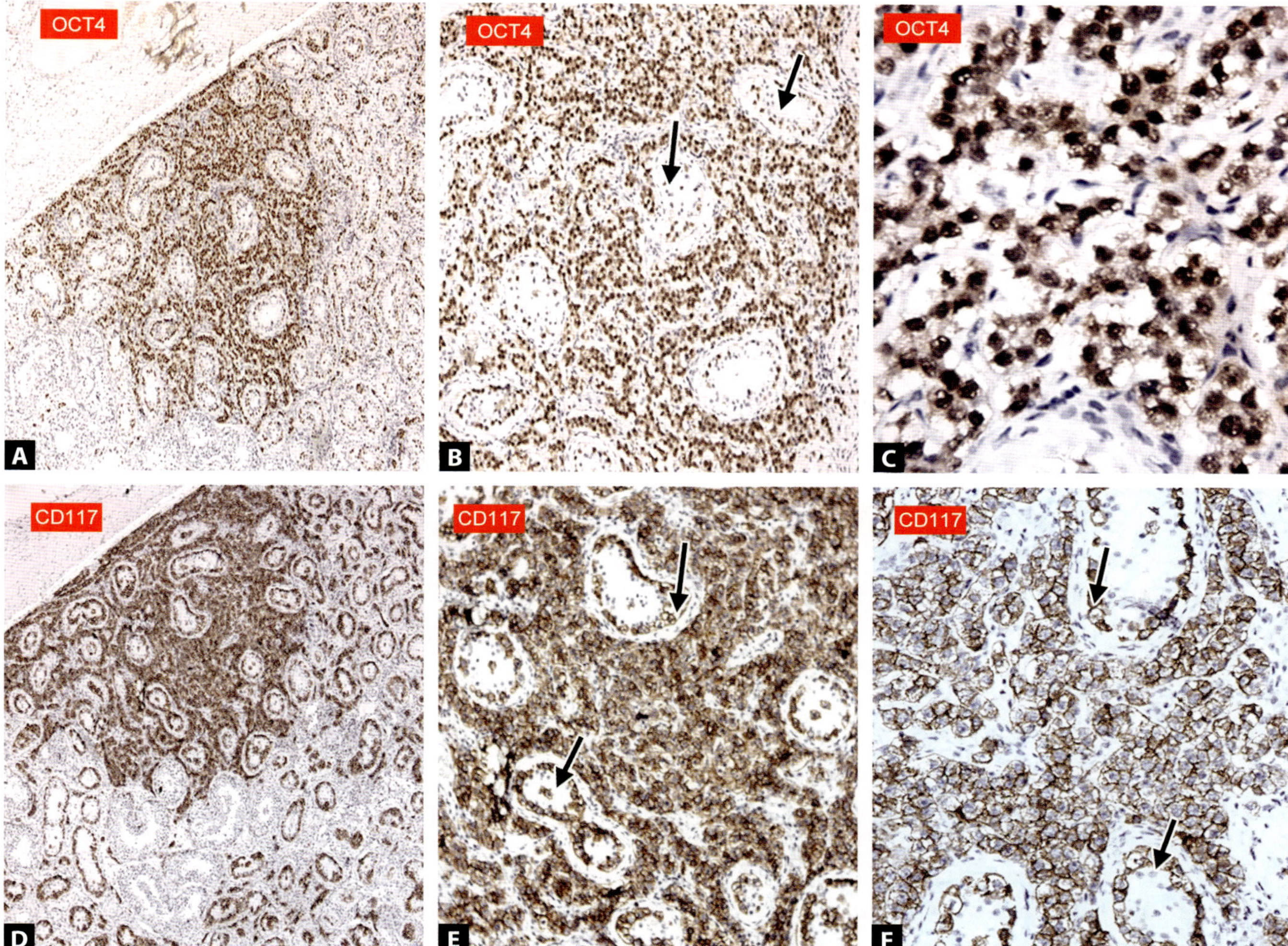

Figs 2A–F: The solitary focus of seminoma in left testis. (A–C) Shows strong nuclear positivity with OCT4 immunostain; (D–F) Shows strong membranous positivity with CD117. Interspersed seminiferous tubules are discernable which also show positivity with both stains indicating the presence of germ cell neoplasia in situ (arrows).

a mass. Microscopically, sections from the lung nodules and lymph nodes (hilar/carinal) revealed a tumor with extensive areas of necrosis. The tumor cells (Fig 5C) were arranged in a papillary, glandular and alveolar pattern with a high mitotic activity. Several Schiller–Duval bodies [Figs 5C–D (arrows)] and intra- and extracytoplasmic periodic acid-Schiff (PAS) positive diastase resistant hyaline globules were seen [Fig 5D-inset]. The morphology was characteristic of a yolk sac or endodermal sinus tumor. Retroperitoneal and para-aortic lymph nodes were enlarged and matted into a mass (8 × 5 × 4), which was encasing the aorta (Fig 6A). Microscopically retroperitoneal, para-aortic, paratracheal and supraclavicular lymph nodes showed a tumor with morphology of an embryonal carcinoma (Figs 6B–C)which showed strong positivity with CD30 [Figs 6C (inset)].

FINAL AUTOPSY DIAGNOSIS: PM 14170

30 Years Male

- Microscopic/occult seminoma with GCNIS, atrophy and Leydig cell hyperplasia in the left testis.
- Extensive nonseminomatous (endodermal sinus type) metastasis to both lungs and lymph nodes (hilar/carinal) and embryonal carcinoma to the para-aortic, retroperitoneal, supraclavicular and paratracheal lymph nodes.

TESTICULAR CANCER

Testicular cancer is amongst the most common solid malignancy affecting males between the ages of 15 years and 35 years, although it accounts for only 1 % of all cancers in men. Germ cell neoplasms[1,2] comprise 90-95% of

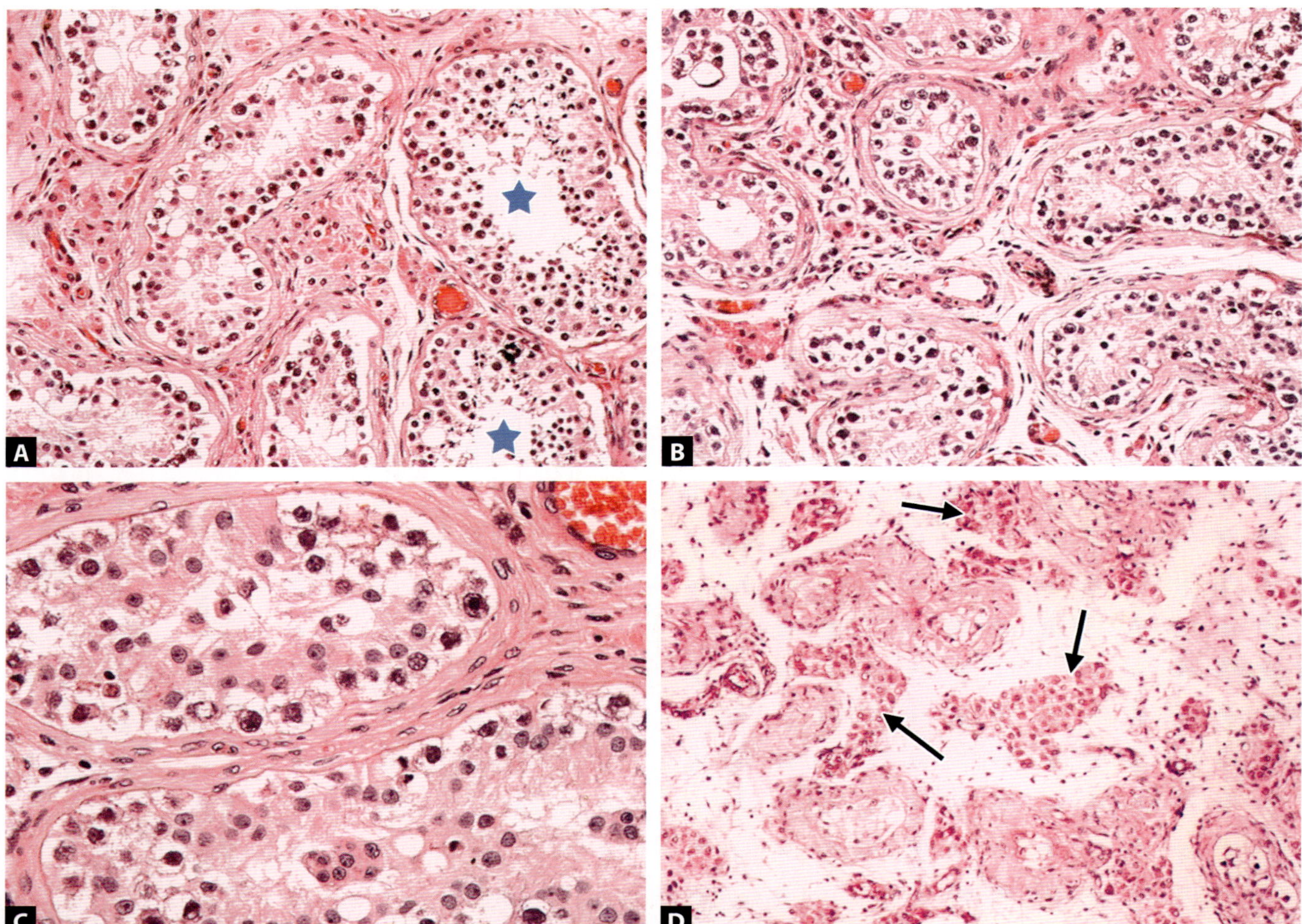

Figs 3A–D: (A–C) Left testis showing germ cell neoplasia in situ (GCNIS) wherein a seminiferous tubule shows large pleomorphic, seminoma-like cells with clear cytoplasm. Few adjacent tubules show normal spermatogenesis (stars). (D) Left testis shows area of atrophic tubules with intervening Leydig cell hyperplasia (arrows).

testicular tumors. Because of the tremendous morphological heterogeneity, several classification systems have come up over the years. The 2016 WHO[3] classification system is the most commonly used wherein testicular germ cell tumors are divided into (1) Non-invasive germ cell neoplasia (GCNIS and Gonadoblastoma) (2) Germ cell tumors derived from GCNIS (Seminoma and Non-seminomatous tumors ie embryonal carcinoma, post-pubertal teratomas, post-pubertal yolk sac tumor and choriocarcinoma/other trophoblastic tumors). (3) Germ cell tumors unrelated to GCNIS (Pre-pubertal teratoma, Pre-pubertal yolk sac tumor and spermatocytic tumor). Epidemiological risk factors[4] include cryptorchidism, hypospadias, previous testicular cancer, impaired spermatogenesis, family history of testicular cancer and testicular dysgenesis syndrome. Endocrine disrupting chemicals ie organochlorine compounds which include dichlorodiphenyl-trichloro-ethane (DDT) and its metabolites have a role to play in testicular cancer. Genetic aberrations associated with testicular germ cell tumors include isochromosome i(12)p.[5] Apart from this KIT and RAS gene family mutations have been implicated in germ cell tumors.

The histogenesis of germ cell tumors of the testes has undergone a change. One of the previous theories was that the seminoma acts as a common precursor lesion (having developed from GCNIS) and may then transform into embryonal carcinoma or more rarely directly into other forms of germ cell tumors like the yolk sac tumor, teratoma and choriocarcinoma.[6] The points which supported this theory were:

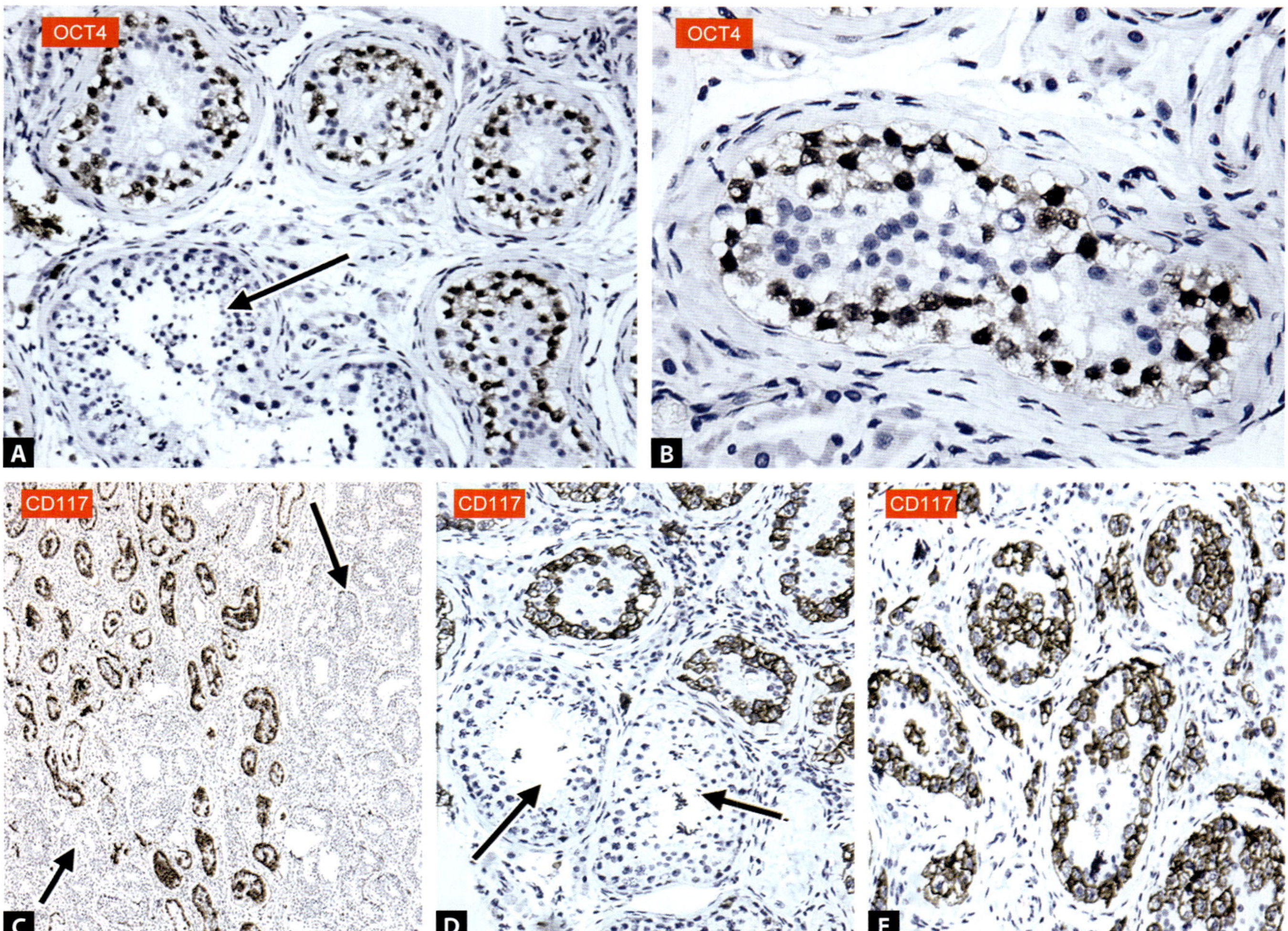

Figs 4A–E: (A–B) Foci of germ cell neoplasia in situ (GCNIS) show strong nuclear positivity with OCT4. A normal adjacent seminiferous tubule is negative for OCT4 (arrow); (C–E) Foci of GCNIS show strong membranous positivity with CD117. Adjacent normal seminiferous tubules in "C and D" are negative for the CD117 (arrows).

(1) The common identification of nonseminomatous metastasis at autopsy in patients who originally had pure testicular seminomas. (2) The light microscopic observation of focal nonseminomatous germ cell tumor differentiation in seminomas (3) The similarities between GCNIS and seminoma. But, now it is hypothesized that the GCNIS is derived from the gonocytes ie the primordial germ cells as they are both morphologically similar, express the same embryonic markers, have closely overlapping transcription profiles and epigenetic features. The fact that GCNIS is closely associated with testicular dysgenesis syndrome (where-in there is aberrant gonadal development) which is a strong risk factor for testicular germ cell tumors, further substantiates the above hypothesis. An early event in the histogenesis of GCNIS is the failure of the gonocytes to shut off expression of OCT3/4, which occurs when the gonocytes shift from the center of the seminiferous tubules to the spermatogonial niche. GCNIS is the precursor of seminomas and non-seminomatous tumors. So, GCNIS progresses to intratubular seminoma and then into invasive seminoma. Non-seminomatous testicular tumors occur when a GCNIS or a seminoma cell (which express OCT3/4 along with SOX 17) gets reprogrammed to an embryonal carcinoma cell (which express OCT3/4 and SOX2 along with pluripotency factors NANOG and LIN28). What causes the neoplastic germ cell to re-programme into an 'embryonal carcinoma cell' is not known. Embryonal carcinoma cell is a pleuipotent stem cell of a non-seminoma and can give rise to other non-seminomatous tumors like yolk

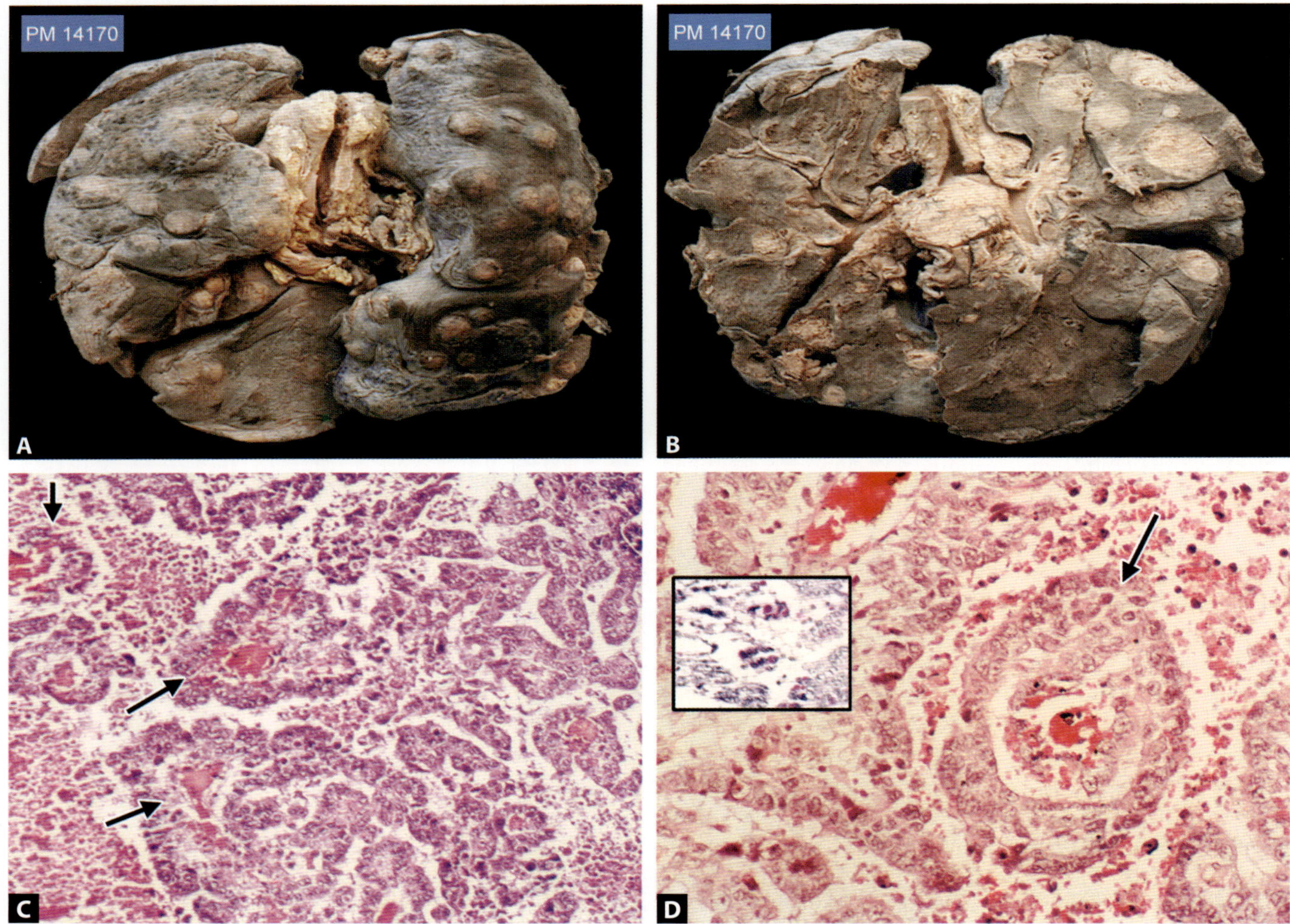

Figs 5A–D: (A) Gross picture of both lungs showing multiple, subpleural, metastatic tumor nodules along with enlarged carinal and paratracheal lymph nodes; (B) Cut section of both lungs showing multiple metastatic tumor nodules present diffusely; (C) Photomicrograph from the lung nodule showing a tumor with a tubulopapillary pattern characteristic of a yolk sac tumor (arrows); (D) Tumor shows the characteristic Schiller–Duval body (arrow) seen in yolk sac tumors. Inset shows periodic acid-Schiff (PAS) positive diastase resistant hyaline globules both within and outside the tumor cells.

sac tumor, choriocarcinoma/ other trophoblastic tumors and teratomas. It is a well documented fact that in malignancies, it is the cancer stem cell that metastasizes. So, it is not surprising that in the testicular germ cell tumors, the embryonal cell metastasizes and gives rise to metastatic tumors different from the ones at the primary site. Thus, it is very much possible that in a pure seminoma, a semonoma cell gets re-programmed to an embryonal carcinoma cell which metastasizes to produce a non-seminomatous metastasis. The level of differentiation at the metastatic site is always less than the primary site, which is proven by the fact that teratomatous components are not seen in the visceral metastatic sites.

It is a well known fact that an apparently pure seminoma of testis can have necropsy evidence of nonseminomatous metastasis. In a large necropsy series[7] (154 patients) with germ cell tumor of testis, there were 16 cases of pure seminomas and 7 out of these i.e. 44% had nonseminomatous metastasis. Similar observations have been made by others.[8] This phenomenon is seen in about 3% patients with apparently pure seminoma of the testis. Thus, seminomas may show striking difference between the morphology of the primary tumor and its metastasis, which may play a major role in treatment failure. The reason however is attributed to the fact that the non-seminomatous element in the seminoma could have escaped detection and thus there is a need for studying adequate sections. An equally plausible explanation to this phenomenon is the above mentioned re-programming theory.

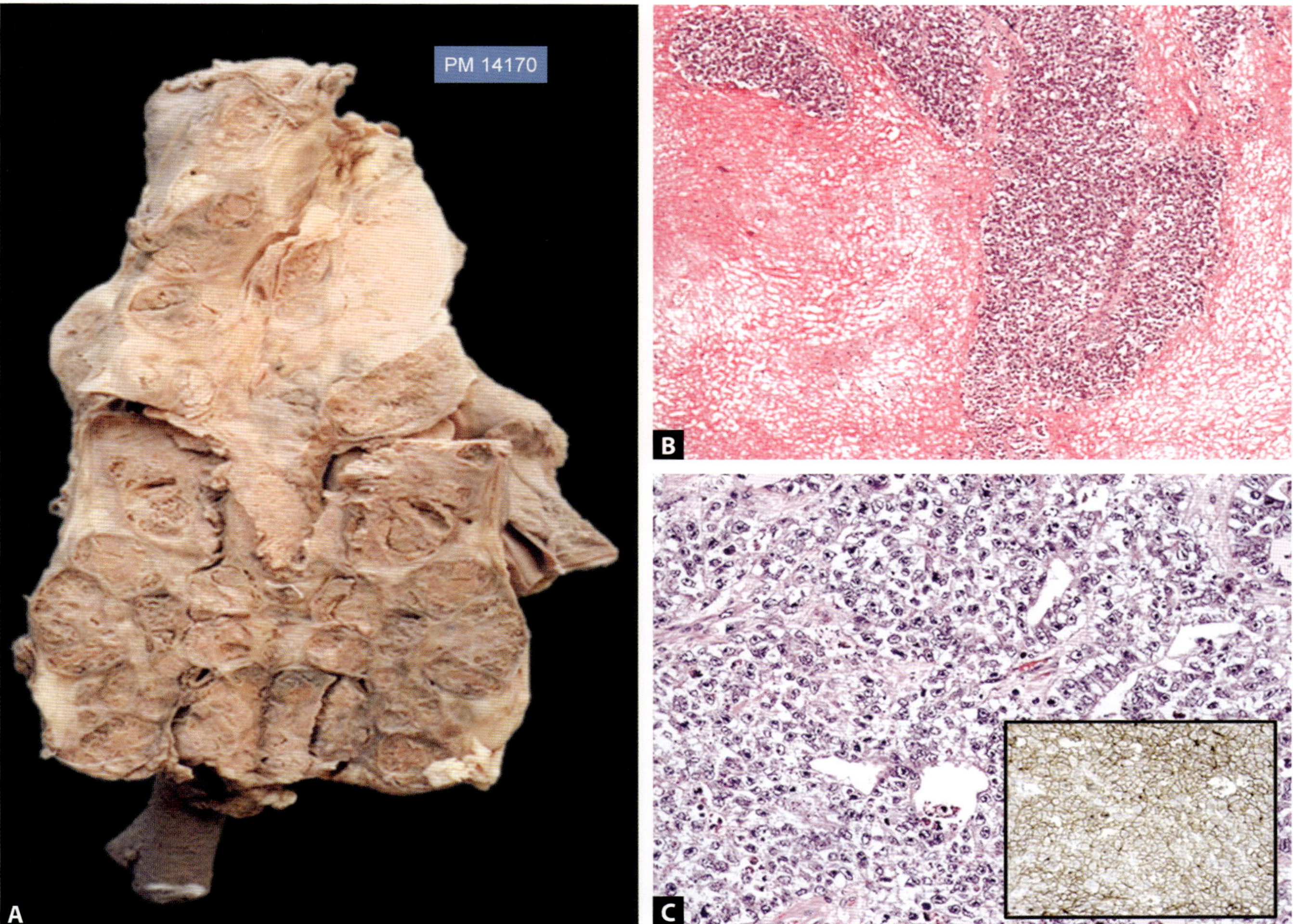

Figs 6A–C: (A) Cut section of the enlarged para-aortic lymph nodes encasing the aorta; (B–C) Low-and high-power photomicrographs from the para-aortic lymph nodes shows sheets of bizarre malignant cells with pleomorphic, hyperchromatic nuclei and large areas of necrosis, morphology consistent with embryonal carcinoma. Inset in "C" shows strong membranous positivity with CD30.

Cases of widespread metastasis with occult testicular tumors or only fibrous scars in the testis, as the only evidence of a germ cell tumor are well known.[9-11] Testicular germ cell tumors, especially choriocarcinoma and seminomas can regress leaving a homogeneous scar. Such scars can be associated with testicular atrophy, shrunken seminiferous tubules with decreased or absent spermatogenesis, GCNIS or residual viable tumor such as teratoma.[12] The metastasis often differs from the residual viable tumor in the testis. Retrogression in testicular seminoma with viable metastases is well known. Seminomas are known to produce an inflammatory host response composed of lymphocytes, histiocytes, plasma cells and a granulomatous reaction, which causes regression of the tumor.

Seminomas are generally localized at presentation and patients present with stage I disease ie limited to the testis. A small number ie approximately 15 percent have stage II disease limited to retroperitoneal nodes. Non-seminomatous germ cell tumors (NSGCT's) spread via the blood stream to distant organs like the liver, lung, bones, or brain. Seminomas do not take this route of spread and less than five percent of patients at presentaion show a spread beyond the retroperitoneal nodes. The International Germ Cell Cancer Collaborative Group (IGCCCG) based on their prognostic model, have grouped the seminomas into the good and intermediate prognosis and only the NSGCT's have been described under the poor prognosis category.

Germ cell neoplasia in situ (GCNIS) is known to be the precursor lesion of all testicular germ cell tumors with the exception of pre-pubertal teratomas, pre-pubertal yolk sac tumors and spermatocytic tumors.[13] Fifty percent of the patients, developed an invasive tumor within 5 years. GCNIS is identified in 2-8% patients with cryptorchidism.[14] It is seen in 5-8% of the contralateral testis of a patient with a testicular germ cell tumor.[15] This explains the need for a biopsy from the contralateral testis while operating for a testicular neoplasm. GCNIS is seen in 1% of patient with infertility[16] and at higher rates in patients with Y chromosome positive gonadal dysgenesis and androgen insensitivity syndrome.[17] It is also observed in virtually all cases of invasive germ cell tumors of the testes in adults, if residual seminiferous tubules are present.[18] Microscopically, germ cells with enlarged hyperchromatic nuclei and clear cytoplasm align along the basal aspect of the seminiferous tubules which are devoid of spermatogenesis, sertoli cells and show a thickened basement membrane. Majority of the cases of GCNIS show PAS positive diastase resistant granules in the cytoplasm, which can however also be seen in sertoli cells and nonneoplastic spermatogonia. Immunostain for placental like alkaline phosphatase (PLAP) which is membrane eccentuated is positive in 97% of the cells of GCNIS.

The diagnosis of testicular tumors can be very problematic at times, but immunohistochemistry[19] has helped tremendously. Embryonal carcinomas are positive for CD30, OCT4, AE1/AE3, SOX2; Yolk sac tumors are positive for Glypican 3, AFP+/-, PLAP+/-; Seminomas are positive for OCT4, CD117, podoplanin, SOX17; Choriocarcinoma is positive for HCG, Glypican 3 +/-, PLAP+/-; Spermatocytic tumors are negative for all including OCT4 and CD117; GCNIS is positive for OCT4, CD117 and PLAP.

COMMENTARY—INDEX CASE: PM 14170

This case was a diagnostic challenge. The young man came with dyspnea and hemoptysis. FNAC of the enlarged supraclavicular lymph node was suggestive of a metastatic embryonal carcinoma and X-ray showed cannonball shadows in both the lung fields. The physical examination of the testes was however normal. In cases with biopsy evidence of metastatic testicular neoplasm and normal physical examination of the testes, ultrasonography of the testes is mandatory. In such a clinical setting, an abnormal echotexture of the testes is virtually diagnostic of a primary tumor in the testes and under such circumstances an orchiectomy is justifiable. Ultrasonography of the left testis revealed an abnormal echotexture, but ultrasound-guided FNAC was still inconclusive. The necropsy, however, clearly demonstrated the presence of a microscopic/occult/regressed seminoma, GCNIS, atrophy and Leydig cell hyperplasia in the left testis. There was widespread nonseminomatous metastasis (yolk sac tumor in the lung and hilar/carinal lymph nodes and embryonal carcinoma in the retroperitoneal/paratracheal/supraclavicular lymph nodes). The left testis revealed marked atrophy with leydig cell hyperplasia, a background, highly susceptible for a germ cell tumor. The cause for this unilateral atrophy in the index case could not be discerned. Amongst the various causes—obstruction, trauma and unilateral cryptorchidism can be responsible.

TAKE HOME MESSAGE

- Germ cell neoplasia in situ is the precursor lesion of all germ cell tumors with the exception of spermatocytic tumor, pre-pubertal teratomas and pre-pubertal yolk sac tumors.
- Occult/microscopic/regressed germ cell tumors/fibrous scars as the only evidence of a germ cell tumor, producing widespread metastasis are rare, but known.
- Nonseminomatous metastasis can be produced by pure seminomas of the testis. The reason is attributed to the fact that the non-seminomatous elements in the seminoma escapes detection due to inadequate sampling or due to the re-programming theory.
- In cases with biopsy evidence of metastatic testicular neoplasm, with normal physical examination of the testis, ultrasonographic detection of an abnormal echotexture of the testes is virtually diagnostic of a primary tumor. An orchiectomy under such circumstances is justifiable.

REFERENCES

1. Williamson SR, Delahunt B, Magi-Galluzzi CM, et al. The WHO 2016 classification of testicular germ cell tumors: A review and update from the International Society of Urological Pathology testis consultation group. Histopathology 2017;70: 335-46.
2. Isabell A Sesterhenn, MD, Charles J Davis, Jr, Pathology of germ cell tumors of the testis. Cancer control 2004;11(6): 374-87.
3. Ulbright TM, Amin MB, Balzer B eta l. Germ cell tumors. In: Moch H, Humphrey PA, Reuter VE, Ulbright TM (eds). WHO classification of tumors of the urinary system and male genital organs, 4th edn. Lyon: IARC Press, 2016;189-226.
4. Ewa Rajpert-De Meyts, Katherine A McGlynn, Keisei Okamoto, et al. Testicular germ cell tumours. Lancet 2016; 387: 1762–74
5. Atkin NB, Baker MC. Specific chromosome change, i(12p), in testicular tumors ? lancet 1982;2:1349.

6. Czaja JT, Ulbright TM. Evidence for the transformation of seminoma to yolk sac tumor with histogenetic considerations. Am J Clin Path 1992;97:468-77.
7. Bradeal JJ, Vugrin D, Whitmore WF. Autopsy findings in 154 patients with germ cell tumors of the testis. Cancer 1982; 50(3):548-51.
8. Johnson DE, Appelt G, Samuels ML, et al. Metastases from testicular carcinoma: Study of 78 autopsied cases. Urology 1976;8:234-39.
9. Holmes AS, Klimberg IW, Stonesifer KJ, et al. Spontaneous regression of testicular seminoma: case report. J Urol 1986;135:795-6.
10. Kebapci M, Can C, Isiksoy S, et al. Burned-out tumor of the testis presenting as supraclavicular lymphadenopathy. Eur Radiol. 2002;12:371-3.
11. S Andhavarapu, BG Low, J Raj, et al. J Armenta-Corona: Regressed Testicular Seminoma with Extensive Metastases. The Internet Journal of Oncology. Number 1. DOI: 2008;10(5):5580/15f5.
12. Balzer BL, Ulbright TM. Spontaneous regression of testicular germ cell tumors: an analysis of 42 cases. Am J Surg Pathol. 2006;30:858-65.
13. Gondos B, Migliozzi JA. Intratubular germ cell neoplasia. Semin Diagn Pathol 1987;4:292-303.
14. Giwercman A Bruun E, Frimodt-Moller Ce et al. Prevalence of Carcinoma-in-situ and other histopathologic abnormalities in testes of men with a history of cyptorchidism. J Urol. 1989; 142:998-1002.
15. Von der Maase H, Rorth M, Walbom-Jorgensen S, et al. Carcinoma in situ of contralateral testis in patients with testicular germ cell cancer: study of 27 cases in 500 patients. Br Med J 1986;293:1398-1401.
16. Pryor JP, Cameron KM, Chilton CP, et al. Carcinoma in situ in testicular biopsies in men presenting with infertility. Br J Urol. 1983;55:780-84.
17. Muller J, Skakkebaek NE, Ritzen M, et al. Carcinoma in situ of the testis in children with 45, X/46 XY gonadal dysgenesis. J Pediatr. 1985;106:431-36.
18. Coffin CM, Ewing S, Dehner LP. Frequency of ITGCN with invasive testicular germ cell tumors. Arch Path Lab Med. 1985;109:555-59.
19. Thomas M, Ulbright TM, Tickoo SK, Berney DM, et al. Best Practices Recommendations in the Application of Immunohistochemistry in Testicular Tumors- Report From the International Society of Urological Pathology Consensus Conference. Am J Surg Pathol. 2014;38(8):e50-59

CONTRIBUTIONS BY:

1. Dr RK Vasishta, Professor and Head, Department of Histopathology (Consultation)
2. Dr Pankaj Kaul, Tutor, Department of Histopathology (Immunohistochemistry)
3. Dr SC Varma, Ex-Professor and Head, Department of Internal Medicine (Clinician In-Charge)

Post Graduate Institute of Medical Education and Research, Chandigarh, India.

CASE 10

Malignant Teratoma, Primary Pulmonary, Containing Yolk Sac Tumor, Associated with Hematologic Neoplasia: PM 13633

Nandita Bharadwaj Kakkar

 HIGHLIGHTS OF THE CASE

This is the first case in the world literature of a primary pulmonary malignant teratoma, containing yolk sac tumor associated with cellular phase of myelofibrosis with extensive extramedullary hematopoiesis/myeloid metaplasia, in a young 20-year-old male. Primary pulmonary teratomas are very rare. The association between mediastinal nonseminomatous germ cell tumors with yolk sac elements and various hematologic neoplasias is well documented in literature.

Keywords: Malignant teratoma, primary pulmonary, yolk sac element, myelofibrosis, myeloid metaplasia, association, hematologic neoplasia autopsy.

 CLINICAL HISTORY

Date of Admission: 19.07.1993, Date of Death: 22.07.1993, Duration of Hospital Stay: 3 Days

A 20-year-old male, nonsmoker, presented with a history of fever and right-sided chest pain for 15 days, dry cough for 6 days and minimal hemoptysis for 2 days. He also complained of breathing difficulty, bleeding from the nose and loss of appetite. On examination, there was mild pallor, petechial spots on the right suprascapular region and bilateral mobile and nontender axillary and inguinal lymph nodes (1 cm each). Liver (4 cm) and spleen (3 cm) were enlarged. Investigations revealed a hemoglobin of 10 g/dL, a total leukocyte count of 8,000/µL with 72% polymorphs and 28% lymphocytes. The platelet count was initially 60 × 10^3/µL and later dropped to 10 × 10^3/µL. Peripheral blood film was normocytic normochromic and the reticulocyte count was 0.8%. Coagulogram and routine blood biochemistry were normal. Fine-needle aspiration of the axillary lymph node showed reactive hyperplasia. Pleural fluid was grossly hemorrhagic and contained few reactive mesothelial cells. Chest X-ray showed a consolidation in the right middle lobe. A clinical diagnosis of consolidation right middle lobe with the possibilities of lymphoma or disseminated tuberculosis was made. The patient continued to deteriorate and died after a hospital stay of 3 days.

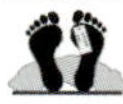 AUTOPSY FINDINGS: PM 13633

A partial autopsy was done. There was 500 mL of hemorrhagic fluid in the right pleural cavity. The ***right lung*** showed a tumor occupying the upper and middle lobes and measuring 12 × 10 × 6 cm (Fig 1A). The tumor was well within the lung and in direct continuity with the lung parenchyma. On cut section, the tumor was variegated and revealed areas of hemorrhage and necrosis. Cystic spaces containing keratinous material and calcification were seen. The left lung showed patchy areas of consolidation but no tumor was found. On microscopic examination the tumor contained elements from all the three germ cell layers, i.e. (1) ectoderm, (2) mesoderm and (3) endoderm. These consisted of cysts lined by squamous/respiratory/bronchial epithelium (Figs 1B–D), cartilage, both mature/immature (Figs 2A and B), bone formation (Fig 2C), glial element (glial fibrillary acidic protein positive) with ganglion cells (Fig 2D), choroid plexus (Fig 2E), meningeal whorls (Fig 2F), vascular spaces (Fig 3A), colonic glands (Fig 3B) and neuroepithelial component (Fig 3C). The teratomatous component was admixed with areas exhibiting extensive extramedullary hematopoiesis/myeloid metaplasia with plenty of megakaryocytes (Figs 3D–F). The malignant component (Figs 4A–B) consisted of glands lined by cells containing hyperchromatic pleomorphic nuclei as well as cells exhibiting a microcystic and alveolar pattern. An occasional Schiller–Duval body (Fig 4C), periodic acid-Schiff positive hyaline globules and alpha-

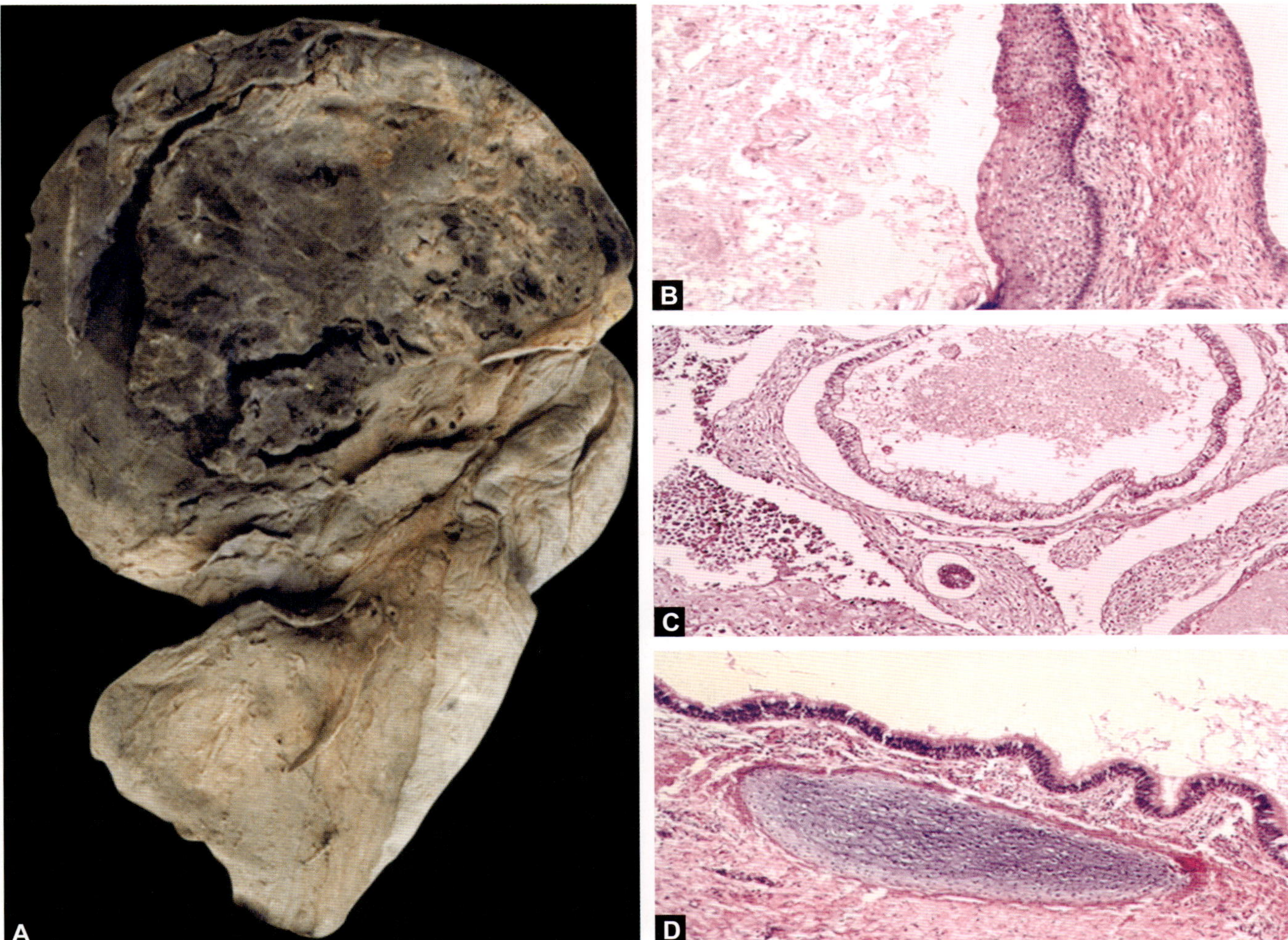

Figs 1A–D: (A) Right lung shows a large variegated tumor measuring 12 × 10 × 6 cm. Photomicrographs of the tumor showing cystic spaces lined by (B) Squamous epithelium containing keratinous material; (C) Respiratory epithelium; and (D) Bronchial epithelium containing cartilage in the wall.

fetoprotein (AFP) positivity were seen in these glands. This confirmed the presence of a yolk sac tumor. Overall features were those of a malignant teratoma, primary pulmonary with yolk sac tumor and extensive myeloid metaplasia. The ***liver*** (Fig 4D) was diffusely enlarged and weighed 2.5 kg. Microscopically it showed expansion of sinusoids due to extensive infiltration by a polymorphic infiltrate composed of giant cells, granulocytic precursors and nucleated red blood cells (Figs 5A–C). Some of the giant cells were atypical, while others conformed to the morphology of megakaryocytes and were periodic acid-Schiff positive. The granulocytic precursors were strongly positive for chloroacetate esterase (Fig 5D). Features were consistent with florid extramedullary hematopoiesis/myeloid metaplasia. Extramedullary hematopoiesis was also seen in the enlarged spleen, hilar lymph nodes, lower lobe of the right lung, left adrenal gland and extensively within the tumor. ***Bone marrow*** revealed panhyperplasia and marked proliferation of typical and atypical megakaryocytes. The reticulin stain demonstrated grade 1 to 2+ fibrosis. The hematological diagnosis was a cellular phase of myelofibrosis with extensive myeloid metaplasia. The testes and other organs were normal. The teratoma was confined to the right lung only and no tumor was detected at any other site in the body.

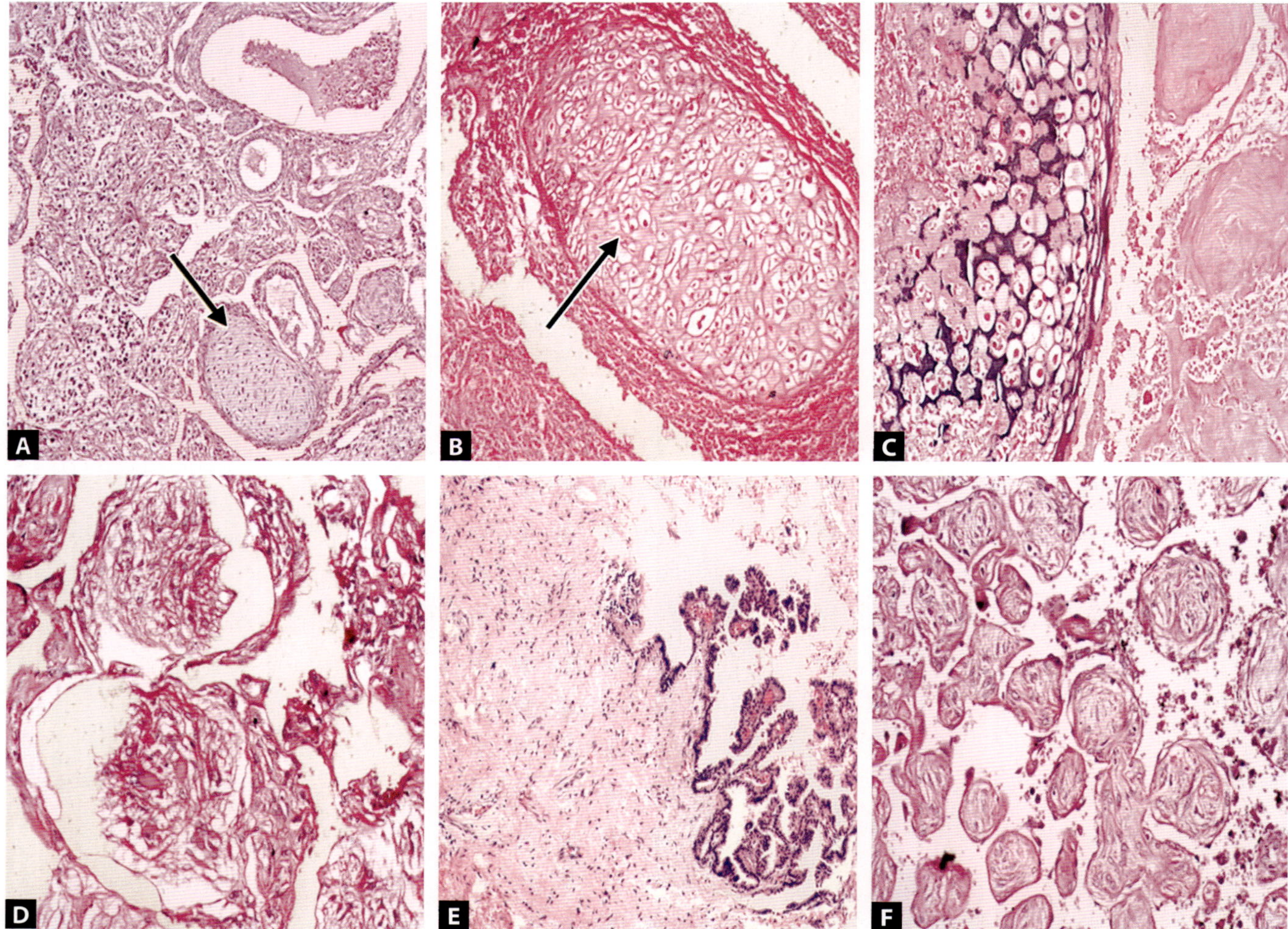

Figs 2A–F: Photomicrographs of the tumor showing (A) Mature cartilage (arrow); (B) Immature cartilage (arrow); (C) Immature bone; (D) Glial tissue with ganglion cells; (E) Choroid plexus; and (F) Meningeal whorls.

FINAL AUTOPSY DIAGNOSIS: PM 13633

20 Years Male

- Malignant teratoma, primary pulmonary with Yolk Sac tumor—Right lung.
- *Myeloproliferative disorder*: Cellular phase of myelofibrosis with extensive extramedullary hematopoiesis/myeloid metaplasia in liver, spleen, lower lobe of the right lung, hilar lymph nodes, adrenal gland and within the tumor itself.

TERATOMAS

Teratomas arise in order of frequency in the ovaries, testes, anterior mediastinum, retroperitoneum, presacral/coccygeal regions, pineal/other intracranial sites, neck and abdominal viscera. Uncommon sites for teratomas are the placenta, heart, lung, intestine, spleen, uterus, fallopian tubes, recto-uterine (cul-de-sac) and kidney. Teratomas arising in the lungs are among the rarest tumors encountered in pathology. To make a diagnosis of pulmonary teratoma two criteria are important: (1) Establishing a physical association between the tumor and the lung; (2) Excluding a teratoma from an extrapulmonary site. In males, the exclusion from the testes is very important. One may find in the testis, a microscopic focus of tumor or just a scar and thus in autopsies both the testes should be blocked in toto and examined meticulously. Mohr is credited with reporting the first case of pulmonary teratoma in 1939. Pulmonary teratomas, occur in young adults, have predilection for females and commonly involve the left upper lobe. Clinical manifestations are cough,

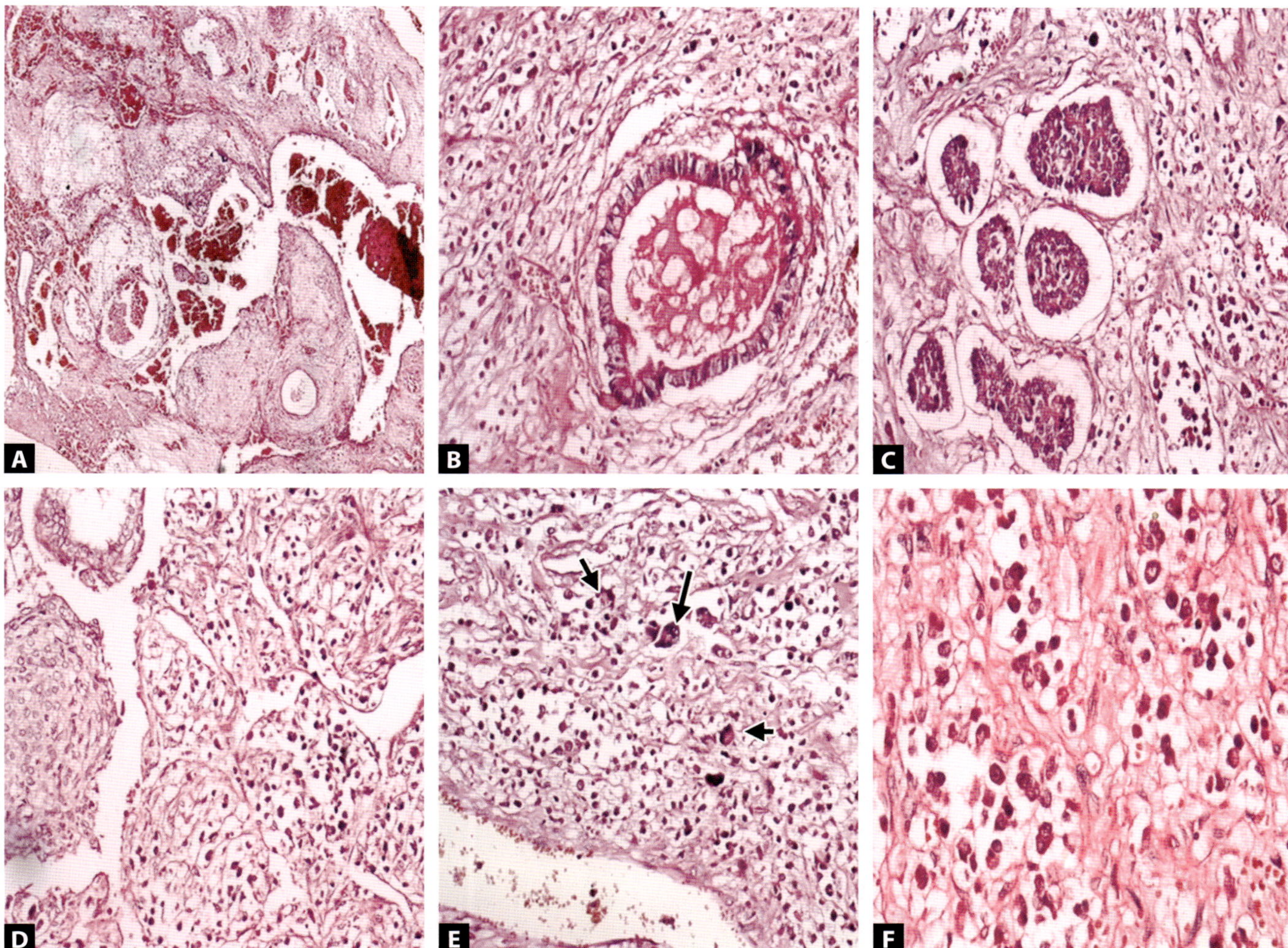

Figs 3A–F: Photomicrographs of the tumor showing: (A) Vascular spaces; (B) Colonic glands; (C) Neuroepithelial component; and (D–F) Extensive myeloid metaplasia with megakaryocytes (arrows).

dyspnea, hemoptysis and at times trichoptysis. Diagnosis is usually made after surgery, but in retrospect calcification or cavitation in the X-rays are said to be diagnostic. One-third of these tumors are malignant. Both mediastinal and pulmonary teratomas develop in relation to the thymus and its anlage, the third pharyngeal pouch. Migration of aberrant tissue from the third pharyngeal pouch along the developing bronchi gives rise to the intrapulmonary teratomas.

Teratomas are neoplasms that originate in the pleuripotent cells and are composed of a wide diversity of tissues, foreign to the organ or anatomic site in which they arise. This definition does not specify the number of germ layers (ectoderm, mesoderm and endoderm) that are represented in a teratoma. Monodermal teratomas composed exclusively of one type of tissue are recognized in the ovary and other organs (carcinoid, struma ovarii). A large number of sections should be studied to document elements from the various germ layers and to catch even the smallest malignant focus. AFP levels should be known to the pathologist and peritoneal/lymph node implants should be submitted for histopathology. Teratomas are classified into mature, immature and malignant teratomas.

Mature Teratomas

They are benign tumors, usually cystic and contain only mature tissue. These are skin and adnexa (predominantly in the ovarian teratomas), glia, fat, fibrous tissue, bone, cartilage and any other mature tissue like thyroid, pancreas, etc. The

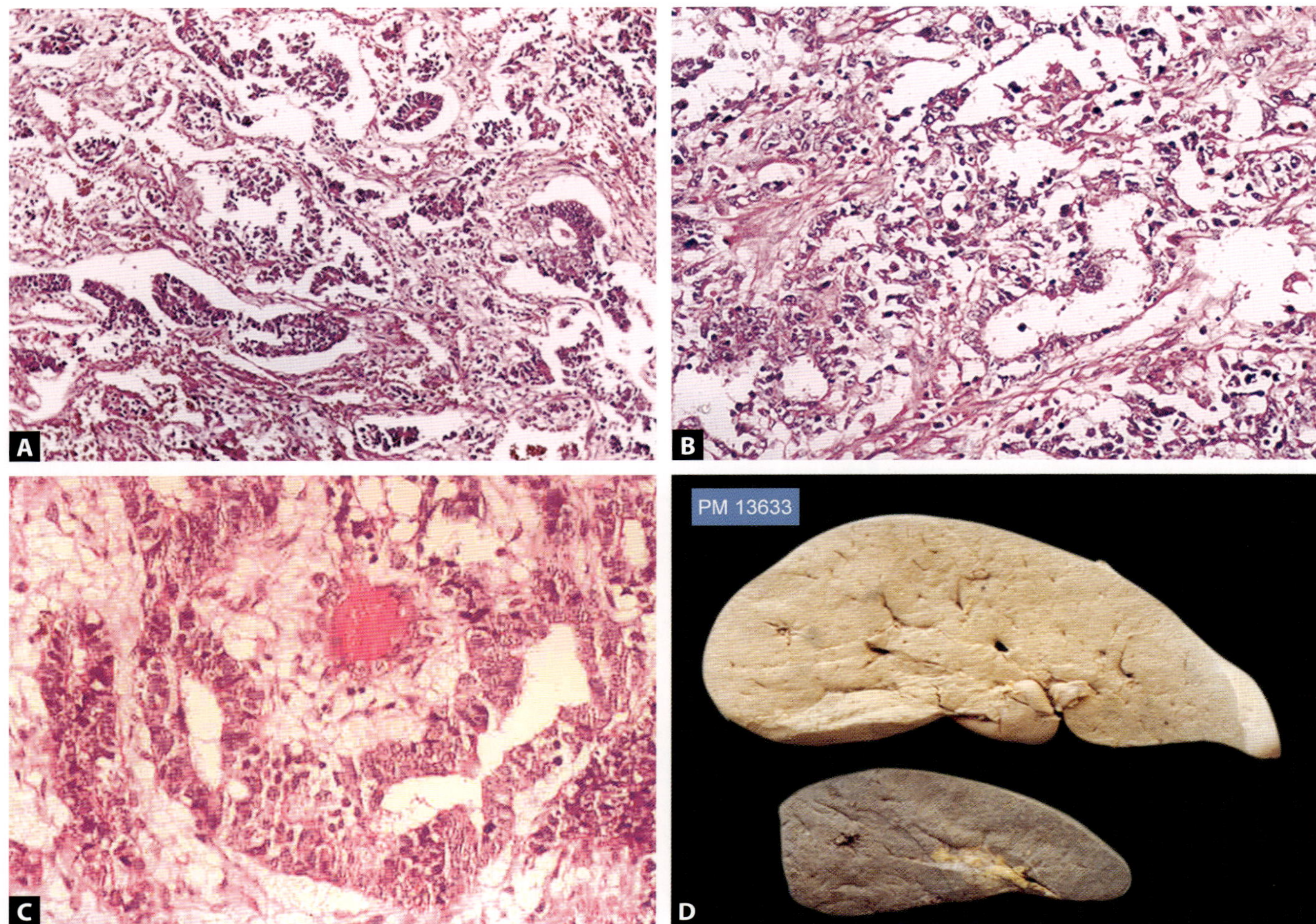

Figs 4A–D: Photomicrographs of the tumor showing: (A–B) Glands lined by cells containing hyperchromatic pleomorphic cells; (C) Schiller–Duval body; and (D) Slice of the enlarged liver and spleen.

reported cases of mature teratomas turning malignant (either metastasis or malignant recurrences) are the ones in which the immature/malignant focus escaped detection at the time of primary diagnosis. In rare instances, a mature teratoma metastasizes, but the metastasis shows only mature tissue. Local recurrence consisting of mature tissue may occur as a result of incomplete resection. Peritoneal implants of mature glial tissue can occur in very large, predominantly solid or partly cystic mature teratoma of the ovary (gliomatosis peritonei).

Immature Teratomas

They contain incompletely differentiated tissues of various types, in varying proportion and varying grades of immaturity. Neuroepithelial component (most common), immature mesenchyme, nephrogenic and lung tissue can be seen. Presence of an occasional small focus of blastema resembling Wilms' tumor can go with a diagnosis of an immature teratoma, but blastema in large amounts labels a tumor as a malignant teratoma. A small focus of yolk sac or any other malignant component however designates a tumor as malignant. Morphologic criteria for incompletely differentiated tissues are not standardized, but increased cellularity, enlarged hyperchromatic nuclei, scanty basophilic cytoplasm are features indicative of immaturity. Mitotic figures can be seen, but atypical mitosis is not noted. The immature teratomas have been graded over the years by many workers, but the grading by Heifetz et al is in use and is based on the semiquantitative assessment of the amount of immature tissue in the various histologic sections of the tumor. Grade 1: immature epithelial (neural or blastema) tissue occupying less than one low power (4X objective) field, Grade II: immature epithelial tissue with or without immature stroma occupying no more than three low

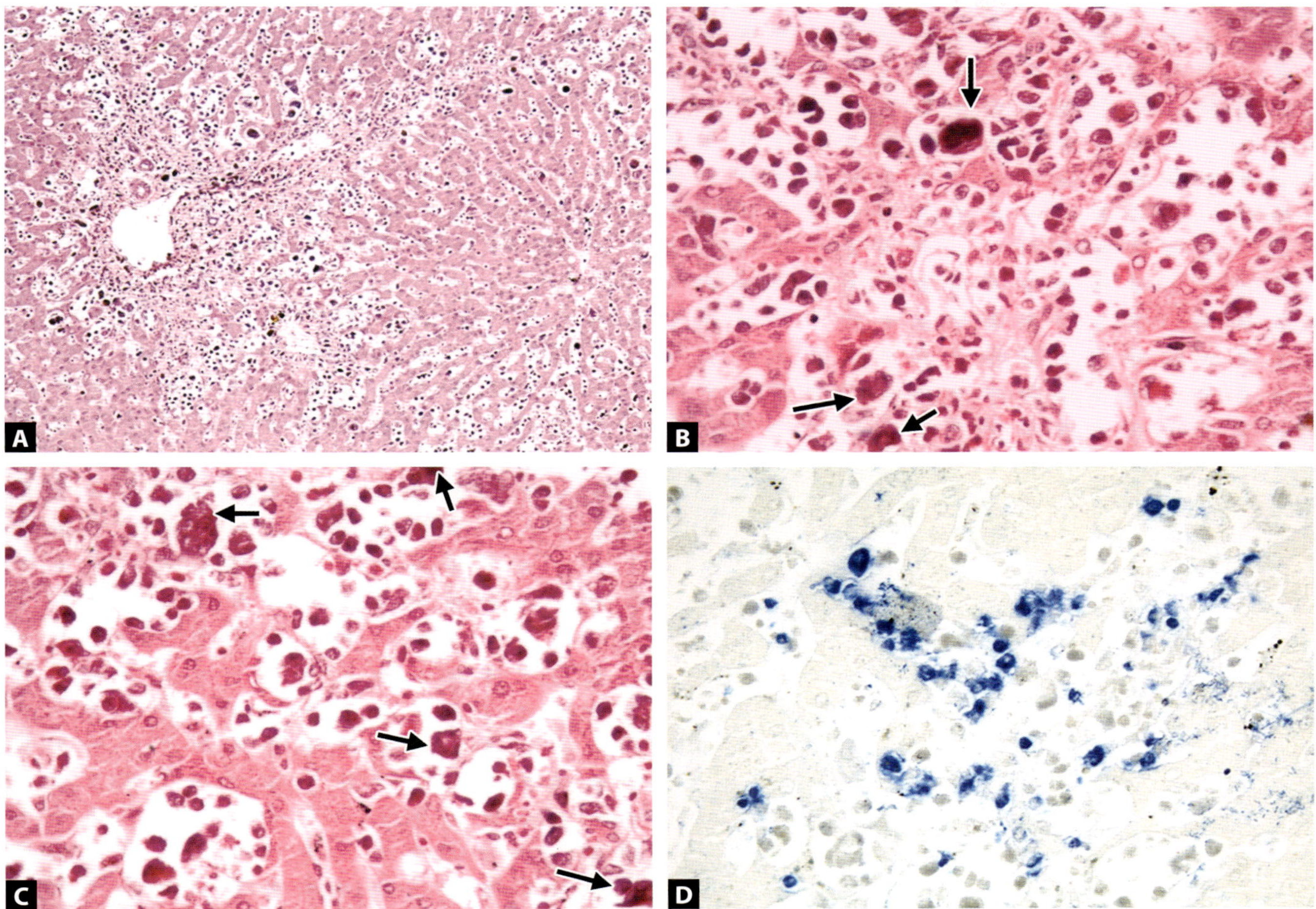

Figs 5A–D: (A) Liver shows expansion of sinusoids due to infiltration by a polymorphic infiltrate with megakaryocytes; (B–C) Liver at high power showing sinusoids packed with megakaryocytes (arrows), myeloid cells and nucleated red blood cells; and (D) The granulocytic precursors are strongly positive for chloroacetate esterase.

power (4X objective) fields, Grade III: immature epithelial tissue with or without immature stroma occupying more than three low power (4X objective) fields. Behavior of immature teratomas is very unpredictable. This is largely due to inadequate sampling and missing out on the small foci of yolk sac/other malignant component, at the time of original diagnosis. Of the 9/35 immature teratomas in Heifetz et al series which recurred, five had foci of yolk sac element in the original tumor and all nine cases had an elevation of serum AFP levels. In the other four, inadequate sampling missed the malignant component. So ideally, these tumors should have been labeled as mixed malignant teratomas at the first instance. Presence of even a small focus of neuroepithelial tubules in a sacrococcygeal teratoma is said to have a very unpredictable behavior and should alert the pathologist and the clinician.

Malignant Teratomas

Malignant teratomas contain germ cells, i.e. yolk sac element, trophoblastic or undifferentiated components exclusively or in combination with mature or immature tissue. Areas resembling seminomas with large polygonal cells with prominent nucleoli, fibrous septae with lymphocytes, granulomas and syncytial giant cells can be seen. Embryonal carcinoma (EC) like areas show cells in sheets or exhibit a tubulopapillary arrangement (no hyaline globules). Choriocarcinomatous (CC) areas are composed of a mixture of hemorrhage, necrosis, cytotrophoblastic and syncytiotrophoblastic cell (hCG positive). Yolk sac (YST) areas where the small tumor cells are arranged in a variety of patterns with Schiller–Duval bodies and intra/extracytoplasmic hyaline globules may be seen. AFP positivity is seen in the tumor cells. Malignant teratomas with non-germ cell elements can also be seen, e.g.

malignant neuroectodermal tumor and sarcomas of various types. Malignant teratomas behave in a malignant fashion and the ones with nonseminomatous elements (EC, CC and YST) behave most aggressively. Metastasis of malignant teratomas at times shows absolute mature elements. The explanation is that the mature elements are remnants persisting following eradication of the malignant component (which is more responsive to chemotherapy). It could also be due to the maturation of the immature elements as a result of chemotherapy.

ASSOCIATION OF MEDIASTINAL GERM CELL TUMORS AND HEMATOLOGIC NEOPLASIA

Coexistance of mediastinal germ cells tumors and hematologic malignancies was first recognized by Sales et al in 1984, in a young male with coexistant mediastinal teratoma and erythroleukemia. Prior to this, there were few reports of this association. Thereafter, Hernández-Nieto et al reported a coexistent malignant mediastinal teratoma and malignant histiocytosis and Hagberg et al reported a blastic myeloproliferative disorder with a mediastinal teratoma. But the breakthrough came in 1990, when Nichols et al further established this unique association in 16 cases of various hematologic neoplasias (AML-M7/M4/M5, acute mixed lineage/undifferentiated leukemia, myelodysplastic syndrome with abnormal megakaryocytes, megakaryocytic myelosis and essential thrombocythemia) and mediastinal nonseminomatous germ cell tumors, particularly those with serologic or histologic evidence of yolk sac element. Nichols et al postulated that the hematologic neoplasia is due to the multipotential differentiation of malignant germ cells. Hartmans and Nichols further published the same association in the year 2000. This theory has been proven by finding a common chromosomal abnormality, i.e. isochromosome of (12p), in both the mediastinal germ cell tumor and the leukemic cells in the bone marrow. Germ cell tumors of the testis also demonstrate this unique chromosomal abnormality, i.e. isochromosome of (12p).

A large comprehensive study was carried out at the Sloan-Kettering Memorial Hospital (New York) wherein 3,500 cases of leukemia, 600 cases of lymphomas and 200 cases of solid tumors were studied. Amongst them, two cases of leukemia were found with an i(12p) and surprisingly both these cases had an associated mediastinal germ cell tumor. This was a clear cut indicator that there is a common progenitor cell giving rise to both the mediastinal germ cell tumor and the associated leukemic blasts. The hematologic malignancies are not due to therapy is evident from the fact that (1) Therapy related neoplasms take an average of 2–5 years for their occurrence; (2) Five of the 16 patients in Nichol's series and 13 others in literature developed hematologic abnormality before the administration of chemotherapy; (3) Therapy-related hematologic neoplasms show a preceding abnormal hematologic picture like pancytopenia, etc. and this was not seen in the above cases. This further proves the fact that there is an association of mediastinal nonseminomatous germ cell tumors and hematologic neoplasia.

COMMENTARY—INDEX CASE: PM 13633

This is the first case reported in world literature where a malignant teratoma, primary pulmonary with yolk sac tumor is associated with a hematologic neoplasia. Histologically mature (from all germ layers), immature and malignant components were found in the pulmonary teratoma. Apart from this a very prominent myeloid metaplasia with plenty of atypical megakaryocytes were seen in the tumor. Physical association between the tumor and the lung was established and an origin from an extrapulmonary site, especially the testes was meticulously ruled out (blocked in toto). The associated hematologic abnormalities in this case were panhyperplasia and abnormal proliferation of predominantly atypical megakaryocytes in the bone marrow. The multiorgan involvement would indicate a megakaryocytic myeloproliferative disease. It bears similarities with the two cases of acute megakaryocytic myelosis reported by Nichols et al Some investigators regard megakaryocytic myelosis as a variant of acute granulocytic leukemia with prominent proliferation of megakaryocytes. Others consider it as an acute form of myelofibrosis with myeloid metaplasia. Most of the cases that have been reported as aleukemic megakaryocytic myelosis, were actually myelofibrosis with myeloid metaplasia that followed a chronic clinical course. The present case is also a case of aleukemic megakaryocytic myelosis or cellular phase of myelofibrosis with myeloid metaplasia wherein, there is a prominent myeloid metaplasia in the sites of fetal extramedullary hematopoiesis. Myeloid metaplasia develops early and may even precede the development of myelofibrosis. Early during the course of the disease, a cellular phase without accompanying myelofibrosis is common and that is what we saw in this case as well.

TAKE HOME MESSAGE

- Pulmonary teratomas are very rare. Before diagnosing a case it is mandatory to establish a physical association between the tumor and the lung and also to rule out metastasis from an extrapulmonary site.

- Association between mediastinal nonseminomatous germ cell tumors, particularly those with serologic or histologic evidence of yolk sac element and various hematologic neoplasias, is well known. This association has been proven by finding a common chromosomal abnormality, i.e. isochromosome of (12p), in both the mediastinal germ cell tumor and the leukemic cells in the bone marrow. Thus, both entities arise from a common progenitor cell.

Acknowledgment

This autopsy case was published as a short case report in the journal "Respiration" as—Kakkar N, Vasishta RK, Banerjee AK, et al Primary pulmonary malignant teratoma with yolk sac element associated with a hematologic neoplasia. Respiration. 1996;63:52-4.

Due permission has been granted by S Karger AG Basel Switzerland to include it in this book. Full credit is given to the original source.

SUGGESTED READING

1. Bosl GJ, Dmitrovsky E, Reuter VE, et al. Isochromosome of chromosome 12: clinically useful marker for male germ cell tumors. J Natl Cancer Inst. 1989;81:1874-8.
2. Chaganti RS, Ladanyi M, Samaniego F, et al. Leukemic differentiation of a mediastinal germ cell tumor. Genes Chromosomes Cancer. 1989;1:83-7.
3. deMent SH, Eggleston JC, Spivak JL. Association between mediastinal germ cells tumors and hematologic malignancies. Am Surg Pathol. 1985;9:23-9.
4. Disaia PG, Saltz A, Kagan AR, et al. Chemotherapeutic retroconversion of immature teratoma of the ovary. Obstet Gynecol. 1977;49:346-50.
5. Gibas Z, Prout GR, Pontes JE, et al. Chromosome changes in germ cell tumor of the testis. Cancer Genet Cytogenet. 1986;19:245-52.
6. Hagberg H, Gustavson KH, Sundstrom G, et al. Blastic phase of myeloproliferative syndrome coexisting with a malignant teratoma. Scand J Hematol. 1983;30:36-42.
7. HartmannJT, NicholsCR, DrozJP, etal. Hematologicdisorders associated with primary mediastinal nonseminomatous germ cell tumors. Natl Cancer Inst. 2000;92:54-61.
8. Hawkins EP, Finegold MJ, Hawkins HK, et al. Non-germinomatous malignant germ cells tumors in children. A review of 89 cases from the Pediatric Oncology Group, 1971-1984. Cancer. 1986;58:2579-84.
9. Heifetz S, Cushing B, Giller R, et al. Immature teratomas in children: pathologic considerations. A Report from the combined Pediatric Oncology Group/Children's Cancer Group. Am J Surg Pathol. 1998;22:1115-24.
10. Hernandez-Nieto L, Bombi JA, Caralps A, et al. Histologic medullary reticulocytosis (Robb-Smith's disease) in a renal transplant patient. Lancet. 1977;2:261-2.
11. Macht M, Mitchell JD, Cool C, et al. A 31-year-old woman with hemoptysis and an intrathoracic mass. Chest. 2010;138:213-9.
12. Meares EM Jr, Briggs EM. Occult seminoma of the testis masquerading as primary extragonadal germinal neoplasm. Cancer. 1972;30:300-6.
13. Nichols CR, Roth BJ, Heerema N, et al. Hematologic neoplasia associated with primary mediastinal germ cell tumors. N Engl J Med. 1990;322:1425-9.
14. Pound AW, Willis RA. A malignant teratoma of the lung in an infant. J Pathol. 1969;98:111-4.
15. Präuer HW, Mack D, Babic R. Intrapulmonary teratoma 10 years after removal of mediastinal teratoma in a young man. Thorax. 1983;38:632-4.
16. Rappaport H. Atlas of Tumor Pathology, sect III, fasc. 8: Tumors of haematopoietic system. Washington, DC: AFIP; 1963.
17. Sales LM, Vontz FK. Teratoma and Di Gulielmo syndrome. South Med J. 1970;63:448-50.
18. Truong LD, Jurro S, McGarran MK. Gliomatosis peritonei: Report of two cases and review of the literature. Am J Surg Pathol. 1982;6:443-9.
19. Zenker D, Aleksic I. Intrapulmonary cystic benign teratoma: a case report and review of the literature. Ann Thorac Cardiovasc Surg. 2004;10:290-2.

CONTRIBUTIONS BY:

1. Dr AK Banerjee, Ex-Professor and Head, Department of Histopathology (Consultation)
2. Dr RK Vasishta, Professor and Head, Department of Histopathology (Consultation)
3. Late SD Deodhar, Professor, Department of Internal Medicine (Clinician In-Charge)

Post Graduate Institute of Medical Education and Research, Chandigarh, India.

CASE 11

Young Male with Metastasis: Do not Waste Time—Look for the Primary in the Testes: PM 19388

Nandita Bharadwaj Kakkar

HIGHLIGHTS OF THE CASE

A 27-year-old male came with pain abdomen, dyspnea on exertion and vomiting. He had cachexia, generalized lymphadenopathy, mass in the epigastrium, deranged liver function tests, cannonball shadows in the chest, multiple hepatic space occupying lesions, ascites with portal vein/inferior vena cava (IVC) thrombosis. Fine-needle aspiration done twice from the supraclavicular lymph node revealed only necrosis. The patient died with a clinical diagnosis of "Young male with disseminated malignancy, ? Primary". Autopsy revealed mixed germ cell tumor (GCT) of the right testis with extensive metastasis to the lymph nodes, liver and lungs.

***Keywords*:** Young male, disseminated malignancy, primary, testis, mixed germ cell tumor, autopsy.

CLINICAL DETAILS

Date of Admission: 03.08.2003, Date of Death: 13.08.2003, Duration of Hospital Stay: 10 Days

A young male (27 years) came with a history of pain abdomen for 2 months. The pain was in the right upper quadrant to begin with and later became diffuse. The pain had no association with meals and posture. There was generalized weakness, loss of weight and appetite. Dyspnea on exertion was present since 20 days, but there was no expectoration, cough or hemoptysis. There was history of vomiting since 20 days and edema feet since 7 days, but no facial puffiness was noted. There was no history of jaundice, gastrointestinal bleed, urinary complaints and bowel symptoms. He was a heavy smoker and a bhang addict since 4 years. On ***examination***, he was cachetic but conscious and alert. He was afebrile with a normal blood pressure. There was pallor, icterus, pedal edema and left supraclavicular lymph node was enlarged (2.5 cm). The abdomen was distended, tense, with an everted umbilicus and prominent veins, with flow from below upward. The liver was enlarged 3 cm below the right costal margin, with a span of 20 cm. There was a vague mass palpable from the epigastrium till the umbilicus. Spleen was not palpable and the bowel sounds were heard.

Investigations

Investigations revealed a normal hemogram, coagulation parameters, blood sugar and renal function tests. The liver function tests were abnormal with a serum bilirubin of 7 mg% with a conjugated fraction of 3.5 mg% and alkaline phosphatase of 120 U/L. HIV serology was negative. ***X-ray chest*** showed multiple cannonball lesions in both lung fields. ***Ultrasonography*** revealed a huge heterogeneous, solid retroperitoneal mass extending from the epigastrium up to the level of the aortic bifurcation. The mass was encasing and lifting the aorta and other major vessels. There was no calcification, cystic change or necrosis. Infrahepatic inferior vena cava (IVC) was chinked and was not visible till the level of aortic bifurcation. The plane between the mass and left lobe of the liver was ill defined. The liver was enlarged and replaced by a mass. The left and middle hepatic veins were not seen, but the right vein was splayed around the mass. The main portal vein was not seen, but the splenoportal confluence was patent. Free fluid was present in the pelvis. CT scan (abdomen and chest) showed multiple hepatic space occupying lesions (SOLs) with thrombosis of the portal vein and IVC, retroperitoneal/hilar lymphadenopathy, multiple nodules in both lungs and ascites. Fine-needle aspiration cytology (FNAC) done twice from the supraclavicular lymph node revealed only necrosis. A clinical diagnosis of retroperitoneal tumor ? nature, portal vein and IVC thrombosis with involvement of the liver and lung was made. In view of the disseminated disease and inconclusive FNAC, an image-guided FNAC from the retroperitoneal mass was planned. But, the patient had a sudden cardiorespiratory arrest from which he could not be revived and died after a hospital stay of 10 days. The unit's final diagnosis was—Young male with Disseminated Malignancy, ? Primary.

AUTOPSY FINDINGS: PM 19388

A partial autopsy was performed. There was two liters of straw colored fluid in the peritoneal cavity. The ***right testis*** was enlarged and measured 6 × 5 × 4 cm (Fig 1A). Cut section (Figs 1B) revealed a 4 cm well circumscribed nodule with adjacent compressed residual testis. The tumor was variegated in appearance and showed areas of hemorrhage and necrosis. On microscopic examination, the right testis revealed a tumor consistent with morphology of mixed GCT with components of embryonal carcinoma comprising 50%, yolk sac component comprising 20% and necrosis comprising 30% of the tumor. The tumor was multinodular with undifferentiated embryonal carcinoma showing highly pleomorphic cells with prominent nucleoli, high mitosis and areas of necrosis (Figs 2A–C). This component was positive for CD30, OCT4 (Figs 2D and E) and negative for CD117 and glypican 3. The yolk sac component was composed of tubulopapillary areas (Fig 3A) with the characteristic Schiller–Duval bodies [Figs 3B and C (arrows)] and periodic acid–Schiff (PAS) positive, diastase resistant globules. This yolk sac component was positive for glypican 3 (Fig 3D). No seminomatous or teratomatous component was noted. The adjacent testes did not show any evidence of germ cell neoplasia in situ or any atrophy. Adjacent seminiferous tubules showed changes due to compression and distant ones showed normal spermatogenesis. The tumor was infiltrating the spermatic cord. The ***left testis*** was within normal limits grossly (Figs 1A–B) and microscopically. The para-aortic ***lymph nodes*** (Fig 4A) were enlarged and formed a large mass 10 × 8 × 6 cm in which the aorta and IVC were caught up. There was a thrombus in the IVC above the level of the kidneys [Fig 4A (long arrow)]. Microscopically the lymph nodes showed a morphology of embryonal carcinoma (Fig 4B) with extensive necrosis and areas of yolk sac differentiation (Fig 4C). Apart from these nodes the hilar, carinal, peripancreatic nodes were enlarged and showed a similar tumor morphology. The ***liver*** weighed 1,200 g. Cut section (Fig 5A) showed multiple tumor nodules getting confluent, the largest measuring 6 cm in diameter, showing foci of necrosis and hemorrhage. Portal vein was occluded by a thrombus. Microscopy of the liver showed metastatic mixed GCT composed of embryonal carcinoma (Figs 5B–E) where the cells were CD30 (membranous) and OCT4 (nuclear) positive and yolk sac component exhibited the typical tubulopapillary component (Fig 5F). ***Lungs*** weighed 600 g and there were multiple tumor nodules (1–2.5 cm in diameter) on the pleural aspect and on cut section (Figs 6A and B). No thromboemboli were seen. Microscopy, showed a tumor with embryonal carcinoma (Fig 6C) along with a tubuloalveolar pattern

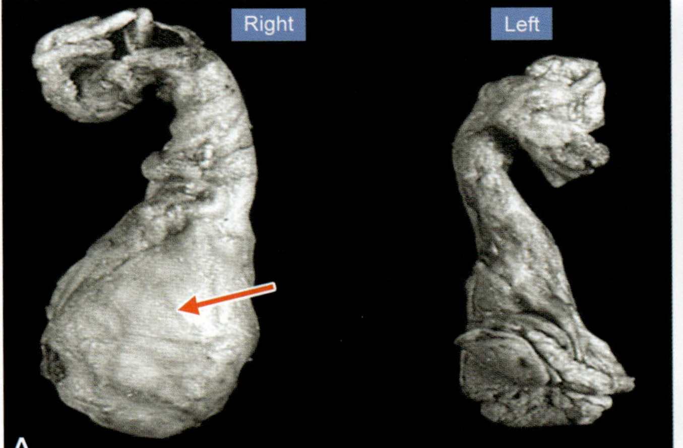

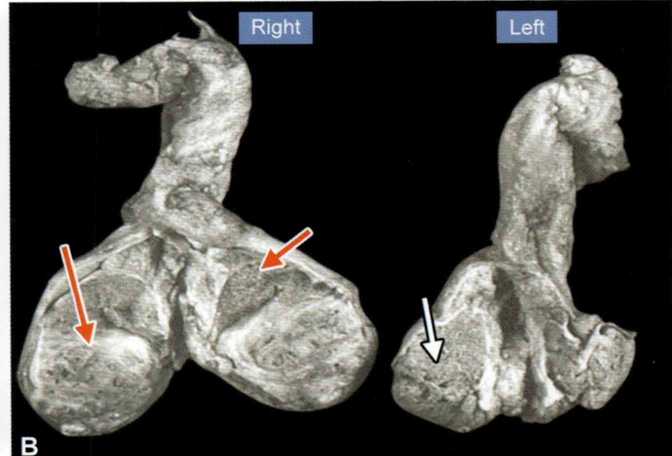

Figs 1A and B: (A) Whole specimens of both the testis with the spermatic cord. The right testis (arrow) is enlarged measuring 6 × 5 × 3 cm. Left testis is within normal limits; (B) Cut open specimens of both the testis. The right testis shows a tumor measuring 4 cm in diameter (long arrow) with the normal testis appreciated at the upper part (short arrow). The left testis is normal grossly (white arrow).

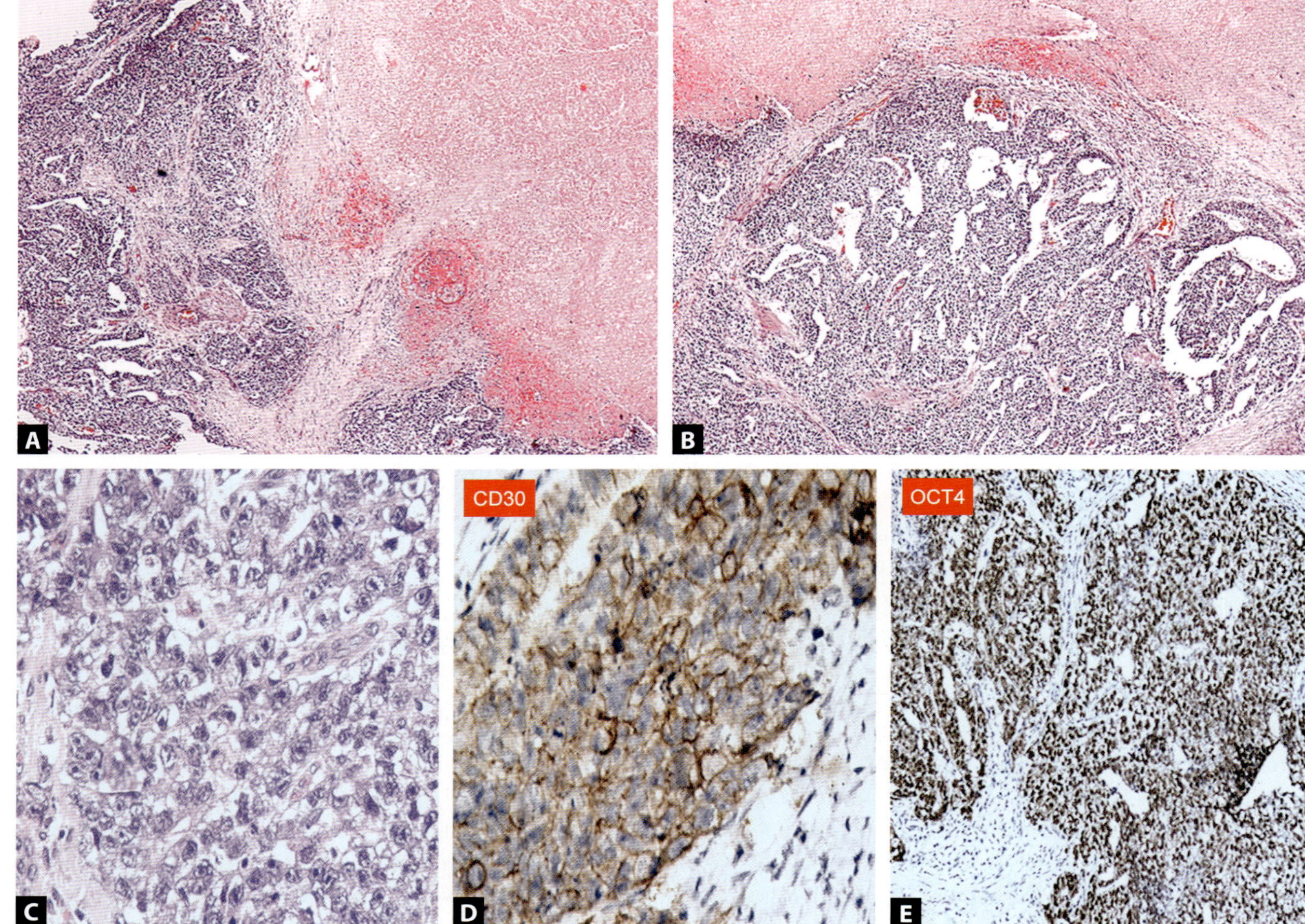

Figs 2A–E: (A–B) Photomicrographs from the testis show a pleomorphic tumor with large areas of necrosis; (C) Testicular tumor shows large pleomorphic cells with prominent nucleoli, consistent with morphology of embryonal carcinoma; (D) Embryonal carcinoma shows CD30 membranous positivity; and (E) Embryonal carcinoma shows nuclear positivity with OCT4.

showing Schiller–Duval bodies (Fig 6D) and PAS positive diastase resistant globules. Peribronchial, intrabronchial, intra-alveolar spread with lymphangitic carcinomatosis (Fig 6E) was seen. In the lungs, the yolk sac pattern was more prominent.

FINAL AUTOPSY DIAGNOSIS: PM 19388

27 Years Male, with Disseminated Malignancy

- Mixed germ cell tumor (embryonal carcinoma 50% and yolk sac tumor 20%)—Right testis.
- Extensive metastasis to the lymph nodes (para-aortic, retroperitoneal, peripancreatic, hilar, carinal and supraclavicular), liver and lungs.
- Direct infiltration of the tumor into the inferior vena cava.
- Portal vein thrombosis.
- Pulmonary hemorrhage and edema.

GERM CELL TUMORS OF THE TESTES

Approximately 90% of testicular neoplasms1-3 originates from the germ cells. Germ cell tumors (GCT) of the testes are a heterogeneous group of neoplasms with varied histopathology, clinical behavior and etiopathogenesis. Cytogenetic studies reveal a different pathogenesis for the different groups of GCT's, i.e. prepubertal, postpubertal and spermatocytic seminoma (now termed Spermatocytic tumor). Only the postpubertal GCT's are said to arise from intratubular germ cell neoplasia. The 2016 WHO[4] classification system divides testicular germ cell tumors into (1) Non-invasive

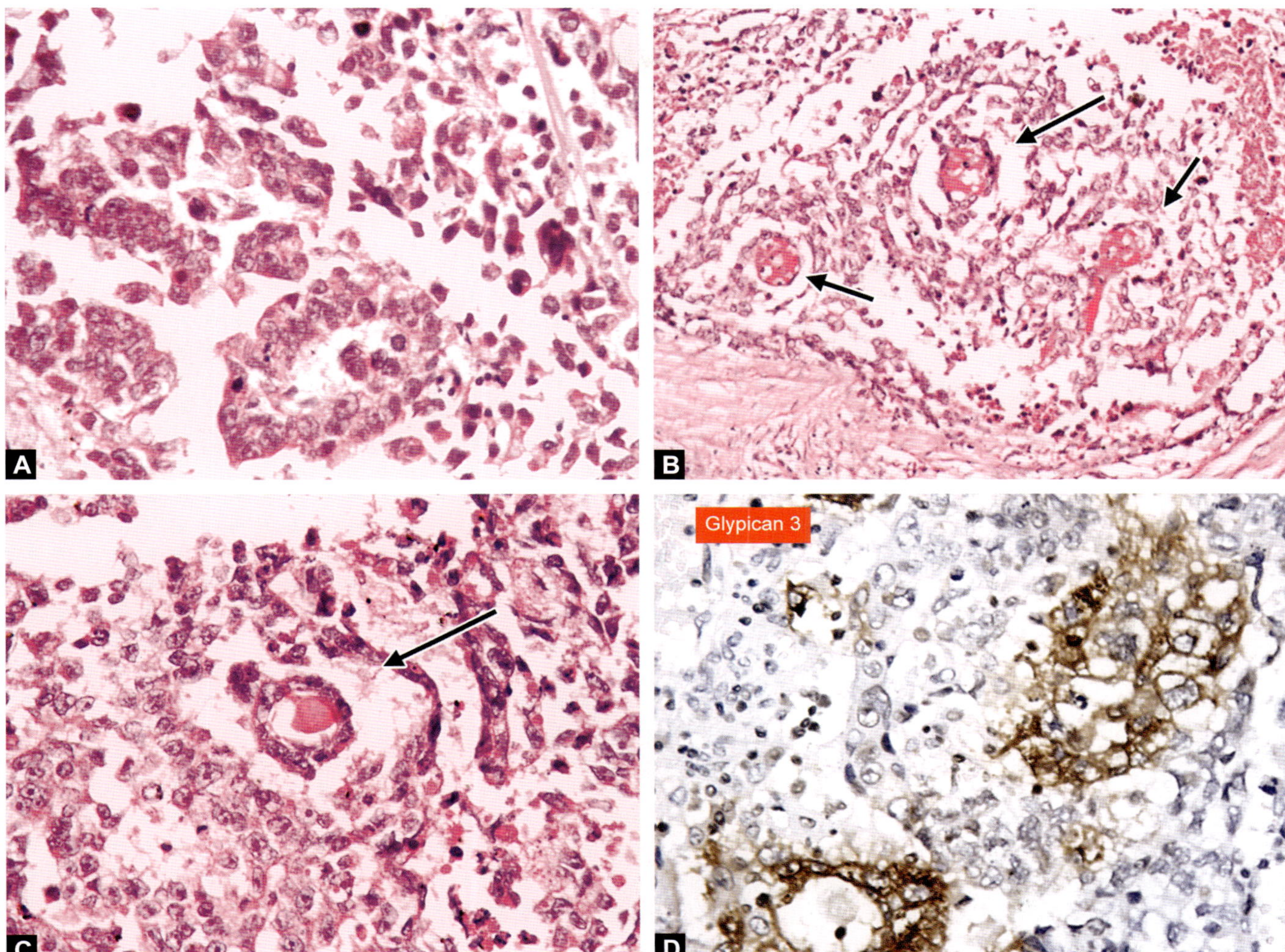

Figs 3A–D: Testicular tumor showing: (A) Tubulopapillary pattern; (B–C) Schiller–Duval bodies (arrows) characteristic of yolk sac differentiation; and (D) Yolk sac component shows positivity with glypican 3.

germ cell neoplasia (GCNIS and Gonadoblastoma) (2) Germ cell tumors derived from GCNIS (Seminoma and Non-seminomatous tumors ie embryonal carcinoma, post-pubertal teratomas, post-pubertal yolk sac tumor and choriocarcinoma/other trophoblastic tumors). (3) Germ cell tumors unrelated to GCNIS (Pre-pubertal teratoma, Pre-pubertal yolk sac tumor and spermatocytic tumor). But the majority of non-seminomatous germ cell tumors (NSGCT) i.e. about 69–91% (in various studies) are of mixed type.[5,6] The recommended term used in such cases is "mixed germ cell tumor", followed by listing of the various components present with an estimate of their relative proportions in percentage. This is because a mixed GCT with a large component of mature teratoma has a better prognosis. Mixed GCT's, with seminomatous component occur at a later age than those without it and are not seen before puberty. Elevated α-fetoprotein and β-hCG correlate with the presence of yolk sac elements and syncytiotrophoblastic cells (singly or as a part of choriocarcinoma) respectively. Grossly, mixed GCTs have a variegated appearance with foci of hemorrhage and necrosis, reflecting their different components. The common morphologic subtypes in a mixed GCT in descending order are embryonal carcinoma, teratoma, yolk sac tumor, seminoma and choriocarcinoma.[7] Elements of teratoma are encountered in the range of 55–77%[8] and confer a better prognosis,[9,10] i.e. such tumors are less aggressive, less likely to progress, respond well to treatment and have better survival rates. Microscopically, the appearance of the various components of mixed GCT's is identical to the various pure neoplasms. The major pitfall is that many pathologists

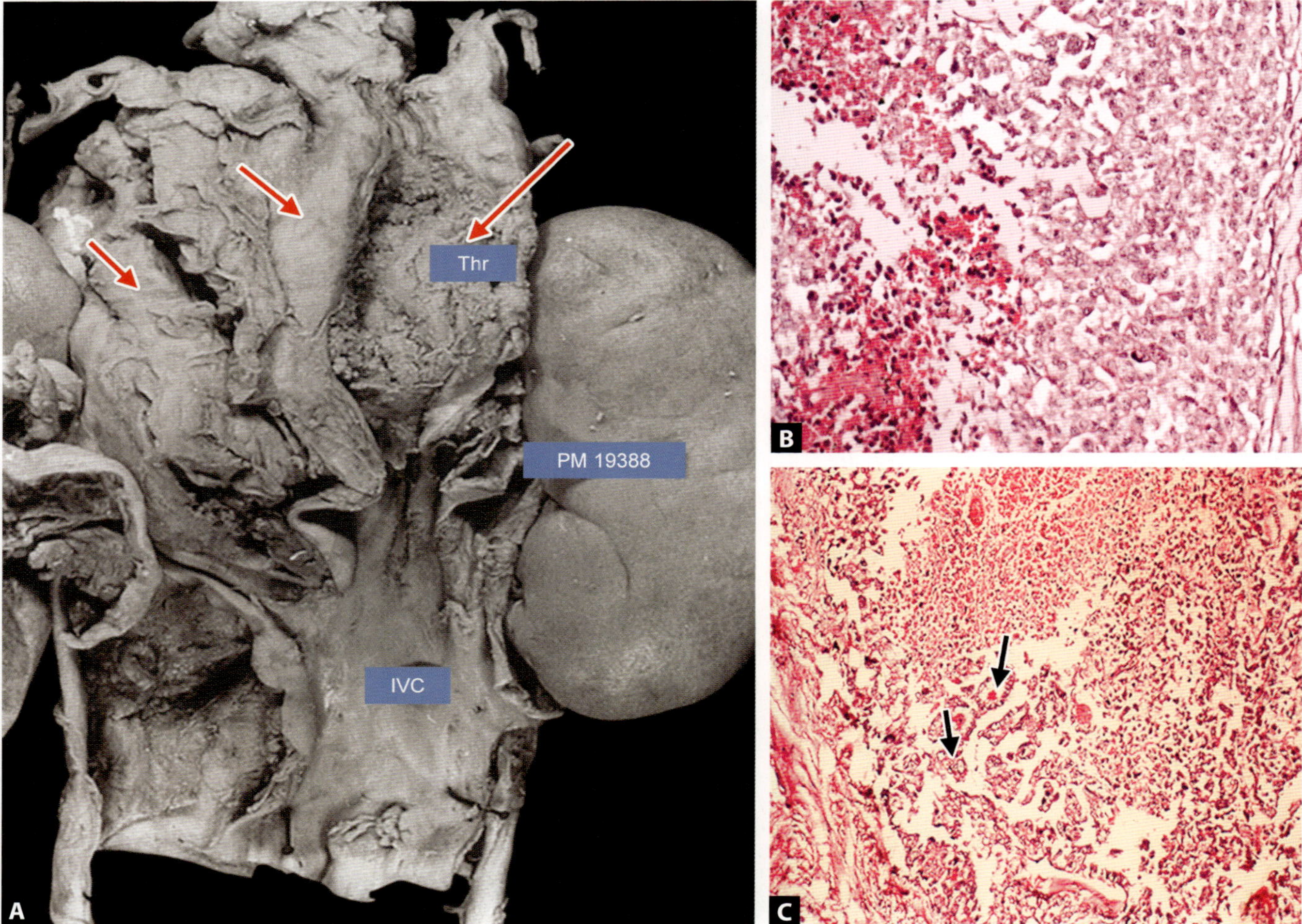

Figs 4A–C: (A) Gross picture of the opened up inferior vena cava showing a large tumor thrombus (long arrow) and enlarged para-aortic lymph nodes (small arrows) forming a mass. Photomicrographs from the enlarged lymph nodes showing: (B) Metastatic embryonal carcinoma along with necrosis; and (C) Yolk sac areas showing Schiller–Duval bodies (arrows) and tubulopapillary pattern and necrosis (upper part).

overlook foci of yolk sac tumor, which characteristically occurs in close association with an embryonal carcinoma component.[11] The double layered pattern of embryonal carcinoma is actually a mixed GCT composed of embryonal carcinoma with yolk sac tumor.[12] Embryonal carcinoma is a germ cell neoplasm composed of primitive epithelial cells arranged in a solid, papillary and glandular patterns. Pure embryonal carcinomas are rare, comprising 10% of GCTs,[5] but an embryonal carcinoma component is present in 87% of mixed germ cell tumors. They occur a decade earlier than seminomas, present with a testicular mass which may be associated with pain and approximately 65–70% of patients with an embryonal carcinoma predominant tumor, have metastasis at the time of diagnosis. This is in contrast to the seminomas where 70% are confined to the testis at diagnosis. In an autopsy study of 78 cases,[13] the sites of metastases in order of decreasing frequency for all cases were lung, retroperitoneal lymph nodes, liver, mediastinal lymph nodes, brain, kidney, gastrointestinal tract, bones, adrenals, peritoneum and spleen. In another autopsy study of 174 cases,[14] for all tumor types, the most common sites of distant metastasis were lung (89%), liver (73%), brain (31%) and bone (30%).

Although morphology of testicular tumors is easy to discern but immunohistochemistry[15] has made the diagnosis more systematic. Embryonal carcinomas are positive for CD30, OCT4, AE1/AE3, SOX2; yolk sac tumors are positive for glypican 3, AFP±, PLAP±; seminomas are positive for OCT4, CD117, podoplanin, SOX17; choriocarcinoma is positive for HCG, glypican 3±, PLAP±; spermatocytic seminomas are negative for all including OCT4 and CD117; ITGCN is positive for OCT4, CD117 and PLAP.

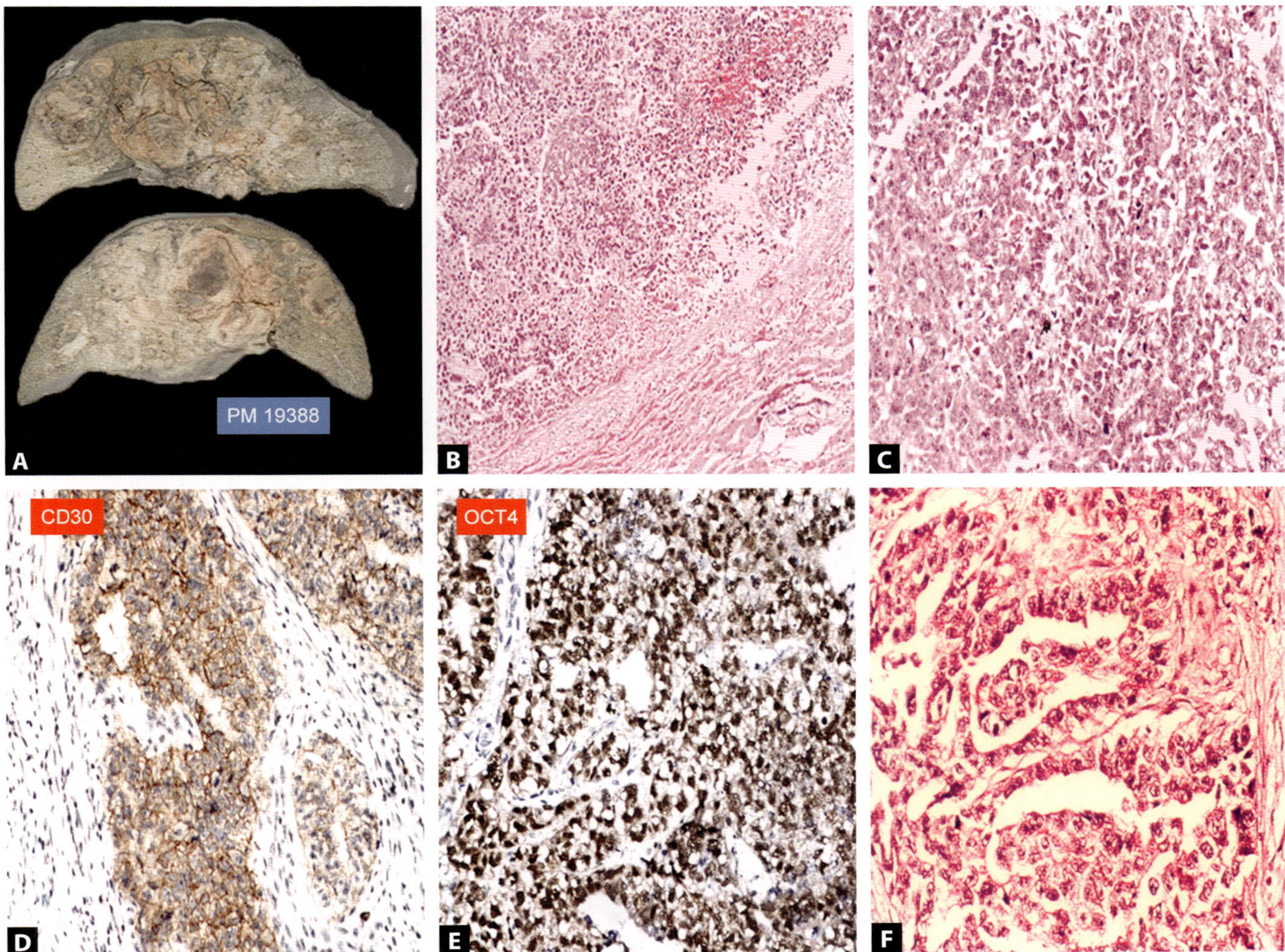

Figs 5A–F: (A) Coronal slices of the liver showing large metastatic tumor nodules getting confluent, replacing the entire liver. The tumor has a variegated appearance with areas of necrosis and hemorrhage. Photomicrographs from the liver shows (B–C) Metastatic embryonal carcinoma showing necrosis with compressed liver cords in the right lower quadrant in "B"; (D) Embryonal carcinoma component shows strong membranous positivity for CD30 immunostain; (E) Embryonal carcinoma component shows strong nuclear positivity for OCT4 immunostain; and (F) Tubulopapillary areas indicative of yolk sac differentiation.

COMMENTARY—INDEX CASE: PM 19388

This young male came with metastatic disease, multiple space occupying lesions in the liver and lung, para-aortic mass and supraclavicular lymph node enlargement. The testes as the primary site of the tumor were not suspected. This brings in the need for a mindset, i,e. young males with metastasis, the testes are the first site to look for the primary. So, a thorough physical examination of the testes and if normal, ultrasonography should be done before ruling out a primary at this site. The primary tumor in the index case was composed of a predominant embryonal pattern with an admixture of yolk sac component, whereas the metastatic site, i.e. the lungs revealed a predominant yolk sac tumor. Necrosis is an important component of embryonal carcinomas and generally gives rise to an inconclusive diagnosis on FNAC. Yet, the necrosis is very suggestive of metastatic carcinoma from the testis in a young male with the above clinical scenario.

TAKE HOME MESSAGE

- In young/middle-aged male with metastatic disease, first rule out a primary in the testes.
- Thorough physical examination of the testis should be done regarding its size, texture and comparison of the two sides.

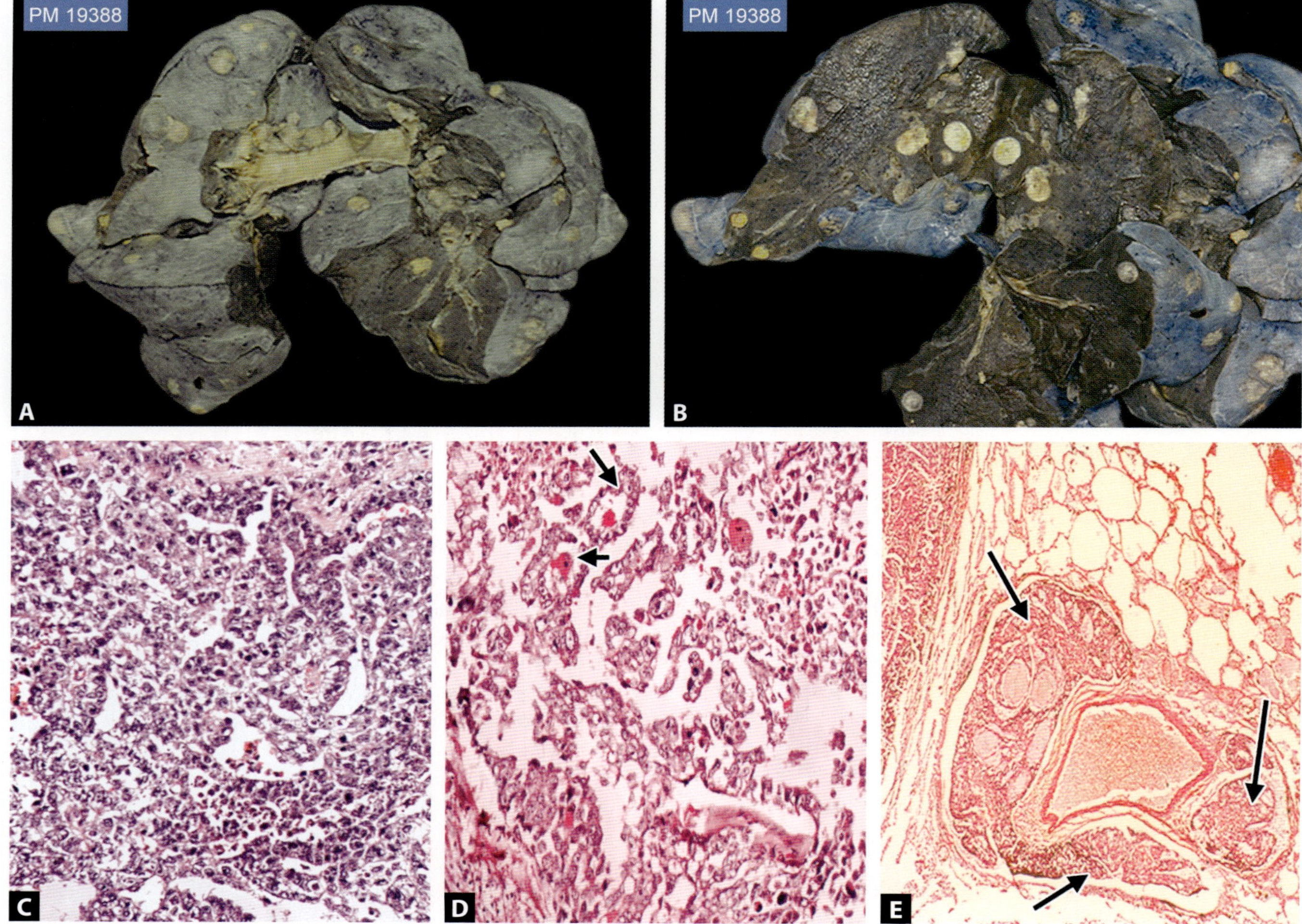

Figs 6A–E: (A–B) Pleural aspect and cut section of the lungs showing metastatic, well-circumscribed whitish nodules scattered all over. Photomicrographs from the metastatic tumor showing (C) Embryonal carcinoma areas; (D) Yolk sac differentiation—tubulopapillary areas with Schiller–Duval bodies (arrows); and (E) Lymphangitic carcinomatosis with tumor clogging the lymphatic channels (arrows).

- Even if the testes are normal on gross examination, do not give up as occult testicular neoplasms occur. These can be picked up by ultrasonography, as an abnormal echotexture is seen in virtually in all such cases. The diagnosis can be clinched.
- If there is a biopsy proven metastatic testicular tumor with a normal physical examination of the testes and ultrasonographic detection of an abnormal echotexture, surgical removal of the testes is justifiable under such circumstances.

REFERENCES

1. Sesterhenn IA, Davis CJ Jr. Pathology of germ cell tumors of the testis. Cancer Control. 2004;11:374-87.
2. Young RH. Testicular tumors—some new and a few perennial problems. Arch Pathol Lab Med. 2008;132:548-64.
3. Ulbright TM. Germ cell neoplasms of the testis. Am J Surg Pathol. 1993;17:1075-91.
4. Ulbright TM, Amin MB, Balzer B eta l. Germ cell tumors. In: Moch H, Humphrey PA, Reuter VE, Ulbright TM (eds). WHO classification of tumors of the urinary system and male genital organs, 4th edn. Lyon: IARC Press, 2016;189-26.
5. Jacobsen GK, Barlebo H, Olsen J, et al. Testicular germ cell tumors in Denmark 1976-1980. Pathology of 1058 consecutive cases. Acta Radiol Oncol. 1984;23:239-47.
6. Barsky SH. Germ cell tumors of the testis. In: Javadpour N, Barsky SH (Eds). Surgical Pathology of Urologic Diseases. Baltimore, MD: Williams and Wilkins; 1987. pp. 224-46.
7. Mosharafa AA, Foster RS, Leibovich BC, et al. Histology in mixed germ cell tumors: is there favorite pairing? J Urol. 2004;171:1471-3.

8. Klepp O, Olsson AM, Henrikson H, et al. Prognostic factors in clinical stage I nonseminomatous germ cell tumors of the testis: multivariant analysis of prospective multicenter study. J Clin Oncol. 1990;8:509-18.
9. Sesterhenn IA, Weiss RB, Mostofi FK, et al. Prognosis and other clinical correlates of pathology review in stage I and II testicular carcinoma: a report from the testicular cancer intergroup study. J Clin Oncol. 1999;10:69-78.
10. Levin HS. Prognostic features of primary and metatastic testis germ-cell tumors. Urol Clin North Am. 1993;20:39-53.
11. Mostofi FK, Sesterhenn IA, Davis CJ Jr. Developments in histopathology of testicular germ cell tumors. Semin Urol. 1988;6:171-288.
12. Jacobsen GK. Histogenetic considerations concerning germ cell tumors. Morphological and immunohistochemical comparative investigation of the human embryo and testicular germ cell tumours. Virchows Archiv A. 1886;408:509-25.
13. Johnson DE, Appelt G, Samuels ML, et al. Metastases from testicular carcinoma. Study of 78 autopsied cases. Urology. 1976;8:234-9.
14. Bredael JJ, Vugrin D, Whitmore WF Jr. Autopsy findings in 154 patients with germ cell tumors of the testis. Cancer. 1982;50:548-5.
15. Ulbright TM, Tickoo SK, Berney DM, et al. Best practices recommendations in the application of immunohistochemistry in testicular tumors: report from the International Society of Urological Pathology consensus conference. Am J Surg Pathol. 2014;38:e50-9.

CONTRIBUTIONS BY:

1. Prof RK Vasishta, Professor and Head, Department of Histopathology (Consultation)
2. Prof Kartar Singh, Ex-Professor and Head, Department of Gastroenterology (Clinician In-Charge)

Post Graduate Institute of Medical Education and Research, Chandigarh, India.

CASE 12

Occult, Peripheral, Mucin-secreting Adenocarcinoma of Lung with Florid Meningeal Carcinomatosis along with Thrombotic Microangiopathy and Disseminated Intravascular Coagulation, Leading to Bilateral Renal Infarction: PM 26226

Nandita Bharadwaj Kakkar

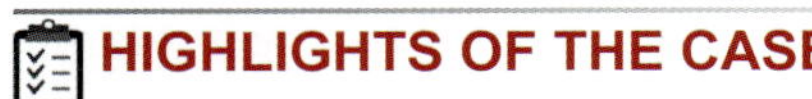

HIGHLIGHTS OF THE CASE

A 51-year-old lady, who had undergone a cholecystectomy 2 months back, was now unwell since a month. She had headache, vomiting, altered sensorium, fever and neck rigidity. There was shortness of breath and history of hematochezia. Investigations revealed lytic/sclerotic multiple bone lesions, a high uric acid, cerebrospinal fluid (CSF) initially suggestive of meningitis and the third tap revealed malignant cells (reported after her demise), leukoerythroblastic picture, microangiopathic hemolytic anemia, thrombocytopenia, deranged coagulogram, markedly deranged renal/liver function tests and high alkaline phosphatase. A clinical diagnosis of metastatic bone disease (occult primary) with meningitis and sepsis was made. Autopsy revealed a microscopic, peripheral, mucin secreting, adenocarcinoma of right lung with florid lymphangitic/meningeal carcinomatosis, disseminated bone metastasis, thrombotic microangiopathy (TMA) with disseminated intravascular coagulation (DIC) leading to total infarction of both kidneys and an early (<24 hours) inferior wall myocardial infarction.

Keywords: Occult, peripheral, mucin-producing adenocarcinoma, lung, meningeal carcinomatosis, thrombotic microangiopathy, disseminated intravascular coagulation, bilateral renal infarction, autopsy.

CLINICAL DETAILS

Date of Admission: 23.08.2014, Date of Death: 27.08.2014, Duration of Hospital Stay: 4 Days

A 51-year-old female was admitted with history of decreased appetite and nausea along with low-grade fever, since 1 month. For the last 5 days, the fever was high grade associated with rigors and chills and she was in a state of altered sensorium, in the form of decreased verbal output and not obeying commands. There were no seizures or any focal deficit and she was moving all four limbs. There was shortness of breath since 3 days, but there was no cough, expectoration, hemoptysis or chest pain. There was history of decreased urinary output since 1 day. No hematuria was however present. There was no history of loose stools, abdominal pain or jaundice. On ***examination***, there was pallor, BP was 120/80 mm Hg, respiratory rate was 32/min, rapid and shallow, bilateral crepitations were present, liver was palpable 3 cm below the right costal margin and there was generalized guarding. Her status was E3V2M4, neck rigidity was present, planters were down going and no apparent cranial nerve palsy was noted.

Investigations and Course of Management

Hematological: Hemoglobin fell from 11.2 to 6.2 g/dL; TLC was 33,000/μL and later came down to 16,900/μL with P68, L18, M8, E4, My2, nRBCs 3/100; platelets fell from 1,58,000/μL to 17,000/μL; peripheral blood film showed microangiopathic changes with 8% schistocytes and a reticulocyte count of 7.6%. Coagulogram was deranged (PT/PTI/INR—24'/58%/1.75) and aPTT was 40'. In view of the leukoerythroblastic picture, thrombocytopenia and 8% schistocytes, an advice to work up for hemolytic uremic syndrome/thrombotic thrombocytopenic purpura (HUS/TTP) was given. D-dimer test could not be done. ***Blood biochemistry*** revealed deranged renal (serum urea/creatinine—144/6.5 mg%), liver function tests (serum bilirubin 1.8 mg%, SGOT/SGPT/ALP—290/130/562 U/L) and uric acid—15.4 mg%. Random blood sugar ranged from 100 to 230 mg%. The *CSF* was done thrice, the first time (high proteins, low sugar and polymorphs) it showed 70 cells with 90% polymorphs, proteins 67 mg%, sugar 25 mg%, ADA 6 IU/L and the second time there were no cells. The third tap was done on the day of her demise and the report was collected after her demise. It revealed CSF positive for metastatic adenocarcinoma. The routine urine examination showed albumin 1+ with nil sugar. Tests for malaria and dengue were negative ***Radiology***: The ultrasonography of the abdomen—liver 14 cm with raised echotexture and grade 2 fatty liver, common bile duct and pancreas were normal, right kidney 9.8 cm, left kidney 10.2 cm and spleen 7.8 cm. No mass lesion identified. Non-contrast computerized tomography of head and contrast enhanced computerized tomography of the chest and abdomen showed multiple lytic and sclerotic lesions in the skull, vertebrae, scapula and pelvis.

She was treated for meningitis, was intubated and put on mechanical ventilation. Bowel sounds were absent and she had not passed stools since 3 days. Third CSF tap was done and hemodialysis was started, soon after which she deteriorated, went into hypotension, EKG monitor showed ST elevation, ventricular fibrillation and she could not be revived. Unit's final clinical diagnosis was—Metastatic bone disease (occult primary), meningitis with sepsis, septic encephalopathy, cause of death being an inferior wall myocardial infarction and cardiac arrhythmia.

AUTOPSY FINDINGS: PM 26226

A complete autopsy was performed on this 51-year-old lady. Both pleural cavities contained 200 mL and the peritoneal cavity contained 250 mL of straw colored fluid. The ***lungs*** (Fig 1A) were heavy and weighed 1200 g. The pleural aspect (Fig 1B) showed tiny whitish specks, more on the right side. Cut section showed a yellowish, well-circumscribed lesion in the right upper lobe (subpleural location) which looked like an old healed focus of tuberculosis. The lung around this area was firm to feel and it was blocked in toto. On gross examination, no tumor was identified in the lungs. The hilar and carinal lymph nodes were not enlarged, but were blocked. Microscopic examination of the sections from the right upper lobe showed a walled off, old healing focus of tuberculosis, composed of caseation necrosis and hyalinization (Fig 1C). No epithelioid cell granulomas were seen and Ziehl–Neelsen stain for AFB was negative. Surrounding this, there were few similar foci of tuberculosis, getting confluent. Sections from the firm area (Fig 1D) around these foci, however showed a tumor amidst the fibrosis, with features of an adenocarcinoma (Figs 1E and 2A) of the type "solid predominant with mucin production". This focus of tumor was 1.5 cm. The malignant cells (Fig 2A) were large with pleomorphic nuclei, many showed prominent nucleoli and cytoplasmic vacuoles pushing the nuclei to the periphery. These cells were positive for Alcian blue stain, indicating mucin production. Lepidic spread of the tumor was evident with presence of tumor cells in the alveoli (Fig 2B) and in areas forming small nodules. Extensive lymphangitic carcinomatosis (Figs 2C and D) in the parenchyma of both lungs, pleura and in the peripancreatic areas was noted. The tumor was infiltrating into the pleura and into the hilar/carinal lymph nodes. Immunohistochemistry revealed positive staining for TTF-1 (Fig 2E), CK-7 (Fig 2F), E-cadherin and negative staining for CD-20, p63, CK5/6, calretinin, WTI, ER and PR. Overall features were consistent with a diagnosis of microscopic, peripheral, mucin producing, adenocarcinoma of the lung with extensive lymphangitic carcinomatosis and pleural spread. The ***brain*** weighed 1,270 g. There was an opalescent exudate (Figs 3A–C), diffusely covering the convexities, inferior orbital surface, brainstem and cerebellum. Meningeal vessels were congested. Uncal and tonsillar herniation was noted. Coronal slicing of the brain did not reveal any focal lesion or hemorrhage. Microscopy revealed florid meningeal carcinomatosis with the malignant cells clogging the leptomeninges (Figs 3D–F). The malignant cells were percolating into the sulci and were also seen in the Virchow–Robin spaces. The leptomeninges around the brain-stem and cerebellum showed a very heavy infiltration. The malignant cells showed a prominent signet ring cell morphology (Fig 3F), were very strongly positive for Alcian blue stain (Fig 4A) and showed a similar immunohistochemistry as seen in the lung, i.e. positive for CK7 (Fig 4B), TTF1 (Fig 4C) and E-cadherin. The oculomotor (Figs 4D–F) and trochlear nerves were also infiltrated by malignant cells and showed destruction and myelin loss. Sections from the ***vertebrae*** showed total replacement of the bone marrow by malignant cells. The ***kidneys*** weighed 280 g. The capsular surface (Fig 5A) showed a moth eaten appearance and on cut section (Fig 5B) both the kidneys were infarcted in toto. The renal artery and veins at the hilum did not contain any thrombus. Microscopy revealed total infarction (Fig 5C), with all levels of arteries, i.e. interlobar, arcuate, intralobular, occluded by fibrin rich thrombi along with fibrinoid necrosis of the wall showing nuclear debris (Figs 5D and 6A). These thrombi were positive (deep red) for Marshall scarlet blue (MSB) stain, indicating them to be fibrin rich (Fig 6B). The glomerular capillaries, afferent and efferent arterioles showed extensive

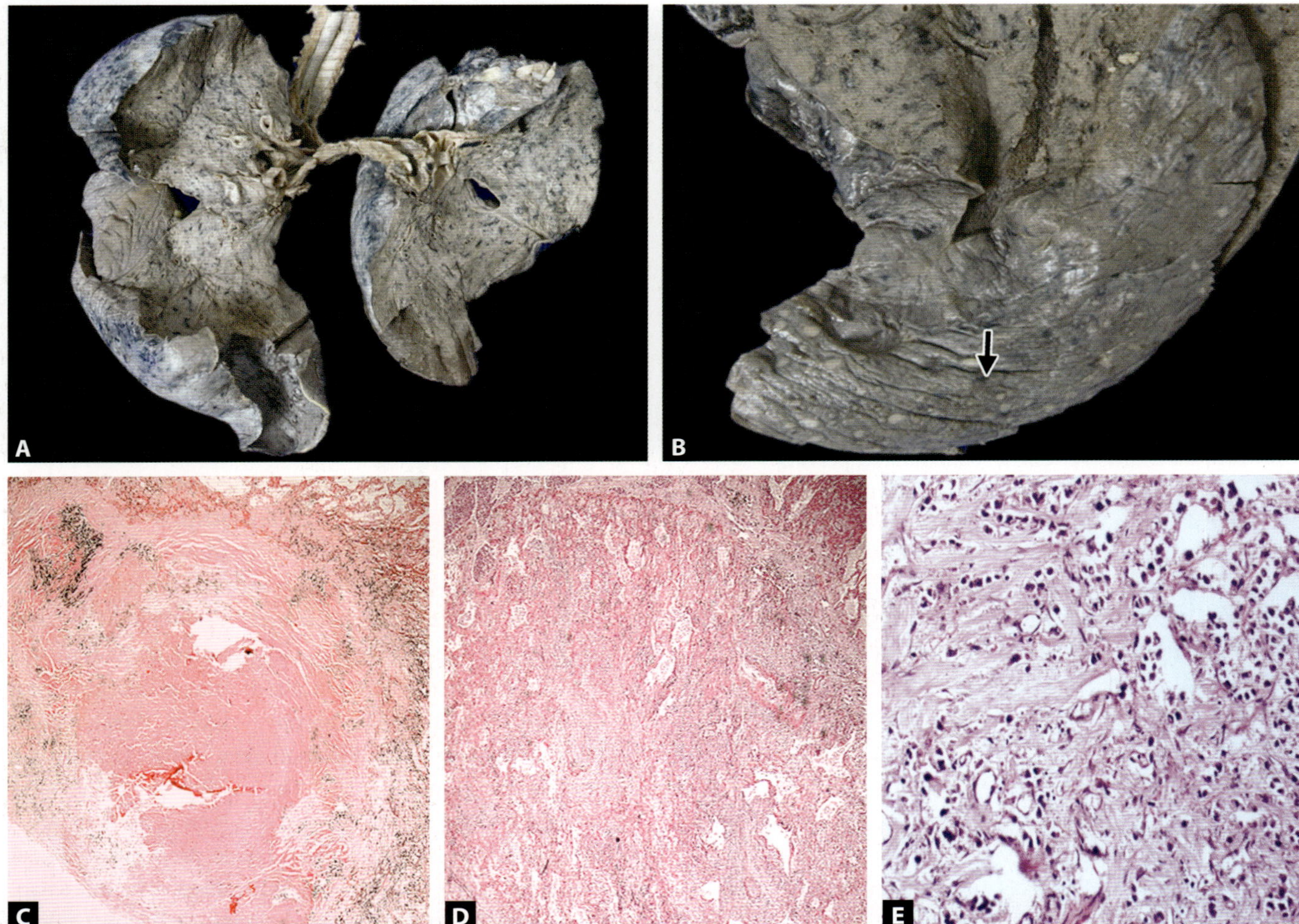

Figs 1A–E: (A) Cut section of both lungs which are subcrepitant and no tumor was identified; (B) Pleural aspect showing whitish specks (arrow); (C) Photomicrograph from the right upper lobe of lung showing old healing focus of tuberculosis; (D) Focus of firm, fibrotic area in the right upper lobe; and (E) Firm area showing tumor cells amidst the fibrosis.

fibrin thrombi with fibrinoid necrosis (Fig 6C) and MSB stain confirmed the fibrin (Fig 6D). Immunofluorescence was positive for fibrinogen in the arteries and in the glomerular capillary loops. Overall features were suggestive of thrombotic microangiopathy (TMA), i.e. atypical hemolytic uremic syndrome (HUS) with extensive infarction. The ***heart*** weighed 250 g. The right ventricular wall was 0.6 cm, indicating a right ventricular hypertrophy. The valves and chambers were normal. The apex of the left ventricle showed hemorrhagic discoloration of the myocardium. Left anterior descending artery, 3 cm from its origin showed a 50% occlusion, right coronary artery showed 30% narrowing with a stiff wall and left circumflex was within normal limits. Microscopy did not reveal any frank myocardial infarction but an early (<24 hours) myocardial infarction remains a possibility. Few smaller arteries in the myocardium, however, showed fibrin thrombi. The ***liver*** was enlarged and weighed 1,400 g. On microscopic examination diffuse macrovesicular steatosis was noted. No features of nonalcoholic fatty liver disease were seen. Other organs, i.e. the gastrointestinal tract, spleen, uterus, ovaries, adrenals and pancreas were within normal limits. The ***gall bladder*** was removed by a laparoscopic cholecystectomy, 2 months prior to the demise of the patient, at an outside health facility. The histopathology report was chronic cholecystitis with cholelithiasis.

FINAL AUTOPSY DIAGNOSIS: PM 26226

51 Years Female

- ***Microscopic adenocarcinoma of lung***: Solid predominant with mucin production with lymphangitic carcinomatosis (lung, peripancreatic area), pleural and lymph node (hilar/carinal) involvement.

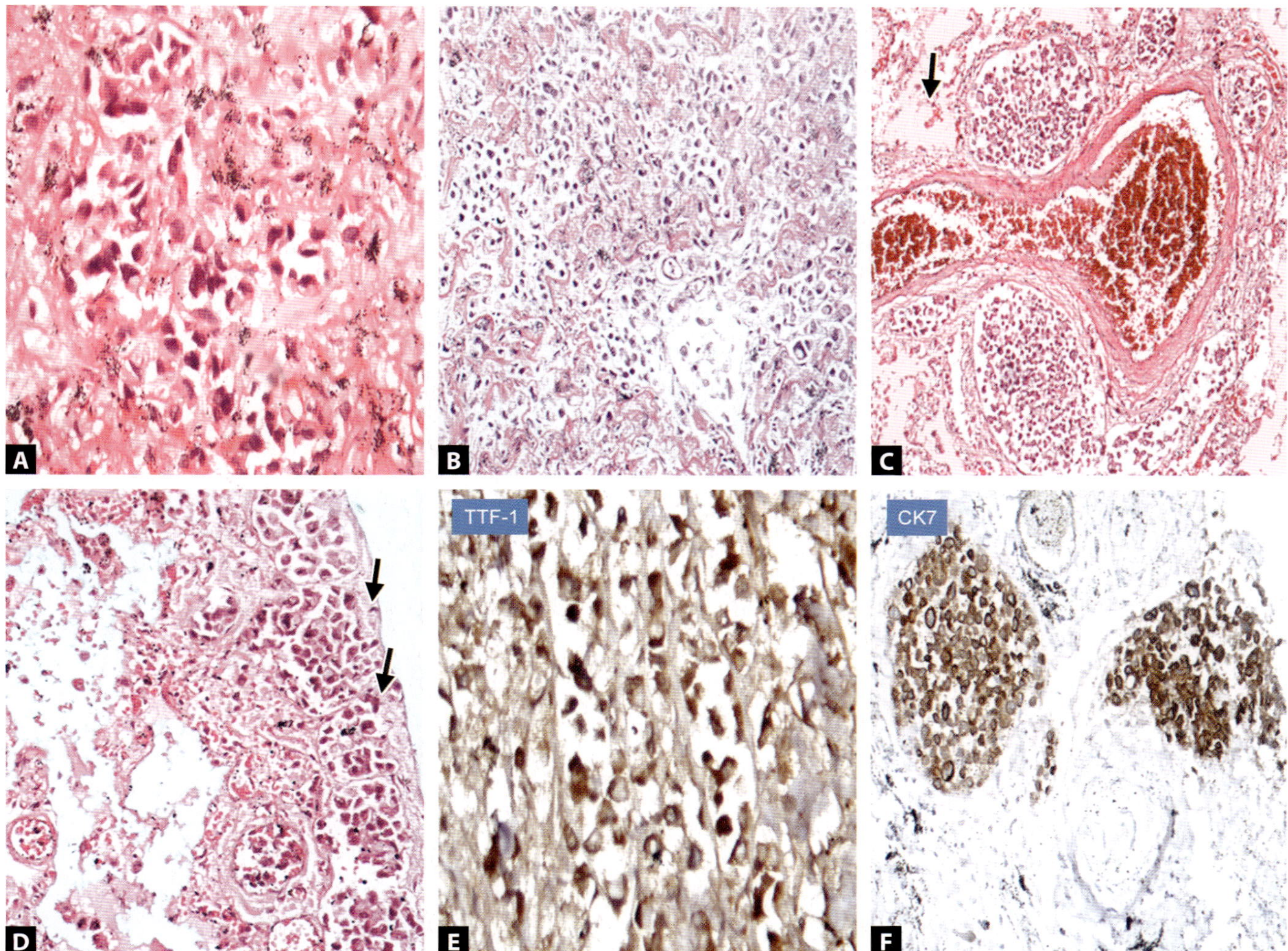

Figs 2A–F: Photomicrographs from the right lung. (A) Clusters of tumor cells seen amidst fibrosis, showing eccentric nucleus and cytoplasmic mucin; (B) Lepidic spread of tumor cells; (C) Lymphangitic spread of the tumor (arrow); (D) Lymphatics in the pleura loaded with tumor cells (arrows); (E) Tumor cells showing strong nuclear positivity for TTF-1; and (F) Tumor cells showing strong positivity for CK7.

- Meningeal carcinomatosis with involvement of oculomotor and trochlear nerves.
- Disseminated bone metastasis.
- Thrombotic microangiopathy—atypical HUS, leading to bilateral renal infarction.
- Early (<24 hours) inferior wall myocardial infarction.
- Diffuse macrovesicular steatosis—liver.
- Old healed focus of tuberculosis—right upper lobe.
- Bilateral pleural effusion and ascites.

ADENOCARCINOMA OF THE LUNG

Lung cancer is one of the most common cause of major cancer incidence and mortality worldwide.[1] Amongst this, adenocarcinoma is the most common histologic subtype, accounting for almost half of all cases of lung cancers.[2] It occurs at a younger age as compared to squamous cell carcinomas and the male to female ratio is approximately 2:1. Adenocarcinomas generally arise in the periphery of the bronchial tree and often disseminates into the pleural cavity leading to effusions. It has a great propensity to spread via the lymphatics, but hematogenous metastasis is also frequent. The incidence of intrapulmonary spread is highest in adenocarcinomas and occurs via the lymphatics, blood vessels and airways.

In 2011, Travis et al[3,4] assimilated the new classification system intended to support clinical practice, which was based on a multidisciplinary approach to the diagnosis of lung adenocarcinoma. The classification was developed by an international core panel of experts representing International

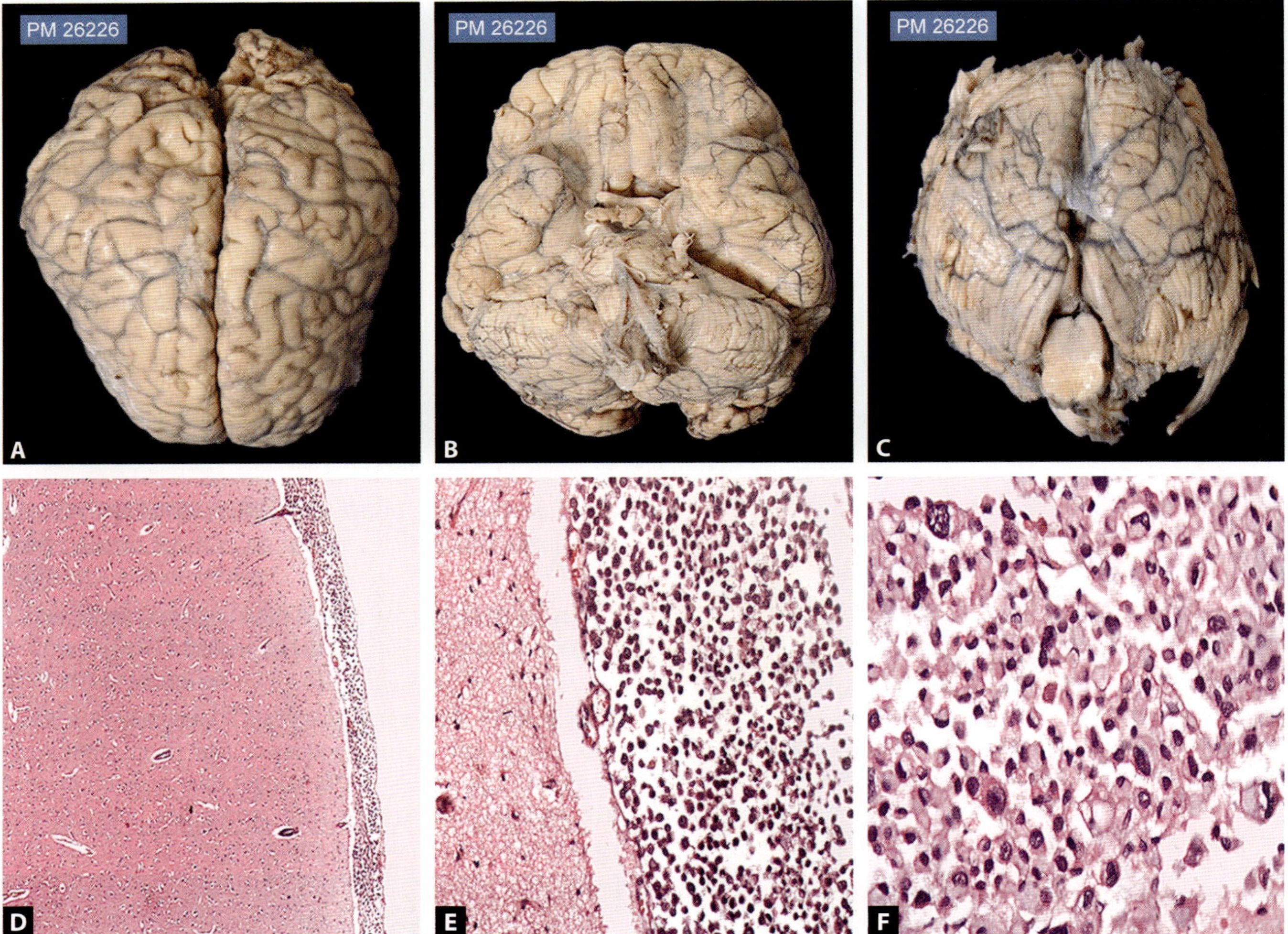

Figs 3A–F: Gross photographs of the brain showing an opalescent exudate diffusely covering the (A) Convexities; (B) Inferior orbital surface; (C) Cerebellum; (D–E) Meningeal carcinomatosis with the malignant cells clogging the leptomeninges; and (F) Tumor cells in the meninges showing signet-ring cell morphology.

Association for the Study of Lung Cancer (IASLC), American Thoracic Society (ATS) and European Respiratory Society (ERS) with contributions by oncologists, pulmonologists, pathologists, radiologists, molecular biologists and thoracic surgeons. This classification has played a very important role in clinical practice, in research investigations and clinical trials. The group recommended that patients with adenocarcinoma of lung, should be tested for epidermal growth factor receptor (EGFR) mutation, as it is a validated predictive marker for response and progression-free survival with EGFR tyrosine kinase inhibitors, in advanced disease. The terms bronchioloalveolar carcinoma (BAC) and mixed subtype adenocarcinoma are not used any more. For resected adenocarcinomas, new concepts of adenocarcinoma in situ and minimally invasive adenocarcinoma have been introduced which define patients having 100% disease-free survival after complete resection. Invasive adenocarcinomas are classified by the predominant pattern, be it lepidic, acinar, papillary or solid. The term "micropapillary" is added as a new histologic subtype with poor prognosis. Former mucinous BACs are now called "invasive mucinous adenocarcinoma". In resection specimens, they divided adenocarcinomas into:

- *Preinvasive lesions*:
  - Atypical adenomatous hyperplasia
  - Adenocarcinoma in situ (≤3 cm, formerly BAC):
    - Nonmucinous
    - Mucinous: Mixed mucinous/nonmucinous.
- *Minimally invasive adenocarcinoma (≤3 cm lepidic predominant tumor with ≤5 mm invasion)*:
  - Nonmucinous

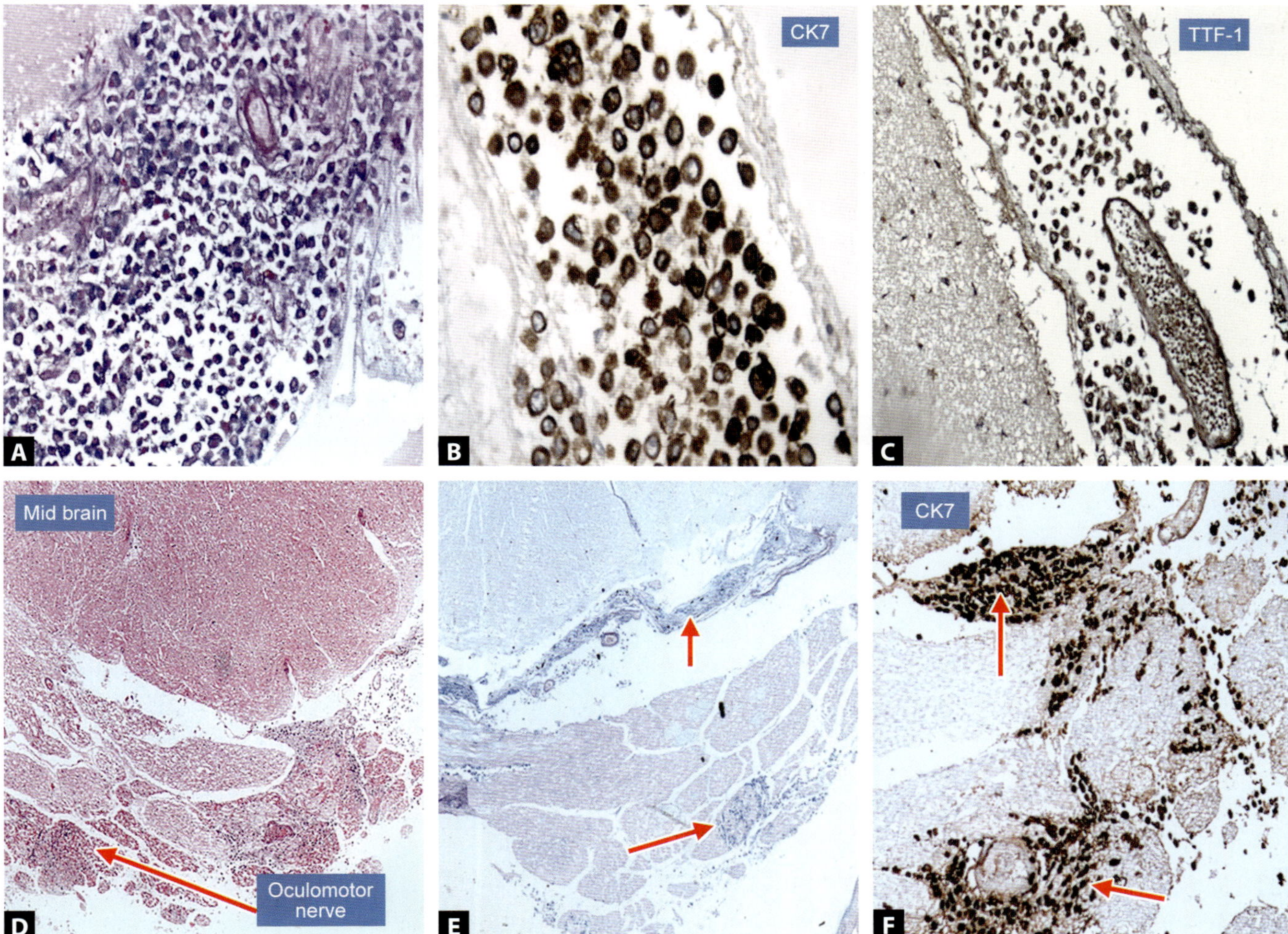

Figs 4A–F: Tumor cells in the meninges show strong positivity with (A) Alcian blue stain; (B) CK-7 immunostain; (C) TTF-1 immunostain; (D) Oculomotor nerve showing infiltration by tumor cells (arrow) which is seen better in (E) Alcian blue stain (arrows); and (F) CK7 immunostain (arrows).

- Mucinous
- Mixed mucinous/nonmucinous.

- *Invasive adenocarcinoma*:
  - Lepidic predominant (formerly nonmucinous BAC pattern, with >5 mm invasion)
  - Acinar predominant
  - Papillary predominant
  - Micropapillary predominant
  - Solid predominant with mucin production.
- *Variants of invasive adenocarcinoma*:
  - Invasive mucinous adenocarcinoma (formerly mucinous BAC)
  - Colloid
  - Fetal (low and high grade)
  - Enteric.

MENINGEAL CARCINOMATOSIS

Involvement of the leptomeninges[5] by metastatic tumors can be seen in solid tumors, where in the term "meningeal carcinomatosis" is used or is seen in lymphoproliferative malignant disease. It is most frequently seen in breast (3%) and lung adenocarcinomas (7%) as well as in melanomas (1.5%).[6] In cases of disseminated malignancy, meningeal carcinomatosis can present as the first manifestation of the disease in 5–10% of patients.[7] Mode of spread is from the blood, CSF or via nerve and vascular sheaths. Signs and symptoms are varied depending on involvement of the cerebral hemisphere, cranial nerves, spinal cord or the roots. Headache tops the list and isolated headache leading to the diagnosis of leptomeningeal metastasis from occult signet-ring cell adenocarcinoma of the transverse colon has

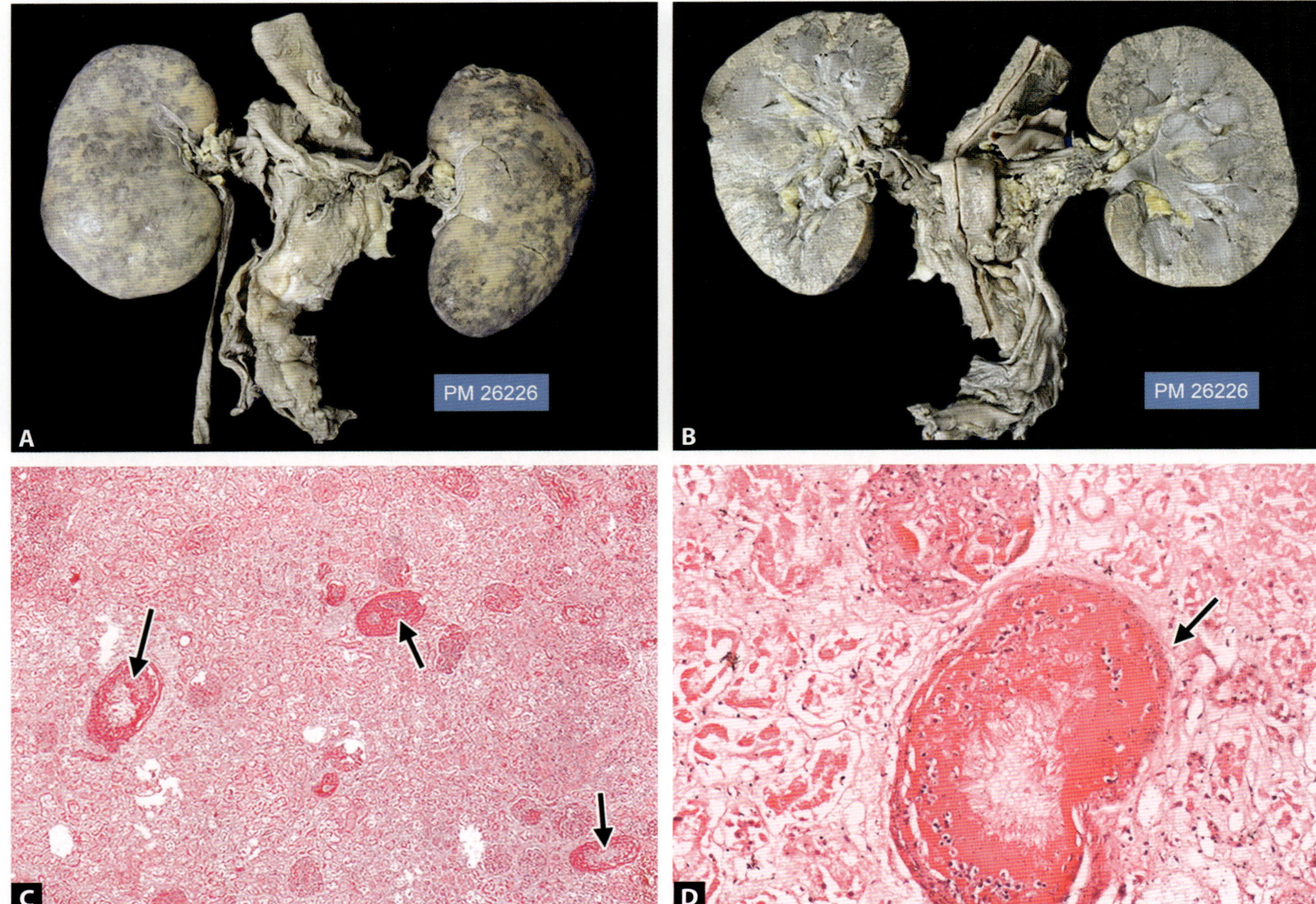

Figs 5A–D: (A) Capsular aspect of the kidneys showing a moth eaten appearance; (B) Cut section of both the kidneys showing infarction; (C) Photomicrograph of the kidney showing total infarction, with arteries occluded by fibrin rich thrombi (arrows); and (D) Intralobular artery occluded by a fibrin rich thrombus along with fibrinoid necrosis of the wall showing nuclear debris (arrow).

been reported.[8] Cranial nerve involvement[9] cause a variety of signs and symptoms depending on which nerve is involved. The most affected cranial nerves are III, IV, VI and VII. Optic nerve involvement leads to loss of vision and diplopia. Magnetic resonance imaging (MRI) shows leptomeningeal enhancement.[10] CSF examination can clinch the diagnosis if malignant cells are detected in the first sample, which happens in only 50% of patients.[11] At times repeat CSF sampling is usually needed, as was in the index case, where malignant cells were caught in the third lumbar puncture. Meningeal carcinomatosis is associated with a bad prognosis with a mean survival rate of 3–6 months.

THROMBOTIC MICROANGIOPATHY

Thrombotic microangiopathy[12-14] is a broad term characterized by microvascular endothelial injury and thrombosis. Under this broad umbrella, comes the typical HUS, atypical HUS and thrombotic thrombocytopenic purpura (TTP). In HUS, there occurs endothelial injury and activation with a secondary prothrombotic state. In typical HUS, the trigger is the shiga and shiga-like toxins produced by enteric pathogens. In atypical HUS, the etiology is multifactorial—nonenteric infections, genetic defects in compliment activation and regulation, drugs, bone marrow transplantation, antibody mediated rejection in transplantation, radiation, pregnancy/postpartum states, systemic sclerosis, autoimmune disorders like antiphospholipid antibody syndrome/SLE, malignant hypertension, neoplasms like mucin-secreting adenocarcinomas, rarely leukemia/lymphoma and idiopathic. TTP occurs due to increased thrombosis and secondary endothelial injury. The etiology is familial [mutations in gene encoding ADAMTS13—a von Willebrand factor (vWF) cleaving

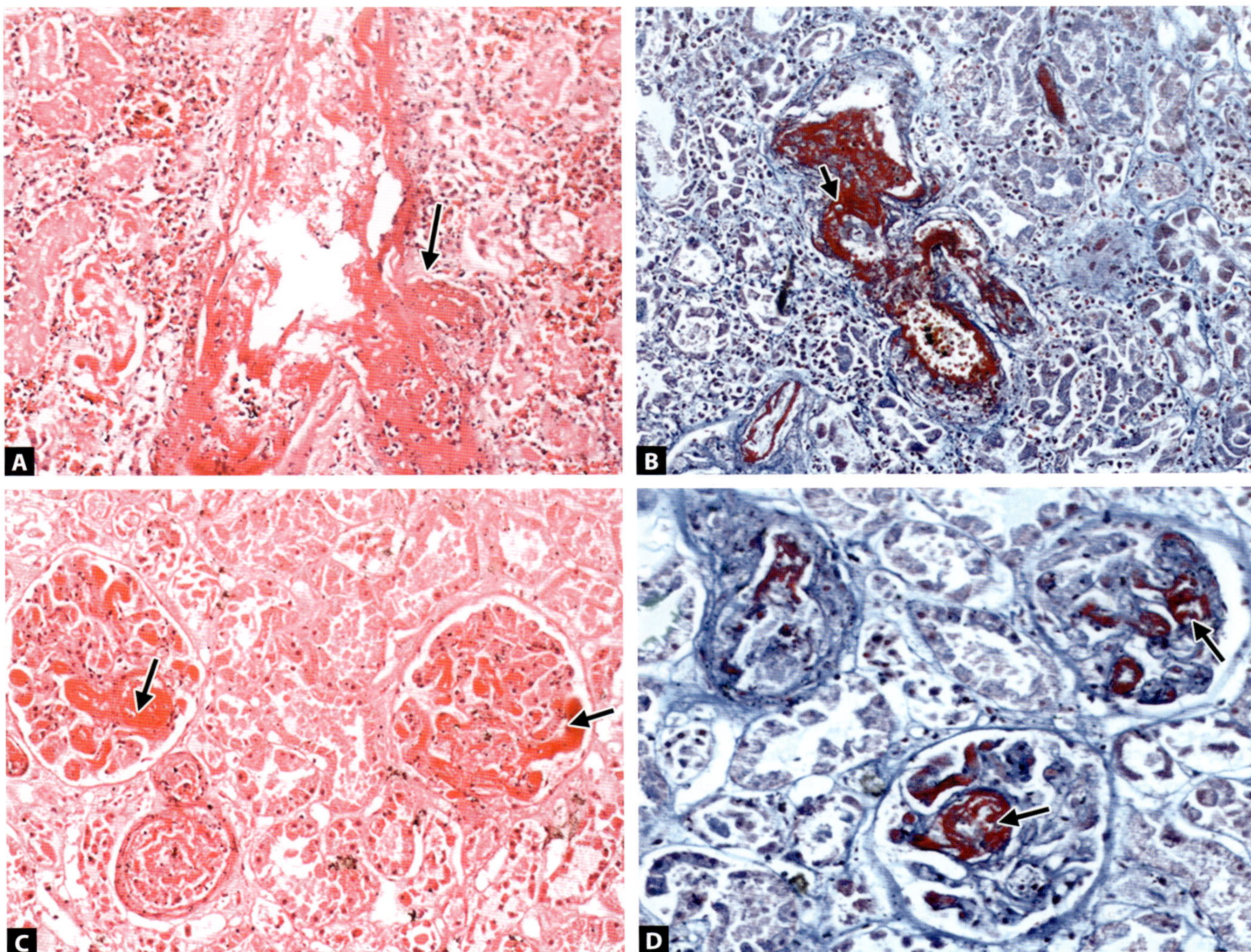

Figs 6A–D: (A) Interlobar artery (arrow) showing thrombus along with fibrinoid necrosis of the wall showing nuclear debris; (B) MSB stain, stains the fibrin deep red (arrow); (C) Glomerular capillaries clogged with fibrin thrombi (arrows) and show fibrinoid necrosis; and (D) MSB stain confirms the fibrin in the glomerular capillaries (arrows).

protease], autoimmune due to autoantibodies against ADAMTS13, drugs and idiopathic. The microscopic features of HUS and TTP seem to be virtually identical, but clinical presentation varies and is based on etiology. Atypical HUS has a significant clinical overlap with TTP and is referred to as, atypical HUS/TTP. TTP is said to have a poorer prognosis, involves multiple organs, affects the CNS significantly, less frequently and less severely involves the kidney and occurs in older individuals. Amorosi et al[15] enumerated the classic pentad of symptoms in TTP, which consists of fever, neurologic manifestations, thrombocytopenic purpura, microangiopathic hemolytic anemia and renal derangement. However, a review of a series of patients with TTP highlighted the fact that the classic pentad is present in only 40% of patients during the course of their illness.[16] This led to a change in the diagnostic criteria and now two principal clinical features, i.e. microangiopathic hemolytic anemia and thrombocytopenia, in the appropriate clinical context, are enough to diagnose TTP and the therapy can be initiated. This has further narrowed the gap between TTP and HUS.[17]

Acute presentation is seen in typical HUS, which presents with fever, watery diarrhea followed by bloody diarrhea, renal insufficiency and hypertension. A subset of atypical HUS (catastrophic APLA syndrome and scleroderma renal crisis) has abrupt onset of symptoms with no prodrome of diarrhea. Insidious presentation is seen in TTP and in a subset of atypical HUS, patients present with fever, microscopic hematuria, mild proteinuria, hypertension and chronic renal insufficiency. Neurological symptoms are prominently seen in TTP. Investigations reveal a microangiopathic hemolytic anemia, due to the RBC fragmentation and platelet consumption, that occurs when the blood flows through injured/narrowed blood vessels. So there is anemia, thrombocytopenia, more than 1% schistocytes in the peripheral blood, negative Coombs test, elevated lactate dehydrogenase and normal prothrombin and partial thromboplastin time. On gross examination, the kidneys in the acute phase are enlarged, show petechial hemorrhages on the surface and patchy cortical necrosis, which at times can be very extensive. In the chronic phase, the kidneys are small and granular. On microscopic examination, in acute TMA, the glomeruli show thickening of the capillary wall due to subendothelial expansion, endothelial swelling, bloodless appearance, thrombi with fibrinoid necrosis and nuclear debris. TTP thrombi are platelet rich, whereas HUS thrombi are fibrinogen rich. Tubulointerstitium shows acute tubular injury, edema and cortical necrosis in severe cases. Blood vessel changes are very prominent, arterioles at the hilum are affected frequently and show endothelial swelling, thrombi, fibrinoid necrosis without inflammatory infiltrate and luminal occlusion. Interlobular and arcuate arteries are also involved and show similar changes. Total infarction of both kidneys, as seen in our index case is rare.

Thrombotic microangiopathy occurs due to a chronic, uncontrolled, excessive activation of complement, which leads to platelet activation, endothelial injury, white cell recruitment and activation. Clinically, TMA from any etiology includes a thrombotic component and is distinct from DIC. However, patients with DIC and TMA share many features, including compliment activation, thrombocytopenia, microangiopathic hemolytic anemia, microvascular thrombosis leading to end organ ischemia, infarction and dysfunction, such as acute kidney injury.[18] But they arise from very different etiologies. Thus, when both TMA and DIC are operating in a given patient, it is difficult to say which mechanism is the dominant one, but the impact of both together would definitely be more catastrophic.

The course of many malignancies, particularly the mucin-secreting metastatic adenocarcinomas of lung, stomach and breast, can be complicated by TMA.[19] These patients present with an abrupt onset hemolytic anemia, with fall of hemoglobin, more than 1% schistocytes in peripheral blood and high reticulocyte count. There can be mild azotemia, but acute renal failure generally does not occur. Sometimes the clinical picture may resemble HUS or TTP. In addition to microangiopathic hemolytic anemia, coagulation studies frequently indicate DIC, which suggests a different pathogenetic mechanism from classic HUS. Usual autopsy findings are tumor emboli and fibrin microthrombi, mostly within small renal/pulmonary vessels, including arterioles and capillaries.[20]

COMMENTARY—INDEX CASE: PM 26226

This 51-year-old female presented with headache, vomiting, altered sensorium, fever and neck rigidity, shortness of breath and history of hematochezia. Investigations revealed disseminated bone metastasis, third CSF tap revealed meningeal carcinomatosis, microangiopathic hemolytic anemia, leukoerythroblastic picture, thrombocytopenia, deranged coagulogram, markedly deranged renal/liver function tests and high alkaline phosphatase. Autopsy revealed a microscopic, mucin producing, adenocarcinoma of right lung with florid lymphangitic/meningeal carcinomatosis, disseminated bone metastasis, TMA with DIC leading to total infarction of both kidneys. The lung adenocarcinoma was an occult one, both radiologically and also on gross examination. It was found adjacent to the healing foci of tuberculosis, possibly arose in a scarred area, as the tumor cells were seen amidst fibrosis. This tiny focus of tumor had produced widespread metastasis. Occult lung carcinomas occur mainly in the larger bronchus, but peripheral location is relatively rare. Tamura et al[21] studied 38 occult lung cancers in a 10-year-period and found only four, i.e. 10.5% in the peripheral region. These four cases of radiologically occult, peripheral lung carcinomas revealed venous invasion, widespread metastasis and thus a bad prognosis. Tamura et al[21] found positive staining in all their four cases of occult peripheral lung cancers with autocrine motility factor receptor (AMFR). This receptor binds autocrine motility factor which is a tumor-secreted cytokine that stimulates both random and directed cell migration.[22] Meningeal carcinomatosis is most frequently seen in breast, lung adenocarcinomas as well as in melanomas and is the first manifestation of systemic cancer in 5–10% of patients. In the index case, third and fourth cranial nerves were infiltrated by the tumor cells and these are the common nerves involved as reported in literature. In this case of mucin secreting, peripheral, occult, lung carcinoma with widespread dissemination, signs of both DIC and TMA (atypical HUS) were present. This combination, i.e. TMA along with DIC in a setting of malignancy has been reported in literature.[23] Blood coagulation parameters were deranged along with clinical sign of bleeding, i.e. hematochezia and this was indicative of overt DIC in the index case. However, the triad of microangiopathic hemolytic anemia, thrombocytopenia and 8% schistocytes in the peripheral blood pointed toward a TMA. In the setting of a mucin-secreting adenocarcinoma, atypical HUS is considered. The postmortem revealed totally infarcted kidneys with fibrin rich, thrombotic occlusion with fibrinoid necrosis, affecting all levels of arteries right from the interlobar to glomerular capillaries. Total infarction of both kidneys is generally not seen in atypical HUS, where cortical necrosis is generally reported. But, in the index case, the severity of the TMA along with superadded DIC, triggered by the underlying malignancy, could have caused this degree of devastation. DIC and TMA are said to be two distinct disorders with different pathogenesis. In cancer-associated DIC, abnormal procoagulant tissue factor produced by the tumor cells, acts on the endothelium, leading to activation of the extrinsic coagulation pathway through a complex binding with factor VII. On the other hand, cancer-associated TMA, caused injury of the endothelium with an enhanced release of ultra-large vWF multimers, which further lead to platelet activation, formation of microthrombi, red cell fragmentation and thrombocytopenia.

TAKE HOME MESSAGE

- Lung cancer is one of the most common cause of major cancer incidence and mortality worldwide and amongst this, adenocarcinoma is the most common histologic sub-type.
- The new classification of lung adenocarcinoma by Travis et al is intended to support clinical practice and is based on a multidisciplinary approach to the diagnosis of lung adenocarcinoma.
- Occult lung adenocarcinoma, both radiologically and on gross examination are very rare.
- The peripheral, occult lung cancers disseminate widely and are said to be positive of AMFR which binds autocrine motility factor, a tumor secreted cytokine that stimulates both random and directed cell migration.
- Meningeal carcinomatosis is most frequently seen in breast/lung adenocarcinomas as well as in melanomas and is the first manifestation of systemic cancer in 5–10% of patients.
- A combination of TMA along with DIC in a setting of malignancy as seen in this case, led to total infarction of both kidneys and acute renal shutdown.

REFERENCES

1. Boyle P, Levin B. World Cancer Report 2008. Lyon: International Agency for Research on Cancer; 2008.
2. Curado MP, Edwards B, Shin HR, et al. Cancer Incidence in Five Continents. Lyon: IARC Scientific Publications; 2007.
3. Travis WD, Brambilla E, Noguchi M, et al. International association for the study of lung cancer/American Thoracic Society/European Respiratory Society International Multi-disciplinary Classification of Lung Adenocarcinoma. J Thorac Oncol. 2011;6:244-85.
4. Travis WD, Brambilla E, Noguchi M, et al. Diagnosis of lung adenocarcinoma in resected specimens: implications of the 2011 International Association for the Study of Lung Cancer/ American Thoracic Society/European Respiratory Society classification. Arch Pathol Lab Med. 2013;137:685-704.
5. Sabater AL, Sadaba LM, de Nova E. Ocular symptoms secondary to meningeal carcinomatosis in a patient with lung adenocarcinoma: a case report. BMC Ophthalmology. 2012;12:65.
6. Gleissner B, Chamberlain MC. Neoplastic meningitis. Lancet Neurol. 2006;5:443-52.
7. Chamberlain MC. Neoplastic meningitis. J Clin Oncol. 2005; 23:3605-13.
8. Kleinfeld K, Peters WH, Stephenson C, et al. Leptomeningeal metastasis from occult signet-ring cell colon adenocarcinoma presenting with isolated headache. J Clin Neurosci. 2013; 20:890-2.
9. Kato Y, Takeda H, Dembo T, et al. Progressive multiple cranial nerve palsies as the presenting symptom of meningeal carcinomatosis from occult colon adenocarcinoma. Intern Med. 2012;51:795-7.
10. Sze G, Soletsky S, Bronen R, et al. MR imaging of the cranial meninges with emphasis on contrast enhancement and meningeal carcinomatosis. AJNR Am J Neuroradiol. 1989;10:965-75.
11. Wasserstrom WR, Glass JP, Posner JB. Diagnosis and treatment of leptomeningeal metastases from solid tumors: experience with 90 patients. Cancer. 1982;49:759-72.
12. Sánchez-Corral P, Melgosa M. Advances in understanding the aetiology of atypical haemolytic uraemic syndrome. Br J Haematol. 2010;150:529-42.
13. Noris M, Remuzzi G. Atypical hemolytic-uremic syndrome. N Engl J Med. 2009;361:1676-87.
14. Schneider M. Thrombotic microangiopathy (TTP and HUS): advances in differentiation and diagnosis. Clin Lab Sci. 2007;20:216-20.
15. Amorosi EL, Ultmann JE. Thrombotic thrombocytopenic purpura: report of 16 cases and review of the literature. Medicine. 1966;45:139-59.
16. Ridolfi RL, Bell WR. Thrombotic thrombocytopenic purpura: report of 25 cases and review of the literature. Medicine. 1981;60:413-28.
17. Terrell DR, Williams LA, Vesely SK, et al. The incidence of thrombotic thrombocytopenic purpura-hemolytic uremic syndrome: all patients, idiopathic patients and patients with severe ADAMTS-13 deficiency. J Thromb Haemost. 2005; 3:1432-6.

18. Kurosawa S, Stearns-Kurosawa DJ. Compliment, thrombotic microangiopathy and disseminated intravascular coagulation. J Intensive Care. 2014;2:65. DOI 10.1186/s40560-014-0061-4.
19. Lesesne JB, Rothschild N, Erickson B, et al. Cancer-associated hemolytic-uremic syndrome: Analysis of 85 cases from a national registry. J Clin Oncol. 1989;7:781-9.
20. Lohrmann HP, Adam W, Heymer B, et al. Microangiopathic hemolytic anemia in metastatic carcinoma. Report of eight cases. Ann Intern Med. 1973;79:368-75.
21. Tamura M, Ohta Y, Oda M, et al. Peripherally located occult lung cancer with AMFR expression. Ann Thorac Cardiovasc Surg. 2003;9:184-7.
22. Kara M, Ohta Y, Tanaka Y, et al. Autocrine motility factor receptor expression in patients with stage I non-small cell lung cancer. Ann Thorac Surg. 2001;71:944-8.
23. Robier C, Neubuer M, Beham-Schmid C, et al. Thrombotic microangiopathy and disseminated intravascular coagulation associated with carcinocythemia in a patient with breast cancer. J Clin Oncol. 2011;29:e825-6.

CONTRIBUTIONS BY:

1. Dr Varun Dhir, Additional Professor, Department of Internal Medicine (Compilation of Clinical Details)
2. Dr KL Gupta, Professor and Head, Department of Nephrology (Clinician In-Charge)
3. Dr Jasmina Ahluwalia, Professor, Department of Hematology (Hematologist In-Charge)
4. Dr Navneet Sharma, Professor, Department of Internal Medicine (Clinician In-Charge)
5. Dr Manphool Singhal, Additional Professor, Radiodiagnosis and Imaging

Post Graduate Institute of Medical Education and Research, Chandigarh, India.

CASE 13

Young Male with Occult, Diffuse Type, Mucin-secreting Adenocarcinoma of the Stomach with Extensive Lymphangitic Carcinomatosis, Presenting with Deep Vein Thrombosis and Pulmonary Embolism: PM 21829

Nandita Bharadwaj Kakkar

HIGHLIGHTS OF THE CASE

This is a case of a 35-year-old male, who came with pain and swelling of lower limbs, abdominal distention, decreased urine output, progressive dyspnea, effusions, renal failure and hyperbilirubinemia. The clinical diagnosis was bilateral deep vein thrombosis (DVT) (femoropopliteal veins) with venous thromboembolism to the inferior vena cava, renal veins and lungs. Autopsy revealed a mucin-secreting adenocarcinoma (diffuse type) of the stomach, pulmonary thromboembolism, florid pulmonary lymphangitic carcinomatosis and non-bacterial endocarditis with splenic and renal infarcts.

***Keywords*:** Occult, adenocarcinoma, mucin secreting, diffuse type, stomach, lymphangitic carcinomatosis, progressive dyspnea, DVT, thromboembolic disease, nonbacterial thrombotic endocarditis.

CLINICAL DETAILS

Date of Admission: 27.01.2007, Date of Death: 05.02.2007, Duration of Hospital Stay: 9 Days

A 35-year-old male came with pain and swelling in lower limbs since one month, abdominal distention since 20 days, decreased urine output and breathlessness since 15 days. The pain and swelling started from the left limb and went on to involve the right side. It began from the ankles and then progressed to involve both lower limbs. He subsequently developed abdominal distention which increased rapidly. There was no vomiting, constipation or diarrhea. There was decreased urine output without any dysuria, pyuria or graveluria. There was yellowish discoloration of urine but no pruritis or passage of clay colored stool. He was also having gradually progressive shortness of breath 2 weeks prior to hospitalization, but there was no orthopnea, paroxysmal nocturnal dyspnea, cough, chest pain, fever or altered sensorium. There was no history of tuberculosis, diabetes mellitus, hypertension or any chronic lung/liver disease. He was a chronic alcoholic, consuming 150–180 g/week and a chronic smoker since 10 years. On ***examination***, he was conscious, afebrile, dyspneic, BP—110/80 mm Hg, pulse rate—84 beats/min, respiratory rate—24 breaths/min, no stigmata of chronic liver disease, axillary lymph node 1×1 cm. Respiratory system examination revealed decreased air entry in bilateral bases. Cardiovascular and central nervous system examination were normal. The abdomen was distended, tense with no visible tortuous veins, organomegaly was difficult to appreciate, free fluid was present and bowel sounds were sluggish.

Investigations

***Hemogram*:** Hb—12.8 g/dL; TLC increased from 8,000 to 27,800/μL; platelets —250,000/μL.

***Blood biochemistry*:** Serum urea—gradually increased from 94 to 228 mg%; serum creatinine—gradually increased from 1 to 4.2 mg%; total protein/serum albumin—5.8/3 gms; serum calcium—10.3 mg%; total bilirubin/conjugated fraction increased from 2.0/1.2 to 9.0/3.9 mg%; SGOT—21 U/L. SGPT—80 U/L; serum alkaline phosphatase—80 U/L.

***Ascitic fluid*:** Cells—440, DLC P60 L40, protein—4.1 g/dL, sugar 82 mg/dL, culture sterile, SAAG—0.8 g/dL, i.e. low, ADA—24 IU/L, i.e. normal, no malignant cells.

***Pleural fluid*:** TLC-410, DLC—predominant polymorphs, protein—4.2 g/dL, sugar—53 mg/dL, i.e. normal, ADA—24 IU/L, i.e. normal, SAAG—0.5 g/dL, i.e. low.

Blood culture x 3 sterile; Serology—HIV, HbsAg, anti-HCV –ve; G6PD—N; urine Hb—nil; routine urine: albumin +, sugar—nil, no pus cells/RBC seen, granular casts present.

***Radiology*:** Chest X-ray—normal; Abdominal X-ray—dilated loops seen; Ultrasonography abdomen—liver, gallbladder, spleen and kidneys normal in size and outline. Gross ascites present; Compression ultrasonography: bilateral femoral and popliteal deep vein thrombosis (DVT); CT angiography: subsegmental pulmonary thromboembolism; Doppler ultrasonography abdomen: attenuated, monophasic flow pattern in hepatic veins and inferior vena cava. MRI and MRV abdomen: hepatomegaly with no focal lesion, thrombosis of suprarenal part of inferior vena cava extending downward with gross ascites and pleural effusion, common hepatic and bile ducts dilated. Spleen, pancreas and kidneys are normal.

***Electrocardiography*:** Sinus tachycardia, echocardiography shows dilated RA/RV, no regional wall motion abnormality (RWMA), clot or effusion.

***Upper gastrointestinal endoscopy*:** Edematous mucosal folds with superficial erosions and ulcers with pigmented base. No growth was identified.

Course in hospital*:** This young male with bilateral DVT (femoropopliteal) and thromboembolism was treated with heparin infusion with regular aPTT monitoring. The patient was dyspneic and ascitic fluid analysis showed high TLC with low SAAG, for which he was started on cefixime and moxifloxacin injection. Meanwhile the patient developed vomiting with altered blood and features of ileus. Abdominal X-ray did not show any perforation and a possibility of mesenteric vein thrombosis with mesenteric ischemia was kept. The patient continued to have fever and antibiotics were changed to piperacillin/tazobactam and linezolid. He had dyspnea, tachypnea and renal failure for which he was on continuous oxygen supplementation and conservative management. The patient however sustained a cardiopulmonary arrest from which he could not be revived. The unit's ***clinical diagnosis was—bilateral DVT of femoropopliteal veins with venous thromboembolism to the inferior vena cava, renal veins and lungs along with acute renal failure.

AUTOPSY FINDINGS: PM 21829

A complete autopsy (abdominothoracic with brain) was performed on this 35-year-old male. The peritoneal and pleural cavities yielded 1,500 mL and 200 mL of straw colored fluid respectively. ***Stomach*** (Figs 1A–D): A firm infiltrative growth was seen in the antrum along the greater curvature, measuring 3 × 2 × 2 cm, which was growing transmurally and could be seen on the serosal aspect. Microscopic sections (Figs 1E and F and Fig 2A) revealed a poorly differentiated adenocarcinoma—diffuse type, with a clear cut origin from the gastric mucosa. There were areas wherein the tumor was present as glands and in islands with prominent mucin production. The mucin stained deep blue with Alcian blue stain (Figs 2B and C). The tumor was seen to extend transmurally and was forming tumor nodules on the serosal aspect. Extensive lymphatic emboli, i.e. lymphangitic carcinomatosis, was noted in the adjacent normal stomach (Figs 2D–F). Immunohistochemistry (Figs 3A–B) revealed positivity with CK7 and CD20, thereby substantiating the foregut origin. The tumor was extending into the duodenum (Fig 3C) and was infiltrating it transmurally to invade the pancreas (Fig 3D). ***Omentum*** (Figs 3E–G) was thick, cake like and microscopy revealed extensive tumor deposits along with tumor packed lymphatics. The loops of the ***small intestine*** were badly adherent and could not be dissected out (Fig 4A). On microscopic examination (Fig 4B) the serosal aspect of the small and large intestine was plastered by the tumor, what is known as peritoneal carcinomatosis. At places the tumor was infiltrating into the muscularis propria of the small and large gut. The external surface of the ***pancreas*** was plastered by a layer of whitish membrane which on microscopy revealed tumor deposits. The serosal aspect of the ***gallbladder*** also showed tumor deposits. The ***lungs*** (Fig 4C) were heavy and weighed 1,010 g. Pleura was thickened and shaggy. Cut section of the lungs was firm but did not reveal any focal lesion. The right lobar artery and its branches were occluded by thrombus. No infarct was noted. Sections from the lung revealed pleural lymphatics (Figs 4D–F) clogged by tumor cells and in areas the pleura was plastered by a thick layer of tumor cells. Florid lymphangitic carcinomatosis with peribronchial and alveolar spread of the tumor was noted (Figs 5A–C). The right lobar artery contained a tumor thrombus (Figs 5D and E) and another branch contained an organizing thrombus (Fig 5F). ***Liver*** (Figs 6A–D) was enlarged, weighed 1,600 g and was bile stained. No focal lesion was noted. No thrombi were seen in the hepatic veins and portal vein. Microscopy revealed expanded portal tracts with tumor occluding the lymphatics. Ductular proliferation with cholestasis in the portal ductules and periportal hepatocytes were noted. ***Spleen*** (Figs 6E and F) was enlarged (250 g) and showed areas of infarction on the capsular aspect and on cut section. On microscopy, showed tumor deposits and areas of infarction. Apart from this, metastasis was seen in the abdominal ***lymph nodes*** [mesenteric, peripancreatic, portal, para-aortic, gastric and celiac (Fig 7A)] and ***bone marrow*** (Fig 7B). The ***heart*** (Fig 7C) weighed 260 g. The mitral valve showed tiny irregular, firm, warty, whitish, vegetations attached above the line of closure of the valve. The valve itself was

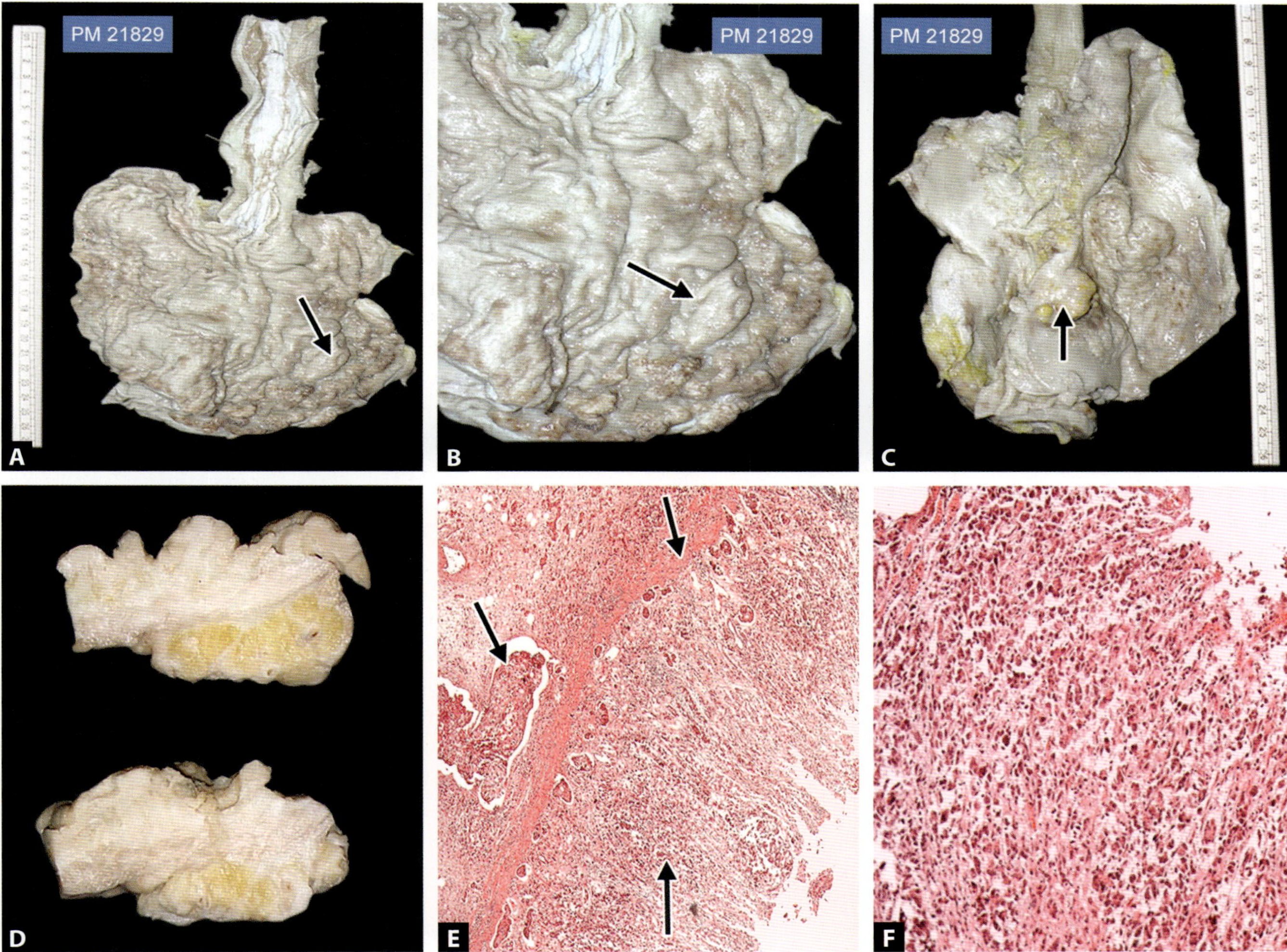

Figs 1A–F: (A and B) Gross specimen of the stomach and esophagus showing a firm mass measuring 3 × 2 × 2 cm (arrows) in the antrum along the greater curvature (arrow); (C) Serosal aspect of the stomach showing the mass protruding out and forming a protuberance on this surface (arrow); (D) Cut section of the stomach at the level of the mass showing firm white thickening of the entire wall. Photomicrograph of the stomach; (E) Showing origin of the tumor from the mucosa (lower arrow) along with extensive lymphatic involvement along the muscularis mucosae (upper arrow) and also seen in the submucosa (middle arrow); and (F) Mucosa of the stomach showing origin of poorly differentiated diffuse type of adenocarcinoma.

normal. Other valves, chambers and the coronaries were normal. Microscopy of the vegetations confirmed the presence of nonbacterial thrombotic endocarditis (NBTE) (Fig 7D). The ***kidneys*** weighed 360 g. The external surface of both kidneys showed blotchy congestion (Fig 7E). The left kidney showed an infarct 2 × 2 × 1 cm (Fig. 7F). The renal vessels and inferior vena cava did not show any thrombus at this point of time. ***Kidney*** showed changes of early acute tubular necrosis. The ***brain*** on gross examination revealed subarachnoid ooze in the left frontoparietal region, measuring 4 × 4 cm. The deep veins of the legs could not be dissected out due to lack of permission.

FINAL AUTOPSY DIAGNOSIS: PM 21829

35 Years Male with Femoropopliteal Deep Vein Thrombosis

- Mucin secreting adenocarcinoma (diffuse type) of stomach with contiguous spread to the duodenum, pancreas and metastasis to the lungs (florid lymphangitic carcinomatosis), lymph nodes (gastric, celiac, mesenteric, peripancreatic, portal, para-aortic), liver, spleen, peritoneum (peritoneal carcinomatosis) and bone marrow.
- Nonbacterial thrombotic endocarditis.
- Infarcts—spleen and kidney.
- Pulmonary thromboembolism with pulmonary hemorrhage.

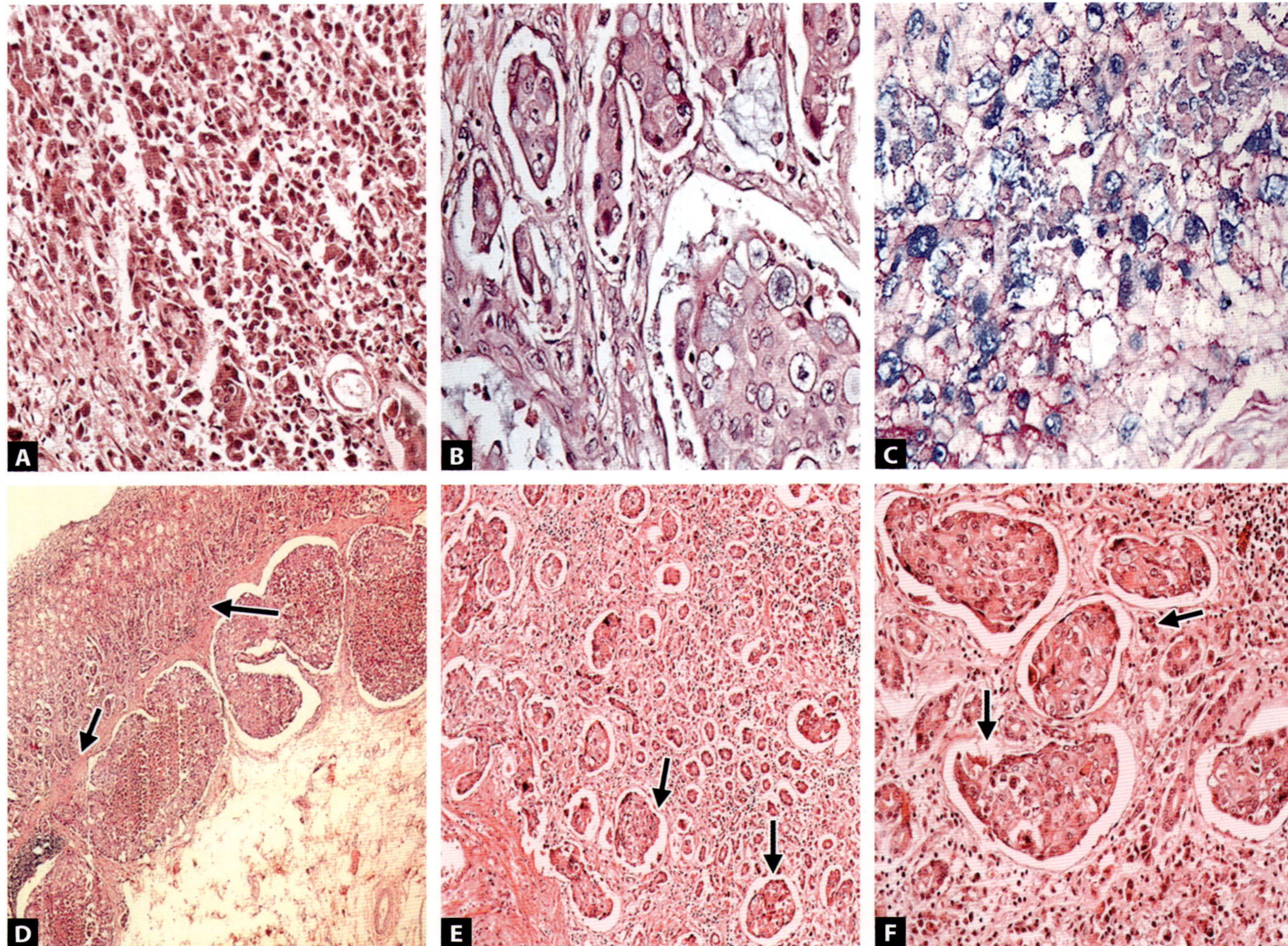

Figs 2A–F: Photomicrographs of the stomach showing (A) Poorly differentiated, diffuse type of adenocarcinoma; (B) Tumor cells in islands and vague glands showing mucin production; (C) Mucin shows strong positivity with Alcian blue stain; and (D–F) Photomicrograph of the adjacent grossly normal stomach showing extensive lymphangitic carcinomatosis (arrows) in the submucosa and mucosa.

LYMPHANGITIC CARCINOMATOSIS

Lymphangitic carcinomatosis as the name suggests, is spread of tumor via the lymphatics, thus leading to their obstruction. It was first described by Gabriel Andrai in 1829. This mode of spread can occur anywhere in the body, but is most commonly seen in the lungs and the patients present with progressively increasing dyspnea and a nonproductive cough. At times, the onset of respiratory symptoms precedes the diagnosis of the primary tumor, as in the index case. The tumor clogs the lymphatics and spreads into the adjacent interstitial tissue, resulting in thickening of the bronchovascular bundles and septae. The tumor cells invoke a desmoplastic reaction and the edema fluid leads to dilatation of the lymphatics, thus contributing to the interstitial widening. The tumor cells can also spread to the adjacent lung parenchyma leading to a nodular pattern. The most common tumors (80% are adenocarcinomas) that spread in this peculiar way are those from the breasts, stomach, lungs, pancreas and prostate. Patients with lymphangitic carcinomatosis have a dismal prognosis with an average survival of approximately 3 months. These patients are mostly misdiagnosed as having interstitial lung disease or sarcoidosis. Thus, in patients with progressive dyspnea, lymphangitic carcinomatosis must be kept in the differential diagnosis and ruled out. A lung biopsy can clinch the diagnosis.

DEEP VEIN THROMBOSIS IN MALIGNANCY

Patients with various cancers are at risk of developing a hypercoagulable state due to release of procoagulants by the

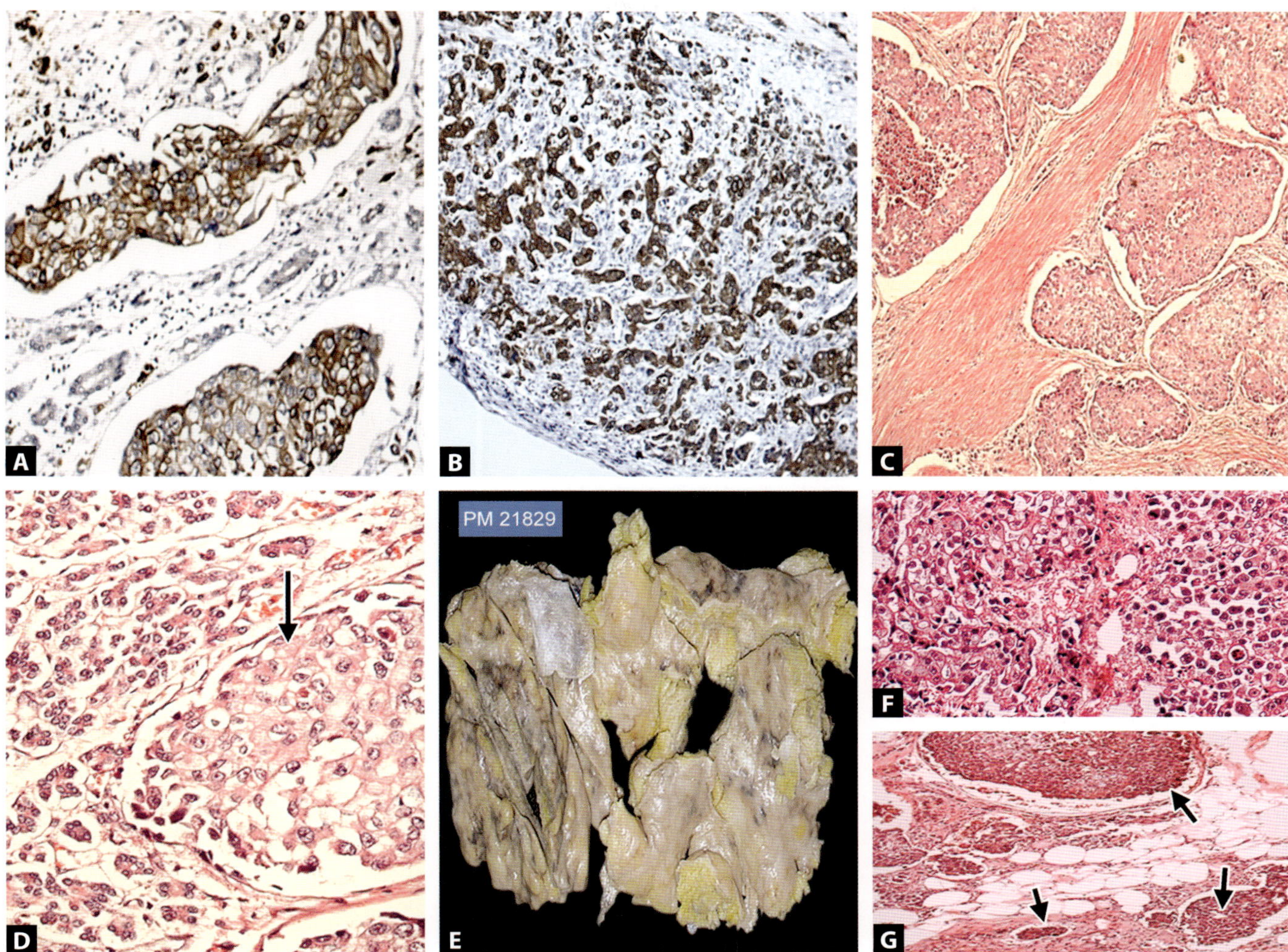

Figs 3A–G: (A) CK7 positivity in the tumor cells; (B) CK20 positivity in the tumor cells; (C) Tumor infiltrating the duodenum; (D) Tumor island (arrow) seen amidst the pancreatic acini; (E) Gross photograph of the omentum which appears thick and cake like with areas of hemorrhage; (F) Photomicrograph of the omentum showing tumor deposits; and (G) Omentum showing extensive lymphatic emboli (arrows).

tumor. This predisposes to DVT and subsequent pulmonary embolism (PE) and death. Brain tumors, multiple myeloma, pancreatic and gastric cancer have the highest risk for DVT and PE. A well-validated tool, i.e. "the Khorana score", is used to calculate risk for DVT and PE in patients with cancer. A score of more than or equal to 3 is the highest risk category, with a 7% chance of DVT/PE within 2.5 months (median). Thus patients with cancer are put on anticoagulation prophylaxis and monitored. At times the DVT is the first sign and after a thorough evaluation the malignancy comes to light. Thus, all patients with idiopathic DVT should be screened for occult malignancy.

The Trousseau sign of malignancy or Trousseau's syndrome was first described by Armand Trousseau in the 1860s, during the course of his own illness with pancreatic cancer. This syndrome describes recurrent signs of thrombophlebitis occurring due to blood clots at different locations in the superficial veins, which appears as a painful nodule under the skin. This is a rare manifestation of venous thromboembolism and is particularly seen with pancreatic, gastric and lung cancers and could be the first manifestation of the disease. This is not to be confused with Trousseau sign of latent tetany occurring due to hypocalcemia.

NONBACTERIAL THROMBOTIC ENDOCARDITIS

As the name suggests, this is a deposition of sterile small masses of fibrin, platelets and blood components usually attached to the heart valves at the lines of closure. Also

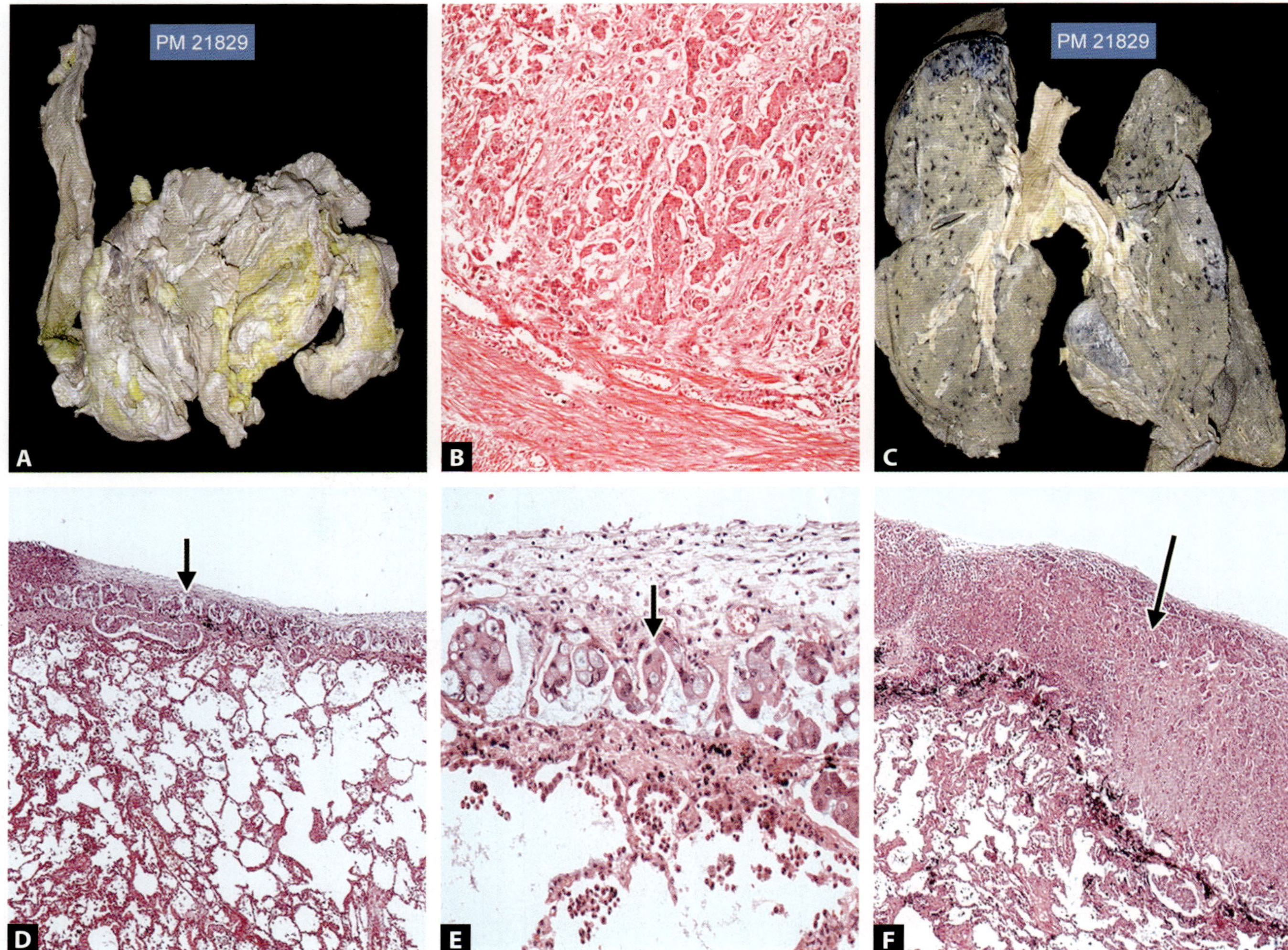

Figs 4A–F: (A) Coiled up loops of the small and large intestine; (B) The serosal aspect of the intestine plastered by the tumor; (C) Gross picture of the cut section of the lungs showing no focal lesion; (D–E) The pleural aspect of the lung showing extensive lymphangitic carcinomatosis (arrows); and (F) Pleural aspect of the lung plastered by a thick band of tumor (arrow). The alveolar spaces can be seen below it.

known as marantic endocarditis or bland vegetations. They are seen in debilitated patients with malignancies or sepsis. They do not cause any problems to the valves, as they are small, nondestructive, but can dislodge and embolize to various organs, thus producing infarcts. In the index case, the NBTE was seen on the mitral valve and they got dislodged and produced infarcts in the spleen and the kidney. Histologically, they are composed of bland fibrin with no inflammation. It is seen that in a large number of cases, NBTE occurs along with PE, thus substantiating the point that a hypercoagulable state is the common denominator. This occurs in cancers, especially mucin secreting adenocarcinomas, proving the point that the circulating mucin has a procoagulant effect. NBTE can be seen in acute promyelocytic leukemia, debilitating states like sepsis, burns, hyperestrogenic states and in endocardial trauma due to indwelling catheters.

COMMENTARY—INDEX CASE: PM 21829

This was a young male, who came with pain and swelling of lower limbs, abdominal distention, decreased urine output and progressive dyspnea. There was ascites, pleural effusion, renal failure and hyperbilirubinemia. Radiologic investigations revealed bilateral femoropopliteal DVT and subsegmental pulmonary thromboembolism. Autopsy revealed an occult, diffuse type, mucin secreting adenocarcinoma of the stomach with florid lymphangitic carcinomatosis (in the

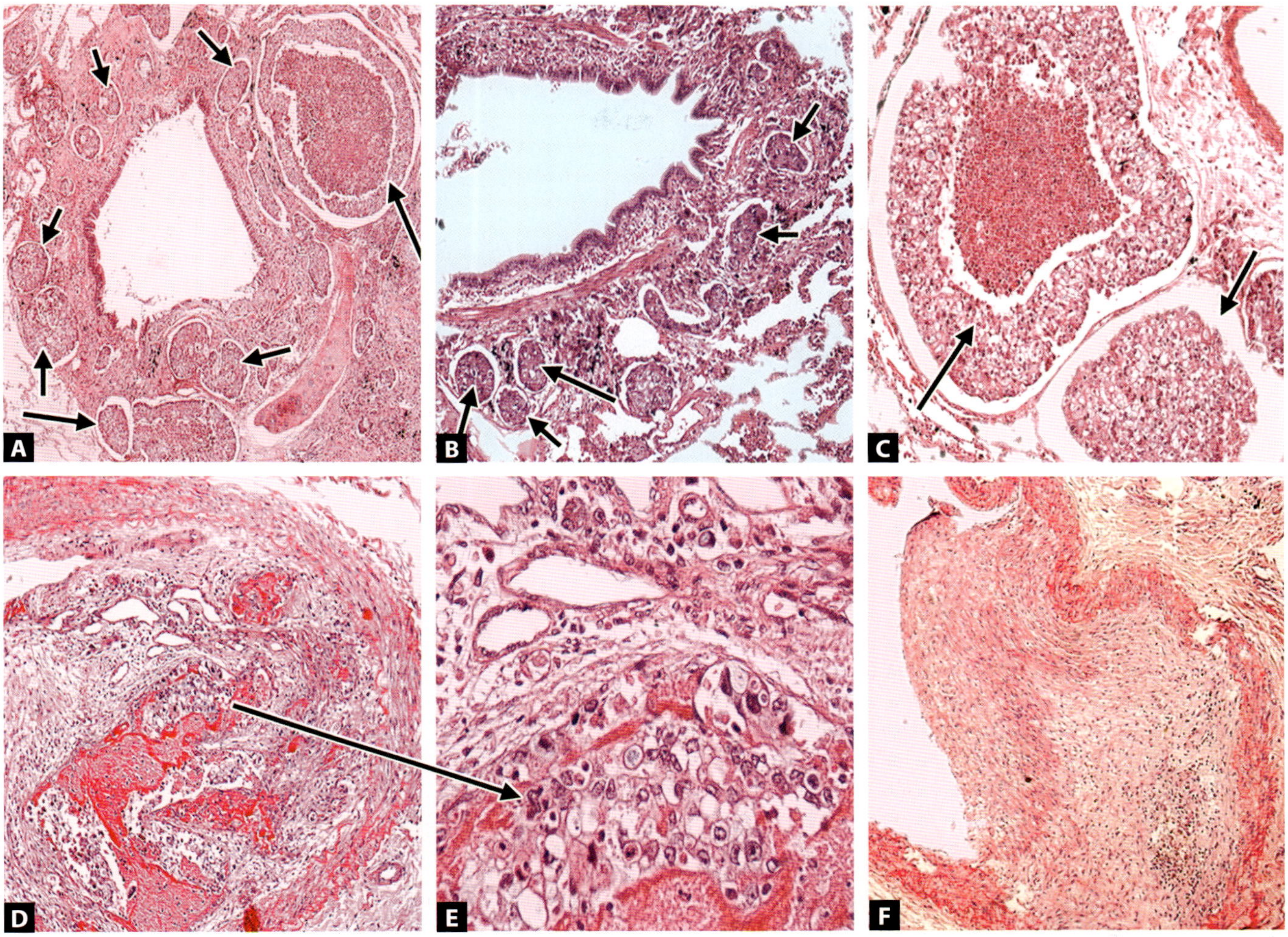

Figs 5A–F: Photomicrographs of the lung (A–C) Showing florid lymphangitic carcinomatosis in the peribronchial location with the tumor cells clogging the lymphatic spaces (arrows); (D–E) Lobar artery clogged by a tumor thrombus (arrow); and (F) A large pulmonary artery clogged by an organizing thrombus composed of fibrin but no tumor.

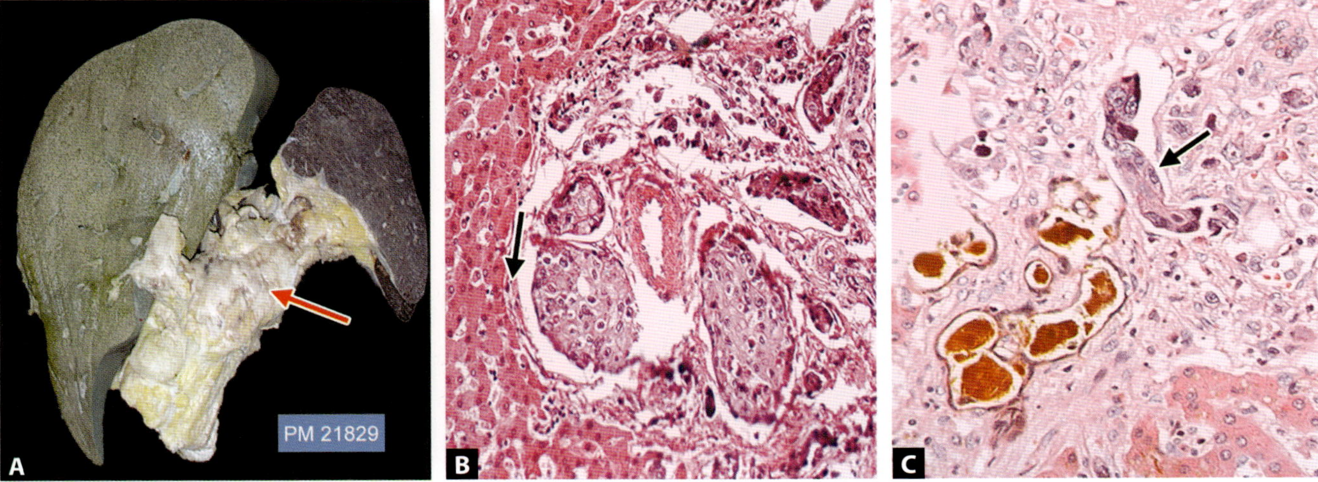

Figs 6A–C:

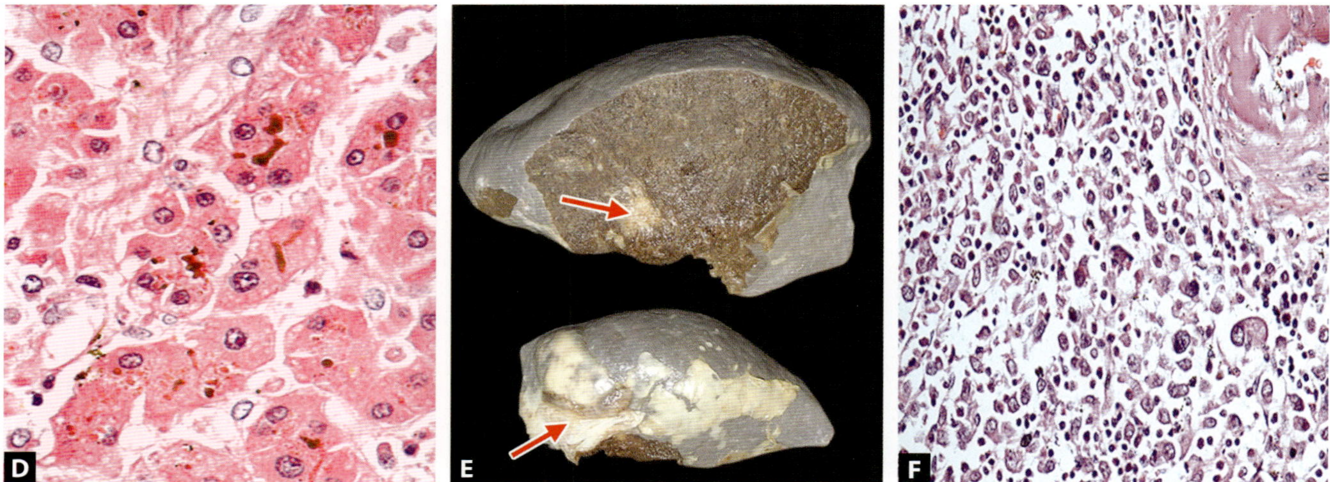

Figs 6A–F: (A) Organ complex of the slice of liver, spleen, and pancreas. The pancreas is covered by a whitish membrane (arrow); (B) Photomicrograph of the liver showing a portal tract with the lymphatics clogged by tumor cells (arrow); (C) Portal tract show cholestasis along with tumor cells (arrow); (D) Periportal hepatocytes show cholestasis; (E) Coronal slice of the spleen showing infarct (upper arrow). The capsular aspect is plastered by tumor cell (lower arrow); and (F) Spleen showing tumor deposits in the periarteriolar area.

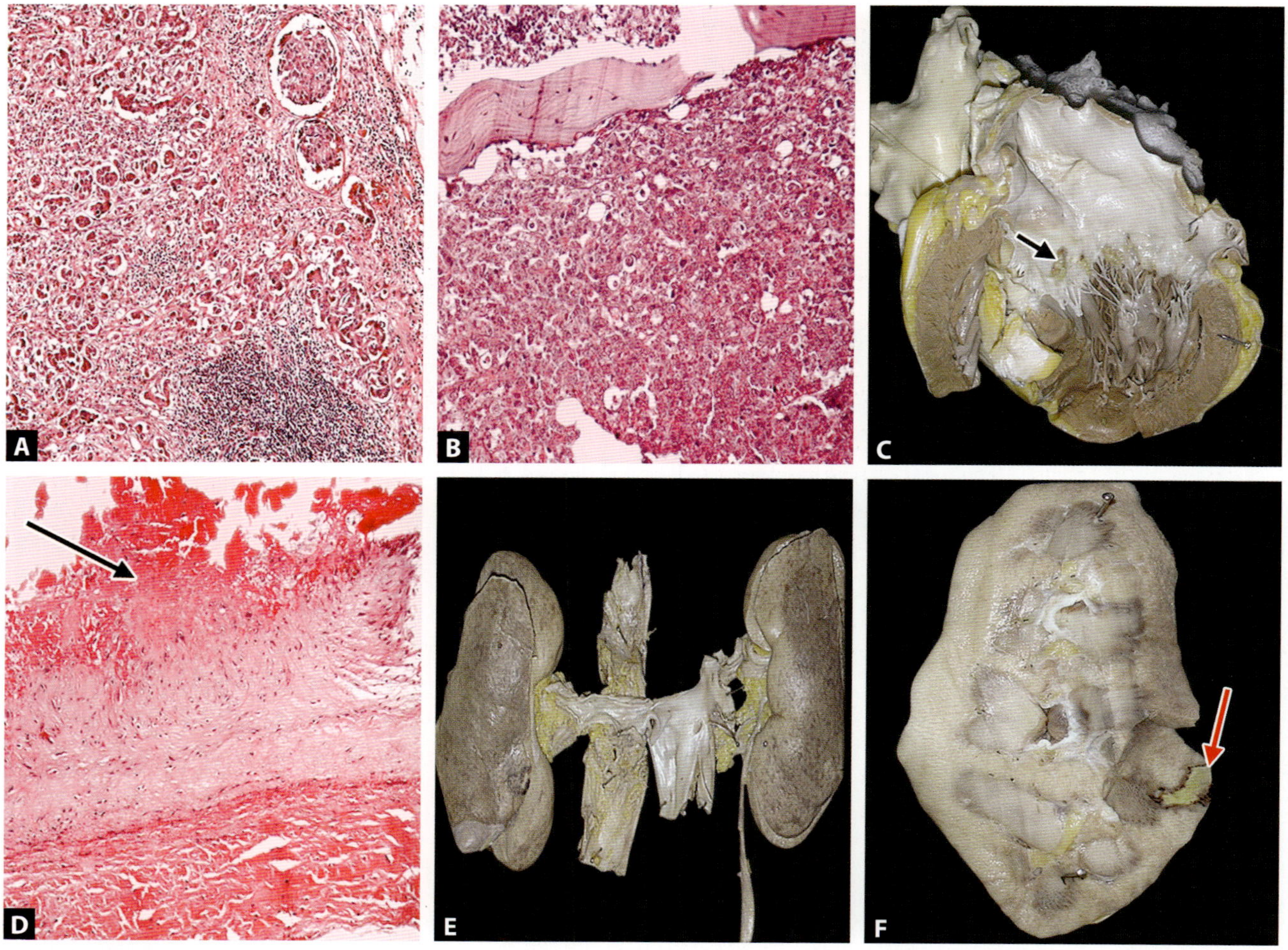

Figs 7A–F: (A) Peripancreatic lymph node replaced by tumor deposits. (B) Section of the bone marrow showing tumor deposits; (C) Gross picture of the left inflow tract of the heart showing small vegetations (arrow) seen at the line of closure of the mitral valve; (D) Photomicrograph of the vegetation showing fibrin (arrow) attached to the valve. No inflammatory cells seen: (E) Gross picture of the kidneys showing blotchy congestion; and (F) Cut section of the kidney showing an infarct (arrow).

Flowchart 1: Sequence of events.

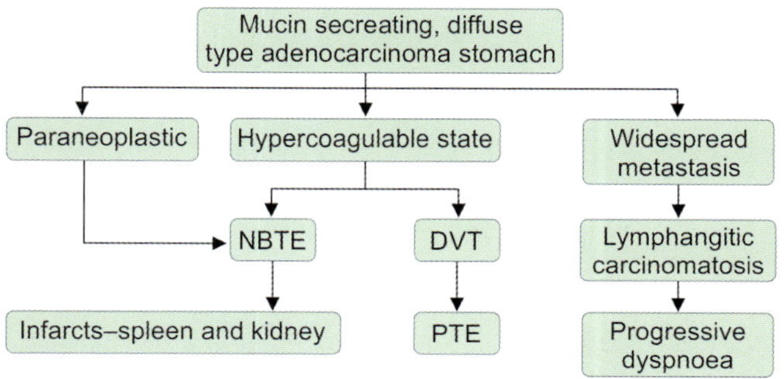

(NBTE: Nonbacterial thrombotic endocarditis; DVT: Deep vein thrombosis PTE: Pulmonary thromboembolism)

adjacent stomach, lungs and liver), pulmonary thromboembolism and NBTE on the mitral valve leading to splenic and renal infarcts. Thus a hypercoagulable state occurred due to the diffuse type of adenocarcinoma of the stomach which led to DVT, thromboembolism and NBTE. The NBTE further led to infarcts in the spleen and kidney. The adenocarcinoma led to lymphangitic carcinomatosis leading on to progressive dyspnea. The pulmonary compromise due to thromboembolism and lymphangitic carcinomatosis led to the death of the patient (Flowchart 1).

TAKE HOME MESSAGE

- Deep vein thrombosis can be the first manifestation of an underlying malignancy.
- Mucin secreting adenocarcinomas produce a hypercoagulable state leading to deep vein thrombosis, thromboembolism and also NBTE.
- Lymphangitic carcinomatosis is a peculiar way of tumor spread via the lymphatics. The most common tumors (80% are adenocarcinomas) that spread in this way are those from the breasts, stomach, lungs, pancreas and prostate.
- Lymphangitic carcinomatosis leads to progressive dyspnea and is misdiagnosed as interstitial lung disease. It may be the first manifestation of an underlying malignancy.

Acknowledgment

This case was published as a clinicopathological conference in our hospital bulletin. Das A, Kakkar N, Mahi S, Lal A, Sakhuja V. Case of adenocarcinoma stomach with extensive thrombotic manifestation. Bulletin PGI. 2007;41:92-102 (non-indexed).

SUGGESTED READING

1. Ai Zheng. Clinical features and diagnosis of pulmonary lymphangitic carcinomatosis. 2006;25:1127-30.
2. Ansari D, Ansari D, Andersson R, et al. Pancreatic cancer and thromboembolic disease, 150 years after Trousseau. Hepatobiliary Surg Nutr. 2015;4:325-35.
3. Dennstedt FE, Greenberg SD, Kim HS. Pulmonary lymphangitic carcinomatosis from occult stomach carcinoma in young adults: an unusual cause of dyspnea. Chest. 1983;84:787-8.
4. Gilchrist FJ, Alton H, Brundler MA, et al. Pulmonary lymphangitic carcinomatosis presenting as severe interstitial lung disease in a 15-year-old female. Eur Respir Rev. 2011;20: 208-10.
5. Kang MJ, Ryoo BY, Ryu MH, et al. Venous thromboembolism (VTE) in patients with advanced gastric cancer: An Asian experience. Eur J Cancer. 2012;48:4492-500.
6. Moubax K, Wuyts W, Vandecaveye V, et al. Pulmonary lymphangitic carcinomatosis as a primary manifestation of gastric carcinoma in a young adult: a case report and review of the literature. BMC Res Notes. 2012;5:638. doi:10. 1186/1756-0500-5-638.
7. Thomas A, Lenox R. Pulmonary lymphangitic carcinomatosis as a primary manifestation of colon cancer in a young adult. CMAJ. 2008;179:338-40.
8. Zhang K, Huang Y. Clinical features and diagnosis of pulmonary lymphangitic carcinomatosis. Ai Zheng. 2006; 25:1127-30.

CONTRIBUTIONS BY:

1. Prof Kartar Singh, Ex-Professor and Head, Department of Gastroenterology, Hepatology and Nutrition (Clinician In-Charge)
2. Dr Anupam Lal, Professor, Department of Radiodiagnosis and Imaging

Post Graduate Institute of Medical Education and Research, Chandigarh, India.

SECTION 3

Infections Adult Cases

CASE 14

Amebic Ileocolitis, Perforation and Liver Abscess: PM 18836

Nandita Bharadwaj Kakkar

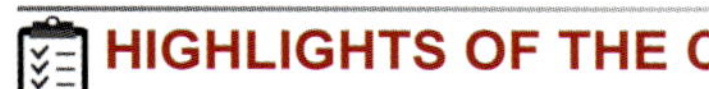

HIGHLIGHTS OF THE CASE

This is a classical case of intestinal and extraintestinal amebiasis in a middle aged male. The patient presented with fever, conjugated hyperbilirubinemia, markedly deranged liver enzymes and coagulopathy. At autopsy there was amebic ileocolitis with serositis and perforation along with amebic liver abscess (ALA).

***Keywords*:** Autopsy, amebic iliocolitis, amebic liver abscess and *Entamoeba histolytica*.

CLINICAL HISTORY

Date of Admission: 10.11.2002, Date of Death: 10.11.2002, Duration of Hospital Stay: 20 Hours

A 40-year-old male from rural Punjab presented with a 15 day history of high-grade intermittent fever with rigors and chills. There were 2–3 spikes a day, each spike lasting for 2–3 hours. The fever lasted for 5–6 days and subsided after the onset of jaundice. Jaundice was present since 10 days and was evidenced by high colored urine, clay colored stools and yellow sclerae. There was an increasing dull aching, continuous, non-colicky, epigastric and right upper quadrant pain. Abdominal distention developed a week prior to admission. He developed non-projectile bilious vomitings (5–6/day). The patient was obstipated and oliguric (200 mL of urine per day) for 3–4 days. There was no pruritis, bleeding, loss of consciousness or seizures. He was a nonsmoker and an occasional alcohol consumer. There was no history of diabetes, hypertension or jaundice. Examination at admission revealed an afebrile, conscious but markedly restless, icteric man with tachycardia (108/min) but with no edema, pallor or stigmata of chronic liver disease. The blood pressure was normal initially (140/90 mm Hg), but subsequently became unrecordable. The abdomen was tensely distended with guarding and rebound tenderness. The liver was enlarged (6 cm below right costal margin), firm with a well-defined margin. Bowel sounds were absent. There was decreased air entry and crepitations at the lung bases. Preliminary investigations revealed a normal Hb (13.6 g/dL), polymorphonuclear leukocytosis with shift to the left (TLC—26,000/μL, DLC–N52, L16, M2, E2, promyelocytes 3, myelocytes 20 and metamyelocytes 5), a normocytic normochromic peripheral blood film and increased platelets with giant forms; normal electrolytes; prerenal azotemia (urea—105 mg%, creatinine 1.1 mg%); hyperbilirubinemia (9.4 mg%—conjugated 7 mg%); raised aspartate transaminase/alanine transaminase (AST/ALT–640/490 U/L); ↑ alkaline phosphatase (2,000 U/L); hypoalbuminemia (2 gms; total protein 6 gms) and deranged coagulogram (PTI 48%, PTTK 45 sec). HbsAg was negative. Ascitic fluid examination: proteins 40 mg%, sugar 76 mg%, TLC 11,800 with 60% polymorphs and 40% lymphocytes. The erect abdominal X-ray revealed paralytic ileus. An ultrasound and a contrast enhanced computed tomogram of the abdomen showed a single large (>10 cm) abscess in the right lobe of the liver with a subcapsular collection, rupture and ascites. The patient was managed initially as a case of fulminant viral hepatitis with an anti-hepatic coma regime. This was changed to ciplox, metrogyl and appropriate pressor support, after the sonogram, a pigtail drainage was planned but the patient succumbed to his illness.

***Units diagnosis*:** Liver abscess ? amebic ? pyogenic, ruptured, bilateral pneumonia, paralytic ileus and septic shock.

AUTOPSY FINDINGS: PM 18836

A partial autopsy was performed on this middle-aged male. The peritoneal cavity yielded one liter of straw colored fluid which was tinged with pus. The pleural and pericardial cavities were within normal limits. The terminal ileum, ***cecum*** and the ascending colon were densely adherent to each other. There were exudates on the serosal aspect. Mucosa of the cecum, ileocecal valve and a small part of the terminal ileum showed congestion and diffuse ulceration (Fig 1A). Discrete ulcers with central opening and hyperemic borders were present in the ascending colon. Microscopy of the large intestine revealed flask-shaped ulcers (Fig 1B) comprising of a mixed inflammatory infiltrate, necrosis and replete with trophozoites of ***E. histolytica*** which showed strong magenta positivity with periodic acid–Schiff (PAS) stain (Fig 1C). Massons trichrome stain pinpointed the trophozoites by staining the ingested RBCs deep red (Fig 1D). The large or the invasive form of trophozoite which range in size from 20–50 μm in diameter, with a clear to granular cytoplasm, eccentrically placed around nucleus with the ingested red blood cells in the cytoplasm (diagnostic hallmark) were well appreciated on H&E stain (Fig 1E). Transmural necrotizing inflammation and dense organizing serositis was seen. The paracolic fat showed abscesses, replete with trophozoites (Figs 2A and B). The terminal part of the small intestine also showed similar ulcers with plenty of trophozoites of E. histolytica. The ***liver*** weighed 2,400 g. There was a large abscess (Fig 2C) in the posterior superior aspect of the right lobe, measuring 12 × 10 × 8 cm with a 3 cm area of

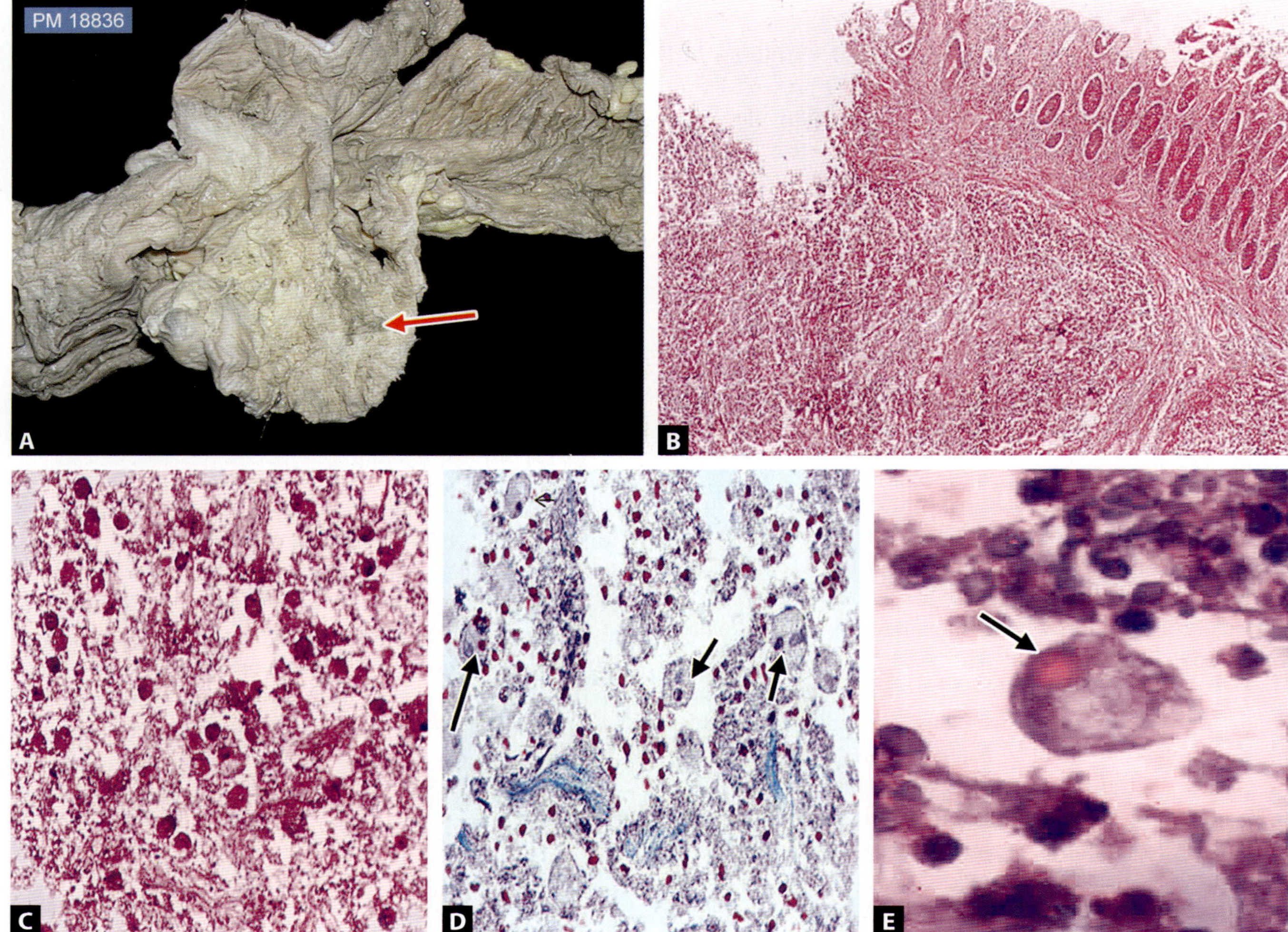

Figs 1A–E: (A) Opened up ileocecal area showing diffuse ulceration (red arrow) of the cecum and the ileocecal valve; (B) Periodic acid–Schiff (PAS) stain shows a typical flask-shaped amebic ulcer; (C) Advancing edge of the cecal ulcer replete with PAS positive trophozoites of *E. histolytica*; (D) Trichrome stain showing plenty of trophozoites (black arrows) and one of them showing an ingested RBC (long arrow); and (E) A trophozoite of *E. histolytica* with an ingested RBC (arrow).

hyperemia around it. The abscess showed a necrotic center and shaggy wall. It was reaching the capsule of the liver to which the diaphragm was firmly adherent. Thus an impending rupture was imminent. The biliary tree and the portal veins were normal. On microscopic examination, the abscess showed the characteristic zonation (Fig 2D) with a central zone of necrotic material (Fig 3A), an intermediate zone consisting of degenerated liver cells, few leukocytes, fibroblasts, *RBCs* and trophozoites (Fig 3B) and a peripheral zone consisting of congested capillaries with varying degrees of liver cell necrosis (Fig 3C) and trophozoites invading the adjoining healthy liver tissue (Fig 3D). Many trophozoites were seen within portal veins (Fig 4A) and few were seen infiltrating the adjacent sinusoids. The surrounding liver showed areas of hepatocytic loss with infiltration by macrophages and florid cholangitis. The liver away from the abscess showed features of septicemia and cholangitis (Fig 4B). The ***lungs*** weighed 780 g. Both the lower lobes showed extensive hemorrhagic consolidation. Microscopy revealed bronchopneumonia and alveolar hemorrhages. The ***kidneys*** showed features of early acute tubular necrosis and the ***spleen*** (220 g) revealed septicemic changes. Other organs were within normal limits.

FINAL AUTOPSY DIAGNOSIS: PM 18836

40 Years Male

- Amebic ileocolitis with serositis and perforation
- Amebic liver abscess with cholangitis

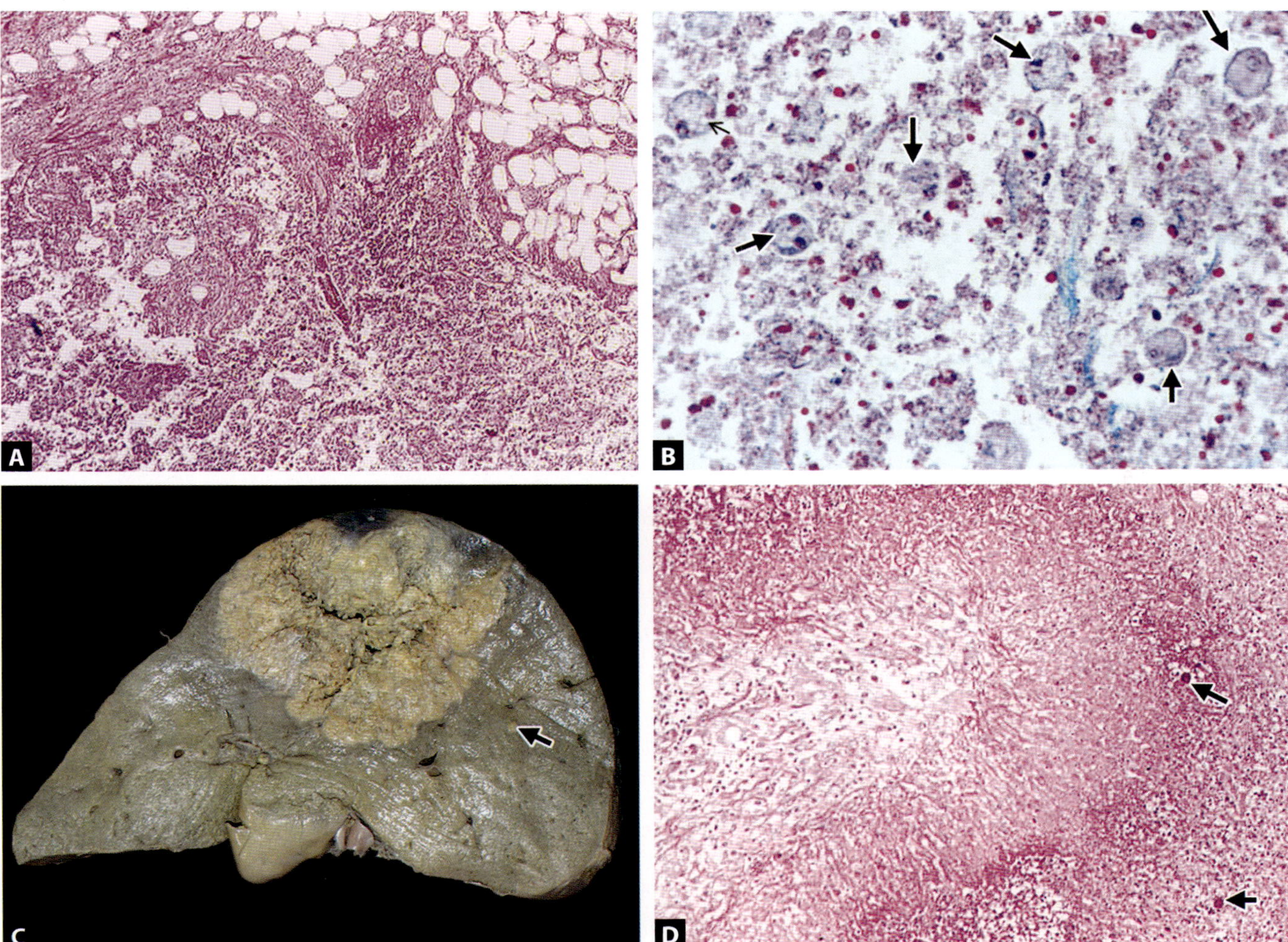

Figs 2A–D: (A) Paracolic abscess showing dense inflammation; (B) Paracolic abscess replete with trophozoites of *Entamoeba histolytica* (arrows) on Massons trichrome stain; (C) Coronal slice of the liver showing a large necrotic abscess reaching the superior aspect. A tiny white nodule 0.5 mm is also seen away from the main abscess (arrow); and (D) Photomicrograph from the hepatic abscess showing a central necrotic area. Few PAS positive trophozoites can be seen in the intermediate zone (arrows).

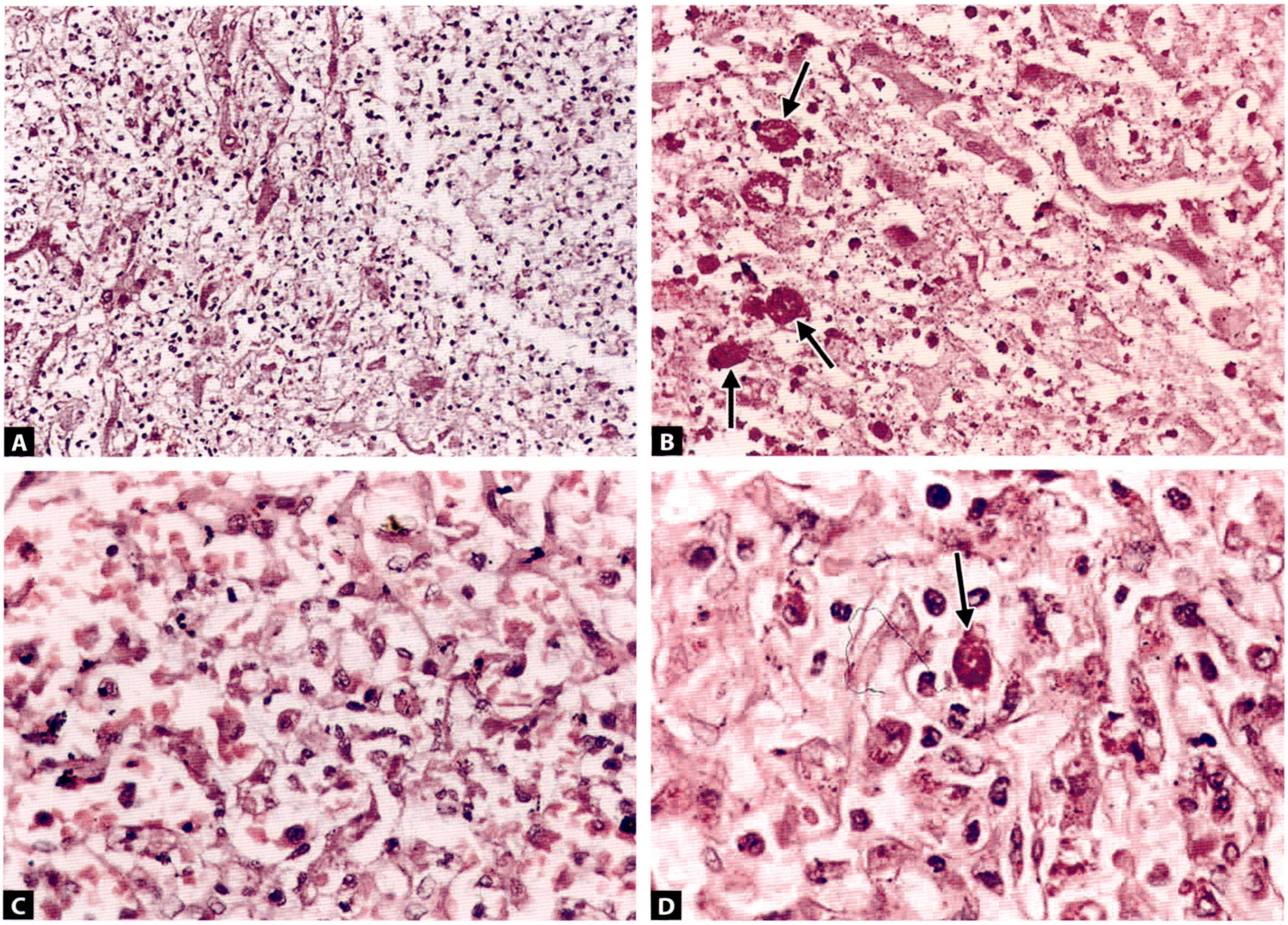

Figs 3A–D: Photomicrograph from the hepatic abscess showing: (A) Central necrotic zone; (B) Intermediate zone showing periodic acid–Schiff (PAS) positive trophozoites (arrows) of *Entamoeba histolytica* along with degenerating hepatocytes; (C) Peripheral zone showing replacement of hepatocytes by macrophages; and (D) A PAS positive trophozoite (arrow) within the sinusoid at the periphery of the abscess.

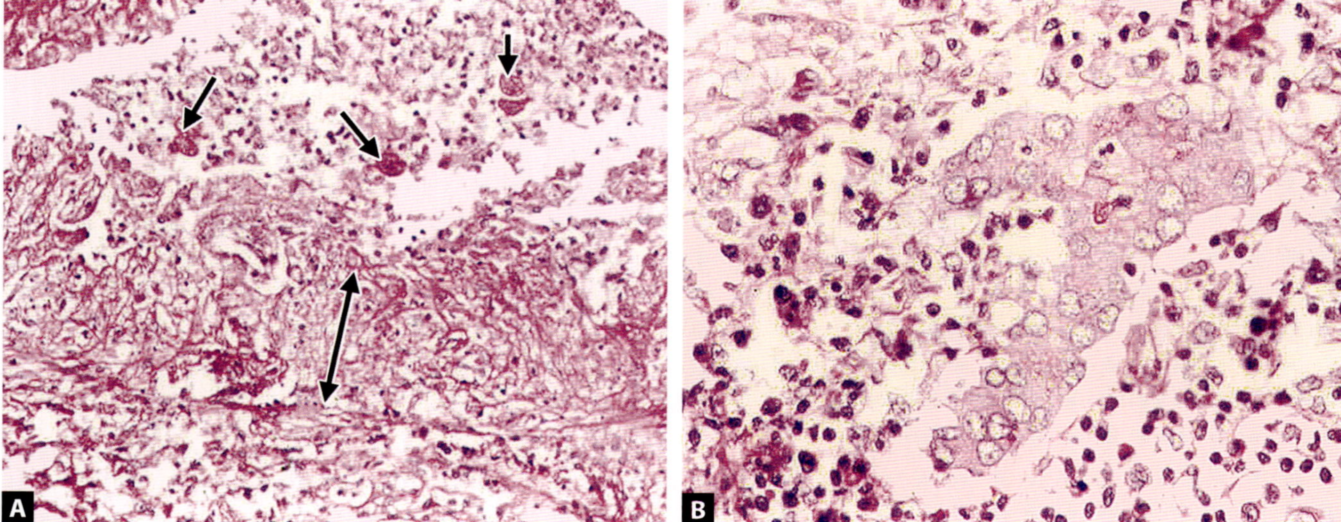

Figs 4A–B: (A) Trophozoites of *Entamoeba histolytica* (black arrows) within a portal vein. The wall of the vein is highlighted by a double headed arrow; and (B) Portal tract showing a bile duct with acute cholangitis.

- Septicemia—liver and spleen
- Pulmonary hemorrhage and bronchopneumonia.

AMEBIASIS

Amebiasis is caused by ***E. histolytica***, a protozoan parasite and is well known for its protean manifestations and can simulate many diseases. It is globally distributed, affects 10% of the world population and only 10% of the infected population develops amebiasis, either intestinal or extraintestinal. The remaining 90% are asymptomatic carriers of trophozoites in the gut. The majority of morbidity and mortality occurs in Asia, Central/South America and Africa. Children are especially vulnerable and can have repeated infections. Amebiasis occurs predominantly in the developing countries like India, Mexico and Columbia, resulting in approximately 40 million cases of dysentery and liver abscess.

Infection with ***E. histolytica*** occurs via the feco-oral route. The mature quadrinucleate cysts are the infective forms of the parasite which are swallowed along with the contaminated food/drink. They pass unaltered through the stomach (the cyst wall is resistant to the action of the gastric juices) and reach the intestine where the cyst wall is digested by the action of trypsin. The excystation however occurs when the cyst reaches the cecum or the lower part of the ileum (neutral or slightly alkaline medium). Each cyst gives rise to eight amebulae, each one of which is capable of developing into a trophozoite. The trophozoites multiply by simple binary fission under anaerobic conditions. The trophic forms are exclusively parasitic in their habit, growing at the expense of the living tissues and multiplying abundantly. The pathogenicity is due to the amoeba proteins which aid in tissue invasion: (a) Cysteine proteinases which breakdown the proteins of the extracellular matrix. (b) A lectin on the parasite surface that binds to the carbohydrates on the surface of the colonic epithelial cells and red blood cells. (c) Amebapore, a channel forming protein which makes holes in the plasma membrane of the host cells and lyses them. The amebapore is a small peptide that has the same structure as the NK—lysine of killer lymphocytes. This leads to necrosis of tissues and thus helps the organism to get its nourishment by the absorption of the dissolved tissue juices. The trophozoites keep receding from the dead tissue and proceed toward the healthy tissue, producing flask-shaped ulcers in the cecum. They find their way into the radicles of the portal vein and get carried away to the liver to produce abscesses. Here the organism grows and multiplies for a while and causes mass destruction. But its further progress is arrested, encystation does not occur and the organism reaches its dead end. Those trophozoites which remain in the intestinal wall produce acute dysentery, where a large number of trophozoites are thrown out along with the slough. The aim of the parasite is to live in harmony with the host, produce strains which are capable of giving rise to cysts and thus to propagate its own species. Hence, a high degree of pathogenicity of the parasite is a disadvantage to itself. After some time when the disease settles down due to host tolerance, the lesions begin to heal. Encystation of the parasite occurs within the lumen of the intestine and these are discharged from the infected individual for transference into another susceptible host, where they can grow and continue their life cycle. Natural infection of ***E. histolytica*** occurs only in man and monkeys. Fecal contamination of drinking water, vegetables/fruits and eating of uncooked vegetables and fruits infected with human feces are the primary causes. Handling of food by carriers (contact or convalescent), i.e. cyst passers or cyst carriers is a common mode of spread.

Pathology of Amebiasis

The incubation period is 4–5 days. The pathogenic lesions may be intestinal or extra-intestinal to the liver, lung, pericardium and brain. The clinical classification is as such:

- *Intestinal amebiasis*:
  - Noninvasive carrier state
  - *Dysentery*: Complicated (perforation, peritonitis and hemorrhage) or uncomplicated
  - Non-dysenteric colonic disease—ameboma, stricture and intussusceptions.
- *Hepatic amebiasis*: Abscess—simple (usually solitary) or complicated (multiple, extension to pleura, pericardium and peritoneum)
- *Other sites*: Skin, lung, brain and genitalia
- *Postinfective sequelae*: Post-dysenteric colitis.

Intestinal Amebiasis

This is strictly confined to the large gut. It may be generalized (whole length of the large gut) or localized to the ileocecal region (cecum, ascending colon, ileocecal valve and appendix) or occasionally to the sigmoido-rectal region. The amebic ulcers are discrete and a healthy mucosa always intervenes between the ulcers even when they are extensive. Early lesion looks like nodular elevations with an opening at the center with hyperemic borders. Ulcers vary from pin head to an inch or more, are round to oval, transverse in large coalescing ulcers, have ragged and undermined margins and the base is filled with necrotic yellow black slough. Superficial ulcers do not extend beyond the muscularis mucosa and deep ulcers go down till the submucosa and extend laterally to communicate with adjacent ulcers. At times, they are transmural and lead to complications like local peritonitis, hemorrhage, perforation, generalized peritonitis, pericecal/pericolic abscesses and gangrene of large gut. The ulcers show neutrophils (early ulcer), macrophages, necrotic debris and trophozoites of ***E. histolytica***. The parasite is seen predominantly along the borders of the ulcers invading into the viable tissue. In advanced lesions they are seen a considerable distance away from the actual ulcer, reaching the serosal aspect. The parasites may also be seen burrowing into the small venules or lying within the lumina of dilated venous radicles. A trophozoite is 20–50 μm in diameter with a clear to granular cytoplasm and an eccentrically placed round nucleus with a sharp nuclear membrane and a prominent central karyosome. Ingested red blood cells seen in the cytoplasm is the diagnostic hallmark. The usual confusion is with a macrophage, which is smaller in size, has a more basophilic nuclei and less granular cytoplasm. Trophozoites are intensely PAS positive due to the glycogen in the cytoplasm.

Amebic Liver Abscess

In 40% patients of amebic dysentery, the trophozoites are carried as emboli by the radicles of the portal veins to the liver, leading to solitary and less often multiple discrete abscesses. The patient presents with pain and tenderness in the right hypochondrium due to the stretching of the capsule of the liver. The pain is sometimes referred to the right acromial region due to the irritation of the phrenic nerve which supplies the undersurface of the diaphragm. The pain may also be referred to the lower abdomen or the right iliac fossa. Fever, to begin with shows a low evening rise and later becomes high and constant. Jaundice is an unusual manifestation. An invasive lesion in the large bowel is mandatory for the parasite to pass into the portal circulation, but only one-third patients with ALA have a history of bowel symptoms. The hepatic complication generally appears when the intestinal symptoms have subsided. In majority of the cases, it appears after about 1–3 months of the disappearance of the dysenteric attack. But cases have been reported where liver abscesses have developed after a lapse of months or even years. However, in a small percentage of cases both the intestine and the liver are involved at the same time and these cases are invariably fatal. Once the trophozoites reach the capillary system of the liver, it acts as an efficient filter and holds the parasites. They multiply and proceed to carry on their cytolytic action. Soon they cause obstruction to the circulation and produce thrombosis of the sinusoids leading to ischemic necrosis of the surrounding liver cells. The process of destruction then goes on in concentric layers and a big sized abscess is formed. The center liquefies by the cytolytic action of the amebae and the liquefaction extends radially. Most amebic abscesses are in the right lobe (posterior-superior lobe) due to its greater portal venous drainage compared to the left lobe. They range in size from 5–20 cm. The earliest macroscopic lesion, which is rarely encountered, is of one or more small nodules of pale necrotic liver tissue. Fully developed abscesses have a ragged margin without a fibrous rim and liquid contents likened to anchovy sauce, being brown-red, at times with a paste like consistency. The abscess gradually merges into the healthy liver with an intervening area of hyperemia. Old lesions can develop a fibrotic capsule up to a centimeter thick. The earliest histological finding is the presence of amebic trophozoites in the sinusoids, associated with coagulative necrosis between the portal tract and the terminal venule of an acinus. Sections from the abscess shows three zones: (1) A central zone of cytolyzed granular material with no amoebae, (2) An intermediate zone consisting of degenerated liver cells, few leukocytes, fibroblasts, RBCs and trophozoites, (3) A peripheral zone consisting of congested capillaries with varying degrees of liver cell necrosis and plenty of trophozoites invading the adjoining healthy liver tissue.

Jaundice in Amebic Liver Abscess

Hyperbilirubinemia is known to occur in cases of ALA, but its incidence and severity is variable. Jaundice occurring in a setting of ALA, heralds danger and points toward an upcoming hepatic coma, various complications (abdominal and extra-abdominal) and a high morbidity/mortality. Alcoholics with ALA have a higher incidence of jaundice. In patients of ALA who develop jaundice, the onset of disease is acute with rigors and sweating. Many factors may contribute to hyperbilirubinemia which include increased load of bilirubin, decreased hepatic uptake and decreased conjugation/excretion of bilirubin. But studies have indicated that patients with ALA and jaundice generally have a massive abscess impinging on the hilum/inferior surface of the liver, thus compressing and distorting the biliary tree leading to intrahepatic cholestasis. There is an improvement after surgical drainage of the abscess, thus proving the obstructive nature of the jaundice. Others have postulated that jaundice in patients with ALA is caused by biliovascular fistula resulting from hepatic necrosis leading to damage to bile ducts and hepatic veins.

COMMENTARY—INDEX CASE: PM 18836

This was a classical and a fatal case of amebiasis in which the intestinal ulcers and the liver abscess occurred at the same time. Diffuse ulceration was seen in the cecum and multiple ulcers in the terminal ileum and ascending colon. The discrete ulcers were typically flask-shaped replete with trophozoites (PAS positive, some of them with engulfed RBCs) seen in large numbers at the advancing edge. There was transmural necrotizing inflammation with dense organizing serositis and abscesses in the paracolic fat, replete with trophozoites. The liver abscess was large, encroaching upon the hilum of the liver and reaching the superior surface, with the overlying capsule adherent to the diaphragm, with an impending rupture. Microscopic examination of the abscess showed the characteristic zonation as described above. There was jaundice with conjugated hyperbilirubinemia, markedly deranged liver enzymes and coagulopathy, a result of the pressure effect as described above.

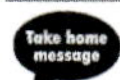

TAKE HOME MESSAGE

- Amebic liver abscess with coexisting amebic intestinal lesions occurs in a small percentage of cases and these cases are invariably fatal.
- Jaundice can occur in cases of amebic liver abscess (ALA) due to pressure and distortion of the biliary tree, which results in intrahepatic cholestasis. It should be regarded as an emergency.

SUGGESTED READING

1. Aikat BK, Bhusnurmath SR, Pal AK, et al. Amoebic liver abscess—A clinicopathologic study. Indian J Med Res. 1978;67:381-91.
2. Aikat BK, Bhusnurmath SR, Pal AK, et al. Pathology and pathogenesis of fatal hepatic amoebiasis—A study based on 79 autopsy cases. Trans R Soc Trop Med Hyg. 1979;73:188-92.
3. Espinosa-Cantellano M, Martínez-Palomo A. Pathogenesis of intestinal amebiasis: from molecules to disease. Clin Microbiol Rev. 2000;13:318-31.
4. Haque R, Huston CD, Hughes M, et al. Amebiasis. N Engl J Med. 2003;348:1565-73.
5. Maltz G, Knauer CM. Amebic liver abscess: a 15-year experience. Am J Gastroenterol. 1991;86:704-10.
6. Nigam P, Gupta AK, Kapoor KK, et al. Cholestasis in amoebic liver abscess. Gut. 1985;26:140-5.
7. Petri WA, Jr, Haque R, Mann BJ. The bittersweet interface of parasite and host: lectin-carbohydrate interactions during human invasion by the parasite Entamoeba histolytica. Annu Rev Microbiol. 2002;56:39-64.
8. Ralston KS, Petri WA, Jr. Tissue destruction and invasion by Entamoeba histolytica. Trends Parasitol. 2011;27:254-63.
9. Sarda AK, Mishra A, Malhotra N, et al. Hyperbilirubinemia in Patients with Amoebic Liver Abscess: A Study of 75 Cases. J Gastroint Dig Syst. 2013;3:138. doi:10.4172/2161-069X.1000138.
10. Singh V, Bhalla A, Sharma N, et al. Pathophysiology of jaundice in amoebic liver abscess. Am J Trop Med Hyg. 2008;78:556-9.
11. WHO/PAHO/UNESCO report. A consultation with experts on amoebiasis. Mexico City, Mexico 28-29 January, 1997. Epidemiol Bull. 1997;18:13-4.

CONTRIBUTIONS BY:

1. Dr Navneet Sharma, Professor, Department of Internal Medicine (Clinician In-Charge)
2. Dr Sadhana Lal, Professor, Department of Gastroenterology (Compilation of Clinical Details)

Post Graduate Institute of Medical Education and Research, Chandigarh, India.

CASE 15

Cerebral Toxoplasmosis in a Human Immunodeficiency Virus Positive Patient: PM 19210

Nandita Bharadwaj Kakkar

HIGHLIGHTS OF THE CASE

This is a classical case of cerebral toxoplasmosis in a young, human immunodeficiency virus (HIV) positive male. The HIV status came to light after the death of the patient. Unfortunately, the diagnosis could not be made antemortem and the patient was treated on the lines of tuberculosis.

Keywords: Autopsy, toxoplasma, meningoencephalitis, AIDS defining illness, unsuspected HIV.

CLINICAL DETAILS

Date of Admission: 07.05.2003, Date of Death: 13.05.2003, Duration of Hospital Stay: 6 Days

A young male (26 years), agriculturist by profession, came with fever of 3–4 months duration, which was intermittent, moderate to high grade with no chills/rigor. It was associated with headache and body aches. He was treated with drugs off and on, with which there were intermittent remissions. Headache was there since 3–4 months, which was bifrontal, continuous and of moderate to severe intensity. There was cough with expectoration since 3 weeks, which was minimal, mucoidy with no blood. There was dysarthria and deviation of angle of mouth to the left side since 15 days. Projectile vomiting, 2–3/day with no relation to food intake was present since 2 weeks. Seizures were present since 4–5 days, were tonic-clonic and 1–2/day. They started as left focal with secondary generalization. There was altered sensorium since 3–4 days with increased intensity of headaches. There was no history of diabetes, hypertension, tuberculosis, trauma, dyspnea, hemoptysis, otitis media or sinusitis. On ***examination,*** he was average built. There was no skin pigmentation, nodules, anemia, cyanosis, clubbing and lymphadenopathy. The pulse was 90 beats/min, regular and the BP was 130/80 mm Hg. Chest, cardiovascular and abdominal examination were normal. CNS examination showed a drowsy, irritable male who did not verbalize or obey commands. Second cranial nerve was involved with dilatation and sluggish reaction of the left pupil. The other pupil was normal. Seventh nerve palsy of upper motor neuron type was present and ? Right VI nerve palsy ? Poor gag was also seen. There was terminal neck stiffness. There was no motor or sensory deficit and deep tendon reflexes revealed bilateral exaggerated biceps (+++). Plantars were bilateral up-going.

Investigations and Course of Management

Investigations revealed a normal hemoglobin and platelet count, raised total leukocyte count (15,000/µL) and a raised ESR (60–95 in the 1st hour). Liver function tests, serum blood sugar, renal function tests, routine urine analysis and electrocardiogram were within normal limits. Serum calcium levels were raised (10.1 mg%). ***CT scan*** (non-contrast and contrast enhanced) of the head showed left thalamic and occipital space occupying lesions with perilesional edema and midline shift. ***Non-contrast computerized tomography, i.e. NCCT*** (Fig 1A) showed an ill-defined lesion in the region of the left striate cortex with gross surrounding perilesional edema. The ipsilateral sylvian fissure, the lateral and third ventricles were compressed with shift to the right. The contralateral right ventricle was distorted and dilated. Effacement of the suprasellar cisterns was present. There was no evidence of calcification in the lesion. ***CECT*** head (Fig 1B) showed a thick-walled ring lesion with gross perilesional edema. Enhancement of the left sylvian fissure was also observed. These findings suggest the presence of an infective lesion with possible etiologies being tuberculosis or toxoplasmosis. However, the presence of lymphoma cannot be entirely ruled out.

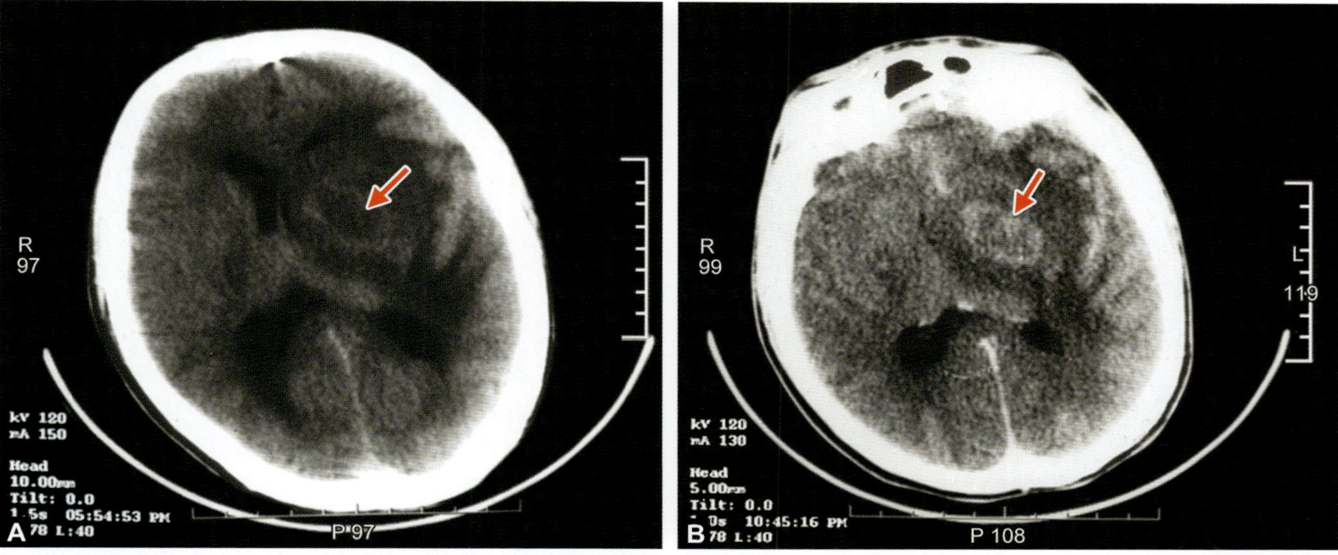

Figs 1A and B: (A) Non-contrast computerized tomography (NCCT) head shows an ill-defined lesion in the region of the left thalamus (arrow) with gross surrounding perilesional edema; and (B) Contrast-enhanced computed tomography (CECT) head shows a thick-walled ring lesion (arrow) with gross perilesional edema.

Patient was started on mannitol, glycerol, pantocid, ceftriaxone and antitubercular treatment. Sample was sent for HIV testing, the report of which was received after his death. There after an ***MRI*** revealed a 3 × 2 cm space occupying lesion in the deep left parietal region with perilesional edema and mass effect. The mass was heterogeneous with irregular peripheral patchy enhancement with chinking of left lateral ventricle and a midline shift to the right. Multiple smaller satellite lesions with peripheral enhancement and perilesional edema were seen posterior to the above lesion in the right cerebellum and the right lentiform nucleus. Altered signal intensity was seen in the left cerebellar hemisphere along with abnormal meningeal enhancement. The impression given was that of a multifocal lesion ? tubercular in etiology. Thereafter, the patient was noted to have improved sensorium and mannitol was stopped. After an ophthalmology opinion ruled out the presence of papilledema, a lumbar puncture was done. The cerebrospinal fluid (CSF) revealed 30 mg/dL of proteins, 54 mg/dL of sugar and no white blood cells. A day after this, the patient was found to be unresponsive, with no respiration and was declared dead. The ***Unit's clinical diagnosis*** was chronic meningitis with multiple tuberculomas.

AUTOPSY FINDINGS: PM 19210

A partial autopsy was performed wherein only the brain was examined. There was no significant external abnormality. The ***brain*** weighed 1,405 g and there was diffuse edema, more in left cerebral hemisphere (Fig 2A). There was no obvious gross exudate. Prominent uncal herniation (Fig 2B) was present, more on left side. On coronal slicing, there were multiple lesions with central necrosis and discoloration. A large 5 × 5 × 6 cm ill-defined lesion was seen in the left frontoparietal region in the region of the left thalamus [Fig 2C (arrow)], a 2 × 2 × 1 cm lesion in the posterior parietal, a 2 × 1.5 × 1 cm lesion in the right lentiform nucleus [Fig 2D (arrows)] and a 1 × 1 cm lesion in the right occipital lobe and left cerebellar hemisphere. Microscopy revealed large necrotizing abscesses with central coagulative necrosis (Fig 3A) containing nuclear debris, vascular thrombosis [Fig 3B (arrows)] and surrounded by inflammation predominating in lymphomononuclear cells, plasma cells and macrophages (Fig 3C). Perivascular lymphomononuclear infiltrate (Fig 3D) and microglial nodules were seen [Fig 3E (arrow)] in the periphery. Meningeal inflammation and borderzone encephalitis was also noted. The necrotic areas showed many rounded cysts and pseudocysts amidst the dense inflammation [Fig 3F (arrows)]. The cysts contained innumerable bradyzoites [Figs 4A and B (arrows)], pseudocysts containing tachyzoites (Fig 4A) and free tachyzoites [Fig 4C (arrows)] were also seen. Semithin sections showed clusters of cysts [Fig 4D (arrows)]. Scanning electron microscopy (Figs 5A–C) shows cysts with bradyzoites and pseudocysts with tachyzoites. Postmortem blood sample and the sample sent preterminally tested strongly positive for HIV.

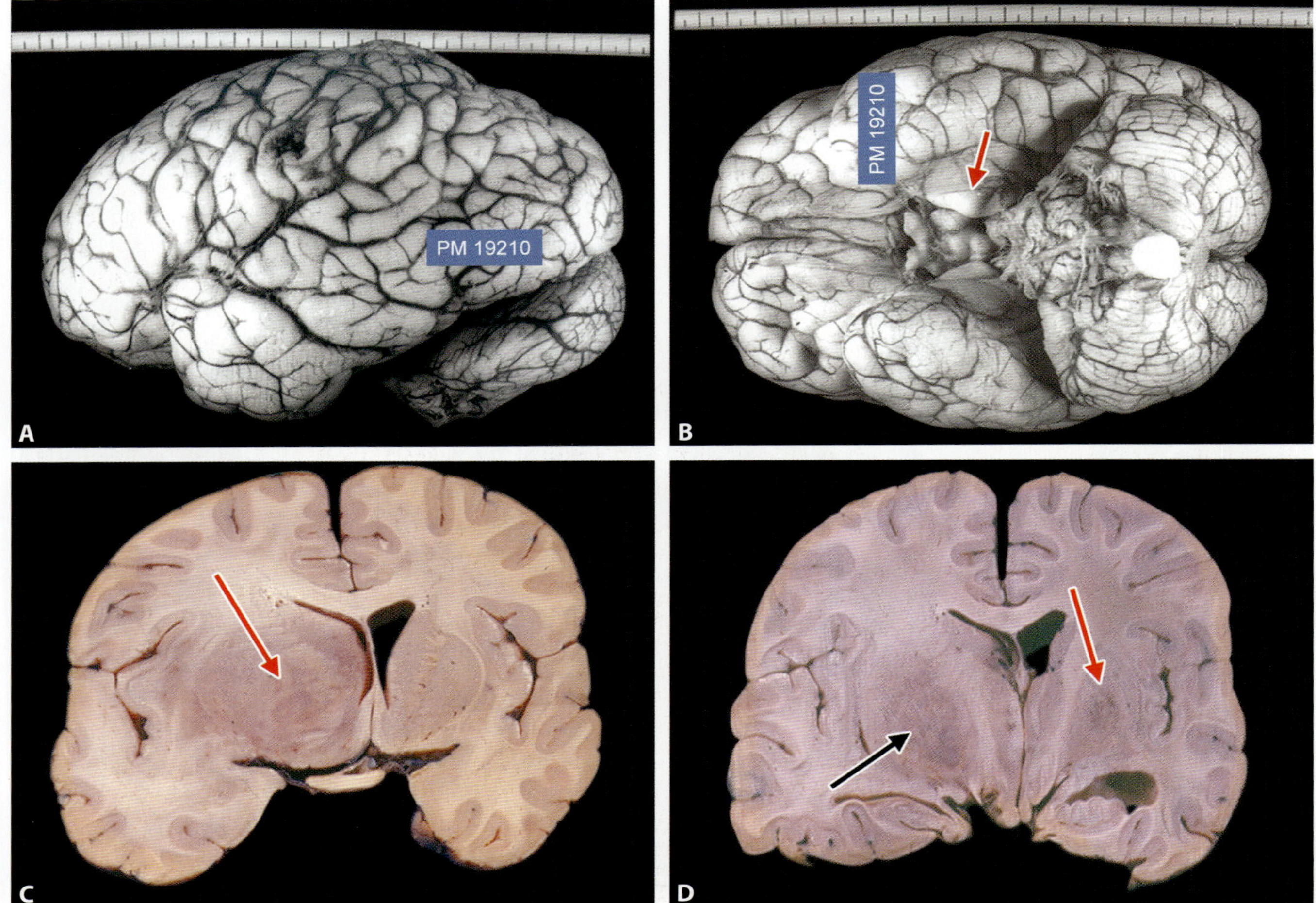

Figs 2A–D: (A) Left lateral aspect of the brain showing edema, flattening of the gyri and narrowing of the sulci; (B) Base of the brain showing uncal herniation more on the left side (arrow); (C) Coronal slice of the brain showing a large 5 × 5 × 6 cm ill-defined lesion in the region of the left thalamus (arrow on the left side); and (D) A more posterior coronal slice showing two lesions, a 2 × 1.5 × 1 cm lesion in the right lentiform nucleus (red arrow) and the same lesion seen in the previous picture (black arrow).

FINAL AUTOPSY DIAGNOSIS: PM 19210

26 Years Male, HIV Positive

Toxoplasma Meningoencephalitis.

TOXOPLASMOSIS

Toxoplasmosis[1] is a parasitic disease caused by *Toxoplasma gondii*. It dwells in the blood and different types of tissue and is widely distributed in man and animals all over the world. It has an intestinal phase in its definitive host, the cat of family Felidae particularly Felis catus, the domestic cat. It also has an extra-intestinal phase in its heterologus host such as mouse, man and other animals. The initial infection is taken care off by the immune system thus preventing the development of disease. This does not lead to the eradication of the parasite, which lies dormant in a cystic form in the muscle and the brain. Humans[2] contact the infection in a number of ways: (1) By eating undercooked/raw meat containing tissue cysts present in the muscles of intermediate hosts such as pigs and sheep, (2) By ingesting the oocysts from food or water contaminated by feces from an infected cat, (3) Through the placenta, (4) Contamination of skin by handling of culture of toxoplasma/contaminated meat. The oocysts contain two sporocysts which on maturation (1–5 days) develop into 4 sporozoites/tachyzoites (resemble the trophozoites) which are infective to man and other animals. After ingestion, the sporozoites/tachyzoites enters the circulation (by invading the wall of the gut) and undergoes an active phase by rapid division of the tachyzoite stage in the mesenteric lymph nodes, predominantly in the macrophages.

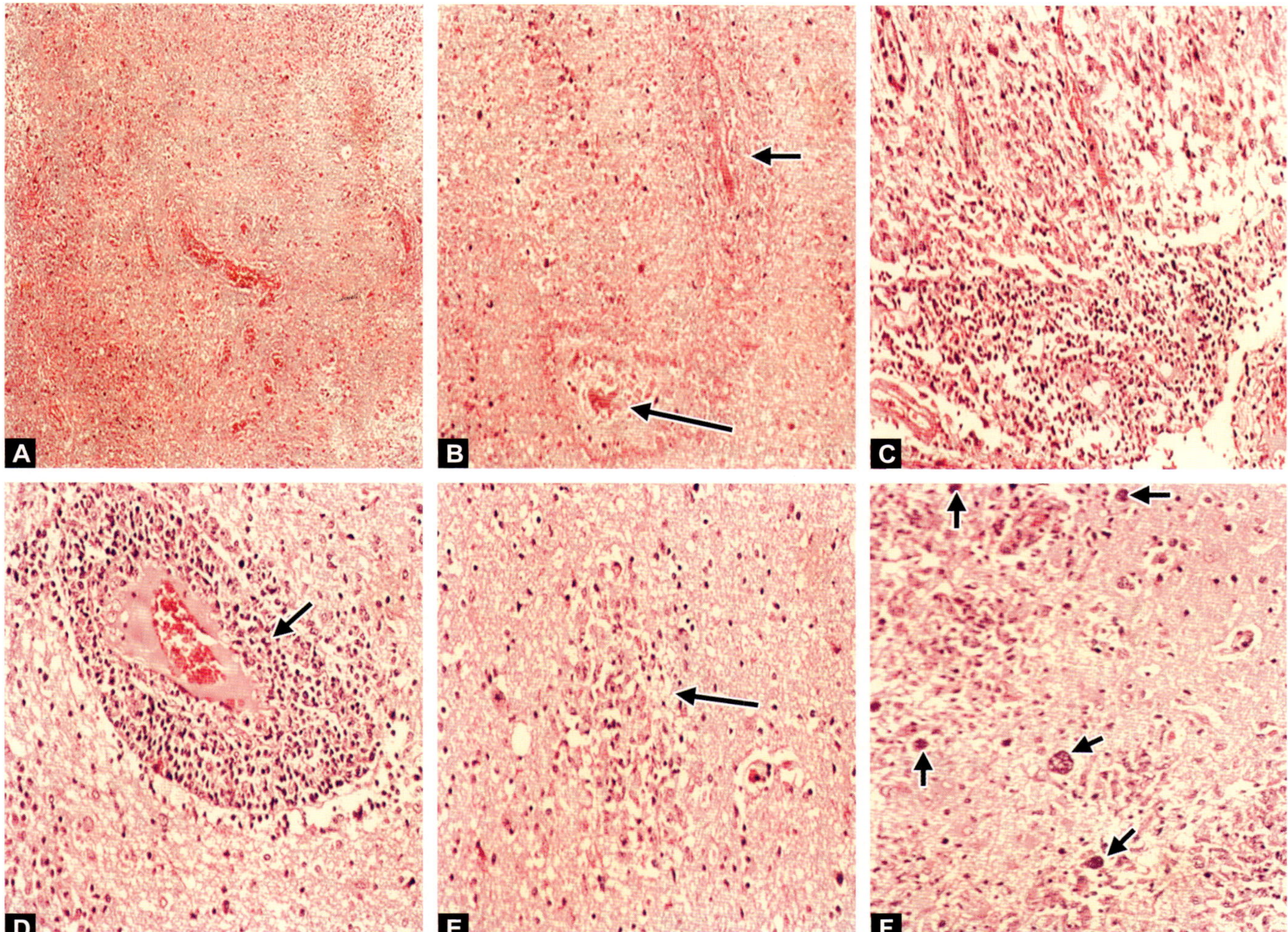

Figs 3A–F: Photomicrographs from the necrotic lesion in the brain shows: (A) Coagulative necrosis with nuclear debris; (B) Vascular thrombosis (arrows); (C) Dense lymphomononuclear cell infiltrate at the periphery of the lesion; (D) Perivascular lymphomononuclear cell infiltrate (arrow); (E) Glial nodule (arrow); and (F) Multiple cysts of toxoplasma (arrows) amidst the inflammatory infiltrate.

The tachyzoite form is crescent shaped, 4–7 µm long, 2–3 µm wide and usually found in intracellular clusters of 8–32 parasites. The tachyzoite form undergoes rapid division by a process of internal budding, termed endodyogeny and repeated divisions occur before the host cell ruptures and releases the parasite. The tachyzoites spread via the bloodstream to a number of different organs like the brain, eyes, liver, spleen, heart, skeletal muscle, lymph nodes and placenta of pregnant mothers. The development of the immune response may eradicate the tachyzoites and brings an end to the acute phase. However, tachyzoites undergo stage conversion into pseudocysts in the above-mentioned places. The parasite inside the pseudocyst is called an endozoite/tachyzoite and has a central nucleus. A pseudocyst may contain 50–100 organisms and represent the proliferative stage of the parasite and is responsible for much of the tissue damage. In the brain and skeletal muscle, the tachyzoites can get converted into tissue cysts, inside which the parasite multiplies slowly. The parasite inside the tissue cyst is known as cystozoite/bradyzoites (nucleus is situated at the periphery in the rounded end). These tissue cysts are most often found in the CNS, skeletal and cardiac muscle and vary in size from 12–100 µm and contain hundreds of bradyzoites. It does not cause any damage to the tissues and is not associated with any signs and symptoms. They persist for years and when the immune system becomes suppressed, they provide a source for reactivation. Both the pseudocysts and tissue cysts are infective. Treatment is very effective against the tachyzoite stage, but nothing works on the tissue cysts and hence they can never be eradicated.

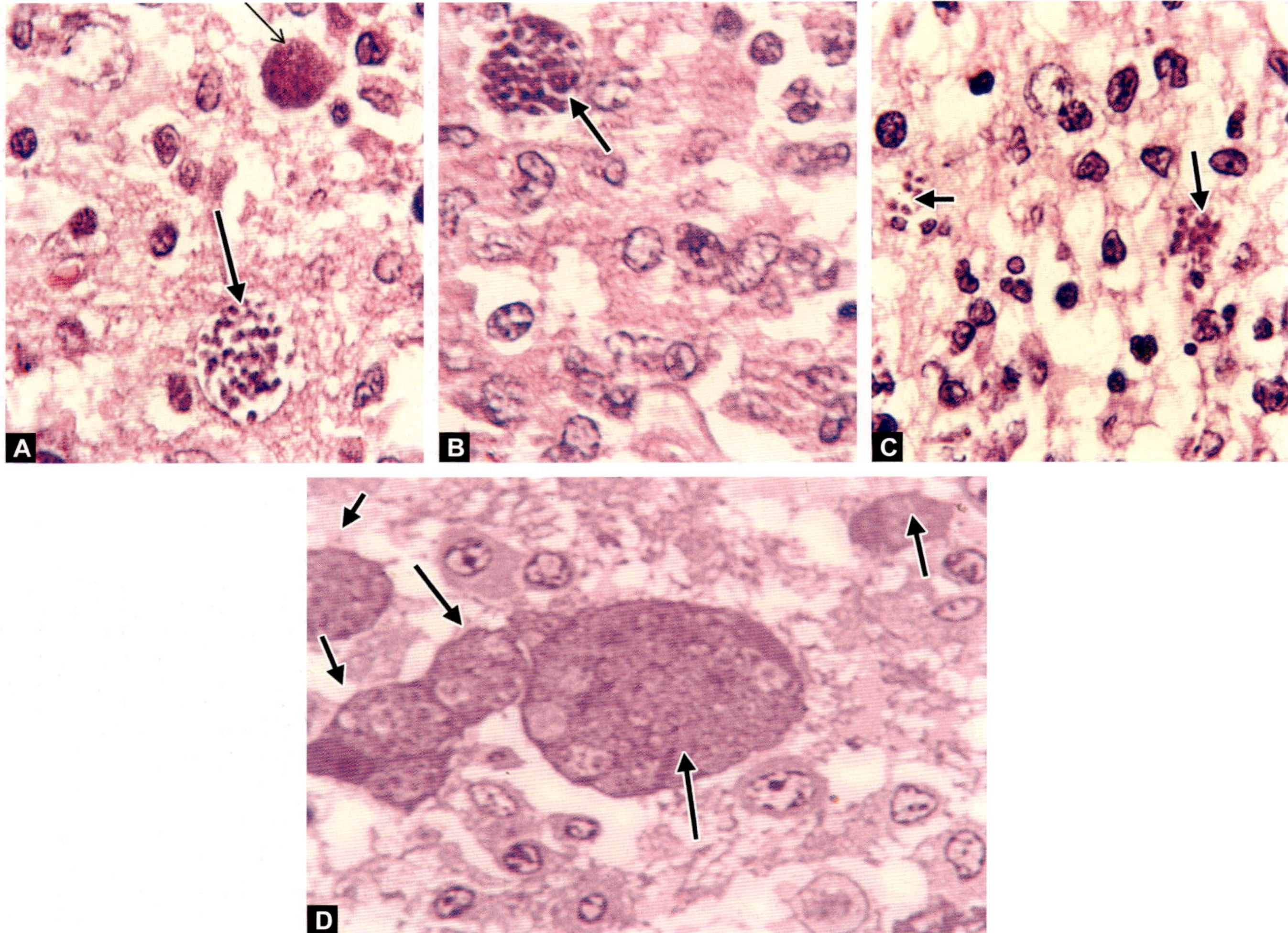

Figs 4A–D: (A and B) Photomicrographs showing cyst of toxoplasma packed with bradyzoites (upper arrows) and a pseudocyst containing fewer tachyzoites (lower arrow); (C) Tachyzoites (arrows) lying free amidst the inflammation; and (D) Semithin section shows plenty of cysts (arrows). .

Toxoplasmosis can present as primary toxoplasmosis in immunocompetent individuals, in immunosuppressed patients (HIV infection, post-transplantation, congenital immunodeficiencies)[3-7] and as congenital toxoplasmosis,[8-9] Occurrence of toxoplasmosis in man depends on the status of the host's immune system, virulence of the organism and genetic polymorphisms in the host. This decides the different patterns and degrees of disease severity that we get to see in toxoplasma infection. In immunocompetent individuals, infection with Toxoplasma is common, but is a subclinical infection and resolves itself, symptoms being of an acute febrile illness. CNS involvement is uncommon and can occur as diffuse meningoencephalitis or rarely with features of a space occupying lesion. Extracranial involvement in acquired toxoplasmosis is more severe, whereas in congenital infection, the primary hit occurs to the brain. Cerebral toxoplasmosis has increased many folds since the emergence of HIV acquired immunodeficiency syndrome (AIDS) and is the most common opportunistic infection involving the brain. The clinical presentation in immunosuppressed varies from mass lesions or seizures. CNS involvement by toxoplasmosis can be the first sign of unsuspected HIV infection and is an AIDS defining illness. The most common pattern is that of a solitary mass. But CNS lymphoma, tuberculoma and progressive multifocal leukoencephalopathy have to be ruled out. CT scan shows multiple, bilateral ring enhancing lesions. MRI is better and a more accurate modality in differentiating toxoplasmosis from other lesions. Other diagnostic aids include anti-Toxoplasma antibody titers, CSF PCR and western blot.

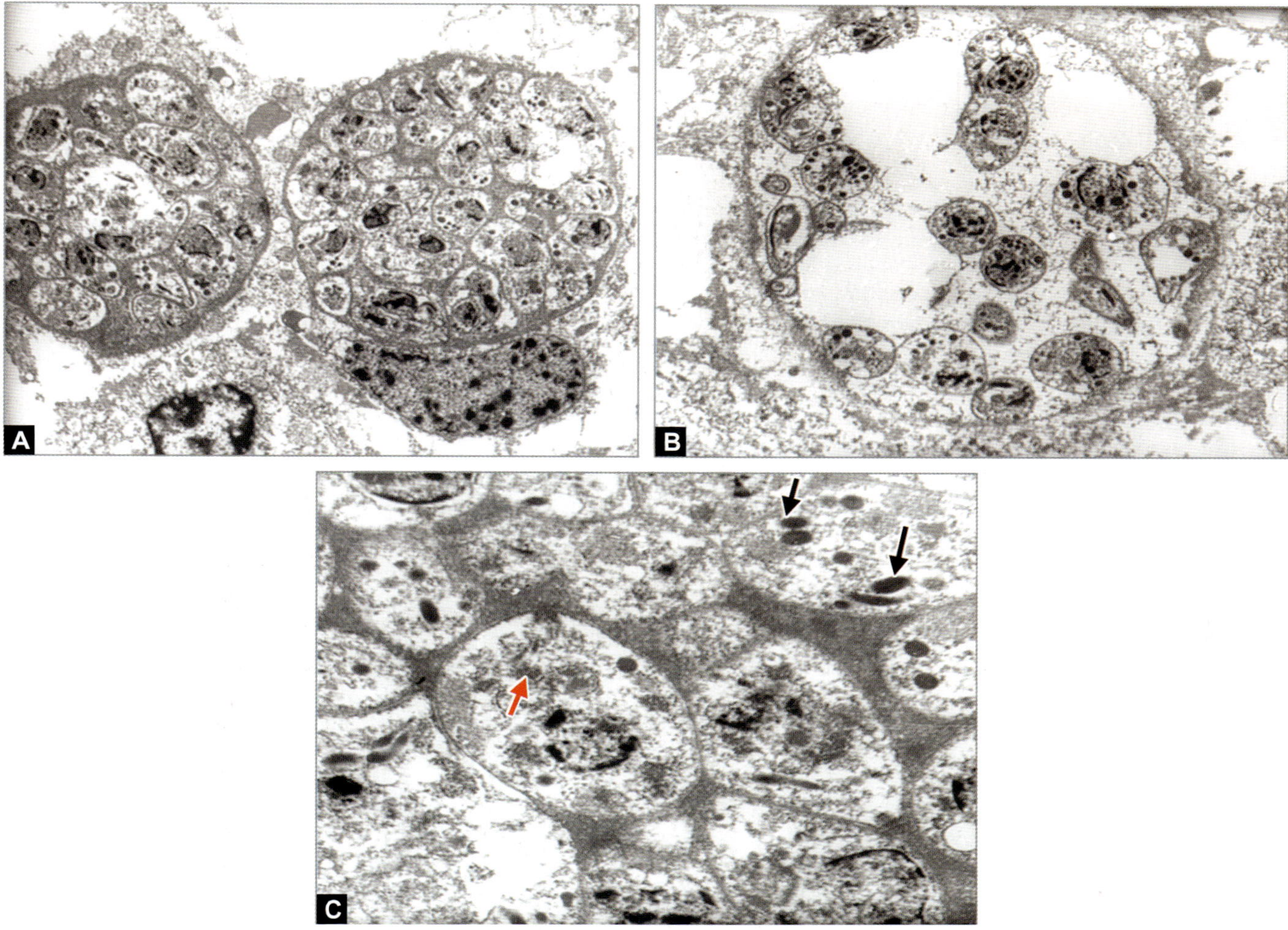

Figs 5A–C: Electron microscopy. (A) Showing cysts packed with bradyzoites (cut horizontally); (B) A pseudocyst containing fewer tachyzoites (cut horizontally); and (C) Higher power shows horizontally cut bradyzoites containing dense granules (black arrows), micronemes (red arrow).

Pathology of cerebral toxoplasmosis in AIDS patients show three main type of lesions: (1) Poorly circumscribed necrotizing abscesses which show inflammatory cells, lipid laden macrophages, newly formed capillaries along with tachyzoites and encysted organisms. The vessels within and around may show vasculitis, necrosis, intimal proliferation and thrombosis. (2) Organizing abscesses may be seen in which a central area of coagulative necrosis is surrounded by macrophages containing organisms. (3) Treated cases show well demarcated non-necrotic or cystic spaces with microglial nodules, astrogliosis and lipid laden macrophages with scanty organisms. These may be seen in the gray or white matter. Congenital toxoplasmosis is transmitted through the placenta and occurs when the maternal infection occurs during pregnancy. ***T. gondii*** has the highest risk of affecting the fetus during the second trimester. After birth, the babies present with convulsions, cerebral calcification, hydrocephalus and chorioretinitis. The pathology too differs in newborns due to the immune status and because of the effect of the organism on the developing brain. Parasites multiply in the subependymal and ependymal tissue and brain shows necrosis (minimal to widespread), vascular thrombosis, periaqueductal and periventricular calcification/necrosis and hydrocephalus due to aqueductal destruction. Severe brain destruction leads to microcephaly.

COMMENTARY—INDEX CASE: PM 19210

This was a 26-year-old agriculturist, who presented with fever, continuous bifrontal headache, vomiting, seizures and altered sensorium. CNS examination revealed an irritable young male with second and seventh (UMN type) cranial nerve involvement. CT scan and MRI of the brain showed multiple, bilateral, varying sized ring enhancing lesions with marked perilesional edema. Although the HIV status (positive) of the individual was not known antemortem, yet a unilateral or a bilateral asymmetrical mass in the basal ganglia region is very characteristic of Toxoplasma. Microscopy revealed characteristic multiple necrotic abscesses replete with inflammatory cells, pseudocysts with tachyzoites, free tachyzoites and tissue cysts with bradyzoites. Massive edema was present in the brain and severe cerebral edema is said to be a hallmark of toxoplasmosis. There was limited overlying meningitis and this was the reason for an acellular CSF. Lumbar puncture should be avoided as 2% patients with space occupying lesions may show a normal fundus, but CSF pressure may still be raised. A unilateral lesion or unequal bilateral lesions in brain may not cause a diffuse rise in CSF pressure and hence papilledema may be missing.

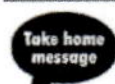

TAKE HOME MESSAGE

- Multiple asymmetrical bilateral ring enhancing lesions in the brain on MRI scan is very diagnostic of toxoplasmosis.
- CNS involvement by toxoplasmosis can be the first sign of unsuspected HIV infection and is an AIDS defining illness.

REFERENCES

1. Krick JA, Remington JS. Toxoplasmosis in the adult—an overview. New Engl J Med. 1978;298:550-3.
2. Rose I. Morphology and diagnostics of human toxoplasmosis. Gen Diagn Pathol. 1997;142:257-70.
3. Luft BJ, Remington JS. Toxoplasmic encephalitis in AIDS. Clin Infect Dis. 1992;15:211-22.
4. Luft BJ, Hafner R, Korzun AH, et al. Toxoplasmic encephalitis in patients with the acquired immunodeficiency syndrome. Members of the ACTG 077p/ANRS 009 Study Team. N Engl J Med. 1993;329:995-1000.
5. Daras M, Koppel BS, Samkoff L, et al. Brainstem toxoplasmosis in patients with acquired immunodeficiency syndrome. J Neuroimaging. 1994;4:85-90.
6. Porter SB, Sande MA. Toxoplasmosis of the central nervous system in the acquired immunodeficiency syndrome. N Engl J Med. 1992;327:1643-8.
7. Navia BA, Petito CK, Gold JMW, et al. Cerebral toxoplasmosis complicating the acquired immune deficiency syndrome: clinical and neuropathological findings in 27 patients. Ann Neurol. 1986;1:224-38.
8. Lowichik A, Siegal JD. Parasitic infections of the central nervous system in children. Part 1: Congenital infections and meningoencephalitis. J Child Neurol. 1995;10:4-17.
9. Swisher CN, Boyer K, McLeod R. Congenital toxoplasmosis. The Toxoplasmosis Study Group. Semin Pediatr Neurol. 1994;1:4-25.

CONTRIBUTIONS BY:

1. Dr RK Vasishta, Professor and Head, Department of Histopathology (Consultation)
2. Dr NK Khandelwal, Professor and Head, Department of Radiodiagnosis and Imaging (Figs 1A and B)
3. Dr RJ Dash, Ex-Professor and Head, Department of Endocrinology (Clinician In-Charge)

Post Graduate Institute of Medical Education and Research, Chandigarh, India.

CASE 16

Pulmonary Hyalinizing Granuloma with Recent Onset Cryptococcal Meningoencephalitis in an Immunocompetent Male: PM 21122

Nandita Bharadwaj Kakkar

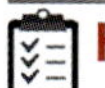

HIGHLIGHTS OF THE CASE

A young male presented with nonspecific symptoms (generalized body aches and malaise) since a year. Fever, off and on was present since 4 months, which became persistent a month before admission. He was diagnosed at an outside facility as a case of tuberculosis, was put on antitubercular treatment, but did not respond to it and it was withdrawn. Headache came a week before admission. At admission, X-ray chest/CT led to a re-diagnosis of tuberculosis and he was started on antitubercular therapy (ATT) again. Contrast-enhanced computed tomography (CECT) head at admission revealed a normal study, 4 days later showed cerebral edema and on the day of demise revealed a left high parietal hypodensity with no basal exudates. The cerebrospinal fluid (CSF) examination at admission revealed features of chronic meningitis, but the last CSF examination, a day prior to death revealed cryptococci. The patient progressively deteriorated and developed right hemiparesis, complex partial seizures and bilateral sixth nerve palsy. Autopsy diagnosis was pulmonary hyalinizing granuloma with recent onset cryptococcal meningoencephalitis in an immunocompetent male. .

Keywords: Autopsy, *Cryptococcus*, meningitis, immunocompetent, pulmonary hyalinizing granuloma.

CLINICAL DETAILS

Date of Admission: 09.12.2005, Date of Death: 20.12.2005, Duration of Hospital Stay: 12 Days

A 35-year-male was admitted in our institute for 12 days. He presented with generalized body aches and malaise since one year. There was fever, off and on since 4 months, which became persistent, one month prior to admission. Fever was low grade with evening rise, no rigors/chills were present and it responded to antipyretics. Chest X-ray was suggestive of pulmonary tuberculosis and he was started on antitubercular treatment, to which he did not respond and the same was discontinued after one month. Dry cough was present and at times, there was mucoid expectoration. A week before the admission, there was high grade persistent fever with headache. The headache was holocranial, intermittent, severe, accompanied with nausea and vomiting. However, there were no seizures, altered sensorium or any focal deficit. There was no history of loose stools, pain abdomen, chest pain, breathlessness, skin lesions, joint swelling, diabetes or hypertension. On ***examination,*** he was fully conscious, oriented, moving all four limbs, afebrile, pulse 100/min, BP 126/80 mm Hg and respiratory rate 20/min. There was no pallor, cyanosis, jaundice, lymphadenopathy, pedal edema or any skin lesion. Both liver and spleen were palpable 5 cm below their respective costal margins. There was no ascites. Cardiovascular and respiratory system were normal. CNS examination revealed a conscious, oriented male, Kernig's sign positive, no papilledema, pupils 4 mm bilateral equal, no cranial nerve/sensory/motor deficit, deep tendon jerks present with down going plantars.

Investigations and Course of Management

Total leucocyte count was 12,000/μL with 90% polymorphs. Hemoglobin, platelets and blood biochemistry were within normal limits. HIV was non-reactive. Chest X-ray revealed bilateral conglomerate miliary infiltrates. CECT (chest and abdomen) revealed multiple discrete (5–15 mm) lymph nodes in the paratracheal, pretracheal, precarinal and bilateral hilar regions. In the lungs, there were bilateral, patchy areas of parenchymal consolidation with a cavity in the left lung with intracavitary soft tissue, suggestive of a fungal ball.

Table 1: Details of cerebrospinal fluid examination.

	At admission	*5 days later*	*One day before death*
Cells	NIL	60	90
DLC		Lymphocytes	Lymphocytes
ADA (IU/L)	ND	5.5	ND
Sugar (mg/dL)	72	15	33
Protein (mg/dL)	20	60	40
India Ink	ND	ND	Cryptococcus ++
Fungal culture	ND	ND	*Cryptococcus neoformans*
Crypto LA	ND	ND	+

(DLC: Differentiated leukocyte count; ADA: Adenosine deaminase).

Features were suggestive of post-primary Kochs with endobronchial spread with superimposed fungal infection. CECT head at admission revealed a normal study, 4 days later showed cerebral edema with no hydrocephalus and on the day of demise, revealed left high parietal hypodensity with no basal exudates. Cerebrospinal fluid examination was done thrice (Table 1).

To begin with, he was treated as a case of tubercular meningitis and was put on antitubercular treatment and steroids. He developed complex partial seizures and bilateral sixth nerve palsy. Repeat CSF examination was suggestive of chronic meningitis. After 5 days, he developed severe headache, altered sensorium and seizures. Repeat CT head disclosed cerebral edema without hydrocephalus/infarcts. The patient however deteriorated and he developed right hemiparesis. At this time, CT head showed a hypodense lesion in the left high parietal area. A third repeat CSF examination showed presence of *Cryptococcus*. He was immediately started on amphotericin, but his condition deteriorated and he succumbed to his illness. Unit's final diagnosis was Cryptococcal Meningitis.

AUTOPSY FINDINGS: PM 21122

A complete autopsy was performed. The serous cavities were within normal limits. The ***lungs*** were bulky, together weighing 1,370 g. The pleura was thickened and firm, stony hard nodules were felt on palpation (Fig 1). The lung parenchyma was stony hard and gritty to cut, making the lung very difficult to slice. Cut section (Figs 2A and B) however revealed diffusely scattered multiple stony hard nodules, many of them confluent and some calcified. A cavity was noted in the left lower lobe, measuring 4 cm in diameter, containing pultaceous material. Bronchiectasis was noted in both lungs. Microscopic examination (Fig 3A-D) showed well-circumscribed granulomas/nodules composed of central whorled deposits of lamellar hyaline collagen, separated by clear spaces and surrounded by sparse lymphocytic infiltrate. The collagen was hypocellular and in areas had a very ropy appearance (Fig 4A). The nodules were getting confluent and few showed calcification. Granulomas were seen in the vicinity of bronchioles leading to their dilatation and causing bronchiectasis (Fig 4B). Sections studied from the cavity in the left lower lobe contained a ball of Aspergillus, with the fungal profiles also infiltrating the adjacent alveolar spaces. The hilar, carinal, paratracheal and pretracheal ***lymph nodes***

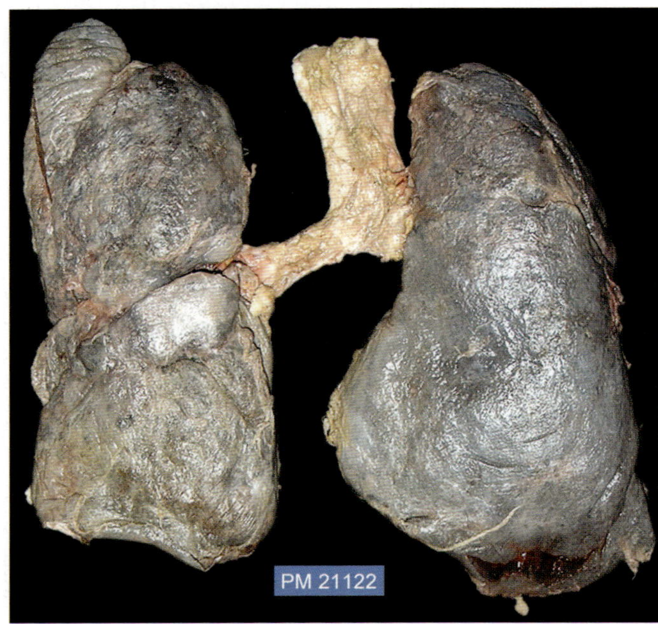

Fig 1: Gross picture of both lungs showing a thickened pleura, puckered at places.

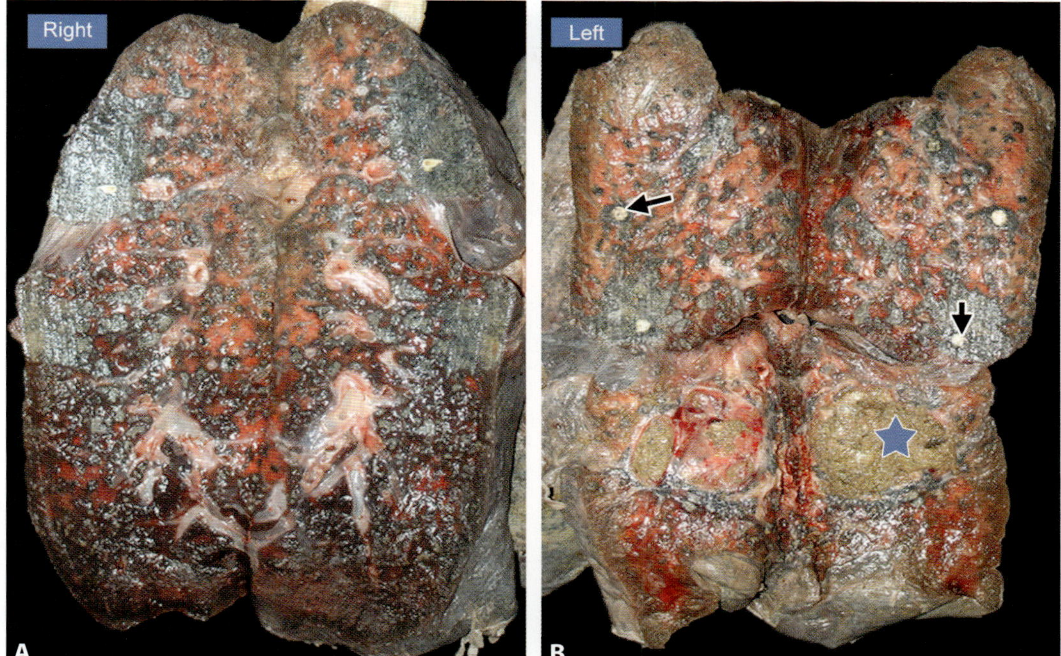

Figs 2A and B: Cut section of both lungs showing diffusely scattered multiple, stony hard nodules, many of them getting confluent. Calcified nodules were seen in the left lung (arrows). A cavity was noted in the left lower lobe, measuring 4 cm in diameter, containing pultaceous material (star).

(Fig 4C) were mildly enlarged and revealed similar hyalinized well-circumscribed granulomas (Fig 4D) as seen in the lung. Periodic acid–Schiff (PAS), Alcian blue, mucicarmine and Grocotts stain, done on multiple sections of the lung and lymph nodes, did not reveal any organisms. Ziehl–Neelsen stain done on multiple sections was negative. Overall features were those of pulmonary hyalinizing granulomas involving the lung and lymph nodes, left lower lobe aspergilloma and bilateral bronchiectasis. The ***brain*** weighed 1,300 g. The convexities were covered with a shiny, slimy exudate (Figs 5A and B). No basal exudates were however visible (Fig 5C). A 4 mm hemorrhagic spot was seen in the left parietal white matter. Microscopy revealed a dense foamy exudate (Figs 6A–D) in the meninges composed of histiocytes, lymphocytes, plasma cells, giant cells, polymorphs, nuclear debris and was replete with encapsulated, refractile, empty looking fungal profiles, ranging in size from 5 to 12 μm and showing prominent budding. The PAS stain showed deep pink staining of the body of the organism and the Alcian blue stain, stained the capsule deep blue (Figs 6E and 7A). Mucicarmine (Figs 7B and C) stained the capsule deep pink and many cryptococci were seen within the giant cells. Morphology and staining characteristics of the fungal profiles conformed to the morphology of cryptococci. A tiny parenchymal lesion was noted in the left parietal white matter, composed of cryptococci. Overall features were those of cryptococcal meningoencephalitis. The ***liver*** (1850 g) and ***spleen*** (420 g) were enlarged and revealed septicemic changes. Liver also showed steatosis.

FINAL AUTOPSY DIAGNOSIS : PM 21122

35 Years Immunocompetent Male

- Bilateral pulmonary hyalinizing granuloma, left lower lobe aspergilloma and bilateral bronchiectasis.
- Hyalinizing granulomas—lymph nodes (hilar, carinal and pre/paratracheal)
- Cryptococcal meningoencephalitis
- Septicemic changes—liver and spleen.

PULMONARY HYALINIZING GRANULOMA

Pulmonary hyalinizing granuloma (PHG)[1-4] is a rare disease wherein the hallmark of diagnosis is extensive fibrosis occurring in a nodular pattern. It affects adults but has no sex predilection.[3-5] Patients present with nonspecific symptoms like fever, cough, fatigue, pleuritic chest pain and dyspnea. However, many patients are completely asymptomatic with lesions found incidentally during routine screening

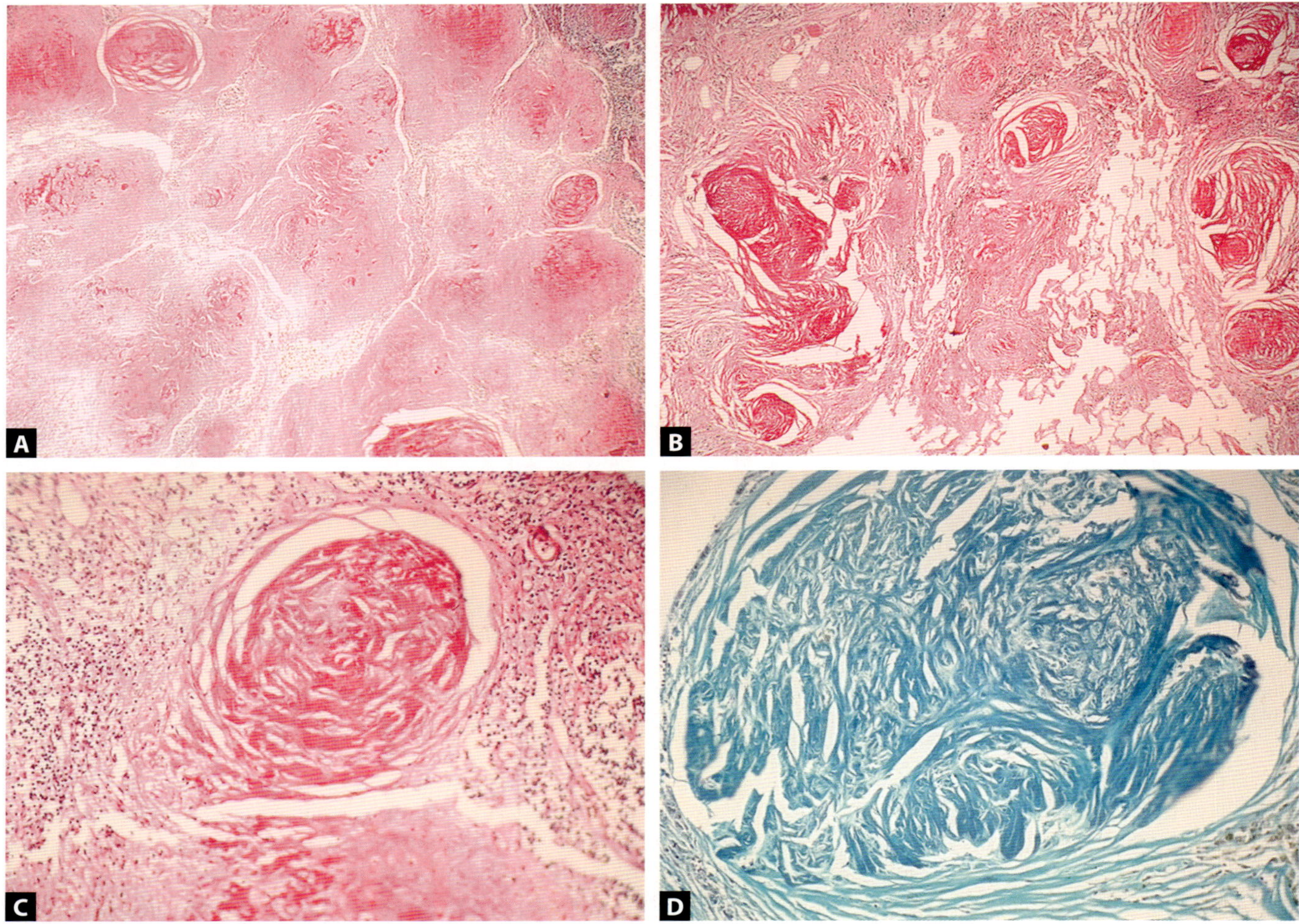

Figs 3A–D: (A to C) Lung showing well-circumscribed granulomas/nodules composed of central whorled deposits of lamellar hyaline collagen, separated by clear spaces and surrounded by sparse lymphocytic infiltrate; and (D) Massons trichrome stains the collagen deep green.

examinations.[5] The etiology of this entity is not known, but it appears to be due to a florid immune response provoked by various infections[4] (*Mycobacterium tuberculosis*, Histoplasma and other fungal infections) and many autoimmune/collagen disorders. Many patients with immune mediated diseases and those afflicted by mycobacterial/fungal infections are diagnosed to have PHG. Other diseases associated with PHG are rheumatoid arthritis, Sjögren's syndrome, posterior uveitis, hemolytic anemia, sclerosing mediastinitis, retroperitoneal fibrosis,[6] lymphomas and Castleman's disease.[7] X-ray chest and CT findings show multiple randomly distributed, unilateral or bilateral nodules and/or masses with well-defined borders. Calcification and rare cavitation can be seen. The nodules range in size from few millimeters to 15 cm in diameter, with an average diameter of 2 cm. Lymphadenopathy is absent. F-18 fluorodeoxyglucose positron emission tomography (FDG-PET/CT) can reveal increased metabolic activity in PHG lesions. This entity enters the differential diagnosis of patients with pulmonary nodules,[4] which includes infections (tuberculosis/fungal infections/histoplasma), malignancy, rheumatoid nodules, amyloidosis, granulomatosis with polyangiitis, sarcoidosis and lymphomatoid granulomatosis. Histopathological examination clinches the diagnosis, but many entities have to be excluded before coming to this diagnosis. Moreover, awareness about PHG is a must, as the eyes cannot see what the mind does not know. On microscopic examination, well-circumscribed nodules composed of central whorled deposits of lamellar hyaline collagen, separated by clear spaces and surrounded by sparse inflammatory cells are seen. Bronchiectasis with fungal colonization can occur as a complication of PHG. There is no definitive treatment, although

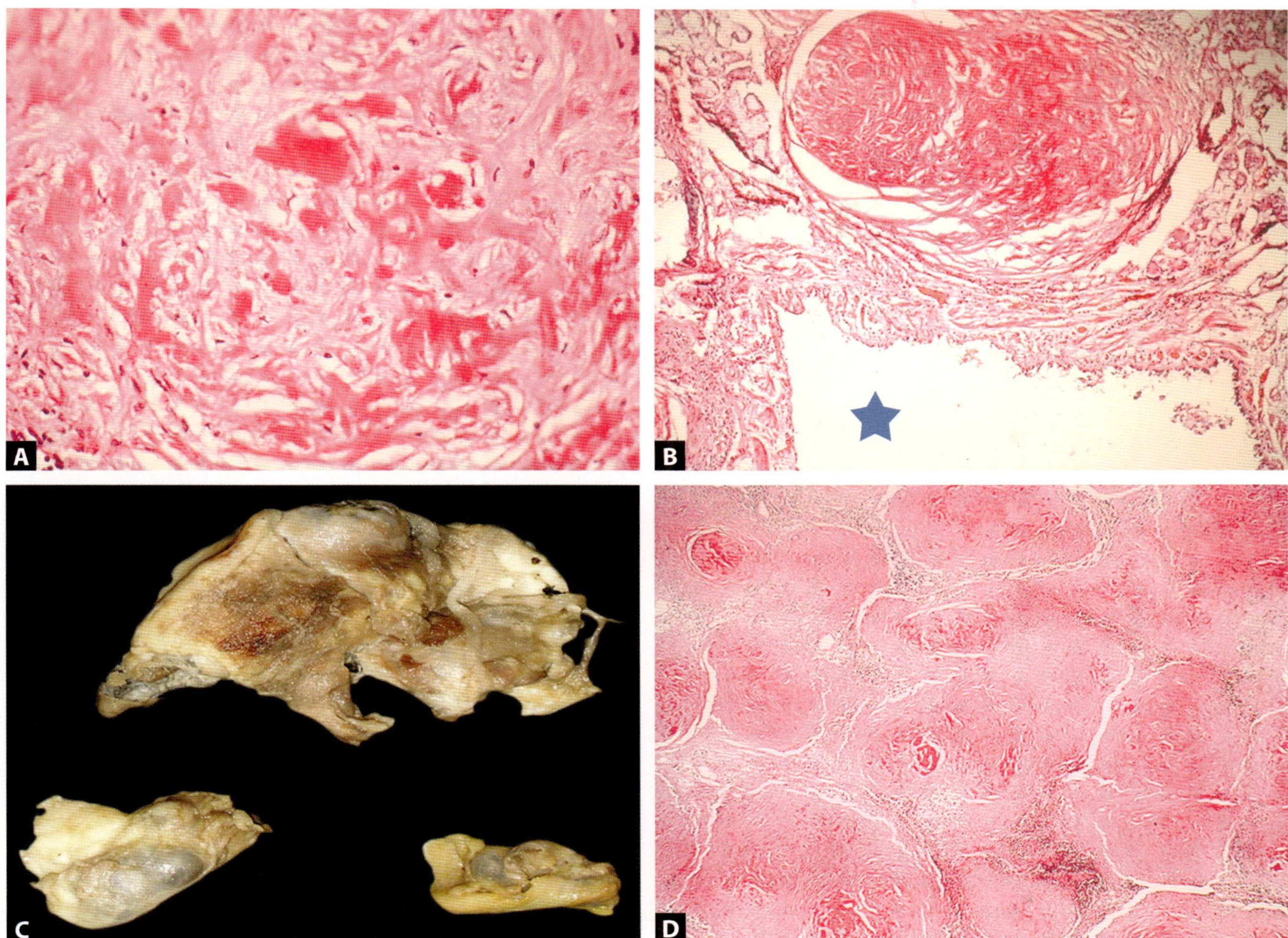

Figs 4A–D: (A) Ropy collagen within the granuloma; (B) A dilated bronchiole (star) adjacent to a hyalinized granuloma; (C) Gross picture of the enlarged carinal, para/pretracheal lymph nodes; and (D) Microphotograph from the lymph node showing similar hyalinized granulomas as seen in the lungs.

successful resolution of the nodules with the administration of glucocorticoids has been reported.

CRYPTOCOCCAL MENINGITIS

Cryptococcal meningitis[8-11] is a common opportunistic infection in the immunocompromised individuals due to impaired cell mediated immunity. It can be seen post-transplant, in acquired immunodeficiency, hematological malignancies, sarcoidosis, connective tissue diseases and in patients on steroid therapy. It can occur in immunocompetent individuals as well. Infection by ***Cryptococcus*** is acquired by inhaling spores, which first leads to pulmonary infection. In immunocompetent individuals as a result of intact cell-mediated and humoral immunity, the infection is either symptomless or leads to a mild pneumonia which resolves on its own. The signs and symptoms of pulmonary cryptococcosis are fever, cough, pleuritic pain, malaise, weight loss and at times a streaky hemoptysis. In the immunocompromised individuals, hematogenous dissemination from the lungs may result in the involvement of other organs, including brain. However, in the immunocompetent hosts, pulmonary infection generally resolves, but may remain dormant in the lungs and lymph nodes or at times, as a mediastinal mass, ready to erupt (even years later) with hematogenous dissemination, when the immune status gets compromised.

Infection with ***Cryptococcus neoformans*** is the most common fungal infection of the CSF and may present as meningitis (most common), chronic or subacute meningoencephalitis or as a space-occupying lesion. In meningitis, sign

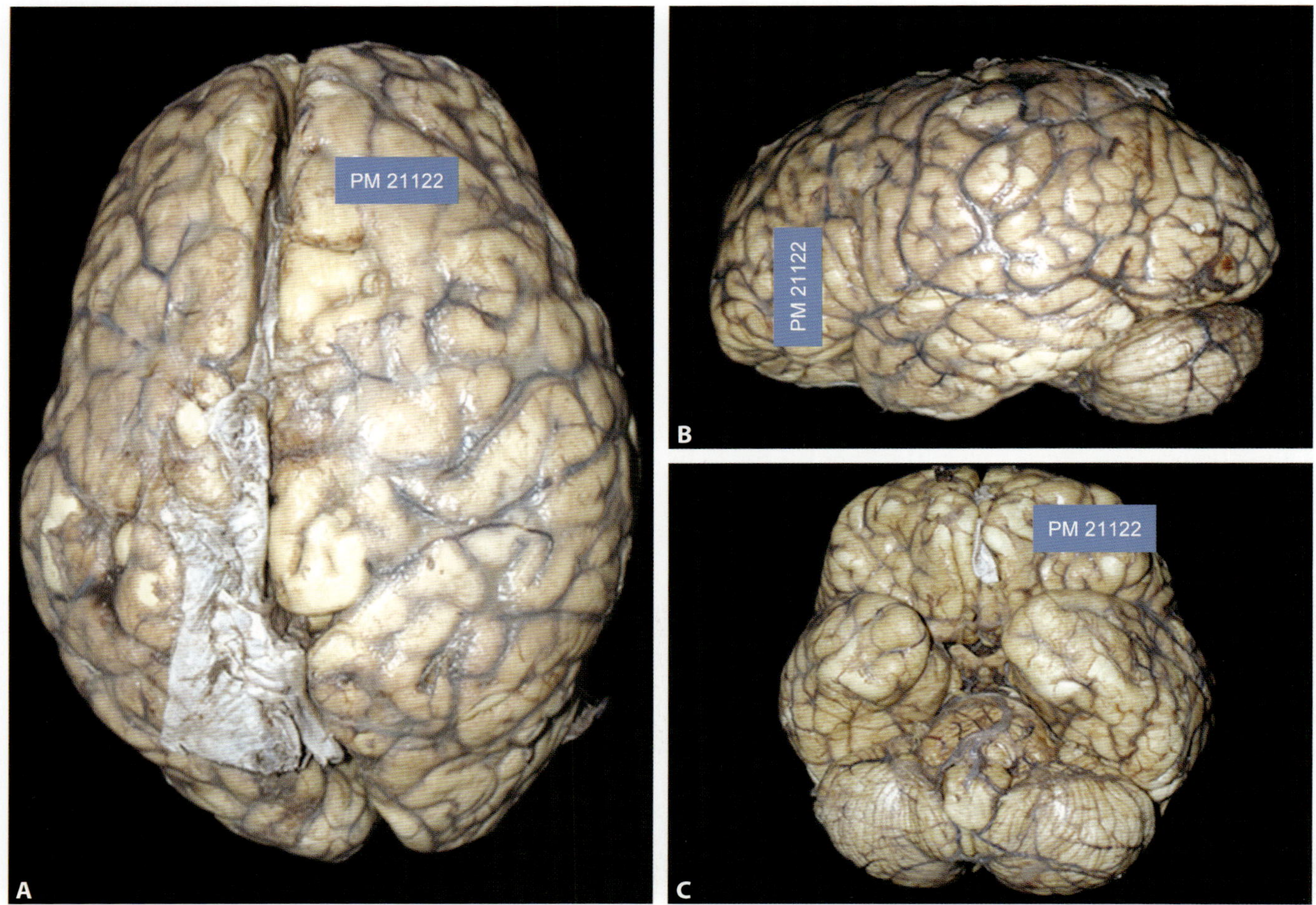

Figs 5A–C: (A and B) Superolateral and left lateral aspect of the brain showing slight opalescence due to a slimy exudate; and (C) Base of the brain is free of any exudate.

and symptoms include fever, headache, altered sensorium, neck rigidity, papilledema, cranial nerve palsies, hearing/visual loss, gait impairment and neurological deficits. In immunodeficiency like HIV infection, cryptococcal infection occurs when the CD4 counts go below 100 cells/μL. Cryptococcus neoformans breaches the blood-brain barrier by transcellular migration across brain endothelial cells.[10-11] The endothelial cells show changes in their organelles, like swelling of mitochondria/endoplasmic reticulum, production of urease and membrane damage leading to a break of the blood-brain barrier. Thereafter, the organism replicates in the subarachnoid space leading to the formation of a slimy leptomeningeal exudate, which first predominates at the base of the brain and later extends over the convexities. This exudate extends into the ventricles and along the Virchow-Robin spaces, where clusters of cryptococci distending the perivascular spaces is seen, thus imparting the characteristic soap bubble appearance. Hydrocephalus may develop. Microscopically[12,13] the meningitic exudate is composed of a minimal inflammatory infiltrate composed of macrophages, giant cells, lymphocytes, polymorphs admixed with cryptococci, perivascular small tubercles (mimics tuberculosis), borderzone encephalitis which may extend deep into the parenchyma and pseudocystic dilatation of Virchow-Robin spaces containing cryptococci. This exudate can further extend into the spinal cord and nerve roots giving rise to myeloradiculitis. Intracerebral abscesses and cryptococcomas (in the cerebrum, cerebellum and spinal cord) may be found in some cases. The meningeal reaction could either be gelatinous (seen in immunocompromised individuals) with minimal inflammation and sheets of cryptococci or granulomatous (seen in immunocompetent hosts) wherein there are giant cells, lymphocytes, histiocytes and fibroblastic response admixed with cryptococci.

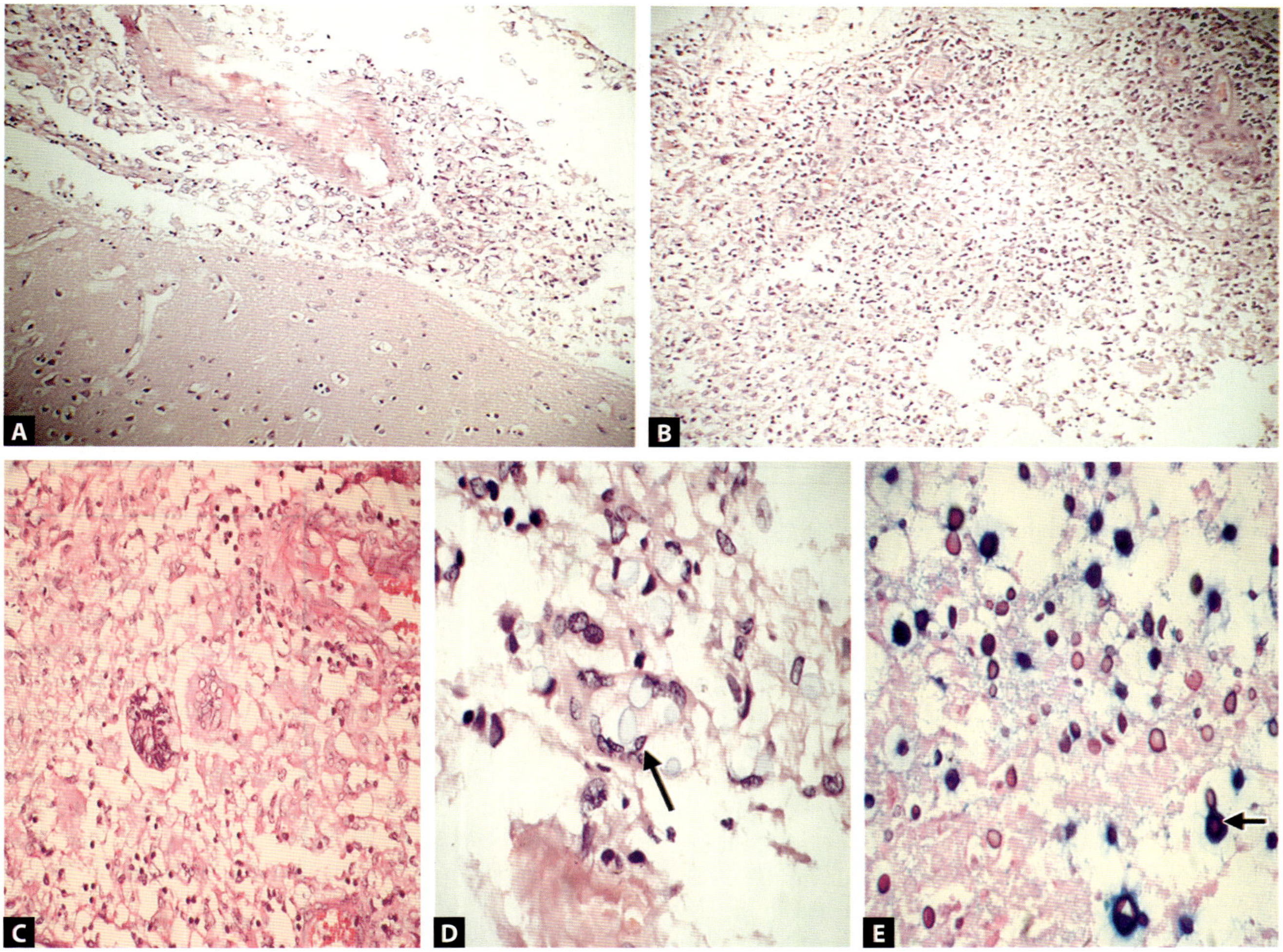

Figs 6A–E: (A and B) Photomicrograph showing a foamy meningeal exudate. Meningeal exudate showing: (C) Histiocytes, polymorphs and giant cells; (D) Encapsulated, refractile, empty looking fungal profiles (arrow), ranging in size from 5 to 12 μm; and (E) Periodic acid–Schiff (PAS) Alcian blue stain showing plenty of cryptococci with some showing prominent budding (arrow).

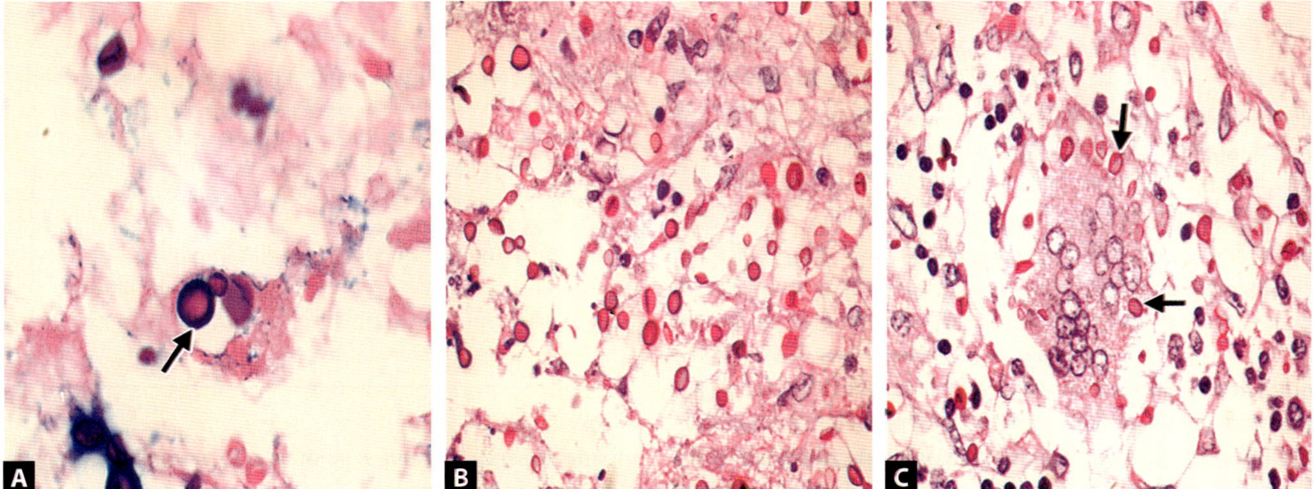

Figs 7A–C: Meningeal exudate. (A) Periodic acid–Schiff (PAS) Alcian blue stain—PAS stains the body of the cryptococci pink and the Alcian blue stains the capsule deep blue (arrow); and (B and C) Mucicarmine stain showing plenty of cryptococci with magenta staining of the capsule, with many cryptococci seen within the giant cell (arrows).

Immunocompromised individuals show more parenchymal brain lesions and a higher incidence of involvement of extracranial sites. The thick gelatinous polysaccharide capsule of the Cryptococcus has tremendous value as it aids in the detection of this fungi. The capsule is stained by mucin stains such as Mayer's mucicarmine (magenta color) and Alcian blue (deep blue color). Periodic acid–Schiff stains the entire organism, i.e. the body and the capsule, deep pink/magenta. Grocotts silver stain, stains the body black. With India ink, the unstained mucoid capsule of the fungi appears as a clear halo against a dark background. Mucicarmine staining of the capsule is diagnostic and this reaction is not given by any other pathogenic yeast like fungus. Cryptococcal antigen (CRAG) test detects the capsular antigen in the plasma or the CSF.

COMMENTARY—INDEX CASE: PM 21122

This young 35-year-old male presented with nonspecific symptoms (generalized body aches, fatigue and malaise) since a year. This was followed by cough and fever. The plausible sequence of events in this case seems to have started with cryptococcal infection of the lung (more than a year ago), which is acquired by inhalation of spores. As happens in immunocompetent hosts, as a consequence of both cell-mediated and humoral immunity, the initial pulmonary infection is generally asymptomatic, although a self-limited pneumonia resolving over several weeks to months in the absence of treatment may be seen. This had happened in the index case as well. Thereafter, the patient developed bilateral pulmonary hyalinizing granuloma as a result of the exaggerated immune response to the antigenic stimuli by the CRAG. The nonspecific symptoms of generalized body aches, fatigue, malaise, followed by cough and fever were the result of the acquisition of bilateral pulmonary hyalinizing granuloma. Fever, off and on, was present for 4 months, which became persistent a month before admission. X-ray chest at this point, done at an outside facility, revealed bilateral miliary infiltrates (as is seen in patients with pulmonary hyalinizing granuloma). The patient was put on antitubercular treatment, did not respond to it and the treatment was withdrawn. Headache, came only a week before admission to our institute. At admission to PGIMER, X-ray chest revealed bilateral miliary tubercles and CT showed 5–15 mm nodes in the hilar and paratracheal region. Tuberculosis was the clinical diagnosis and he was restarted on ATT. CECT head at admission to PGI revealed a normal study, 4 days later showed cerebral edema and on the day of demise revealed a left high parietal hypodensity with no basal exudates. The CSF examination at admission revealed features of chronic meningitis, but the last CSF examination, a day prior to death revealed cryptococci. The patient progressively deteriorated and developed right hemiparesis, complex partial seizures and bilateral sixth nerve palsy. The cryptococcal meningitis was of recent onset, as the organism can get reactivated from the sites of initial infection, years later. Pulmonary hyalinizing granuloma can bring down a patient's immune status, as happened in the index case. So, in the index case the cryptococci got reactivated from the lungs/lymph nodes and led to the occurrence of cryptococcal meningoencephalitis, which ultimately led to the demise of the patient. Autopsy diagnosis was pulmonary hyalinizing granuloma with recent onset cryptococcal meningoencephalitis in an immunocompetent male.

In conclusion, the young immunocompetent male first contacted a self-limited cryptococcal infection of the lungs, followed by bilateral pulmonary hyalinizing granuloma along with involvement of the lymph nodes. Later due to the dip of immunity and reactivation of the dormant cryptococci, cryptococcal meningoencephalitis led to the demise of the patient.

TAKE HOME MESSAGE

- Pulmonary hyalinizing granuloma is a rare disease wherein the hallmark of diagnosis is extensive fibrosis occurring in a nodular pattern.
- The etiology of this entity is not known, but it appears to be due to a florid immune response to various infections and autoimmune/collagen disorders.
- Radiology shows multiple randomly distributed well-defined nodules.
- Cryptococcal meningitis is a common opportunistic infection in the immunocompromised individuals but can occur in immunocompetent individuals as well.
- *Cryptococcus neoformans* has a predilection for the lung and the CNS.
- Cryptococcal thick gelatinous polysaccharide capsule has a tremendous value as it aids in the detection of this fungi.
- The cryptococcal capsule is stained by Mayer's mucicarmine (magenta color) and Alcian blue (deep blue color), PAS stains the entire organism deep pink/magenta, Grocott's silver stain, stains the body black and in India ink preparation, the unstained mucoid capsule of the fungi appears as a clear halo against a dark background.
- Mucicarmine staining of the capsule is diagnostic and this reaction is not given by any other pathogenic yeast-like fungus.

REFERENCES

1. Brandão V, Marchiori E, Zanetti G, et al. Hyalinizing granuloma: an unusual case of a pulmonary mass. Case Rep Med. 2010;2010:984765.
2. Yousem SA, Hochholzer L. Pulmonary hyalinizing granuloma. Am J Clin Pathol. 1987;87:1-6.
3. Lvovsky D, Rosman J, Iliescu ME. Pulmonary hyalinizing granuloma (PHG) presenting as bilateral dense apical masses. Chest. 2004;126:950S-1S.
4. Chalaoui J, Gregoire P, Sylvestre J, et al. Pulmonary hyalinizing granuloma: a cause of pulmonary nodules. Radiology. 1984;152:23-6.
5. Agrawal D, Deshpande R, Maheshwari S, et al Pulmonary hyalinizing granuloma with ureteric fibrosis: a case report and review of relevant literature. Indian J Chest Dis Allied Sci. 2006;48:283-5.
6. Atagi S, Sakatani M, Akira M, Yamamoto S, et al. Pulmonary hyalinizing granuloma with Castleman's disease. Intern Med. 1994;33:689-91.
7. Shinohara T, KanekoT, Miyazawa N, et al. Pulmonary hyalinizing granuloma with laryngeal and subcutaneous involvement: report of a case successfully treated with glucocorticoids. Intern Med. 2004;43:69-73.
8. Murthy JM, Sundaram C. Fungal infections of the central nervous system. Handb Clin Neurol. 2014;121:1383-401.
9. Eisenman HC, Casadevall A, McClelland EE. New insights on the pathogenesis of invasive *Cryptococcus neoformans* infection. Curr Infect Dis Rep. 2007;9:457-64.
10. Chang YC, Stins MF, McCaffery MJ, et al. Cryptococcal yeast cells invade the central nervous system via transcellular penetration of the blood-brain barrier. Infect Immun. 2004; 72:4985-95.
11. Chen SH, Stins MF, Huang SH, et al. *Cryptococcus neoformans* induces alterations in the cytoskeleton of human brain microvascular endothelial cells. J Med Microbiol. 2003; 52:961-70.
12. Lee SC, Dickson DW, Casadevall A. Pathology of cryptococcal meningoencephalitis: analysis of 27 patients with pathogenetic implications. Hum Pathol. 1996;27:839-47.
13. Benesová P, Buchta V, Cerman J, et al. Cryptococcosis—a review of 13 autopsy cases from a 54-year period in a large hospital. APMIS. 2007;115:177-83.

CONTRIBUTIONS BY:

1. Dr RK Vasishta, Professor and Head, Department of Histopathology (Consultation)
2. Dr Vivek Lal, Professor and Head, Department of Neurology (Compilation of Clinical Details)
3. Dr SC Varma, Ex-Professor and Head, Department of Internal Medicine (Clinician In-Charge)

Post Graduate Institute of Medical Education and Research, Chandigarh, India.

CASE 17

Leptospirosis with Multiorgan Involvement: PM 22793

Nandita Bharadwaj Kakkar

HIGHLIGHTS OF THE CASE

This is a classical case of leptospirosis, clinically and at autopsy. Patient presented acutely with fever, pain in abdomen, respiratory distress and conjunctival suffusion. Investigations revealed deranged renal and liver function tests, hypokalemia, deranged coagulogram, leukocytosis, anemia and low platelets. Autopsy showed classic features of leptospirosis—tubulointerstitial nephritis, acute hepatitis, pancarditis and widespread hemorrhages. Warthin–Starry stain brought out the spirochetes in the renal tubular epithelium and the postmortem blood sample serology was positive for Leptospira.

Keywords: Leptospira, tubulointerstitial nephritis, acute hepatitis, pancarditis, hemorrhages, Warthin–Starry stain, serology, multiorgan.

CLINICAL DETAILS

Date of Admission: 2.9.2008, Date of Death: 4.9.2008, Duration of Hospital Stay: 2 days

A 42-year-old female came with high grade, intermittent fever with rigors and chills, present since 10 days. There was a dull aching pain in the epigastric region and in the right upper quadrant since 7 days. Difficulty in breathing and a mild decrease in urinary output was present since the past 2 days, probably because of inadequate fluid intake. There was no history of any drug intake, surgery, blood transfusion or any such illness in the family. There was no past history of jaundice. She was non-alcoholic and was married with five children. On ***examination,*** she was febrile, icteric, pale and pedal edema was present. There was no lymphadenopathy. Pulse was 80/min regular, BP—90/60 mm Hg, jugular venous pressure was normal and conjunctival suffusion was present. The abdomen was distended, there was no free fluid and the right hypochondrium was tender. There was mild hepatosplenomegaly and the bowel sounds were present. The central nervous system (CNS) and cardiovascular system (CVS) were normal. On chest examination there was vesicular sounds and crepitations.

Investigations and Course of Management

Hemogram: Hb—9.4 g/dL, TLC—24,000/μL, DLC—N75, L21, M3, E1, platelets—35,000/μL, peripheral smear—no malarial parasite, coagulogram—PTI 35%, aPPT 50' (N: 25'–32'), D-dimers + and fibrinogen—0.68 g/L (N: 2–4 g/L). ***Blood biochemistry:*** Na^+/K^+—144/3.4 mEq/L, serum urea/creatinine—143/3.8 mg%, serum bilirubin, total/conjugated—5.8/5.3 mg%, SGOT/SGPT—169/58 U/L, alkaline phosphatase—193 U/L, total proteins/albumin/globulins—4.8/2/2.8 g, random sugar—80 mg%; ABG—PaO_2: 50.1, $PaCO_2$: 39.9, pH: 7.2, HCO_3: 16.7, SaO_2: 75.8; routine urine—albumin traces, sugar negative, RBCs more than 50/HPF, pus cells: 2–4/HPF, epithelial cells: 1–2/HPF, blood culture—sterile; viral markers—negative; dengue serology—negative, malaria: QDx negative; ***ECG*:** sinus rhythm; ***Ultrasound abdomen*:** Liver 17 cm with mildly increased echotexture, gallbladder contracted with multiple stones, kidneys normal and minimal fluid present with mildly enlarged spleen.

This 42-year-old female came with an acute presentation with fever, respiratory distress, deranged liver and renal function tests and disseminated intravascular coagulation. She had hypotension, was intubated and put on a ventilator, was given inotropes and broad spectrum antibiotics. She was being worked up for gallbladder perforation and leptospirosis. But she had a cardiorespiratory arrest and could not be revived. ***Units final clinical diagnosis*** was gallbladder perforation, ? leptospirosis, ? scrub typhus, ? dengue, ? Hantavirus and hepatopulmonary syndrome.

AUTOPSY FINDINGS: PM 22793

A complete autopsy was performed after due permission. The peritoneal cavity contained 250 mL of straw-colored fluid. The ***kidneys*** (Figs 1A and B) were enlarged, together weighed 498 g and the capsular aspect was dusky with petechial hemorrhages. Cut section (Fig 1C) was dusky with medullary congestion and petechial hemorrhages. The renal veins were within normal limits. Microscopic examination revealed multiple areas of hemorrhage (Figs 1D and E), florid tubulointerstitial nephritis (Figs 2A–C) with dense inflammation composed of lymphomononuclear cells, plasma cells along with neutrophils, acute tubular necrosis and fibrin thrombi (Fig 2D) in the glomerular capillaries (DIC like changes). Warthin–Starry stain done on multiple sections showed plenty of characteristic *Leptospira* in the tubular epithelium and in the interstitium, amidst the inflammation (Figs 2E and F). The ***heart*** (Fig 3A) weighed 350 g and hemorrhages could be seen on the pericardial surface. It was flabby, but on cutting open, the chambers and valves appeared normal. Microscopy (Figs 3B–D) revealed a florid pancarditis with mixed inflammation (lymphocytes, plasma cells and neutrophils) leading to significant myocytolysis. The section from the mitral valve (Fig 3E) showed inflammatory infiltrate and the left anterior descending artery (Fig 3F) revealed intimitis. The ***liver*** (Fig 4A) was enlarged and weighed 3,125 g, was bile stained with a nutmeg

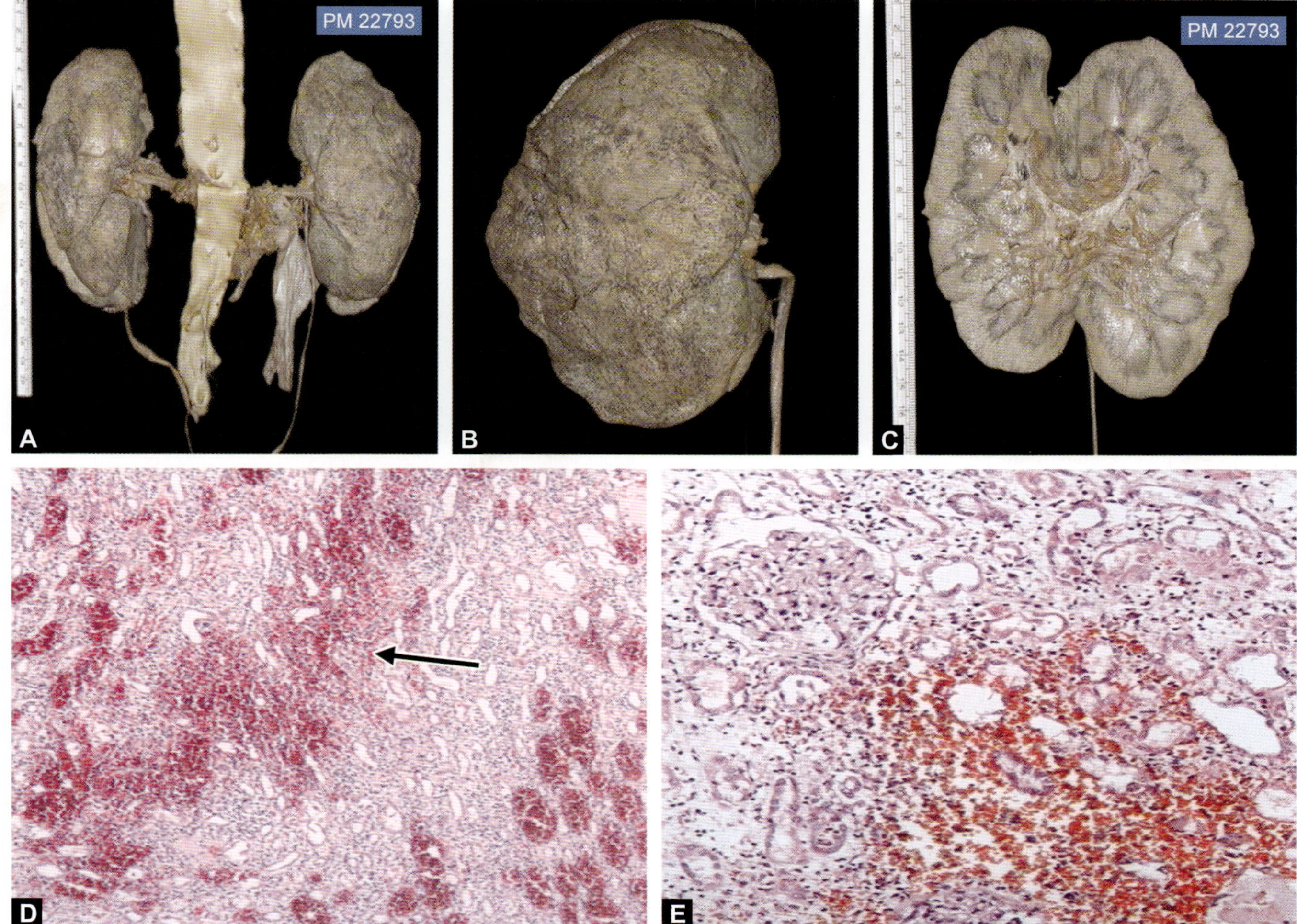

Figs 1A–E: (A and B) Gross photographs of the kidneys showing dusky discoloration with petechial hemorrhages present diffusely; (C) Cut section of the kidney is dusky. Medulla shows congestion. Photomicrographs of the kidney showing (D) Congestion of vasa recta and interstitial hemorrhage; (E) Hemorrhage in the cortex.

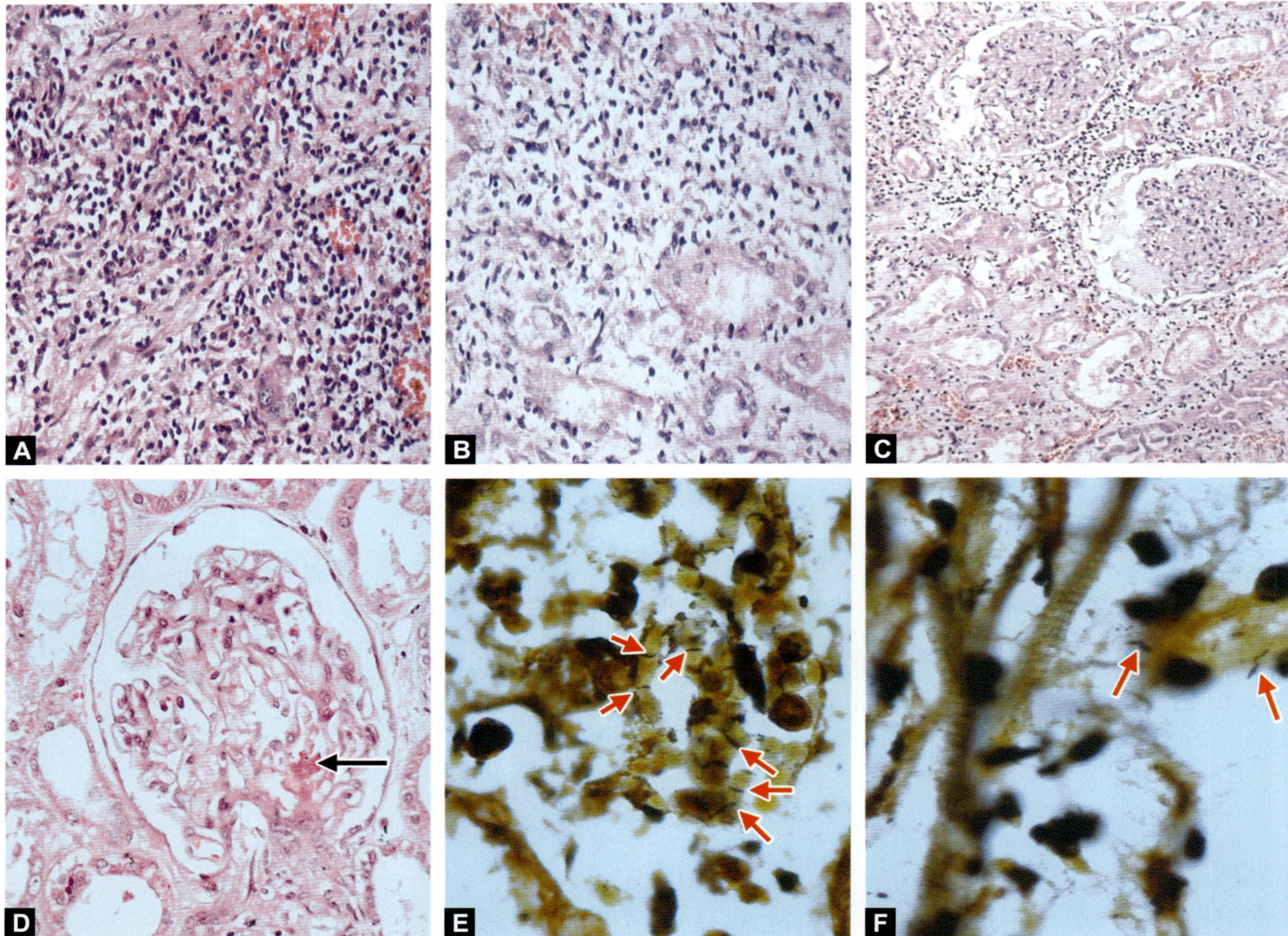

Figs 2A–F: Photomicrographs of the kidney. (A and B) Medulla showing dense inflammation composed of lymphocytes, plasma cells and polymorphs. Destruction of tubules noted; (C) Interstitial inflammation in the cortex around the glomeruli; (D) Glomerulus showing fibrin thrombi (arrow); (E and F) Warthin–Starry stain shows slender *Leptospira* in the tubular epithelial cells (arrows).

appearance. Microscopy showed features of acute hepatitis with bridging hepatic necrosis. The portal tracts (Figs 4B–D) were expanded with dense inflammatory infiltrate, which was spilling into the adjacent liver parenchyma. Foci of lobular inflammation (Fig 4E), centrizonal hemorrhagic necrosis (Fig 4F) and steatosis were noted. The ***spleen*** (Fig 5A) was enlarged, weighed 370 g and was defluent. Microscopy showed septicemic changes (Fig 5B). The ***gallbladder*** (Fig 5C) did not show any perforation. On opening a single stone was present and the mucosa showed large areas of hemorrhage. Microscopic examination (Fig 5D) showed features of acute-on-chronic cholecystitis with mixed inflammation, present transmurally. The ***lungs*** weighed 1,088 g together and cut section were firm with areas of hemorrhage which were confirmed on microscopy (Fig 5E). Apart from this, there was edema and early bronchopneumonia. Hemorrhages were noted in the diaphragm, adrenals (Fig. 5F) and lymph nodes (mildly enlarged). The ***brain*** weighed 1,050 g and on coronal slicing exhibited petechial hemorrhages in white matter and cerebral peduncles. The ***lymph nodes*** showed foci of hemophagocytosis. The para-aortic nodes showed healed and healing epithelioid cell granulomas with Langhans type of giant cells (AFB negative). The ***gastrointestinal tract*** revealed submucosal inflammation in esophagus, acute gastritis and foci of transmural lymphocytic inflammation in small intestine and large intestine. The ***pancreas*** showed features of chronic pancreatitis. The postmortem PCR done for parvovirus and adenovirus were negative. Postmortem serology for hepatitis C virus (HCV), parvovirus, Epstein–Barr virus and dengue were negative. Postmortem serology was

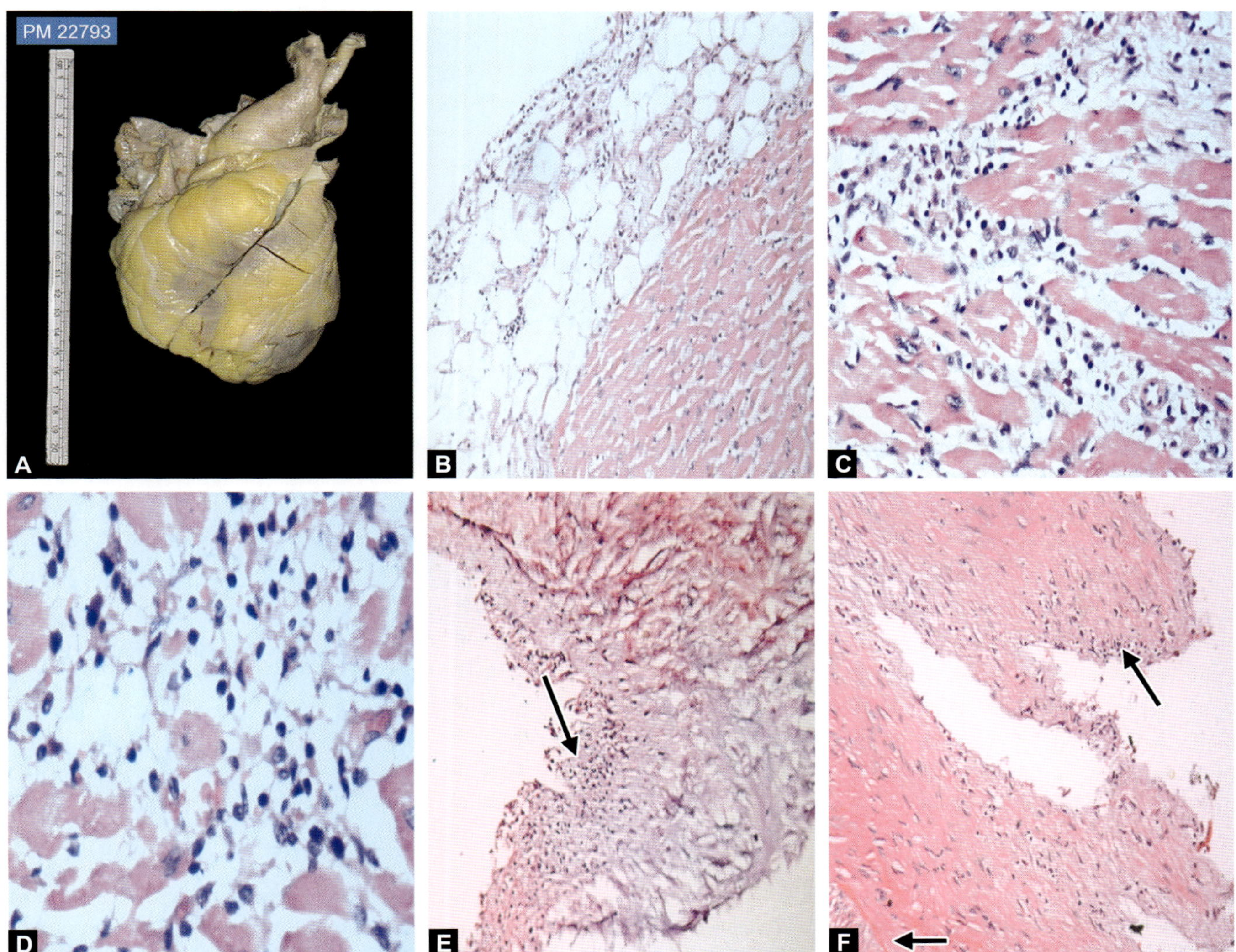

Figs 3A–F: (A) Gross picture of the heart which is flabby. Photomicrographs of the heart showing (B) Mild inflammation in the pericardium; (C and D) Florid mixed inflammation in the myocardium causing myocytolysis; (E) Mitral valve leaflet showing inflammation (arrow); (F) Intima of the left anterior descending coronary artery showing intimitis with a sprinkle of polymorphs and nuclear debris (long arrow). The internal elastic lamina is seen in the left lower corner (arrow).

sent (Dr Lal Path Labs) for *Leptospira* as there was a strong suspicion and *Leptospira* IgM was strongly positive.

FINAL AUTOPSY DIAGNOSIS: PM 22793

42 Years Old Female

Acute leptospirosis (Postmortem serology for *Leptospira*: IgM positive 30 U/mL, Warthin-Starry stain shows *Leptospira* in tubular epithelial cells with:

- Acute interstitial nephritis, acute tubular necrosis, hemorrhages and DIC-like changes—kidney
- Florid pancarditis with hemorrhages
- Acute hepatitis with hemorrhages and centrizonal necrosis
- Septicemic spleen
- Acute-on-chronic cholecystitis with cholelithiasis
- Pulmonary hemorrhages, edema and bronchopneumonia
- Hemorrhages in the adrenals, brain, diaphragm and lymph nodes
- Gastrointestinal tract—nonspecific inflammation
- Granulomatous inflammation—para-aortic nodes
- Chronic pancreatitis.

LEPTOSPIROSIS

Leptospirosis is an acute infectious illness occurring in humans and the animals and is caused by the pathogenic

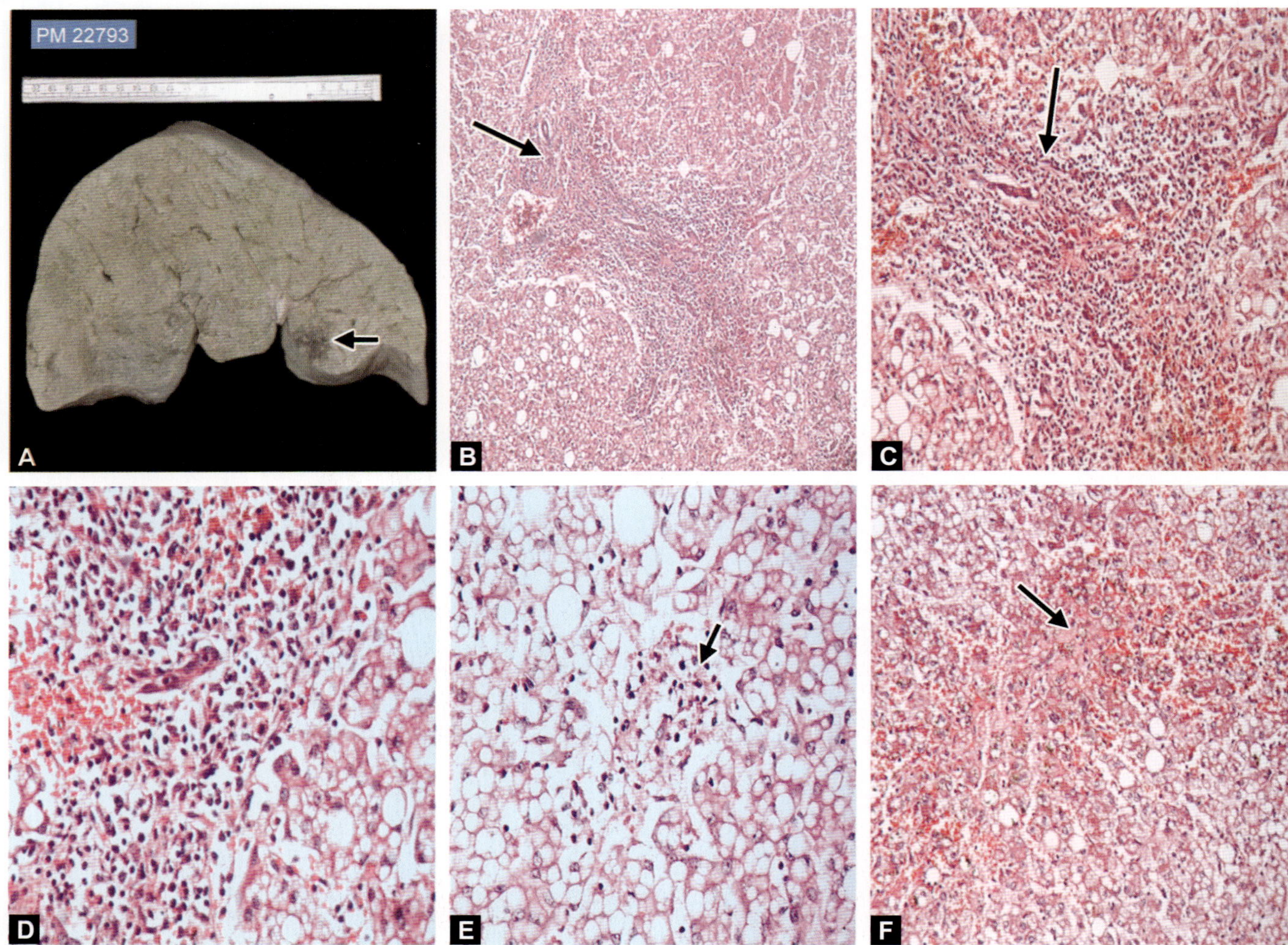

Figs 4A–F: (A) Coronal slice of the enlarged liver, which is bile stained with a nutmeg appearance. Areas of hemorrhage are seen (arrow). Photomicrographs of the liver showing (B and C) expansion of the portal tracts (arrows) with dense inflammation along with bridging hepatic necrosis. Bile ducts can be seen amidst the inflammation; (D) Portal tract shows dense inflammation composed of lymphocytes, plasma cells, and few polymorphs. Piecemeal necrosis can be seen; (E) Foci of lobular inflammation (arrow) with loss of hepatocytes. Steatosis is prominent in the surrounding hepatocytes; (F) Centrizonal hemorrhagic necrosis (arrow) indicating shock.

spirochetes of the genus *Leptospira*. Twenty-one species of *Leptospira* have been identified and about 13 of these cause disease in the humans. Leptospires are tightly coiled, helical spirochetes, 6–20 µm long and 0.1 µm in diameter. It is the most common zoonosis, occurs worldwide, has a greater incidence in the tropical regions and is known by a number of names, i.e. Weil's disease, European swamp fever, mud fever, pea picker's disease, swineherd's disease etc. It is known as an "***emerging infectious disease***" and there have been large outbreaks in Nicaragua, Brazil, India, Southeast Asia and United States. Leptospirosis occurs in the animals particularly the rodents (like the rats) and some domesticated animals too, who secrete the live or virulent organisms in their urine. The leptospires can live in the environment, i.e. in fresh water for many weeks. Humans get infected by direct contact with the urine or from the contaminated food and water. The portal of entry is the mucous membranes (nose, eye, mouth) and skin abrasions. The infection is acquired from water while swimming/wading/rice growing or by direct contact with the animals (rats, other rodents, cattle, dogs and pigs). There are reports of acquiring leptospirosis by drinking cola directly through the cans, on which the rats have urinated. Infection occurs due to poor sanitation in low socioeconomic strata, in farmers and in people who indulge in water sports. It varies in severity from a mild illness to a devastating multiorgan system syndrome, with some unique

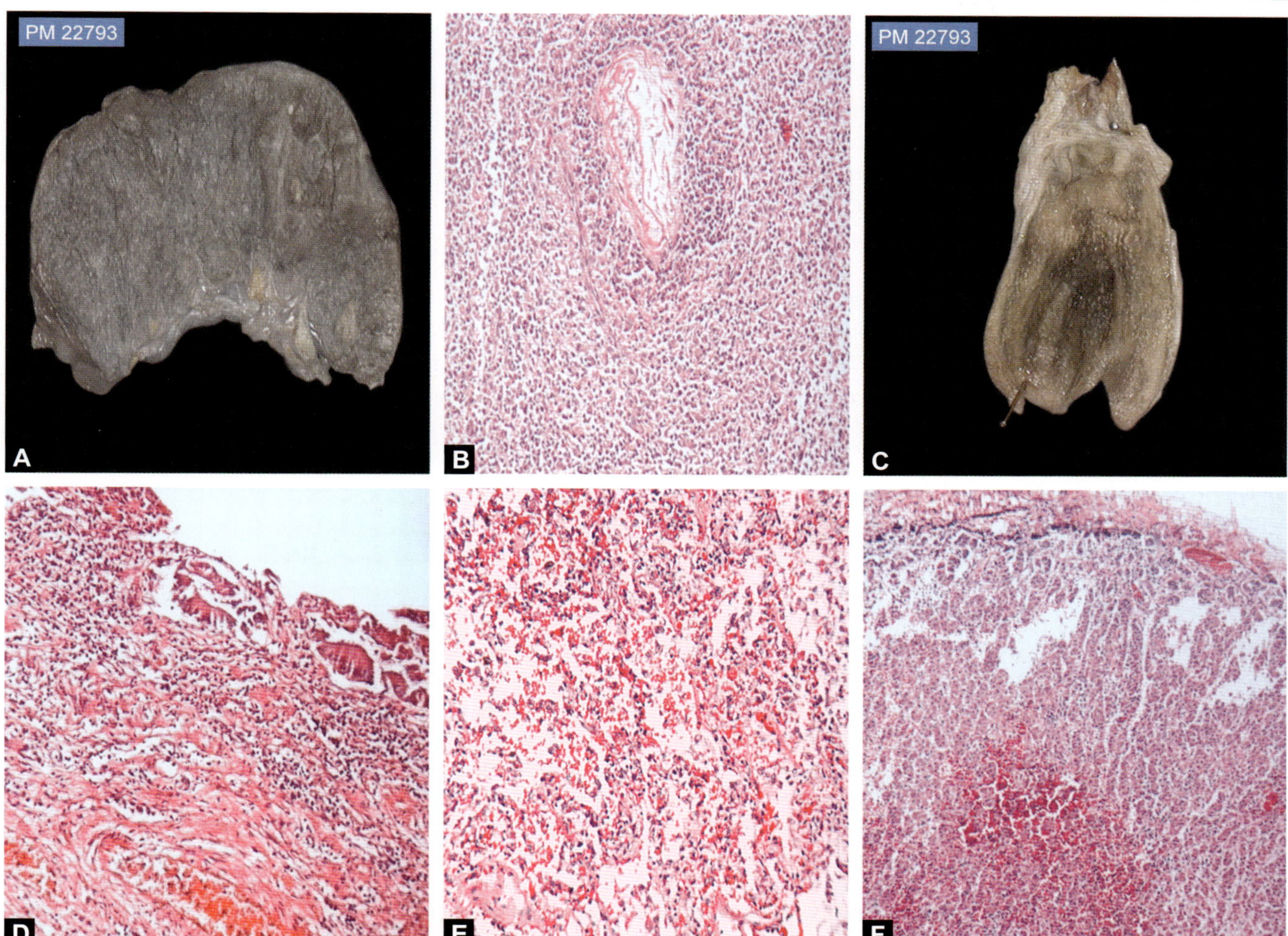

Figs 5A–F: (A) Coronal slice of the enlarged spleen; (B) Spleen show septicemic changes with polymorphs in the sinuses and around the vessels; (C) Gross picture of the gallbladder showing hemorrhage on the mucosal aspect; (D) Gallbladder showing lining epithelium and transmural inflammation; (E) Photomicrograph of the lungs showing hemorrhages; (F) Adrenal gland showing hemorrhage.

features. Severe disease occurs in 10–15% of humans who get infected with *Leptospira*. These patients develop fever, rigors or chills, headache, body aches, retro-orbital pain, photophobia, abdominal pain, nausea, vomiting, conjunctival suffusion or hemorrhages, hemorrhagic rash, jaundice, acute kidney injury (non-oliguric with hypokalemia), pulmonary hemorrhage or edema, acute respiratory distress syndrome, hemorrhagic features, shock and have a high mortality. Early diagnosis and early initiation of antibiotic therapy is of utmost importance for saving life.

Leptospirosis involves multiple organs. It leads to widespread hemorrhages. The kidneys show hemorrhages, tubulointerstitial nephritis, the *Leptospira* proliferate in the proximal tubular epithelium and there is acute tubular necrosis. Liver shows a picture of acute hepatitis with dense portal inflammation, piecemeal necrosis, bridging necrosis, lobular inflammation, bile plugs and hemorrhages. The heart shows severe pancarditis with lymphomononuclear cells composed of lymphocytes and plasma cells. Myocyte necrosis can be seen. Meninges may show a sparse exudate composed of lymphocytes and plasma cells. Hemorrhages can be seen in the brain parenchyma. Lungs show hemorrhage and sparse inflammation. Serological tests are sensitive and specific, but become positive after 7 days of infection. The gold standard is the microscopic agglutination test (MAT). The other tests available are enzyme-linked immunsorbent assays (ELISA) and indirect hemagglutination tests.

COMMENTARY—INDEX CASE: PM 22793

This was a 42-year-old female who came with an acute presentation. She had high grade fever with rigors and chills, abdominal pain, respiratory distress, jaundice, pallor, pedal edema, conjunctival suffusion and mild hepatosplenomegaly. Investigations revealed anemia, polymorphonuclear leukocytosis, low platelets, conjugated hyperbilirubinemia, deranged liver enzymes, low serum proteins with hypoalbuminemia, deranged coagulogram, d-Dimers positive, low fibrinogen, hypokalemia, deranged urea or creatinine and hematuria. Autopsy revealed classical features of fatal leptospirosis. There was florid tubulointerstitial nephritis, acute tubular necrosis, fibrin thrombi in the glomerular capillaries and the Warthin–Starry stain showed *Leptospira* in the renal tubular epithelial cells. Liver showed features of acute hepatitis with bridging hepatic necrosis. Pancarditis was present with florid myocarditis leading to myocytolysis. The mitral valve leaflet showed inflammation and intimitis was seen in the left anterior descending artery. The gall bladder showed acute-on-chronic cholecystitis. Hemorrhages were seen in the kidneys, liver, lungs, adrenals, brain and diaphragm. The postmortem sample sent by the pathologist was strongly positive for *Leptospira* IgM. Thus, this case has a perfect clinicopathological–serological correlation. Leptospirosis was a clinical possibility. This was the first autopsy case of acute leptospirosis that was presented in the "Wednesday Staff Clinicopathological Conference" routinely held in PGIMER. This brought awareness amongst the clinicians and after this many more cases came into light and led to emergence of a well-equipped laboratory.

TAKE HOME MESSAGE

- Leptospirosis is a zoonosis and severe fatal disease occurs in 10–15% cases.
- Early diagnosis and treatment can save many. Awareness is the key to success.
- Autopsy shows acute tubulointerstitial nephritis, acute hepatitis, myocarditis and hemorrhages in many organs, particularly the lungs.

SUGGESTED READING

1. Andrade L, de Francesco Daher E, Seguro AC. Leptospiral nephropathy. Semin Nephrol. 2008;28(4):383-94.
2. Seguro AC, Andrade L. Pathophysiology of leptospirosis. Shock. 2013;39(Suppl 1):17-23.
3. Sethi S, Sharma N, Kakkar N, et al. Increasing trends of leptospirosis in Northern India: a clinico-epidemiological study. PLoS NEGL Trop Dis. 2010;4(1):e579.

CONTRIBUTIONS BY:

1. Dr Gurpreet Singh, Professor and Head, Department of Surgery (Clinician In-Charge)
2. Mr Charan Singh, Technical Assistant, Department of Histopathology (Warthin Starry stain)
3. Dr Baijayantimala Mishra, Department of Virology

Post Graduate Institute of Medical Education and Research, (PGIMER), Chandigarh, India.

CASE 18

Silicotuberculosis: PM 26075

Nandita Bharadwaj Kakkar

HIGHLIGHTS OF THE CASE

An 83-year-old male, stone cutter by profession, with no previous comorbidities, presented with on and off fever and cough for 4 months with intermittent episodes of hemoptysis and altered sensorium for 12 days. On examination he had hypotension, tachycardia and neck rigidity. Cerebrospinal fluid (CSF) analysis was exudative with elevated proteins, low sugars and 300 cells, predominantly polymorphs. Noncontrast computed tomography (NCCT) and contrast-enhanced computed tomography (CECT) head were within normal limits. Chest X-ray showed fine nodular opacities in both the lungs. A clinical diagnosis of pulmonary tuberculosis with tubercular meningitis was made. Autopsy revealed chronic silicosis (lung and hilar lymph nodes), disseminated miliary tuberculosis (AFB ++) involving the lungs (silicotuberculosis), lymph nodes (hilar, mediastinal), liver, spleen, kidneys and bone marrow, tubercular meningitis with borderzone encephalitis, choroid plexitis and tuberculoma (AFB +++), superadded bronchopneumonia, crossed fused renal ectopia, prostate hyperplasia and complicated atherosclerosis.

Keywords: Silicotuberculosis, tubercular meningitis, miliary tuberculosis, crossed fused renal ectopia, autopsy.

CLINICAL DETAILS

Date of Admission: 22.5.2014, Date of Death: 24.5.2014, Duration of Hospital Stay: 2 Days

An 83-year-old male with no previous comorbidities presented with fever (on and off) and persistent cough of 4 months duration along with altered sensorium since 12 days. The fever was not associated with any rigors and chills. The cough was associated with mild expectoration with intermittent blood streaking. There was no diurnal variation. There was altered sensorium in the form of decreased responsiveness. However, no neurological deficits were seen. There was no history of seizure, jaundice, petechiae, diabetes, hypertension and pulmonary tuberculosis. He was a nonsmoker and did not consume alcohol. On physical examination, blood pressure was 90/50 mm Hg, pulse 150/min, respiratory rate 24/min and SpO_2—90% on room air. There was no pallor, icterus, cyanosis or lymphadenopathy. The abdomen was soft and nontender. There was no hepatomegaly. Respiratory and cardiovascular systems were within normal limits. Central nervous system (CNS) examination revealed E1VTM3, neck rigidity was present, pupils were both equal and reacting to light, deep tendon reflexes were +1 and plantars were mute. NCCT and CECT head were within normal limits. Features of raised intracranial tension were present. Chest X-ray showed fine nodular opacities in both the lungs.

Investigations and Course of Management

Investigations revealed—Hb 11.3 g/dL, TLC 19300/µL and platelets 1,30,000/uL. Blood biochemistry revealed normal electrolytes, renal and liver function tests. CSF analysis was exudative with elevated proteins and low sugars and 300 cells, predominantly polymorphs (300 cells/with P80 L20, RBCs + and protein/sugar: 260/37 mg/dL). Arterial blood gas (ABG) showing hypoxia, CO_2 retention. Occupational history was found out after the autopsy and it came out that this man was a laborer and had worked for many years as a stone cutter. He was started on antibiotics and intravenous fluids after which his hypotension and tachycardia improved. But the next day he had bradycardia followed by sudden cardiac arrest and could not be revived. Units final diagnosis was pulmonary tuberculosis with tubercular meningitis. Cause of death being refractory septic shock, type II respiratory failure and pulmonary thromboembolism.

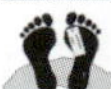 AUTOPSY FINDINGS: PM 26075

Date of Admission: 22.05.2014, Date of Death: 24.05.2014, Duration of Hospital Stay: 2 Days

A complete autopsy was performed. All serous cavities were within normal limits. The ***lungs*** (Fig 1A) were voluminous and together weighed 1,026 g. The pleural surface was dull with fibrinous tags and focal pleural thickening. The cut surface was blackish and subcrepitant to feel. No thrombus was identified. Numerous intimately admixed, blackish and yellowish nodules ranging in size from 0.2 cm to 0.5 cm were identified (Fig 1B). On microscopic examination, the black nodules were composed of acellular concentric lamellar bundles of collagen in the center, with numerous black pigment laden macrophages at the periphery (Figs 2A–D). On polarizing, these nodules showed brightly birefringent, needle-shaped crystals, indicating these to be silicate crystals (Fig 2E). Many of these silicotic nodules were present in the subpleural location leading to pleural thickening. The white millet sized nodules were composed of central area of caseation necrosis bordered by epithelioid cells, lymphocytes and Langhans type of giant cells (Figs 3A–C). The Ziehl–Neelsen stain showed strong positivity for acid-fast bacilli (AFB) (Fig 3D). Many of these small tubercular millet sized nodules were coalescing to form larger nodules. Few of the silicotic nodules showed signs of necrosis in the center. The adjacent lung parenchyma shows emphysematous change and superadded bronchopneumonia. The hilar and mediastinal ***lymph nodes*** also revealed typical silicotic nodules (Fig 4A) along with tubercular granulomas (Fig 4B) which were positive for AFB. Overall features were suggestive of chronic silicosis with miliary tuberculosis. The ***brain*** weighed 1,130 g. The external surface showed a thin meningeal exudate over the ventral aspect of temporal lobe (Fig 5A). In addition, basal exudates were also present. Bilateral tonsilar herniation was noted, supporting the presence of raised intracranial tension. On coronal slicing, a small tuberculoma was identified in the parahippocampal gyrus (Fig 5B). Lateral ventricles were mildly dilated. Microscopy revealed multiple epithelioid cell granulomas in the subarachnoid space (Fig 5C), many of which were surrounding the meningeal vessels causing fibrinoid necrosis and endarteritic changes (Figs 6A and B). This infiltrate was extending into the adjacent brain parenchyma leading to borderzone encephalitis (Fig 6B). The tuberculoma was sampled and showed extensive caseation necrosis surrounded by epithelioid cells, lymphocytes and

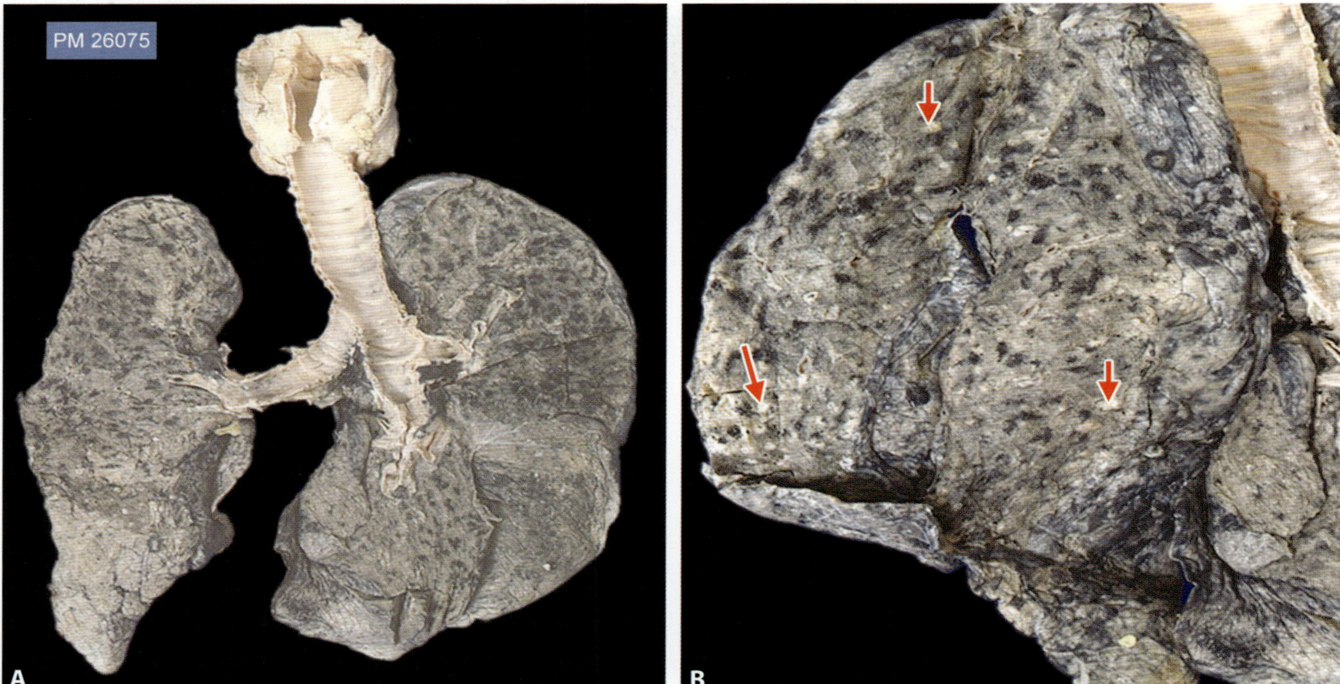

Figs 1A and B: (A) Gross picture of the voluminous lungs with the tracheobronchial tree; and (B) Close up of the cut section of the lung showing small white (red arrows) and black nodules.

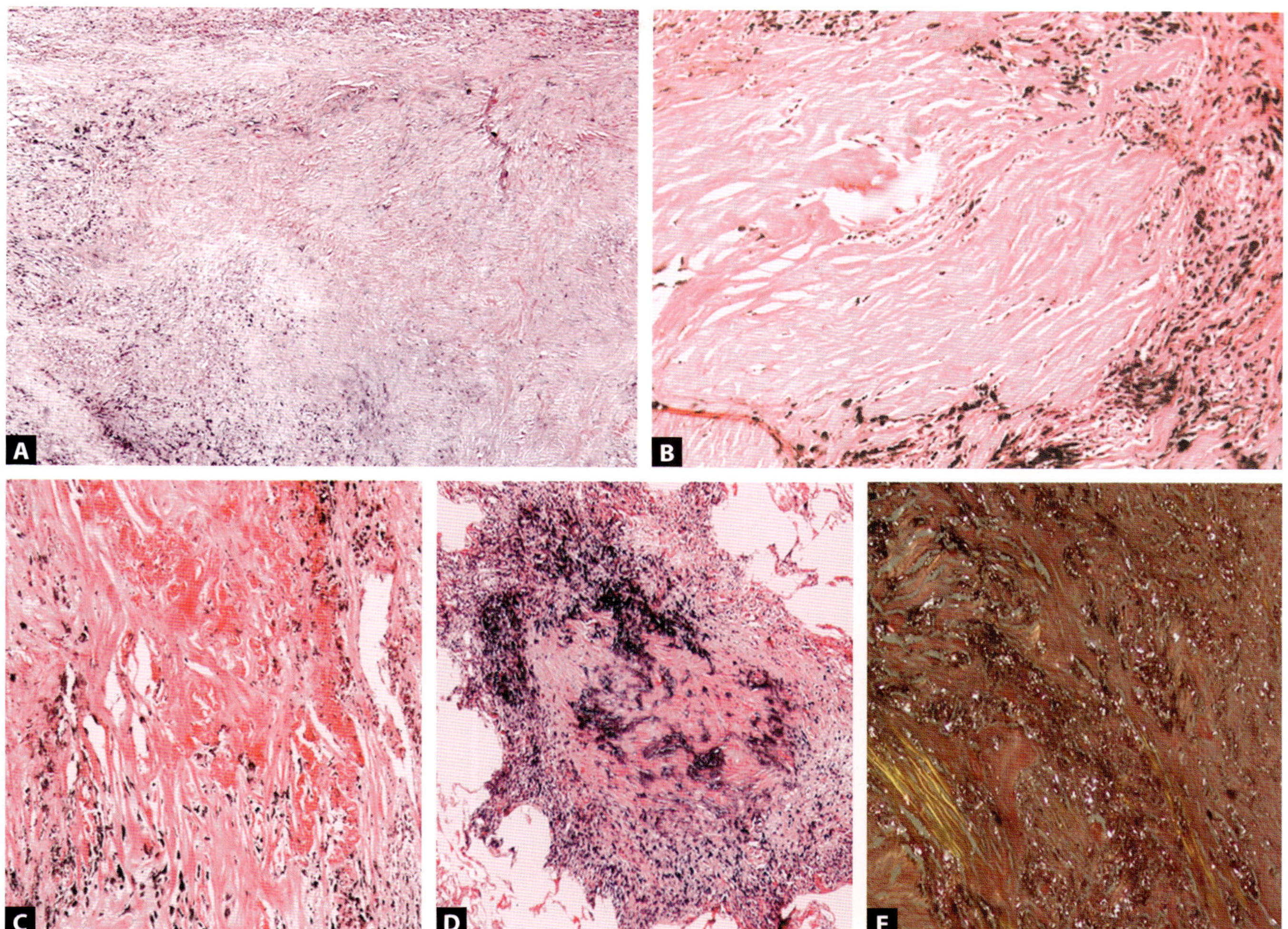

Figs 2A–E: (A to C) Low and high power of a large silicotic nodule with acellular concentric lamellar bundles of collagen in the center with numerous black pigment laden macrophages at the periphery; (D) A smaller silicotic nodule; and (E) Polarized light showing birefringent, needle-shaped crystals of silica.

Langhans giant cells. Choroid plexitis was noted in the form of inflammation and multiple granulomas (Fig 6C). Stain for AFB was very strongly positive in the meningeal exudate (Fig 6D). Features were those of tubercular meningitis with borderzone encephalitis, choroid plexitis and tuberculoma. Multiple epithelioid cell granulomas were noted in the ***liver*** (portal tracts and lobules) (Fig 7A), ***spleen*** and the ***bone marrow*** (Fig 7B). Both the ***kidneys*** (weighed 290 g) were fused and were placed on right side of the aorta, consistent with the diagnosis of crossed fused renal ectopia (Figs 7C and D). They showed vascular splaying with three different branches arising from the abdominal aorta and supplying one each at both the poles of kidney and third one was entering the middle portion of the kidney. There were two separate venous draining channels one from each pelvis and two ureters. On microscopic examination, multiple epithelioid cell granulomas were noted in the cortex and medulla (Fig 7E). The ***heart*** weighed 338 g and was unremarkable. The coronaries revealed atherosclerosis and calcification of the vessel wall, with 30–40% occlusion. The arch and descending thoracic aorta revealed complicated atherosclerosis. There was adenoleiomyomatous hyperplasia seen in the ***prostate*** and adrenals showed hemorrhage. Other organs were within normal limits. Occupational history was found after the autopsy diagnosis was made. The fact came to light that this man was a laborer, who had worked for many years as a stone cutter.

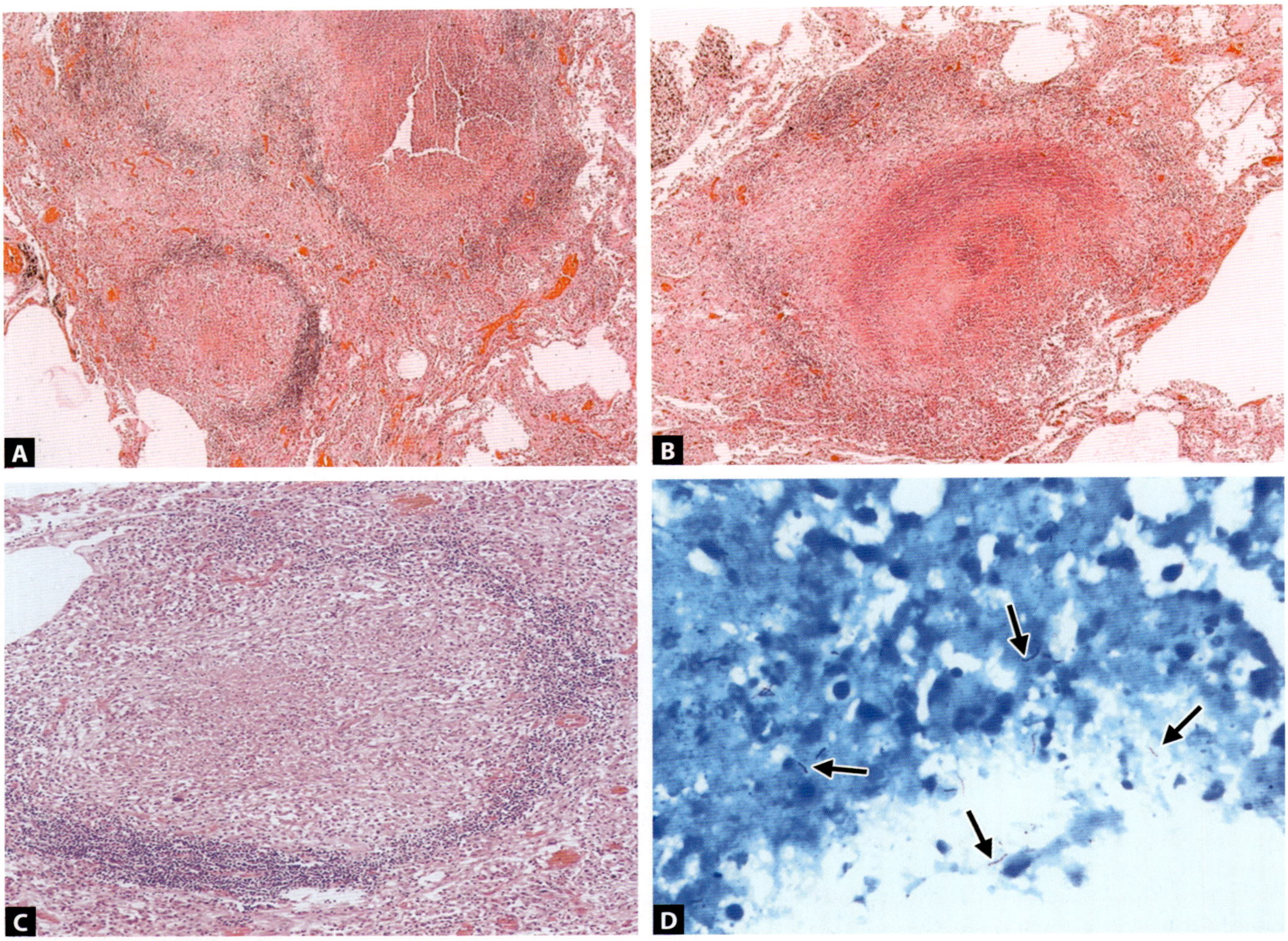

Figs 3A–D: (A to C) Photomicrographs of the lung showing granulomas with central area of caseation necrosis bordered by epithelioid cells, lymphocytes and few Langhans type of giant cells; and (D) Ziehl–Neelsen stain showing plenty of acid fast bacilli (arrows).

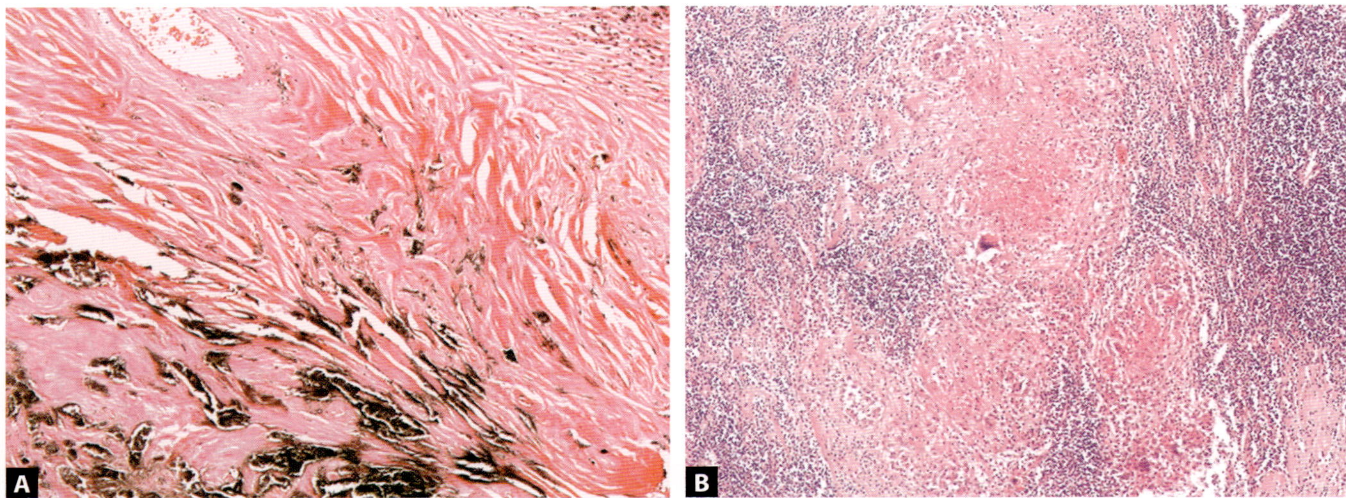

Figs 4A and B: (A) Silicotic nodule in the mediastinal lymph node; and (B) Epithelioid cell granulomas in the lymph node.

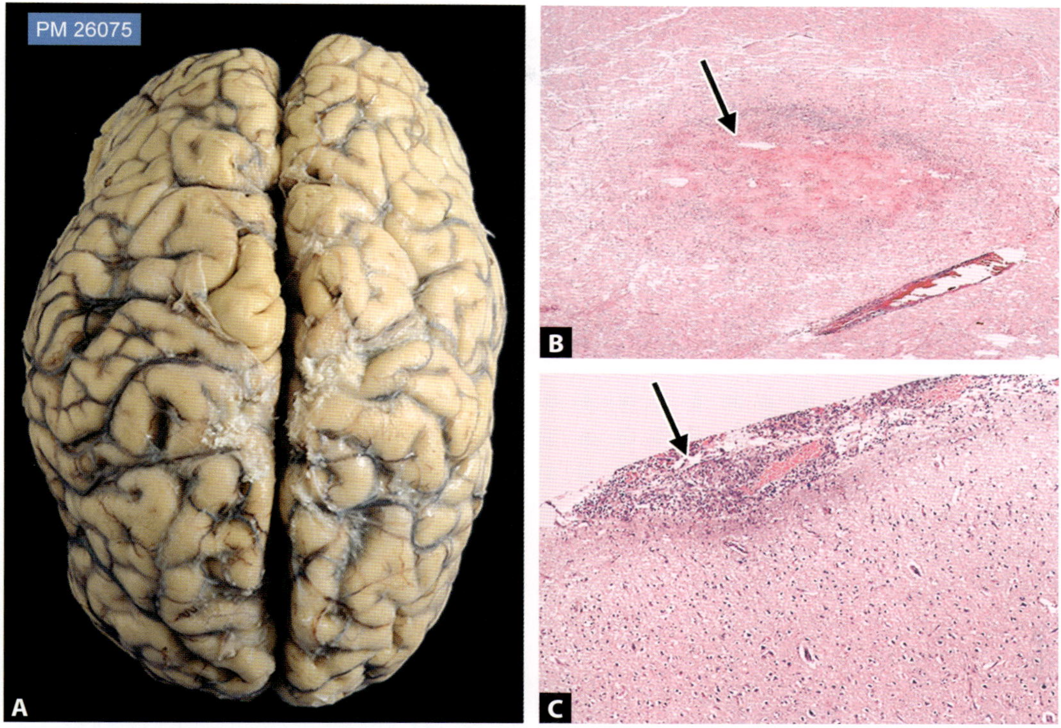

Figs 5A–C: (A) Superolateral surface of the brain showing a mild meningeal exudate; (B) Tuberculoma (arrow) in the parahippocampal gyrus; and (C) Granulomatous inflammation in the subarachnoid space (arrow).

FINAL AUTOPSY DIAGNOSIS: PM 26075

83 Years Old Male

- Chronic silicosis—lung and hilar lymph nodes
- Disseminated miliary tuberculosis (AFB ++) involving the lungs (silicotuberculosis), lymph nodes (hilar, mediastinal), liver, spleen, kidneys and bone marrow
- Tubercular meningitis with borderzone encephalitis, choroid plexitis and tuberculoma (AFB +++)
- Superadded bronchopneumonia
- Crossed fused renal ectopia
- Adenoleiomyomatous hyperplasia—prostate
- Complicated atherosclerosis—arch and descending thoracic aorta.

SILICOSIS AND ITS SEQUELAE

Silicosis is the most prevalent chronic occupational lung disease that occurs due to inhalation of free crystalline silicon-dioxide also known as silica. Silica, i.e. SiO_2 is the oxidized form of silicon and it occurs either in an amorphous noncrystalline form or as a crystalline form. The histopathologic changes commonly occur postexposure, after a latent period of 25–30 years. It leads to respiratory impairment due to the occurrence of a slowly growing nodular fibrosing pneumoconiosis. This further predisposes the lung to various infections which can be catastrophic. The principal sources of industrial exposure to free silica are hard rock mining, quarrying, tunneling, metal casting work, stone cutting, polishing and cleaning monumental masonry. The crystalline form of silica is more fibrogenic and it includes quartz (most commonly implicated form in silicosis), cristobalite and tridymite. After inhalation the particles interact with epithelial cells and are phagocytosed by the macrophages. Ingested silica particles cause activation and release of mediators by pulmonary macrophages and these include interleukin-1 (IL-1), IL-18, TNF, fibronectin, lipid mediators, oxygen-derived free radicals and fibrogenic cytokines. However, when mixed with other minerals, quartz has been thought to reduce the fibrogenic effect. Pulmonary fibrosis due to silica exposure is dose-dependent and occurs after many years of exposure.

There are two main types of silicosis–(1) Acute silicosis occurs after heavy exposure to high concentrations of silica. The symptoms can develop within a few weeks or as long as 5 years after the exposure. This is characterized by the accumulation of lipoproteinaceous material within the alveo-

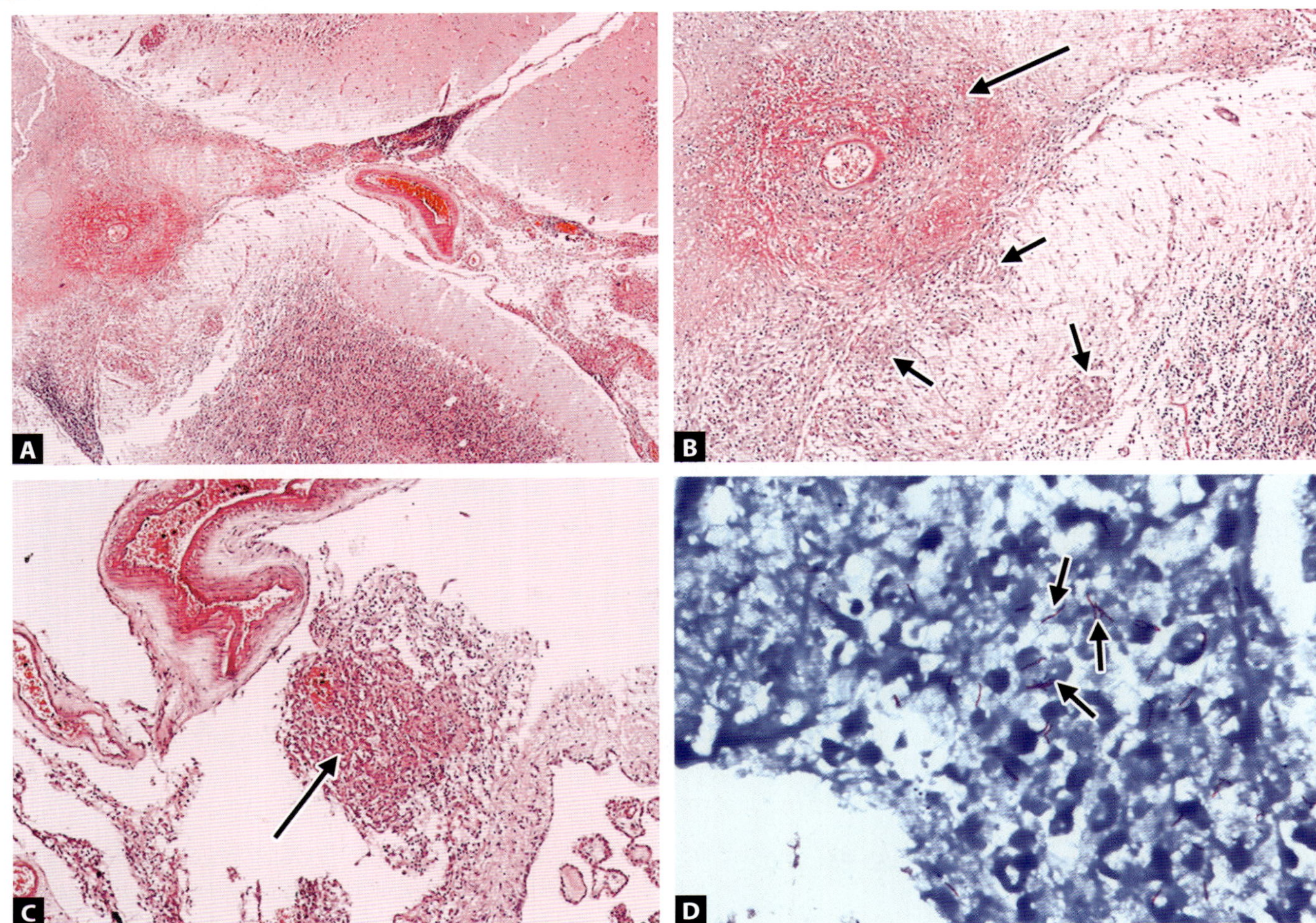

Figs 6A–D: (A) Florid granulomatous inflammation over the cerebellar folia; (B) Caught up vessel in the exudate showing endarteritic changes (long arrow) with granulomas in the molecular layer (small arrows); (C) Granuloma in the choroid plexus (arrow); and (D) Meningeal exudate replete with acid fast bacilli (Ziehl–Neelsen stain) (arrows).

lar spaces, morphologically similar to alveolar proteinosis. (2) Chronic silicosis occurs after a long-term exposure of low concentrations of silica dust. This is the most common form of the disease and is often undetected after many years. A chest X-ray does not reveal the disease for as long as 20 years after exposure. This type of the disease severely hinders the ability of the lung to fight infections, making the person more susceptible to lung infections, including tuberculosis. A third hyperacute variety of silicosis, which is rare, occurs very rapidly within weeks or months after intense exposure to fine dust, high in silica. Extrathoracic silicotic lesions (in spleen, liver, bone marrow and abdominal nodes) may also be found, especially in cases with heavy and prolonged exposures. Plain chest X-rays or CT may show fine nodular infiltrates in upper zones of the lungs along with hilar/mediastinal lymphadenopathy. Five to 15% have eggshell calcification outlining the peripheral margin of mediastinal lymph nodes.

Typical microscopic picture of silicotic nodules shows dense, concentric, acellular, whorled collagen with a peripheral zone of black, dust laden macrophages. Under polarized light, fine birefringent particles are seen throughout the nodule. No giant cells or necrosis is seen. These nodules may be confused with fibrotic/collagenized healed granulomas. Examination of sections with polarized light is of limited use in this regard, because silica particles are weakly birefringent and small particles in tissue sections may be difficult or impossible to visualize. In simple silicosis, the lung parenchyma between nodules is normal or near normal. Giant cells are uncommon. With disease progression, the

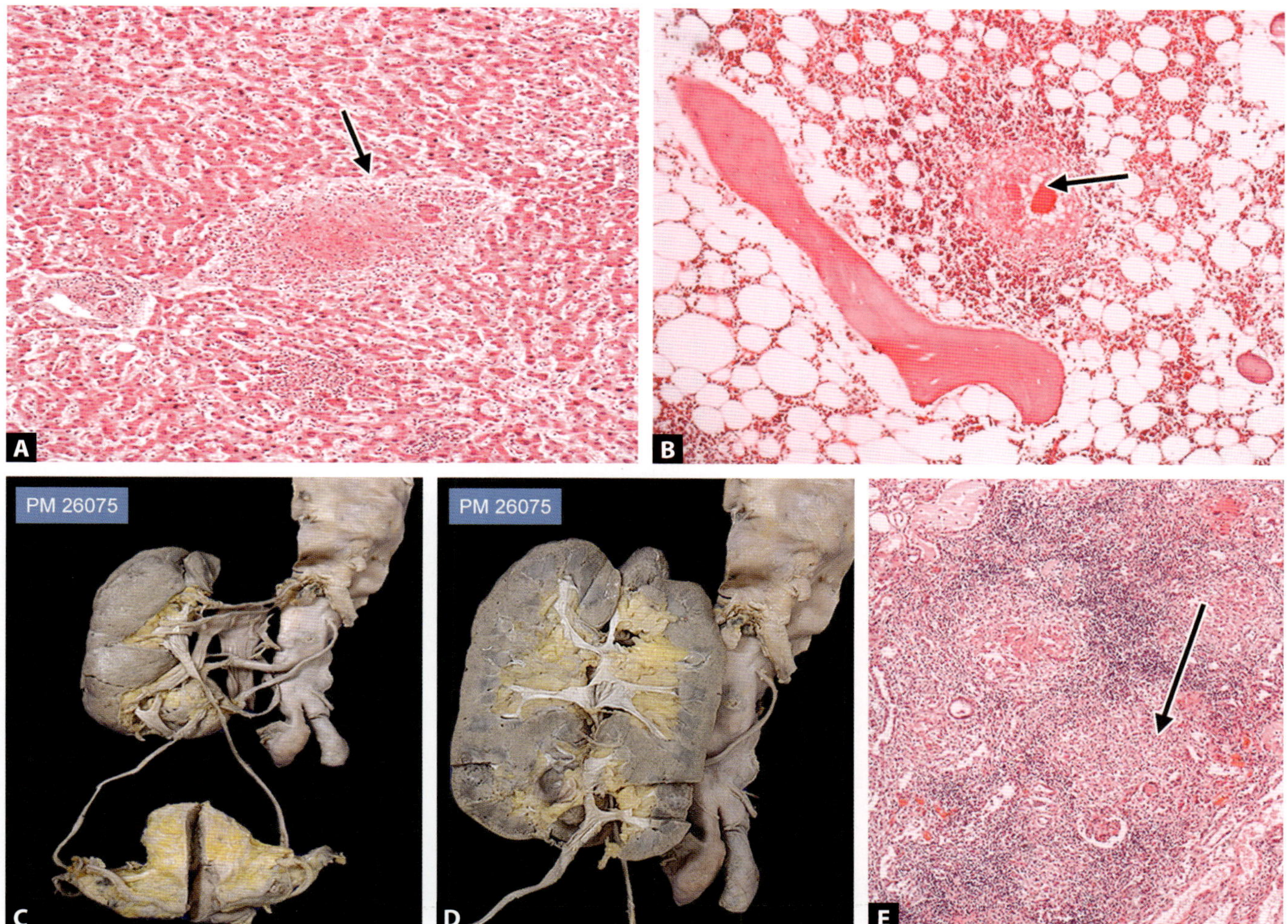

Figs 7A–E: (A and B) Epithelioid cell granuloma in the liver and bone marrow (arrows); (C and D) Kidneys showing crossed fused renal ectopia; and (E) Multiple epithelioid cell granulomas in the kidney (arrow).

individual nodules may coalesce into hard, collagenous scars, eventually leading to progressive fibrosis. The intervening lung parenchyma may be compressed or over expanded and a honeycomb pattern may develop. The coalescent lesions are referred to as conglomerate silicosis. Such masses may cavitate centrally as a result of ischemia, although when this occurs, superinfection chiefly caused by *Mycobacterium tuberculosis* should be suspected.

Silicosis predisposes to tubercular infection by lowering the cell-mediated immunity. The silica particles contribute by disabling the pulmonary macrophages to kill the ingested mycobacteria. Silicotuberculous nodules show central caseation necrosis. Under polarizer, brightly birefringent needle-shaped crystals about 7–15 µm are observed.

COMMENTARY—INDEX CASE: PM 26075

An 83-year-old male, stone cutter by profession, with no previous comorbidities, presented with on and off fever and cough for 4 months with intermittent episodes of hemoptysis and altered sensorium. There was hypotension and neck rigidity. CSF analysis was suggestive of tubercular meningitis. The NCCT and CECT head were within normal limits. Chest X-ray showed fine nodular opacities in both the lungs. A clinical diagnosis of pulmonary tuberculosis with tubercular meningitis was made. In this 83-year-old male, occupational history did reveal a history of stone cutting and at autopsy there was chronic silicosis in the lungs and lymph nodes, which is the most common form of this disease. The chronic silicosis had predisposed the lung to tuberculosis, which showed wide spread miliary dissemination with a heavy bacillary load. The brain involvement eventually led to his demise due to tonsillar herniation. Crossed fused renal ectopia was an incidental finding.

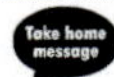

TAKE HOME MESSAGE

- Silicosis is the most common chronic occupational lung disease that occurs due to inhalation of proinflammatory, crystalline, silicon-dioxide also known as silica.
- Silica occurs, either in an amorphous noncrystalline form or as a crystalline form. The latter is more fibrogenic and it includes quartz (most commonly implicated in silicosis), cristobalite and tridymite.
- Ingested silica particles cause activation and release of inflammatory mediators by pulmonary macrophages particularly IL-1 and IL-18.
- Silicosis predisposes to tubercular infection by lowering the cell-mediated immunity.

SUGGESTED READING

1. Diseases associated with exposure to silica and nonfibrous silicate minerals. Silicosis and Silicate Disease Committee. Arch Pathol Lab Med. 1988;112:673-720.
2. Gibbs AR, Wagner Jc. Diseases due to silica. In: Churg A, Green FHY (Eds). Pathology of Occupational Lung Disease, 2nd edition. Baltimore: Williams and Wilkins, 1998.
3. Heppleston AG. Pulmonary repair and fibrosis. In: Glynn LE (Ed). Tissue Repair and Regeneration. Amsterdam: Elsevier/North Holland, 1981. pp. 393-456.
4. Kleinerman J, Green F, Laquer WM, et al. Pathology standards for coal workers pneumoconiosis. Arch Pathol Lab Med. 1979;103:375-432.
5. Kleinerman J. The pathology of some familiar pneumoconiosis. Semin Roentgenol. 1967;2:244-64.
6. McDonald JW, Roggli VL. Detection of silica particles in lung tissue by polarized light microscopy. Arch Pathol Lab Med. 1995;119:242-6.
7. Slavin RE, Swedo JL, Brandes D, et al. Extrapulmonary silicosis: A clinical, morphologic and ultrastructural study. Hum Pathol. 1985;16:393-412.
8. Travis WD, Colby TV, Koss MN, Rosado-de-Christenson ML, Muller NL, King TE Jr. Non-neoplastic disorders of the lower respiratory tract. Occupational lung diseases and pneumoconioses. In: King DW (Ed). Atlas of Nontumor Pathology, First Series, Fascicle 2. Washington, DC: American Registry of Pathology, 2002.
9. Watanabe S, Shirakami A, Takeichi T, et al. Alterations in lymphocyte subsets and serum immunoglobulins in patients with silicosis. J Clin Lab Immunol. 1987;23:45-51.

CONTRIBUTIONS BY:

1. Dr Pavithra HN, Junior Resident, Department of Pathology (In taking gross photographs)
2. Dr Sumita Bhogal, Junior Resident, Department of Internal Medicine (Compilation of Clinical Details)
3. Dr Ashish Bhalla, Professor, Department of Internal Medicine (Clinician In-Charge)

Post Graduate Institute of Medical Education and Research, Chandigarh, India.

CASE 19

Rabies Meningoencephalitis, Post-Pet Dog Bite: PM 27786

Nandita Bharadwaj Kakkar

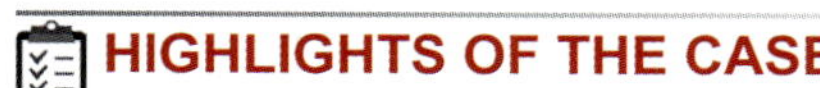

HIGHLIGHTS OF THE CASE

A 25-year-old male came with history of fever since 1 week, altered sensorium since a day, bouts of agitated behaviour/ excessive anger, hydrophobia and history of pet dog bite followed by its death, 4 months back (denied initially). He did not take any post-bite prophylaxis. Contrast-enhanced magnetic resonance imaging initially revealed a normal study followed by features suggestive of viral encephalitis. The clinical diagnosis was viral encephalitis ? rabies encephalitis. Autopsy revealed a classical case of rabies meningoencephalitis, replete with Negri bodies.

Keywords: Rabies, encephalitis, Negri body, hydrophobia, pet dog, bite.

CLINICAL DETAILS

Date of Admission: 28.10.16, Date of Death: 06.11.16, Duration of Hospital Stay: 8 Days

A 25-year-old male came with history of fever for 7 days and altered sensorium since 1 day. The fever was high grade, continuous, and temporarily relieved with analgesics. There was associated headache and multiple nonbilious vomitings. There were no chills, rigors, night sweats or any other B-symptoms. The fever was not associated with joint pain, rash or any other localizing signs. There was altered sensorium since 1 day along with decreased activity. There were bouts of agitated behavior and excessive anger. There were two episodes of marked disorientation followed by drowsiness. There was history of inability to drink water and there was history of death of his pet dog 4 months back. Initially the mother denied any history of dog bite, but subsequently it came to light that the pet dog had bitten the patient and died after 3 days. No post-bite prophylaxis was taken. On *examination* the pulse was 116/min, BP 64/30 mm Hg, internal jugular vein was collapsed, and 1.5 liters fluid rush, increased the BP to 124/70 mm Hg. His temperature was 39.5°C, patient was drowsy, Glasgow coma score was E4V2M6 and the pupils were equal and reactive to light. Abnormal continuous movements of eyes and lower facial muscles were present. Neck rigidity was absent. Deep tendon reflexes were 2+ across all joints along with the presence of bilateral plantar reflex withdrawal. Higher mental functions and sensory examination could not be performed. Examination of the cardiovascular/respiratory systems and abdomen were within normal limits. He was intubated.

Investigations

Blood work-up: During the hospital stay, the hemoglobin fell from 13.7 g/dL to 10.9 g/dL, TLC was 7,100/μL, platelets were 170,000/μL, Na^+ was initially 122 mEq/L and then was corrected to 167 mEq/L, K^+—4.3 mEq/L, serum creatinine/urea—1.06/36 mg%, serum bilirubin—0.47 mg%, AST/ALT/ALP—151/266/256 U/L, total proteins/albumin—5.3/2.3 g, blood/tracheal aspirate culture—sterile, Widal—negative, serology for dengue/malaria/scrub typhus/ leptospira were negative, routine urine examination—within normal limits, and procalcitonin—1.73 ng/mL.

CSF examination: 27.10.2016—WBC Nil, protein—63 mg%, sugar—75 mg%, ADA—2 IU/L, culture—sterile. 02.11.2016—WBC 120 cells (L90, P10, RBCs ++), protein 105 mg%, sugar 103 mg%, ADA—2 IU/L, HSV PCR—negative, work-up for autoimmune encephalitis—negative.

Contrast-enhanced magnetic resonance imaging (CEMRI) on 29.10.16: Grossly normal study. CEMRI on **05.11.16:** Presence of diffuse T2/FLAIR hyperintensities involving cortex/subcortical white matter along with diffuse gyral and sulcal effacement involving bilateral frontal, parietal, temporal, occipital regions, caudate nuclei, putamen and internal capsule with no post-contrast enhancement. Mass effect seen in the form of surrounding edema, transthalamic and left uncal herniation with chinking of third ventricle. Features suggestive of viral encephalitis.

Electroencephalogram (EEG)—29.10.17: Suggestive of diffuse encephalopathy.

Course in hospital: This 25-year-old male, with no prior comorbidities, presented to the Emergency services with complaints of fever for 1 week, altered sensorium since 1 day, history of hydrophobia, and presence of hallucinations. There was history of death of a pet dog 4 months back, but dog bite was initially denied. Neurology and Psychiatry consultation were sought and a possibility of ? viral encephalitis (? dengue) was kept and ceftriaxone along with acyclovir were started. On 28.10.16, at 3 AM, he had one episode of generalized tonic-clonic seizure, was intubated and put on ventilatory support. Eptoin along with levetiracetam were added in view of persistent uprolling of eyes. This persisted and valproate was further added. Due to rapidity of deterioration and normal MRI, a possibility of autoimmune encephalitis was also kept, and he was started on 1 g intravenous methylprednisolone. Fever work-up was sent along with cerebrospinal (CSF) for all infectious possibilities. He developed three episodes of hypotension, which normalized by itself. Continuous twitching movements of eyelids and perioral muscles were present. Repeat CSF was normal and paraneoplastic panel sent to an outside laboratory at Kochi was also negative. Corneal smear and nape of neck biopsy could not be done. He developed persistent hypotension with low central venous pressure (CVP), but responded to fluids. Later on his fiancée revealed the information that the patient had informed her that his pet dog had bitten him, after which the dog died within 2–3 days. No post-bite prophylaxis was taken. He soon developed hypotension and the urine output worsened. Noradrenaline was started, adrenaline was added by evening, and vasopressin added by night. The urine output decreased drastically and finally became nil. Dobutamine was added but the hypotension persisted. Patient developed cardiac arrest, cardiopulmonary resuscitation was done as per protocol, but he could not be revived and declared dead at 2:30 PM on 06.11.2016. ***Units clinical diagnosis*** was viral encephalitis, ? rabies encephalitis.

AUTOPSY FINDINGS: PM 27786

A complete autopsy was performed with abdominothoracic and bitemporal incisions. Spinal cord was not removed due to lack of permission. The brain was overweight and weighed 1,746 g. External examination (Figs 1A and B) and coronal slicing (Figs 2A and B) revealed diffuse edema, leading to narrowing of sulci, flattening of gyri, narrowing of ventricles, and bilateral uncal herniation. The meningeal vessels were congested. No focal lesion was visible grossly. The brain stem (Figs 2C and D) was normal grossly. On microscopic examination, the meninges showed lymphocytic infiltrate (Fig 3A) with congested blood vessels. The cortex was edematous and this was appreciated in the form of rarefaction of the brain parenchyma (Fig 3B). Hypoxia was a predominant feature and the brain was replete with hypoxic

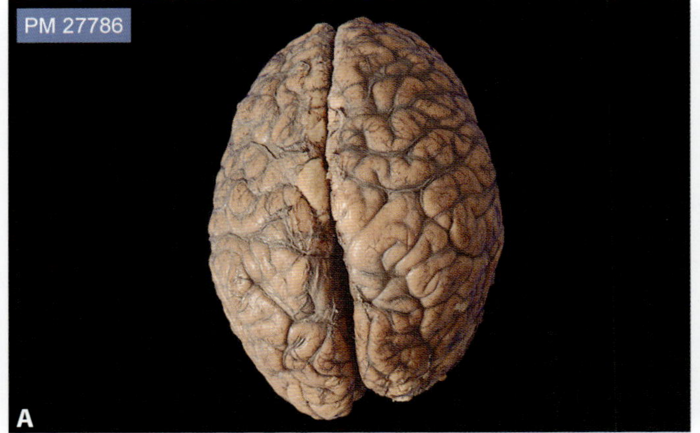

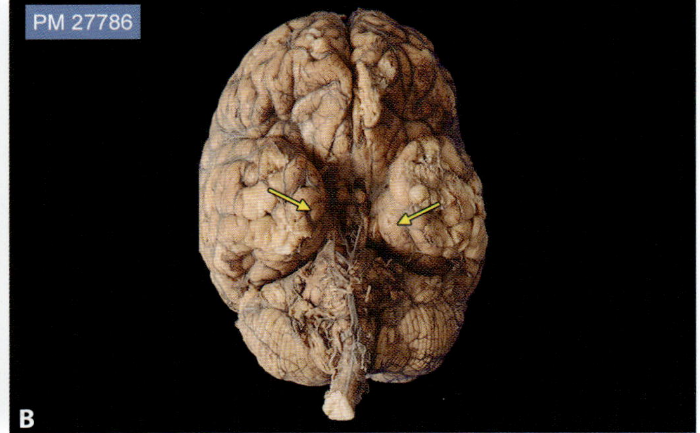

Figs 1A and B: (A) Brain from the superolateral aspect shows narrowing of sulci and flattening of gyri due to significant edema. Congested vessels are noted. No exudate or hemorrhage is seen; (B) Base of the brain shows bilateral uncal herniation (arrows). No exudate or hemorrhage is seen.

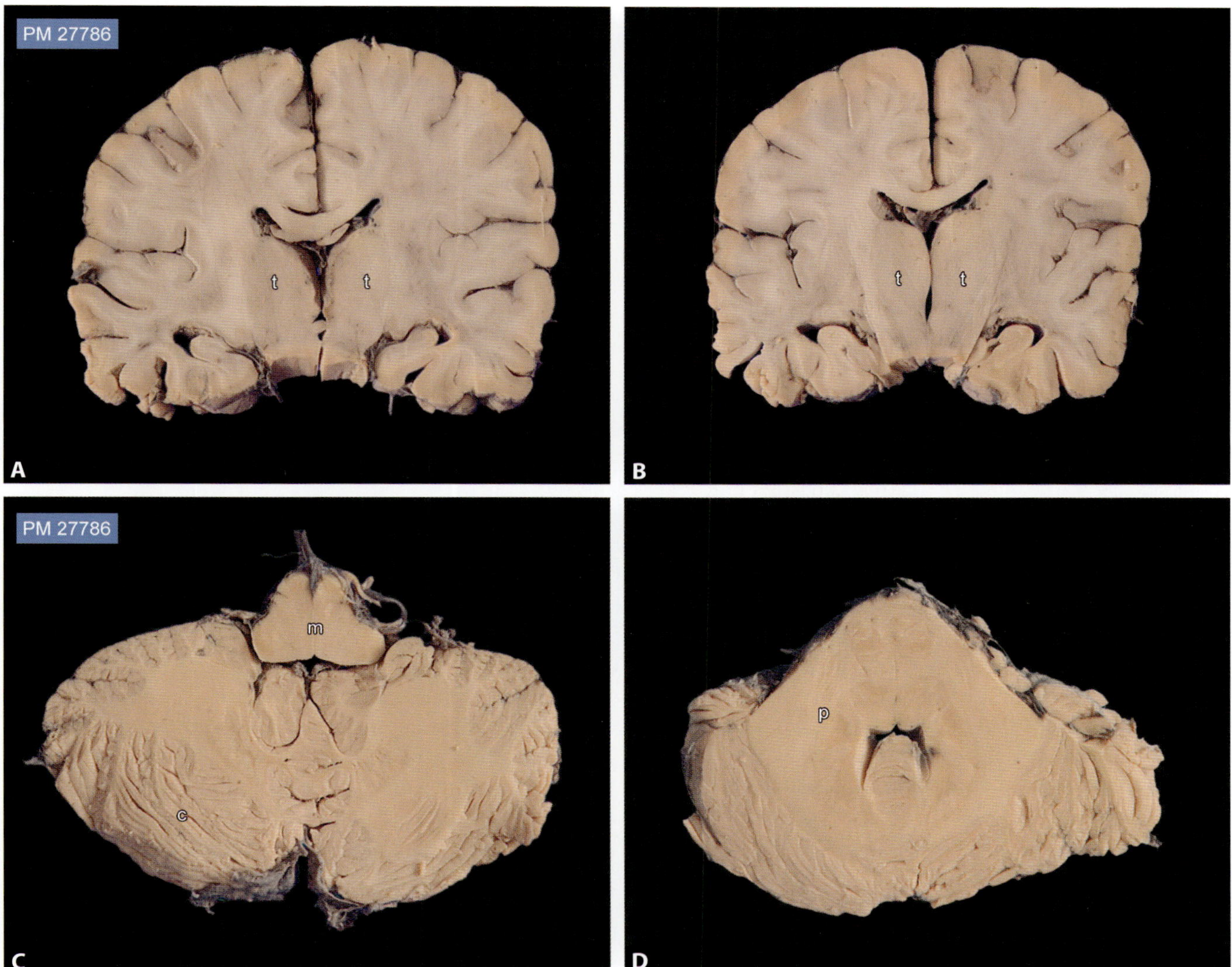

Figs 2A–D: (A and B) Coronal slices of the brain, at different levels of the thalami (t), showing narrowing of ventricles. No focal lesion is seen; (C) Cut section of the cerebellum (c) and midbrain (m) which is normal grossly; (D) Cut section of the pons (p) which is normal grossly.

neurons (Fig 3C) showing shrinkage of cytoplasm/cell processes and a pyknotic nucleus in which chromatin pattern could hardly be discerned. Sections from the midbrain, pons, medulla, cerebellum, and basal ganglia showed features of viral encephalitis in the form of microglial nodules (Fig 3D) highlighted by the macrophage marker CD68 (Fig 3E), perivascular lymphocytic infiltrate (Fig 3F), diffuse edema, perineuronal edema, and neuronophagia. There was loss of Purkinje cells in the cerebellum. The pyramidal cells in the hippocampus (Figs 4A–C) and the Purkinje cells in the cerebellum (Figs 4D–F) contained the pathognomonic Negri bodies, seen as sharply demarcated round to oval eosinophilic inclusions in the cytoplasm, which were single or multiple. Anti-rabies antibody (Figs 5A–C) showed strong positivity in the Negri bodies along with diffuse granular positivity in the cytoplasm of pyramidal/Purkinje cells and also along the neuronal processes. Features were those of rabies meningoencephalitis. The ***lungs*** weighed 890 g together and cut section revealed thrombi in sub-segmental arteries along with hemorrhagic consolidation (Fig 5D). On microscopic examination, pulmonary edema, alveolar hemorrhage, thrombi in sub-segmental arteries, and early bronchopneumonia were noted. The ***adrenal gland*** (Figs 5E and F). revealed a florid lymphocytic adrenalitis. All other organs were within normal limits.

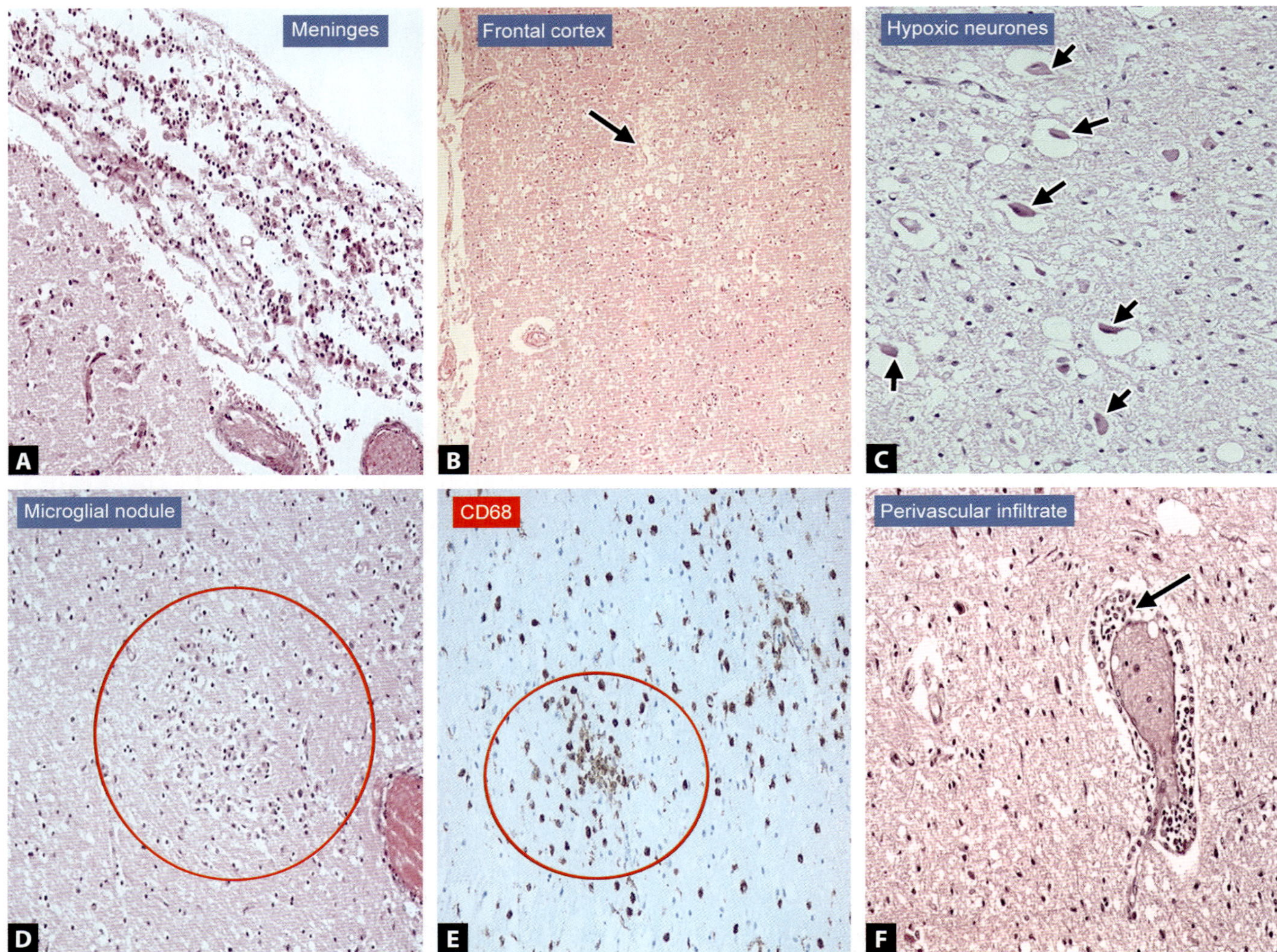

Figs 3A–F: Photomicrographs of the brain. (A) Meninges show lymphocytic infiltrate in the subarachnoid space. (B) Frontal cortex shows edema in the form of rarefaction (arrow). (C) Hypoxic neurons (arrows) showing shrinkage of cytoplasm/cell processes and a pyknotic nucleus. (D) Microglial nodule (red circle). (E) CD68 immunostain highlights the microglial nodules (red circle). (F) Perivascular lymphomononuclear cell infiltrate (arrow)..

FINAL AUTOPSY DIAGNOSIS: PM 27786

25 Years Male with History of Pet Dog Bite

- Rabies meningoencephalitis with global hypoxia/ischemia
- Bronchopneumonia, pulmonary hemorrhage, and edema
- Pulmonary thromboembolism
- Lymphocytic adrenalitis.

RABIES ENCEPHALITIS

Rabies is a rapidly progressive, highly infectious, fatal disease of central nervous system occurring in both humans and animals. It is caused by infection with rabies virus, which is a neurotropic, RNA virus that belongs to genera Lyssavirus and family Rhabdoviridae. Rabies virus particles have a bulleted structure of 75 nm by 200 nm, with a helical nucleocapsid surrounded by a thin protein-studded membrane. It has a nonsegmented, linear, negative sense, single-stranded RNA genome. Humans are susceptible to rabies and the risk is maximum for the laboratory staff, doctors, veterinarians, dog handlers, hunters and public who gets bitten by a stray rabid dogs (especially in India). Dogs are responsible for majority of urban human rabies cases. Cats are also effective vectors of transmission. Jackal, fox, wolves, hyena, mongoose are vectors for wildlife rabies. Bats are the primary reservoirs of rabies on all the inhabited continents. The bite of a rabid animal is the most common mode of transmission. Licks on abraded skin or mucosa can

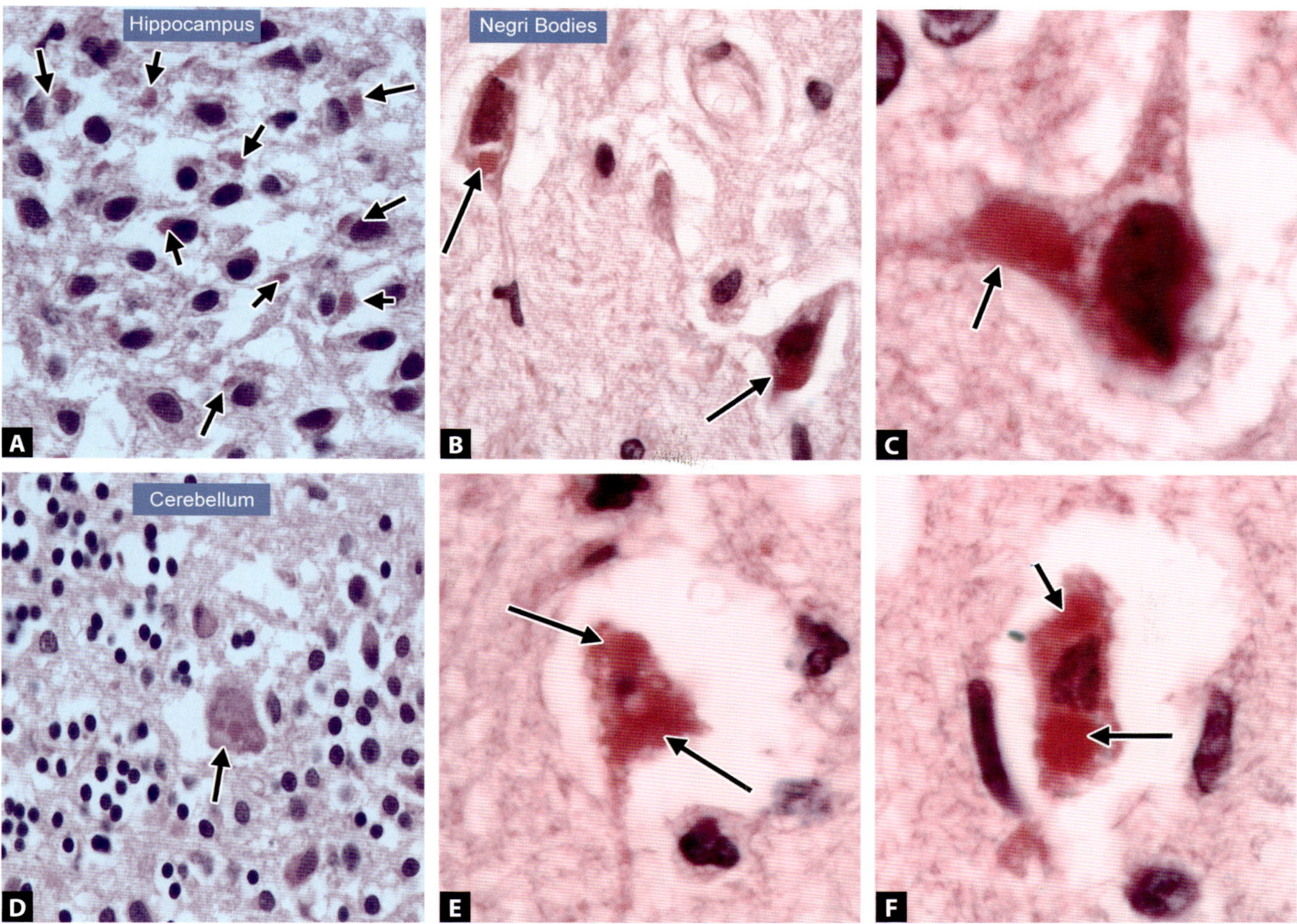

Figs 4A–F: Photomicrographs of the brain. (A to C) Pyramidal cells in the hippocampus showing the classical Negri bodies, seen as sharply demarcated round to oval eosinophilic inclusions in the cytoplasm (arrows). (D to F) Purkinje cells of the cerebellum showing the classical Negri bodies (arrows). In "A" the eosinophilic inclusions are granular.

also transmit the rabies virus. Transmission by aerosols has also been documented, e.g. persons visiting caves harboring rabies-infected bats. Human to human transmission has been reported in the setting of infected corneal transplant and organ transplant. After a bite, the virus enters the neural tissues and travels to the brain by axonal transport. It infects the neurons of the brain, and then the virus travels back to the parenchymal organs. The infection of the brain largely depends on the role of microglial cells.

The clinical features of rabies infection can be divided into five stages—the incubation period, the prodrome, acute neurological phase, coma, and death. The ***incubation period*** of rabies ranges from 1 week to greater than 6 years. Incubation period is shorter in severe exposures and in bites on face, head/neck, upper extremities, and in those by wild animals. The ***prodromal stage*** begins when the virus moves centripetally from the periphery to dorsal root ganglia and then to the central nervous system. Prodromal symptoms last a few days, generally not more than a week. Patients experience local symptoms or neuropathic pain at the bite site, presumably due to ganglioneuritis, described as burning, numbness, tingling, itching or pruritus. Nonspecific symptoms like malaise, fever, headache along with wound site paresthesias is diagnostic. The ***acute neurological phase*** of rabies can be distinguished as classic (encephalitic/furious and paralytic/dumb forms) and nonclassic forms. It marks the dysfunction of the nervous system. Patients with encephalitic form and paralytic form die within 7 days and 2 weeks, respectively. In the encephalitic or furious rabies, the earliest feature is hyperactivity which is aggravated by thirst, fear, light, noise and by other stimuli. Within 24 hours, three cardinal signs appear, fluctuating consciousness, phobic or

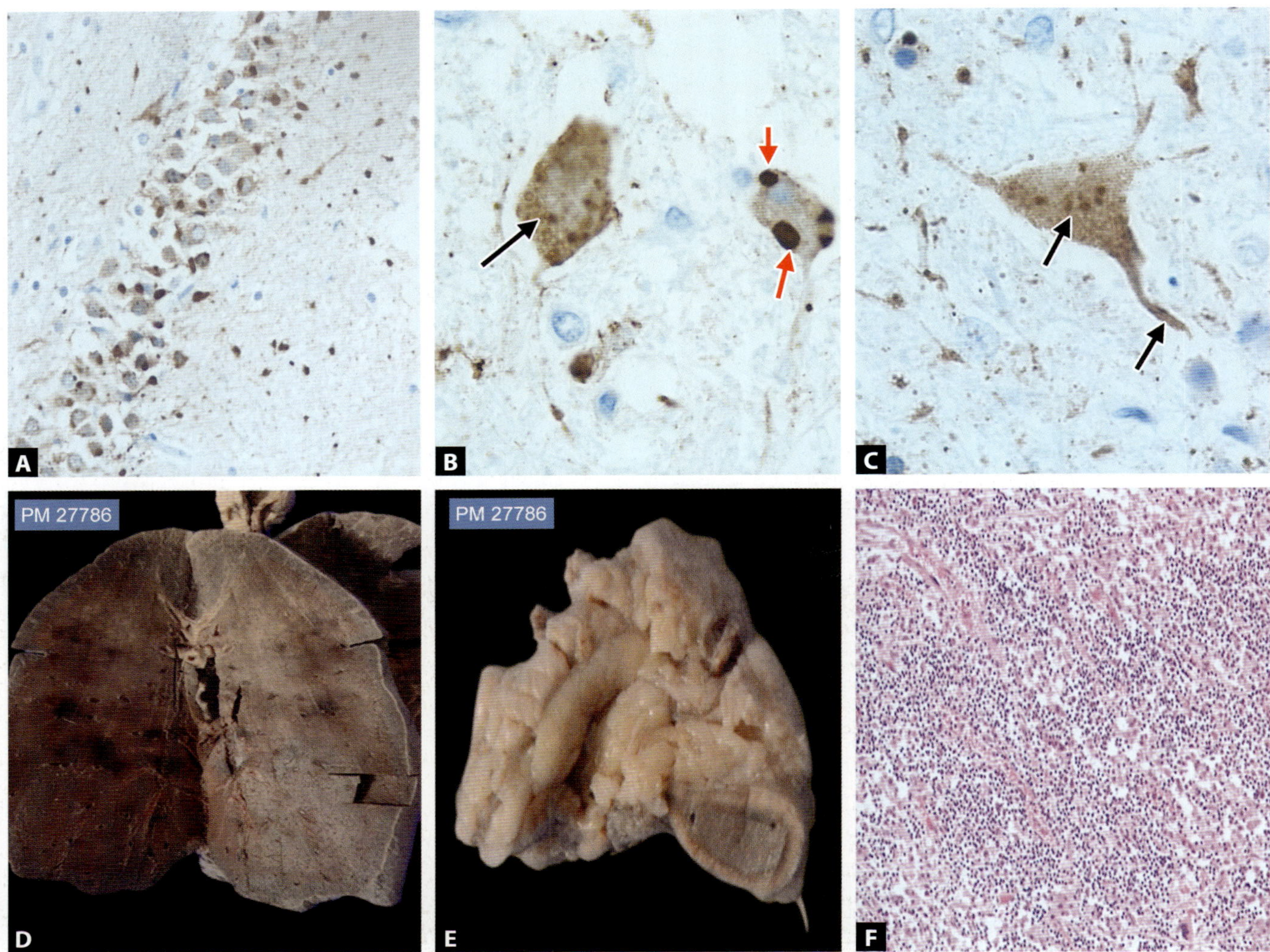

Figs 5A–F: Immunohistochemistry with anti-rabies antibody. (A) Shows strong cytoplasmic positivity in the pyramidal cells of the Ammon's horn. (B and C) Show diffuse granular positivity in the cytoplasm of pyramidal and Purkinje cells and also seen along the neuronal processes (black arrows). One neuron in "B" shows multiple brown-colored Negri bodies (red arrows). (D) Cut section of the right lung showing hemorrhagic consolidation. (E) Cut section of the adrenal gland which is normal. (F) Photomicrograph of the adrenal gland showing florid lymphomononuclear cell infiltrate.

inspiratory spasms, and signs of autonomic stimulation. Mental status alternates between normal periods and bouts of progressively increasing agitation and depression. Pharyngeal muscle contracture leads to hydrophobia. Meningismus occurs followed by flaccid paralysis, deterioration of consciousness and coma. Paralytic (Dumb) rabies is difficult to diagnose because of the lack of aggression. Phobic spasms occur in about 50% of the cases. Weakness usually starts in the bitten limb and then spreads to all limbs, the bulbar and the respiratory muscles. Nonclassic rabies is the bat-related rabies and they have clinical features different from those of dog-related cases. In addition to neuropathic pain, which is much more common, radicular pain, sensory/motor deficits and choreiform movements of the bitten limb occur during the prodromal phase. Focal brainstem signs and myoclonus are common.

Once rabies virus is successfully inoculated into wounds, the viral glycoprotein binds to nicotinic acetylcholine receptor on the muscle. After budding from the plasma membrane of muscle cells, the virus is taken up into unmyelinated nerve endings at the neuromuscular junctions or at the muscle spindles. Rabies virus is transported to the CNS via retrograde axoplasmic flow. The virus then infects and replicates the dorsal root ganglia and anterior horn cells. At the dorsal root ganglia, viral replication may be recognized and attacked by immune effectors, resulting in ganglioneuritis and a clinical prodrome of neuropathic pain at the bite site. Travel from the peripheral nerves to the CNS, occurs at a fairly constant rate of 8–20 mm/day and the time taken depends on the distance of the inoculation site from the CNS. Once the virus is in a neuronal cell, rapid amplification takes place. Virus disseminates via plasma membrane budding, direct cell-to-cell transmission or by trans-synaptic propagation. Rabies virus preferentially localizes in the brainstem, thalamus, basal ganglia and spinal cord irrespective of clinical presentation or bite site. Replication of the virus in the CNS is followed by centrifugal movement of the rabies virus, along the peripheral nerve axons, back to the peripheral tissues. Jogai et al. demonstrated rabies virus antigen in the adrenal and lacrimal glands.

Pathology of rabies: The brain is edematous and herniations occur. Microscopically, changes of viral encephalomyelitis are seen, predominantly in the brain stem and spinal cord. There is vascular congestion and perivascular cuffing by inflammatory exudate, composed of lymphocytes and plasma cells. Microglial hyperplasia, neuronophagia, and microglial nodules are seen. The Negri bodies seen as round or oval inclusions within the cytoplasm of nerve bodies are characteristic and a hallmark of rabies. Negri bodies may vary in size from 0.24 μ to 27 μ. They are found most frequently in the Purkinje cells of the cerebellum, pyramidal neurons of the hippocampus, medulla, pontine nuclei and spinal cord. Only 50–80% of brain tissue samples found positive by virus isolation methods show Negri bodies. Negri body represents surplus viral nucleoprotein that selectively accumulates in subpopulations of neurons during infection with rabies. Another form of inclusion body, are the Lyssa bodies. These are irregular and less sharply demarcated from the surrounding neuronal cytoplasm. Immunohistochemistry with anti-rabies antibodies is very helpful and show cytoplasmic positivity in the neurons, even in cases where no Negri bodies are found, thus clinching the diagnosis.

COMMENTARY—INDEX CASE: PM 27786

A 25-year-old male came with history of fever since 1 week, altered sensorium since a day, bouts of agitated behavior or excessive anger, hydrophobia, and history of pet dog bite followed by its death, 4 months back (denied initially). He did not take any post-bite prophylaxis. Contrast-enhanced magnetic resonance imaging initially revealed a normal study followed by features suggestive of viral encephalitis. The clinical diagnosis was viral encephalitis, ? rabies encephalitis. Autopsy revealed a classical case of rabies meningoencephalitis, replete with Negri bodies, showing strong positivity with anti-rabies antibody. The problem in clinical diagnosis.

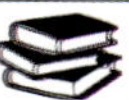

TAKE HOME MESSAGE

- Rabies is a rapidly progressive, highly infectious, fatal disease caused by rabies virus which is a neurotropic RNA virus.
- The Negri bodies seen as round or oval eosinophilic inclusions within the cytoplasm of nerve bodies are characteristic and a hallmark of rabies infection.
- The Negri bodies are found most frequently in the Purkinje cells of the cerebellum, pyramidal neurons of the hippocampus, medulla, pontine nuclei, and spinal cord.

SUGGESTED READING

1. Burton EC, Burns DK, Opatowsky MJ, et al. Rabies encephalomyelitis: clinical, neuroradiological, and pathological findings in 4 transplant recipients. Arch Neurol. 2005; 62:873-8.
2. Conomy JP, Leibovitz A, McCombs W, et al. Airborne rabies encephalitis: demonstration of rabies virus in the human central nervous system. Neurology. 1977;27:67-9.
3. Hemachudha T, Laothamatas J, Rupprecht CE. Human rabies: A disease of complex neuropathogenetic mechanisms and diagnostic challenges. Lancet Neurol. 2002;1:101-9.
4. Houff SA, Burton RC, Wilson RW, et al. Human-to-human transmission of rabies virus by corneal transplant. N Engl J Med. 1979;300:603-4.
5. Jogai S, Radotra BD, Banerjee AK. Immunohistochemical study of human rabies. Neuropathology. 2000;20:197-203.
6. Jogai S, Radotra BD, Banerjee AK. Rabies viral antigen in extracranial organs: a post-mortem study. Neuropathol Appl Neurobiol. 2002;28:334-8.
7. Lahaye X, Vidy A, Pomier C, et al. Functional characterization of Negri bodies (NBs) in rabies virus-infected cells: Evidence that NBs are sites of viral transcription and replication. J Virol. 2009;83:7948-58.

CONTRIBUTIONS BY:

1. Dr Shilpi Thakur, Junior Resident, Department of Pathology (In working up the Case)
2. Dr Setu Gupta, Junior Resident, Department of Internal Medicine (Compilation of Clinical Details)
3. Dr BD Radotra, Professor, Department of Histopathology (Consultation)
4. Dr Navneet Sharma, Professor, Department of Internal Medicine (Clinician In-Charge)

Post Graduate Institute of Medical Education and Research, Chandigarh, India.

SECTION 4

Hepatobiliary and Pancreatic Disorders Adult Cases

CASE 20

Extrahepatic Portal Venous Obstruction due to Cavernomatous Transformation of Portal Vein and Portal Cavernoma Cholangiopathy: PM 22260

Nandita Bharadwaj Kakkar

 HIGHLIGHTS OF THE CASE

This is a case of a 38-years female who first presented in childhood with repeated hematemesis starting at the age of 7 years. At the age of 19-years, she was diagnosed to have extrahepatic portal venous obstruction with dilated left intrahepatic biliary radicals. She underwent 3 sessions of endoscopic sclerotherapy and was then lost to follow-up. She resurfaced at the age of 38-years with jaundice, malena, hematemesis, altered sensorium, massive splenomegaly, marked conjugated hyperbilirubinemia, coagulopathy and renal failure. Autopsy revealed cavernomatous transformation of portal vein with portal cavernoma cholangiopathy and phlegmonous inflammation of the gut.

Keywords: Cavernous transformation, portal vein, cavernoma, portal vein thrombosis, portal cavernoma cholangiopathy, phlegmonus inflammation.

 CLINICAL DETAILS

Date of Admission: 13.10.2007, Date of Death: 16.10.2007 and Duration of Hospital Stay: 3 Days.

Background History

This 38-years female, is a known case of extrahepatic portal venous obstruction (EHPVO). At the age of 7-years, she had 3 episodes of upper gastrointestinal bleed. At the age of 15-years she had jaundice and fever lasting for 7 day. At the age of 19-years in 1988, she again had hematemesis. Ultrasonography (USG) and standardized perfusion value (SPV) confirmed EHPVO involving distal portal vein and splenic vein with short gastric, retroperitoneal and splenorenal collaterals. She underwent 3 sessions of endoscopic sclerotherapy (EST) in December 1988. During this admission she had a brief episode of decompensation with ascites. Investigations revealed Hb of 4.3 g/dL, TLC 2,300/uL, platelets- 60,000/uL. The liver function tests were normal. She received 5-units of blood transfusion. Endoscopic retrograde cholangiopancreaticography (ERCP) done in January, 1989 showed a smooth narrowing of common hepatic duct with dilated left intrahepatic biliary radicals (IHBR). After January 1989, she was lost to follow-up.

Present Illness

She was admitted on 13th October, 2007 with complaints of jaundice and pruritis since 3 months, malena since 7 days and hematemesis since 2 days. The jaundice was progressive, associated with high colored urine, pruritus and progressive abdominal distension. There were 2–3 episodes of hematemesis, ½–1 L in 2 days, associated with postural hypotension. There was altered sensorium since one day. There was a change in sleep pattern for 2 months and history of biliary colics.

General Physical Examination

Malnourished with muscle wasting, pulse —128/min, feeble, BP— 90/60 mm Hg, RR 28/min, afebrile, icterus 3+, pallor+, no cyanosis/clubbing, drowsy and irritable. The abdomen was distended with distended veins, liver and spleen were palpable 3 cm and 6 cm below their respective costal margins, shifting dullness was present, bilateral crepts present in basal areas, she was drowsy, flaps were present and her status was E3M2V1.

Investigations and Course of Management

Hemogram: Hb—8.8 g/dL, TLC— 33,000/μL, DLC P48, L40, M10, E2, platelets—59,000/μL, random blood sugar—101 mg%, urea—305 mg%, creatinine—8.4 mg%, $Na^+/K^+/Cl^-$—133/2.1/88 mEq/L, serum bilirubin—total/conjugated— 54.4/31.3 mg%, SGOT/SGPT—66/120 U/L, PTI—29%, INR—2.5, PTTK greater than 2 min, d-DIMER—positive, fibrinogen—3.24 g/L, fibrin monomer-negative, blood culture—grew ***E. Coli***. Leptospria, HBsAg, anti HCV serology negative, Ascitic fluid: Protein 750 mg/dL, sugar 12 mg/dL, TLC—3,200/cmm, DLC—morphology distorted, SAAG and ADA—not done. ***Radiology*****:** Chest X-ray—normal, ***USG abdomen*** (13.10.07): ***Liver***: 14.2 cm, mildly coarsened in echotexture, smooth surface, bilobar intrahepatic biliary radicals dilated (IHBRD) upto confluence of right and left hepatic ducts; portal vein replaced by collaterals which are also seen in mesentry, retroperitoneum and in the lienorenal ligament, splenic vein prominent and patent, gallbladder—multiple calculi present, CBD—not dilated, moderate ascites present, bilateral kidneys show increased cortical echogenicity. Impression—EHPVO with portal hypertensive biliopathy, cholelithiasis, bilateral renal parenchymal disease and ascites.

The patient was treated for gastrointestinal bleed, spontaneous bacterial peritonitis and for hepatic encephalopathy. She received intravenous somatostatin/tazobactum/piperacillin/noradrenalin/dopamine, fluid replacement, potassium and lactulose. Peritoneal dialysis was planned but the patient had cardiac arrest and could not be revived. ***Units final diagnosis*****:** Extrahepatic portal venous obstruction, portal hypertensive biliopathy, hepatitis B related chronic liver disease, cholangitis with sepsis and septic shock, upper GI bleeding? Variceal, acute renal failure.

AUTOPSY FINDINGS: PM 22260

A complete autopsy was performed. The pleural cavity contained 500 mL and peritoneal cavity 3,000 mL of straw colored fluid. The stomach contained 500 mL of altered blood. The ***portal vein, splenic vein and superior mesenteric veins*** were markedly dilated (Fig 1A). About 1 cm distal to the confluence of the portal vein, till its entry into the hilum of the liver, the vein structure was not identified and was composed of a loose meshwork of connective tissue (Figs 1A and B). Multiple sections from here revealed cavernomatous transformation of portal vein. The portal vein was made up of a cluster of different sized venous channels, arranged haphazardly within a connective tissue support and the original portal vein was not discernable (Figs 1C and D; 2A and B). The ***liver*** (Figs 1A and B) weighed 800 g and was deeply bile stained. The common hepatic duct and the intrahepatic bile ducts were dilated. The intrahepatic bile ducts were tortuous and contained bile sludge (Figs 3E and F). On microscopic examination the liver (Figs 2C–E and 3A–D) showed expansion of portal tracts with bile ductular proliferation, fibrosis, proliferation of small branches of the portal vein, portal bridging fibrosis and focal cholangitis. The larger portal tracts showed marked bile ductular proliferation and bile plugging. Periportal canalicular and hepatocytic cholestasis was seen. Overall features were those of extrahepatic portal venous obstruction with cavernomatous transformation of portal vein and portal cavernoma cholangiopathy. The ***spleen*** (Fig 4A–D) was markedly enlarged and weighed as much as the liver i.e. 800 g. Microscopy revealed a congestive splenomegaly replete with Gamna-Gandy bodies. The submucosa of the lower end of the ***esophagus*** (Figs 5A–C) was replete with markedly dilated varices. The ***stomach*** (Fig 5A) contained altered blood and microscopic examination revealed superficial erosions. Focal areas showed a phlegmonous inflammation, where in large areas of the submucosa contained dense neutrophilic infiltrate with an overlying normal mucosa (Figs 5D and E). The ***large gut*** showed areas of thickening with submucosal hemorrhages. Microscopy showed focal areas of phlegmonous colitis with a dense neutrophilic infiltrate in the submucosa. The ***lungs*** (Figs 5F and G) showed bone marrow emboli and foci of terminal aspiration. The ***kidneys*** were bile stained and revealed features of acute tubular necrosis. Rests of the organs including the brain were within normal limits.

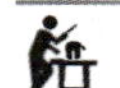

FINAL AUTOPSY DIAGNOSIS : PM 22260

38 Years Female

Recurrent Hematemesis Since 7-year of Age

- *Extrahepatic portal venous obstruction*: Cavernomatous transformation of portal vein.
- Portal cavernoma cholangiopathy.
- Portal hypertension: Congestive splenomegaly, esophageal varices, ascites.
- Phlegmonous inflammation of the stomach and colon.
- Bone marrow emboli in lungs with terminal aspiration.
- Early acute tubular necrosis-kidneys.

HEPATIC MICROCIRCULATION

Portal Circulation

The portal veins do not directly feed the sinusoidal circulation and divide into successive branches of conducting/distributing veins, named according to hierarchy as interlobar/segmental/interlobular portal veins. Interlobular veins further branches into preterminal portal venules, terminal

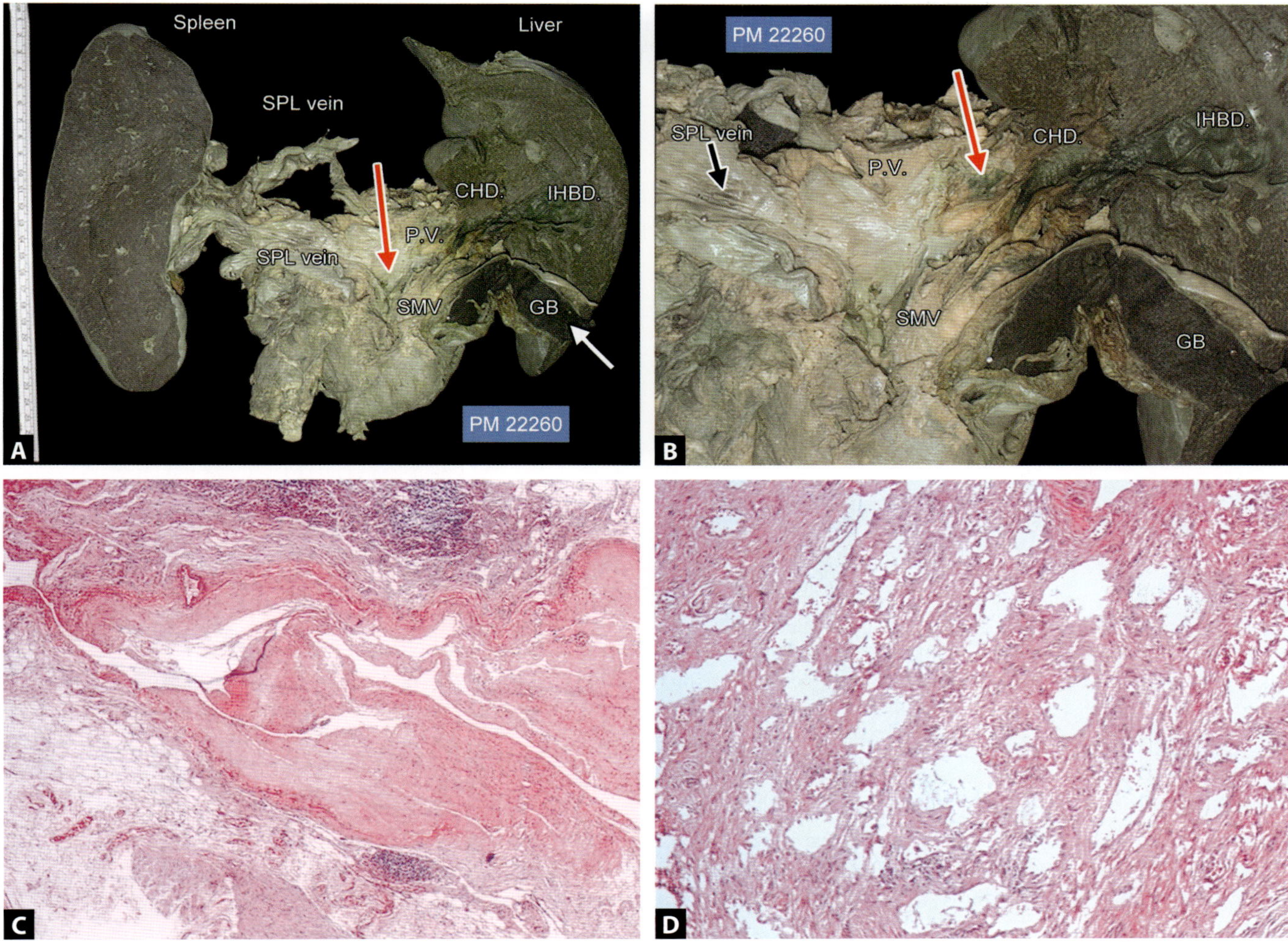

Figs 1A–D: (A) Organ complex comprising of slice of enlarged spleen, slice of the bile stained liver, gallbladder (lower arrow), confluence of splenic vein and superior mesenteric vein (red arrow); (B) Close-up view to show splenic vein (SPL vein), superior mesenteric vein (SMV) forming the portal vein (PV) discernable for one cm beyond, which it is composed of a loose meshwork of connective tissue i.e. the cavernoma (long red arrow). Also seen is the dilated common hepatic duct (CHD) which further communicates with the markedly dilated intrahepatic bile ducts (IHBD). The opened up gallbladder is also seen (GB); (C) Cross section of the portal vein just proximal to the cavernoma; (D) Photomicrograph of the cavernoma composed of a cluster of different sized vessels arranged haphazardly within a connective tissue support.

portal venules and the inlet venules, which pass through the periportal limiting plate and open into the sinusoids. The ***inlet venules*** are guarded by sphincters composed of sinusoidal lining cells called ***inlet sphincters***.

Arterial Circulation

The common hepatic artery supplies the liver and the hepatic artery branches follow the portal veins. Each portal tract has two or more branches. Terminally the arteries follow three routes:

- The periportal plexus seen in the portal area around the portal vein branches and it drains into the sinusoids.
- The peribiliary plexus—as the name suggests supplies all the intrahepatic bile ducts and finally drains into the hepatic sinusoids. This plexus develops parallel with the intrahepatic bile ducts.
- The terminal hepatic arterioles—drain into the periportal sinusoids via the arteriosinus branches. They possess an internal elastic lamina and a layer of smooth muscle cells.

Venous Circulation

The blood reaching the sinusoids via the portal and arterial circulation perfuses the parenchyma and then enters the terminal hepatic venules (central veins of the classic

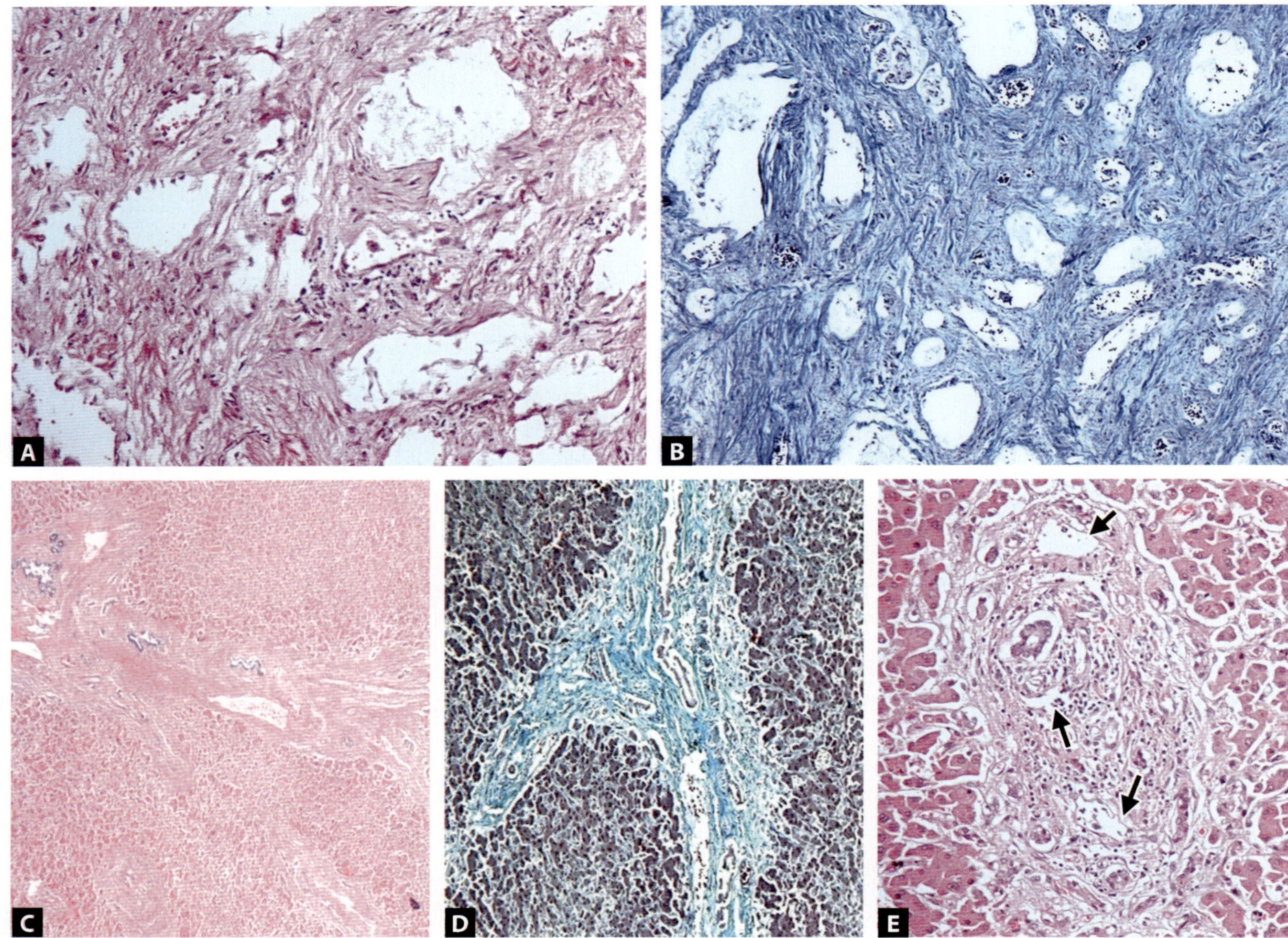

Figs 2A–E: (A and B) Photomicrograph of the cavernoma composed of endothelial lined spaces within a connective tissue support (H&E and Massons's trichrome stain). Photomicrographs of the liver showing (C and D) Expansion of portal tracts and porto-portal bridging fibrosis (H&E, Massons's trichrome stain); (E) Expanded portal tract showing fibrosis, mild inflammation and proliferation of small branches of the portal vein (arrows).

lobule) for onward transmission. The walls of the veins have fenestrations through which the sinusoids open. The terminal veins join to form the larger hepatic veins. The blood that flows through the sinusoids is arterial, venous or mixed. The classic lobule, which is hexagonal, has at its centre, a central vein which is the terminal tributary of the hepatic vein.

Diseases of the Portal Vein, Extrahepatic Portal Venous Obstruction and Cavernomatous Transformation of Portal Vein

Portal vein is formed by the union of the splenic vein and the superior mesenteric vein. Its diameter is 0.6–1.2 cm and in portal hypertension it can go up till 1.9 cm. Portal hypertension occurs due to obstruction of the hepatic blood flow. It can be presinusoidal, sinusoidal and postsinusoidal. Commonest cause of portal hypertension is cirrhosis, but non-cirrhotic portal hypertension is also common worldwide and very much seen in India. When splenomegaly and varices occur without cirrhosis it is usually a portal vein disease and when hepatomegaly and ascites occur, it points towards a hepatic vein disease. ***Portal vein disease*** encompasses many entities, which include:

- ***Thrombosis*** of large portal vein which comprises of the extrahepatic portal vein obstruction and cavernomatous transformation of portal vein. Thrombosis could be due to various conditions:
  - Hypercoagulable states (polycythemia vera, myeloproliferative disorders, oral contraceptives, lupus

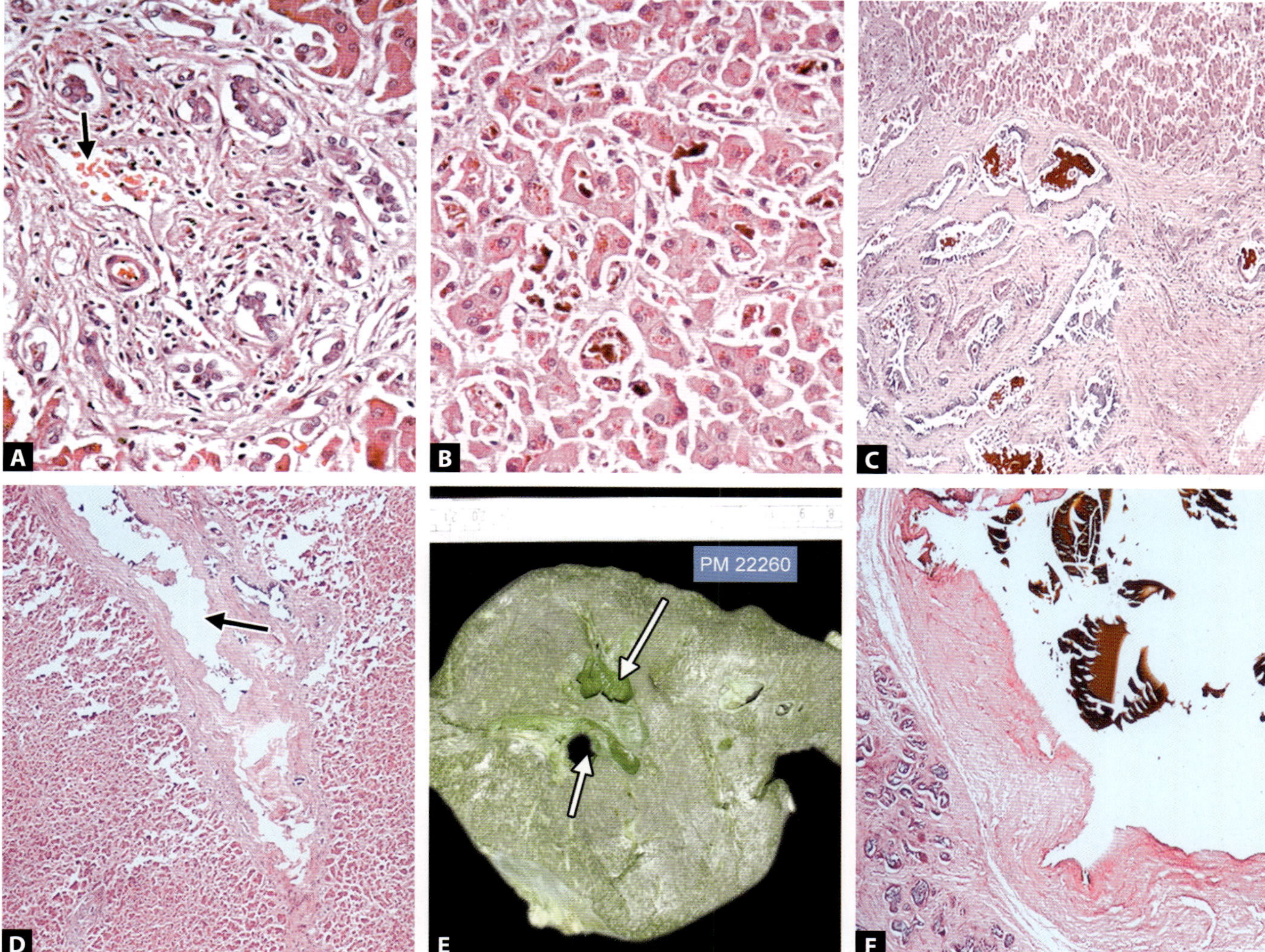

Figs 3A–F: Photomicrographs of the liver showing (A) Portal tract with bile ductular proliferation, fibrosis and a portal vein (arrow); (B) Periportal hepatocytes show canalicular cholestasis; (C) A large portal tract shows ductular proliferation and cholestasis; (D) Large portal tract shows dilated portal vein (arrow); (E) Slice of the liver which is deeply bile stained showing markedly dilated intrahepatic bile ducts (arrows) containing sludge; (F) Photomicrograph of the dilated intrahepatic bile duct containing sludge.

anticoagulant, deficiencies of protein C and protein S, antithrombin, factor II, factor V leiden, etc.)
  - Mass lesion/stasis (cirrhosis, hepatocellular carcinoma, carcinoma pancreas, etc.)
  - Vascular injury like pylephlebitis etc.
- ***Primary hypoplasia/agenesis*** of the portal vein (congenital shunts and childhood cavernomatous transformation).
- ***Local portal tract disease*** (primary portal phlebitis/arteritis/bile duct disease).

In India, extrahepatic portal vein obstruction is the cause of portal hypertension in 40% adults and in 80–85% of children, who present with hematemesis. Portal vein thrombosis occurs and is followed by compensatory mechanism of recanalization, by virtue of formation of collaterals around the obstructed portal vein, leading to the formation of ***cavernoma***. These collaterals also engulf the bile ducts and the gallbladder. Cavernous transformation of the portal vein thus occurs as a reparative/recanalizing process and is a complication of portal vein thrombosis. Eventually, the portal vein gets converted into a cluster of different sized venous channels, arranged haphazardly, within a connective tissue support and the original portal vein is not discernable. Recanalization occurs to a greater extent in patients without cirrhosis or in disorders where there is increased resistance to portal flow. Thus, it occurs more commonly in healthy livers. This entity was for the first time, described in 1869

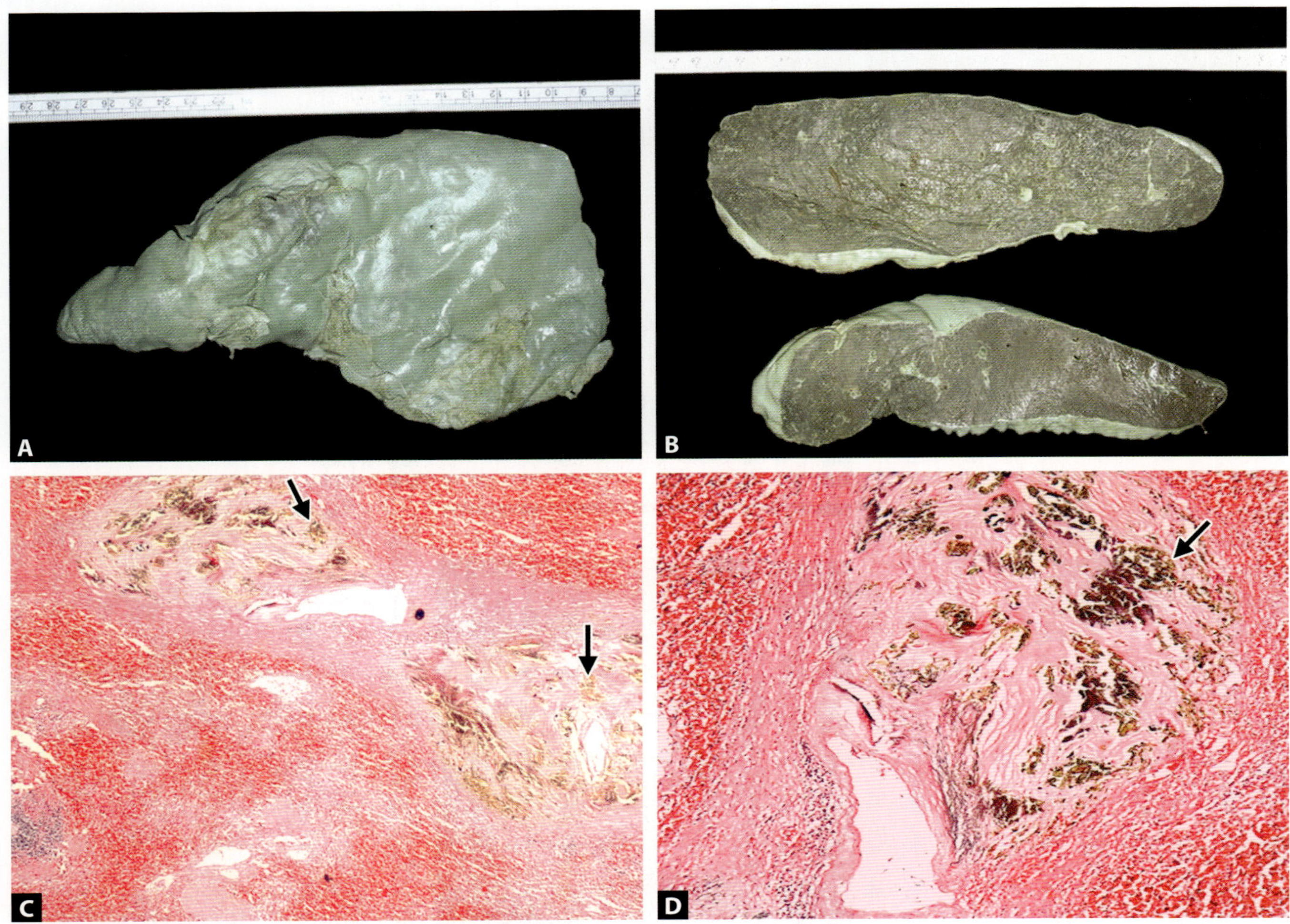

Figs 4A–D: (A) Capsular aspect of the markedly enlarged spleen, showing capsular wrinkling; (B) Coronal slices of the spleen showing diffuse congestion; (C and D) Photomicrographs of the spleen showing marked red pulp congestion and formation of Gamna-Gandy bodies (arrows).

by Balfour and Stewart. It was in 1928 that Köbrich used the term ***cavernoma*** to define the newly developed network of small vessels. Portal vein thrombosis, partial or complete leads to decreased blood supply to the liver, with active formation of collaterals, starting within a few days of the obstruction and forming a ***cavernoma*** within 3–5 weeks. The cavernoma is usually located at the hilum of the liver extending for a variable length inside and outside the liver. Patients present with portal hypertension, variceal bleed (gastroesophageal), massive splenomegaly and portosystemic collaterals. Abdominal ultrasonography, color Doppler ultrasonography, computed tomography angiography (CTA) and magnetic resonance imaging (MRI) are used to confirm its diagnosis.

Cavernous transformation of the portal vein leads to changes in the biliary tree and pancreatic ducts. Biliary abnormalities are reported in 81–100% cases of CTPV, but only a small percentage present with symptoms. Pathogenesis is unclear, but postulated mechanisms include extrinsic compression by portal collaterals and ischemic stricture of the bile duct due to injury at the time of portal venous thrombosis. Shunt surgery results in regression of some of the cholangiographic changes associated with CTPV and relieves symptoms.

PHLEGMONOUS INFLAMMATION OF THE GUT

Bacterial cellulitis of the gastrointestinal tract is known as phlegmonous inflammation. It has a predilection for the stomach, but other parts of the GIT can also be affected. Predisposing factors are alcoholism with or without liver disease, cirrhosis of any etiology, fulminant hepatitis, chronic renal failure, septicemia (due to bacterial endocarditis,

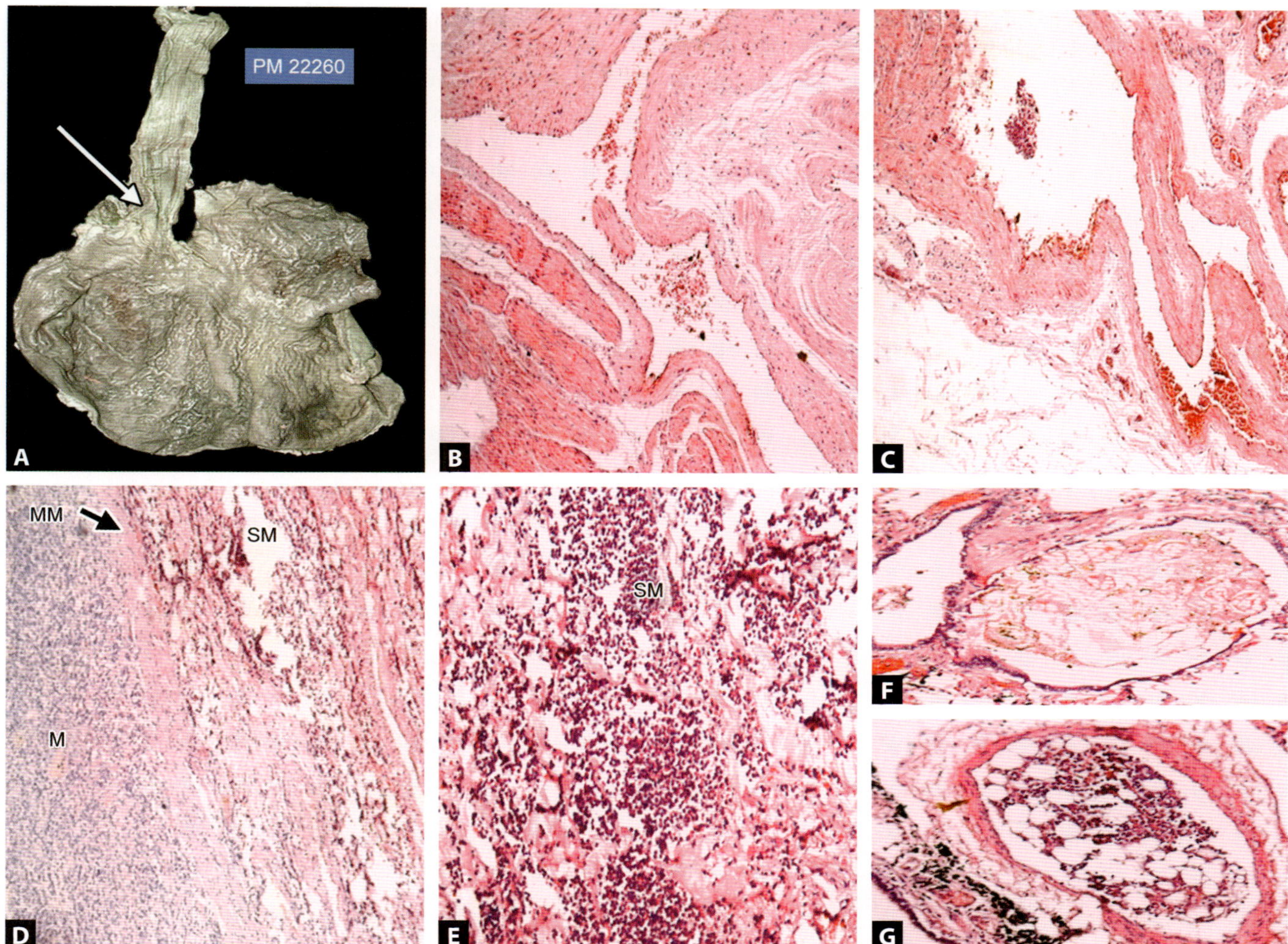

Figs 5A–G: (A) Gross photograph of the stomach and esophagus. Mucosa of the stomach is discolored. Gastroesophageal (GE) junction shows varices (arrow); (B and C) GE varices show dilated and tortuous veins with a thickened wall; (D and E) Photomicrograph of the stomach showing intact mucosa (M), muscularis mucosae (MM) and submucosa (SM). Submucosa is widened and shows dense neutrophilic infiltrate; (F) Photomicrograph of the lung showing aspirated material in the bronchiole; (G) Lung showing bone marrow emboli.

osteomyelitis, puerperal sepsis etc.), AIDS, peritoneovenous shunt, peptic ulcer, gastric surgery or idiopathic. Organisms implicated are **streptococci** (commonest), ***E. coli, Staphylococcus aureus, Diplococcus pneumoniae, Clostridium welchii, Proteus vulgaris, B. subtitis,*** etc. Grossly, the wall of the gut shows thickening, but no ulceration. On microscopic examination the mucosa is normal. The submucosa is expanded with a dense neutrophilic exudate. Bacteria can be identified amidst the polymorphs. Localization of the organisms and the neutrophilic reaction in the submucosa is a mystery. Various theories are:

- Bacteria may enter via a damaged mucosa.
- In portal hypertension, the gut is edematous and the loose connective tissue of the submucosa could provide an excellent soil for the rapid and diffuse spread of bacteria, during an episode of bacteremia.
- Hematogenous spread.

COMMENTARY—INDEX CASE

This 38-years female, first presented in childhood with hematemesis at the age of 7-years, episode of jaundice at the age of 15 years and again hematemesis at the age of 19 years. At this point of time (December 1988) ultrasonography confirmed EHPVO with short gastric, retroperitoneal and splenorenal collaterals and ERCP detected dilated left intrahepatic biliary radicals. She underwent 3 sessions of endoscopic sclerotherapy and was then lost to follow-up.

In October 2007, at the age of 38 years, she was readmitted with jaundice, malena, hematemesis, altered sensorium, massive splenomegaly, marked conjugated hyperbilirubinemia, coagulopathy, renal failure, bilobar intrahepatic biliary radical dilatation and cavernomatous transformation of portal vein. Autopsy confirmed cavernomatous transformation of portal vein with portal cavernoma cholangiopathy, portal hypertension (congestive splenomegaly, esophageal varices, ascitis) along with phlegmonous inflammation of the stomach and colon. Thus, this patient lived with EHPVO with cavernomatous transformation of portal vein (CTPV) for 31-years of her life. Since she presented at 7-years of life with hematemesis, there is a possibility of a developmental malformation of the portal vein leading to EHPVO.

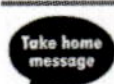

TAKE HOME MESSAGE

- In India, extrahepatic portal vein obstruction is the cause of portal hypertension in 40% adults and in 80–85% of children, who present with hematemesis.
- Major cause of EHPVO is portal vein thrombosis which in due course gets converted to a ***cavernoma***.
- Biliary abnormalities are reported in 81–100% cases of cavernomatous transformation of portal vein but a small percentage present with symptoms.
- Phlegmonous inflammation of the GIT tract is a bacterial cellulitis of the submucosa.

SUGGESTED READING

1. De Gaetano AM, Lafortune M, Patriquin H, et al. Cavernous transformation of the portal vein: patterns of intrahepatic and splanchnic collateral circulation detected with Doppler sonography. AJR Am J Roentgenol. 1995;165(5):1151-5.
2. Kakkar N, Vashista RK, Banerjee AK, et al. Phlegmonous inflammation of GIT: An autopsy study of 3 cases. Indian Jour Path Micro. 1999;42(1):101-5.
3. Kumar M, Saraswat VA. Natural history of portal cavernoma cholangiopathy. J Clin Exp Hepatol. 2014;4(Suppl 1):S62-6.
4. Ramos R, Park Y, Shazad G, et al. Cavernous transformation of portal vein secondary to portal vein thrombosis: A case report. J Clin Med Res. 2012;4(1):81-4.

CONTRIBUTIONS BY:

1. Dr YK Chawla, Former Director PGI, Ex-Professor and Head, Department of Hepatology (Clinician In-Charge)
2. Dr RK Dhiman, Professor and Head, Department of Hepatology (Clinician In-Charge)
3. Dr NK Khandelwal, Professor and Head, Department of Radiodiagnosis and Imaging

Post Graduate Institute of Medical Education and Research, Chandigarh, India.

CASE 21

Chronic Budd-Chiari Syndrome with Mesoatrial Shunt, Venocentric Cirrhosis, Hepatocellular Carcinoma Infiltrating into the Hepatic Duct Causing Obstruction and Hemobilia: PM 27800

Nandita Bharadwaj Kakkar

HIGHLIGHTS OF THE CASE

This is a 50-year male with chronic Budd-Chiari syndrome with mesoatrial shunt, venocentric cirrhosis and multinodular hepatocellular carcinoma arising in its background. The hepatocellular carcinoma had invaded into the extrahepatic biliary tree, leading to tumor bleed causing hemobilia, rupture of the gallbladder (due to a large blood clot), hemoperitoneum, extrahepatic bile duct obstruction and cholangitis.

Keywords: Budd-Chiari syndrome, chronic, venocentric cirrhosis, mesoatrial shunt, hepatocellular carcinoma, invasion, biliary tract, extrahepatic bile duct obstruction, gallbladder perforation, hemoperitoneum.

CLINICAL DETAILS

Past History

In December 2003 (at the age of 37-year) patient had hematemesis and hepatic encephalopathy. He was diagnosed as Budd-Chiari syndrome (BCS) at an outside facility. In July 2004, he had recurrence of hematemesis, hepatic encephalopathy and ascites, was admitted and evaluated in PGIMER. At that time the USG Doppler showed non-visualized left hepatic vein at the cavoatrial junction. Inferior vena cava angiography showed narrowing of intrahepatic IVC, 4 cm from cavoatrial junction and nonopacification of all three hepatic veins. In September 2004, eradication of esophageal varices was done and he was put on propranolol and diuretics. Mesoatrial shunt was advised, but then he was lost to follow-up. In October 2005, mesoatrial shunt was done. Thereafter, till 2011, he was on irregular follow-up in the OPD and after 2011 till 2016, he was lost to follow-up.

Present Admission—Date of Admission—09.11.2016; Date of Death— 11.11.2016, Duration of Hospital Stay: 2 Days

A 50-year old male came with yellowish discoloration of the eyes since 5 days, which was insidious in onset, gradually progressive, associated with cholestatic symptoms but not associated with any prodrome. There was no malena, hematemesis, fever and loss of appetite/weight. There was pain abdomen since 3 days, which was acute in onset, located in the right hypochondrium/umbilical region, was moderate to severe in intensity, nonradiating, not related to food intake, no aggravating factors present, not associated with nausea/vomiting, lasting for 2–3 hours and partially relieved with medication. There was no history of diabetes, hypertension, coronary artery disease or any cerebrovascular accident. He was a reformed alcohol consumer since 2003 and a smoker.

Examination

On ***examination*** he was conscious, alert, cooperative, PR: 90/min, RR: 20/min, BP: 130/80 mm Hg, no pallor, icterus was present, no cyanosis/clubbing, no pedal edema, afebrile at admission, SpO_2: 98% at room air, no lymphadenopathy, JVP not raised and onychomycosis was present. Abdominal examination revealed a midline scar and another scar seen along the right costal margin, hepatomegaly (4 cm below RCM), moderate splenomegaly, tenderness in the right upper quadrant, no free fluid/shifting dullness and bowel sounds were present. Respiratory, cardiovascular and central nervous systems were within normal limits.

Investigations and Course of Management

***Hemogram*:** Hb: 7.8 g/dl, TLC— 16,100/uL, Platelets— 164,000/uL; deranged coagulogram (PT— 49', PTI— 26%, aPTT— 46'); Liver function tests—serum bilirubin

T/C—17.95/10.26 mg%, SGOT/SGPT—345/81 U/L, ALP—536 U/L, total proteins/albumin—6.2/2.1 gms; amylase—378 U/L; lipase— 575 U/L; serum procalcitonin—1.58 ng/mL; viral markers: HbsAg/HIV/anti-HCV—nonreactive; blood C/S—sterile.

Radiology

- *Chest X-ray*: Normal study.
- *Ultrasonography abdomen*: Edematous and thickened GB wall ? Gangrenous cholecystitis, bilateral intrahepatic biliary radical dilatation with nonpatent confluence, patent mesoatrial shunts with suspicious area of liver ? Nodule and mild ascites.
- *Contrast-enhanced CT abdomen with CT angiography* of abdominal vessels—Chronic liver disease with large peripheral wedge shaped hypodense areas ? infarct with surface discontinuity at places ? rupture. Bilobar intrahepatic biliary radical dilatation (IHBRD) is seen with hyperdense soft tissue at the confluence of right and left hepatic ducts extending into CBD till its lower end ? etiology. A large soft tissue measuring 10.5 × 9.5 cm with heterogeneous attenuation and hyperdense contents with tortuous vessels, with evidence of active extravasation s/o active bleed. Hyperdense contents in the intrahepatic biliary radicles and CBD likely hemorrhagic. Multiple peripheral wedge shaped hypodense lesions in bilateral kidney? Infarcts. Nodular lesions in right lobe of liver ? Nodular regenerative hyperplasia, moderate ascites ? hemoperitoneum, normally opacified mesoatrial shunt.

In view of clinical deterioration of the patient and the USG suggestive of suspicious gangrenous cholecystitis, urgent CECT abdomen was done in the night and patient was shifted to GE ICU. Repeat CECT showed heterogeneously enhancing soft tissue lesion at the confluence, with bilobar IHBRD with nonpatent confluence. Another soft tissue mass (10.5 × 9.5) with evidence of active bleed was seen. Repeat hemoglobin dropped to 6.3 g/dL, resuscitated with FFP and PRBC transfusion. Planned for digital subtraction angiography (DSA) but deferred due to coagulopathy (INR—3.37). Patient developed increase in pain abdomen, tachycardia, tachypnea and increase in the abdominal girth. He developed hypotension and was given IV fluids and inotropic support. He was intubated in view of drop in saturation and was put on ventilatory support. He had persistent hypotension and hence second inotrope (vasopressin) was added. Patient sustained cardiac arrest and despite best efforts, could not be revived.

Clinical Diagnosis

Refractory septic shock, chronic Budd-Chiari syndrome, mesoarterial shunt (2005), extrahepatic biliary obstruction (EHBO) with a hilar mass? Cholangiocarcinoma with hepatic metastasis, ? Cholangitic abscess, disseminated intravascular coagulation.

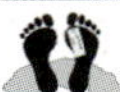

AUTOPSY FINDINGS: PM 27800

A partial autopsy was performed after due permission. Patient was of average built, abdomen was distended, skin showed yellowish discoloration and multiple ecchymotic patches. The skin of both lower limbs was discolored and thick. The peritoneal cavity yielded 1,000 mL of brownish fluid. Other serous cavities are within normal limits.

Liver

***Gross*:** Liver was enlarged and weighed 2,200 g. The capsule showed nodularity in most areas and was smooth in some parts. Cut section of the liver (Figs 1A and B; 2A and B) was bile stained and showed multiple tumor nodules ranging in size from 0.5–5 cm in diameter, getting confluent and occupying a major part of the right lobe. The left lobe appeared to be shrunken. The surrounding liver showed a variety of changes i.e. areas of diffuse fibrosis, vague nodularity and nutmeg appearance. The intrahepatic bile duct and the common hepatic duct contained a greenish mass reaching uptill the formation of the common bile duct and protruding a little into the common bile duct (Figs 1A–D). The smaller intrahepatic bile ducts showed presence of blood clots (Fig 2A). The intrahepatic part of the inferior vena cava was narrow and showed obliteration of the opening of the hepatic veins (Fig 2C). The portal vein was mildly dilated (Fig 2D). The gallbladder (Figs 1A and C) was enlarged, ruptured and a large blood clot was seen to be coming out of the ruptured site. The mesoatrial shunt composed of a Dacron graft, connecting the superior mesenteric artery and the right atrium (attached at the right auricle) was patent (Fig 2E).

***Microscopy*:** Microscopic examination of the liver revealed a markedly distorted lobular architecture. Numerous small and large hepatic veins showed organizing thrombi leading to fibrous obliteration of their lumen (Figs 3A–E). Large areas of fibrosis were seen. Reversed lobulation cirrhosis i.e. venocentric cirrhosis, wherein there is sparing of the portal tracts, was prominently seen (Figs 4A–D). Cirrhotic nodules containing the central vein in the center were appreciated. All these features suggest a Budd-Chiari syndrome (BCS). Apart from this, the multiple nodules seen more in the right lobe, revealed features of hepatocellular carcinoma (Figs 5A–E). Nodule in nodule appearance was noted. The tumor cells were arranged in a trabecular pattern (sinusoidal, plate like) with plates more than 3-cells thick, showed marked

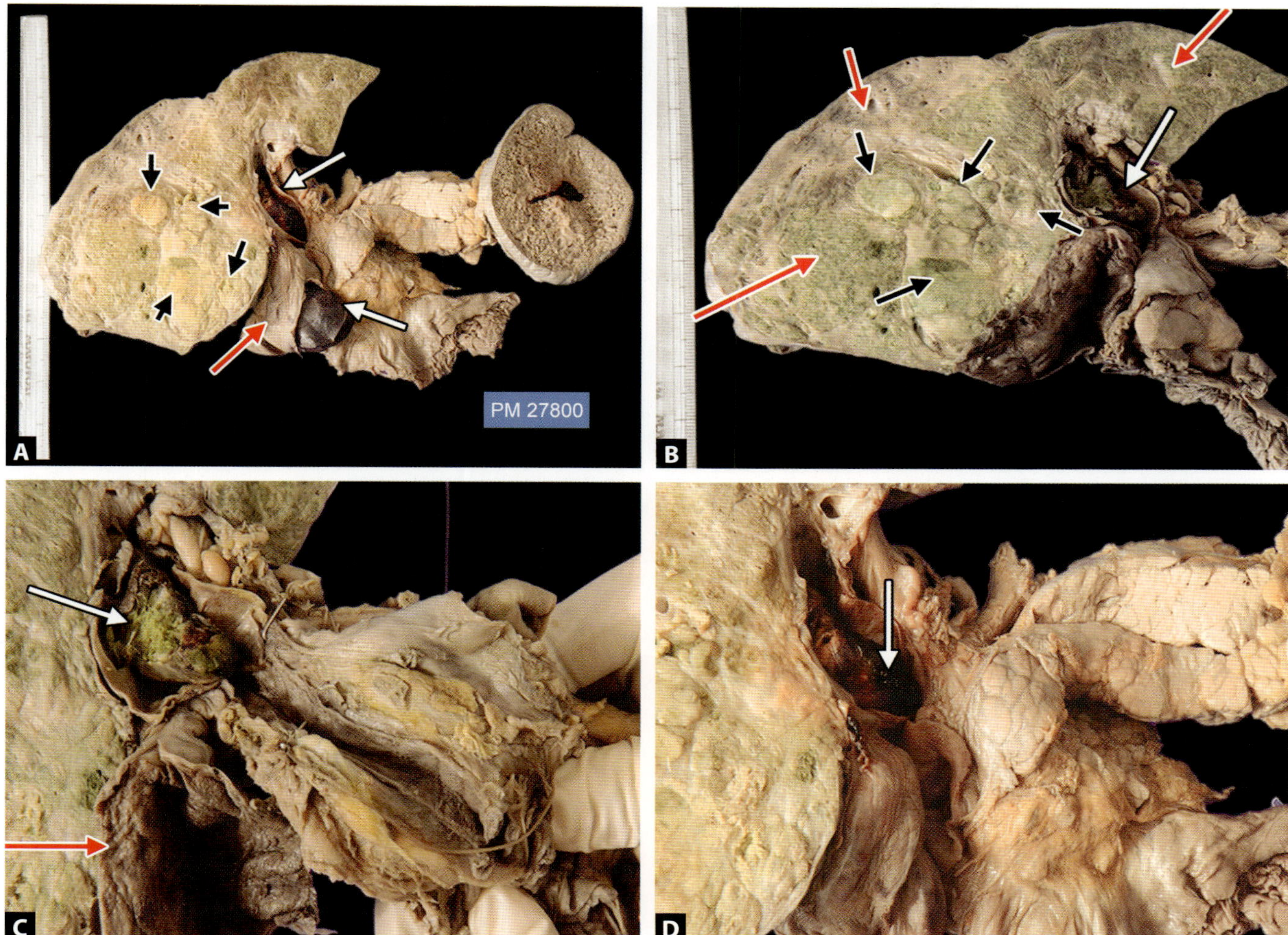

Figs 1A–D: (A and B) Coronal slice of the liver which is bile stained and shows multiple tumor nodules (black arrows) getting confluent, occupying a major part of the right lobe. The left lobe appears to be more shrunken. The gallbladder in A (red arrow) shows a rupture with a blood clot peeping out (lower white arrow). The surrounding liver in B shows a variety of changes, diffuse fibrosis, vague nodularity and nutmeg appearance (red arrows). The intrahepatic bile duct (upper white arrow in A and white arrow in B) and the common hepatic duct contained a greenish mass, mixed with blood clot; (C) Close-up view of the intrahepatic bile duct (white arrow) and the common hepatic duct containing a greenish mass which was reaching uptill the formation of the common bile duct. The ruptured gallbladder can be seen (red arrow), its mucosa is rough and shows blackish discoloration. The clot has been removed; (D) The intrahepatic bile duct (white arrow) containing greening mass admixed with blood clot.

pleomorphism, enlarged hyperchromatic nuclei and moderate cytoplasm. Tumor cells showed prominent bile secretion with formation of bile plugs and intracytoplasmic cholestasis. The greenish mass present in the right intrahepatic bile duct, common hepatic duct and early part of the common bile duct, on microscopy revealed a tumor with features of hepatocellular carcinoma (Figs 6A and B). Thus, the hepatocellular carcinoma was invading into the biliary tract and was reaching up till the CBD. This mass in the extrahepatic biliary tract was causing extrahepatic biliary obstruction along with tumor bleed, leading to hemobilia (Fig 6C). The tumor bleed inside the biliary tract led to hemobilia (bile ducts of all sizes contained red blood cells) and the blood made its way into the gallbladder, which contained a large blood clot measuring 5 × 4 × 3 cm and this led to its rupture. Microscopy of the blood clot in the gallbladder confirmed the blood clot and no tumor cells were found in it. The extrahepatic biliary obstruction (Figs 6D–F) due to the infiltrating hepatocellular carcinoma could be appreciated in the liver, in the form of portal tract expansion due to edema and bile ductular proliferation, bilirubinostasis seen as bile plugs and within the hepatocytes, pseudo acinar transformation and cholangitis.

The ***spleen*** (Fig 1A) weighed 190 g and showed congestive splenomegaly. No esophageal varices were seen as a mesoatrial shunt was done.

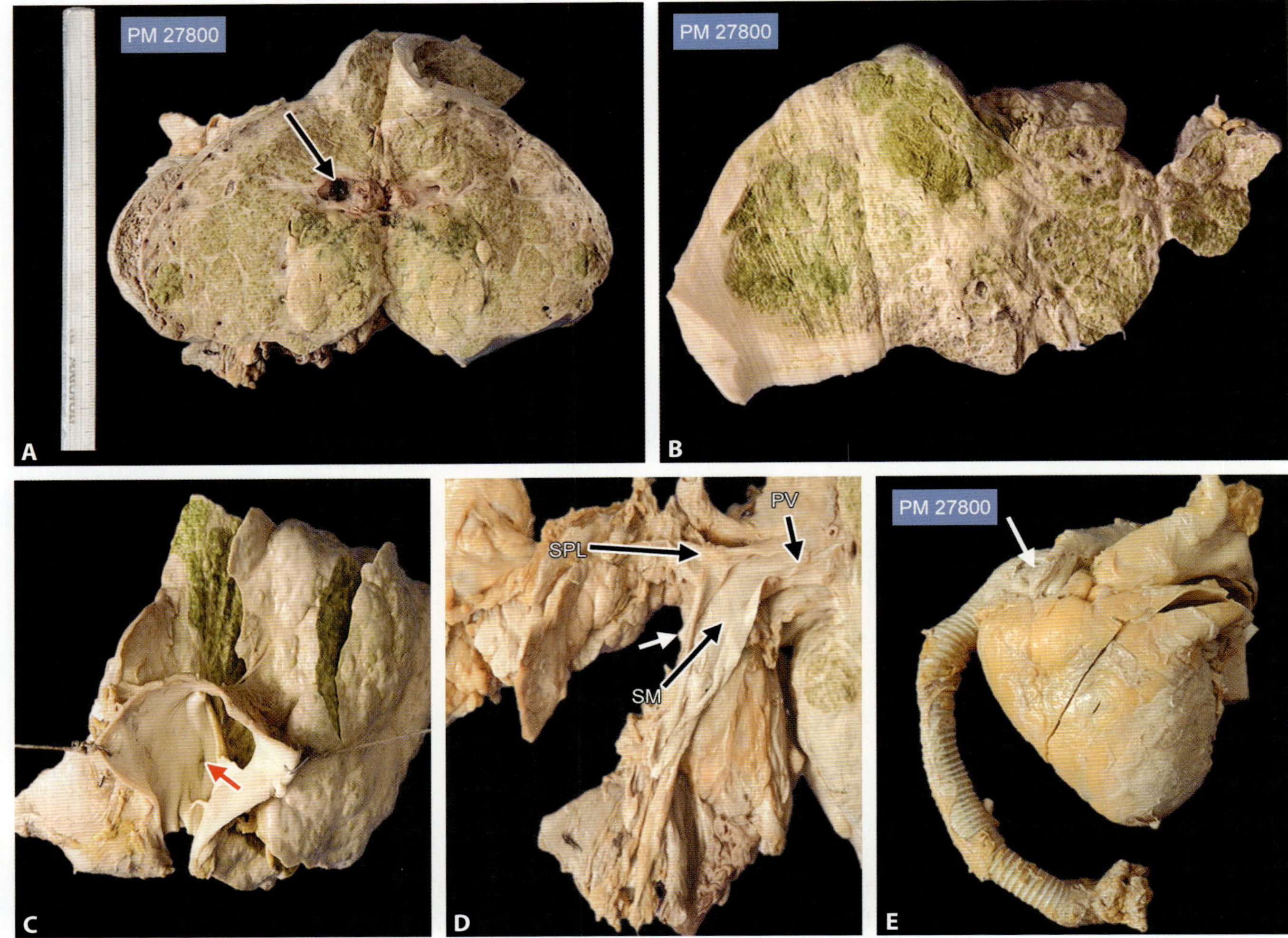

Figs 2A–E: (A) Coronal slice of the liver shows blood clot in the branch of the intrahepatic bile duct; (B) Coronal slice of the liver is bile stained, shows confluent areas of fibrosis and nodules separated by fibrous septa; (C) The opened up intrahepatic part of the inferior vena cava is narrow and shows obliteration of the opening of the hepatic vein (arrow). The capsular aspect of the liver shows nodules; (D) The splenic vein (SPL), superior mesenteric vein (SM) joins to form the portal vein (PV) which is mildly dilated. No thrombus is seen; (E) The heart showing the mesoatrial shunt opening into the right atrium at the right auricle (white arrow).

The ***heart*** (Figs 7A and B) weighed 480 g. A patent mesoatrial shunt was present and right ventricular hypertrophy was noted (wall measured 0.8 cm). The left ventricular wall measured 2 cm indicating left ventricular hypertrophy. The ***lungs*** (Fig 7C) revealed features of pulmonary arterial hypertension along with edema. Bile casts were noted in the kidneys.

FINAL AUTOPSY DIAGNOSIS: PM 27800

A 50-year male, case of chronic BCS with mesoatrial shunt, hilar mass leading to extrahepatic biliary obstruction.

- Chronic Bud-Chiari syndrome with venocentric cirrhosis and patent mesoatrial shunt.
- Hepatocellular carcinoma.
- Hepatocellular carcinoma invasion into the intrahepatic duct, common hepatic duct, common bile duct leading to following conditions:
  - Tumor bleed causing hemobilia and perforation of gallbladder due to a large blood clot.
  - Hemoperitoneum.
  - Features of extrahepatic biliary obstruction, cholangitis.
- Biventricular hypertrophy of heart.
- Pulmonary arterial hypertension.
- Bile casts in kidney.

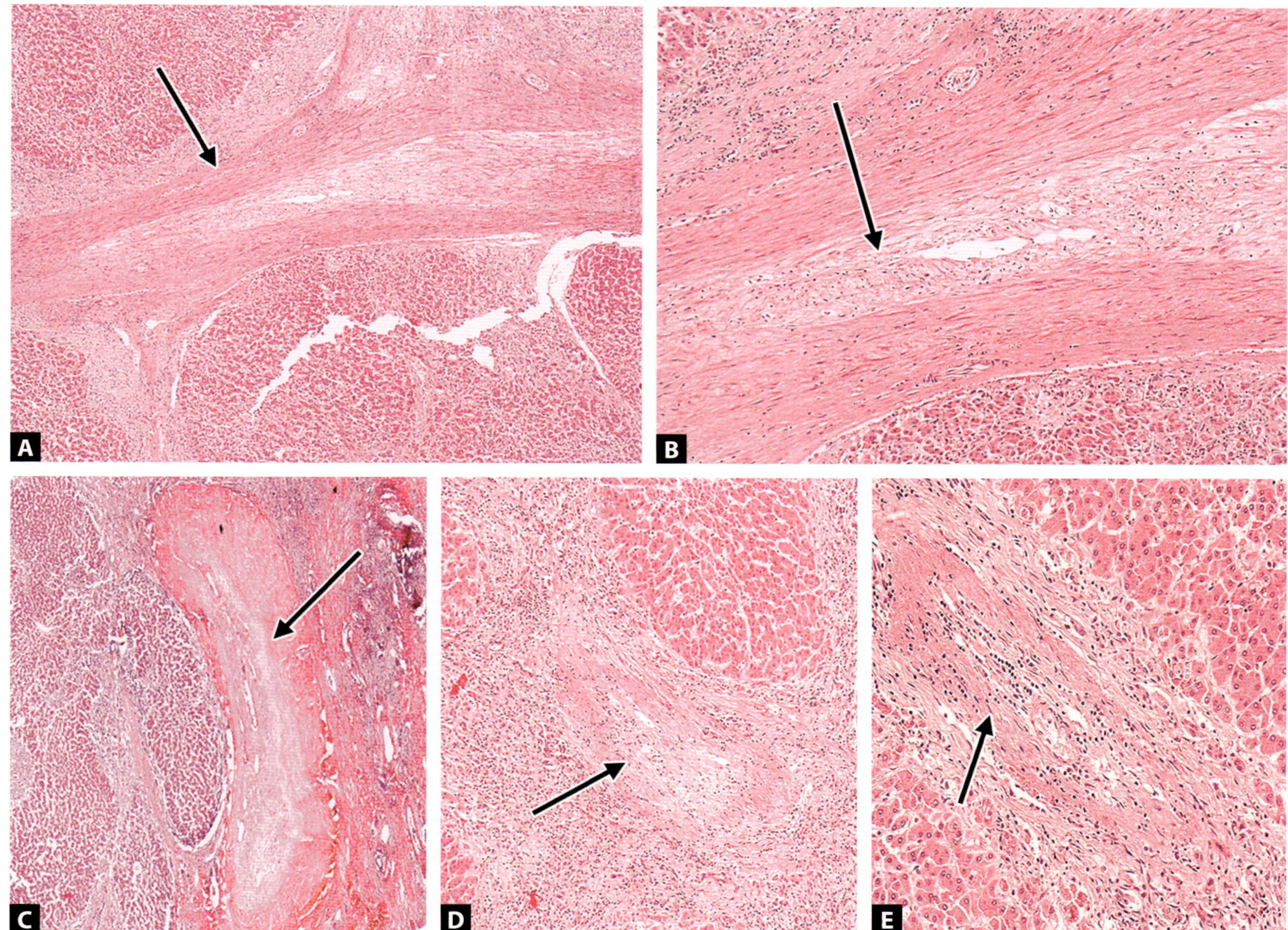

Figs 3A–E: Photomicrographs of the liver showing fibrous obliteration of the large and small hepatic veins (arrows).

BUDD-CHIARI SYNDROME

The Budd-Chiari syndrome encompasses a large group of disorders, wherein there is obstruction of the hepatic venous outflow at various levels i.e. at the level of the right atrium, inferior vena cava, large hepatic veins and hepatic venules. Hepatic venous outflow obstruction causes a back pressure, leading to sinusoidal congestion which causes ischemic injury to the liver cells. Eventually portal vein hypertension ensues, further leading to congestion and necrosis of hepatocytes, regeneration, fibrosis and cirrhosis. Patients present with enlarged liver/spleen, abdominal pain, liver dysfunction and ascites. If the surgical treatment is not carried out, patients survive for less than 2 years. When all major hepatic veins are thrombosed, patients present with fulminant hepatic failure. The etiology of BCS is a hypercoagulable state (myeloproliferative disorders, pregnancy, oral contraceptives, factor V Leiden, Protein C/S deficiency etc.), stasis/mass lesions (membranous constrictive pericarditis, congestive heart failure, membranous obstruction of inferior vena cava, cirrhosis, HCC, epithelioid hemangioendothelioma, hydatid cyst etc.), vascular injury (trauma, vasculitis, Behçet's disease, sarcoidosis, ventriculoatrial shunt etc.) and miscellaneous uncertain disorders (mixed connective tissue disease, celiac disease, etc).

Microscopically, the acute lesions of BCS show sinusoidal congestion with red blood cells in the space of Disse, dilatation of veins, organizing thrombi in the small hepatic veins/portal veins, varying degree of hepatocytic necrosis and eventually parenchymal extinction. With time, the sinusoids get collagenized, hepatocytes get necrosed and the small hepatic veins are not discernable, as they get embedded in the septa which connect the hepatic veins, leading to

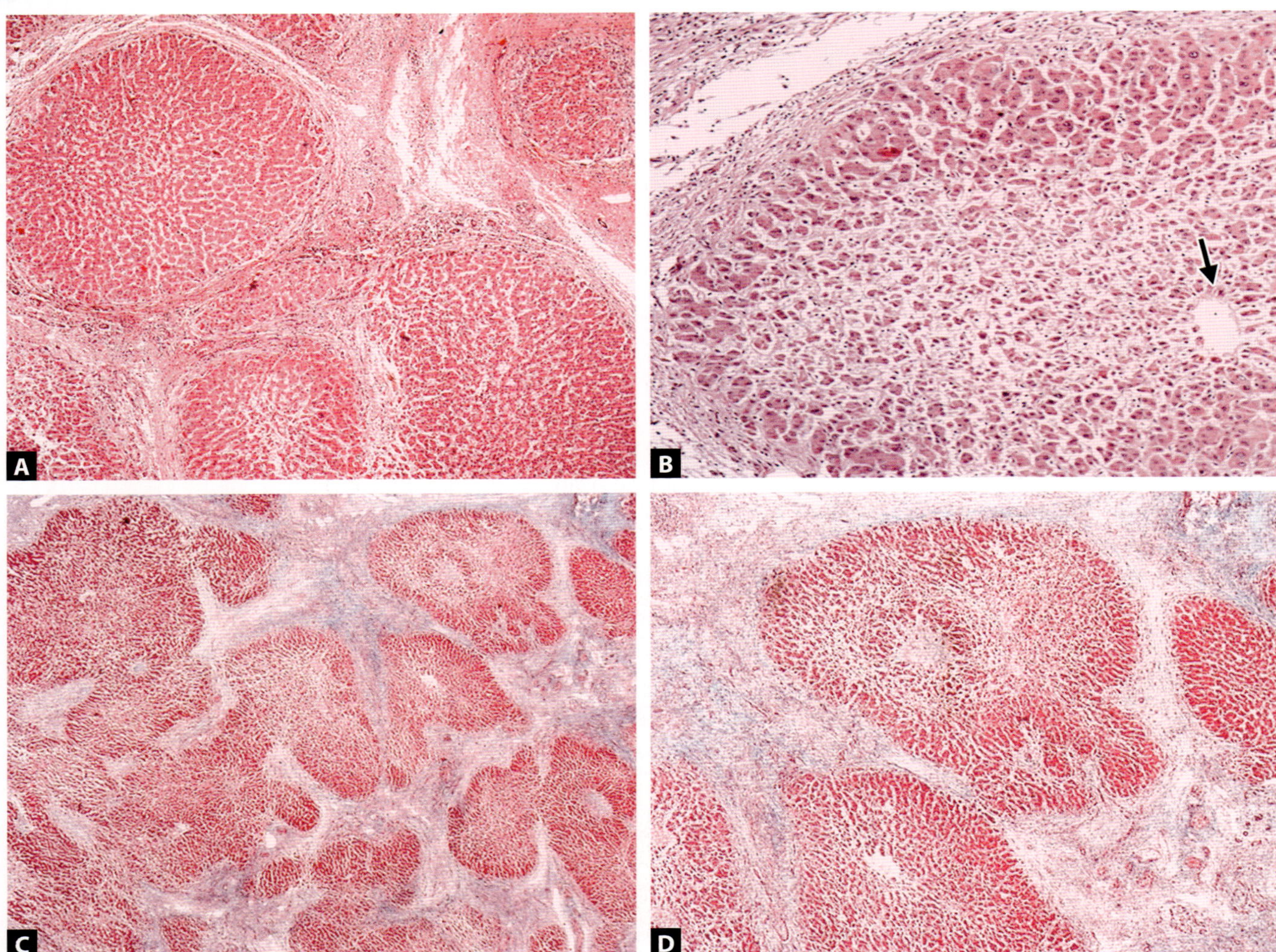

Figs 4A–D: (A and B) Photomicrographs from the liver shows reversed lobulation/venocentric cirrhosis, wherein there is sparing of the portal tracts and the central vein is appreciated at the center of the nodule (arrow in B); (C and D) Masson's trichrome stain demonstrating the prominent *reversed lobulation*.

cirrhosis, with sparing of portal tracts. The cirrhosis which ensues is designated as venocentric cirrhosis or reversed lobulation cirrhosis, which occurs when the obstruction is limited to the hepatic veins. Portal vein thrombosis can occur in BCS and when it occurs, the cirrhosis is predominantly of venoportal type. Remodeling of the liver occurs, caudate lobe hypertrophy occurs when caudate lobe veins are spared or left lobe is hypertrophied when the left hepatic vein is patent and so on. Thus, grossly the liver in advanced stages is bile stained with hypertrophy of the lobes depending upon the patency of their veins, nodules surrounded by fibrous septa are appreciated and significant confluent fibrosis can be seen. Hepatocellular carcinoma can be seen in the background of chronic BCS as was seen in the index case. They are diagnosed at imaging (USG, CT, MRI) in combination with clinical findings. Once a diagnosis of hepatocellular carcinoma in a background of BCS is established, transcatheter arterial chemoembolization i.e. TACE is resorted to.

COMMENTARY—INDEX CASE: PM 27800

This is the story of a man, who was diagnosed with Budd-Chiari syndrome at the age of 37-year (in 2003). Eradication of esophageal varices was done in 2005 and soon after that a mesoatrial shunt was put. He was on irregular follow-up and was then lost to follow-up. In 2016, at the age of 50 years, he was readmitted with jaundice along with cholestatic symptoms and severe pain abdomen. On investigating, he had

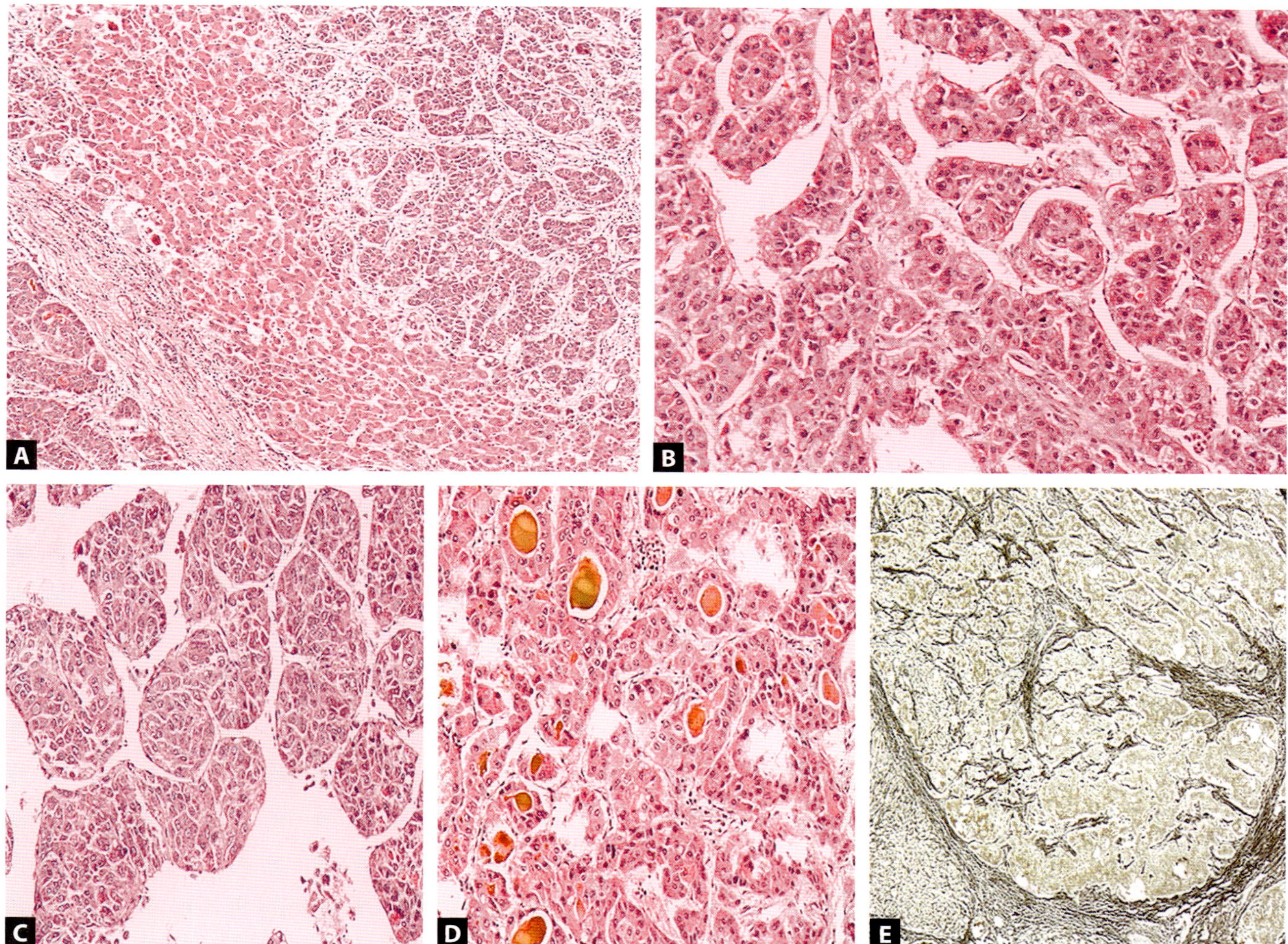

Figs 5A–E: Photomicrographs of the liver (A) Hepatocellular carcinoma arising within a nodule giving a nodule in nodule appearance; (B and C) Tumor cells arranged in a trabecular pattern with plates more than 3 cells thick; (D) HCC cells producing bile; (E) Reticulin stain shows paucity of reticulin fiber in the tumor nodule.

low hemoglobin, conjugated hyperbilirubinemia, raised liver enzymes, alkaline phosphatase and coagulopathy. Radiology revealed a hilar mass. A clinical diagnosis of chronic Budd-Chiari syndrome with mesoarterial shunt and extrahepatic biliary obstruction with a hilar mass ? Cholangiocarcinoma ? with hepatic metastasis ? Cholangitic abscess, disseminated intravascular coagulation was made. At autopsy there was a multinodular hepatocellular carcinoma arising in the background of chronic Budd-Chiari syndrome with venocentric cirrhosis. The mesoatrial shunt done 11 years ago was patent. The hepatocellular carcinoma had invaded into the hepatic ducts and then grown into the common hepatic duct, reaching uptill the common bile duct. This mass on CECT abdomen was seen as a hyperdense soft tissue at the confluence of right and left hepatic ducts extending into CBD till its lower end and clinically a possibility of cholangiocarcinoma was kept. Further there was tumor bleed from the invading HCC mass in the biliary tract leading to the following conditions:

- Blood in the small and large intrahepatic bile ducts (hemobilia).
- The blood had traversed into the gallbladder and formed a large blood clot leading to rupture of the gallbladder and causing hemoperitoneum.
- The invading HCC mass in the biliary tract led to features of extrahepatic bile duct obstruction and cholangitis. The mesoatrial shunt was patent.

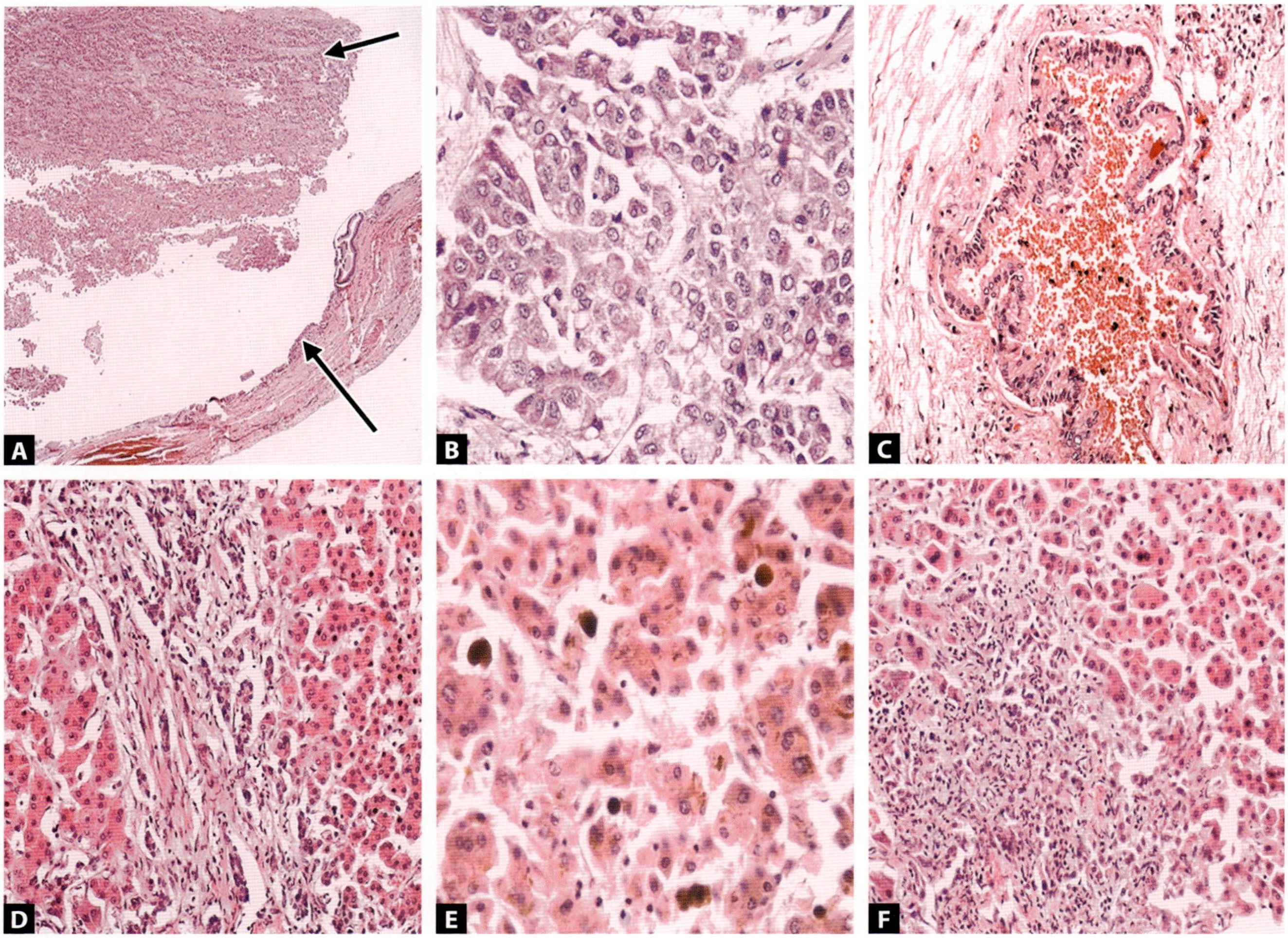

Figs 6A–F: (A) Photomicrograph from the common hepatic duct shows the wall lined by columnar epithelium (lower arrow). The tumor is present in the lumen of the duct (upper arrow); (B) Mass in the hepatic duct shows a tumor with features of HCC; (C) Medium-sized bile duct shows hemobilia; (D) Photomicrographs of the liver shows porto-portal bridging fibrosis with bile duct proliferation; (E) Perivenular hepatocytes show cholestasis both ductular and hepatocytic; (F) Portal tract shows acute inflammation with cholangitis.

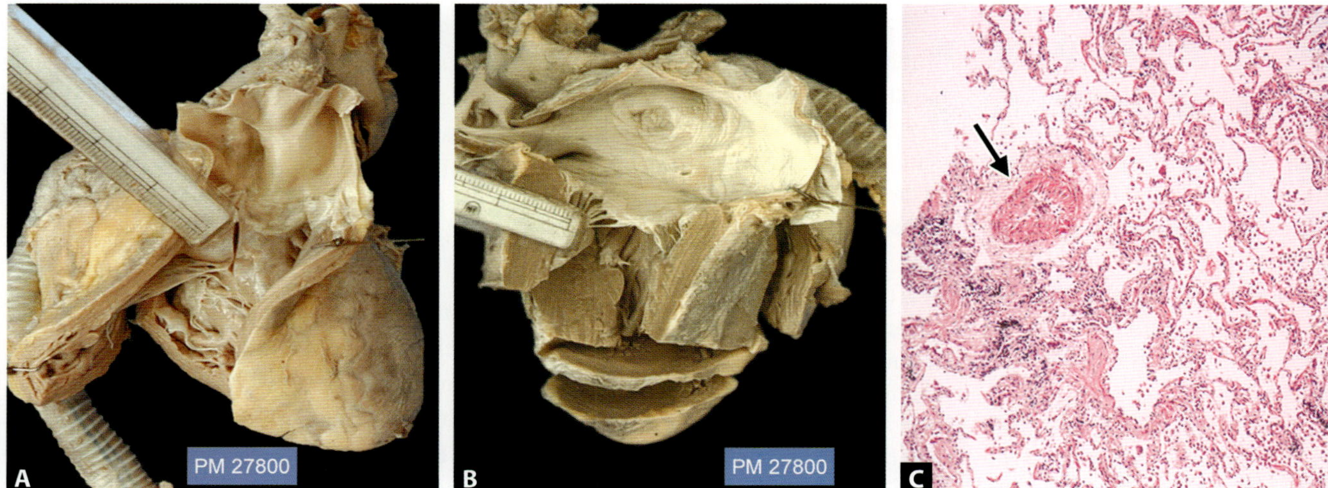

Figs 7A–C: (A) Gross photograph of the heart showing right outflow tract. The right ventricular wall shows hypertrophy; (B) Left inflow tract showing normal mitral valve. The left ventricular wall shows hypertrophy; (C) Photomicrograph of the lung showing a small vessel with medial hypertrophy.

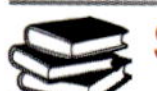

TAKE HOME MESSAGE

- The Budd-Chiari syndrome encompasses a large group of disorders, wherein there is obstruction of the hepatic venous outflow at various levels.
- Chronic BCS leads to reversed lobulation cirrhosis or venocentric cirrhosis.
- Hepatocellular carcinoma can arise in the background of chronic BCS.

SUGGESTED READING

1. Aydinli M, Bayraktar. Budd-Chiari syndrome: Etiology, pathogenesis and diagnosis. World J Gastroenterol. 2007; 13(19):2693-6.
2. Havlioqlu N, Brunt EM, Bacon BR. Budd-Chiari syndrome and hepatocellular carcinoma- a case report and review of literature. Am J Gastroenterol. 2003;98(1):201-4.

CONTRIBUTIONS BY:

1. Dr Anand Bardia, Junior Resident, Department of Pathology (In taking gross Photographs)
2. Dr Gurwinder Kaur, Senior Resident, Department of Pathology (In taking gross Photographs)
3. Dr Jawaharlal G, Junior Resident, Department of Internal Medicine (Compilation of Clinical Details)
4. Dr RK Kochhar, Professor and Head, Department of Gastroenterology, Hepatology and Nutrition (Clinician In-Charge).
5. Dr NK Khandelwal, Professor and Head, Department of Radiodiagnosis and Imaging.

Post Graduate Institute of Medical Education and Research, Chandigarh, India.

CASE 22

Acute on Chronic Pancreatitis Leading to Portal Vein Pyemia, with Multiple Liver Abscesses and Life-threatening Sepsis Shock: PM 25975

Nandita Bharadwaj Kakkar

 HIGHLIGHTS OF THE CASE

A 46-year-old male was diagnosed with anterior wall myocardial infarction (MI) and a stent was placed in the left anterior descending artery. Two weeks later, he was readmitted with congestive cardiac failure (CCF). He was diagnosed with sepsis, antibiotics were administered, his condition improved and he was discharged. Five weeks later, he was readmitted with high grade fever and breathlessness. Clinical diagnosis was recent MI with stenting, CCF, left ventricular systolic dysfunction, liver abscesses with cholangitis, shock ? septic ? cardiogenic. Autopsy revealed old healed MI with stent in situ, acute on chronic pancreatitis with abscesses leading to portal vein pyemia and multiple liver abscesses.

Keywords: Pylephlebitis, infective suppurative thrombosis of portal vein, portal vein pyemia, acute pancreatitis, pyogenic liver abscesses, autopsy.

 CLINICAL DETAILS

Date of Admission: 14.03.2014, Date of Death: 17.03.2014, Duration of Hospital Stay: 3 Days

A 46-year-old male was admitted in January of 2014 with acute onset chest pain, was diagnosed to have an acute anterior wall myocardial infarction with electrocardiogram showing ST↑ and T↓ in V 1–4, along with left ventricular hypertrophy. Thrombolytic therapy was not administered due to late presentation. Coronary angiography revealed a double vessel disease, involving the left anterior descending (LAD) and left circumflex arteries (LCA). He underwent percutaneous coronary intervention (PCI) and a stent was placed in the left anterior descending artery. He was readmitted 2 weeks later with features of congestive cardiac failure. Echocardiography showed an ejection fraction of 35–40% with hypokinesia in LAD territory and moderate left ventricular systolic dysfunction. The total leukocyte count was raised (27,900/uL) with polymorphonuclear leukocytosis. Ultrasonography of the abdomen revealed a fatty liver with a portal vein of 13 mm and gallbladder containing sludge. He was treated with antibiotics, his condition improved and he was discharged again. Five weeks later, he was readmitted with complaints of high grade fever accompanied with rigors and chills since one month. There was breathlessness, dry cough and abdominal distension since 3 days. There was no history of loose stools, malena, jaundice or rash. He was an alcoholic and a smoker. On examination, he was conscious, cooperative, there was pallor, no jaundice, cyanosis, clubbing or any lymph node enlargement was noted. He was febrile (temp—38°C), there was bilateral pitting edema, pulse—115 beats/min, BP— 80/50 mmHg on noradrenaline infusion of 3 mL/h, respiratory rate— 36/min, SpO_2—96% on FiO_2—0.4 and CVP—18 cm. Chest examination revealed decreased breath sounds in both basal areas. A pigtail was inserted on the left side which brought out straw-colored fluid. Cardiovascular system revealed normal S1/S2 and there were no added sounds. The abdomen was tense, distended and shifting dullness was present. The liver and spleen were not enlarged.

Investigations

Hemogram revealed Hb of 7.5 g/dL, TLC of 35,500/uL with 90% neutrophils, platelets: 101,000/uL and ESR: 114 (1st hour). Blood biochemistry—serum electrolytes $Na^+/K^+/Cl^-$—126/3.1/91 mEq/L, serum bilirubin (T/C)—2.4–3.1/0.7–1.6 mg%, SGOT/SGPT—129/97 U/L, alkaline phosphatase 107 U/L, total proteins/albumin 5.8/1.9 gms, INR 1.32 and normal renal function tests. Ascitic fluid analysis revealed—proteins

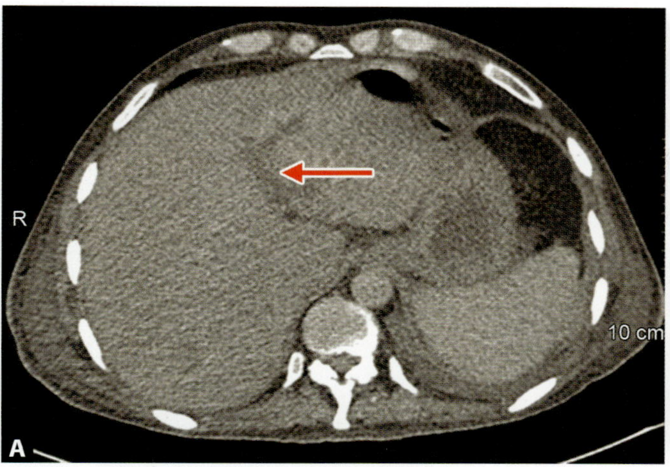

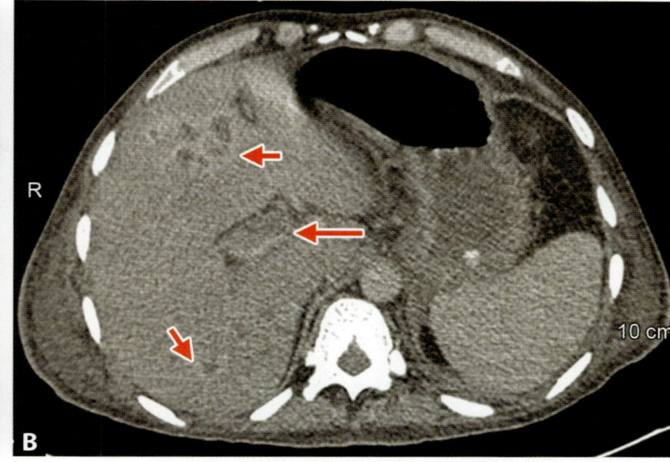

Figs 1A and B: (A and B) Axial contrast enhanced CT scans shows hypoattenuating thrombus in the intrahepatic portal vein and its left branch (large arrows) with conglomerating peripheral enhancing lesions in liver (small arrows) suggestive of abscesses.

0.9 g/dL, sugar 51 mg/dL (serum blood sugar levels being 59 mg/dL), cells 1,000/uL predominantly polymorphs and culture was sterile. Pleural fluid analysis—proteins 0.9 g/dL, sugar 59 mg/dL, cells 1,000/uL predominantly polymorphs and RBC's. Widal, peripheral blood for malarial parasite and blood culture were negative. ***Echocardiography*** done at this time showed stent in LAD, mild left ventricular systolic dysfunction, mild mitral regurgitation (MR), no pericardial effusion or vegetation and ejection fraction of 48%. ***Ultrasonography*** revealed a liver span of 13 cm, few hypoechoic lesions in left lobe, portal vein 1.1 cm and no intrahepatic biliary radical dilatation. ***Contrast-enhanced computed tomography (CECT)*** chest and abdomen showed bilateral pleural effusion (right more than left) with loculations on left side and underlying collapse/consolidation of lungs, portal vein thrombosis (intrahepatic and left branch) (Fig 1A), conglomerate abscesses in liver (segment II, IV and VI) (Fig 1B), dilated left cardiac chambers and dilated, air distended bowel loops ? Paralytic ileus. Patient developed acute respiratory failure, shock and expired. ***Final clinical diagnosis*** was— recent MI with post PCI with stent to LAD, CCF, left ventricular systolic dysfunction, liver abscess with cholangitis, shock ? septic ? cardiogenic.

AUTOPSY FINDINGS: PM 25975

A partial autopsy was performed on this 46-year-old male. The pleural cavity and peritoneal cavity yielded 600 mL and 2.5 liters of straw-colored fluid respectively. The ***heart*** weighed 380 g and right atrium, right ventricle, tricuspid valve and right outflow tract were normal. The left atrium and left ventricle were dilated. The mitral and aortic valve however were normal and the ascending aorta showed grade 1 atherosclerosis. There was a whitish firm area of fibrosis in the apical wall of the left ventricle indicating an old healed infarction, which on microscopy showed fibrosis along with hypertrophied myocytes (Figs 2A and B). Left anterior descending artery revealed a stent in situ with no luminal occlusion, left and right circumflex arteries (RCA) were 50% and 15% occluded respectively by atheromatous plaques (Fig 2C). The ***pancreas*** (Fig 3A) was firm to feel and showed areas of discoloration, with few dilated ducts and loss of normal acinar architecture. Few chalky-white deposits were also seen. Microscopic examination (Fig 3B) revealed dilatation of predominantly small to medium-sized ducts which contained inspissated secretions. Variable (in amount and distribution) degree of interlobular, intralobular and periductal fibrosis was seen with variable loss of acinar structures. Lymphomononuclear cell infiltrate was noted. Features were those of chronic pancreatitis. Over and above this, there were multiple acute neutrophilic abscesses (Fig 3C–arrows) causing extensive pancreatic destruction. An occasional abscess (Fig 3D) appeared to be arising in a dilated duct, as it also contained the remnant of the pink inspissated secretion. Areas of acute inflammation destroying the pancreatic parenchyma (Fig 4A) and fat necrosis (Fig 4B) were noted. Overall features in the pancreas were of an acute on chronic pancreatitis. The ***liver*** weighed 1,200 g. Coronal slices were bile stained, discolored and revealed multiple abscesses (Figs 5A and B) ranging in size from 0.2–5 cm. Some of the abscesses were getting confluent in

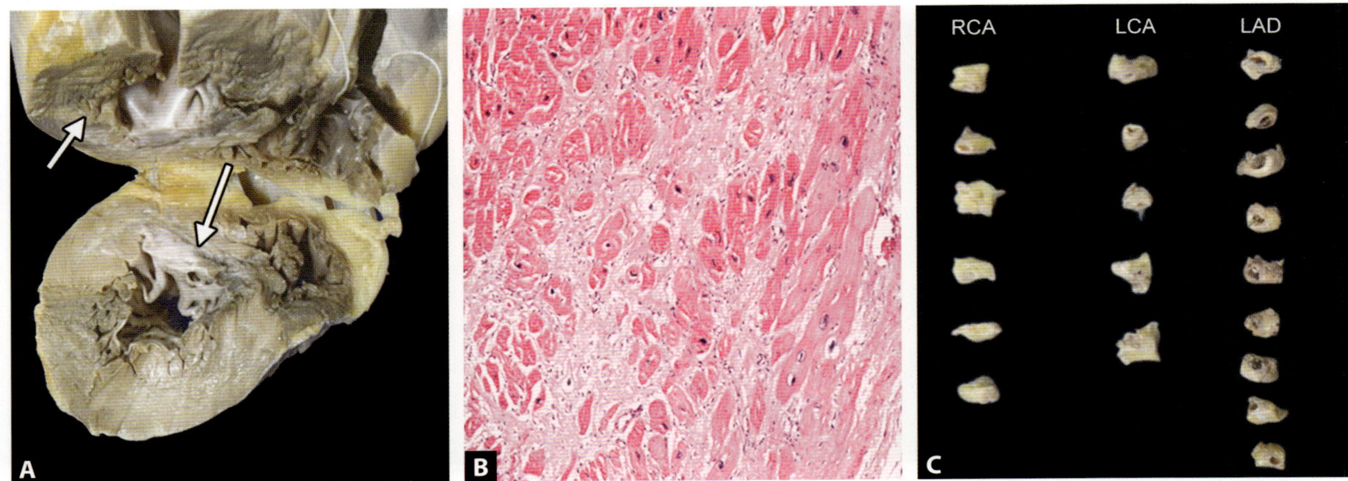

Figs 2A–C: (A) Apical slice of the heart showing whitish areas of fibrosis (arrows) indicating old infarction in the anterior wall; (B) Photomicrograph from these whitish areas in the anterior wall show areas of fibrosis and hypertrophied myocytes; (C) Serial sections of the coronaries—LAD showing stent in situ, LCA 50% and RCA 15% occlusion. (LAD: Left anterior descending; LCA: Left circumflex artery; RCA: Right circumflex artery)

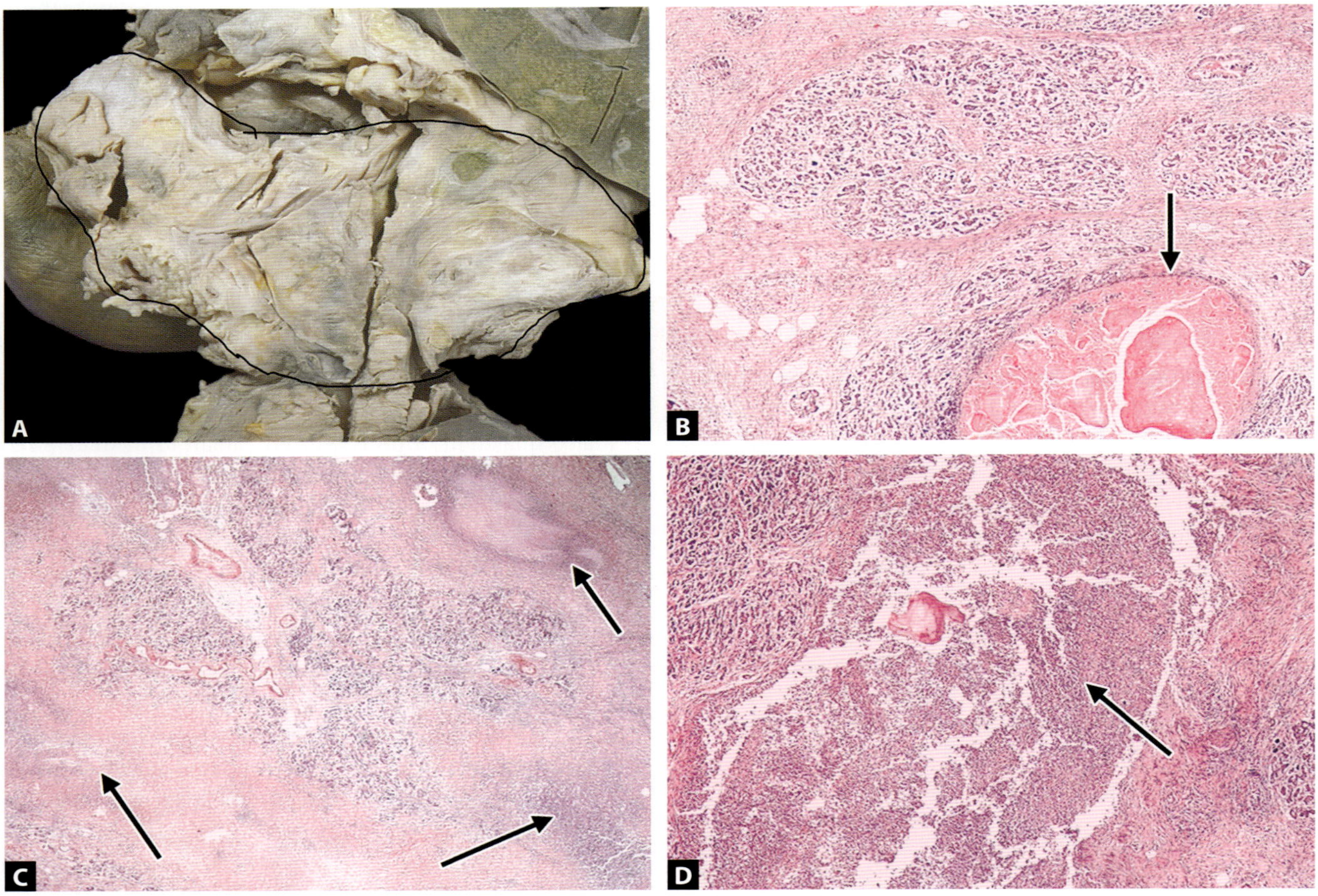

Figs 3A–D: (A) Gross photograph of the cut open pancreas (marked) which is firm in consistency with loss of the normal architecture; (B) Photomicrograph of the pancreas showing dilated ducts containing inspissated pink secretions (arrow), fibrosis, inflammation and loss of pancreatic parenchyma; (C) Multiple acute neutrophilic abscesses (arrows) amidst the pancreatic parenchyma; (D) Pancreatic abscess (arrow) containing the remnant of the pink inspissated secretion, indicating its origin from within a duct.

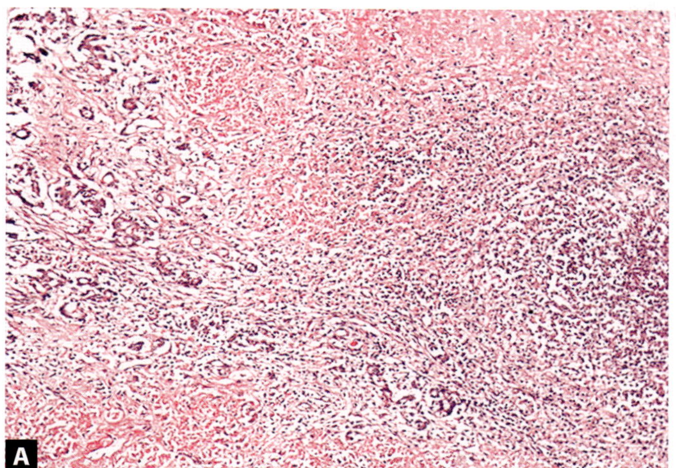
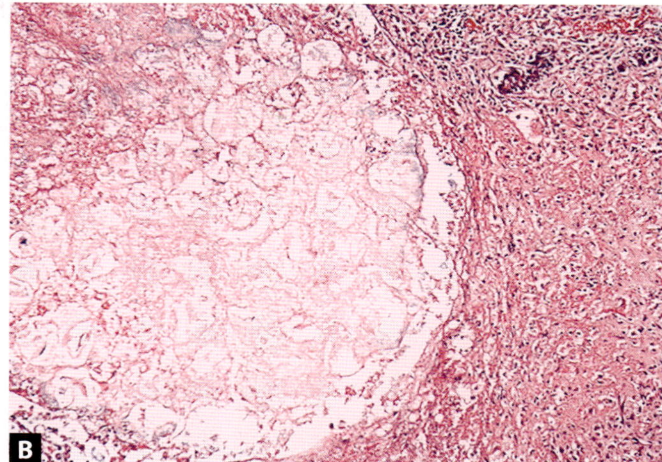

Figs 4A and B: (A) Acute inflammation causing extensive destruction of the pancreatic parenchyma; (B) Pancreas showing areas of fat necrosis with surrounding acute inflammation.

areas, forming a conglomerate mass. Few of them showed breaking down with shaggy necrotic material inside (Fig 5C). The biliary tract was dissected and was within normal limits. No stones were present in the gallbladder. The area of the confluence of portal vein contained adhesions and the vein was difficult to discern. On opening the portal vein, it contained a thrombus in the intrahepatic part and in its left branch, correlating well with the computed tomography (CT) scan. On microscopic examination the portal vein (Figs 5D and E) revealed a septic thrombus with florid acute vasculitis. The liver abscesses contained acute neutrophilic exudate with nuclear debris (Figs 6A and B). The portal tracts (Fig 6C) were expanded and portal vein branches were dilated containing septic thrombi with vasculitis. The bile ducts and hepatic artery seen in the vicinity were within normal limits. In some portal tracts, small acute abscesses were seen originating from the focus of septic thrombus in the portal vein and this transition was very well apparent (Fig 6D). The biliary tract (Figs 7A and B) at all levels (common bile duct, hepatic duct, its branches, small bile ducts in the portal tracts) did not reveal any inflammation. Gallbladder was within normal limit and no stones were identified. Florid centrizonal/perivenular necrosis was seen, indicating severe shock (Fig 7C). Periodic acid-schiff (PAS) and Gram's stain did not reveal any organism. Overall features in the liver were of multiple pyogenic liver abscesses (more in the right lobe) secondary to portal pyemia with portal vein septic thrombosis/ vasculitis and features of shock. The ***lungs*** weighed 760 g and the pleural cavities contained 600 mL of straw-colored fluid. The pleurae were puckered and cut section revealed consolidation, more on the right side and in the lower lobes (Fig 7D). No thromboembolism was noted. Microscopy revealed features of chronic passive venous congestion in the form of pulmonary edema and hemosiderin laden macrophages (Fig 7E), secondary to left ventricular systolic dysfunction and subsequent congestive cardiac failure. Apart from that bronchopneumonia was noted (Fig 7F). The ***spleen*** weighed 90 g and showed features of septicemia. The gastrointestinal tract (GIT) was studied extensively but was within normal limits.

FINAL AUTOPSY DIAGNOSIS : PM 25975

A 46 Year Old Male

- Old-healed myocardial infarction with mild left ventricular dilatation and congestive cardiac failure.
- Chronic passive venous congestion—lungs.
- Coronary artery disease—LAD—stent in situ—no abnormality detected, LCA—50% occluded, RCA—15% occluded, Grade 1 atherosclerosis.
- Acute on chronic pancreatitis with acute abscesses.
- Pylephlebitis/infective suppurative thrombosis of portal vein/portal vein pyemia.
- Multiple pyogenic liver abscesses with features of severe shock (centrizonal hemorrhagic necrosis).
- Bronchopneumonia, bilateral pleural effusion, septicemic spleen, ascites.

PYLEPHLEBITIS/PORTAL VEIN PYEMIA/ INFECTIVE SUPPURATIVE THROMBOSIS OF THE PORTAL VEIN

The term pylephlebitis,[1-5] is also known as portal vein pyemia or infective suppurative thrombosis of the portal

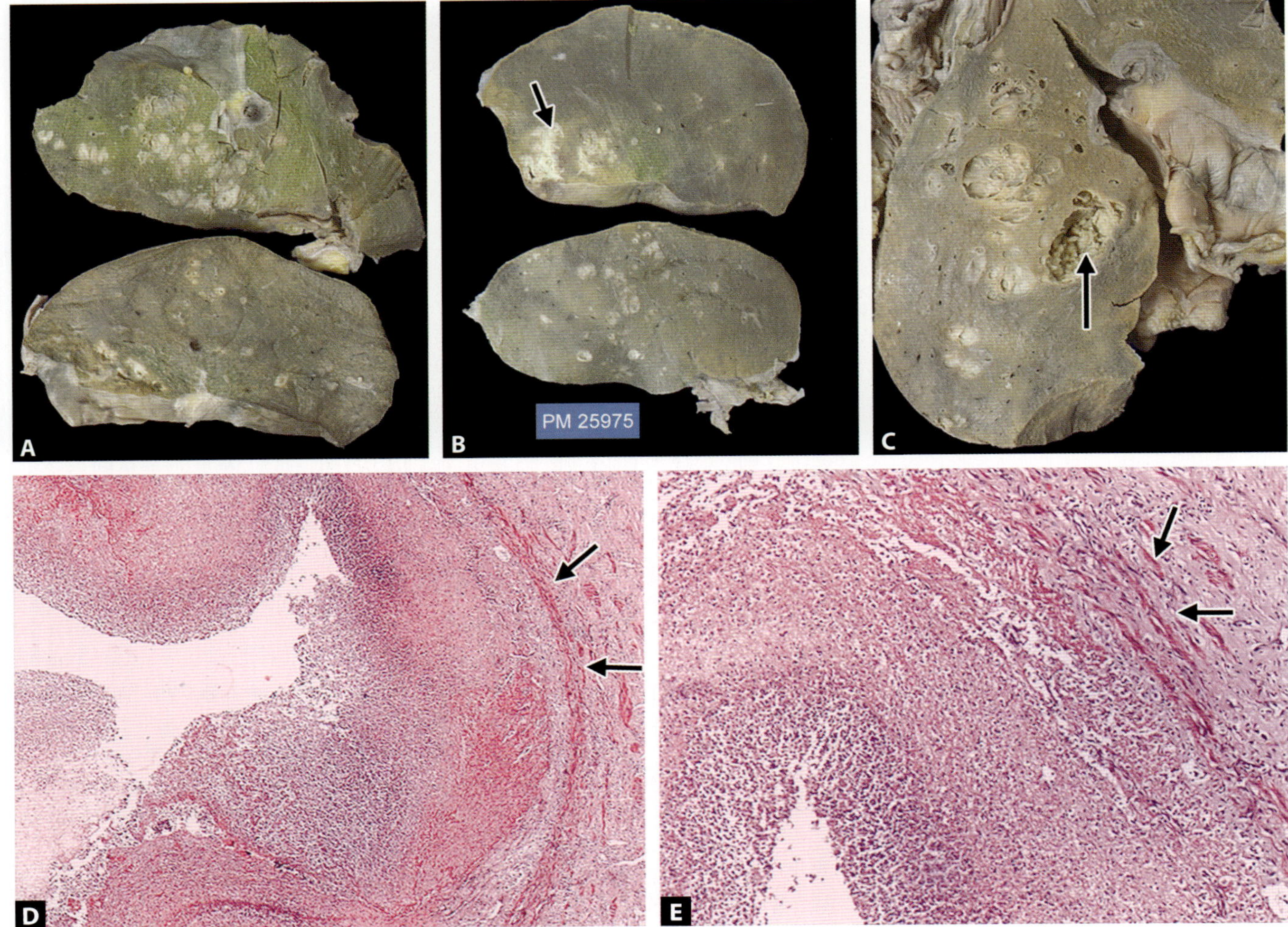

Figs 5A–E: (A–C) Coronal slices of the bile stained liver showing multiple liver abscesses getting confluent in areas and forming a conglomerate mass (arrow in B). Few abscesses show breaking down with shaggy necrotic material (arrow in C); (D and E) Photomicrograph of the portal vein shows a septic thrombus with florid acute vasculitis of the wall. Arrows indicate the wall of the portal vein.

vein or septic thrombophlebitis of the portal venous system. Secondary involvement of the branches of the portal veins may occur. It is an uncommon and life-threatening complication of intra-abdominal sepsis,[6] occurring in parts of the gastrointestinal tract, drained by the portal vein or by contiguous spread from the biliary tree.[7] It most often follows diverticulitis,[8,9] perforated appendicitis,[10-12] peritonitis, intestinal obstruction and infected acute pancreatitis.[13,14] Other causes cited in literature are contiguous infection due to cholangitis[14] or infected choledocholithiasis, cholecystitis,[13] inflammatory bowel disease (colitis and ileitis), amoebic colitis, hemorrhoidal banding, as a complication of the intragastric migration of a silicone gastric band, following a CT-guided liver biopsy, recent abdominal surgery and post flexible sigmoidoscopy.[15] An underlying hypercoagulable state[16] is often diagnosed after presentation with this condition. Amongst all causes, the most common etiology of pylephlebitis is diverticulitis followed by appendicitis, cholecystitis and infected acute pancreatitis. Plemmons et al[2] found no underlying cause in 32% cases, whereas Waxman et al[9] could not find a primary source of infection in 70% cases. The superior mesenteric and splenic veins, drains blood from the abdominal portion of the gastrointestinal tract, with the exception of the lower part of the rectum and then join to form the portal vein. The process that leads to pylephlebitis, starts as thrombophlebitis of small veins draining an area of infection, which extends into the larger veins, finally leading to septic thrombophlebitis of the portal

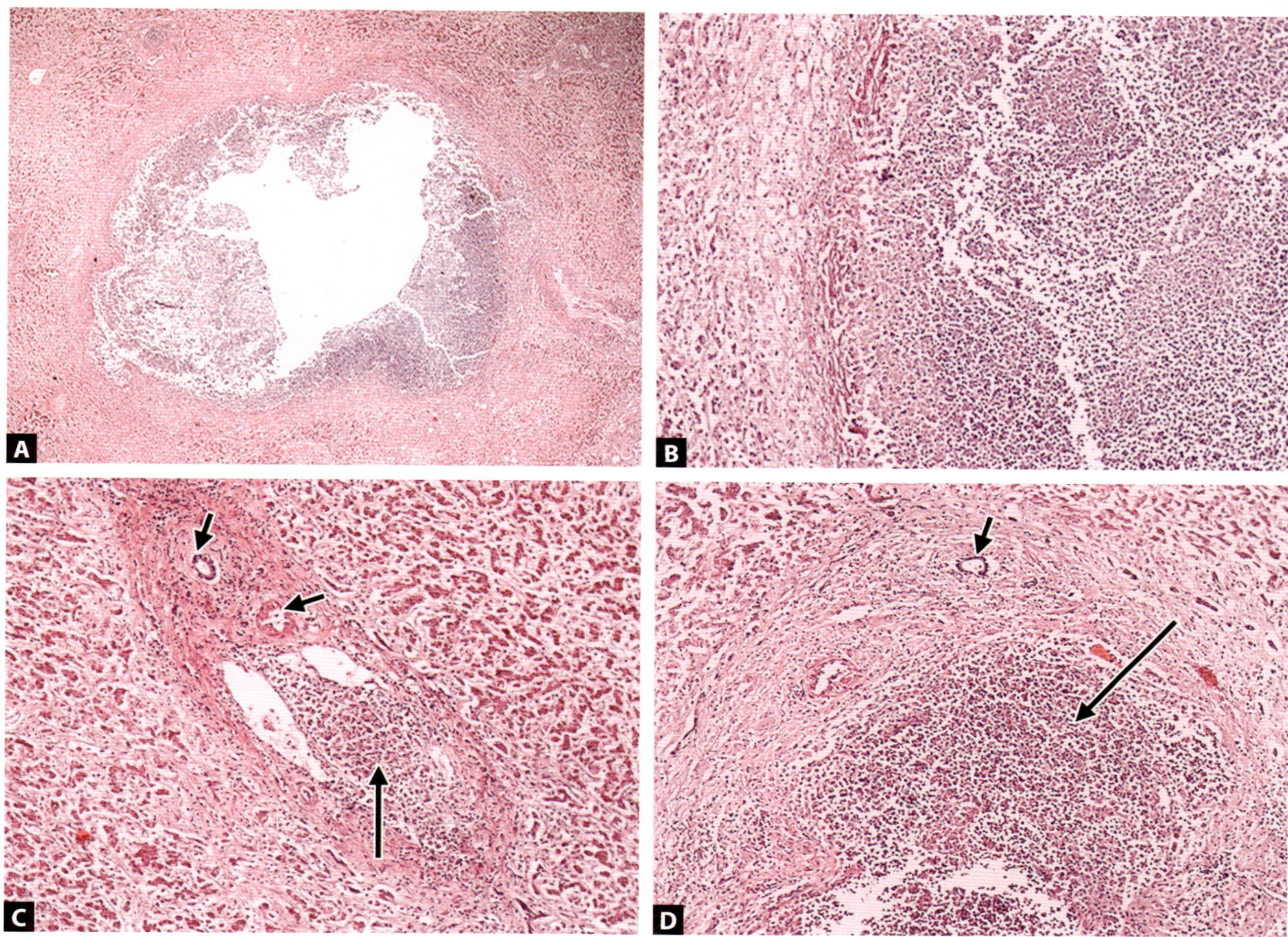

Figs 6A–D: (A and B) Low and high power view of a liver abscess containing acute neutrophilic exudate and nuclear debris; (C) Portal tract showing a septic thrombus in the portal vein (long arrow). The bile duct and the hepatic artery are seen in the vicinity and are normal (small arrows); (D) Portal tract showing a small acute abscess originating from the focus of septic thrombus in the portal vein (long arrow). The bile duct seen is normal (small arrow).

vein. The superior mesenteric vein shows thrombophlebitis in a larger number of cases (40–45%) as compared to the splenic vein (12% cases). Once pylephlebitis occurs, there is extension of the infection into the intrahepatic branches of the portal vein in 40% case. Mesenteric vein involvement can lead to bowel ischemia, infarction and death.

The symptoms of pylephlebitis are nonspecific and confusing, but a high index of suspicion clinches the diagnosis. Patients may present with an acute abdomen, with symptoms related to the primary intra-abdominal event or may be asymptomatic. It typically presents with fever accompanied with rigors/chills, signs of sepsis, leukocytosis, deranged liver function tests and upper quadrant abdominal pain, which at times may be absent. Other clinical features include malaise, fatigue, nausea, vomiting, diarrhea, anorexia and weight loss. There may be hepatomegaly and jaundice. It is a potentially fatal condition, but a timely diagnosis and aggressive treatment can save many. Complications include multiple liver abscesses,[9-11,17] infarction of the bowel due to thrombophlebitis of the superior mesenteric vein and portal hypertension. It is diagnosed by experienced radiologists[18] on modern imaging techniques like Doppler ultrasonography, CECT of the abdomen and reports of the diagnosis have increased in the last decade. Ultrasound has its limitations due to the interference with bowel gas, but may show portal vein thrombosis and the primary intra-abdominal focus. CECT is a better modality, as it can well delineate the intra-abdominal primary infection like appendicitis, diverticulitis along with the mesenteric and portal vein thrombosis, liver abscesses and bowel ischemia. Gas in the portal vein[19] can be seen

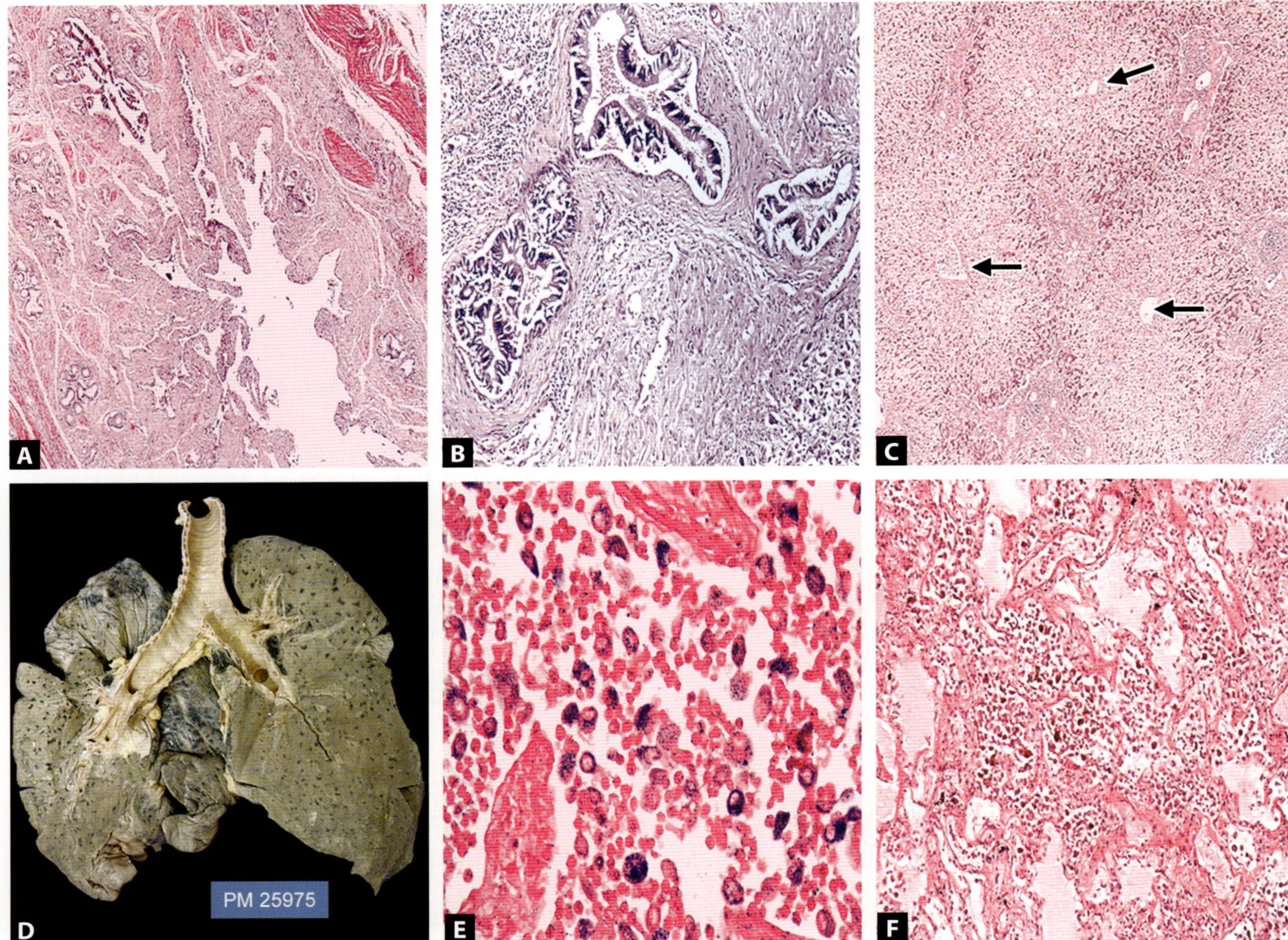

Figs 7A–F: (A) Photomicrograph from the common bile duct showing normal morphology; (B) Larger portal tracts show normal bile ducts. No inflammation is seen; (C) Liver showing extensive centrizonal/perivenular necrosis, a feature of shock. Central veins are demarcated by arrows; (D) Cut section of the lung showing consolidation, more on the right side and in the lower lobes; (E) Prussian blue stains show blue-colored hemosiderin in the macrophages—heart failure cells; (F) Alveolar spaces showing edema and polymorphs mixed with macrophages.

in fulminant abdominal sepsis or trauma and can be seen in cases of pylephlebitis. Blood cultures may be positive in 50–88% of cases and the organisms found are generally polymicrobial. Anaerobic bacteroides species top the list but *E. coli* and *Klebsiella pneumoniae* are also seen. Treatment should be immediate and very aggressive. Broad spectrum antibiotics, which cover gram-negative bacilli, anaerobes and aerobes should be started at once for duration of at least a month to prevent development of hepatic abscesses, which is a very common complication. An underlying hypercoagulable state may be present in some and hence, anticoagulants are also administered. The role of anticoagulation is debatable but it prevents extension of the thrombus, which can lead to bowel ischemia and infarction. In the study by Plemmons et al[2] and Kanellopoulo et al[20] patients who were given anticoagulation did much better. Drainage of pericolonic and large liver abscesses can be done to resolve the focus of infection. Mortality is very high, ranging between 30% and 80% and it is due to severe sepsis, secondary to the overwhelming intra-abdominal infection. Many cases are however diagnosed postmortem. In the present era, with the awareness of this condition, new imaging modalities, better expertise, aggressive antibiotic therapy and administration of anticoagulation, the mortality has come down to 20–30% in most places. Pylephlebitis has to be differentiated from the bland portal vein thrombus, which is more common than pylephlebitis and is managed in a different way.

PYOGENIC LIVER ABSCESS

In pyogenic liver abscess, the infection may reach the liver through the biliary tract, portal vein, hepatic artery or by direct extension. The commonest portal of entry is the ***biliary tract*** and this mode of entry is seen in 30–50% of the cases. The end result is cholangitis which leads to multiple liver abscesses. The various causes include choledocholithiasis, strictures (benign or malignant) and various interventions like endoscopic retrograde cholangiopancreatography (ERCP) or percutaneous transhepatic procedures. Infection via the ***portal vein*** (i.e. pylephlebitis/portal vein pyemia) is a common route of entry, but is now less common in the industrialized countries. The source of sepsis is generally intra-abdominal infection due to diverticulitis, appendicitis, peritonitis and infected acute pancreatitis. This leads to septic portal thrombophlebitis leading to the formation of multiple pyogenic hepatic abscesses. Septicemia from any cause may disseminate via the ***hepatic artery***, giving rise to multiple liver abscesses. ***Direct extension*** of infection leading to liver abscesses can occur due to liver trauma or empyema of the gallbladder. However, in a large percentage of cases the cause cannot be ascertained. The presenting sign and symptoms include fever, loss of appetite, weakness and enlarged/tender liver and pleural effusion may be present. At times patients present with features of septic shock. Diagnosis is clinched by ultrasonography and CT scan of the abdomen which determine the size, characteristics, number and anatomical location of the liver abscesses. A chest X-ray may show an elevated diaphragm or a pleural effusion. Further tests such as an ERCP or a colonoscopy can determine the source of infection.

COMMENTARY—INDEX CASE: PM 25975

This 46-year-old male was diagnosed with anterior wall MI and a stent was placed in LAD artery. Two weeks later, he was readmitted with congestive cardiac failure, ejection fraction of 35–40%, with moderate left ventricular systolic dysfunction. There was some source of infection at this point of time, as the TLC was high with polymorphonuclear leukocytosis. He improved on antibiotics and was discharged. But within a week he became febrile again. Five weeks later, he was readmitted with high grade fever and breathlessness. The abdomen was tense, distended and shifting dullness was elicited. There was anemia and polymorphonuclear leukocytosis. CECT showed bilateral pleural effusion (right more than left) with consolidation of lungs, conglomerate abscesses in liver, portal vein thrombosis, dilated left cardiac chambers and dilated, air distended bowel loops ? paralytic ileus. Echocardiography done at this time revealed a better cardiac status with ejection fraction of 48% and only a mild left ventricular systolic dysfunction. But despite all measures the patient succumbed to his illness. Autopsy revealed no abnormality in the stent or any fresh myocardial infarction. There was acute on chronic pancreatitis with pancreatic abscesses leading to pylephlebitis/infective suppurative thrombosis of portal vein/portal vein pyemia which further led on to multiple pyogenic liver abscesses.

The patient was an alcoholic and an undiagnosed case of chronic pancreatitis that was elicited at autopsy. So two-week post-PCI, he developed acute infection which initially subsided with antibiotics and reerupted within a week, when he became febrile again. This was the setting of an acute on chronic pancreatitis, which later erupted into a full-blown acute pancreatitis with acute abscesses, which led on to pylephlebitis. Pylephlebitis is life-threatening and in the index case it went on to produce multiple varying sized pyogenic liver abscesses. The small portal veins in the portal tracts contained septic thrombi and small abscesses could be seen originating from them, enlarging and forming large abscesses. The gallbladder did not reveal any stones. The entire biliary tract, from the common bile ducts till the small bile ducts in the portal tracts did not show any inflammation, indicating that the biliary tract was not the cause of pyogenic liver abscesses in this case. There was no source of infection in the GIT as well, which could have contributed to the portal pyemia.

TAKE HOME MESSAGE

- Pylephlebitis, also known as portal vein pyemia or infective suppurative thrombosis of the portal vein or septic thrombophlebitis of the portal venous system is an uncommon life-threatening complication of intra-abdominal sepsis.
- It most often follows diverticulitis, perforated appendicitis, peritonitis, intestinal obstruction and infected acute pancreatitis.
- The symptoms of pylephlebitis are nonspecific and confusing, but a high index of suspicion and modern imaging techniques, clinch the diagnosis.
- Complications of pylephlebitis include multiple liver abscesses, infarction of the bowel due to thrombophlebitis of the superior mesenteric vein and portal hypertension.
- Blood cultures may be positive in 50–88% of cases and the organisms found are generally polymicrobial.

- The underlying cause of pylephlebitis may remain unknown in 30–50% of cases.
- In pyogenic liver abscess, the infection may reach the liver through the biliary tract, portal vein, hepatic artery or by direct extension.

REFERENCES

1. Wireko M, Berry PA, Brennan J, et al. Unrecognized pylephlebitis causing life-threatening septic shock: a case report. World J Gastroenterol. 2005;11(4):614-5.
2. Plemmons RM, Dooley DP, Longfield RN. Septic thrombophlebitis of the portal vein (pylephlebitis): diagnosis and management in the modern era. Clin Infect Dis. 1995;21(5):1114-20.
3. Case records of the Massachusetts General Hospital. Weekly clinicopathological exercises. Case 18-1977. N Engl J Med. 1977:296(18):1051-7.
4. Kasper DL, Sahani D, Misdraji J. Case records of the Massachusetts General Hospital. Case 25-2005. A 40-year-old man with prolonged fever and weight loss. N Engl J Med. 2005;353(7):713.
5. Saxena R, Adolph M, Zeigler JR, et al. Pylephlebitis: a case report and review of outcome in the antibiotic era. Am J Gastroenterol. 1996;91(6):1251-3.
6. Wong K, Weisman DS, Patrice KA. Pylephlebitis: a rare complication of an intra-abdominal infection. J Community Hosp Inter Med Perspect; 2013. [Online] Available from http//.dx.doi.org/10.3402/jchimp.v3i2.20732. [Accessed on April, 2018]
7. García-Gutiérrez M, Luque-Márquez R, Rodríguez-Suárez S. Portal vein thrombosis associated with biliary tract infection. Gastroenterol Hepatol. 2012;35(9):644-8.
8. Al Hajjar N, Crişan D, Grigorescu M, et al. Acute diverticulitis—an unusual cause of liver abscesses in a young man: a case report. Chirurgia (Bucur). 2012;107(2):267-72.
9. Waxman BP, Carvanagh LL, Nayman J. Suppurative pylephlebitis and multiple hepatic abscesses with silent colonic diverticulitis. Med J Aust. 1979:2(7):376-8.
10. Chang TN, Tang L, Keller K, et al. Pylephlebitis, portal-mesenteric thrombosis and multiple liver abscesses owing to perforated appendicitis. J Pediatr Surg. 2001;36(9):E19.
11. Márová K, Chochola M, Golán L, et al. Liver abscesses with portal and mesenteric vein thrombosis in combination with late onset of appendicitis. Cas Lek Cesk. 2005;144(7): 489-93.
12. Castro R, Fermamdes T, Oliveira MI, Castro Miguel. Acute appendicitis complicated by pylephlebitis: A case report. Case reports in Radiology; 2013. [Online] Available from http://dx.doi.org/10.1155/2013/627521. [Accessed on April, 2018].
13. El-Wahsh M. A case of portal vein thrombosis associated with acute cholecystitis/pancreatitis or coincidence. Hepatobiliary Pancreat Dis Int. 2006;5(2):308-10.
14. Cheung DY, Kim JK, Jo DH, et al. A case of portal vein thrombosis associated with acute pancreatitis and cholangitis. Korean J Gastroenterol. 2005;46(1):60-5.
15. Patel RT, Deen KI, Fielding JW. Portal pyemia following flexible sigmoidoscopy. Br Jour Surg. 1994;81(9):1337.
16. Baril N, Wren S, Radin R, et al. The role of anticoagulation in pylephlebitis. Am J Surg. 1996;172(5):449-52.
17. Hoffman HL, Partington PF, DeSanctis AL. Pylephlebitis and liver abscess Am J Surg 1954;88(3):411-6.
18. Harch JM, Radin RD, Yellin AE, et al. Pylethrombosis: serendipitous radiologic diagnosis. Arch Surg. 1987;122(10): 1116-9.
19. Kluge S, Hahn KE, Lund CH, et al. Pylephlebitis (septic thrombophlebitis of the portal vein) with portal venous gas: an unusual focus of infection in a patient with septic shock. Dtsch Med Wochenschr. 2003;128(25-26):1391-4.
20. Kanellopoulou T, Alexopoulou A, Theodossiades G, et al. Pylephlebitis: an overview of non-cirrohotic cases and factors related to outcome. Scand J Infect Dis. 2010;42(11-12): 804-11.

CONTRIBUTIONS BY:

1. Dr Navneet Sharma, Professor, Department of Internal Medicine (Compilation of Clinical Details)
2. Dr Manphool Singhal, Additional Professor, Department of Radiodiagnosis and Imaging (Contributing Figs 1A and B)
3. Dr SK Jindal, Ex-Professor and Head, Department of Pulmonary Medicine (Clinician In-Charge)

Post Graduate Institute of Medical Education and Research, Chandigarh, India.

CASE 23

Lipomatous Pseudohypertrophy of the Pancreas with Polyglandular Autoimmune Syndrome Type II and Inflammatory Myopathy: PM 22590

Nandita Bharadwaj Kakkar

HIGHLIGHTS OF THE CASE

A 53-year-old, postmenopausal female came with a 4-months history of watery diarrhea, anasarca, weight loss, weakness in both limbs and progressively increasing breathlessness. She was diabetic since one year. Investigations revealed anemia, marked hypoproteinemia/hypoalbuminemia, hypothyroidism and obstructive jaundice. The clinical diagnosis given was, chronic diarrhea with severe malabsorption, protein losing enteropathy, anemia ? Celiac disease ? Immunoproliferative small intestinal disease (IPSID) ? GI lymphoma with hypothyroidism. Autopsy revealed lipomatous pseudohypertrophy of the pancreas with stigmata of chronic calcific pancreatitis, cholestasis, lymphocytic thyroiditis and adrenalitis—polyglandular autoimmune syndrome type II, inflammatory myopathy, isolated splenic tuberculosis, bronchopneumonia, pulmonary edema and aspiration.

Keywords: Lipomatous pseudohypertrophy, pancreas, neoplasm, pseudotumor, calcific pancreatitis, polyglandular, autoimmune syndrome, autopsy.

CLINICAL DETAILS

Date of Admission: 29.04.2008, Date of Death: 10.05.2008 and Duration of Hospital Stay: 7 days

A 53-year-old-female presented with diarrhea of 4-months duration along with anasarca, progressively increasing breathlessness, fatigue and weakness in both limbs since 2 months. The frequency of stools was 8–10 times/day with presence of nocturnal diarrhea. The stools were large in volume, semisolid to watery, not associated with blood/mucus/foul-smell and contained undigested food. They however decreased in frequency as well as amount with fasting. There was history of passage of undigested food and occasional non-bilious vomiting, not associated with abdominal pain at any time. There was no history of decreased urine output or jaundice. The patient also complained of gradually increasing weakness in both the limbs with difficulty in getting up from squatting position, as well as difficulty in climbing stairs. There were no sensory symptoms. The patient had progressively increasing breathlessness of 2-months duration with history of orthopnea, but no history of chest pain/palpitation/cough/fever or paroxysmal nocturnal dyspnea. She had also noticed a pruritic rash over left elbow and on both the lower limbs for the last 15 days. There was anorexia and history of loss of weight, her current weight being 32 kg. Twelve-years back she had diarrhea of similar nature and was diagnosed as a case of hyperthyroidism. Antithyroid drug, neo-mercazole was started and she improved, but then left the treatment on her own. She also had a similar episode of diarrhea 4-years back and that was accompanied with swelling of the body. She was treated by a local practitioner, the swelling subsided, but the treatment records were not available. A year ago she developed diabetes mellitus and was on treatment. She was postmenopausal, homemaker by profession and a vegetarian, with no addictions. On ***examination*** she was conscious, oriented and short-statured. There was pallor, pedal edema and alopecia. The pulse was 100 beats/min regular and the BP (100/70 mm Hg) was on the lower side. There was no lymphadenopathy, goiter and the jugular venous pressure (JVP) was not raised. There was no hepatosplenomegaly, ascites and per rectal examination was normal. Both plantars were down going, power in upper limbs was 4/5 and in the lower limbs was 2/5, weakness being more in the proximal muscles. The cubital and popliteal fossa showed ill-defined erythema with brownish scaling and few erosion. Xerosis was present on lower back with minimal scaling. Skin lesions were suggestive of tinea incognita.

Investigations

Hematological: Hb- 8.2 g/dL; TLC- 10,500/uL; Platelets-72000/uL; ESR (1st hour) - 52 mm; PTI 86%.

Biochemistry/Microbiology: Total serum bilirubin/conjugated fraction- 2.9/1.8 mg%; SGOT/SGPT—64/47 U/L; alkaline phosphatase 56 U/L; total serum proteins/albumin/globulin—3.7/2/1.7 gm; random blood sugar 71 mg%; Lipid profile: cholesterol 43 mg%, LDL-C 1.0, HDL-C 0.3, triglycerides 90 mg/dl; Thyroid function tests: free T3 0.88 pg/ml (low) free T4- 0.51 ng/dL (low); T3: 0.29 (N: 0.7-2), T4: 133.6 (N), TSH: 4.10 (N: 0.17-4.05); Sudan III stain for decalcified fat was greater than 200 globules/HPF with largest globule greater than 40 μ in size; Stool—C difficile toxin present; CRP—positive; IgA tTG: negative; Blood culture: Sterile; Urine albumin: traces; 24 hours urinary proteins: 90 mg; Urine C/S: Growth of E coli; Abdominal fat pad: negative for amyloid; Stool R/E: no ova or cyst or atypical organisms, pus cells and mucus present, no fungus; HIV serology: negative; Mantoux test: Negative .

Radiology: Chest X ray (admission): Left pleural effusion. One week later - No evidence of pleural effusion; ***USG Abdomen***: Normal study for abdomen, moderate left pleural effusion; ***Compression USG B/L lower limbs***: No evidence of deep vein thrombosis;

Others: ***ECG***: Sinus tachycardia, low voltage; ***2-D ECHO***-coronary artery disease, regional wall motion abnormality in left anterior descending artery territory, ejection fraction 47%, moderate LV systolic dysfunction, mild pericardial effusion and mild mitral regurgitation; ***Upper GI Endoscopy***: normal esophagus, atrophic mucosa in stomach and duodenum, duodenal folds decreased in height and number; **Duodenal biopsy** - chronic nonspecific inflammation.

Units Clinical Diagnosis: Chronic diarrhea with severe malabsorption, protein losing enteropathy, anemia, ? celiac disease ? IPSID ? GI lymphoma, hypothyroidism, disseminated tinea infection, coronary artery disease, Type 1 respiratory failure, Cause of death - cardiac arrhythmia.

AUTOPSY FINDINGS: PM 22590

A partial autopsy was performed. The pleural and peritoneal cavities contained 500 mL and 900 mL of straw-colored fluid respectively. The antemortem duodenal biopsy (5785/08) revealed no evidence of celiac disease or amyloid. Grossly, the ***pancreas*** weighed 240 g, was enlarged, lipomatous, but maintained its basic shape (Fig 1A). On cut section, it was totally lipomatous with dilated ducts containing concretions (Figs 1B and C). On microscopic examination (Figs 1D, 2A and B), the exocrine pancreas was totally wiped-out and replaced by mature fat, which contained isolated clusters of Islets of Langerhan's. An occasional cluster of acini (Figs 2C and D) devoid of secretary granules was seen and few clusters of acini could be seen around the dilated ducts. Focal areas of lymphocytic infiltration (Fig 2E) were also noted, destroying the pancreatic acini. The ducts were dilated and contained concretions, metaplastic lining at places, subepithelial mucous glands and fibrosis (Fig 2F). Overall features were those of lipomatous pseudohypertrophy of the pancreas with stigmata of chronic calcific pancreatitis. The ***liver*** (Fig 3A) weighed 1,100 g, cut section was bile stained with a nutmeg appearance. On microscopic examination there was a lymphomononuclear infiltrate in the portal tracts and prominent canalicular cholestasis (Fig 3B). The ***thyroid*** gland was atrophic and microscopic examination showed a florid lymphocytic thyroiditis with marked destruction of the thyroid follicles by lymphocytes (Figs 4A–C). ***Adrenal glands*** revealed a picture of lymphocytic adrenalitis (Fig 4D). ***Skeletal muscle*** (Figs 5A–D) revealed a picture of a florid inflammatory myopathy with dense lymphocytic infiltrate, degeneration, regeneration of muscle fibers, muscle infarct, presence of plenty of myoblasts, basophilia of the sarcoplasm, perifascicular atrophy, endothelial prominence in blood vessels and hemorrhage. The ***spleen*** (Fig 6A) weighed 50 g and cut section showed tiny, white, millet-sized lesions (0.1–0.5 cm). Microscopy revealed multiple epithelioid cell granulomas with caseation necrosis and Langhans type of giant cells (Fig 6B). Stain for acid-fast bacillus (AFB) was negative. The ***lungs*** together weighed 950 g, pleura were dull and areas of consolidation were noted. Microscopy revealed a confluent pneumonia (Fig 6C), edema, aspiration and bone marrow emboli. Aorta revealed grade 2 atherosclerosis. Left anterior descending artery was 20% occluded by an atheromatous plaque. The heart, kidneys, GIT and bone marrow did not reveal any abnormality.

FINAL AUTOPSY DIAGNOSIS: PM 22590

53 Years Female

- Lipomatous pseudohypertrophy (diffuse) of the pancreas with stigmata of chronic calcific pancreatitis.
- Cholestasis
- Lymphocytic thyroiditis and adrenalitis—Polyglandular autoimmune syndrome type II
- Inflammatory myopathy
- Isolated tuberculosis of the spleen
- Bronchopneumonia, pulmonary edema, aspiration—lungs
- Atherosclerosis — grade 2
- Pleural effusion and ascites.

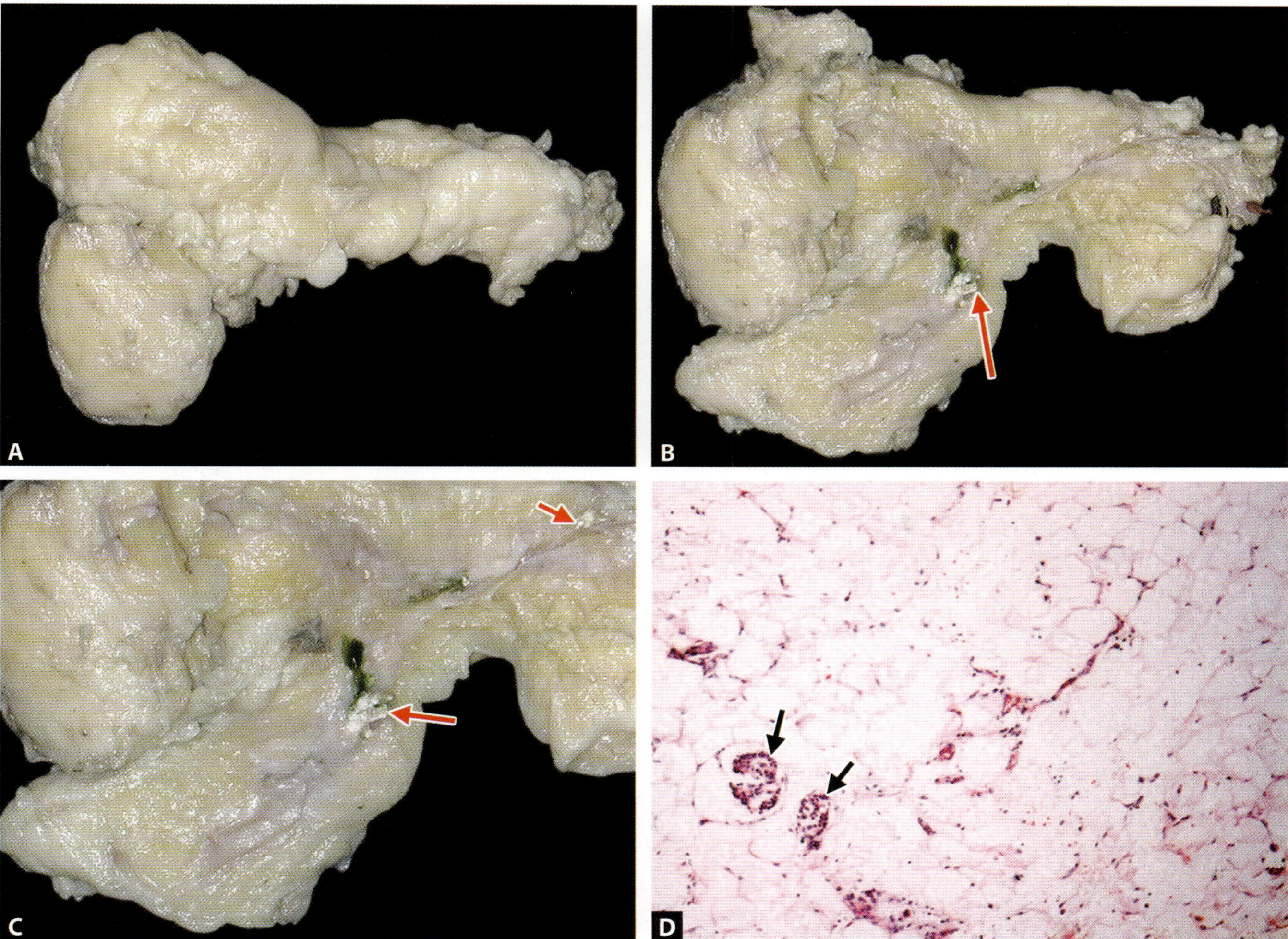

Figs 1A–D: (A) Pancreas is enlarged, lipomatous and maintains its basic shape; (B and C) Cut section of the pancreas is totally lipomatous, no pancreatic tissue is identified, ducts are dilated and contain concretions (arrows); (D) Microscopic section of the pancreas shows total replacement of the acinar tissue by mature adipose tissue. A few islets are however seen (arrows).

LIPOMATOUS PSEUDOHYPERTROPHY OF THE PANCREAS

Lipomatous pseudohypertrophy of the pancreas[1-2] is a rare (only case reports available in literature) and a distinct clinico-pathologic entity. It was first reported in 1931 by Hantelmann.[3] It shows a localized or diffuse fat replacement of acinar pancreas with preservation of the pancreatic ducts and endocrine islets. The exocrine pancreas[4,5] can commonly show focal replacement with mature fat and this correlates with diabetes mellitus, pancreatitis and the basal metabolic index (BMI). The term lipomatous pseudohypertrophy is applied to those cases where there is a tumor-like formation by mature fat, which replaces the acinar pancreas. This pseudotumor clinically mimics pancreatic carcinoma[6] and should be kept in the differential diagnosis while evaluating patients with a hypodense pancreatic neoplasm on imaging. Since pancreatic biopsy is cumbersome and challenging, this entity can be diagnosed by typical imaging findings, for which awareness of this entity is the key to success. Although the etiology and pathogenesis of lipomatous pseudohypertrophy is still unclear, literature suggests that this condition is associated with chronic hepatitis B[7] or other advanced chronic hepatic lesions.[8] This entity has been seen in association with Hashimoto's disease,[2] chronic pancreatitis, biliary strictures, Shwachman-Diamond,[9] Bannayan,[10] and Blizzard-Johanson[11] syndromes and in juvenile Parkinson's disease.[12] It can be a cause of a new-onset upper abdominal pain. It is incidentally detected. The tumor is often large, can attain a large size

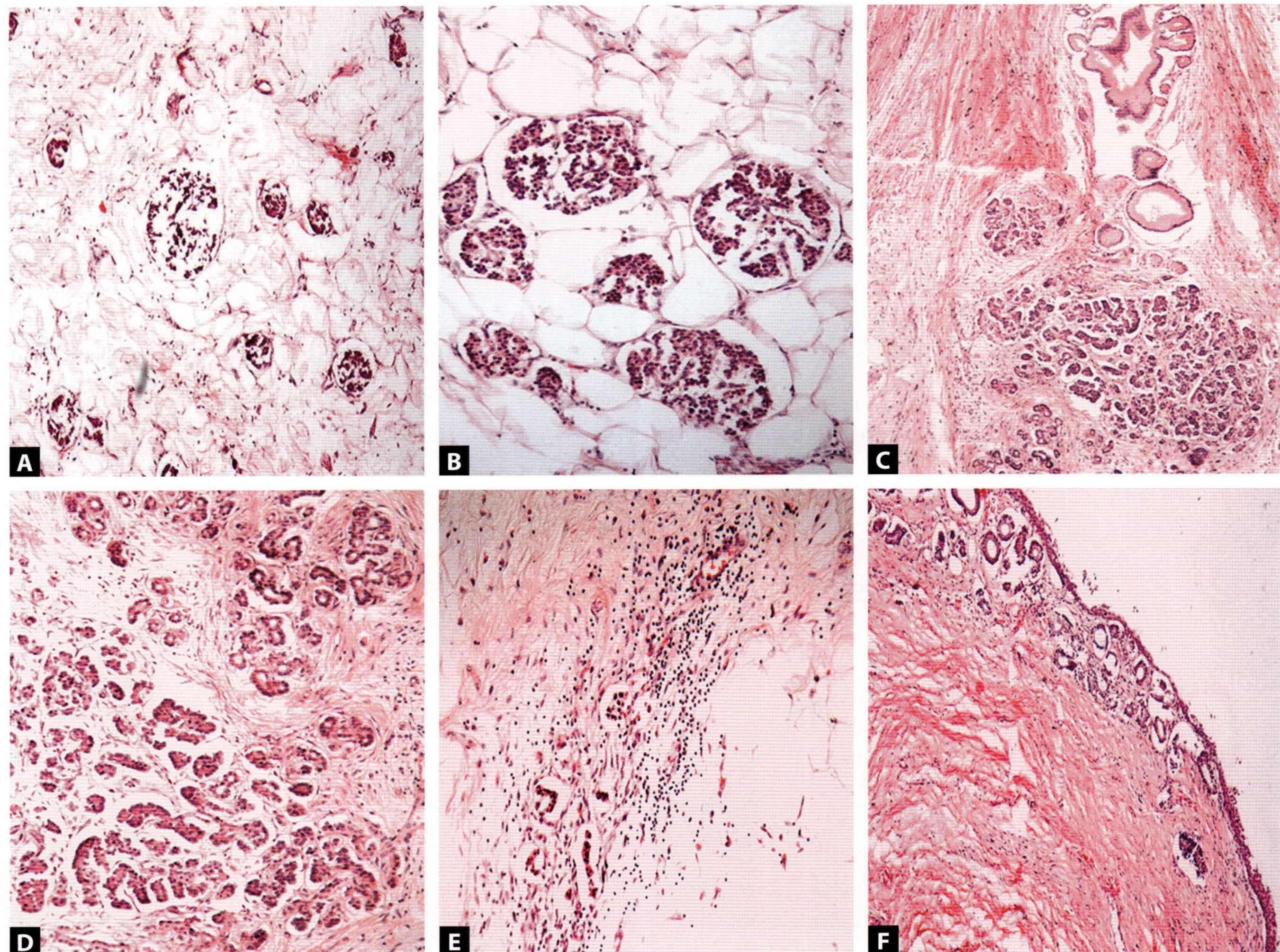

Figs 2A–F: Photomicrographs of the pancreas (A and B) High power of the preserved islets amidst the adipose tissue; (C and D) Occasional focus of acini around ducts. The acinar cells are devoid of secretory granules; (E) Focal area of lymphocytic infiltration; (F) Dilated duct with sub-epithelial mucous glands and fibrosis.

uptill about 24 cms and since it forms a mass, it is often mistaken for a malignancy. Endoscopic ultrasound guided, FNA biopsy showing mature fat cells.

On gross examination, LPH shows a diffuse or localized involvement. Diffuse involvement occurs in 70% cases where in the entire pancreas is enlarged, lipomatous, but maintains its basic shape. In localized involvement, well-circumscribed masses can be found predominantly in the head, but can also be seen in the body and tail. On microscopic examination the pancreatic acinar tissue is replaced by mature adipose tissue, leaving only scattered clusters of Islets of Langerhan's and ducts. An occasional cluster of pancreatic acini devoid of secretary granules can be seen. Stigmata of burnt out chronic pancreatitis can be appreciated at times. Differential diagnosis includes a well-differentiated liposarcoma, but awareness of this entity, absence of lipoblasts, presence of mature adipose tissue, sharp demarcation of the lesion and presence of normal pancreatic parenchyma within the lesion clinches the diagnosis. The pathogenesis of this entity is uncertain and various plausible causes like viral infection and an abnormal metabolism have been postulated in the literature. It appears to be an acquired condition possibly due to injury by infective or toxic agents. Some authors say that it possibly occurs due to duct obstruction leading to secondary parenchymal damage and subsequent replacement by mature fat. LPH could be a form of a lipoma, has been suggested[7], but since there is extensive fat replacement with preservation of the shape, this is less likely. The distribution

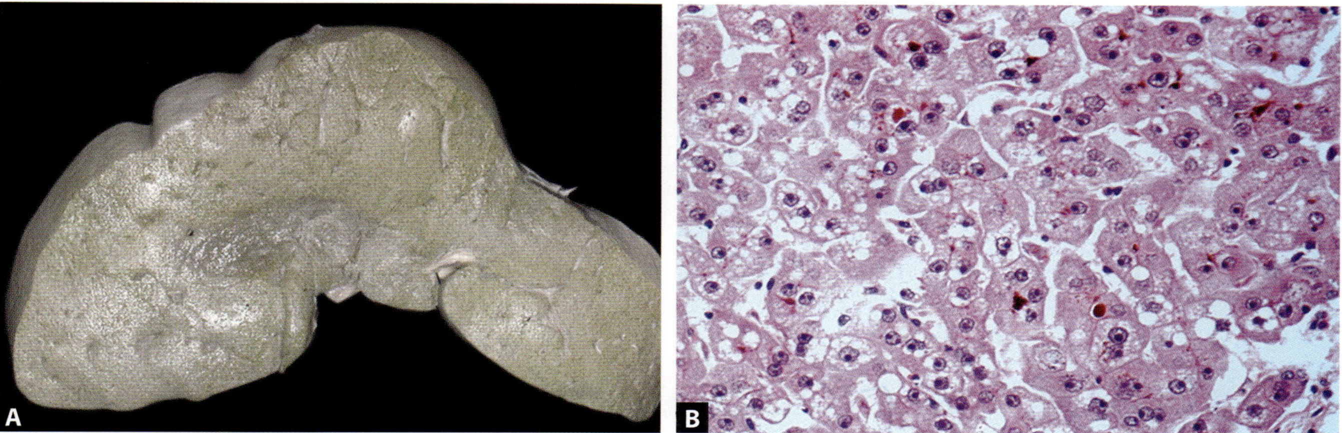

Figs 3A and B: (A) Slice of the bile stained liver; (B) Liver showing prominent canalicular cholestasis.

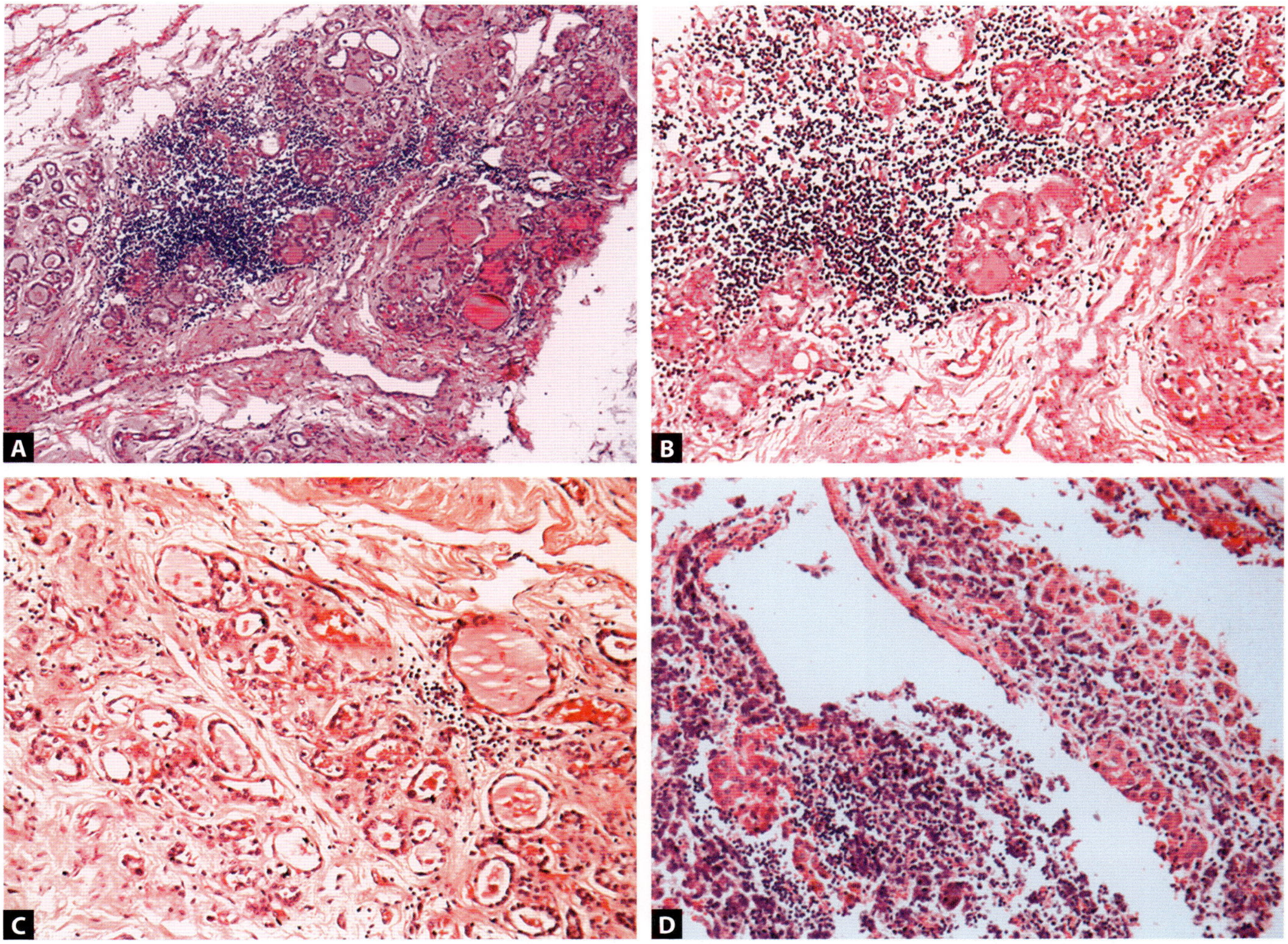

Figs 4A–D: (A–C) Thyroid showing florid lymphocytic thyroiditis with marked destruction of the thyroid follicles; (D) Lymphocytic infiltration in the adrenal gland.

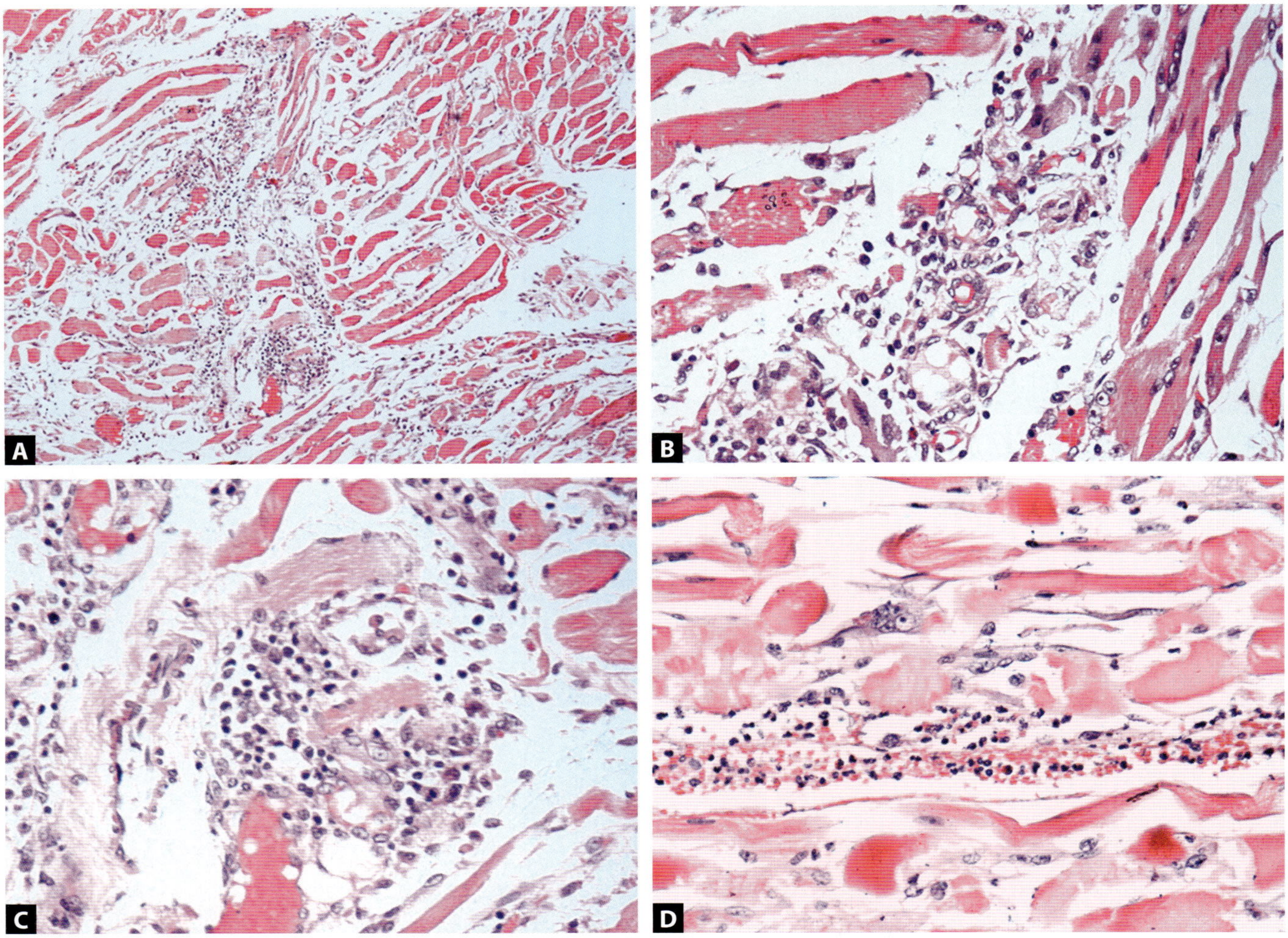

Figs 5A–D: (A–C) Skeletal muscle showing dense lymphocytic infiltrate, degeneration, regeneration of muscle fibers; (D) Muscle shows presence of plenty of myoblasts and perifascicular atrophy.

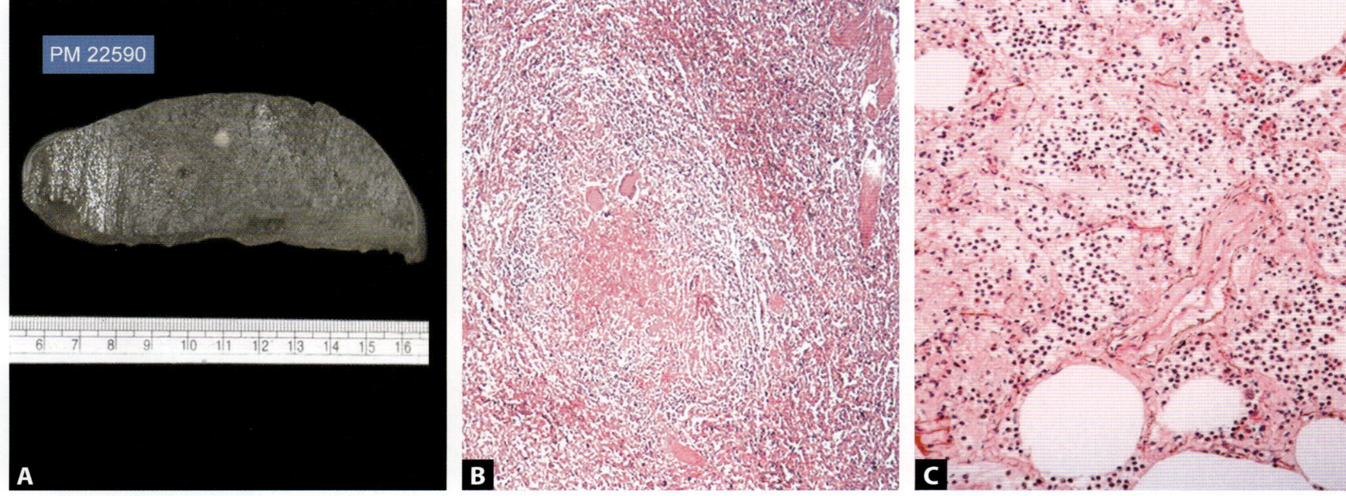

Figs 6A–C: (A) Cut section of the spleen showing a tiny 0.4 mm white nodule and many 0.1 mm white specks; (B) Caseating epithelioid cell granuloma with Langerhan's giant cells; (C) Section of the lung showing bronchopneumonia.

of pancreatic islets within the lesion indicates that it is not an entrapment, but an integral part of the process. Viruses and certain toxic agents like ethionine have been used in experimental animals and can produce replacement by fat, without any inflammation, just like what is seen in LPH of the pancreas in humans.[13] The differential diagnosis of LPH, it is necessary to rule out obesity, diabetes, age-related pancreatic fat infiltration and liposarcoma. Henkinbrant et al[14] reported a case of pseudo-hypertrophy of the pancreas, in a 70-year-old male, with malabsorption and type 2 diabetes, wherein compression of the main bile duct by the enlarged lipomatous pancreas, demonstrated by percutaneous cholangiography, caused a cholestatic jaundice. Altinal et al[15] reported five cases of LPH (3 focal and 2 diffuse) of the pancreas, who underwent a major surgery due to a preoperative diagnosis of ductal adenocarcinoma on radiology.

Thus, LPH is a distinct clinico-pathologic entity, of undetermined etiology and pathogenesis. It mimics a carcinoma and awareness is the key to success in making a diagnosis on radiology. It can also present as new onset pain abdomen, incidental finding at ultrasound, with exocrine insufficiency and as obstructive jaundice. Making a correct diagnosis is mandatory to avoid unnecessary surgery and subsequent morbidity.

POLYGLANDULAR AUTOIMMUNE SYNDROME[16-19]

Autoimmune polyglandular syndrome type II i.e. Schmidt syndrome is one of the most common immunoendocrinopathies. It constitutes a combination of a number of autoimmune disorders like Addison's disease and those affecting the thyroid gland and/or type 1 diabetes mellitus. Celiac disease, hypopituitarism, hypogonadism and myasthenia gravis may occur along with. Other associated disorders which can be seen are seronegative arthritis, idiopathic thrombocytopenic purpura, vitiligo, parkinson's disease and alopecia. Addison's disease with Hashimoto's thyroiditis is the commonest combination and Addison's disease/Graves' disease/type 1 diabetes mellitus the least common. The complete triglandular syndrome is sometimes referred to as Carpenter syndrome. Thyroid involvement can be seen in the form of hypothyroidism (lymphocytic/Hashimoto's thyroiditis) or as hyperthyroidism (Graves' disease). The clinical manifestations are not always simultaneous and one may follow the other. This syndrome occurs in middle-aged women in the third and fourth decades of life. It is associated with HLA-DR3 and/or HLA-DR4 haplotypes and the pattern of inheritance is autosomal dominant with variable expressivity. A genetic susceptibility probably causes an autoimmune trigger, leading to production of organ specific autoantibodies causing an ongoing destruction of the glands. The patient may still be asymptomatic to begin with and later land-up with overt disease. The affected organ demonstrates a lymphocytic infiltrate, leading to partial or complete destruction. Diagnosis is made by estimation of hormone levels and autoantibodies against affected endocrine glands. Treatment includes replacement of deficient hormones and immunosuppressants.

COMMENTARY—INDEX CASE: PM 22590

This 53-year-old, postmenopausal female presented with a 4-months history of watery diarrhea, generalized anasarca, anorexia, weight loss, weakness in both limbs, low blood pressure, skin pigmentation and progressively increasing breathlessness. Investigations revealed anemia, marked hypoproteinemia/hypoalbuminemia, hypothyroidism and mildly elevated liver function tests. The clinical diagnosis given was, chronic diarrhea with severe malabsorption, protein losing enteropathy and anemia ? Celiac disease ? IPSID ? GI lymphoma with hypothyroidism. Around 12 years back she had diarrhea of similar nature and was diagnosed to be a case of hyperthyroidism, for which the antithyroid drug, neo-mercazole was given. How long she was on this therapy was not known. She was diabetic since a year and was on treatment. She was short statured with pallor, pedal edema and alopecia. Motor power was less in all limbs, lower had greater than upper and proximal muscles had greater than distal muscles. Autopsy revealed diffuse lipomatous pseudohypertrophy of the pancreas leading to obstructive jaundice manifesting as marked cholestasis that was seen in the liver. The acinar tissue was totally wiped out, which led to exocrine pancreatic deficiency leading on to severe malabsorption. Stigmata of chronic calcific pancreatitis were seen indicating that the LPH arose in its background. There was florid lymphocytic thyroiditis and moderate adrenalitis along with a florid inflammatory myopathy. The lymphocytic thyroiditis had completely destroyed the thyroid gland leading to severe hypothyroidism. During life, she was not suspected to have Addison's disease, but retrospective analysis of the signs and symptoms, like the presence of fatigue, diarrhea, vomiting, muscle weakness, skin pigmentation and low blood pressure could point towards it. The presence of lymphocytic adrenalitis seen at autopsy is indicative of an ensuing Addison's disease. The index case showed a low platelet count/alopecia and PGA type II can be associated with idiopathic thrombocytopenic purpura and alopecia. Thus, there seems to be a clustering of autoimmune disorders i.e. hypothyroidism due to lymphocytic thyroiditis and setting in of Addison's disease due to the lymphocytic adrenalitis seen at autopsy. Hence, it could fit into a polyglandular autoimmune syndrome type II, which is the most common of the immunoendocrinopathy syndromes. It is characterized by the occurrence of autoimmune Addison's disease in combination with thyroid autoimmune diseases and/or type 1 diabetes mellitus.

Isolated tuberculosis of the spleen is rare. In the present setting of lipomatous pseudohypertrophy of the pancreas, malabsorption and hypoproteinemia made the patient more susceptible to infection.

TAKE HOME MESSAGE

- Lipomatous pseudohypertrophy of the pancreas is a rare and a distinct clinico-pathologic entity.
- Lipomatous pseudohypertrophy of the pancreas shows replacement of the pancreatic acinar tissue by mature adipose tissue with preservation of the pancreatic ducts and Islets of Langerhans. At times, stigmata of burnt out chronic pancreatitis can be appreciated in the background.
- Lipomatous pseudohypertrophy of the pancreas clinically mimicks a pancreatic carcinoma, but can be diagnosed by its typical imaging findings. Making a correct diagnosis is mandatory, to avoid unnecessary surgery.
- The pathogenesis of LPH is uncertain and various plausible causes like viral infection and an abnormal metabolism, have been postulated. .
- Polyglandular autoimmune syndrome type II (PGA-II) is the commonest among the immunoendocrinopathy syndromes. It consists of autoimmune Addison's disease in combination with thyroid autoimmune diseases and/or type 1 diabetes mellitus. The clinical manifestations are not always simultaneous and one may follow the other.

REFERENCES

1. Yasuda M, Niina Y, Uchida M, et al. A case of lipomatous pseudohypertrophy of the pancreas diagnosed by typical imaging. JOP. 2010;11(4):385-8.
2. Hantelmann W. Fettsucht und Atrophie der Bauch specicheldruse bei Jungendlichen. Virchows Arch. 1931; 282(2):630-42.
3. Stamm BH. Incidence and diagnostic significance of minor pathologic changes in the adult pancreas at autopsy: a systematic study of 112 autopsies in patients without known pancreatic disease. Hum Pathol. 1984;15(7):677-83.
4. Olsen TS. Lipomatosis of the pancreas in autopsy material and its relation to age and overweight. Acta Pathol Microbiol Scand. 1978;86A(5):367-673.
5. Adsay NV, Basturk O, Klimstra DS, et al. Pancreatic pseudotumors: non-neoplastic solid lesions of the pancreas that clinically mimic pancreas cancer. Semin Diagn Pathol. 2004; 21(4):260-7.
6. Sasaki M, Nakanuma Y, Ando H. Lipomatous pseudohypertrophy of the pancreas in a patient with cirrhosis due to chronic hepatitis B. Pathol Int. 1998;48(7):566-8.
7. Kuroda N, Okada M, Toi M, et al. Lipomatous pseudohypertrophy of the pancreas: further evidence of advanced hepatic lesion as the pathogenesis. Pathol Int. 2003;53(2):98-101.
8. MacMaster SA, Cummings TM. Computed tomography and ultrasonography findings for an adult with Shwachman syndrome and pancreatic lipomatosis. Can Assoc Radiol J. 1993;44(4):301-3.
9. Okumura K, Sasaki Y, Ohyama M, et al. Bannayan syndrome—generalized lipomatosis associated with megalencephaly and macrodactyly. Acta Pathol Jpn. 1986;36(2):269-77.
10. Maunoury V, Nieuwarts S, Ferri J, et al. Pancreatic lipomatosis revealing Johanson-Blizzard syndrome [in French]. Gastroenterol Clin Biol. 1999;23(10):1099-101.
11. Yoshimura N, Hayashi S, Fukushima Y. Diffuse Mallory bodies in the liver, diffuse Lewy bodies in the brain and diffuse fat replacement (lipomatous pseudohypertrophy) of the pancreas in a patient with juvenile Parkinson's disease. Acta Pathol Jpn. 1992;42(11):826-31.
12. Kojima K. Current Encyclopedia of Pathology. 13B. Metabolic Disturbances of the Pancreas. Tokyo, Japan: Nakayama-Shoten; 1983. pp. 183-95.
13. Henkinbrant A, Khalek W, Farchakh E, et al. Cholestatic jaundice complicating lipomatous pseudo-hypertrophy of the pancreas [in French]. Acta Gastroenterol Belg. 1990;53(3): 315-22.
14. Betterle C, Lazzarotto F, Presotto F. Autoimmune polyglandular syndrome Type 2: the tip of an iceberg? Clin Exp Immunol. 2004;137(2):225-33.
15. Altinel D, Basturk O, Sarmiento JM, et al. Lipomatous pseudohypertrophy of the Pancreas. A Clinicopathologically distinct entity. Pancreas. 2010;39(3):392-7.
16. Schatz DA, Winter WE. Autoimmune polyglandular syndrome II. Clinical syndrome and treatment. Endocrinol Metab Clin N Am. 2002;31(2):339-52.
17. Cutolo M. Autoimmune polyendocrine syndromes. Autoimmun Rev. 2014;13(2):85-9.
18. F Magitta N, Pura M, S Bøe Wolff A, et al. Autoimmune polyendocrine syndrome type I in Slovakia: relevance of screening patients with autoimmune Addison's disease. Eur J Endocrinol. 2008;158(5):705-9.

CONTRIBUTIONS BY:

1. Dr Kartar Singh, Ex-Professor and Head, Department of Gastroenterology (Clinician In-Charge)
2. Dr Surinder Rana, Additional Professor, Department of Gastroenterology (Compilation of Clinical Details)

Post Graduate Institute of Medical Education and Research, Chandigarh, India.

CASE 24

Young Male with Early Onset Micronodular Cirrhosis due to Synergistic Hepatotoxic effect of Alcohol and Hepatitis C Virus Infection along with Cryoglobulinemic Vasculitis: PM 27791

Nandita Bharadwaj Kakkar

HIGHLIGHTS OF THE CASE

A 25-year-old male came with jaundice, ascites, swelling of lower limb, large ulcer on the right foot, oliguria with history of alcohol intake in cirrhogenic doses since 3–4 years. Investigations revealed deranged liver/renal function tests, coagulopathy, anti-HCV reactive with HCV RNA– 1.86 × 102 IU/mL, polymorphonuclear leukocytosis, spontaneous bacterial peritonitis, cholelithiasis, liver showing heterogeneous echotexture and antemortem skin biopsy showing small vessel vasculitis due to ? HCV-related cryoglobulinemia. At autopsy there was micronodular alcoholic cirrhosis with disseminated fungal infection. Synergistic effect of alcohol intake and HCV-infection led to setting in of alcoholic cirrhosis, with out of proportion fibrosis, within a short period of time.

Keywords: Cirrhosis, alcohol, HCV-infection, synergism, dual fungal infection, cryoglobulinemia, mucormycosis, aspergillus.

CLINICAL DETAILS

Date of Admission: 24.10.2016, Date of Death: 09.11.2016, Duration of Hospital Stay: 15 days

A 25-year-old male came with jaundice, progressive abdominal distension and swelling of the leg since one-month along with oliguria for the past 7 days. Jaundice was associated with high colored urine and anorexia. There was an ulcer over the right foot which had progressed to a very large size and for which debridement was done. He had off and on low-grade fever, history suggestive of encephalopathy and constipation. There was no history of diabetes, hypertension, ischemic heart disease and blood transfusions. He was taking alcohol in cirrhogenic doses i.e. 150–200 g/day since 3–4 years. On examination there was pallor, icterus, bilateral pedal edema along with ulcers and bullae over feet and ankle. There was no cyanosis, clubbing or lymphadenopathy and no signs of chronic liver disease. Chest and cardiovascular systems were normal. The abdomen was distended, free-fluid was present and the liver/spleen were not palpable. Bowel sounds were present. He was conscious, oriented and flaps were present.

Investigation and Course of Management

Investigations: ***Hemogram***—Hb ranged from 11.4–6.1 g/dL; TLC from 38,400–22,800/uL with polymorphonuclear leucocytosis, platelets from 151–44 × 10^3, coagulogram was deranged; PT: 37 sec, PTI: 50–35%, PTTK: 55 sec, fibrinogen: 2.03 g/dL, D-dimer: 9,081 ng/mL. ***Blood biochemistry*****:** Total serum bilirubin/conjugated: 16.3/8.2–11.4/5.3 mg%; SGOT/SGPT: 82/42–185/69 U/L; alkaline phosphatase: 142–98 U/L; Total proteins/albumin: 7.5/2.1–6.0/1.3 gms; Ca/Po_4: 7.9/2.5–6.1/5.4 mg%; Na^+ 131–138 mEq/L; K^+ 3.4–4.3 mEq/L; urea: 235 mg%; creatinine: 3.2–5.4 mg%; ***Ascitic fluid analysis:*** At admission—TLC: 800/mm^3, DLC predominantly lymphocytes, SAAG: 1.6 g/dL, protein: 1.5 g/dL, ADA: 7 IU/L, C/S—sterile. Terminally—TLC: 16,000/mm^3, DLC: P80L20, protein: 1.4 g/dL, C/S: E. coli +. Oxygen saturation: 77–90%. **Serology** - HbsAg: Negative, anti-HCV—reactive, HCV-RNA—1.86 × 102 IU/mL, anti-HAV and HEV (IgM)—negative, serology for dengue/leptospira/scrub typhus: Negative. Peripheral blood smear negative for malarial parasite, Widal: Negative. Routine urine examination—sugar/protein: Nil, pus cells—4–6/hpf, urine/blood culture—sterile, pus c/s – ***E. coli*** sensitive to tetracycline, galactomannan: 0.78, C-reactive proteins: 346 mg/L, arterial ammonia: 49 mmol/L, ANA: Negative, ANCA (IF):

Negative, C3 level: 29 mg% (N-50–150 mg%), C4 level: 7 mg% (N-20–50 mg%). ***Radiology***: Ultrasound lower limb—suggestive of cellulitis in right lower limb. No evidence of deep vein thrombosis or any collection noted. Ultrasound abdomen: Liver — Heterogenous echotexture, normal outline, Span 13 cm, no IHBRD, PV 10 mm, GB: Calculus +, wall edema +, kidneys normal, spleen: 17 cm, ascites +++. ***Impression***: Chronic liver disease, cholelithiasis. ***Skin biopsy***: Left lower limb (26,550/16)—small vessel vasculitis (Fig 1A), ***ECG***: Nonspecific changes.

Patient was started on antihepatic coma regime and antibiotics (ceftriaxone/clindamycin initially which was later changed to meropenem and targocid). He was seen by Dermatology, Rheumatology and Nephrology services. He received two sessions of hemodialysis, packed-cell transfusion, fresh-frozen plasma and salt-free human albumin. Debridement (Figs 1B and C) was done in right foot because of extensive ulceration and necrosis. Patient could not afford intravenous immunoglobulin (IVIG) or rituximab. Continued to deteriorate and developed respiratory failure. Antibiotics were changed to colistin and targocid. Fungal sepsis was also considered, but antifungals could not be started due to nonaffordability. Sofosbuvir and daclatasvir were started for HCV infection and related vasculitis. Due to progressive deterioration and progressive hypoxemia, he was put on ventilator and despite all efforts, expired on 09.11.2016. ***Unit's clinical diagnosis***: Acute on chronic liver failure—alcohol and HCV-related, spontaneous bacterial peritonitis, acute kidney/liver injury, small vessel vasculitis ? HCV-related cryoglobulinemia, cholelithiasis ? Fungal sepsis, ***Cause of death***: Multi-organ failure.

AUTOPSY FINDINGS: PM 27791

A complete autopsy was performed. On external examination there was a sinus at the lateral aspect of right mid-thigh, with right leg/left-hand cellulitis, debridement done on the dorsal aspect of the right foot, abdomen was distended, icterus+++, peritoneal cavity yielded 4 litres of reddish brown fluid, each pleural cavity yielded 700 mL and pericardial cavity yielded 100 mL of similar fluid. The ***liver*** (Figs 2A–D) weighed 1,150 g, was shrunken, bile-stained and micronodules were present on the capsular surface. Cut section revealed classical micro-nodular cirrhosis with bile stained nodules separated by fibrous septae. Portal vein was mildly dilated. The gallbladder contained three stones, but the common bile duct was normal. On microscopic examination the liver (Fig 3A) showed a markedly distorted architecture with broad fibrous bands dividing the parenchyma into micronodules less than 3 mm. The regenerative micronodules were better highlighted by reticulin and Masson's trichrome stain (Figs 3B–D). The septae (Fig 4A) showed extensive fibrosis and ductular proliferation. The fibrosis was extending into the nodules leading to prominent pericellular fibrosis (Figs 4B and C). Apart from this there were areas of extensive fibrosis where only a few surviving hepatocytes could be appreciated (Fig 4D). Macrovesicular steatosis, feathery degeneration and marked hepatocytic cholestasis were seen (Figs 4E and F). The central veins revealed a prominent perivenular fibrosis with near total occlusion of many of them (Figs 5A and B). Mallory's bodies (Fig 5C) and satellitosis (liver cell necrosis with neutrophil infiltrate) was seen. No hepatocyte necrosis or sclerosing hyaline necrosis noted.

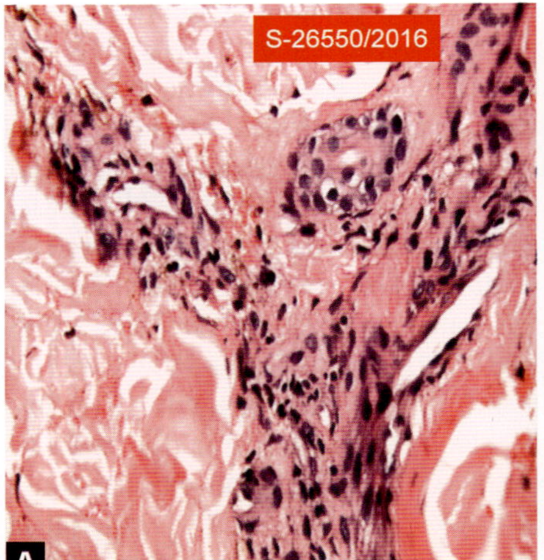

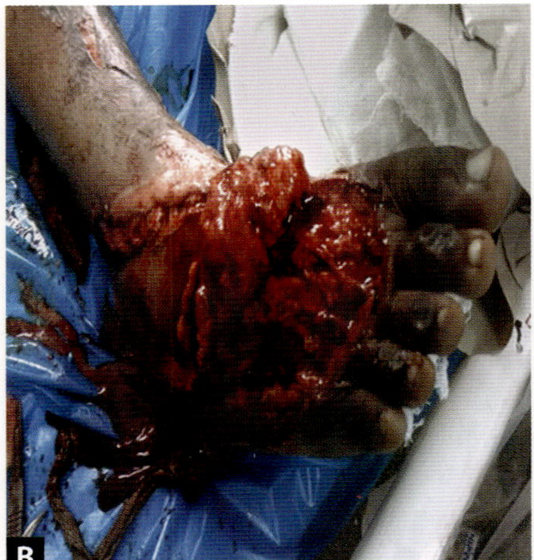

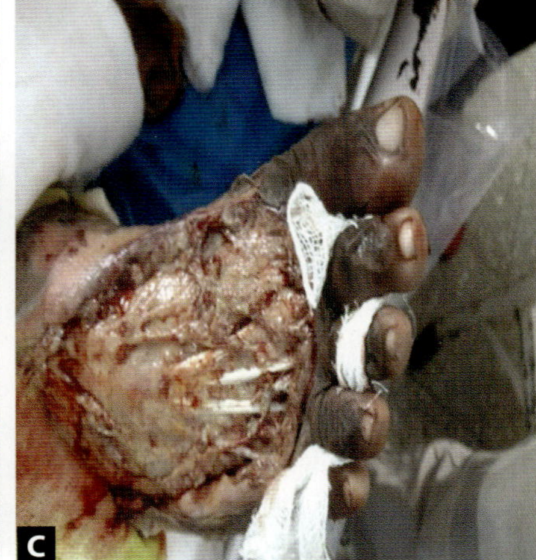

Figs 1A–C: (A) Antemortem skin biopsy from the right leg shows small vessel vasculitis with presence of nuclear debris and RBC extravasation; (B) Large ulcer on the right foot; (C) The ulcer after debridement.

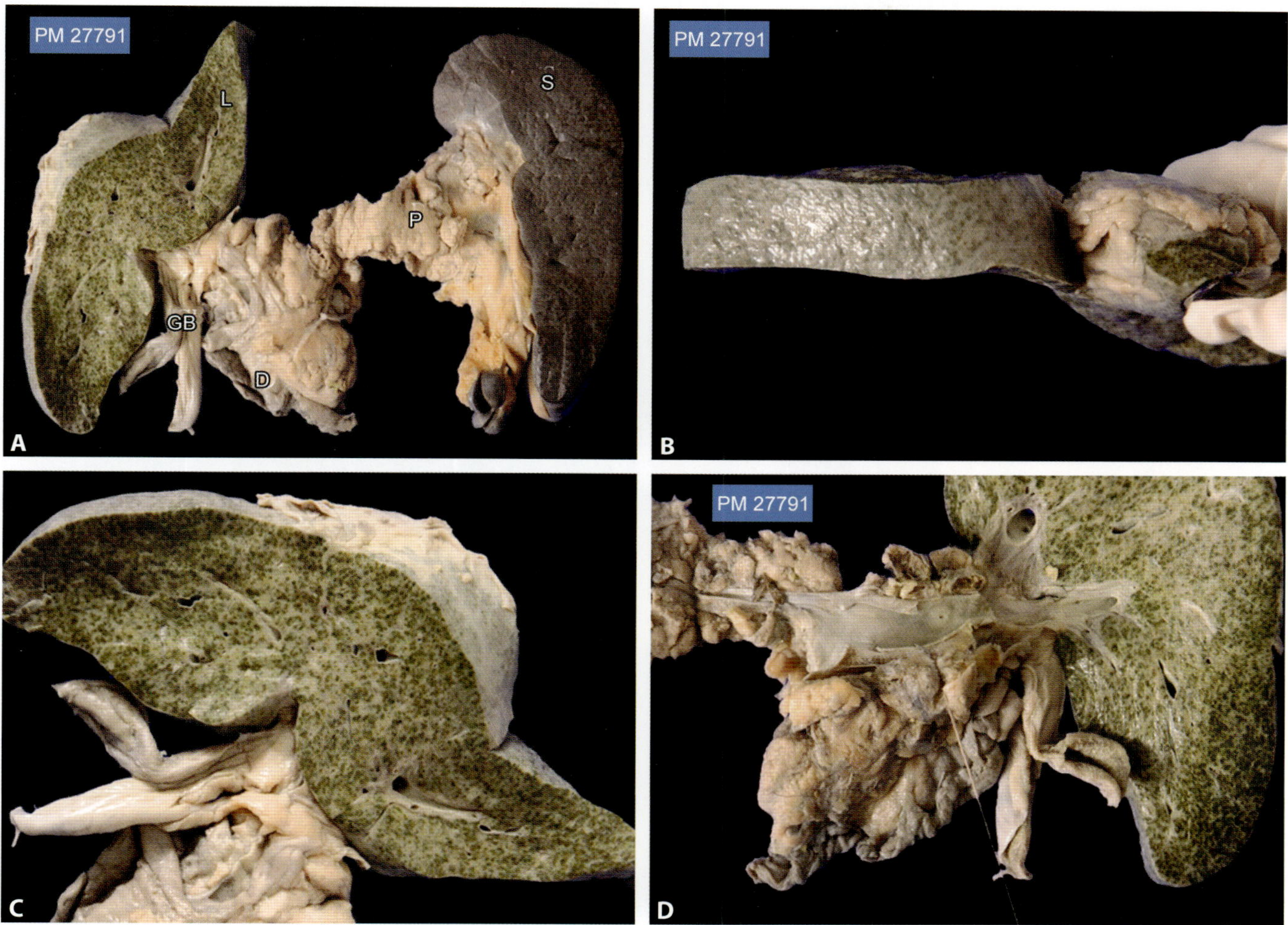

Figs 2A–D: (A) Organ complex of the slice of the shrunken cirrhotic liver (L), pancreas (P), c loop of duodenum (D), gallbladder (GB) and enlarged spleen (S); (B) Capsular aspect of the liver showing micronodules; (C) Cut-section of the liver showing small micronodules separated by white fibrous bands; (D) Opened-up portal vein which is mildly dilated.

Discernable portal tracts appeared normal. No lymphoid follicles, lymphoplasmacytic infiltrate, bile duct damage or any necrosis around terminal hepatic venules was seen, to suggest morphological evidence of Hepatitis C infection. Iron stores were within normal limits. Immunohistochemistry for HbC and HbsAg were negative. Overall features were those of alcoholic micronodular cirrhosis in a case with positive HCV serology. There was congestive splenomegaly with the ***spleen*** weighing 780 g. Altered blood was found in the stomach and esophageal varices were noted (Fig 6A). The pleural aspect of the ***lungs*** showed fibrinous tags, visible nodules and hemorrhages (Fig 6B). The cut section was firm and scattered, small whitish nodules measuring 0.5–1 cm were seen all over (Figs 6C and D). These nodules on microscopic examination (Figs 6E, F and 7A–C) were small abscesses composed of polymorphs, giant cells, areas of necrosis, ill-formed granulomas and were replete with fungal profiles with morphology consistent with both aspergillus and mucormycosis. The ***heart*** (Figs 7D–F and 8A–F) showed areas of myocardial discoloration which revealed myocardial abscesses and areas of coagulative necrosis, replete with fungal profiles with morphology of aspergillus and mucormycosis. Angioinvasion was very prominent. ***Kidneys*** (Figs 9A–C) showed bile cast nephropathy with multiple fungal abscesses replete with hyphae of both aspergillus and mucromycosis. Calcification was noted in the kidney (tubules) and in the myocardium.

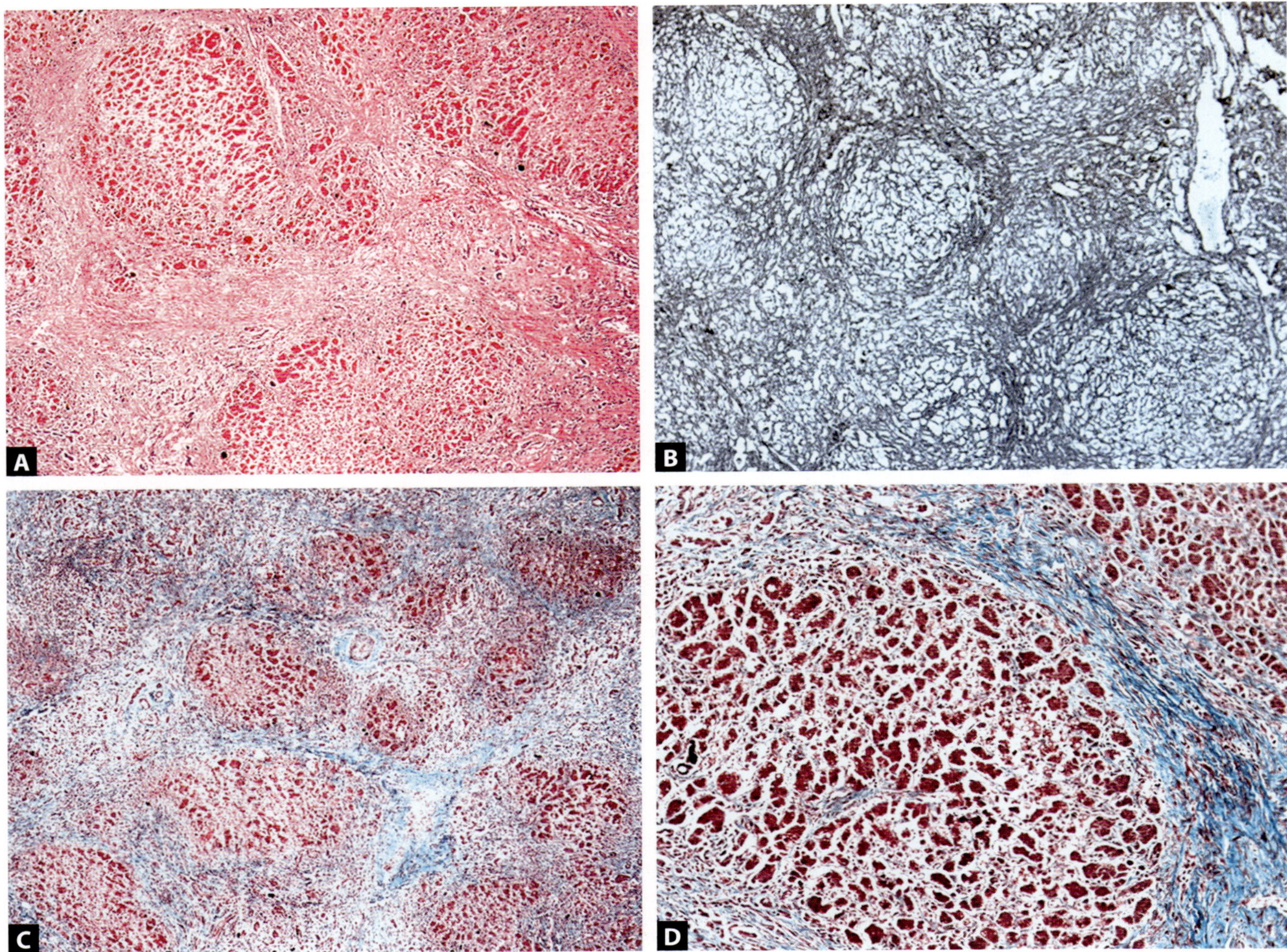

Figs 3A–D: Photomicrographs of the liver showing a distorted architecture. (A) Micronodules of regenerating hepatocytes separated by fibrous septae; (B) Micronodules better highlighted by the reticulin stain; (C) Micronodules better highlighted by the Masson's trichrome (MT) stain; (D) MT stain showing a nodule surrounded by fibrous septa.

FINAL AUTOPSY DIAGNOSIS: PM 27781

A 25-year-old male—Alcoholic in Cirrhogenic Doses and HCV + (HCV-RNA: 1.86 × 102 IU/mL) with Cryoglobulinemia

- Micronodular cirrhosis—alcohol and HCV-related.
- Portal hypertension—ascites, congestive splenomegaly, esophageal varices.
- HCV-related cryoglobulinemia leading to vasculitis and foot ulcer.
- Cholelithiasis with chronic cholecystitis.
- Pulmonary fungal abscessess (Aspergillus and mucormycosis) with dissemination to the heart and kidneys.
- Fibrinous pleuritis with pleural effusion.
- Bile cast nephropathy, subarachnoid hemorrhage.
- Calcification—heart and kidney.
- Pericardial effusion.

HEPATITIS C VIRUS

Hepatitis C virus is a single stranded RNA virus (30–38 nm) with a lipoid envelop, is globally prevalent and chronically infects 170 million people worldwide, is a subgenus of family Flaviviridae, contains 9,400 nucleotides and six viral genotypes, which further contain many subtypes. Different geographic areas have different genotype prevalence. This virus was identified in the year 1989 and was the cause of most of the sporadic and post-transfusion hepatitis, previously labeled as non-A and non-B hepatitis. In approximately 65% cases it spreads by the parenteral route. So intravenous drug

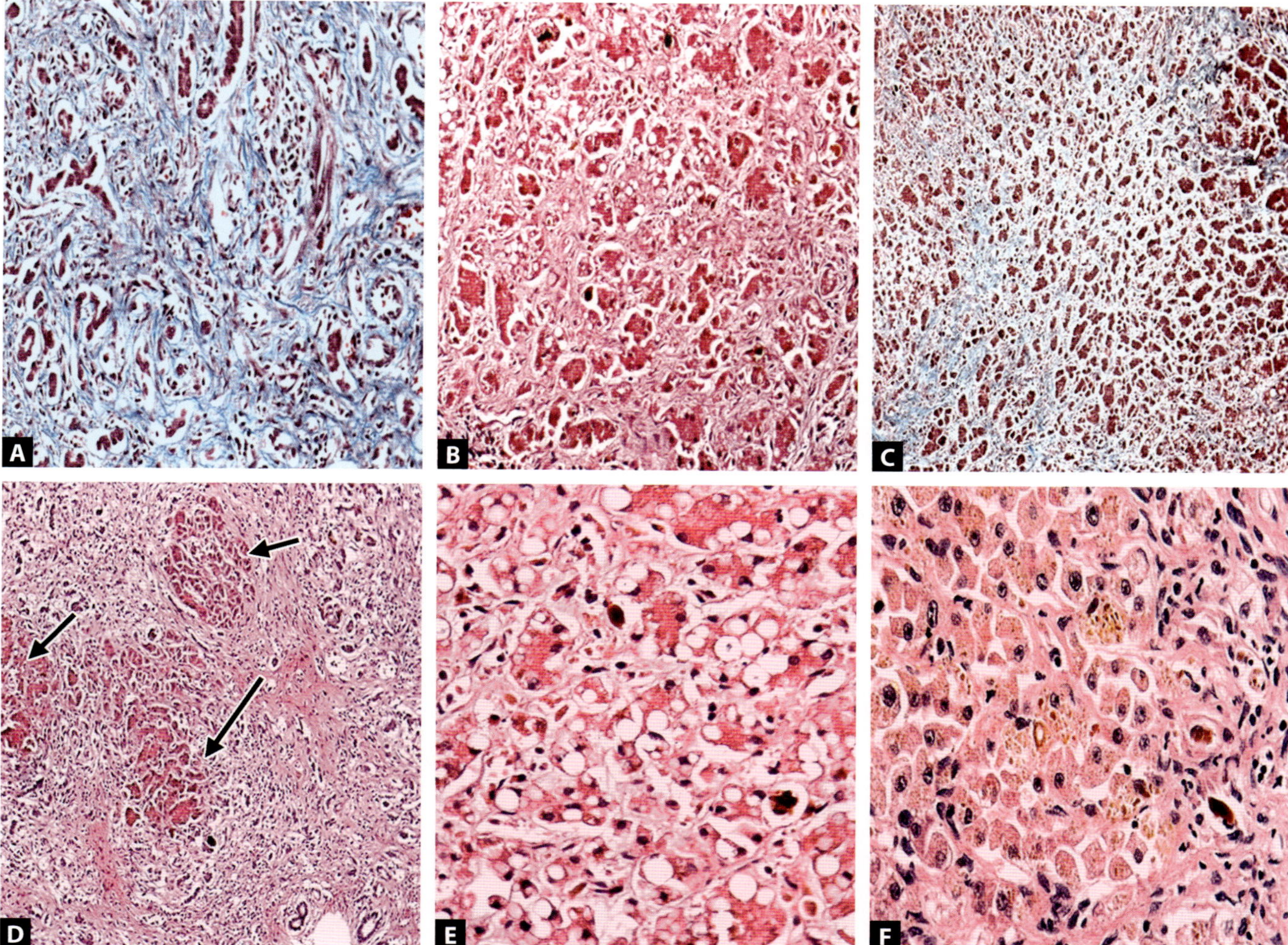

Figs 4A–F: Photomicrographs of the liver. (A) Septa showing fibrosis, minimal inflammation and bile duct proliferation (MT stain); (B and C) Extensive pericellular fibrosis (H&E and MT stains); (D) Showing extensive fibrosis with few left-over nodules of hepatocytes (arrows); (E) Macro-vesicular steatosis; (F) Hepatocytes show feathery degeneration along with hepatocytic and canalicular cholestasis.

use and blood transfusions/blood products is the major mode of spread. Apart from this needle stick injuries in healthcare workers, scarifications, tattoos and intranasal cocaine are the modes of acquisition. In about 33% of victims the means of infection is uncertain. The acute phase is generally asymptomatic and the viral marker found is HCV-RNA and between 2½–6 months, C100-3 (anti-HCV) antibody is detected. After the acute infection, more than 90% cases proceed to a chronic infection of varying degree and a quarter of these will further develop cirrhosis. There is a higher incidence of hepatocellular carcinoma in post-HCV cirrhosis. Known factors for acquiring chronicity are, age greater than 40 at the time of infection, male gender and alcohol intake of more than 50 g/day. Histopathological features of acute-HCV infection is nonspecific and include acidophil bodies scattered near the central vein and mild to moderate lymphoplasmacytic infiltrate in the portal tracts/lobules. In cases of chronic hepatitis C, the histopathology does not correlate well with the deranged liver enzymes or with the symptoms. However, in a case of chronic hepatitis with HCV infection, prominent bile duct damage, steatosis (mixed micro/macrovesicular) and prominent lymphoid aggregates or lymphoid follicles with germinal centers are considered characteristic. Varying degrees of fibrosis is seen which is graded. In severe cases, perivenular confluent necrosis and bridging hepatic necrosis may be seen. Iron stores are generally increased. Extrahepatic complications associated with HCV infection include mixed cryoglobulinemia,

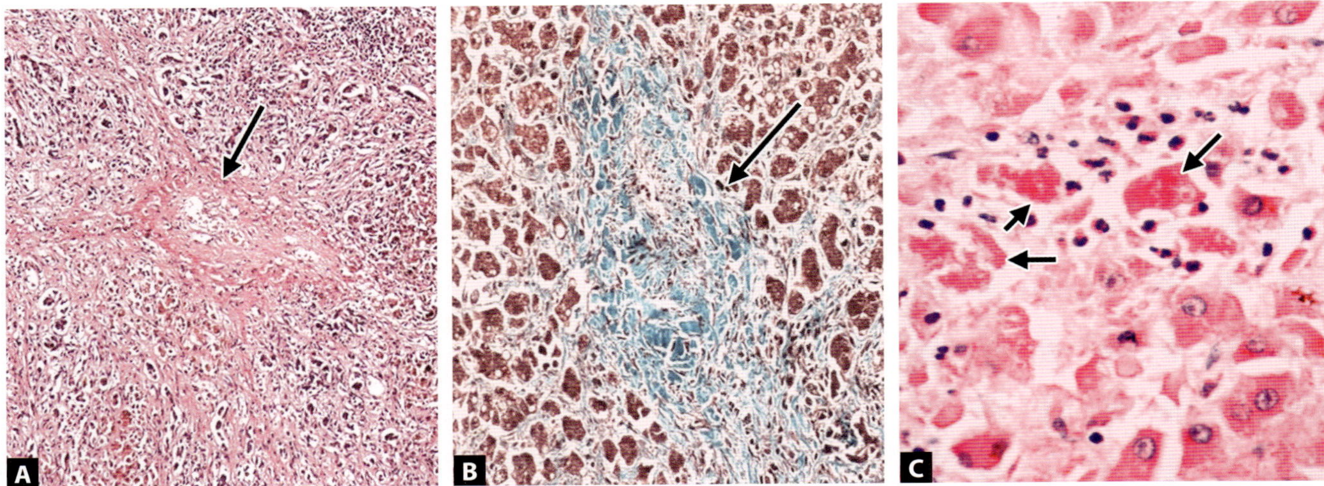

Figs 5A–C: Photomicrographs of the liver (A and B) Prominent perivenular fibrosis—arrows (H&E and MT stains); (C) Hepatocytes containing Mallory's bodies (arrows) surrounded by neutrophils.

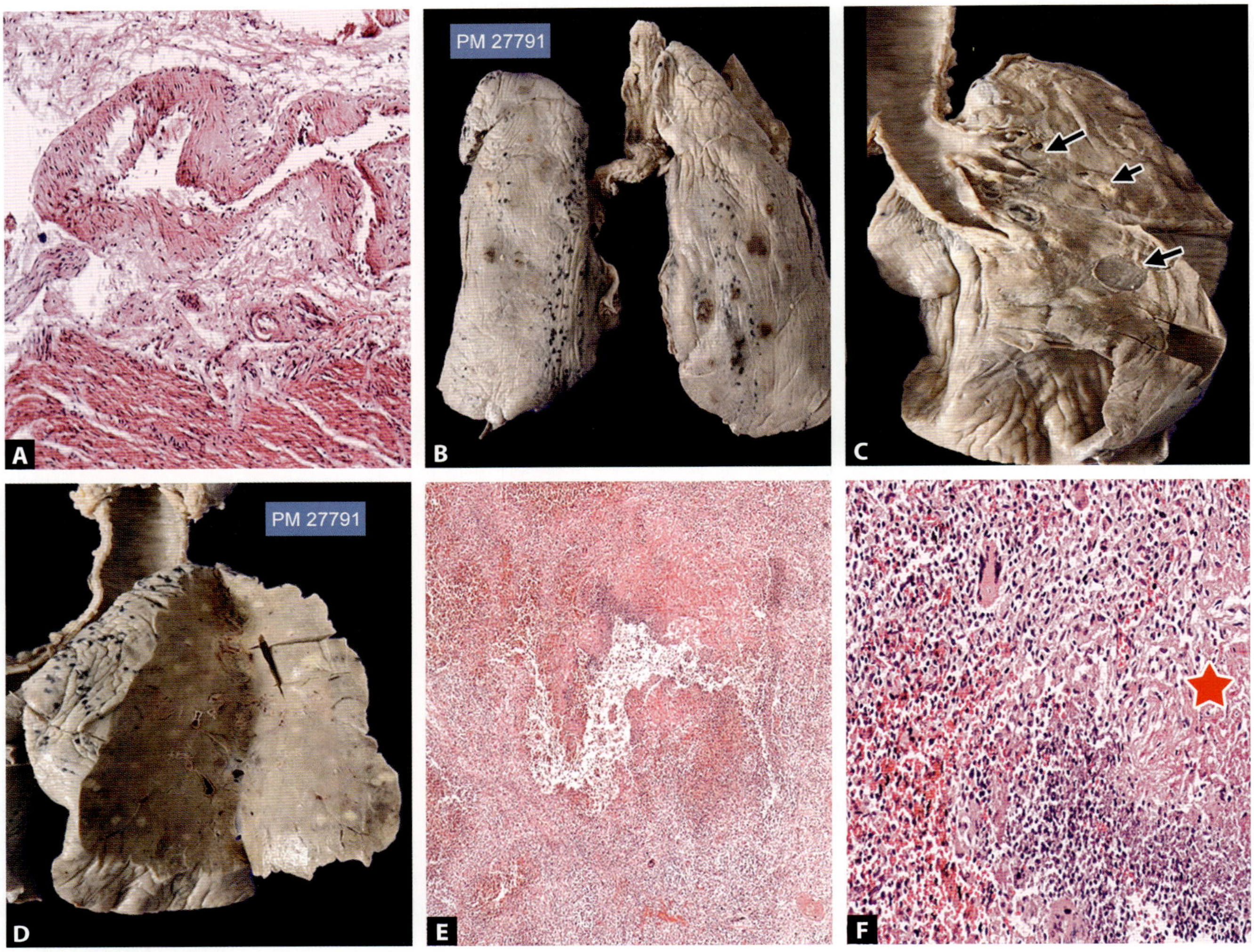

PM 27791

PM 27791

Figs 6A–F: (A) Photomicrograph of the esophagus shows a varix; (B) Gross picture of the lungs with pleura showing visible nodules and hemorrhages; (C and D) Cut-section of the lung shows small abscesses (arrows). Photomicrographs of the lung showing; (E) Abscess with central cavitation; (F) Lung showing ill-formed granulomas with giant cells, dense inflammation and necrosis (red star).

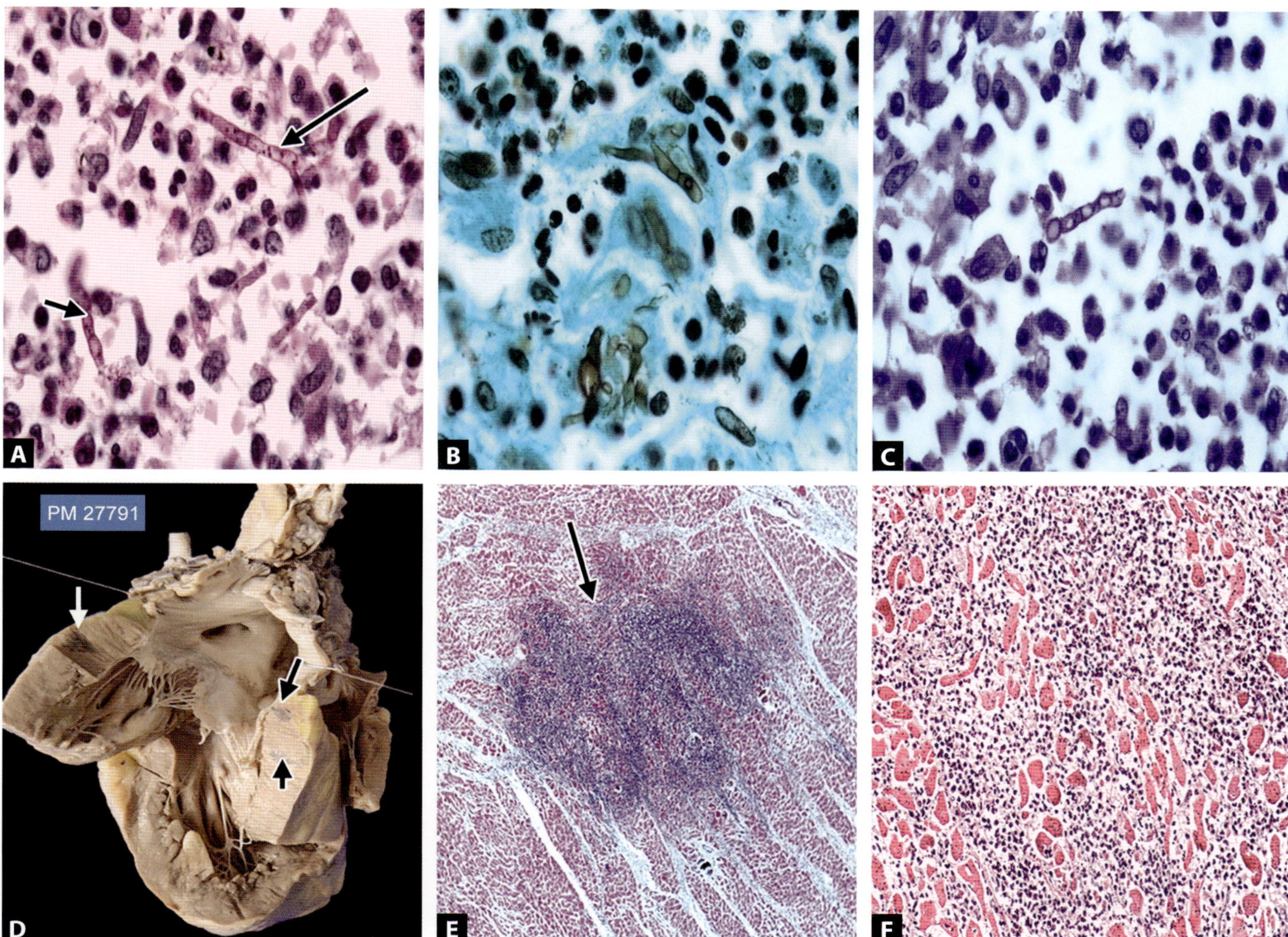

Figs 7A–F: Photomicrographs of the lungs (A) H&E stain shows fungal hyphae both septate (short arrow) and nonseptate (long arrow); (B) Grocott's stain showing fungal hyphae some within the giant cell; (C) PAS stain showing septate hyphae; (D) Left inflow tract of the heart showing areas of discoloration in the myocardium (arrows); (E) Myocardial abscess at low power (arrow); (F) Myocardial abscess showing degenerating myocytes and dense inflammation.

glomerulonephritis, porphyria cutaneous tarda, lichen planus, Sjogren's syndrome and polyarteritis nodosa.

Hepatitis C virus infection is a major cause of chronic liver disease and is now being implicated as a stimulator of B-cell lymphoproliferative disorders like mixed cryoglobulinemia and non-Hodgkin's lymphoma. In cryoglobulinemia there is a clonal expansion of B-cells which express rheumatoid factor in the lymph nodes, liver and peripheral blood. Thus, there is presence of circulating cryoglobulins, which are immune complexes composed of rheumatoid factor, IgG, compliment and HCV-RNA. These get deposited on the endothelium of small/medium sized arteries and veins in the skin, kidneys and peripheral nerves leading on to vasculitis.

PATHOLOGY OF ALCOHOLIC LIVER DISEASE

The pathology of alcoholic liver disease includes fatty change i.e. steatosis, perivenular fibrosis, alcoholic foamy degeneration also known as microvesicular fatty change, alcoholic hepatitis and cirrhosis. ***Steatosis***, predominantly macrovesicular is the first to manifest, begins in the perivenular area and is seen in 90% patients with chronic alcoholism. At this stage the liver cells do not show any necrosis or inflammation, but lipogranulomas due to rupture of the fat containing hepatocytes may be seen. ***Alcoholic foamy degeneration*** also known as microvesicular fatty change is a hallmark of alcohol induced hepatocytic injury, wherein the patients present with hepatomegaly

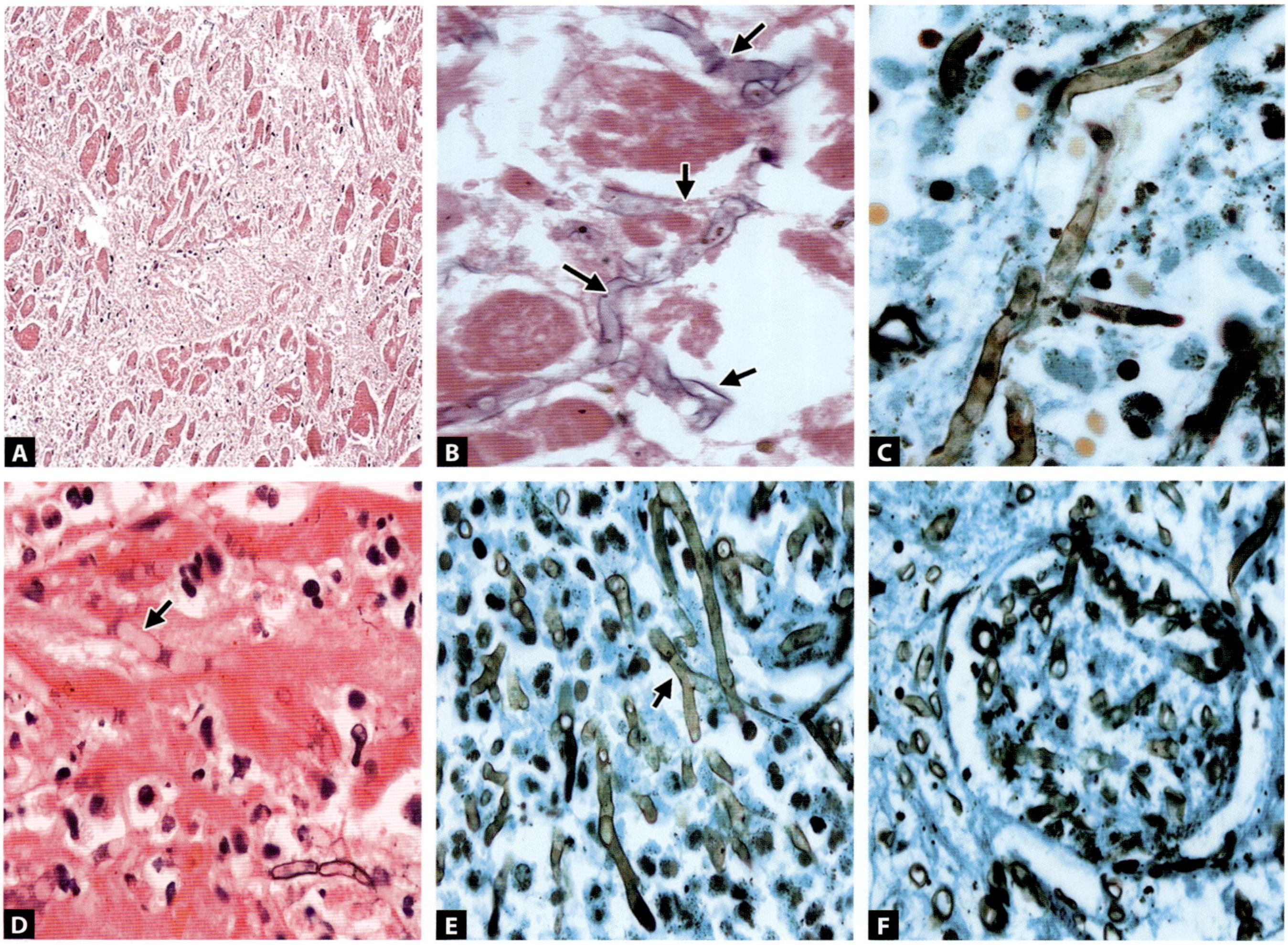

Figs 8A–F: Photomicrographs of the heart showing (A) Areas of infarction; (B) Fungal profiles of mucor amidst the myocytes (arrows); (C) Broad aseptate profiles of mucor on Grocott's stain; (D) Septate hyphae of aspergillous (arrow); (E) Septate profiles of aspergillus with acute angle branching (arrow)–Grocott's stain; (F) Grocott's stain shows angioinvasion by the fungus.

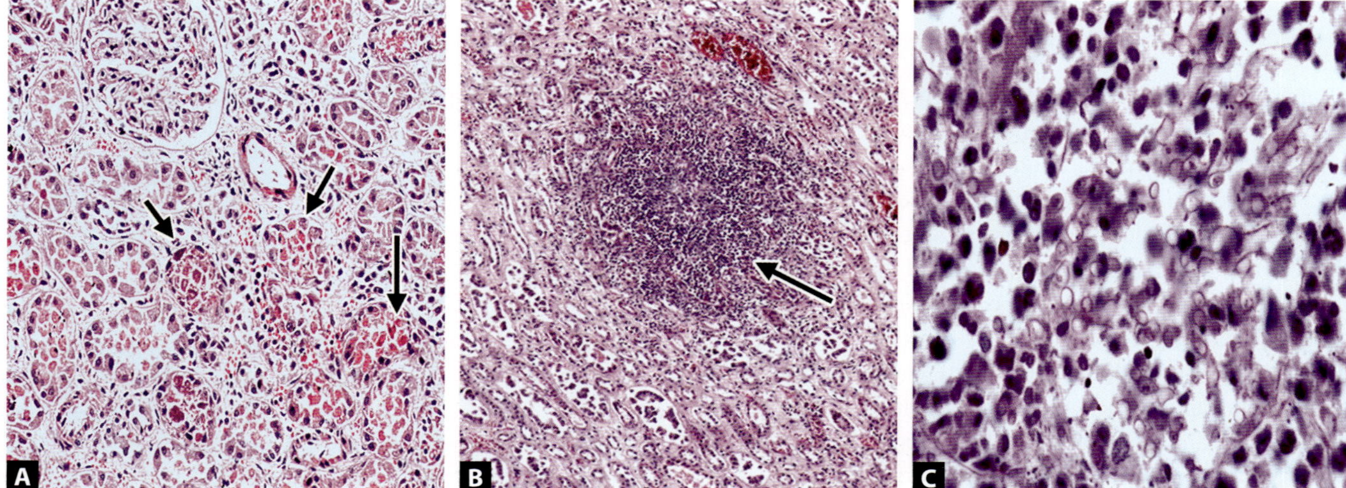

Figs 9A–C: Photomicrographs of the kidney (A) Shows a normal glomerulus and tubules (arrows) containing bile casts with shedding of the tubular epithelium; (B and C) Small abscess (arrow) in the medulla replete with fungal profiles of mucor (H&E and PAS stain).

with elevation of serum bilirubin and marked elevation of aminotransferases and alkaline phosphatase. Biopsy shows predominantly microvesicular fatty change in the perivenular region extending on to zone 2, perivenular hepatocytic cholestasis, canalicular cholestasis, occasional Mallory's bodies/satellitosis and perivenular fibrosis. ***Perivenular fibrosis*** is a feature of alcoholic liver disease which is first in the path of development of cirrhosis and morphologically shows as fibrosis greater than 4 mm around the terminal hepatic venule, extending greater than two-thirds of its circumference. Once detected on a biopsy at an early stage, these patients progress to more severe disease and finally cirrhosis, if the patient continues to take alcohol. ***Alcoholic hepatitis*** clinically presents with hepatomegaly and raised transaminases. Biopsy shows fatty change, satellitosis i.e. hepatocyte necrosis with neutrophils, hepatocytes containing Mallory's bodies (intracytoplasmic eosinophilic irregular masses) surrounded by neutrophilic infiltrate and giant mitochondria which are globular eosinophilic cytoplasmic inclusions. Alcoholic hepatitis can be mild with few foci of satellitosis present in the perivenular locations, occasional Mallory's bodies and minimal pericellular fibrosis. In severe alcoholic hepatitis there is very prominent hepatocytic necrosis with enlarged liver cells containing Mallory's bodies (in approximately two-third cases) and the degree of fibrosis, both pericellular and perivenular is more prominent. Apart from this cholestasis, lipogranulomas, apoptosis, Kupffer cell proliferation and portal tract inflammation can be seen. Sclerosing hyaline necrosis can be seen in alcoholic hepatitis wherein due to florid perivenular necrosis and subsequent replacement by fibrous tissue, the terminal hepatic venules can get occluded, thus producing portal hypertension without cirrhosis. In alcoholic hepatitis, the factors which indicate progression to cirrhosis are foamy degeneration/microvesicular steatosis, fibrosis if present in the fatty liver stage, degree of pericellular/perivenular fibrosis, degree of hepatocytic necrosis, elastic fiber deposition in septae, distortion of liver architecture, terminal hepatic venule occlusion, widespread Mallory's bodies and diffuse parenchymal disease. Bouchier et al in their 10 year follow-up of liver biopsy study of over 500 patients diagnosed with alcoholic liver disease, concluded that, over 70% of those with a diagnosis of fatty liver were alive compared to 37% diagnosed with alcoholic hepatitis. Pares et al stated that the risk of progression to cirrhosis in alcoholic hepatitis can be judged by three factors i.e. initial degree of liver damage, females and continuation of alcohol ingestion. In ***alcoholic cirrhosis***, the liver architecture is distorted by fibrous septae which surround small (is less than 3 mm) uniform sized, regenerative nodules. There can be concomitant features of alcoholic hepatitis indicating continued drinking. The cirrhosis takes over a mixed micro/macronodular appearance if alcohol ingestion is stopped. ***Bile ductular proliferation*** is a regular feature of alcoholic liver disease and has been considered to be due to ductal metaplasia occurring in regenerating hepatocytes or as a progeny of proliferating hepatic stem cells. At times the liver biopsy in a patient taking alcohol shows a picture of both alcoholic liver disease and chronic viral hepatitis, the latter at times being the predominant feature but with disproportionate fibrosis. This indicates a concomitant hepatitis C infection and to a lesser degree hepatitis B infection. This discrepancy in fibrosis is related to a potentiating effect of alcohol. At times all viral markers are negative and there is a possibility that some unknown virus may emerge over time. ***Severe cholestasis*** can be seen in alcoholic liver disease, be it fatty liver, microvesicular steatosis, alcoholic hepatitis or cirrhosis. Portal tract fibrosis is generally not seen in alcohol injury and if seen probably indicates a previous viral hepatitis or acute pancreatitis. Mild (grade 1/2) ***siderosis*** is seen in alcohol liver injury, but at times grade 3/4 siderosis is seen, in which situation there is always some other additive cause like hereditary hemochromatosis. ***Hepatocellular carcinoma*** is seen in approximately 10% patients with alcoholic cirrhosis usually when it is macronodular.

ALCOHOL AND HEPATITIS C VIRUS INFECTION: SYNERGISTIC HEPATOTOXIC EFFECT

Hepatitis C virus is an important cause of chronic liver disease leading to fibrosis, cirrhosis and further hepatocellular carcinoma. Transforming growth factor-β1 (TGF-β1) is said to play a key pathogenetic role in liver fibrosis. This is proven by in vitro studies which report that TGF-β1 levels are elevated in HCV-infected hepatocytes and in liver tissue of HCV patients. These studies have also highlighted that the levels of TGF-β1 in media from in vitro-cultured HCV-infected hepatocytes, activated the primary hepatic stellate cells isolated from rats. This further endorses that TGF-β1 secreted by HCV-infected hepatocytes is likely to play a key role in the liver fibrosis.

Hepatitis C virus infection and alcohol intake have a synergistic hepatotoxic effect and when seen together, leads to early onset of advanced liver disease, leading on to cirrhosis. The pathogenetic mechanism behind this synergism is complex, but the onus lies on the acquisition of an altered immune response, which in the presence of a genetic predisposition leads to increased viral proliferation. Hepatitis

C virus has a higher propensity to infest alcoholic patients as compared to the general population. The figures quoted in the 1990's were to the tune of 40–50%. But over years this number has come down. Novo-Veleiro et al have documented the prevalence of HCV-infection in alcoholics to be 16.32% as compared to the general population, where it is said to be about 1.5–2%. Alcohol and HCV-infection, occurring together, contribute approximately 10–14% cases of cirrhosis and 10% cases of liver transplantation. In patients with HCV-infection the quantity of alcohol required for production of alcoholic liver disease is a matter of debate and ranges from 30–120 g/day. The pathogenesis of the synergism is still a question of ongoing research. But many mechanisms are pointed at. Both alcohol and HCV can bring about alteration in the cell-mediated immunity by adversely affecting the functions of the dendritic cells. Alcohol can alter the antigen-presenting function and the hepatocytes lose their competence to combat the hepatitis C virus, or in other words alcohol helps the HCV to evade the immune response. The following pathogenetic mechanisms are listed:

- Both alcohol and HCV have the propensity to increase the expression of cyclooxygenase 2 i.e. COX2 (which increases oxidative stress) and also augment the production of oxygen free radicals.
- Both alcohol and HCV have a deleterious effect on the functioning of the mitochondria leading to inhibition of hepatic regeneration.
- Both alcohol and HCV alter the functioning of *FOXO3* which is part of the hepatic antioxidant system, thus leading to uncontrolled proliferation.
- Alcohol upregulates miR-122 which promotes the replication of HCV.
- Alcohol is further said to reduce the response to HCV treatment.
- Both alcohol and HCV lead to liver steatosis and their presence together augment fibrosis leading to advanced liver damage.
- Iron overload occurs in alcoholic liver disease and to a minor extent in HCV infection. This excess of iron causes an increase in the reactive oxygen radicals, leading to an increase in the liver inflammatory response and an impaired immune response against HCV virus infection.
- Genetic factors are also said to play a role in the augmentation of liver disease in alcoholics with concomitant HCV infection. There is strong evidence which supports the association of the rs738409 SNP in the *PNPLA3* gene with both ALD and HCV-related advanced liver disease.

COMMENTARY—INDEX CASE: PM 27791

A 25-year-old male came with jaundice, ascites, swelling of both lower limbs, ulcer on the right foot for which debridement was done and oliguria, with history of alcohol intake in cirrhogenic doses since 3–4 years. Investigations revealed deranged liver/renal function tests, coagulopathy and anti-HCV reactive with HCV-RNA: 1.86×10^2 IU/mL, polymorphonuclear leucocytosis, spontaneous bacterial peritonitis, cholelithiasis, liver showing heterogeneous echotexture and skin showing small vessel vasculitis? HCV-related cryoglobulinemia. The test for cryoglobulins was negative (there are fallacies) but the C3 and C4 levels were low. At autopsy there was micronodular alcoholic cirrhosis with excessive fibrosis and disseminated fungal infection. Synergistic effect of alcohol intake and HCV-infection led to setting in of advanced cirrhosis, within a short period of time at a very young age. The liver showed classical features of alcoholic liver disease like macrovesicular steatosis, perivenular fibrosis, pericellular fibrosis, occasional Mallory's hyaline and satellitosis. No lymphoid follicles, lymphoplasmacytic infiltrate, bile duct damage or any necrosis around terminal hepatic venules was seen to suggest morphological evidence of hepatitis C infection. The extensive fibrosis seen in the liver was due to the synergistic hepatotoxic effect of both alcohol and HCV infection. Further there was a large ulcer on the dorsum of the right foot which was debrided. An antemortem skin biospy done, revealed small vessel vasculitis due to HCV-related cryoglobulinemia. The vasculitis further led to the deep ulcer on the dorsum of the foot. Apart from the above basic disease, there was a florid dual fungal infection starting from the lungs (granulomas were seen with giant cells containing fungal profiles) with dissemination to the heart and kidneys.

TAKE HOME MESSAGE

- Hepatitis C virus infection is a major cause of chronic liver disease worldwide.
- Alcohol and hepatitis C virus infection has a synergistic hepatotoxic effect leading to advanced liver disease in a short period of time.
- Mixed cryoglobulinemia is an extrahepatic complication of HCV infection and leads to small/medium vessel vasculitis in the skin, nerves and kidneys.

SUGGESTED READING

1. Armstrong GL, Wasley A, Simard EP, et al. The prevalence of hepatitis C virus infection in the United States, 1999 through 2002. Ann Intern Med. 2006;144(10):705-14.

2. Bouchier IA, Hislop WS, Prescott RJ. A prospective study of alcoholic liver disease and mortality. J Hepatol. 1992;16(3):290-7.
3. Charles ED, Dustin LB. Hepatitis C virus-induced Cryoglobulinemia. Kidney Int. 2009;76(8):818-24.
4. Clouston AD, Jonsson JR, Powell EE. Steatosis as a cofactor in other liver diseases: hepatitis C virus, alcohol, hemochromatosis and others. Clin Liver Dis. 2007;11(1): 173-89.
5. Hou W, Bukong TN, Kodys K, et al. Alcohol facilitates HCV-RNA replication via upregulation of miR-122 expression and inhibition of cyclin G1 in human hepatoma cells. Alcohol Clin Exp Res. 2013;37(4):599-608.
6. Ignacio Novo-Veleiro, Lucía Alvela-Suárez, Antonio-Javier Chamorro, et al. Hepatitis C Virus: Global view Alcoholic liver disease and hepatitis C virus infection. World J Gastroenterol. 2016;22(4):1411-20.
7. Min Hyeok Jee, Ka Young Hong, Ji Hoon Park, et al. (2015). A new mechanism of hepatic fibrogenesis: hepatitis C virus infection induces TGF-β1 production through glucose-regulated protein 94. [Online] Available from doi: 10.1128/JVI.02976-15 [Accessed on April, 2018].
8. Mueller S, Millonig G, Seitz HK. Alcoholic liver disease and hepatitis C: A frequently underestimated combination. World J Gastroenterol. 2009;15(28):3462-71.
9. Nalpas B, Thiers V, Pol S, et al. Hepatitis C viremia and anti-HCV antibodies in alcoholics. J Hepatol. 1992;14(2-3):381-4.
10. Pares A, Caballeria J, Bruguera M, et al. Histological course of alcoholic hepatitis- influence of abstinence, sex and extent of hepatic damage. J Hepatol. 1986;2(1):33-42.
11. Singal AK, Guturu P, Hmoud B et al. Evolving frequency and outcomes of liver transplantation based on etiology of liver disease. Transplantation. 2013;95(5):755-60.
12. Trujillo-Murillo K, Alvarez-Martínez O, Garza-Rodríguez L, et al. Additive effect of ethanol and HCV subgenomic replicon expression on COX-2 protein levels and activity. J Viral Hepat. 2007;14(9):608-17.
13. Wiley TE, McCarthy M, Breidi L, et al. Impact of alcohol on the histological and clinical progression of hepatitis C infection. Hepatology. 1998;28(3):805-9.

CONTRIBUTIONS BY:

1. Dr SK Sinha, Professor, Department of Gastroenterology (Compilation of Clinical Details)
2. Dr RK Kochhar, Professor and Head, Department of Gastroenterology (Clinician In-Charge)
3. Dr Narendra Dhaka, Assistant Professor, Department of Gastroenterology (Clinician In-Charge)
4. Dr TD Yadav, Professor, Department of General Surgery (Clinician In-Charge)

Post Graduate Institute of Medical Education and Research, Chandigarh, India.

CASE 25

Diffuse Hepatocellular Carcinoma Arising in a Setting of Mixed Nodular Cirrhosis, Hepatitis C Virus and Alcohol Related: PM 26695

Nandita Bharadwaj Kakkar

 HIGHLIGHTS OF THE CASE

A 44-year-old male, a follow-up case of cirrhosis, hepatitis C virus and alcohol-related, null responder to pegylated interferon (Peg-IFN) and ribavirin, with multifocal hepatocellular carcinoma (HCC), Barcelona clinic liver cancer-D (BCLC-D), post-transarterial chemoembolization {TACE—3 sessions)} decompensation, on antiviral dual therapy with sofosbuvir and ribavirin, presented with multiple episodes of upper gastrointestinal bleeding for one day. He was found to have anemia, icterus, spontaneous bacterial peritonitis, ascites, conjugated hyperbilirubinemia, thrombocytosis and esophageal varices. Autopsy revealed mixed nodular cirrhosis, hepatitis C virus/alcohol related with diffuse pattern of moderately differentiated hepatocellular carcinoma, with portal vein tumor thrombosis and florid lymphangitic carcinomatosis in the lung.

Keywords: Cirrhosis, hepatitis C, alcohol, multifocal, diffuse, hepatocellular carcinoma, lymphangitic carcinomatosis, incidental renal cell carcinoma and autopsy.

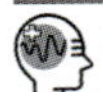 CLINICAL DETAILS

Date of Admission: 12.06.2015, Date of Death: 13.06.2015, Duration of Hospital Stay: 36 Hours

A 44-year-old male, who was on follow-up in our institute for hepatitis C virus and alcohol related cirrhosis since 2013, came with complaints of hematemesis and melena since one day. There were 5–6 episodes (one liter) of hematemesis in a single day associated with melena. There were no postural symptoms, altered sensorium, analgesic intake, pain abdomen, or any oliguria. In 2013 (October), he became symptomatic with weight loss and was detected to have cirrhosis, hepatitis C virus and alcohol related. In January 2014, HCV-RNA was 3.47×10^4 IU/mL, Genotype 1 and he was started on interferon and ribavirin. There was however no response and they were discontinued. In June 2014 the AFP was raised ($>$280 IU/mL). Contrast-enhanced MRI abdomen showed a single, space-occupying lesion {hepatocellular carcinoma (HCC)} in segment V, VI, VII of the liver. In November 2014 the patient underwent the first transarterial chemoembolization followed by a second one in December 2014. At the same time fluorodeoxyglucose positron emission tomography (FDG-PET) showed an uptake in right adrenals and a guided fine needle aspiration revealed a metastatic hepatocellular carcinoma. In February 2015, he was detected to have multi-centric HCC. The third TACE was done in March 2015 after which there was post-TACE decompensation in the form of jaundice and ascites. In April 2015, he was started on sofosbuvir and ribavirin. In May 2015, HCV-RNA levels were 4.9×10^4 IU/mL and he developed anemia, after which ribavirin was stopped. In May 2015, he developed decompensation in the form of ascites and spontaneous bacterial peritonitis. He was a chronic alcoholic since 10 years, consuming alcohol in cirrhogenic doses (100–120 g/day). He was a nonsmoker with no other addiction. On ***examination***: He was conscious, coherent, afebrile, pallor+, icterus+, cyanosis–, clubbing–, pulse 84/min, regular, BP– 110/80 mm Hg, respiratory rate– 22/min, JVP– Normal. The abdomen was distended, shifting dullness was present and bowel sounds were heard. Chest revealed bilateral vesicular breath sounds. Cardiovascular system and central nervous systems were within normal limits.

Investigations

Hematological: Hb-6.9 g/dL, TLC—9500/uL, platelets—584000/uL, Prothrombin time—100 secs.

Biochemistry/Microbiology/others—Na^+/K^+ 130/5.0 mEq/L, S.urea/ creatinine—84/1.5 mg%, S.bilirubin—6.8 mg% with conjugated fraction of 3.8 mg%, SGOT/SGPT—233/63 U/L, alkaline phosphatase—489 U/L; ***Blood/urine culture***: sterile; ***Routine urine examination***—normal; Serology—HIV non-reactive, HBsAg negative, total anti HB negative, anti HCV positive; ***Ascitic fluid***: (4.6.2015) - TLC 850, Polymorphs 50%, lymphocytes 50%, SAAG-2.5 g/dL, sugar 163 mg%, ADA-8 IU/L; ***FNAC*** right adrenal (8/1/15): metastatic HCC; ***ECG*** (1.6.2015): Within normal limit; ***Upper GI Endoscopy*** (29.9.13): Grade 1 x 2 esophageal varices, mild porto-hypertensive gastropathy in fundus.

Radiology: ***Triphasic CT*** (11/12/13): Findings suggestive of chronic liver disease, no hypervascular lesion seen; ***Contrast enhanced MRI*** (June 2014) of the abdomen showed a single, space occupying lesion (hepatocellular carcinoma- HCC) in segment V,VI,VII of the liver. ***FDG PET*** (30/12/14): FDG avid hypodense lesions with reticular calcification seen in the liver. Post TACE changes noted. FDG avid lesion seen in the right adrenal region. No definite evidence of abnormal hyper metabolism elsewhere in the body; ***Contrast enhanced MRI*** (12/2/15): chronic liver disease with portal vein thrombosis, portal hypertension with collaterals. Multiple small nodular hypervascular lesions in both lobes of liver with wash out in portal venous phase? Multicentric HCC .

On the day of admission, he had a cardiorespiratory arrest from which he could not be revived. ***Unit's Final Clinical Diagnosis*:** Cirrhosis - HCV and Alcohol related, PEG IFN Ribavirin null-responder, on Sofosbuvir-Ribavirin, Multifocal HCC (BCLC- Barcelona Clinic Liver Cancer- D), Post 3 TACE sessions, decompensated ascites, spontaneous bacterial peritonitis, metastatis to right adrenal gland, portal vein thrombosis, upper gastrointestinal bleeding ? Variceal.

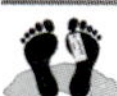

AUTOPSY FINDINGS: PM 26695

A partial autopsy was performed. Both pleural cavities and peritoneal cavity contained 1,000 mL and 2,000 mL of straw colored fluid respectively. There was blood around the nose, body was icteric, moderately built with facial and pedal edema. The ***liver*** was enlarged and weighed 2,800 g. Capsular aspect showed multiple nodules, ranging in size from 0.2–1.5 cm in diameter (Fig 1A). Coronal slices of the liver were firm, bile-stained and showed varying sized nodules, ranging in size from 0.2–2 cm in diameter and few of the larger nodules (red arrows) showed central necrosis (Figs 1B and C). The portal vein contained a thrombus (Fig 1D). There was a large tumor nodule in the liver (Fig 1D, black circle), just above the entry of the portal vein measuring 2 cm in diameter and it also showed central necrosis. This was the point at which the tumor was seen to infiltrate the major branch of the portal vein and then continued into the portal vein as the tumor thrombus (Fig 1D). Microscopic examination (Fig 2A) revealed varying sized regenerative nodules separated by fibrous septae, which were better brought out by reticulin and Masson's trichrome stain (Figs 2B and C). The septae contained lymphomononuclear infiltrate and at places showed bile ductular proliferation (Fig 2A). No lymphoid aggregates or any bile duct damage was noted. Focal piece meal necrosis was however seen. The hepatocytes showed focal macrovesicular steatosis and cholestasis (Fig 2D). Focal perivenular and pericellular fibrosis was seen. No Mallory's hyaline or any neutrophilic satellitosis was seen. Thus, on morphology there was no morphologic evidence of hepatitis C virus infection. Morphology suggestive of alcoholic etiology was however seen. Both alcohol usage and hepatitis C infection, due to their well-known synergistic effect led to cirrhosis in the index case. Apart from the background cirrhosis, there were diffusely scattered nodules (Figs 3A and B) showing frank features of a moderately differentiated hepatocellular carcinoma (HCC). The HCC showed a transition from small tumor nodules (Fig 3C) arising in the center of the cirrhotic nodules (nodule in nodule) to the entire cirrhotic nodule getting converted into a tumor nodule (Figs 3A and B). About 40% of the cirrhotic nodules contained HCC either as a nodule within a nodule, or occupying the entire cirrhotic nodule or as larger nodules ranging in size from 0.5–2 cm in diameter. The reticulin stain showed loss of reticulin fibers in the tumor nodules (Fig 3D). The tumor cells exihibited a trabecular pattern (sinusoidal, plate-like) with plates more than 3-cells thick (Figs 4A and B) and in few areas a compact pattern was noted. In areas, the tumor cells (Figs 4C–F) were large with pronounced nuclear atypia and hyperchromasia, prominent nucleoli, giant cells, mitosis greater than 5/10 HPF along with atypical mitosis, areas of necrosis conforming to the morphology of poorly differentiated HCC. No bile was seen in the tumor cells. Immunohistochemistry done for HbsAg and HbcAg was negative, HepPar-1 (Fig 5A) showed focal positivity in the tumor cells and CD34 (Figs 5B and C) showed diffuse sinusoidal positivity indicating capillarization of the sinusoids, which is a feature seen in HCC. Overall features were those of a diffuse pattern of trabecular, moderately differentiated HCC, arising in a background of cirrhosis (both hepatitis C and alcohol related) along with portal vein infiltration. The ***spleen*** (Fig 1C) was enlarged (250 g) and showed features of congestive splenomegaly. The ***gastro-esophageal*** junction (Figs 5D and E) revealed varices and the

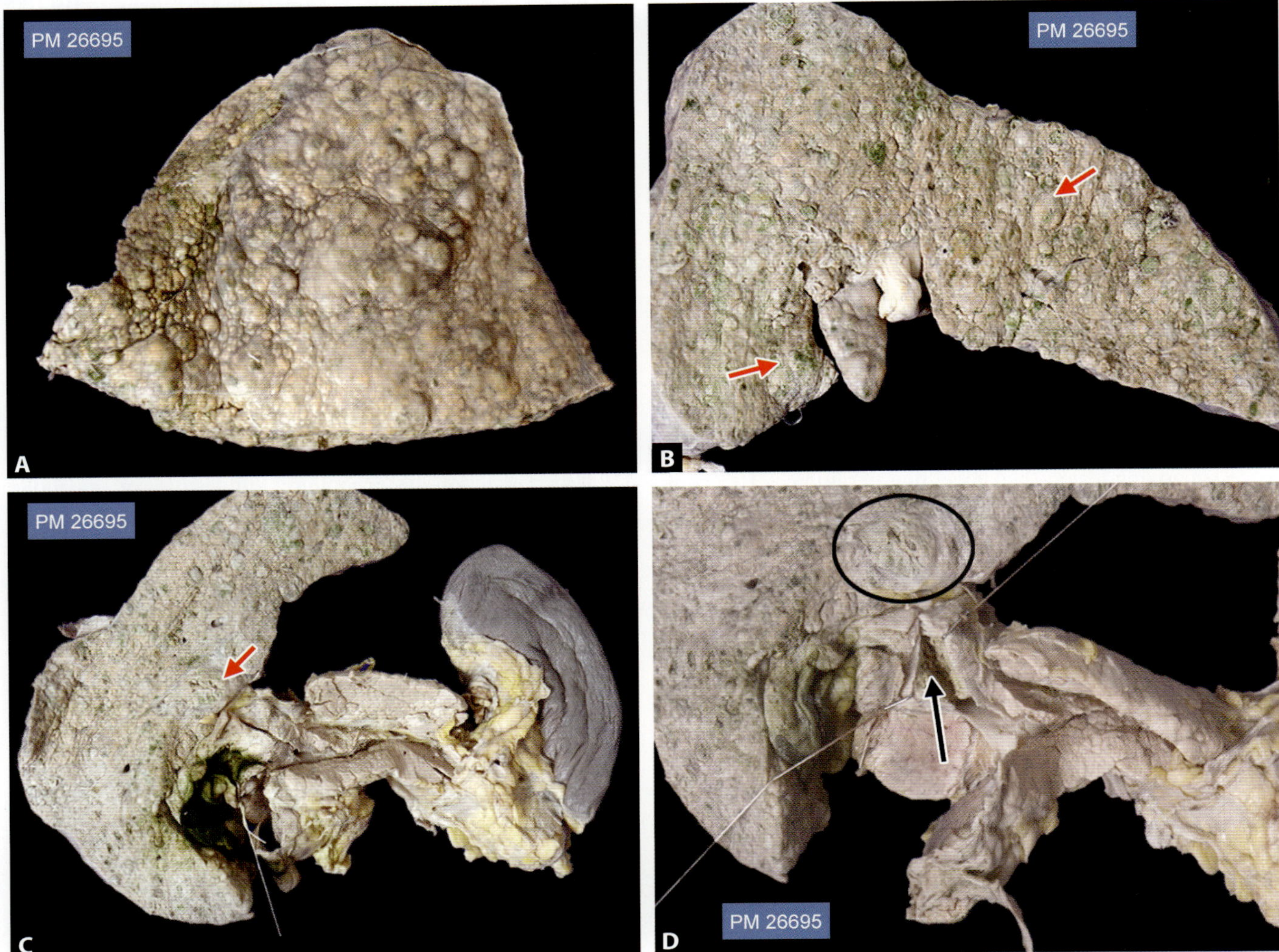

Figs 1A–D: (A) Capsular aspect of the liver shows varying sized nodules; (B) Cut section of the liver shows mixed nodular cirrhosis, few larger nodules (arrows) are seen, some with central areas of necrosis; (C) Organ complex of the slice of liver showing cirrhosis and a large nodule with central necrosis (arrow), gallbladder, cut open pancreas and slice of enlarged spleen; (D) The opened-up portal vein at the porta hepatis showing a thrombus (long black arrow). A large nodule (circle) is seen just above the point of entry of the portal vein which shows central necrosis.

fundus of the stomach showed features of portal gastropathy. Rest of the GIT was normal. The ***lungs*** (Fig 6A) together weighed 1,000 g. The pleura were dull and there was 500 mL of straw-colored fluid in each pleural cavity. Cut section was subcrepitant with areas of hemorrhage. Microscopic examination revealed alveolar hemorrhage, edema and prominent lymphangitic carcinomatosis with lymphatic spaces clogged with tumor, with morphology of hepatocellular carcinoma (Fig 6B). The hilar lymph nodes were free of tumor. The ***kidneys*** together weighed 450 g. Capsular aspect was unremarkable. Cut-section showed a yellowish tumor nodule in the upper pole of the left kidney (Fig 6C-arrow), measuring 1.3 cm in diameter. Sections from the nodule showed a tumor with features of a clear cell, conventional renal cell carcinoma (RCC) (Fuhrman grade 1). The tumor cells were arranged in a tubulopapillary pattern and showed abundant clear cytoplasm (Fig 6D). Immunohistochemistry reveled strong membranous positivity with CD10 (Fig 6E) and a very focal positivity with CK7, thus negating a clear cell papillary carcinoma. No capsular, sinus or vascular invasion was noted. Overall features were those of an incidental, clear cell RCC. The adjacent kidney showed normal glomeruli, blood vessels and tubular calcification. The ***heart*** weighed 385 g. The valves and chambers were normal. The left anterior descending and left circumflex artery showed 45%

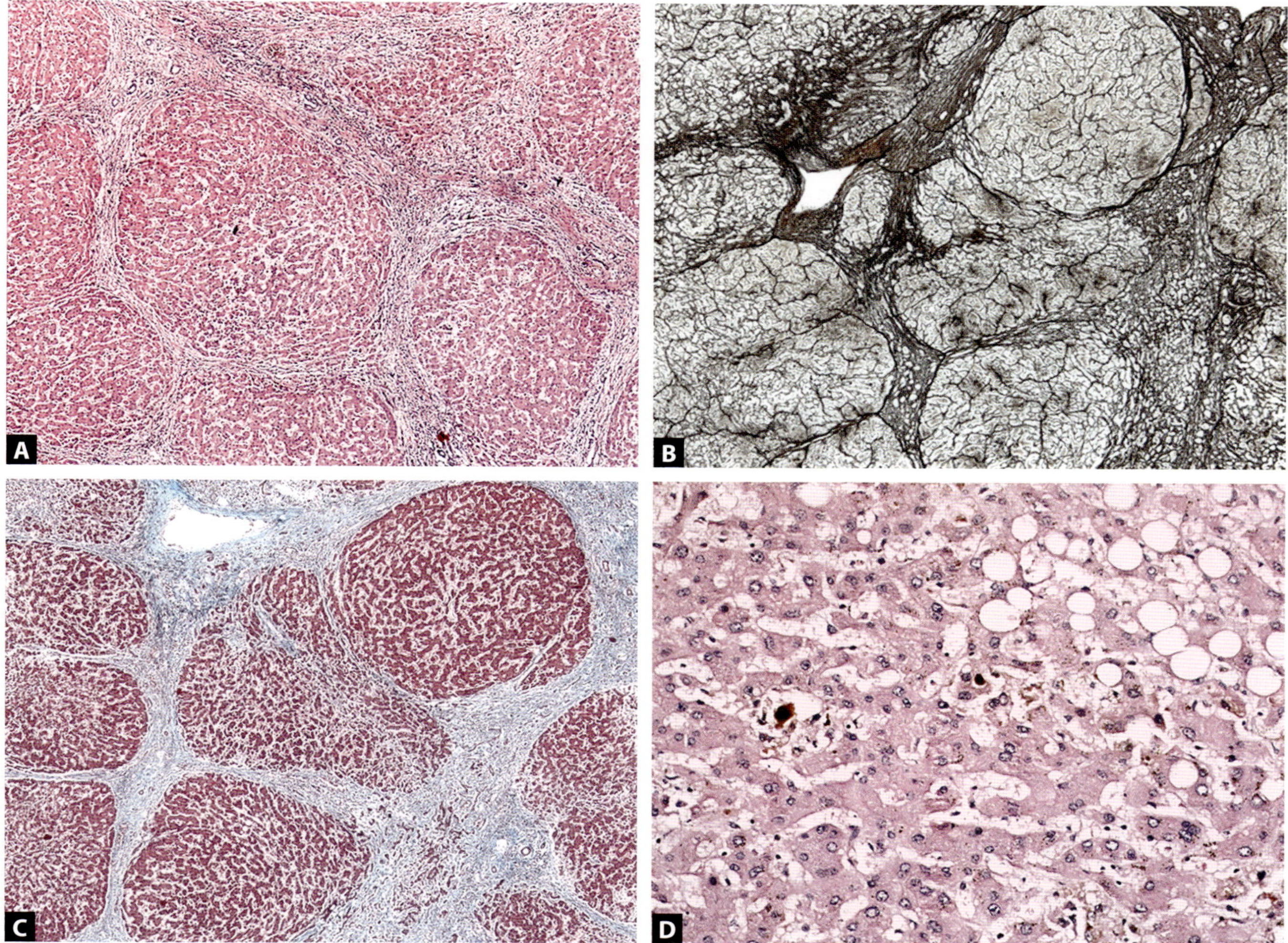

Figs 2A–D: (A–C) Microphotographs of the liver shows loss of architecture and varying sized nodules surrounded by fibrous septae in (A) H&E stain; (B) Reticulin stain; (C) Masson's trichrome stain; (D) Hepatocytes showed focal macrovesicular steatosis and cholestasis.

atherosclerotic narrowing. The right coronary artery showed 25% narrowing. Both the adrenals were blocked in toto and did not reveal any metastasis.

FINAL AUTOPSY DIAGNOSIS : PM 26695

44 Years Male

- Mixed nodular cirrhosis, hepatitis C virus/alcohol-related, with diffuse pattern of moderately differentiated hepatocellular carcinoma.
- Portal hypertension—congestive splenomegaly, ascites, esophageal varices.
- Pulmonary edema, alveolar hemorrhage, pleural effusion and lymphangitic carcinomatosis.
- Incidental renal cell carcinoma: Clear cell conventional—left kidney.

HEPATOCELLULAR CARCINOMA AND CIRRHOSIS

Hepatocellular carcinoma, the fifth most common cancer worldwide, constitutes approximately 80–90% of primary hepatic malignancies in adults. Any chronic liver injury especially associated with cirrhosis, particularly due to hepatitis B, hepatitis C virus infections, alcohol and non-alcoholic steatohepatitis, predisposes to HCC. High-risk etiologies for HCC include HBV, HCV, hereditary hemochromatosis, tyrosenemia, intermediate risk include alcohol, α-1 antitrypsin deficiency, glycogen storage disorder, autoimmune hepatitis and low risk include primary biliary cirrhosis, primary sclerosing cholangitis, fructose intolerance, paucity of intrahepatic bile ducts, congenital hepatic fibrosis, Wilsons disease etc. Earlier, HCC was seen more in HBV-infections, but since now the number of cases of HCV have gone up

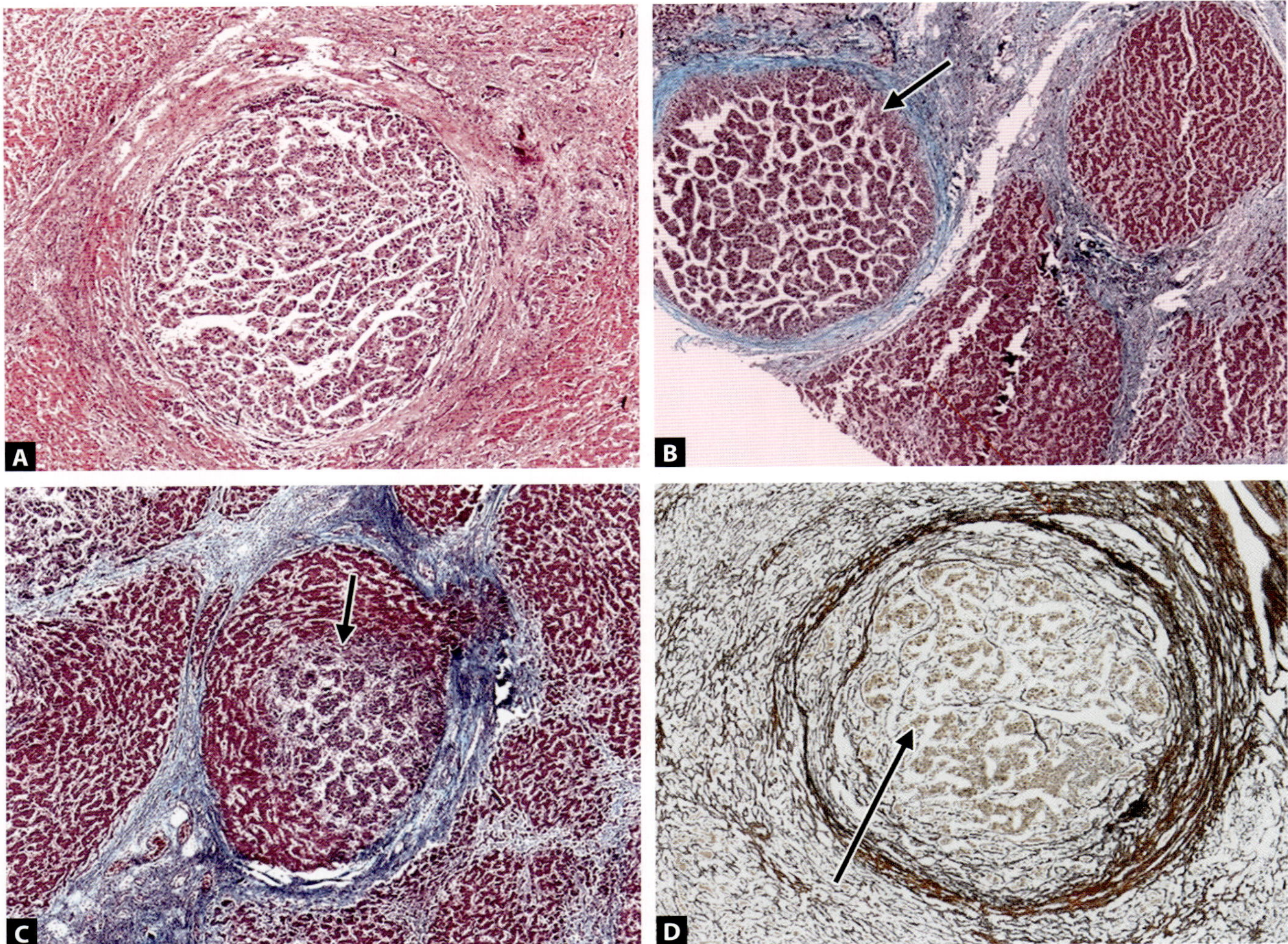

Figs 3A–D: Microphotographs of the liver. (A) Small tumor nodule with morphology of HCC; (B) Masson's trichrome stain shows a tumor nodule (arrow) with adjacent regenerative cirrhotic nodules; (C) HCC (arrow) arising in a regenerative nodule i.e. *nodule within a nodule* (D) Reticulin poor tumor nodule (arrow).

worldwide, HCC is seen more with HCV. HBV is carcinogenic as it can integrate into the host genome leading to chromosomal instability, causes insertional mutations leading to activation of genes involved in cell proliferation and the HBX viral protein modulates cell proliferation and inactivates p53 activities. HCV is a single-stranded RNA virus and does not get integrated into the hepatocytic genome, but leads to HCC through indirect pathways which include chronic inflammation, cell death and proliferation. But transgenic mouse models postulate that HCV has a direct carcinogenic effect on the hepatocytes.

Hepatitis C virus infection was identified in 1989, when patients given blood transfusions acquired a peculiar type of *non-A*, *non-B* hepatitis. HCV has a tremendous effect on the community health, as its incidence is rampantly going up. A diagnosis of having acquired-HCV is not possible in the acute phase i.e. in the first 6 months after infection, as it is asymptomatic. This single-stranded virus belongs to the flaviviridae family, has three major genotypes, each having many subtypes. Subtype 1b carries the greatest risk of chronicity and finally HCC. Majority of the acute infections however progress to chronic HCV, although a small number resolves itself. Acquisition of HCV is through blood and blood products, intravenous drug usage, occupational blood exposure, hemodialysis and transplantation of infected organs. In the western world, HCV is the commonest cause of chronic liver disease and cirrhosis. HCV-infected individuals have a 17-fold increased risk of developing HCC, which

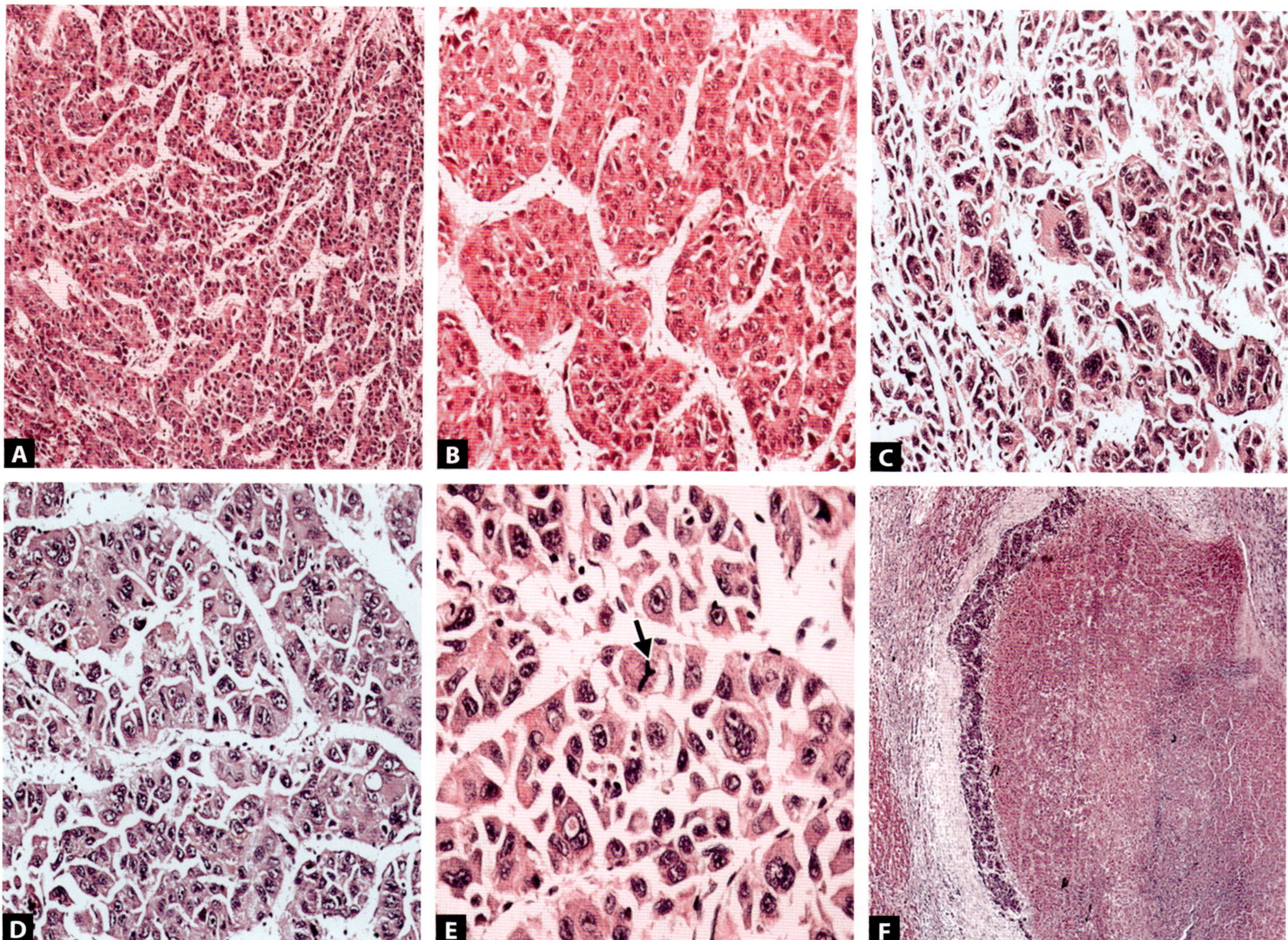

Figs 4A–F: (A and B) HCC shows a trabecular pattern; (C and D) HCC shows pronounced nuclear atypia and hyperchromasia; (E) HCC shows atypical mitosis (arrow); (F) Tumor nodule shows central area of necrosis.

develops within 10–20 years of acquiring HCV infection. This increased risk is directly proportional to the presence of cirrhosis/advanced fibrosis. Hepatitis C virus infection and alcohol intake have a synergistic hepatotoxic effect and when seen together, leads to early onset of advanced liver disease, leading on to cirrhosis and further HCC (*see* PM case no. 27791).

COMMENTARY—INDEX CASE: PM 26695

A 44-year-old male, a follow-up case of cirrhosis, hepatitis C virus and alcohol related, null responder to PEG-IFN and ribavirin, with multifocal HCC, BCLC-D, post-TACE (3 sessions) decompensation, on antiviral dual therapy with sofosbuvir and ribavirin, presented with multiple episodes of upper gastrointestinal bleeding for one day. He was found to have anemia, icterus, spontaneous bacterial peritonitis, ascites, conjugated hyperbilirubinemia, thrombocytosis and esophageal varices. Autopsy revealed mixed nodular cirrhosis, hepatitis C virus/alcohol-related with diffuse pattern of moderately differentiated hepatocellular carcinoma, with portal vein tumor thrombosis and florid lymphangitic carcinomatosis in the lung. This middle-aged man was consuming alcohol in cirrhogenic doses and was also hepatitis C positive (January 2014, HCV-RNA was 3.47×10^4 IU/mL and May 2015 HCV-RNA levels were 4.9×10^4 IU/mL). He developed cirrhosis at a young age because of the synergistic action of both alcohol and hepatitis C virus infection. The cirrhosis was mixed nodular, but signs of alcoholic etiology were discernable, like presence of micronodules, macrovesicular steatosis and focal perivenular/pericellular fibrosis.

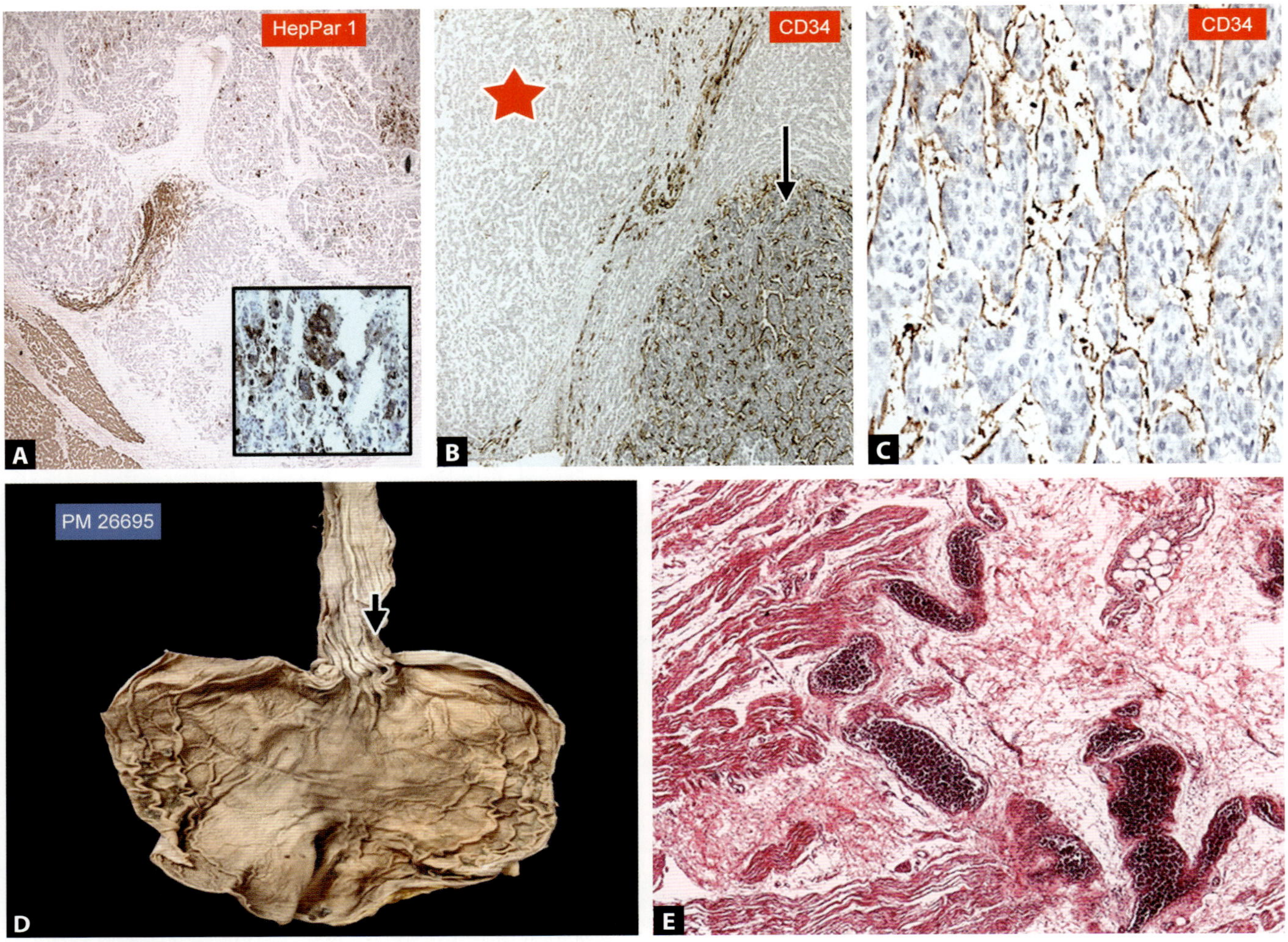

Figs 5A–E: (A) Hep-Par 1 immunostain shows focal positivity in the tumor cells; (B and C) CD34 immunostain shows diffuse sinusoidal positivity in the tumor nodule (arrow), a feature seen in HCC. Adjacent cirrhotic nodules in B (star) do not show this pattern with CD34; (D) Gross photograph of the esophagus and stomach showing varices (arrow); (E) Varices confirmed on microscopy.

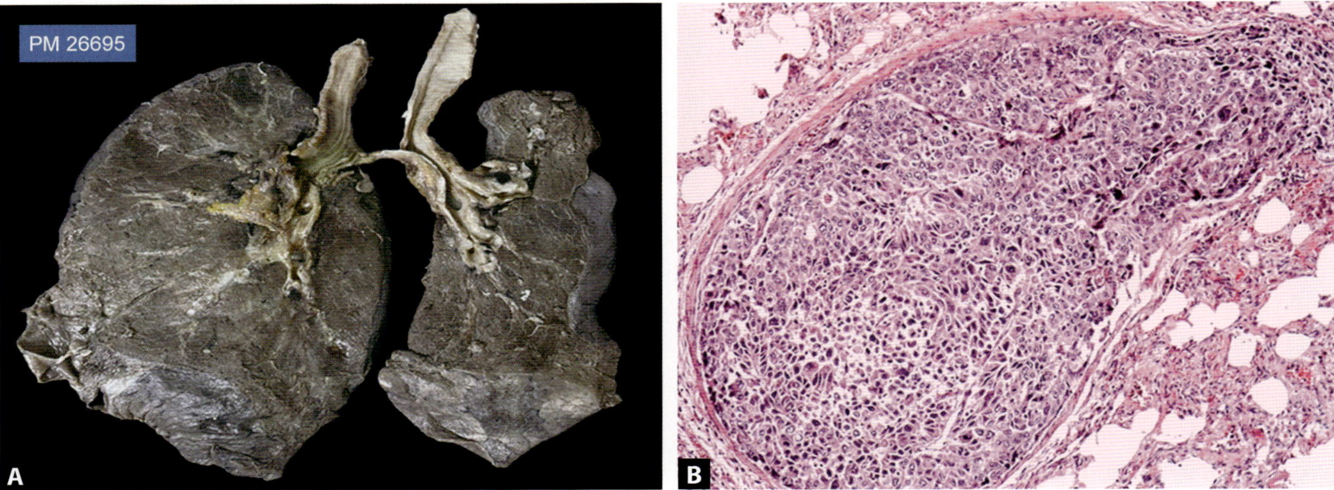

Figs 6A and B:

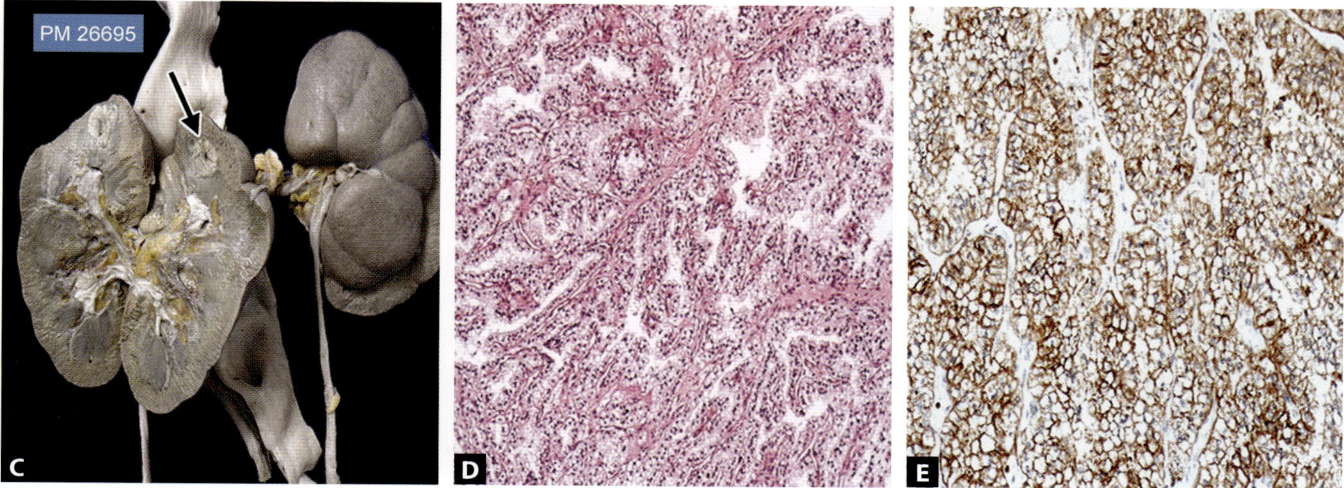

Figs 6A–E: (A) Gross photograph of both lungs. No focal lesion seen; (B) Lymphangitic carcinomatosis in the lungs; (C) Gross photograph of the kidneys. Left kidney shows a well-circumscribed tumor nodule (arrow); (D) Kidney tumor nodule shows features of clear cell RCC; (E) Kidney tumor shows strong positivity with CD10 immunostain.

No lymphoid aggregates or any bile duct injury was noted to suggest morphological evidence of HCV infection. The HCC present in the index case was of the diffuse type with numerous nodules present all over and a large number of them with *nodule in nodule* morphology as explained above, where-in the tumor is indiscernable from the cirrhotic nodule and is referred to as *cirrhotomimetic*.

TAKE HOME MESSAGE

- Hepatitis C virus infection and alcohol intake have a synergistic hepatotoxic effect and when seen together, leads to early onset of advanced liver disease, leading on to cirrhosis and further HCC.
- Both HCV and alcoholic liver injury is a risk factor for acquiring hepatocellular carcinoma.

SUGGESTED READING

1. Andrade LJDO, D'Oliveira A, Melo RC, et al. Association between hepatitis C and hepatocellular carcinoma. J Glob Infect Dis. 2009;1(1):33-7.
2. Koike K. Hepatitis C virus contributes to hepatocarcinogenesis by modulating metabolic and intracellular pathways. J Gastroenterol Hepatol. 2007;22(Suppl. 1):501-2.
3. Takano S, Yokosuka O, Imazeki F, et al. Incidence of hepatocellular carcinoma in chronic hepatitis B and C: A prospective study of 251 cases. Hepatology. 1995;21(3):650-5.

CONTRIBUTIONS BY:

1. Dr Virender Singh, Professor, Department of Gastroenterology (Compilation of Clinical Details)
2. Dr Naveen Kalra, Professor, Department of Radiodiagnosis and Imaging
3. Dr Ashish Bhalla, Professor, Department of Internal Medicine (Clinician In-Charge)
4. Dr RK Kochhar, Professor and Head, Department of Gastroenterology (Clinician In-Charge)

Post Graduate Institute of Medical Education and Research, Chandigarh, India.

CASE 26

Acute Liver Failure and Encephalopathy in a Case of Dengue Shock Syndrome: PM 25035

Nandita Bharadwaj Kakkar

HIGHLIGHTS OF THE CASE

A 23-year-old male, nonalcoholic, came with fever, rash, jaundice, encephalopathy, ascites and acute liver failure. There was hepatomegaly, conjugated hyperbilirubinemia, marked elevation of transaminases (AST > ALT in thousands), coagulopathy, anemia, thrombocytopenia, leukocytosis and dengue by IgM capture ELISA was positive. All viral/autoimmune markers were negative. Autopsy revealed ascites, pleural effusion, extensive bland zonal coagulative hepatocytic necrosis in zone 2 extending on to zone 3, however sparing the periportal hepatocytes (zone 1), along with a confluent necrotizing pneumonia.

Keywords: Dengue infection, zonal necrosis, acute liver failure, autopsy.

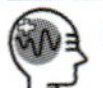

CLINICAL HISTORY

Date of Admission: 29.09.2012, Date of Death: 02.10.2012, Duration of Hospital Stay: 3 days

A 24-year-old male came to PGIMER Chandigarh, with a sudden onset of an acute febrile illness with jaundice and altered sensorium. He came with complaints of fever and rash for 10 days. There was nausea, vomiting, jaundice since 6 days and altered sensorium for the last 2 days. There was no previous history of jaundice, surgery or blood transfusions. He was a nonsmoker and did not consume alcohol. On general physical examination he was drowsy, not arousable with a status of E3M3V1. The pulse was 120/min, regular, blood pressure 102/70 mm Hg and respiratory rate 20/min. There was pallor, icterus and erythematous, non-blanchable maculopapular rash over trunks, axilla and extremities. The liver (span 16 cm) was palpable 1 cm below right costal margin, was soft, nontender, nonpulsatile with no bruit or hum, with regular margins and a smooth surface. On central nervous system examination there were no meningeal signs but the reflexes were sluggish with mute plantars and a decerebrate posturing.

Investigations

Investigations revealed hemoglobin of 14.7 g/dL which within 3 days fell to 7.4 g/dL. The TLC was 15,000/µL with a polymorphonuclear leukocytosis and the platelet count decreased from 1,95,000/µL to 31000/µL within the four-days of hospital stay. ***Liver function tests*** were markedly deranged with elevated serum bilirubin (11.2 mg% with conjugated fraction of 8.18 mg%), aspartate aminotransferase (AST – 3,760 U/L), alanine aminotransferase (ALT – 2,890 U/L) and alkaline phosphatase (252 U/L). Total proteins were 6.2 gms which fell to 4.5 gms and albumin went down from 3.8 to 2.3 gms. The ***coagulogram*** was also deranged with a PT of 28 sec, PTI—50%, INR 1.91, aPTT 60 sec, fibrinogen 1.18 mg/dL and D-dimers were positive. Serum electrolytes, urea, creatinine, uric acid, lipase and amylase were within normal limits. ***Ultrasound abdomen*** showed a liver span of 15 cm with normal echotexture and intrahepatic biliary radicles. Minimal ascites and bilateral pleural effusion was noted. ***Non-contrast CT scan (NCCT)*** head revealed cerebral edema. Hemolytic workup was normal. Markers for autoimmune hepatitis and serology for hepatitis A virus (HAV), hepatitis E virus (HEV), hepatitis B surface antigen (HBsAG), hepatitis C virus (HCV), human immunodeficiency virus (HIV), Epstein-Barr virus (EBV), cytomegalovirus (CMV) and leptospira was negative. Widal/peripheral smear for malarial parasite/QDXMP/malarial antigen/Weil-Felix were negative. Routine urine analysis, urine culture, blood culture and CSF were within normal limits. ***Dengue*** serology was done 6 days after the onset of fever wherein NS1, antigen was negative but dengue by IgM capture ELISA was positive (supplied by National Institute of Virology Pune). On the fourth-day of hospital stay the patient had an episode of bradycardia followed by cardiac arrest, CPR was done but the patient could not be revived. ***Unit clinical diagnosis*** was dengue shock syndrome with acute liver failure, rash, coagulopathy and encephalopathy.

AUTOPSY FINDINGS: PM 25035

A partial autopsy was performed on this 24-year-old male who died after a hospital stay of 3 days. On external examination the body was icteric. The peritoneal and pleural cavities contained 500 mL and 100 mL of straw-colored fluid respectively. The ***liver*** weighed 1,500 g and was deeply bile stained (Fig 1A). Microscopic examination revealed extensive areas of bland coagulative hepatocytic necrosis in zone 2 and zone 3, however sparing the periportal hepatocytes (zone 1) (Figs 1B and C). The necrotic areas (Fig 1D) showed condensation of reticulin framework, RBC's, macrophages, acidophil bodies and scanty inflammatory infiltrate composed of polymorphs, lymphocytes and plasma cells. The periportal hepatocytes revealed microvesicular steatosis and canalicular cholestasis. Viral inclusions were not seen and immunostains for herpes simplex virus was negative. Detection of dengue virus RNA by reverse transcription polymerase chain reaction (RT-PCR) was done on the postmortem liver sample but

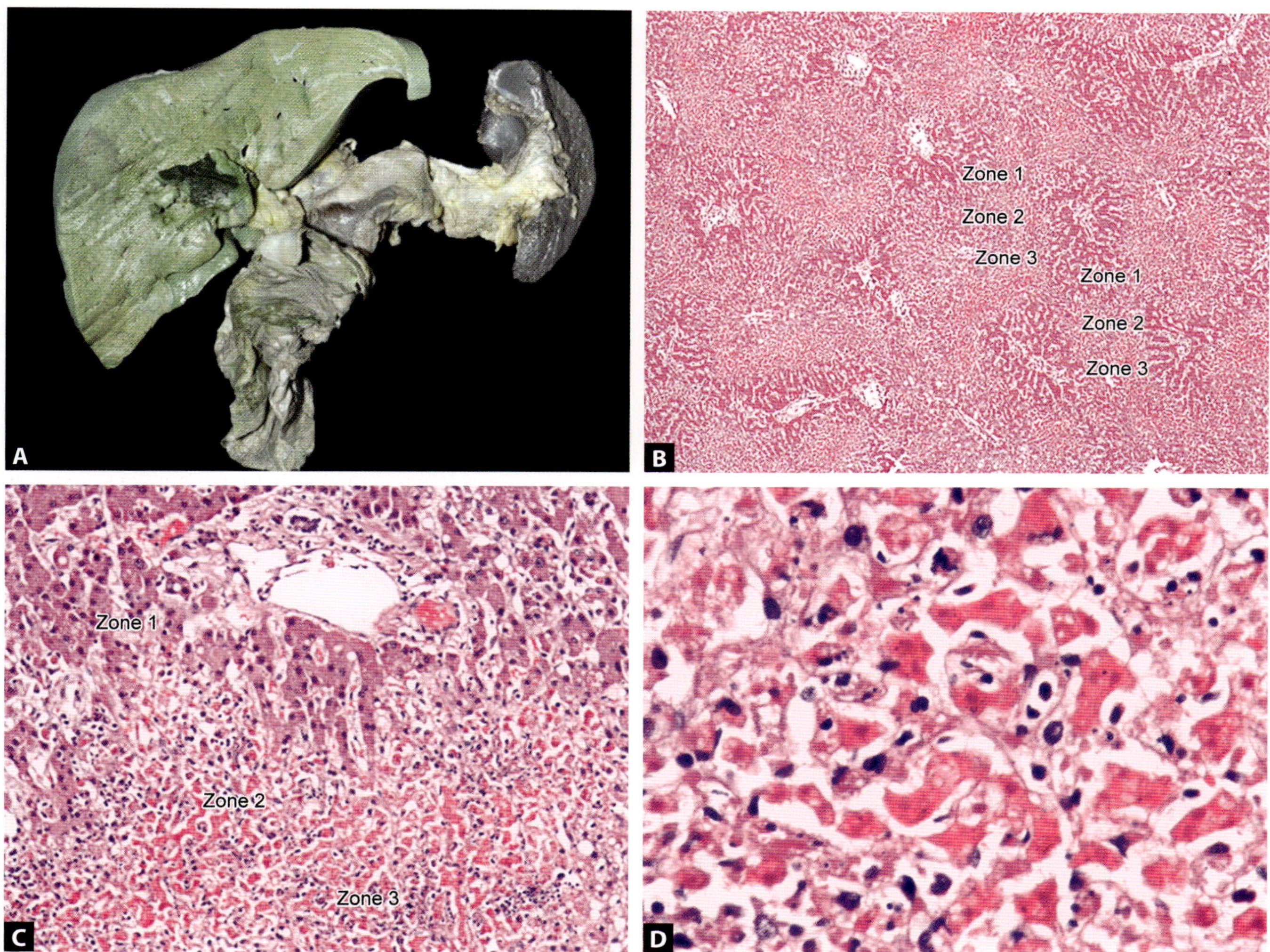

Figs 1A–D: (A) Organ complex comprising of slice of liver, spleen, gallbladder, c loop of duodenum, and pancreas. Liver is bile stained and weighed 1,500 g; (B and C) Microphotograph of the liver at low, and high power showing zonal (zone 2, 3) hepatocytic necrosis, sparing periportal i.e. zone 1 hepatocytes; (D) Areas of necrosis showing nuclear debris and hypereosinophilic necrosed hepatocytes.

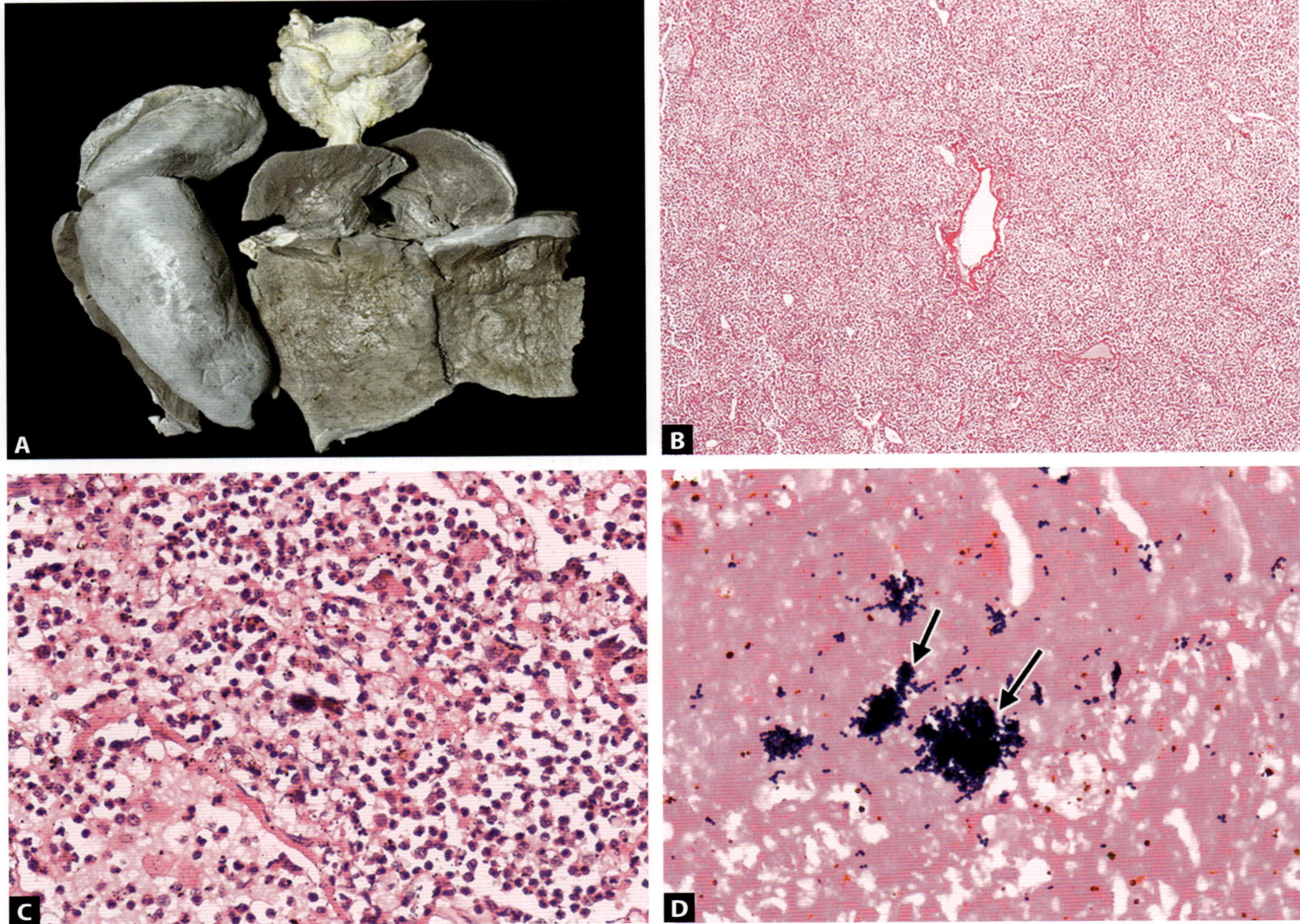

Figs 2A–D: (A) Lungs show areas of discoloration on the pleural aspect and cut section shows consolidation; (B) Low power of the lungs showing alveolar spaces packed with inflammatory infiltrate; (C) High-power view shows polymorphs, nuclear debris and fibrin; (D) Grams stain shows gram-positive cocci (arrows).

was found to be negative. Both ***lungs*** (Fig 2A) on cut section revealed areas of consolidation. On microscopic examination (Figs 2B–D) there was evidence of acute necrotizing pneumonia replete with gram-positive cocci. ***Kidneys*** were normal grossly but exhibited early acute tubular necrosis. Other organs were grossly and microscopically normal.

FINAL AUTOPSY DIAGNOSIS: PM 25035

23 Years Male—Dengue by IgM Capture ELISA Positive

- Extensive zonal hepatic necrosis (zone 2 and 3) consistent with dengue shock syndrome.
- Confluent necrotizing pneumonia—bacterial.
- Early acute tubular necrosis in the kidney.

DENGUE INFECTION

Dengue virus is a RNA virus, member of the genus ***flavivirus*** and family flaviviridae. It is transmitted by the mosquito, Aedes aegypti which is the principal vector and Aedes albopictus which is the secondary vector. The diagnosis of dengue infection (DI) is based on clinical presentation with fever of short duration ($<$15 days) and thrombocytopenia (platelet count $< 100 \times 10^9$/L), irrespective of the presence or absence of hemorrhagic manifestations. Patients are grouped into dengue fever (DF), dengue hemorrhagic fever (DHF) and dengue shock syndrome (DSS) using the WHO criteria. Dengue fever (DF) is defined as fever with constitutional symptoms and the only hemorrhagic manifestation is a positive tourniquet test. In addition, in DHF, there are bleeding manifestations and in DSS there is circulatory collapse with hypotension. In India, dengue infection is a major health problem, has high mortality and multiple serotypes are seen i.e. DEN-1, DEN-2, DEN-3 and DEN-4. Further sequencing has brought out the presence of multiple genotypes for each serotype. Spread of virus serotypes and genotypes to new areas increases the risk of dengue hemorrhagic fever and dengue shock syndrome. A second-episode of infection with DF increases the susceptibility of developing DHF or DSS. At present DEN-1 and DEN-2 are widespread in India and these two serotypes have a higher incidence of involvement of the liver.

Hepatocellular damage does occur in dengue infection but acute liver failure is a rare occurrence. Serum transaminases are elevated in 90% cases of dengue infection. Kularatne et al found moderate serum transaminase elevation (2 times the normal) in 88% of their patients, Nguyen et al found 5 times elevation in transaminase levels and Itha et al found levels exceeding 5 times the upper limit being present in 22% of DF, 27% of DHF and 86% of DSS patients. Liver involvement has been reported to be more profound in DHF/DSS. ALT elevation exceeding 5-fold the normal, represents a greater degree of liver damage. The biochemical pattern of liver injury in patients with dengue infection is similar to that observed among patients with acute viral hepatitis i.e. marked elevation of serum aminotransferases. The magnitude of elevation of ALT and AST levels is comparable and no preferential elevation of one of these enzymes is observed. In view of this biochemical pattern, it is possible to confuse liver involvement in dengue infection (DI) with typical acute viral hepatitis, especially in countries where outbreaks of hepatitis A and E are common. However, the presence of low platelets and persistence of fever after the appearance of jaundice, takes us towards a diagnosis of DI and serological tests help further. The severity of liver injury is unlikely to be a pointer to the diagnosis, since liver disease can be very severe even in DI. Ascites occurs in DI and based on high ascitic fluid protein concentration, it has been attributed to excessive leakage of plasma. SAAG greater than 1.1 g/dL is seen in patients with DI and this indicates that portal hypertension contributes to the development of ascites. Microscopic examination of the liver in DSS shows a characteristic zonal, bland coagulative hepatocytic necrosis in zone 2 extending on to zone 3, however sparing the periportal hepatocytes (zone 1).

The mechanism of liver injury in DI remains unclear. Hepatocytic damage occurs due to any or a combination of the following:

- Direct hepatopathic effect of the virus.
- Host-immune response eliminates the hepatocytes packed with the virus.
- A non-specific effect of shock and hypotension.

A high frequency of liver injury among patients with uncomplicated DI, in the absence of hypotension suggests that the injury is specific. The presence of dengue virus antigens and nucleic acid has been shown in liver tissue using immunohistochemistry, in situ hybridization and in situ polymerase chain reaction technique. In recent years, dengue-specific CD4+ and CD8+ T cells have been shown to play a part in the pathogenesis of severe forms of DI. Occurrence of more severe liver injury in patients with complicated dengue may thus suggest a role for host-immune responses in the causation of liver injury.

Diagnosis of dengue is confirmed by the detection of dengue-specific IgM antibodies, but these are detected only after 5–10 days of fever in case of primary dengue and 4–5 days in secondary dengue. Recently, the detection of non-structural protein 1 (NS1) antigen by ELISA has brought in a revolution in the early/quick diagnosis of dengue, which can be detected on first day of fever by this method (sensitivity 65–100%). Singh et al in a study from India have reported NS1 antigen sensitivity of 71–100% till D3 of fever with corresponding IgM sensitivity of 0–50%. They reported that at D4, both IgM capture ELISA (MAC-ELISA) and NS1 done together, increases the sensitivity of diagnosis. After D5, MAC-ELISA IgM antibody detection gives 100% positivity. Dengue Duo test (NS1/IgM/IgG) is now available as a strip test. Early diagnosis is also possible by detection of dengue virus RNA by RT-PCR which is positive till about 5 days after the onset of fever. However, this requires a sophisticated molecular diagnostic laboratory and also the maintenance of cold chain during sample transport.

COMMENTARY—INDEX CASE: PM 25035

The index case is a proven case of dengue shock syndrome presenting with acute liver failure, rash and encephalopathy. The liver function tests were markedly deranged, there being a conjugated hyperbilirubinemia, marked elevation (in thousands) of transaminases (AST > ALT) and coagulopathy. ALT elevation exceeding 5-fold the normal, represents a greater degree of liver damage. All viral/autoimmune markers were negative. Dengue serology done 6 days after the onset of fever showed non-structural protein 1 (NS1) antigen to be negative, but dengue by IgM capture ELISA was positive (supplied by National Institute of Virology, Pune). Dengue serology by NS1 antigen is positive as early as day 1 till day 5 after the onset of fever and IgM capture ELISA gives 100% result beyond day 5. Detection of dengue virus RNA by RT-PCR was done on the postmortem liver sample (day 14 of fever) but was found to be negative. Autopsy revealed ascites, pleural effusion, extensive bland coagulative hepatocytic necrosis in zone 2 extending on to zone 3, however sparing the periportal hepatocytes (zone 1) which is very typically seen in liver involvement in DSS.

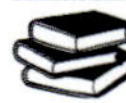

TAKE HOME MESSAGE

- Patients of dengue infection are grouped into dengue fever, dengue hemorrhagic fever and dengue shock syndrome using the WHO criteria.
- Acute liver failure occurs rarely in dengue infection.
- Serology for dengue—NS1 antigen is positive from day 1 till day 5 after onset of fever and IgM capture ELISA is positive after day 5 of fever.
- Detection of dengue virus RNA by RT-PCR is positive from day 1 till day 5, after onset of fever.
- Microscopic examination of the liver in dengue shock syndrome shows a characteristic zonal, bland coagulative hepatocytic necrosis in zone 2 extending on to zone 3, however sparing the periportal hepatocytes (zone 1).

SUGGESTED READING

1. Besoff K, Delorey M, Sun W, et al. Comparison of two commercially available dengue virus (DENV) NS1 capture enzyme linked immunosorbant assays using a clinical sample for the diagnosis of acute DENV infection. Clin Vaccine Immunol. 2008;15(10):1513-8.
2. Dussart P, Labeau B, Lagathu G, et al. Evaluation of an enzyme immunoassay for the detection of dengue virus NS1 antigen in human serum. Clin Vaccine Immunol. 2006; 13(11):1185-9.
3. Gasperino J, Yunen J, Guh A, et al. Fulminant liver failure secondary to hemorrhagic dengue in an international traveler. Liver Int. 2007;27(8):1148-51.
4. Huerre M, Lan N, Marianneau P, et al. Liver histopathology and biological correlates in five cases of fatal dengue fever in Vietnamese children. Vichows Arch. 2001;438(2):107-15.
5. Itha S, Kashyuap R, Krishnani N et al. Profile of liver involvement in dengue virus infection. Natl Med J India. 2005;18(3):127-30.
6. Kabra SK, Jain Y, Pandey RM, et al. Dengue hemorrhagic fever in children in the 1996 Delhi epidemic. Trans R Soc Trop Med Hyg. 1999;93(3):294-8.
7. Kularatne SA, Gawarammana IB, Kumarasiri PR. Epidemiology, clinical features, laboratory investigations and early diagnosis of dengue fever in adults: a descriptive study in Sri Lanka. Southeast Asian J Trop Med Public Health. 2005;36(3):686-92.
8. Kumarasamy V, Chua SK, Hassan Z, et al. Evaluating the sensitivity of a commercial dengue NS1 antigen-capture ELISA for early diagnosis of acute dengue virus infection. Singapore Med J. 2007;48(7):669-73.
9. Malavige GN, Fernando S, Fernando DJ, et al. Dengue viral infections. Postgrad Med J. 2004;80(948):588-601.
10. Nguyen TL, Nguyen T, Tieu NT. The impact of dengue hemorrhagic fever on liver function. Res Virol. 1997;148(4): 273-7.
11. Singh MP, Goyal K, Ratho RK. Nonstructural protein NS1: giving a new structure to dengue diagnosis. J Clin Microbiol. 2010;48(12):4688-9.
12. Singh MP, Majumdar M, Singh G, et al. NS1 antigen as an early diagnostic marker in dengue: report from India. Diagn Microbiol Infect Dis. 2010;68(1):50-4.
13. Wilder-Smith A, Schwartz E. Dengue in travelers. N Engl J Med. 2005;353(9):924-32.
14. World Health Organization. Criteria for grading dengue hemorrhagic fever and dengue shock syndrome. Adapted from WHO guide for diagnosis, treatment and control of dengue hemorrhagic fever. Geneva: World Health Organization; 1980.

CONTRIBUTIONS BY:

1. Dr Shreya Shrivastava, Junior Resident, Department of Pathology (In taking gross photographs)
2. Dr Niranjan Khaire, Junior Resident, Department of Internal Medicine (Compilation of Clinical Details)
3. Dr Mini P Singh, Professor, Department of Virology (Confirming Dengue Infection)
4. Dr Kartar Singh, Ex-Professor and Head, Department of Gastroenterology (Clinician In-Charge)

Post Graduate Institute of Medical Education and Research, Chandigarh, India.

CASE 27

Postpartum, Hyperacute, Fulminant Hepatic Failure due to Hepatitis E Virus: PM 26595

Nandita Bharadwaj Kakkar

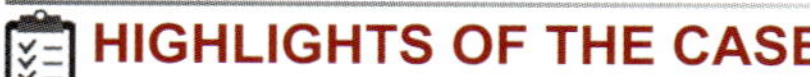

HIGHLIGHTS OF THE CASE

A 22-year-old, day 3 postpartum female, was referred from an outside facility, where she was admitted with sudden onset of jaundice in her 38th week of gestation and then underwent a lower segment emergency cesarean section, after which she deteriorated. She was referred to our institute on the third postoperative day with history of jaundice and altered sensorium (Glasgow Coma Score - E2M5V1). On evaluation there was conjugated hyperbilirubinemia, greater than 5-fold elevated transaminases, markedly deranged coagulogram, hypoalbuminemia, leukocytosis, grade III hepatic encephalopathy, cerebral edema, acute kidney injury and ascites. Markers for hepatitis B virus surface antigen (HBsAg) and anti-HCV were negative. Tests for IgM anti-HAV and IgM anti-HEV were not done antemortem. She was managed as a case of hyperacute liver failure with sepsis, but she developed hypotension followed by cardiac arrest. Autopsy revealed acute viral hepatitis E (RT-PCR-proven) with confluent and bridging hepatic necrosis and ascites.

Keywords**:** Postpartum, fulminant hepatic failure, acute liver failure, acute viral hepatitis, hepatitis E virus, autopsy.

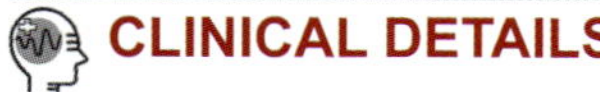

CLINICAL DETAILS

Date of Admission: 24.04.2015, Date of Death: 25.05.2015, Duration of Hospital Stay: 34 Hours

A 22-year-old female, day 3 postpartum was referred to PGIMER, Chandigarh, with history of jaundice since 6 days and altered sensorium since 3 days. She was admitted at an outside facility with sudden onset of jaundice in her 38th week of gestation, was detected to have oligohydramnios and a lower segment caesarian section was done within 2-days of admission. Thereafter, she deteriorated and was referred to the liver ICU of our institute. There was no history of any fever, ascites, upper GI bleed or any drug intake. On general ***physical examination***, she was drowsy and disoriented. The patient was hypotensive (BP: 110/64 mm Hg), pulse rate was 106/min and respiratory rate was 24/min. She was afebrile with an oxygen saturation of 94%. There was deep icterus and bilateral pitting edema. No pallor, cyanosis or clubbing was however noted. There were no peripheral stigmata of chronic liver disease. The abdomen was soft, nontender, lower segment cesarean section (LSCS) wound was healthy and there was no organomegaly or ascites. On CNS examination she was E2M5V1, pupils were normal and reacting to light and deep tendon reflexes were 2+.

Investigations

Hb: 9.8 g/dL; TLC was 18,300/uL; platelets: 440000/uL; liver function tests—total serum bilirubin/conjugated—15.0/11.1 mg%; SGOT/SGPT—1155/786 U/L; alkaline phosphatase: 314 U/L; total serum proteins/serum albumin: 5.5/2 gms; Na^+/K^+—141/4.4 meq/L; serum urea: 45 mg%; serum creatinine—1.8 mg%; deranged coagulogram (PT: 39', PTI: 36%, INR: 2.7, aPPT: 55'); negative viral markers (HIV, HBsAg and anti-HCV), IgM anti-HAV and IgM anti-HEV were not done; ***USG abdomen***: Liver—12 cm, normal echotexture, normal hepatic veins, no intrahepatic biliary radical dilatation, portal vein—normal, uterus—bulky (postpartum), no free fluid. Impression: Grossly normal study; ***NCCT head:*** cerebral edema; ***Chest X-ray:*** Right mid-zone patch. The clinical diagnosis was hyperacute liver failure with sepsis. She developed hypotension, was put on ionotropes and later suffered a cardiac arrest from which she could not be revived.

AUTOPSY FINDINGS: PM 26595

A complete autopsy was performed. The peritoneal cavity yielded 1.5 liters of straw-colored fluid. Other serous cavities were within normal limits. The ***liver*** weighed 720 grams, was soft, foldable and the capsule was wrinkled. The cut surface showed diffuse bile staining of liver parenchyma and a mottled appearance (Figs 1A and B). No nodularity was identified. The portal vein (Fig 1C) and biliary tract (Fig 1D) were within normal limits. Microscopically, there was extensive confluent and bridging hepatic necrosis (Figs 2A and B). Areas of hepatocytic loss showed mild lymphomononuclear cell infiltrate (Fig 2C) and macrophages containing PAS positive material (Fig 2D). Reticulin stain (Fig 3A) highlighted the distortion and condensation of reticulin fibers indicating loss of hepatocytes. Masson's trichrome stain (Figs 3B and C) did not show any overlaying of collagen and elastic fibers in areas of hepatocytic loss, indicating it to be an acute process. In addition intracanalicular cholestasis along with bile plug formation and pseudorosetting were noted (Fig 3D). Serum sample was collected at the time of autopsy and subjected to ELISA, which showed very high titer for IgM anti-HEV. Nested reverse transcriptase—PCR (Fig 3E) was done on paraffin embedded liver tissue targeting ***ORF-1*** gene and hepatitis E was confirmed. Thus, the overall features in the liver were of acute viral hepatitis E with confluent and bridging hepatic necrosis. The ***spleen*** weighed 110 g and showed red pulp congestion. The ***kidneys*** weighed 210 g. Capsular surface was pale and the cut surface showed mild bile staining. Microscopically, glomeruli were normal. Tubules showed

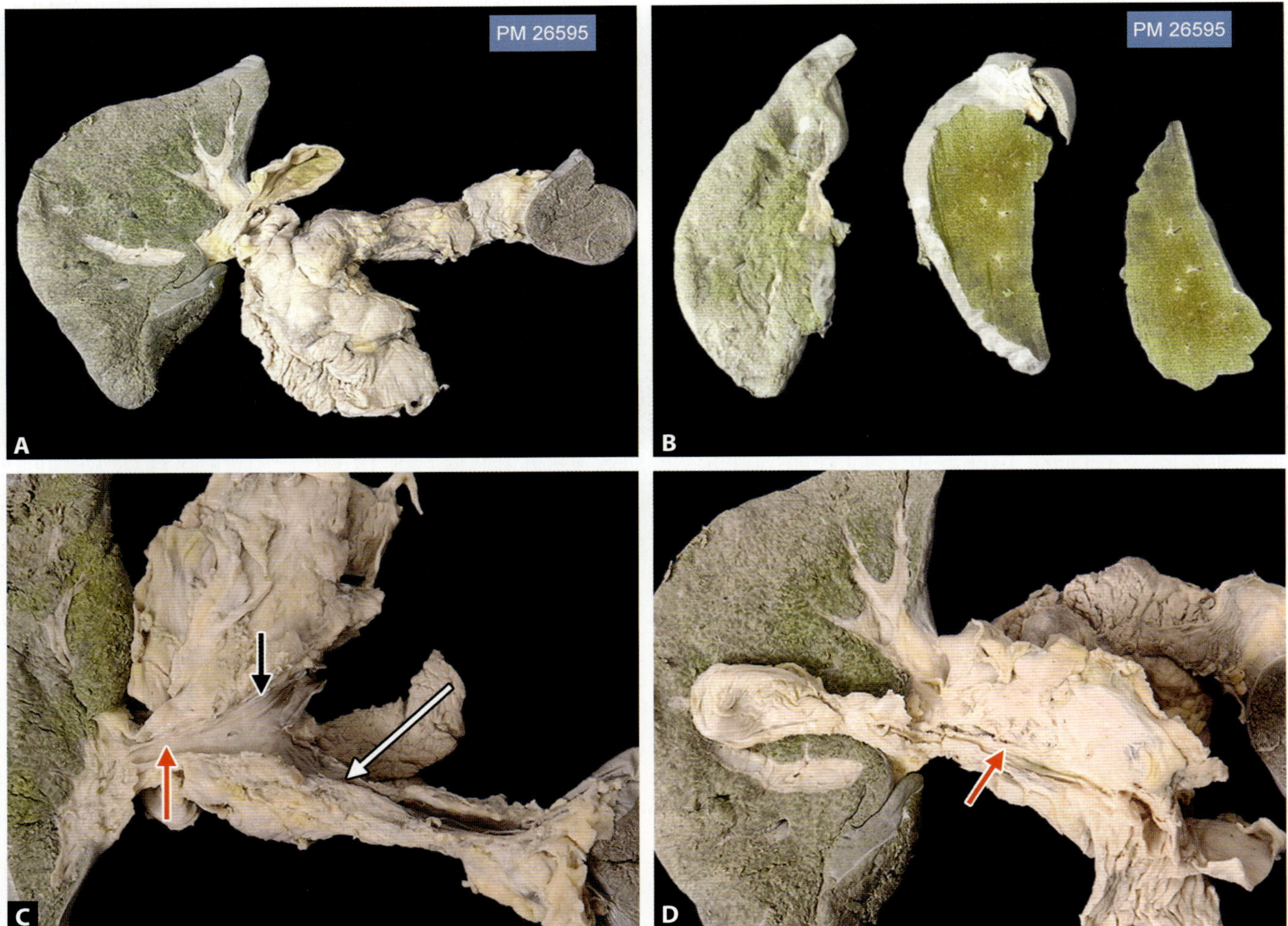

Figs 1A–D: (A) Organ complex of the slice of liver, spleen, pancreas, gallbladder and c loop of duodenum. The liver is bile stained and shrunken; (B) Coronal slices of the shrunken, bile stained liver; (C) Splenic (white arrow) and superior mesenteric (black arrow) veins forming the portal vein (red arrow) which is normal; (D) Opened up common bile duct (red arrow) which is normal.

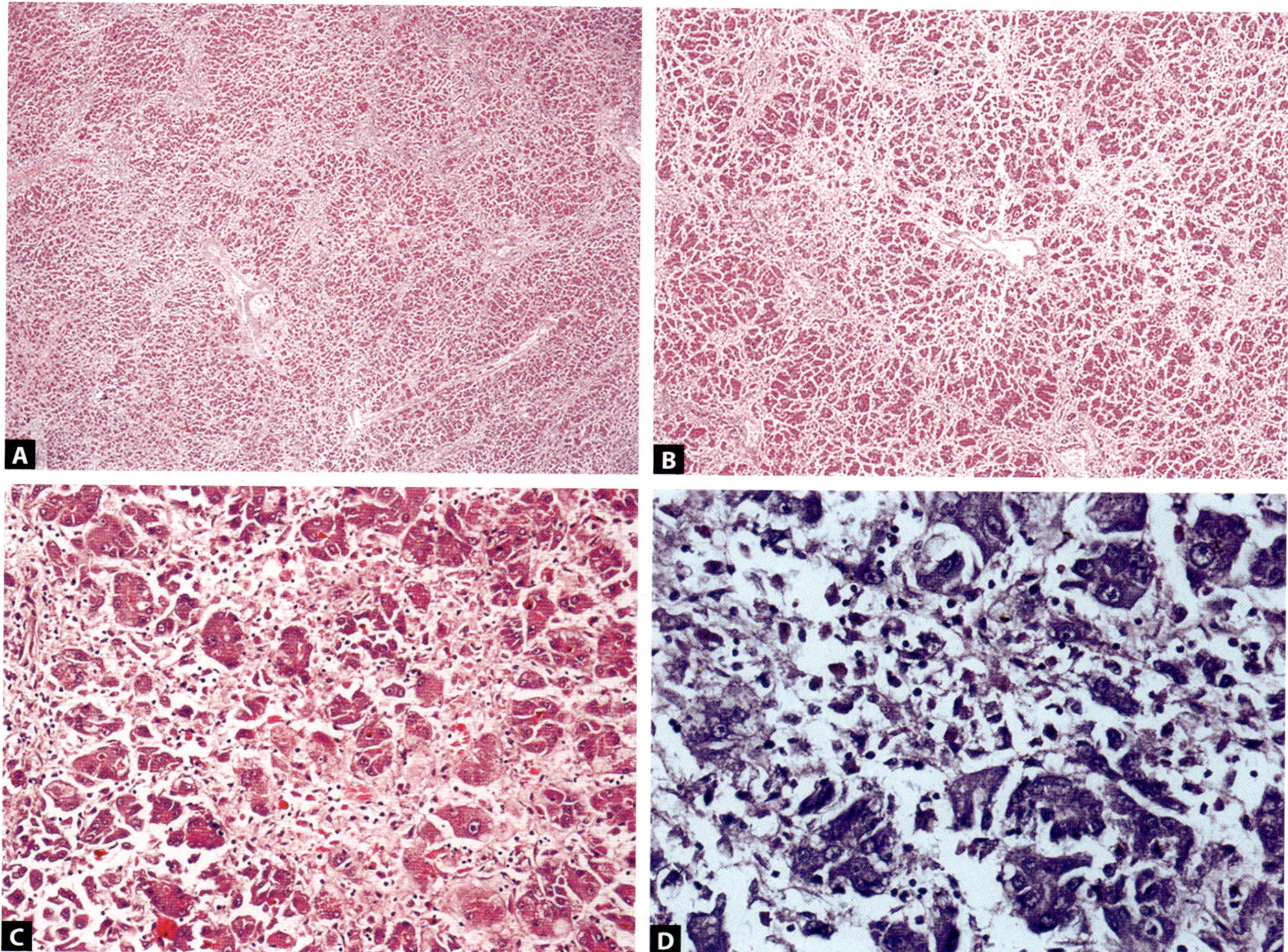

Figs 2A–D: Photomicrographs of the liver showing (A and B) Confluent and bridging hepatic necrosis; (C) Areas of hepatocytic loss with mild lymphomononuclear infiltrate and macrophages; (D) Macrophages show PAS positive material.

focal acute tubular necrosis and bile casts indicating a bile cast nephropathy. ***Lungs*** weighed 482 g. Right pleural (Fig 4A) aspect showed fibrinous tags and the lower part of right lung was adherent to the diaphragm. Microscopically, pleura shows fibrinous pleuritis and organizing inflammation (Fig 4B). There was no evidence of bronchopneumonia. ***Carinal lymph nodes*** (Fig 4C) showed caseous necrosis and multiple epitheloid cell granulomas with a positive stain for AFB. ***Uterus*** showed postpartum changes, but no inflammation. Other organs were within normal limits.

FINAL AUTOPSY DIAGNOSIS : PM 26595

22 Years Female Three Days Postpartum

- Acute viral hepatitis E with confluent and bridging hepatic necrosis.
- Right-sided fibrinous pleuritis.
- Tuberculous lymphadenopathy (carinal lymph nodes).
- Ascites.

PREGNANCY AND HEPATITIS E INFECTION

Acute viral hepatitis[1-4] (AVH) still remains a major health problem in India. It often leads to acute liver failure, wherein the patient develops hepatic encephalopathy due to severe derangement of liver function, in the absence of any previous hepatic disease, with evidence of coagulopathy, within four-weeks of having a typical bout of acute hepatitis (five-fold increase of serum aspartate aminotransferase/ clinical jaundice or both). If the duration of symptoms to encephalopathy is less than a week it is termed as hyperacute liver failure. AVH can be caused by six known viruses i.e. A, B, C, D, E and G, each having a distinct

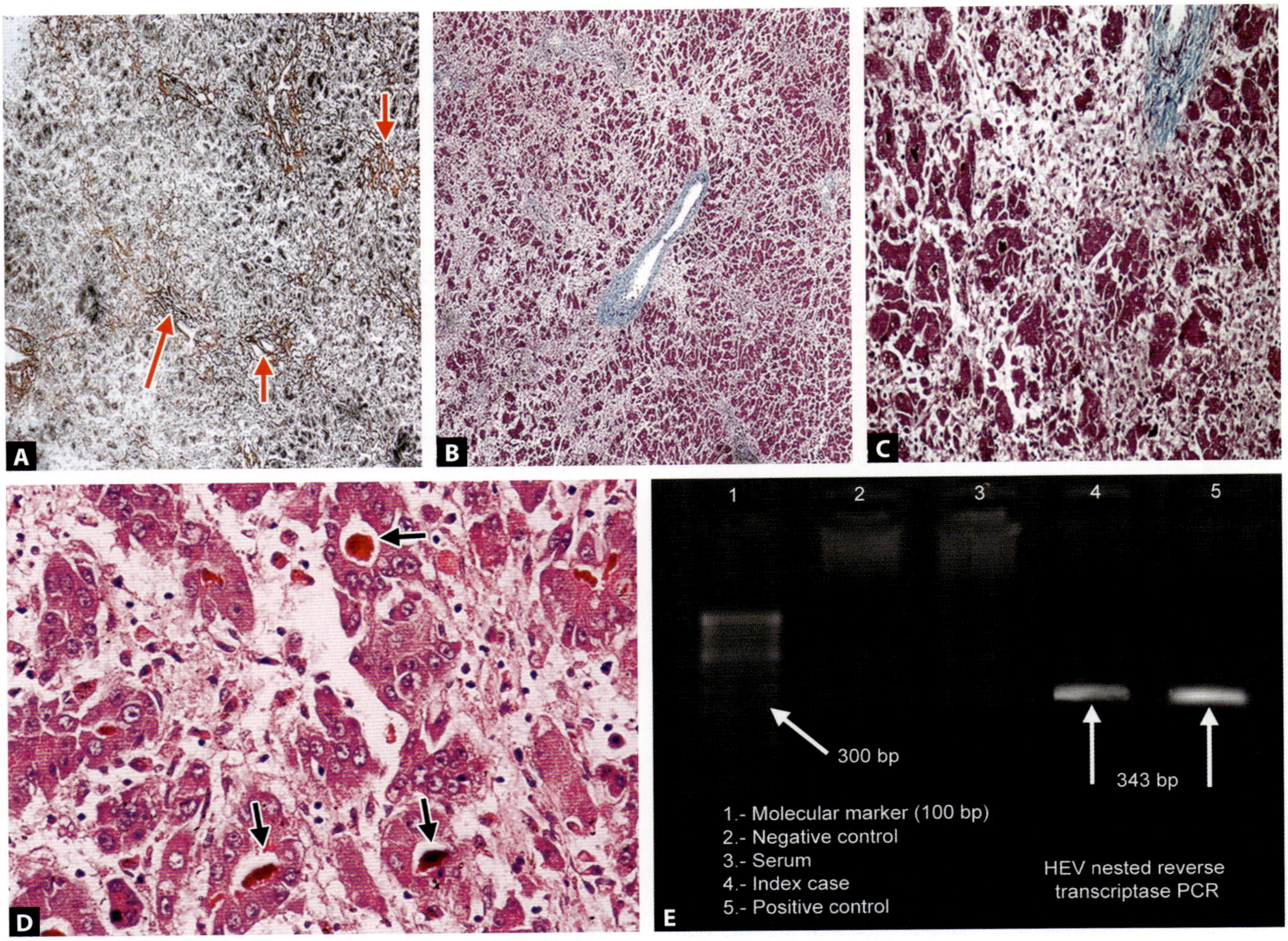

Figs 3A–E: Photomicrographs of the liver. (A) Reticulin stain shows condensation of reticulin fibers (arrows); (B and C) Masson's trichrome stain does not show any collagen deposition; (D) Pseudorosettes with canalicular cholestasis (arrows); (E) Nested reverse transcriptase PCR showing HEV band at 343 bp (arrows).

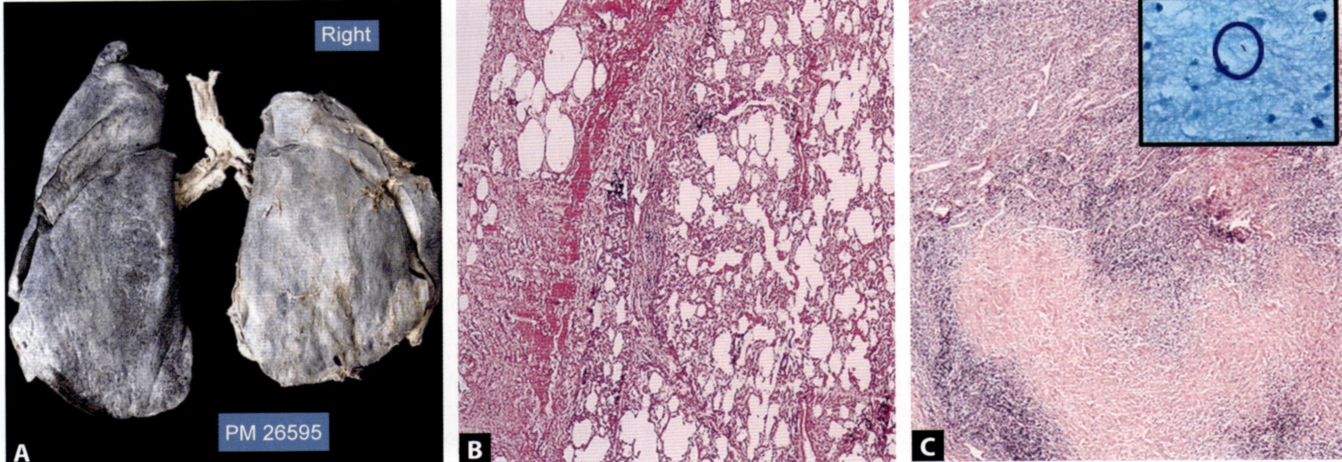

Figs 4A–C: Gross photograph of the pleural aspect of the lungs showing fibrinous tags and haziness on the right side; (B) Photomicrograph showing fibrinous pleuritis; (C) Carinal lymph node showing caseous necrosis, positive for acid-fast bacilli (Inset Ziehl-Neelson stain).

pattern of involvement, severity and prognosis. Normal physiological changes in pregnancy mimic changes which occur in patients with decompensated chronic liver disease. In pregnancy, women are more prone to hepatitis E virus infection, especially in the second/third trimester. Normal demands of pregnancy, malnutrition and inversion of T and B lymphocytes in early pregnancy, have been postulated to be the contributing factors. HEV is endemic in parts of Asia and Africa and is the commonest cause of acute liver failure in pregnancy, wherein it follows a more severe and stormy course, leading to fulminant hepatic failure, especially in the Indian subcontinent. Pregnancy as such predisposes to viral infections, due to the high levels of steroid hormones that promote viral replication. Steroid hormones directly inhibit the hepatocytes, which when exposed to infectious agents, causes their dysfunction. Steroid hormones suppress immunity and lead to apoptosis of lymphocyte. Pregnancy complicated with liver failure due to HEV has a paucity of CD4 positive cells. It is proposed that hormonal changes in pregnancy and associated immunological responses play a role in fulminant hepatic failure after HEV infection. The Indian subcontinent is highly endemic for hepatitis A virus which affects the children and hepatitis E virus which affects the adults. HEV is enterically transmitted (feco-oral route), is a single-stranded RNA virus, a member of the genus ***Herpevirus*** in the family Hepeviridae.

Hepatitis E virus-related infection during pregnancy has a very high maternal and fetal mortality, to the tune of 41–54% and 69% respectively. The prognosis is poor once grade III or IV hepatic encephalopathy sets in and the delivery does not affect the maternal outcome. Khuroo et al[5] have reported that approximately 70% of pregnant women with acute hepatitis E, progress to acute liver failure with a short pre-encephalopathy period, rapid development of cerebral edema and high occurrence of disseminated intravascular coagulation. In our country, ALF leading to death in pregnant women is reported to be 21% with rates going as high as 44% in the third trimester.[5,6] There are high rates of preterm labor, abortions and intrauterine deaths. Vertical transmission to the infant is rare, but has been reported in literature. Various studies (Khuroo et al[5] 86%, Jaiswal et al[7] 58%, Aziz et al[8] 62%, Singh et al[8] 45%, Kumar et al[9] 37%) have shown that HEV is responsible for a major percentage of acute viral hepatitis in pregnant women. Acute hepatitis due to HEV has worse obstetric outcomes and a higher maternal mortality, as compared to acute hepatitis caused by other viruses. There are 4 mammalian genotypes of HEV i.e. Genotypes 1–4 with type 1 and 2 being more virulent and the former being the Asian and African strain.

COMMENTARY—INDEX CASE: PM 26595

The index case was a 22-year-old, three days postpartum female, who was referred from an outside facility, where she was admitted with sudden onset of jaundice in her 38th week of gestation and then underwent a lower segment emergency cesarean section, after which she deteriorated. She came to our institute with jaundice and altered sensorium. There was conjugated hyperbilirubinemia, greater than 5-fold elevated transaminases, markedly deranged coagulogram with INR greater than 2, hypoalbuminemia, leucocytosis, grade III hepatic encephalopathy, cerebral edema, acute kidney injury and ascites. Markers for HIV, HBsAg and anti-HCV were negative. Tests for IgM anti-HAV and IgM anti-HEV were not done antemortem. She was managed as a case of hyperacute liver failure with sepsis, but she developed hypotension followed by cardiac arrest. Autopsy revealed acute viral hepatitis E (Postmortem ELISA—high titer for IgM anti-HEV and postmortem nested reverse transcriptase PCR positive for HEV) with confluent/bridging hepatic necrosis and ascites. The liver morphology shows features of a classical acute viral hepatitis — confluent and bridging hepatic necrosis with cholestasis. There was no lying down of collagen fibers, hence it was an acute process.

TAKE HOME MESSAGE

- Pregnant women are highly prone to hepatitis E virus infection with a large number going into acute liver failure.
- It is proposed that hormonal changes in pregnancy and associated immunological responses play a role in fulminant hepatic failure after HEV infection.

REFERENCES

1. Kamar N, Bendall R, Legrand-Abravanel F, et al. Hepatitis E. Lancet. 2012;379(9835):2477-88.
2. Navaneethan U, Al Mohajer M, Shata MT. Hepatitis E and pregnancy: understanding the pathogenesis. Liver Int. 2008; 28(9):1190–9.
3. Kar P. Hepatitis E virus infection during pregnancy: Why is the disease stormy? Medicine update. 2012;2(2):459-62.
4. Shalimar, Acharya Sk. Hepatitis E and acute liver failure in pregnancy. J Clin Exp Hepatol. 2013;3(3):213-24.
5. Khuroo MS, Teli MR, Skidmore S, et al. Incidence and severity of viral hepatitis in pregnancy. Am J Med. 1981;70(2):252-5.
6. Dahiya M, Kumar A, Kar P, et al. Acute viral hepatitis in third trimester of pregnancy. Indian J Gastroenterol. 2005; 24(3):128-9.
7. Jaiswal SP, Jain AK, Naik G, et al. Viral hepatitis during pregnancy. Int J Gynecol Obstet. 2001;72(2):103-8.

8. Aziz AB, Hamid S, Iqbal S, et al. Prevalence and severity of viral hepatitis in Pakistani pregnant women: a five year hospital based study. J Pak Med Assoc. 1997;47(8): 198-201.
9. Kumar RM, Uduman S, Rana S, et al. Sero-prevalence and mother-to-infant transmission of hepatitis E virus among pregnant women in the United Arab Emirates. Eur J Obstet Gynecol Reprod Biol. 2001;100(1):9-15.

CONTRIBUTIONS BY:

1. Dr Vikarn Vishwajeet, Junior Resident, Department of Pathology (In taking gross photographs)
2. Dr Vikram Thakur, PhD Student, Department of Virology (RT-PCR)
3. Dr Prasanna Kumar, Junior Resident, Department of Internal Medicine (Compilation of Clinical Details)
4. Dr YK Chawla, Former Director PGI and Ex-Professor and Head, Department of Hepatology (Clinician In-Charge)

Post Graduate Institute of Medical Education and Research, Chandigarh, India.

CASE 28

Sporadic, Hepatitis E-related Massive Hepatic Necrosis in a Young Female: PM 26254

Nandita Bharadwaj Kakkar

HIGHLIGHTS OF THE CASE

A 20-year-old female with no prior comorbidities and no stigmata of chronic liver disease, came with history of jaundice since 15 days and altered sensorium since 2 days. Investigations revealed anemia, conjugated hyperbilirubinemia, raised transaminases and alkaline phosphatase, moderate-gross ascites and right-sided pleural effusion. She was intubated, started on anti-hepatic coma measures but suffered a cardiorespiratory arrest, despite best efforts and could not be revived. A clinical diagnosis of fulminant hepatic failure ? Viral ? Autoimmune ? Wilson's disease was kept. Autopsy revealed acute viral hepatitis E (RT-PCR-proven) with massive hepatic necrosis and bronchopneumonia.

Keywords: Hepatitis E, massive hepatic necrosis, fulminant hepatic failure, autopsy.

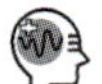

CLINICAL DETAILS

Date of Admission: 13.09.14, Date of Death: 15.09.14, Duration of Hospital Stay: 2 days

A 20-year-old unmarried female, resident of Ganganagar, Rajasthan, presented to the emergency OPD, PGIMER Chandigarh on 13th September, 2014 with clinical presentation of jaundice for 15 days and altered sensorium for the last 2 days. Jaundice was gradually progressive with history of yellow-colored urine and abdominal distension for the past 3 days. There was no history of clay-colored stools or pruritus. No prodromal symptoms or upper GI bleed was present. Altered sensorium was present in the form of repetition of sentences, incoherent talk and reduced food intake. There was no history of seizures, drug intake, previous hospitalization or blood transfusion. There were no previous comorbidities or similar episodes in the past. ***Examination***: Patient was unconscious with Glasgow Coma Scale (GCS) of E4V1M3, pupils bilaterally equal and reacting to light, decorticate posturing present, deep tendon reflexes exaggerated, plantars bilateral extensor; pallor +; icterus ++; pedal edema +; BP: 110/80 mm Hg; PR: 100/min; RR: 24/min; abdomen distended and soft; liver margins palpable, soft and regular; ascites +, CVS/chest — within normal limits.

Investigations

Investigations: Hb— 7.9 g%; TLC: 11,300/uL; Platelets: 377000/uL; PBF: Microcytic hypochromic anemia; total serum bilirubin/conjugated—20.1/14 mg%; SGOT/SGPT/alkaline phosphatase-112/58/243 mEq/L; deranged coagulogram (PT 56 s (c-14 s), PTI— 25%, INR— 3.89, aPPT—52 s), Na^+/K^+—131/4.5 mEq/L; serum urea/creatinine—19/0.5 mg%; card test negative for malarial parasite; serology for dengue, HBsAg, HIV, HCV and widal—negative; X-ray chest—right-sided pleural effusion; USG abdomen—Liver size 13.2 cm with increased periportal echogenicity and moderate to gross ascites. She was intubated, put on AMBU and started on anti-hepatic coma measures, NAC infusion, mannitol, vitamin K, dextrose infusions and FFP transfusions. However, patient had a cardiorespiratory arrest on 15/09/14 and could not be revived. A clinical diagnosis of fulminant hepatic failure (coagulopathy, jaundice, encephalopathy, ascites and right-sided pleural effusion) was kept in this patient. Possible etiologies being ? viral ? Autoimmune ? Wilson's disease. Cause of death being— raised intracranial tension.

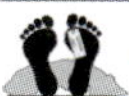

AUTOPSY FINDINGS: PM 26254

A partial autopsy was performed in this patient. The prosector noted 1,500 mL bile-stained fluid in the peritoneal cavity and 250 mL fluid in the right pleural cavity. The ***liver***

(Fig 1A) was grossly shrunken, weighing 800 g, was soft and easily foldable. Microscopic examination showed distorted architecture with approximation of portal tracts. There was massive hepatic necrosis which was confluent and multiacinar (Figs 1B and C). Almost all the hepatocytes were necrosed and these areas showed mild lymphomononuclear cell infiltrate (Fig 1D) and cholangiolar proliferation (Fig 2A). The portal tracts were expanded with lymphoplasmacytic infiltrate. However, no interface hepatitis was seen and there was no fibrosis. Reticulin stain (Fig 2B) showed collapse of reticulin fibers and Masson's trichrome stain (Fig 2C) did not show lying down of collagen fibers, thus indicating the massive hepatocytic loss to be an acute process. Nested reverse transcriptase— PCR (Fig 2D) was done on paraffin embedded liver tissue targeting ORF-1 gene and hepatitis E was confirmed. Overall features were those of massive hepatic necrosis secondary to acute viral hepatitis E infection. The ***spleen*** was mildly enlarged and showed congestion. ***Lungs*** were normal in weight with dullness of pleural surface. Cut surface showed patchy areas of consolidation which were subcrepitant to feel. Sections examined from the consolidated areas showed evidence of bronchopneumonia. Both ***kidneys*** weighed 265 grams and on microscopy showed mild lymphoplasmacytic inflammatory cell infiltrate in the interstitium, tubules showed evidence of vacuolar nephropathy, possibly secondary to intravenous mannitol and bile casts. All other organs were within normal limits.

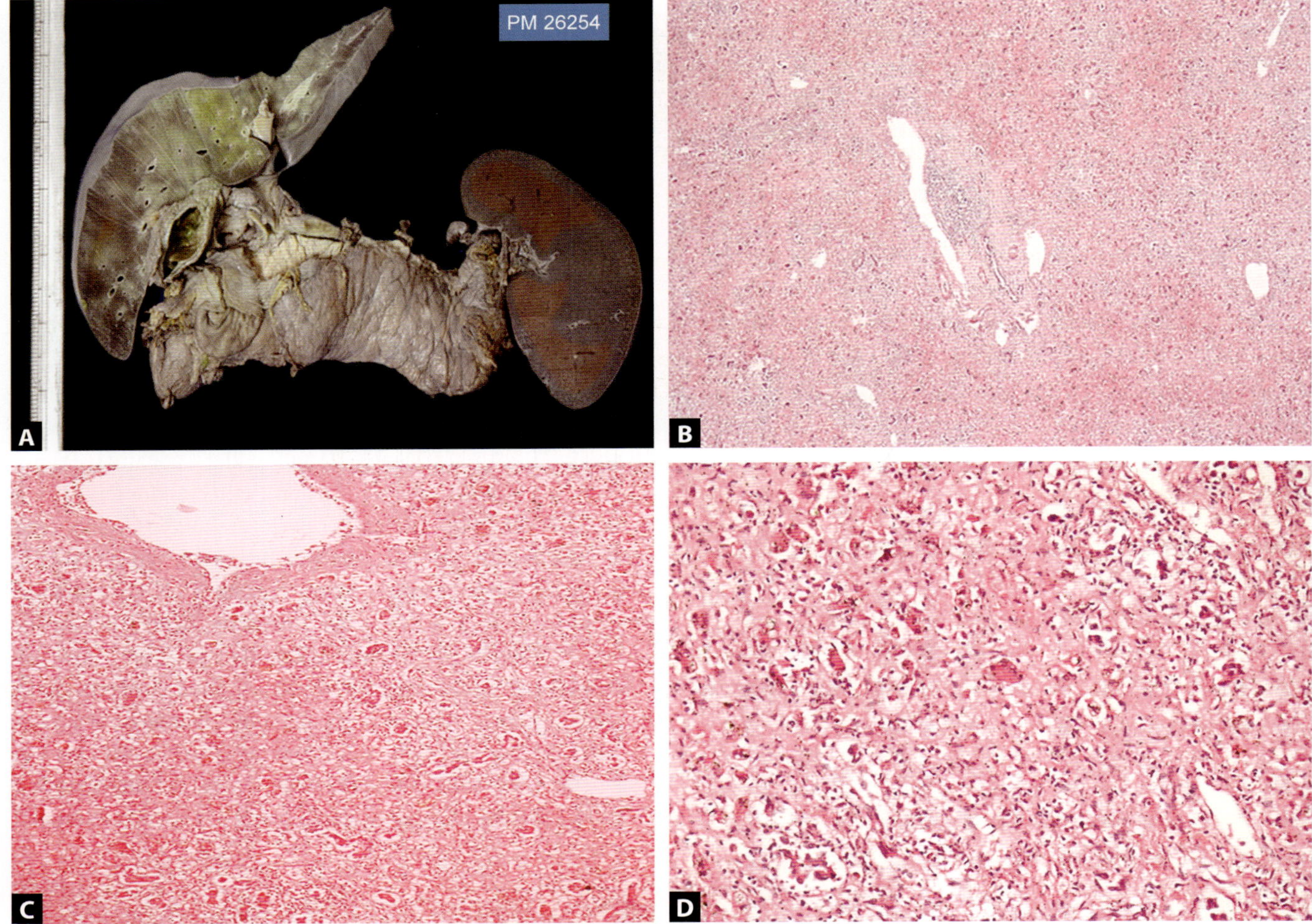

Figs 1A–D: (A) Organ complex of the slice of liver which is bile stained and shrunken, spleen which is slightly enlarged and the pancreas. (B and C) Microphotographs of the liver show massive hepatic necrosis with approximation of the portal tracts. Not a single hepatocyte is discernable. (D) Liver showing total loss of hepatocytes with few cholangioles and a mild lymphomononuclear cell infiltrate.

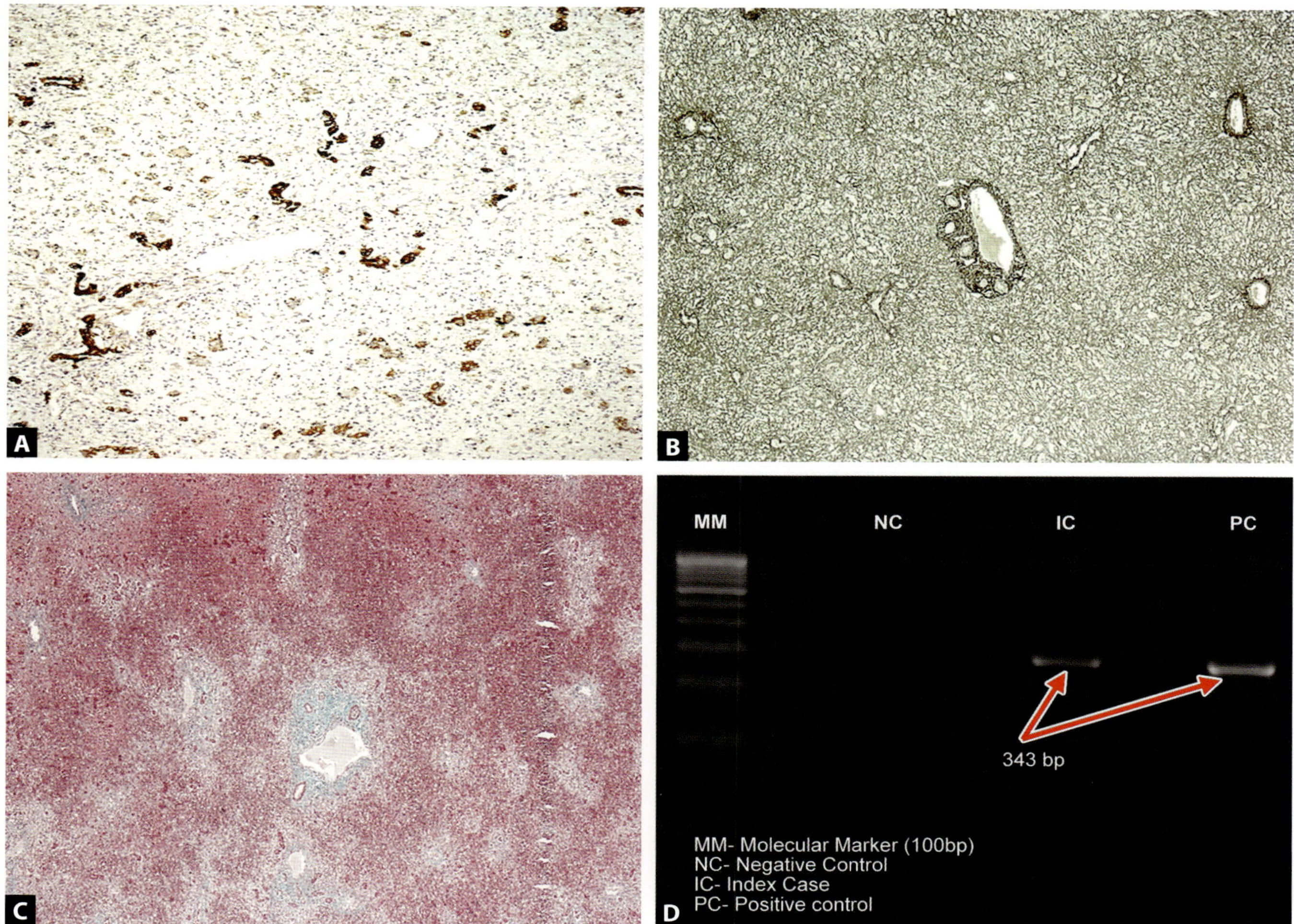

Figs 2A–D: (A) CK7 immunohistochemistry on the section of the liver shows cholangiolar proliferation; (B) Reticulin stain shows collapse of reticulin framework; (C) Masson's trichrome stain does not show laying down of any collagen fibers; (D) Nested reverse transcriptase PCR showing HEV band at 343 bp.

FINAL AUTOPSY DIAGNOSIS : PM 26254

20 Years Old Female

- Acute viral hepatitis E with massive hepatic necrosis (PCR-proven)
- Bronchopneumonia

ACUTE VIRAL HEPATITIS E

Hepatitis E is a major health problem in developing countries and is emerging as a zoonotic disease in developed countries too.[1] It usually presents in the form of an acute self-limited hepatitis. However, in some persons, the illness is more severe and may present as acute liver failure with a high mortality rate. This is more common in pregnant women.[2] The infection is endemic in South, Southeast and Central Asia, the Middle East, parts of Africa and Mexico.[1-3] In India, hepatitis E virus (HEV) infection has accounted for several large outbreaks,[2-4] 50% to 70% of cases with sporadic viral hepatitis and a large proportion of cases with acute liver failure.[5-7] Four HEV genotypes are known and of these, genotypes 1 and 2 cause human disease in endemic areas and do not infect animals.[7] Genotypes 3 and 4 predominantly infect animal species with occasional zoonotic transmission to humans in non-endemic areas and mostly affect elderly persons with other coexistent diseases.[7]

Fulminant hepatic failure is defined as the rapid development of hepatocellular dysfunction and encephalopathy in a person with no prior history of liver disease.[8] The etiological factors of FHF, vary according to the geographical area and age. In children, the commonest cause of acute liver failure is infection with hepatitis A virus, but in India hepatitis E virus is also implicated.[9] There are limited published data on the liver biopsy appearances of acute hepatitis E,[10-12] as these cases usually have a self-limiting illness and a liver biopsy is not clinically indicated.

COMMENTARY—INDEX CASE: PM 26254

A young 20-year-old female with no prior comorbidities and no stigmata of chronic liver disease presented with jaundice (15 days), altered sensorium (2 days), anemia, conjugated hyperbilirubinemia, raised transaminases/alkaline phosphatase, moderate-gross ascites and right-sided pleural effusion. A clinical diagnosis of fulminant hepatic failure ? Viral ? Autoimmune, ?? Wilson's disease was kept. She was intubated, started on anti-hepatic coma measures, but suffered a cardiorespiratory arrest and despite best efforts could not be revived. Autopsy revealed acute viral hepatitis E (nested reverse transcriptase PCR-proven) with massive hepatic necrosis and bronchopneumonia. The transaminases were not greater than 5 times raised, but there was encephalopathy, marked conjugated hyperbilirubinemia and markedly deranged coagulogram with an INR of 3.89. Serology for hepatitis E for some reason was not done antemortem. Hepatitis E is a major health issue in developing countries and why the illness is more severe and presents with acute liver failure with a high mortality rate, is still under scanner. Hepatitis E virus infection has a stormy and devastating course in pregnant women.

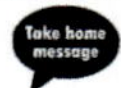

TAKE HOME MESSAGE

- Hepatitis E viral infection is a major health issue in India.
- In some persons, the illness is more severe and may present as acute liver failure with a high mortality rate. This is more common in pregnant women.

REFERENCES

1. Aggarwal R, Naik S. Epidemiology of hepatitis E: Current status. J Gastroenterol Hepatol. 2009;24(9):1484-93.
2. Khuroo MS. Study of an epidemic of non-A, non-B hepatitis. Possibility of another human hepatitis virus distinct from post-transfusion non-A, non-B type. Am J Med. 1980;68(6): 818-24.
3. Naik SR, Aggarwal R, Salunke PN, et al. A large waterborne viral hepatitis E epidemic in Kanpur, India. Bull World Health Organ. 1992;70(5):597-604.
4. Khuroo MS, Rustgi VK, Dawson GJ, et al. Spectrum of hepatitis E virus infection in India. J Med Virol. 1994; 43(3):281-6.
5. Acharya SK, Dasarathy S, Kumer TL, et al. Fulminant hepatitis in a tropical population: Clinical course, cause and early predictors of outcome. Hepatology. 1996;23(6):1448-55.
6. Khuroo MS, Kamili S. Etiology and prognostic factors in acute live failure in India. J Viral Hepat. 2003;10(3):224-31.
7. Acharya SK, Panda SK, Saxena A, et al. Acute hepatic failure in India: A perspective from the East. J Gastroenterol Hepatol. 2000;15(5):473-9.
8. Lu L, Li C, Hagedorn CH. Phylogenetic analysis of global hepatitis E virus sequences: Genetic diversity, subtypes and zoonosis. Rev Med Virol. 2006;16(1):5-36.
9. Williams R. Classification, etiology and considerations of outcome in acute liver failure. Semin Liver Dis. 1996; 16(4):343-8.
10. Khuroo MS, Kamali S. Etiology and prognostic factors in acute liver failure in India. J Viral Hepat. 2003;10(3):224-31.
11. Agrawal V, Goel A, Rawat A, et al. Histological and immunohistochemical features in fatal acute fulminant hepatitis E. Indian J Pathol Microbiol. 2012;55(1): 22-7.
12. Peron JM, Danjoux M, Kamar N, et al. Liver histology in patients with sporadic acute hepatitis E: a study of 11 patients from South-West France. Virchows Arch. 2007;450(4): 405-10.
13. Das P, Jain D, Das A. A retrospective autopsy study of histopathologic spectrum and etiologic trend of fulminant hepatic failure from north India. Diagn Pathol. 2007;2:27.

CONTRIBUTIONS BY:

1. Dr Gurwinder Kaur, Junior Resident, Department of Pathology (In taking gross photographs)
2. Dr Rimesh Pal, Junior Resident, Department of Internal Medicine (Compilation of Clinical Details)
3. Dr Sudha Sharma, Senior Resident, Department of Pathology (In working up the case)
4. Dr Mini P Singh, Professor, Department of Virology (RT-PCR)
5. Dr Ashish Bhalla, Professor, Department of Internal Medicine (Clinician In-Charge)

Post Graduate Institute of Medical Education and Research, Chandigarh, India.

CASE 29

A Classical Case of Wilson's Disease with Hepatic and Neuropsychiatric Manifestations: PM 26195

Nandita Bharadwaj Kakkar

HIGHLIGHTS OF THE CASE

This is the story of a young boy who first came at the age of 13-years with hematemesis and variceal ligation was done. At the age of 15-years he was diagnosed as a case of Wilson's disease and was put on treatment. At the age of 17-years he was readmitted. He had ascites, neuropsychiatric manifestations, low serum ceruloplasmin, high 24-hour urinary copper excretion, Kayser-Fleischer ring, positive D-penicillamine challenge test and altered mixed signal intensity in bilateral putamen, thalami, midbrain, superior cerebellar peduncles and pons, consistent with a diagnosis of Wilson's disease. Autopsy revealed features consistent with Wilson's disease i.e. macronodular cirrhosis with orcein-positive granules and myelinolysis in bilateral putamen.

Keywords: Wilson's disease, macronodular cirrhosis, hepatolenticular degeneration, lenticular myelinolysis, Kayser-Fleischer ring.

CLINICAL DETAILS

Date of Admission: 02.08.2014, Date of Death: 06.08.2014, Duration of Hospital Stay: 5 Days

This 17-years old male had three admissions in our institute.

First admission: In 2010, at the age of 13-years, he was admitted with hematemesis. Ultrasonography at that time revealed a coarse liver echotexture and splenomegaly. Upper gastrointestinal endoscopy revealed grade II varices and variceal ligation was done. There was no history of neonatal jaundice and he had normal developmental milestones. The patient was then lost to follow-up.

Second admission: In 2012 (15 years) he came with ascites, irritable behavior and abnormal posturing of limbs. Ascitic fluid revealed a high SAAG and a growth of Enterobacter fecalis. Serum ceruloplasmin was 16 mg/dL i.e. low (N-25-35 mg/dL), 24-hour urinary copper excretion was 172 μg i.e. high (N-10 to 30 μg/24 hours), Kayser-Fleischer ring was present (on slit-lamp examination) and the D-penicillamine challenge test was positive (1,054 μg in 24 hours). ***MRI brain***—altered mixed signal intensity (T2 hyperintense, T1 hypointense) was seen in bilateral putamen, thalami, midbrain, superior cerebellar peduncles and pons, consistent with a diagnosis of Wilson's disease. HBsAg and Anti-HCV were nonreactive and autoimmune hepatitis work-up was negative. A diagnosis of Wilson's disease was made. Neurology consultation was taken and he was started on D-penicillamine and zinc sulfate 250 mg three times a day each. There was no neurological worsening and he was followed-up on OPD basis. The 24-hour urinary copper excretion came down to normal levels. The upper GI endoscopy was repeated on 28/7/13 and the varices were found to be eradicated.

Third admission: In 2014 at the age of 17-years, he came with history of blunt trauma to right-side of chest and altered sensorium since one day. There was somnolence and decreased verbal response. There was no head injury, ear/nose bleed or seizures. There was no hematemesis, melena, swelling of feet, decreased urine output, constipation, hypertension, diabetes mellitus or tuberculosis. He was a nonsmoker and did not consume alcohol. On ***examination*** he was E2V2M5, conscious, irritable, non-cooperative, afebrile, pulse—104/min, BP—110/70 mm Hg, respiratory rate- 24/min, SpO_2 - 97% on room air, Kayser-Fleischer ring present and there was icterus. There was no pallor, cyanosis, edema, clubbing or any lymphadenopathy. The abdomen was distended, there was ascites, liver was not palpable, spleen was palpable 5 cm below the left costal margin, was firm and bowel sounds were present. CNS examination — patient was E2V2M5, irritable, non-cooperative, there was no neck rigidity, he was moving all limbs and bilateral plantars were flexor. There was an ecchymotic patch over right side of chest extending to axilla and deltoid region.

Investigation and Course of Management

Investigations: Hemogram — Hb was 11.2 g/dL and came down to 10.6 g/dL; total leukocyte count went up from 13,300 to 36,600/uL, with N80, L05, M05, metamyelocytes 10, nRBC's 02; platelets were 45,000/uL; ***renal function tests/electrolytes***: S. urea—91 mg%; S. creatinine: 1–1.1 to 2.1 mg%, Na^+/K^+: 141/2.7 mEq/L; Ca^{+2}/PO_4: 9.3/2.3 mg%; amylase: 24 U/L; ***liver function tests***: Total serum bilirubin/conjugated fraction—37.5/27.8 mg%; OT/PT: 169/73 U/L; alkaline phosphatase: 75 U/L; total proteins/albumin: 4.5/2.6 gms; coagulogram: PT—28 seconds; PTI: 50%; aPTT: 37 seconds; INR-2; blood culture grew E. coli; ***serology***: HBsAg, anti-HCV, IgM anti-HAV, IgM anti-HEV—negative; ***EEG***: suggestive of severe diffuse encephalopathy; arterial ammonia: 146.2 µmol/L (raised); ***ultrasound abdomen*** (2/8/14): Liver 12 cm, echotexture coarse, heterogeneous and nodular, splenomegaly (20 cm), right kidney: 10.6 cm, left kidney: 10.8 cm with bilateral raised cortical echogenicity. Few hyperechoic foci seen in the medulla of right kidney, no free fluid present; ***ultrasound chest*** (5/8/14): No evidence of effusion.

This 17-years male, a known case of Wilson's disease with chronic liver disease (child C, decompensation in 2009) came with blunt trauma chest and altered sensorium (E2V2M5). There was systemic inflammatory response syndrome, fever, tachycardia, tachypnea, splenomegaly, deranged liver function tests with conjugated hyperbilirubinemia and raised transaminases SGOT/SGPT greater than 1, coagulopathy, thrombocytopenia, hypokalemia, E. coli sepsis and a large ecchymotic patch on right-side of chest. He was started on anti-hepatic coma measures (lactulose, rifaximin), oral and IV potassium supplementation and empirical antibiotic (inj. ceftriaxone). Four-units of fresh frozen plasma were transfused and injection vitamin k was administered. During the hospital stay there was progressive leukocytosis, antibiotics were upgraded and a gram-positive coverage was given. There was progressive worsening of sensorium, arterial ammonia was raised and he developed hypotension (BP: 80/60 mm Hg) unresponsive to fluids, high anion gap metabolic acidosis and raised serum creatinine. He was intubated and started on inotropes. He soon developed cardiac arrest from which he could not be revived. ***Units clinical diagnosis*** was Chronic liver disease—Cirrhosis of liver with portal hypertension (child C)—Wilson's disease (hepatic and neuropsychiatric) with acute on chronic liver failure, jaundice, coagulopathy, hepatic encephalopathy, acute kidney injury, severe sepsis (? infected chest wound) and refractory septic shock.

AUTOPSY FINDINGS: PM 26195

A complete autopsy was performed on this 17-year-old male. On external examination he was moderately built, icteric with unhealthy scar over right side of trunk measuring 30 × 15 cm, with unhealthy scars on both knees. The peritoneal cavity yielded 2-liters of bile stained fluid. The pleural and pericardial cavities were within normal limits. The ***liver*** weighed 920 g. The external surface showed numerous macronodules ranging in size from 0.5–1.5 cm in size. Cut surface was bile stained with macronodules separated by fibrous septae (Figs 1A and B). The portal vein was dilated (Fig 1B). Microscopy revealed a distorted lobular architecture with formation of complete nodules separated by predominantly porto-portal bridging fibrosis (Figs 1C and D). The nodules were better appreciated by reticulin and Masson's trichrome stains (Figs 1E and 2A). Portal tracts (Fig 2B) were expanded with dense fibrosis, moderate lymphomononuclear infiltrate and bile ductular proliferation. Nuclear glycogenation was prominent (Fig 2C). Presence of macro/microvesicular steatosis and predominantly centrizonal intracytoplasmic and sinusoidal cholestasis were noted (Figs 2D and E). Increased intrahepatocytic copper associated proteins i.e. coarse cola-colored granules on orcein stain were present (Fig 2F). Overall features were consistent with Wilson's disease. The ***spleen*** was markedly enlarged and weighed 1,030 g (Figs 1A and 3A). Microscopy revealed congestion of red pulp with capillarization of sinusoids and relative depletion of white pulp (Fig 3B). The ***lungs*** (Fig 3C) weighed 750 g. The plurae were dull and opaque and there were small petechial hemorrhages ranging in size from 2 to 5 mm in size. Cut surface was subcrepitant to feel and no focal lesions were seen. On microscopic examination (Fig 3D), there was intra-alveolar hemorrhage and fibrin deposition. The ***kidneys*** weighed 318 g and were swollen. External surface was bile stained with few tiny depressed scars. Cut surface (Fig 3E) showed an indistinct corticomedullary junction and mild increase in intrapelvic fat. On microscopy, tubules contained bile casts (Figs 3F and G) with few intratubular calcifications. The ***brain*** on external aspect showed dilated and congested meningeal blood vessels with bilateral tonsillar herniation. No hemorrhage or exudates were seen. Basal ganglia (Fig 4A) architecture was preserved. The putamen part of the lentiform nucleus appeared soft. On microscopy,

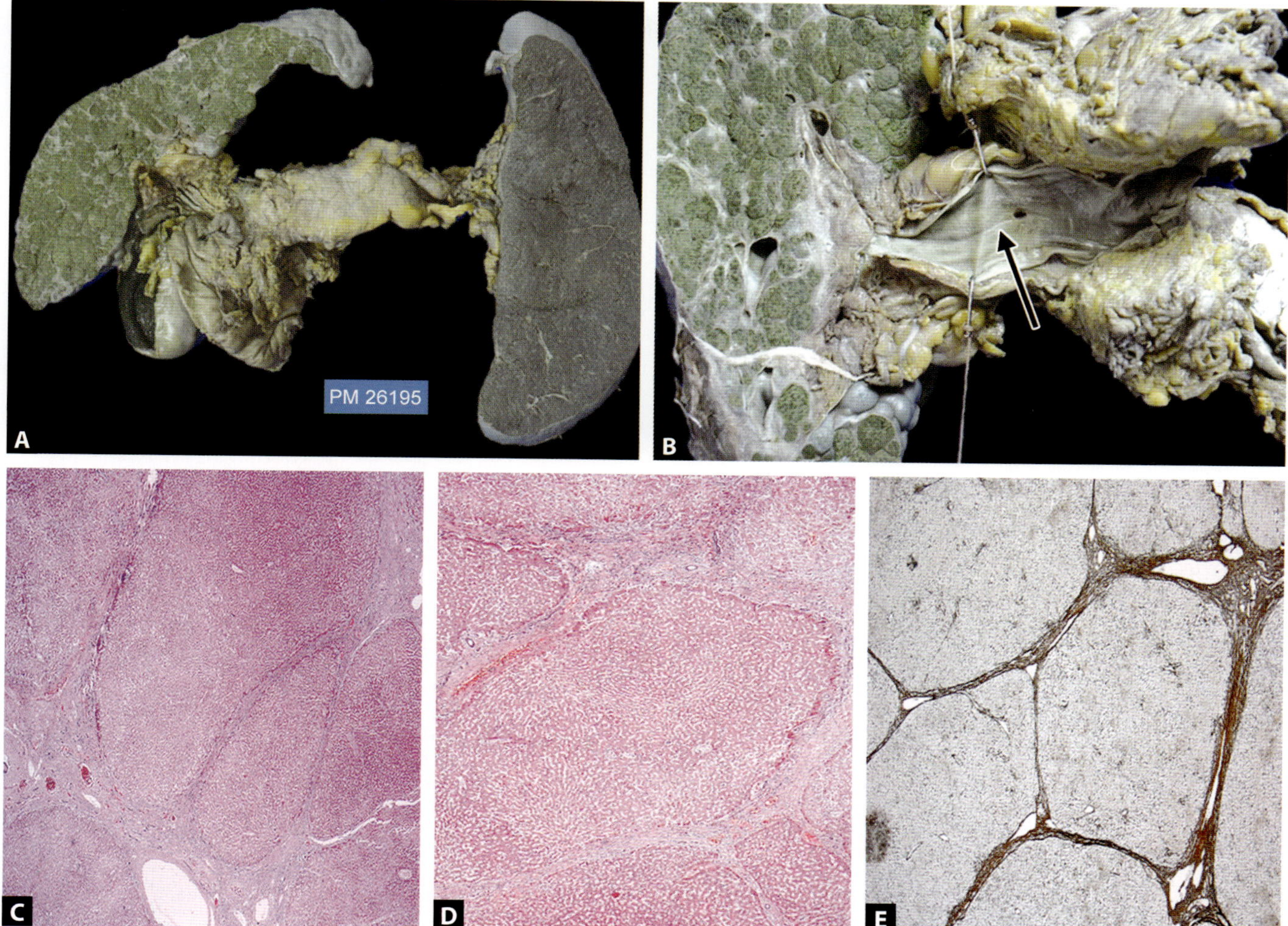

Figs 1A–E: (A) Organ complex of the slice of the shrunken liver with macronodules, enlarged spleen (bigger than the liver), pancreas, gallbladder and the duodenum; (B) Gross picture showing opened up portal vein (arrow) and the bile stained liver showing macronodules; (C and D) Low power photomicrographs of the liver showing varying sized nodules separated by fibrous septae; (E) Reticulin stain highlights the nodules better.

sections (Figs 4B–F) studied from both the putamen revealed irregular areas of rarefaction leading to extensive myelinolysis and cystic change. Sections studied form the thalamus, other parts of the globus pallidus, midbrain, pons, medulla, cerebellum and multiple sections from the cortex, however, did not reveal this kind of change.

FINAL AUTOPSY DIAGNOSIS: PM 26195

17 Year Old Male with Wilson's Disease

- Features consistent with Wilson's disease:
  - Macronodular cirrhosis with increased intrahepatocytic copper associated proteins and nuclear glycogenation.
  - Portal hypertension—ascites, splenomegaly.
  - Myelinolysis: Bilateral Putamen.
- Pulmonary hemorrhages
- Bile casts

WILSON'S DISEASE

Wilson's disease is an inherited and autosomal recessive disease characterized by abnormal accumulation of copper in different organs like liver, brain and eyes.[1] It occurs due to mutation in ***ATP7B*** gene, resulting in reduced excretion of copper in the bile.[2] Its annual incidence is estimated to be 1 in 30,000. It can present at any age, being more common in patients below 35-years of age. The ***ATP7B*** gene, located

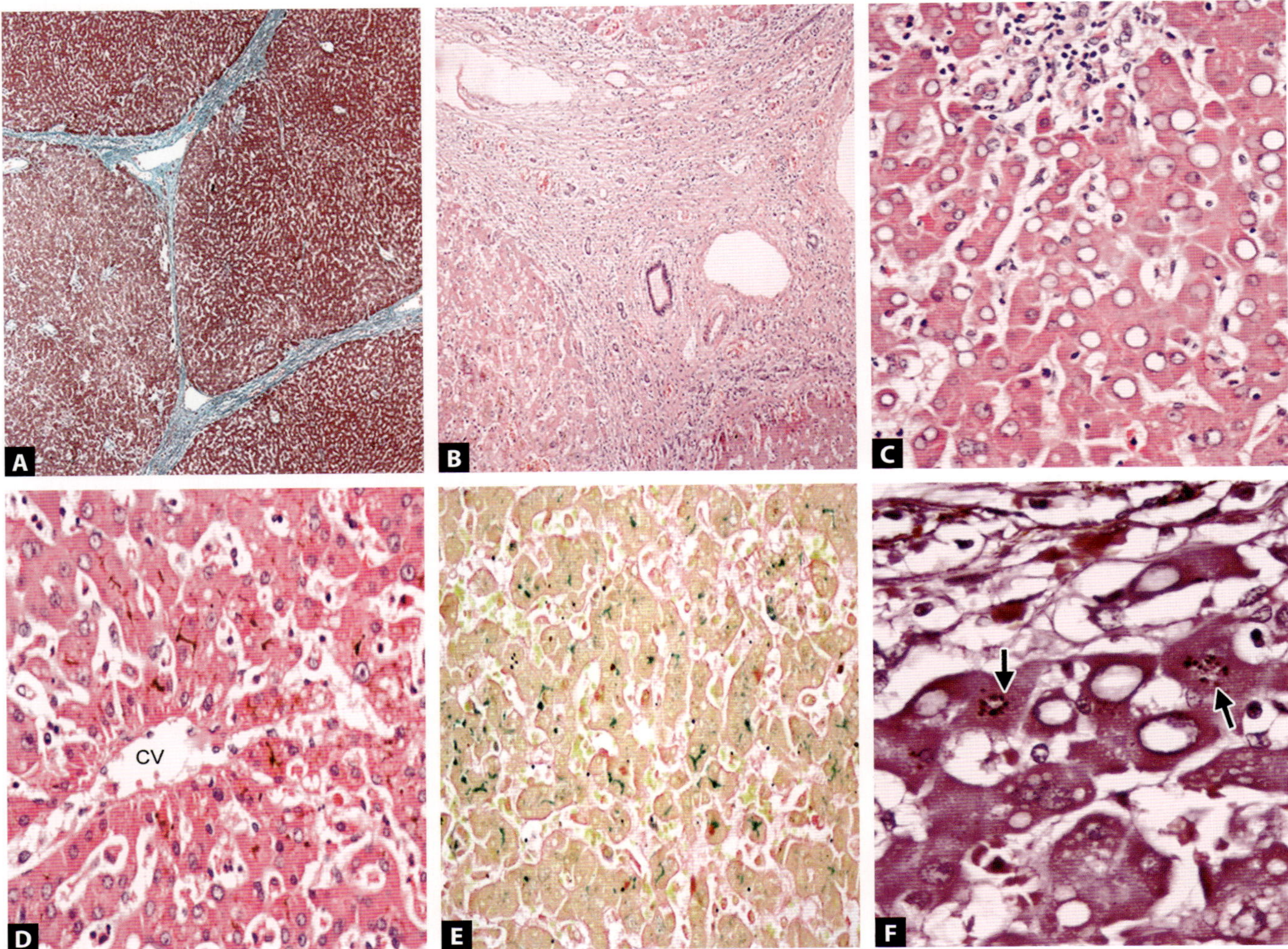

Figs 2A–F: Photomicrographs of the liver (A) Masson's trichrome stain highlights the septae dividing the liver into macronodules; (B) Expanded portal tract showing lymphomononuclear cell infiltrate; (C) Hepatocytes showing glycogenation of the nuclei; (D) Hepatocytes showing cholestasis around the central vein (CV); (E) Cholestasis (green color) in the hepatocytes, better appreciated in the Fouchet's stain; (F) Orcein stain shows coarse cola-colored granules in the hepatocytes (arrows).

on chromosome 13, encodes ***ATP7B*** (P type ATPase), a copper-transport protein, that is located in the golgi apparatus within hepatocytes.[2] This protein transports copper from chaperones into the secretory pathway inducing excretion of copper into bile.[2] Additionally, it also helps in binding of copper into apoceruloplasmin which gets converted into functional ceruloplasmin.[2]

Excessive accumulation of copper results in oxidative damage to the hepatocytes, toxic neuronal damage and impairment of metabolic functions that is manifested in varied clinical signs and symptoms of the disease. Liver disease may manifest as acute liver failure, acute hepatitis, cirrhosis, Coomb's negative hemolytic anemia and portal hypertension. Neurological manifestations, seen in around 50% of the cases, include akinetic-rigid syndrome, cerebellar ataxia and dystonias leading to difficulty in speech, swallowing, abnormal posturing and pseudosclerosis with tremors. Various psychiatric and behavioral changes are also encountered in the form of depression, schizophrenia, cognitive impairment, decreased work and school performance, labile mood and impulsive behavior. Kayser-Fleischer ring, the clinical hallmark of neurological Wilson's disease, occurs due to excessive accumulation of copper in the descemet's membrane of cornea and is detected on slit-lamp examination as a golden layer in the limbus.[3] Several routine tests used for diagnosis of Wilson's disease include serum ceruloplasmin (< 50% of lower normal limit), serum free copper (> 200 mcg/L), hepatic copper estimation on liver biopsy

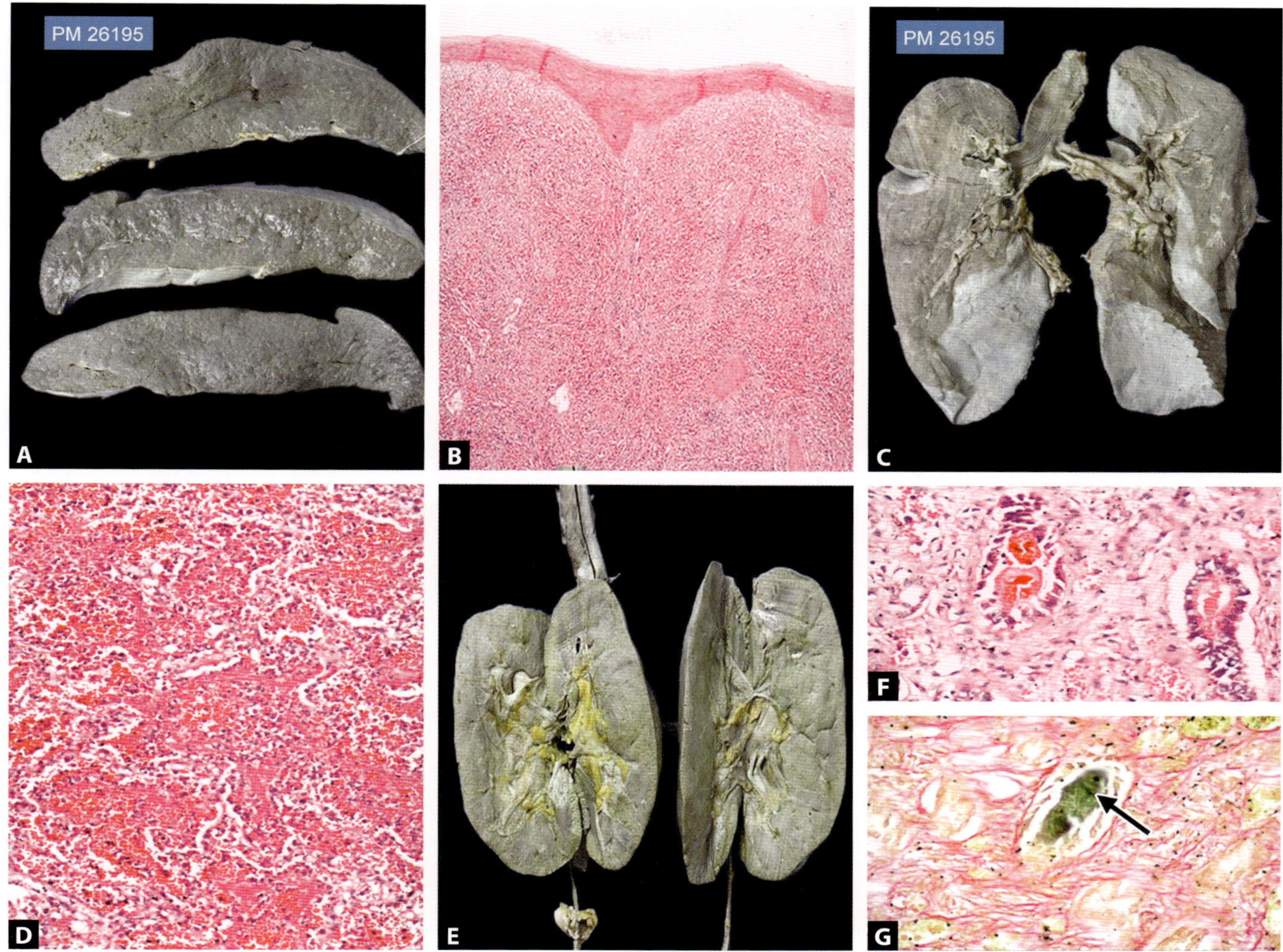

Figs 3A–G: (A) Coronal slices of the diffusely enlarged spleen; (B) Spleen shows red pulp congestion; (C) Cut section of both lungs showing consolidation; (D) Photomicrograph of the lung showing pulmonary hemorrhage; (E) Gross picture of the bile stained kidneys; (F and G) Kidneys showing bile casts stained with Fouchet's stain (arrow).

(>250 mcg/g dry weight), 24-hour urinary copper (>100 mcg/24 hours and >40 mcg/24 hours in children) and K-F rings.[3]

Histomorphological changes on liver biopsy are useful in the diagnosis of Wilson's disease. Liver shows a variety of changes: Fatty change, glycogenated nuclei, acute hepatitis like picture, chronic hepatitis and cirrhosis (usually macronodular, but can be mixed or even micronodular). Occasionally massive hepatic necrosis occurs just like that seen with viruses and drugs. Early changes include non-specific macrovesicular and microvesicular fatty change and nuclear glycogenation/vacuolation.[4] Mallory's bodies are also noted. The intermediate stage is characterized by portal and periportal inflammation, limiting plate breakdown, hepatocytic necrosis and portal fibrosis, while advanced stages are characterized by bridging fibrosis and cirrhosis (macronodular or mixed).[4] In addition, ductular proliferation and cholestasis are the other significant findings. Histochemical demonstration of positive rhodanine staining in biopsy and/or autopsy specimens is a reliable method for identification of copper overload.[5] It stains copper as red-brown granules within the hepatocytes, kupffer cells and portal tract macrophages.[5] Another well-known histochemical technique is orcein staining of copper binding protein within hepatocytes.[5] Imaging modalities like MRI brain are highly sensitive in delineating brain atrophy and hypointensities on T1-weighted image and hyperintensities on T2-weighted images in bilateral basal ganglia, brain-stem, thalamus and cortex. These changes

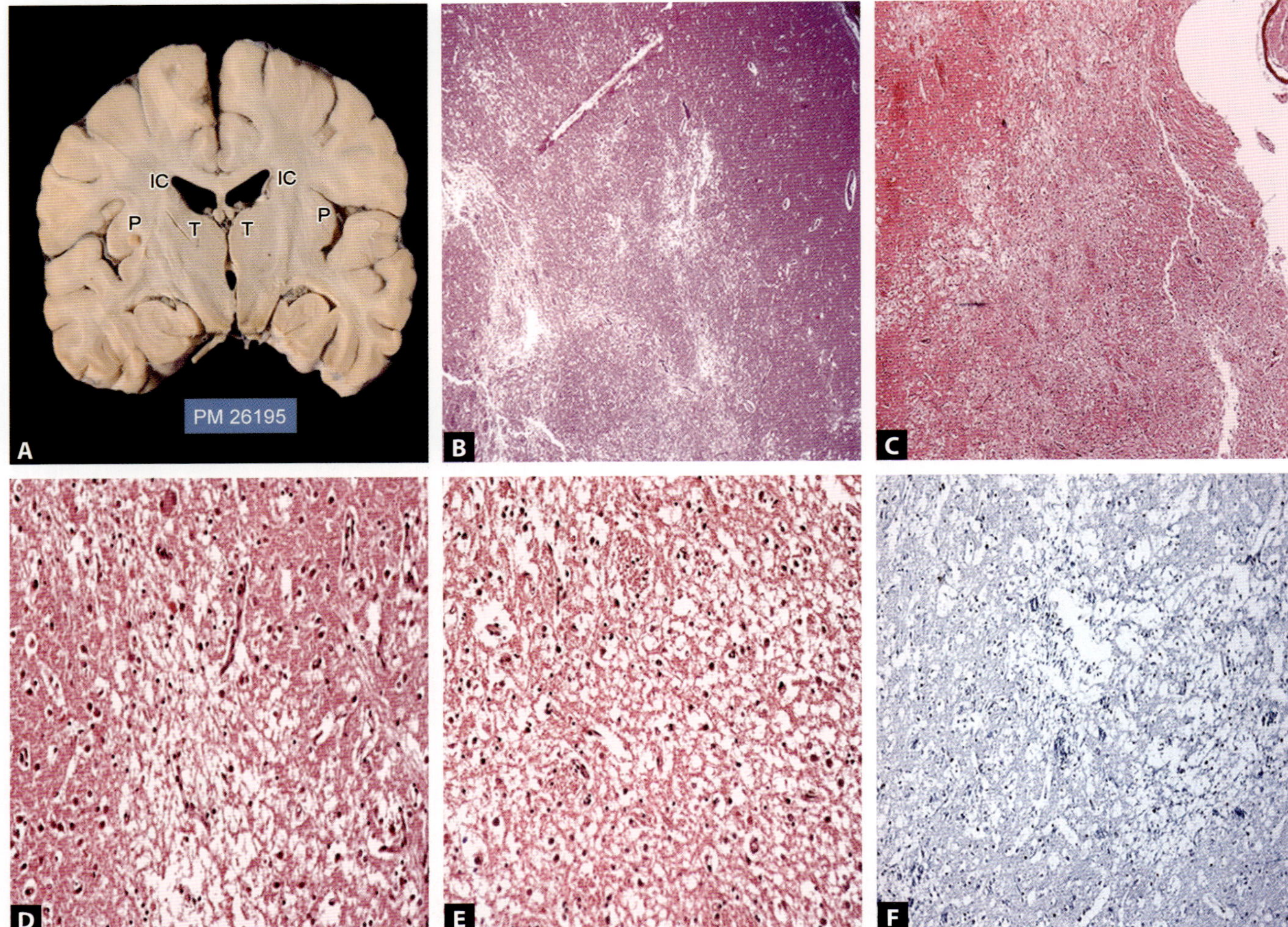

Figs 4A–F: (A) Coronal slice of the brain at the level of the basal ganglia (T- thalamus , P - putamen, IC - internal capsule). There was softening of the putamen, better felt than seen; (B and C) Low power photomicrographs from right and left putamen showing irregular areas of rarefaction; (D and E) The areas of rarefaction in the putamen at high power showing extensive myelinolysis; (F) Myelin stain shows extensive myelin loss with cystic change.

reflect the underlying toxic neuronal damage which are histopathologically characterized by neuronal loss, liquefaction and spongiform degeneration accompanied by gliosis and increase in astrocytes.[4] Opalski cells, arising from degenerating astrocytes, are large cells with granular cytoplasm.[4] Sundaram et al[6] studied eight patients of Wilson's disease at autopsy and highlighted the neuropathological findings of six of these patients who had presented with neurological manifestations. They found central pontine myelinolysis and subcortical white matter cavitations in 5/6 cases, putamen involvement in four and ventricular dilatation in all six cases. They pointed out that pontine myelinolysis and opalski cells correlate well with the neurological form of Wilson's disease.

The medical treatment of Wilson's disease includes initial chelation therapy with penicillamine or trientine. There is an increasing trend of using trientine over penicillamine for neurological and hepatic form of the disease.[4] Maintenance therapy can be offered in the form of reduced dose of chelating agent or zinc. Liver transplantation is indicated in patients with acute fulminant liver failure or those who are nonresponsive to medical therapy.[4] These patients need to be kept on close and long-term follow-up along with monitoring of copper levels.

COMMENTARY—INDEX CASE: PM 26195

This is the story of a young boy, who first came at the age of 13-years with hematemesis and variceal ligation was done. At the age of 15-years he was diagnosed as a case of Wilson's disease and was started on treatment. At the age of

17-years he was readmitted. He had ascites, neuropsychiatric manifestations (behavioral problems, abnormal posturing), low serum ceruloplasmin, high 24-hour urinary copper excretion, Kayser-Fleischer ring, positive D-penicillamine challenge test and altered mixed signal intensity in bilateral putamen, thalami, midbrain, superior cerebellar peduncles and pons, consistent with a diagnosis of Wilson's disease. Autopsy revealed features consistent with Wilson's disease i.e. macronodular cirrhosis with orcein positive granules and myelinolysis in bilateral putamen.

TAKE HOME MESSAGE

- Wilson's disease is an inherited and autosomal recessive disorder due to mutation in ATP7B gene and is characterized by abnormal accumulation of copper in different organs like liver, brain and eyes.
- Liver in Wilson's disease show a variety of changes—fatty change, glycogenated nuclei, Mallory's body, acute hepatitis like picture, chronic hepatitis and cirrhosis which is usually macronodular, but can be mixed or even micronodular.
- Pontine myelinolysis and opalski cells correlate well with the neurological form of Wilson's disease.

REFERENCES

1. Gitlin JD. Wilson disease. Gastroenterology. 2003;125(6):1868-77.
2. Tao TY, Gitlin JD. Hepatic copper metabolism: insights from genetic disease. Hepatology. 2003;37(6):1241-7.
3. Patil M, Sheth KA, Krishnamurthy AC, et al. A review and current perspective on Wilson's disease. J Clin Exp Hepatol. 2013;3(4):321-36.
4. Ala A, Walker AP, Ashkan K, et al. Wilson's disease. Lancet. 2007;369(9559):397-408.
5. Davies SE, Williams R, Portman B. Hepatic morphology and histochemistry of Wilson's disease presenting as fulminant hepatic failure: a study of 11 cases. Histopathology. 1989; 15(4):385-94.
6. Meenakshi-Sundaram S, Mahadevan A, Taly AB, et al. Wilson's disease: A clinicopathological autopsy study. J Clin Neurosci. 2008;15(4):409-17.

CONTRIBUTIONS BY:

1. Dr Vishrut, Junior Resident, Department of Pathology (In taking gross Photographs)
2. Dr Saniya Sharma, Senior Resident, Department of Pathology (Working up the Case)
3. Dr BD Radotra, Professor, Department of Histopathology (Consultation)
4. Dr RK Vasishta, Professor and Head, Department of Histopathology (Consultation)
5. Dr RK Kochhar, Professor and Head, Department of Gastroenterology (Clinician In-Charge)
6. Dr NK Khandelwal, Prof and Head, Department of Radiodiagnosis and Imaging.

Post Graduate Institute of Medical Education and Research, Chandigarh, India.

SECTION 5

Cardiovascular System Adult Cases

CASE 30

Silent Healed Myocardial Infarction and its Complications—Infarct Expansion, Mural Thrombosis, Aneurysm Formation, Extensive Arterial Embolization, Deep Vein Thrombosis and Subsequent Fatal Venous Thromboembolism: PM 21817

Nandita Bharadwaj Kakkar

 HIGHLIGHTS OF THE CASE

A 40-year-old male was admitted with gangrene of the right leg, left toe and dyspnea on exertion since 2 months. His lower limb pulses were not palpable, pedal edema was present, jugular venous pressure (JVP) was raised, liver was palpable, diffuse crepts were present and ECG revealed presence of Q wave with ST ↑ in V2–V5 with poor progression of "R" wave. Doppler of the lower limb revealed thrombus in both the femoral arteries and no spontaneous flow in both sided popliteal, posterior tibial and dorsalis pedis arteries. There was evidence of deep vein thrombosis (DVT). Autopsy revealed a large, healed, transmural, anteroseptal myocardial infarct with infarct expansion, aneurysm formation, mural thrombosis and extensive arterial embolization to the brain, left kidney and both lower limbs. This was further complicated by DVT, extensive venous embolization and fatal bilateral pulmonary embolism.

Keywords: Myocardial infarction, complications, asymptomatic, infarct expansion, aneurysm formation, mural thrombosis, systemic embolization, autopsy.

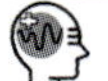 CLINICAL DETAILS

Date of Admission: 01.02.2007, Date of Death: 01.02.2007.

A 40-year-old male came to the emergency ward with presenting complaint of progressive blackening (gangrene) of the right leg, below the knee since 2 months. There was dyspnea on exertion for the same duration of time. He was a smoker. On examination he was conscious, oriented, there was pallor, pedal edema, no cyanosis or fever, radial pulse was 104/min, bilateral popliteal, posterior tibial and dorsalis pedis arteries were not palpable, BP 130/80 mm Hg, RR 22/min, JVP ↑, liver was palpable 2 cm below right costal margin, bilateral diffuse crepts were present but no wheeze was heard. No murmurs were audible. The CNS examination was within normal limits.

Investigation

Investigation revealed a normal hemogram, coagulogram—PT 11 seconds (C-10 seconds), PTI 91%, aPTT 34 seconds (C-25-32), normal blood glucose, lipid profile, electrolytes, renal and liver function tests. The anti-ds DNA antibody (ELISA), sputum for acid-fast bacilli (AFB), HIV, HbSAg and HCV were all negative. ***ECG*** revealed sinus tachycardia, Q wave with ST ↑ in V2–V5, poor progression of "R" wave and left atrial enlargement. X-ray chest showed bilateral consolidation (Rt> Lt), right pleural effusion with cardiomegaly. ***Doppler*** of the lower limb revealed a normal flow velocity and biphasic wave form in left femoral artery, but lumen showed partial thrombosis. Very sluggish flow was seen in right femoral artery in its central part and thrombus was seen along the walls. No spontaneous flow was seen in both popliteal, posterior tibial and dorsalis pedis arteries. Acute thrombosis of both femoral arteries with severe reduction of flow, more on right side was noted. There was evidence of DVT. Both kidneys showed enhanced echogenicity. The patient succumbed to his illness within 5 hours of emergency admission. An echocardiography could not be done. ***Units final diagnosis*** was—thrombosis of both femoral arteries, right lower limb gangrene, left toe gangrene, pneumonia and septicemia.

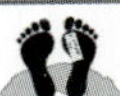

AUTOPSY FINDINGS: PM 21817

A complete autopsy was performed. The body was thin built. The right foot and left toe were gangrenous. Both pleural cavities yielded 250 mL of hemorrhagic fluid. The ***heart*** weighed 485 g (Fig 1A). The right atrium and ventricle were mildly dilated. The tricuspid valve and pulmonary valve were normal. The right atrial appendage contained a thrombus. The root of the pulmonary artery was dilated. The left atrium and ventricle were markedly dilated (Figs 1B and C), but the mitral and aortic valves were normal. The anterior wall of the left ventricle was markedly thinned out with a prominent bulge on the exterior (Fig 1D). A large mural thrombus (Figs 1E and F) was seen in the apical region of the left ventricle measuring 2 × 2 × 1 cm. Coronal slices (Fig 2A) of the heart exhibited thinned out wall of the left ventricle with a large transmural anteroseptal healed infarct. The left anterior descending artery (LAD) showed a 75% atherosclerotic occlusion in its lower part. Left circumflex artery (LCA) and the right coronary artery revealed 15% and 10% occlusion, respectively. The aorta however did not show any significant atherosclerosis. Microscopic examination confirmed the mural thrombus and the transmural anteroseptal old myocardial infarct (Fig 2B) with expansion and aneurysm formation (Fig 2C). Extensive embolization from the mural thrombus to the systemic circulation was noted. The ***brain*** weighed 1,464 g. The circle of Willis did not reveal any thrombus. Multiple cystic infarcts (Fig 2D) were noted in the territory of the left middle cerebral artery, i.e. in the left posterior temporal area measuring 2 × 1 × 1 cm, in the left trigone measuring 3 mm and in the left superior temporal gyrus. Mild ventricular dilatation was noted. On microscopic examination, these were old cystic infarcts with abundant macrophages (Figs 2E and F). There was embolization and total occlusion of ***left renal artery*** with the embolus jutting out and plastering the aorta for about 2.5 cm (Figs 3A–E), right common iliac artery, right internal/external iliac arteries (Figs 3B and 4B) and right femoral artery. Left common iliac artery and its branches internal/external iliac and femoral were partially occluded by thrombus. Right adrenal gland (Figs 4C and D) showed a thrombus in an artery along with infarction. On the venous side there was thrombosis of right internal/external iliac vein, right common iliac vein, left renal vein (Fig 4A), splenic vein, superior mesenteric vein, smaller mesenteric veins, right hepatic vein, right and left pulmonary arteries (saddle thrombus) and their segmental/subsegmental branches (Figs 5A–C). The left ***kidney*** was small in size, measuring 4 × 3 × 2 cm and showed multiple infarcts (Fig 3A and B, 5D). The left renal artery was occluded by a thrombus which was jutting on the aorta at its ostia for a distance of 3 cm. The left renal vein was also occluded by a thrombus. On microscopic examination (Figs 5E and F) the infarcts were seen and the lobar/arcuate arteries were thrombosed by organizing thrombi. The ***right kidney*** was normal grossly and on microscopic examination. The ***liver*** weighed 1,210 g. On cut section, the right hepatic vein was partially thrombosed. On microscopic examination, centrizonal passive venous congestion was seen. The ***spleen*** weighed 210 g and was congested. The ***lungs*** weighed 1,310 g. Both pulmonary arteries (saddle thrombi), segmental and lobar vessels were thrombosed. Cut section of both the lungs revealed multiple wedge-shaped infarcts, some of which were breaking down (Figs 6A–C). Microscopy (Figs 6D–F) revealed organizing thrombi in all caliber vessels, hemorrhage, infarcts, pulmonary arterial hypertension Grade 2 and bronchopneumonia (Fig. 6G).

FINAL AUTOPSY DIAGNOSIS : PM 21817

40 Years Old Male

- Old healed transmural, anteroseptal myocardial infarction with:
  - Left ventricular infarct expansion, aneurysm formation and mural thrombosis.
  - Extensive arterial embolization and occlusion of left renal artery, both common iliac arteries (right > left), internal/external iliac and femoral arteries (right > left).
  - Multiple cystic infarcts—left middle cerebral artery territory.
- Deep vein thrombosis with embolization to the right internal/external iliac vein, right common iliac vein, left renal vein, splenic vein, superior mesenteric vein, smaller mesenteric veins, right hepatic vein, right and left pulmonary arteries (saddle thrombus) and their segmental and subsegmental branches.
- Left renal infarcts.
- Multiple pulmonary infarcts, bronchopneumonia and pulmonary arterial hypertension Grade 2.
- Passive venous congestion—lungs and liver.

MYOCARDIAL INFARCTION AND ITS COMPLICATIONS[1]

Death of cardiac muscle fibers as a result of ischemia is known as myocardial infarction (MI). It is the most common ischemic heart disease and affects a very large population of the world. Myocardial infarcts can be transmural or subendocardial. In transmural infarcts, the entire wall of

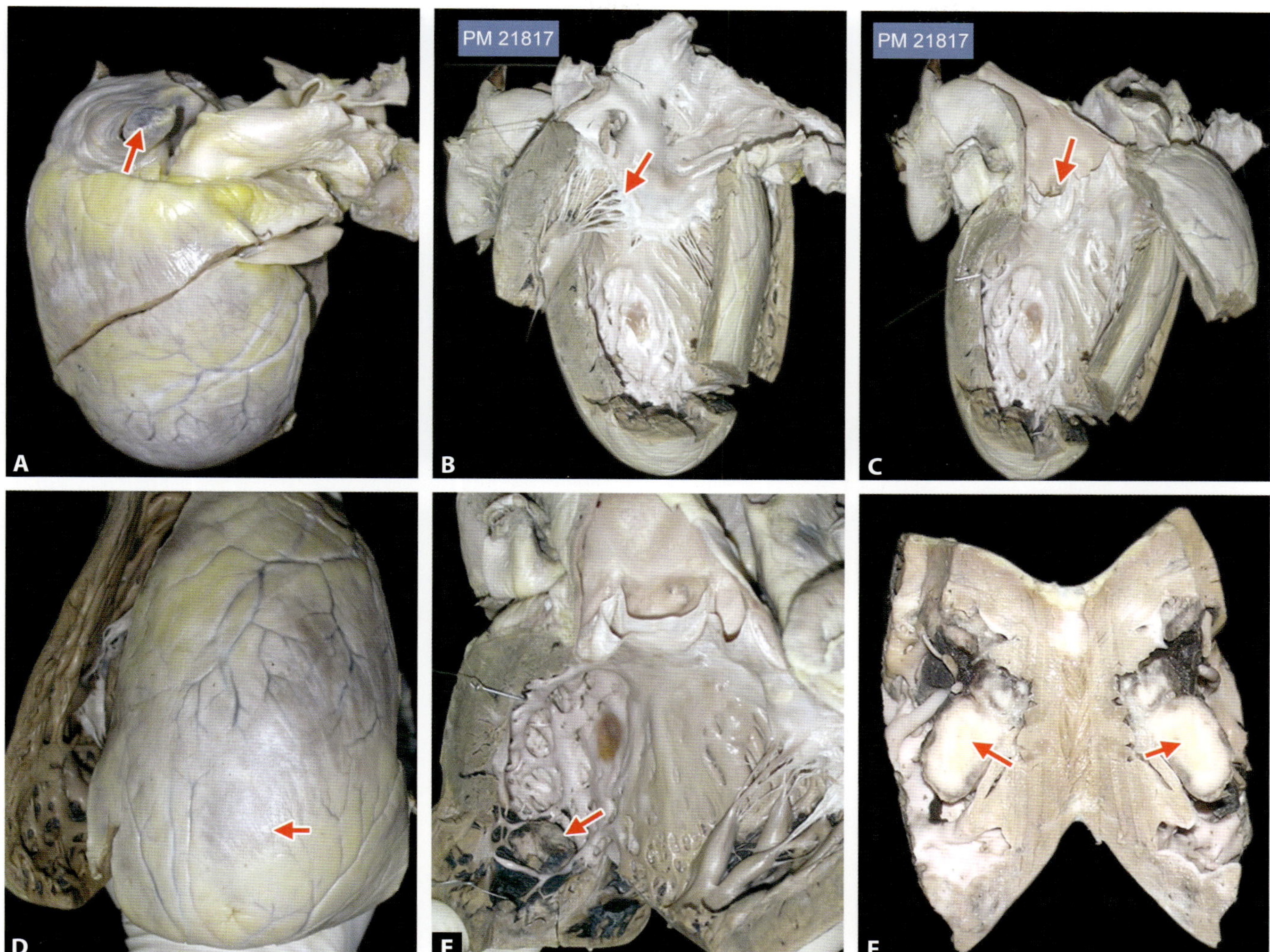

Figs 1A–F: (A) Gross picture of the enlarged heart. The right atrial appendage shows a thrombus (arrow); (B) Opened up left side of the heart showing left atrial dilatation. Mitral valve (arrow) is normal; (C) Left outflow tract showing left ventricular dilatation. Aortic valve (arrow) is normal; (D) Bulge (arrow) on the anterior wall of the left ventricle; (E) Left ventricular mural thrombus in the apical region (arrow); (F) Cut section of the mural thrombus (arrows).

the ventricle, supplied by a single coronary artery undergoes ischemic necrosis. The subendocardium is most vulnerable to any reduction in coronary flow. In subendocardial infarcts, inner one third or at the most half of the ventricular wall gets affected. Extension beyond the perfusion territory of a single coronary artery can occur. Subendocardial infarcts occur when timely thrombolysis is done, before the entire wall gets affected by ischemic necrosis. They also occur in the setting of shock, when there is a severe reduction in the systemic blood pressure. Major risk factors for ischemic heart disease include constitutional/non-modifiable factors like age, sex, genetics and modifiable factors like hyperlipidemia, hypertension, cigarette smoking and diabetes mellitus. Other factors include homocystinuria, elevated plasminogen activator inhibitor-1 and increased C reactive proteins indicating the presence of inflammation and increased lipoprotein (Lp) A levels. Factors where there is difficulty in assessing the risk include sedentary life, type A personality with a stressful lifestyle and obesity. Postmenopausal estrogen deficiency, high carbohydrate and hardened unsaturated fat intake are other risk factors. About 10% of myocardial infarcts occur in people below 40 years and 50% occur below the age of 65 years. Women are protected in the reproductive years due to the estrogen protective mechanism. But after menopause, there can be rapid development of coronary artery disease. Transmural acute MI in 90% cases, occur due to interplay of a number of factors like coronary atherosclerosis, acute atheromatous plaque changes (rupture, ulceration,

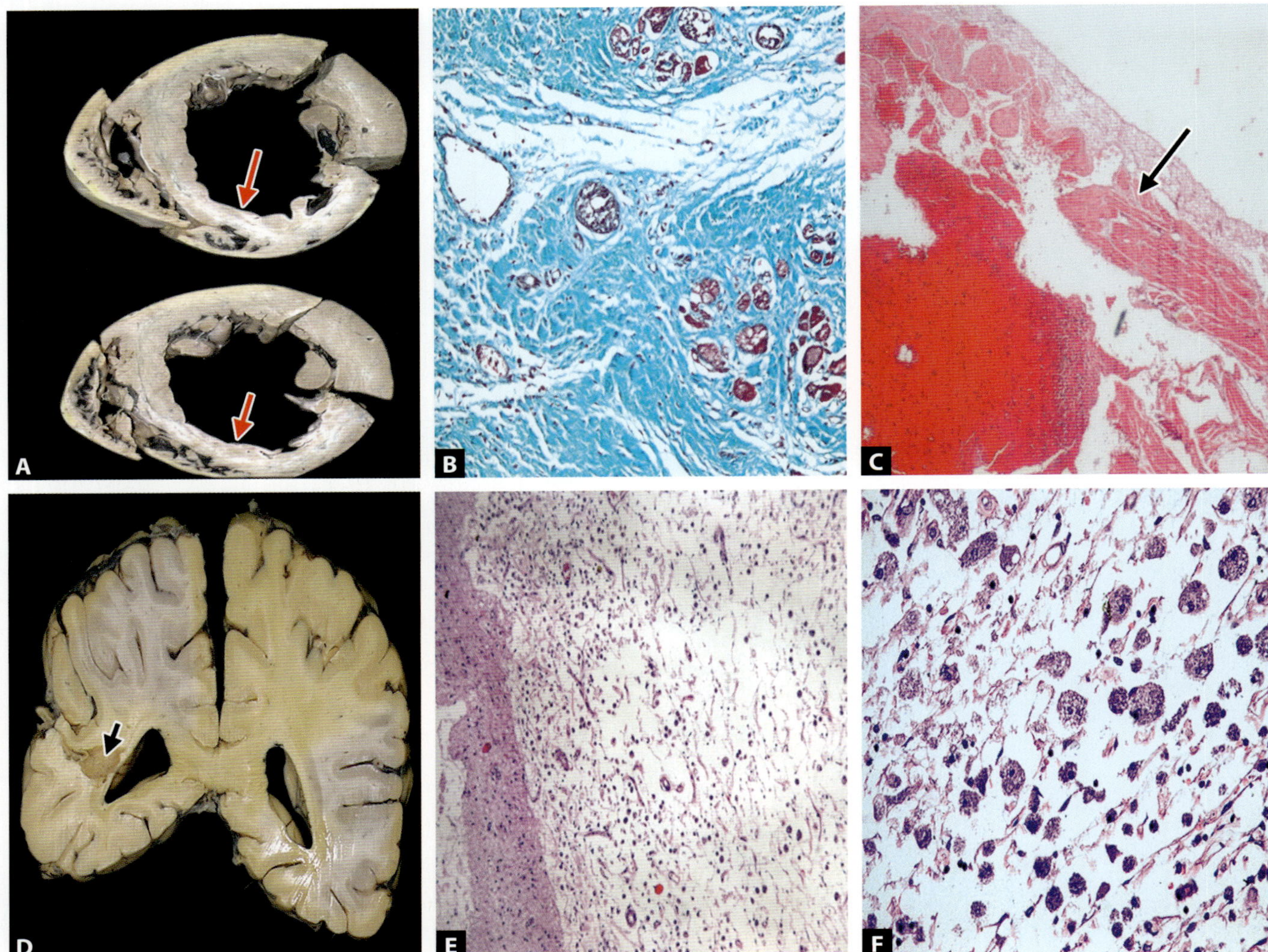

Figs 2A–F: (A) Coronal slices of the heart showing a large transmural anteroseptal infarct (arrows). The myocardium in this area is thinned out and fibrotic; (B) Infarct stained with Masson's trichrome, showing extensive fibrosis (green colored) with few hypertrophied viable myocytes (red colored); (C) Anteroseptal infarct with markedly thinned out wall showing disruption (arrow); (D) Coronal slice of the brain showing a cystic infarct (arrow); (E and F) Photomicrographs from the brain infarct showing abundant macrophages.

erosion, hemorrhage), thrombosis, platelet activation and vasospasm which leads to an occlusive thrombus that overlies a plaque. The situation can be worsened by increased myocardial demand (tachycardia or hypertrophy) or with drop in blood pressure. In 10% cases, acute MI is not associated with thrombosis of an atherosclerotic plaque and here other factors like vasospasm (intense and prolonged) and emboli (from left atrium due to atrial fibrillation) are the etiological factors. MI is diagnosed by typical symptoms (precordial pain, rapid weak pulse, profuse sweating and dyspnea), electrocardiogram and biochemical evidence. After acute MI, levels of cardiac troponin I and T rise at 2–4 hours, peak at 24 hours and remain elevated for 7–10 days. The other alternative is creatine kinase (CK-MB) which rises within 2–4 hours of acute MI, peaks at 24 hours and returns back to normal within 72 hours. So in the initial hours, rise in troponins and CK-MB are similar, but the former remain elevated for a longer duration. In 15% cases of MI, the patients are asymptomatic (especially in the elderly and in diabetics) and the disease is detected later by the advent of complications and ECG changes consisting of new "Q" waves.

The LAD coronary artery is affected in 40–50% of cases (in right dominant heart) and infarcts involve the anterior wall of the left ventricle at the apex, anterior part of the interventricular septum and the apex in a circumferential manner. The left circumflex coronary artery (LCX) is affected

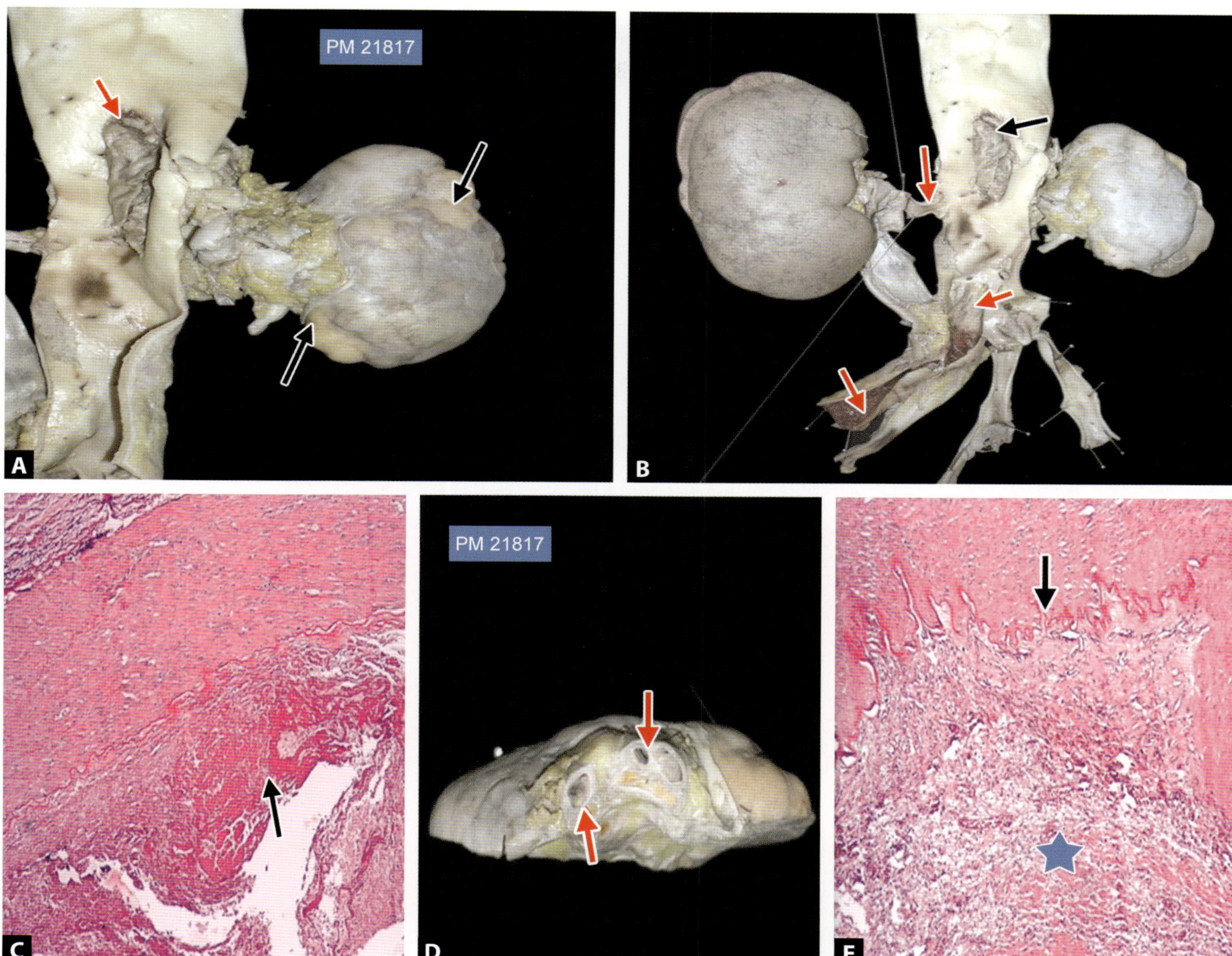

Figs 3A–E: (A) Thrombus in the aorta present at the origin of the left renal artery (red arrow). The left kidney is small and shows multiple infarcts (arrows); (B) Gross picture of the abdominal aorta showing a thrombus in the left renal artery which is jutting out and plastering the aorta (black arrow). The right renal artery is opened up and shows no thrombus (top red arrow). Thrombus is also noted in the right common iliac artery and the external iliac (lower red arrows); (C) Microphotograph of the aortic thrombus shows firm attachment to the wall (arrow); (D) Coronal slice of the left kidney at the hilum showing occlusion of the renal artery and vein by thrombi (arrows); (E) Left renal artery with the organizing thrombus (star). The internal elastic lamina is seen (arrow).

in 15–20% cases and the infarct involves the lateral wall of the left ventricle, sparing the apex. The right coronary artery is affected in 30–40% cases and the infarct involves the posterior part of the ventricular septum, inferior–posterior wall of the left ventricle and the inferior–posterior right ventricular free wall in some cases. The main left coronary artery and the secondary branches like the diagonal branches of the LAD and marginal branches of the LCX, may at times undergo critical occlusions. Gross and microscopic assessment of an infarct, both grossly and microscopically depends on the duration of survival of the patient, after the MI. On gross examination, an infarct of less than 12 hours duration is not visible. On immersing the tissue of the heart in a solution of triphenyltetrazolium chloride, the normal tissue stains brick red, due to the preserved dehydrogenase enzymes, whereas areas of ischemic necrosis due to the depleted dehydrogenases, look like unstained pale zones. An infarct of more than 12–24 hours can be identified on formalin fixation as it elicits a congested look due to the stagnated blood. By 10–14 days, it becomes better defined due to the rimming by a reddish zone. Thereafter, it turns into a fibrous scar. An infarct heals from the borders toward

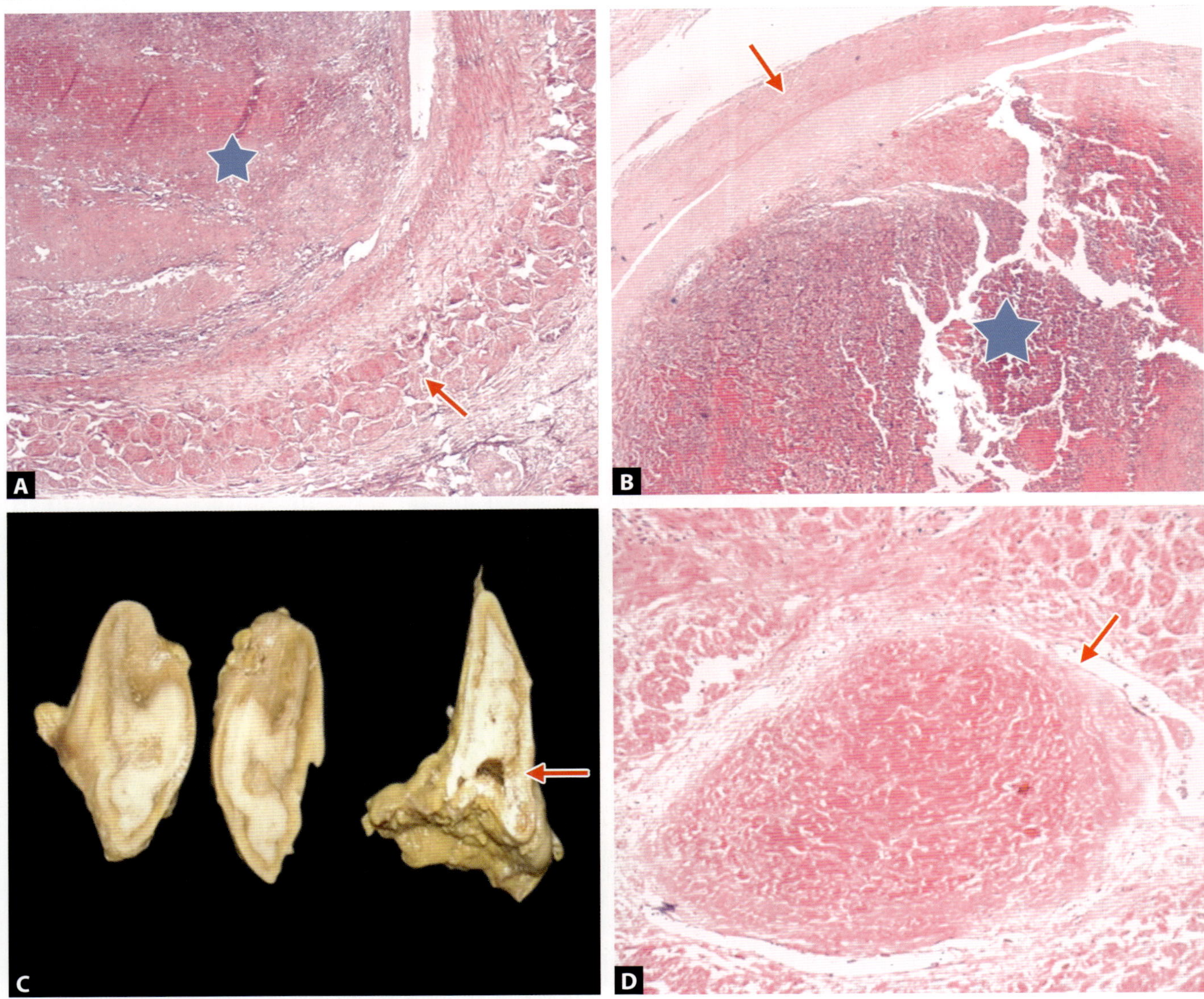

Figs 4A–D: Thrombus (blue stars) in the (A) left renal vein and (B) right common iliac artery. Red arrows point at the vessel wall; (C and D) Gross and microphotograph of the right adrenal gland showing infarction (red arrow in C) with a vessel showing thrombus (red arrow in D).

the center, as it utilizes the inflammatory cells which enter the damaged areas through the proliferating vessels at the margins. Healing further depends on the size of the infarct and a smaller one heals faster. On histopathologic examination in the first 4 hours, there are no changes except for some waviness of fibers at the border zone; between 4–12 hours there is beginning of coagulation necrosis and hemorrhage; between 12–24 hours there is an ongoing coagulation necrosis, hypereosinophilia of the myocytes, nuclear clumping, marginal contraction band necrosis and neutrophils begin to infiltrate; between 1–3 days there is complete necrosis with polymorphonuclear infiltrate; between 3–7 days the dead myofibers disintegrate, neutrophilic debris is seen and macrophages appear at the borders which engulf the dead cells; between 7–10 days macrophages appear in large numbers and are seen to phagocytose the dead cells and granulation tissue appears in the border zone; between 10–14 days the granulation tissue becomes well-developed and collagen deposition begins; between 2–8 weeks the cellularity decreases and the collagen increases and beyond 2 months, dense collagenous scar tissue is seen. At the margins of the infarcts and in the thin zone of viable subendocardium (which is profused by the blood in the cavity), vacuolar degeneration or myocytolysis is seen, wherein large vacuolar spaces are

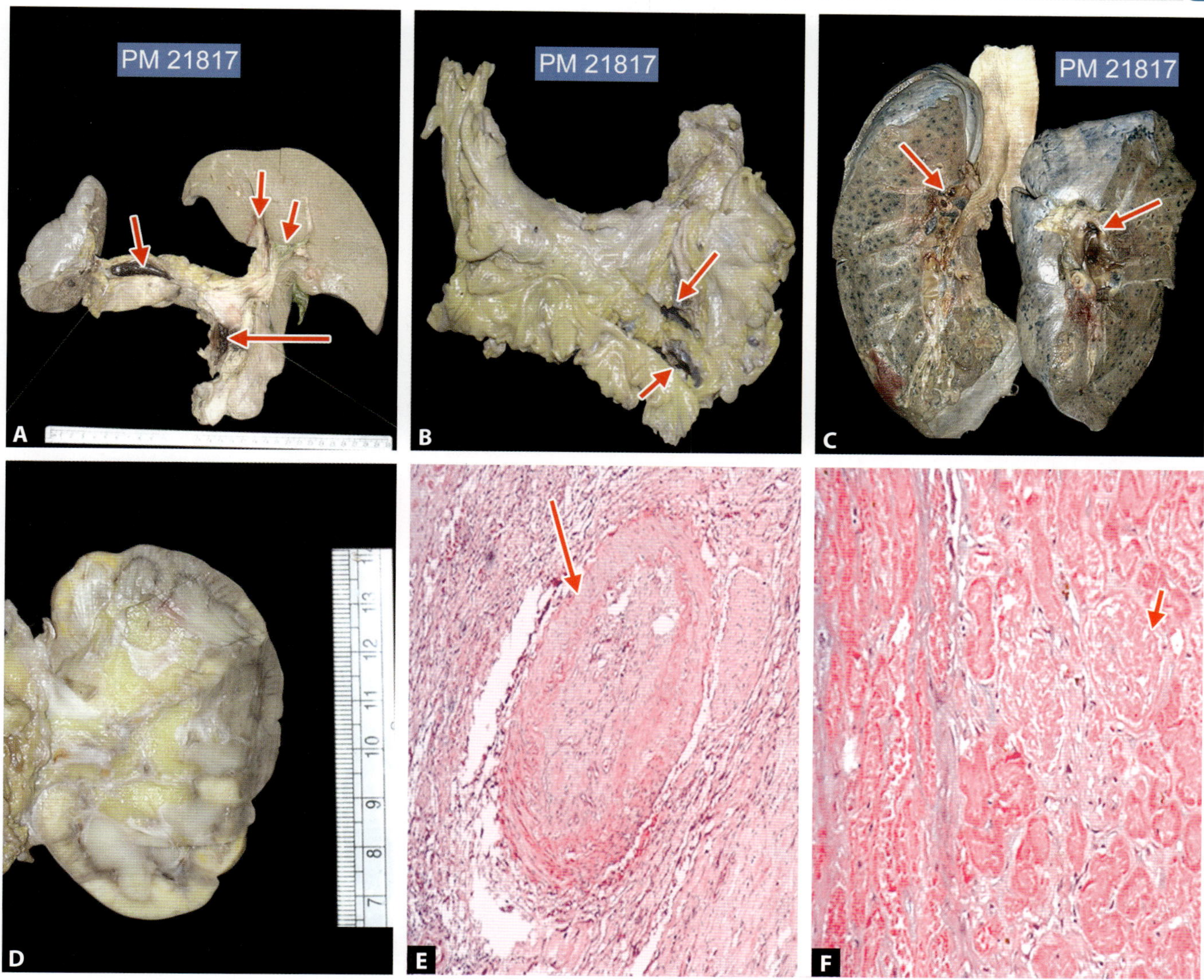

Figs 5A–F: Thrombi (arrows) in the (A) Splenic vein (extreme left arrow), superior mesenteric vein (long arrow), and right hepatic vein (upper arrows); (B) Branches of the mesenteric vein (red arrows); (C) Both pulmonary arteries (red arrows); (D) Cut section of the left kidney showing infarcts; (E) Lobar artery occluded with a thrombus (arrow); (F) Kidney showing infarct with coagulative necrosis of the tubules and glomeruli (arrow).

seen in the cytoplasm. Acute inflammation is most prominent at 2–3 days, phagocytizing macrophages are abundant at 5–10 days, granulation tissue is prominent at 2–4 weeks and scar tissue is well-established by the end of 45 days. The age of a completely healed infarct is impossible to discern.

In the present era, due to the advancements in cardiology, a substantial progress has been made in the prognosis of patients with acute MI. Rapid reversal of coronary flow, i.e. reperfusion can be done by streptokinase thrombolysis, balloon angioplasty (percutaneous transluminal coronary angioplasty—PTCA) and coronary arterial bypass graft (CABG). Reperfusion within 15–20 minutes after the onset of ischemia prevents all necrosis, within 2–4 hours, there is a partial salvage and beyond that there is complete infarction. On microscopic examination, reperfused infarct shows hemorrhage because the injured vasculature (due to ischemia) becomes leaky on restoration of blood flow. Myocyte necrosis, with intensely eosinophilic transverse contraction bands produced due to the exaggerated contraction of myofibrils (once the perfusion is reestablished) can be seen. Reperfusion can lead to new cellular injury, better known as reperfusion injury which prevents the myocardial reperfusion

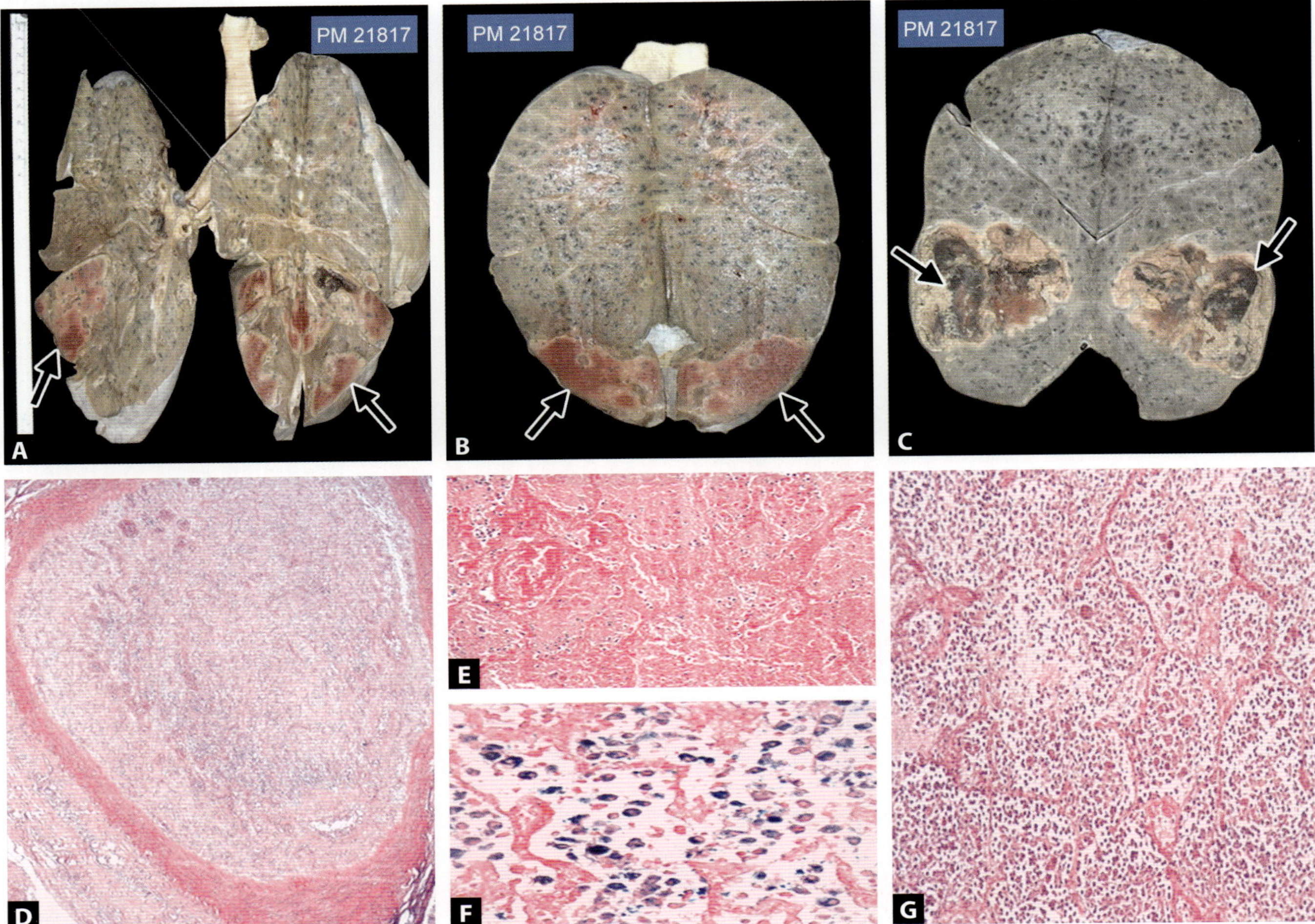

Figs 6A–G: (A–C) Gross photographs of the lungs showing large multiple peripheral infarcts, (arrows in A and B) breaking down in areas (arrows in C); (D) Right pulmonary artery occluded by a thrombus; (E) Photomicrograph of the pulmonary infarct; (F) Perls' stain of lung showing hemosiderin laden macrophages (chronic passive venous congestion); (G) Lung showing bronchopneumonia with polymorphs in sheets.

by occluding the microvasculature leading to the phenomenon of no-reflow. Reperfusion can salvage the myocardium, but critical abnormalities remain at the cellular level leading to prolonged post ischemic ventricular dysfunction or stunned myocardium.

But despite all this, 75% of the patients with MI have one or more complications[2-13] like contractile dysfunction, pericarditis, arrhythmias, right ventricular infarction, extension or expansion of the infarct, dysfunction of the papillary muscle, thrombus in the cavities of the heart, ventricular aneurysm and progressive heart failure leading to chronic ischemic heart disease. Occurrence of complications is related to the size/site of the infarct and whether it is transmural or subendocardial. Cardiogenic shock, arrhythmias and late congestive cardiac failure are seen in cases with large transmural infarcts. Infarct expansion, mural thrombi, aneurysm and free wall rupture are seen with transmural anterior wall infarcts. Conduction defects and right ventricular involvement complicate posterior transmural infarcts. Anterior infarcts have a worse prognosis than the posterior or inferior infarcts.

Complications of acute MI are: (1) Ischemic which include angina, extension of infarct and reinfarction. (2) Mechanical which include cardiogenic shock, heart failure, dysfunction of the mitral valve, expansion of the infarct, aneurysms and cardiac rupture. (3) Arrhythmic which include atrial or ventricular arrhythmias and sinus or atrioventricular node dysfunction. (4) Embolic which include emboli to the brain or to the periphery. (5) Inflammatory i.e. pericarditis. Of all complications, circulatory failure from severe left ventricular dysfunction accounts for most fatalities. Infarct extension is occurrence of fresh necrosis adjacent to an existing infarct. Timely fibrinolytic therapy restores the coronary flow, but in 7–10% of cases within 10 days and in 20–25% cases by 1 year, reocclusion occurs. This leads to infarct extension and these patients have a poorer prognosis. Reinfarction is seen to a larger extent in diabetics or those with prior MI. But now with advancements in coronary care (like stents), repeat infarction occurs in a very small number within 3 months. ***Post-infarction angina*** is angina occurring within few hours to one month after an attack of acute MI. Its incidence is higher in patients who have received streptokinase and in those with non-ST-elevation MI (approximately 25%). ***Infarct expansion*** occurs because the weak myocardial muscle undergoes stretching, thinning and dilatation of the infarcted region and this is often complicated by mural thrombus. Anteroseptal infarcts are more prone to undergo infarct expansion. After acute MI, the myocardium is vulnerable and is more prone to develop stress in the wall, leading to expansion of the infarct. Subacute cardiac rupture is an extreme form of infarct expansion, whereas the chronic form is ventricular aneurysm. ***Ventricular aneurysm*** usually results from a large transmural anteroseptal infarct in 10% of cases. This complication occurs more (10–30%) in patients in whom treatment for reperfusion has not been given. Ventricular aneurysm can lead to arrhythmias, mural thrombus, embolization, heart failure or may be clinically silent. Rupture of the ventricular wall however does not occur. ECG may show persistently elevated ST segments and X-ray of the chest may show an enlarged heart with an abnormal protuberance at the left heart border. Patients with transmural MIs of the apex are at the highest risk for aneurysm formation, followed by those with baso-posterior infarcts. ***Mural thrombus*** occurs in a setting of myocardial contractility abnormality associated with endocardial damage, thus producing a thrombogenic surface, where a mural thrombus can form. Post MI mural thrombus occurs in 20% cases and anterior wall MI especially large ones may show it in over 50% cases. Mural thrombus can dislodge and embolize to the brain and systemic circulation, causing devastation. Cases of MI show clinically evident systemic ***embolism*** in less than 2% cases and most episodes occur 10 days post MI. Anterior wall MI is the biggest culprit due to motion abnormalities and aneurysm formation. Muscle ischemia with superadded atrial fibrillation can lead to systemic embolization. Emboli can manifest as stroke, ischemia, renal infarction, or mesenteric ischemia. Healed MI with aneurysm formation and mural thrombus also predisposes to embolization. Visser et al[14] in their study found left ventricular thrombus complicating myocardial infarction by two-dimensional echocardiography in 119 patients, of which the infarct site was anterior in 98 patients and inferior in 11. Systemic embolism occurred in 26 patients (stroke in 18, lower limb embolism in 7 and mesenteric embolism in 1). Asinger et al[15] evaluated 70 patients after transmural myocardial infarction and found left-ventricular thrombosis in 12 of 35 patients with anterior wall infarction and no thrombus in the other 35 patients with inferior wall infarction. Thrombi were diagnosed on an average of 5 days after the infarction (range, 1 to 11 days). All patients with left ventricular thrombi had severe apical wall motion abnormalities (akinesis or dyskinesis). Asinger et al concluded that patients with severe apical wall motion abnormalities during acute transmural anterior MI are at high risk for left ventricular thrombosis.

COMMENTARY—INDEX CASE: PM 21817

A 40-year-old male was admitted with a history of gangrene of the right leg, left toe and dyspnea on exertion since 2 months. His lower limb pulses were not palpable, pedal edema was present, JVP ↑, liver was palpable, diffuse crepts were present and ECG revealed presence of Q wave with ST ↑ in V2-V5, poor progression of "R" wave and left atrial enlargement. Doppler of the lower limb revealed thrombus in both the femoral arteries and no spontaneous flow in both sided popliteal, posterior tibial and dorsalis pedis arteries. There was evidence of DVT. Autopsy revealed old healed transmural, anteroseptal myocardial infarct with infarct expansion, aneurysm formation, mural thrombosis and extensive arterial embolization to the brain, left kidney and both lower limbs. This was further complicated by DVT and extensive embolization as cited above. Knitting up the sequence of events, this middle-aged male had a healed, large transmural anteroseptal myocardial infarct (in the territory of LAD) which was definitely more than 2 months old. The history of myocardial infarction and treatment was however not forthcoming. It is known that in approximately 15% cases of MI, the patients are asymptomatic and the disease is detected later by the advent of complications and ECG changes consisting of new "Q" waves. The presence of ST elevation seen in the ECG, in the absence of a fresh myocardial infarct correlates well with the aneurysm formation. This is what happened in the index case as well. This anteroseptal transmural infarct underwent infarct expansion. The weak myocardial muscle underwent stretching, thinning and dilatation of the infarcted region leading to aneurysm of the left ventricle. This was the perfect setting for formation of left ventricular mural thrombus which embolized to the brain, left renal artery, right adrenal gland, both lower limbs, leading to infarcts and gangrene. The patient after the myocardial infarction must not have been ambulatory. This led on to the DVT with embolization to the venous side as cited above. Major bilateral pulmonary thromboembolization, i.e. saddle thrombi were present along with infarcts in the lung which was the terminal event. This patient had a biventricular failure. The left heart failure was because of the transmural myocardial infarct and its complications. This subsequently led on to a right heart failure, which led to an increased JVP, centrizonal passive congestion, congestive splenomegaly and pleural effusion.

TAKE HOME MESSAGE

- Approximately 15% cases of MI are asymptomatic and the disease is detected later by the advent of complications and ECG changes consisting of new "Q" waves.
- The presence of ST elevation seen in the ECG, in the absence of a fresh myocardial infarct, correlates well with the aneurysm formation.
- Despite all advancements in cardiology, 75% of the patients with MI have one or more complications which are ischemic, mechanical, arrhythmic, embolic or inflammatory.
- Infarct expansion occurs due to stretching, thinning and dilatation of the infarcted myocardium and this is often complicated by mural thrombus. Large transmural anteroseptal infarcts are more prone to undergo infarct expansion.
- Mural thrombus occurs in a setting of myocardial contractile abnormality associated with endocardial damage which produces a thrombogenic surface.
- Mural thrombus can dislodge and embolize to the brain and systemic circulation, causing devastation.

REFERENCES

1. Kumar V, Abbas AK, Fausto N, et al. Robbins and Cotran Pathologic Basis of Disease, 8th edition. Philadelphia: Saunders Elsevier; 2009.
2. French JK, Hellkamp AS, Armstrong PW, et al. Mechanical complications after percutaneous coronary intervention in ST-elevation myocardial infarction (from APEX-AMI). Am J Cardiol. 2010;105:59-63.
3. Kutty RS, Jones N, Moorjani N. Mechanical complications of acute myocardial infarction. Cardiol Clin. 2013;31:519-31.
4. Wehrens XH, Doevendans PA. Cardiac rupture complicating myocardial infarction. Int J Cardiol. 2004;95(2-3):285-92.
5. Anzai T. Post-infarction inflammation and left ventricular remodeling: a double-edged sword. Circ J. 2013;77(3):580-7.
6. Stokman PJ, Nandra CS, Asinger RW. Left ventricular thrombus. Curr Treat Options Cardiovasc Med. 2001;3:515-21.
7. Osherov AB, Borovik-Raz M, Aronson D, et al. Incidence of early left ventricular thrombus after acute anterior wall myocardial infarction in the primary coronary intervention era. Am Heart J. 2009;157(6):1074-80.
8. Porter A, Kandalker H, Iakobishvili Z, et al. Left ventricular mural thrombus after anterior ST-segment-elevation acute myocardial infarction in the era of aggressive reperfusion therapy--still a frequent complication. Coron Artery Dis. 2005;16(5):275-9.
9. Nihoyannopoulos P, Smith GC, Maseri A, et al. The natural history of left ventricular thrombus in myocardial infarction: a rationale in support of masterly inactivity. J Am Coll Cardiol. 1989;14(4):903.
10. Küpper AJ, Verheugt FW, Peels CH, et al. Left ventricular thrombus incidence and behavior studied by serial two-dimensional echocardiography in acute anterior myocardial infarction: left ventricular wall motion, systemic embolism and oral anticoagulation. J Am Coll Cardiol. 1989;13(7):1514.
11. Weinreich DJ, Burke JF, Pauletto FJ. Left ventricular mural thrombi complicating acute myocardial infarction. Long-term follow-up with serial echocardiography. Ann Intern Med. 1984;100(6):789.
12. Greaves SC, Zhi G, Lee RT, et al. Incidence and natural history of left ventricular thrombus following anterior wall acute myocardial infarction. Am J Cardiol. 1997;80(4):442.
13. Keren A, Goldberg S, Gottlieb S, et al. Natural history of left ventricular thrombi: their appearance and resolution in the posthospitalization period of acute myocardial infarction. J Am Coll Cardiol. 1990;15(4):790.
14. Visser CA, Kan G, Meltzer RS, et al. Embolic potential of left ventricular thrombus after myocardial infarction: a two-dimensional echocardiographic study of 119 patients. J Am Coll Cardiol. 1985;5(6):1276.
15. Asinger RW, Mikell FL, Elsperger J, et al. Incidence of left-ventricular thrombosis after acute transmural myocardial infarction. Serial evaluation by two-dimensional echocardiography. N Engl J Med. 1981;305(6):297.

CONTRIBUTIONS BY:

1. Dr Ashish Bhalla, Professor, Department of Internal Medicine (Clinician In-Charge)
2. Dr Sanjay Bhadada, Additional Professor, Department of Endocrinology (Compilation of Clinical Details)

Post Graduate Institute of Medical Education and Research, Chandigarh, India.

CASE 31

Coexistence of Acute-on-Chronic Rheumatic Heart Disease and Acute Poststreptococcal Glomerulonephritis: PM 21119

Nandita Bharadwaj Kakkar

HIGHLIGHTS OF THE CASE

A 15-year-old male, known case of chronic rheumatic heart disease (RHD) on penicillin prophylaxis, came with swelling of face and feet, gross hematuria, oliguria, shortness of breath, progressive pallor and easy fatigability since 1 month. A clinical diagnosis of chronic RHD, mitral regurgitation (MR)/aortic regurgitation (AR)/pulmonary arterial hypertension (PAH), rapidly progressive renal failure, ? infective endocarditis, hematuria, ? disseminated intravascular coagulation (DIC) and sepsis was made. The patient fulfilled the Jones criteria of acute rheumatic fever with evidence of preceding group A streptococcal infection, i.e. raised antistreptolysin O (ASO) titers. Autopsy revealed a coexistence of acute-on-chronic rheumatic heart disease and acute poststreptococcal glomerulonephritis.

Keywords: Acute or chronic rheumatic heart disease, Aschoff bodies, pancarditis, coexistent, acute poststreptococcal glomerulonephritis, autopsy.

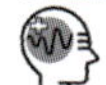

CLINICAL DETAILS

Date of Admission: 19.12.2005, Date of Death: 19.12.2005

A 15-year-old male, a known case of chronic rheumatic heart disease on penicillin prophylaxis, came with history of facial swelling, edema feet, gross hematuria and shortness of breath since 1 month. The facial swelling did not have any diurnal variation or any aggravating or relieving factors. There was oliguria (not quantified), gross hematuria with passage of clots, but no pyuria or graveluria. There was shortness of breath on exertion, but there was no orthopnea, paroxysmal nocturnal dyspnea, expectoration or any wheezing. He complained of progressive pallor and easy fatigability. There was right-sided pleuritic chest pain. There were no complaints of joint pains, sore throat, skin lesions or fever. On examination, he was emaciated, there was anemia, facial puffiness, raised jugular venous pressure (JVP), BP 140/80 mm Hg, pulse rate 110 beats/min and bilateral diffuse crepitations over the lungs. Cardiovascular examination revealed a left parasternal heave, cardiac apex was in the 6th intercostal space in the midaxillary line, S1 and S2 were audible, pulmonary component of the second sound was palpable and a pansystolic murmur was heard at the apex and in the parasternal areas, radiating to the left axilla. ECG showed a prolonged PR interval along with left atrial enlargement and left ventricular hypertrophy. X-ray revealed enlarged kidneys with increased cortical echogenicity and corticomedullary distinction, consistent with renal parenchymal disease. There was cardiomegaly with right atrial/ventricular and left ventricular enlargement, right ventricular hypertrophy and pulmonary arterial hypertension.

Investigations

Hemogram: Hb—3.4 g/dL, TLC—22,000/μL with polymorphonuclear leukocytosis, platelet count 2,21000/uL, ESR—85 in the first hour, peripheral blood film—anisocytosis with microcytes, macrocytes and hypersegmented polymorphs. Coagulogram was markedly deranged—PTI 14%, PTTK 67', fibrinogen 4.43 g/dL and D-dimer positive.

Blood biochemistry: Serum urea—180 mg%, serum creatinine—8.4 mg%, Na^+—120 mEq/L, random blood sugar—65 mg% and liver function tests normal. The blood and urine cultures (done four times) were sterile, ASO titer was raised (800 IU/mL) and CRP was positive. Routine urine examination showed albumin 2+, occasional pus cell and RBCs full field.

He was admitted at an outside health facility for 15 days. Echocardiography done there, revealed RHD with severe MR, mild AR, PAH and pericardial effusion. The ASO was raised, CRP was positive and a diagnosis of acute rheumatic carditis was considered and he was treated with antibiotics. A throat swab grew commensals and one blood culture grew ***Enterobacter*** species. He was given multiple blood transfusions and was referred to our institute. Hematuria persisted and the urine was grossly red in color. Frank passage of blood was also noted. Fresh frozen plasma was administered and hemodialysis was started, during which he had a generalized tonic–clonic seizure. Thereafter, he had respiratory distress and epistaxis. He was intubated but he suffered cardiac arrest and could not be revived. ***Units final diagnosis*** was—chronic RHD, MR/AR/PAH, rapidly progressive renal failure ? infective endocarditis, hematuria, ? DIC and sepsis.

AUTOPSY FINDINGS: PM 21119

A complete autopsy was performed. The heart was enlarged and weighed 440 g (Fig 1A). The pericardium was markedly thickened and the pericardial cavity contained 200 mL of blood tinged fluid along with blood clots. The visceral pericardium revealed the classic bread and butter, i.e. fibrinous pericarditis (Figs 1B and C). The tricuspid, pulmonary valves, right atrium and right ventricle were normal. There was no right ventricular hypertrophy. The left atrium was dilated and subendocardial irregular thickening produced as a result of regurgitant jet, known as MacCallum patch was noted. The mitral valve (Fig 1D) was distorted, free margin was slightly thick, commissural fusion was present, chordae tendineae were short, thick and papillary muscles were hypertrophied. No vegetations or verrucae were however noted. The aortic valve appeared normal grossly, although the free margins were slightly thickened. Microscopic section from the heart revealed an acute pancarditis. Acute fibrinous pericarditis (Fig 2A) with fibrin, acute inflammatory cells and plenty of histiocytes was seen. Classic perivascular Aschoff bodies (Figs 2B–D, Fig 3A—between four arrows) were seen in the interstitial connective tissue of the myocardium, endocardium and also in the mitral valve. The Aschoff body was composed of T lymphocytes, plasma cells and the characteristic macrophages known as Anitschkow cells which are pathognomic of rheumatic fever. These cells were of two types: (1) Caterpillar cells (Figs 2C and D) in which the chromatin has condensed into a central, slender wavy ribbon reminiscent of a caterpillar. (2) Owl eye type with round to ovoid nucleus with prominent nucleoli (Fig 2D—black arrows). Aschoff nodules were also noted in the endocardium (Fig 3A). Dense acute inflammation was noted in the myocardium, endocardium (Fig 3B) and in the mitral valve (Fig 3C). The mitral valve in addition showed changes of chronic rheumatic valvulitis (Fig 3D) in the form of hyalinization, fibrosis, neovascularization and calcification. The aortic valve was normal histologically. So, in the heart there was acute-on-chronic rheumatic heart disease with involvement of the mitral valve along with acute pancarditis (with characteristic Aschoff bodies), with classic bread and butter pericarditis and hemopericardium. The ***kidneys*** weighed 500 g, were enlarged with the capsular aspect being flea bitten (Fig 3E). The renal artery, veins, ureters and the urinary bladder were normal. Microscopic examination (Figs 3F and 4A–E) revealed features of a florid crescentic glomerulonephritis with plenty of RBC casts and interstitial inflammation. No necrotizing lesion or any vasculitis was noted. Many glomeruli showed frank blood in the Bowman's space (Fig 3F). Electron microscopy showed subendothelial (Fig 4D) and subepithelial (Fig 4E) electron dense deposits. Overall features thus suggested an immune complex-mediated crescentic glomerulonephritis. The lungs revealed extensive pulmonary hemorrhage (Fig 4F), early bronchopneumonia and grade 1 PAH. Lymph nodes showed features of reactive hemophagocytosis (Fig 4G).

FINAL AUTOPSY DIAGNOSIS : PM 21119

15 Years Old Male

- Chronic RHD (with mitral valve involvement grossly/histologically) with acute-on-chronic rheumatic pancarditis and hemopericardium.
- Immune complex-mediated crescentic glomerulonephritis—Infectious.
- Pulmonary hemorrhage, bronchopneumonia and grade 1 PAH.
- Infection associated hemophagocytosis.

RHEUMATIC FEVER AND RHEUMATIC HEART DISEASE

Infection with group A ***Streptococcus*** (pharyngitis or skin infection) leads to two serious autoimmune disorders—acute rheumatic fever (ARF) and acute poststreptococcal glomerulonephritis (APSGN). The acute infection generally subsides by the time the sequelae come up. Recurrences are seen in ARF, but not so in APSGN.

Acute rheumatic fever[1-4] is a systemic, immune-mediated, nonsuppurative inflammatory disease, which generally

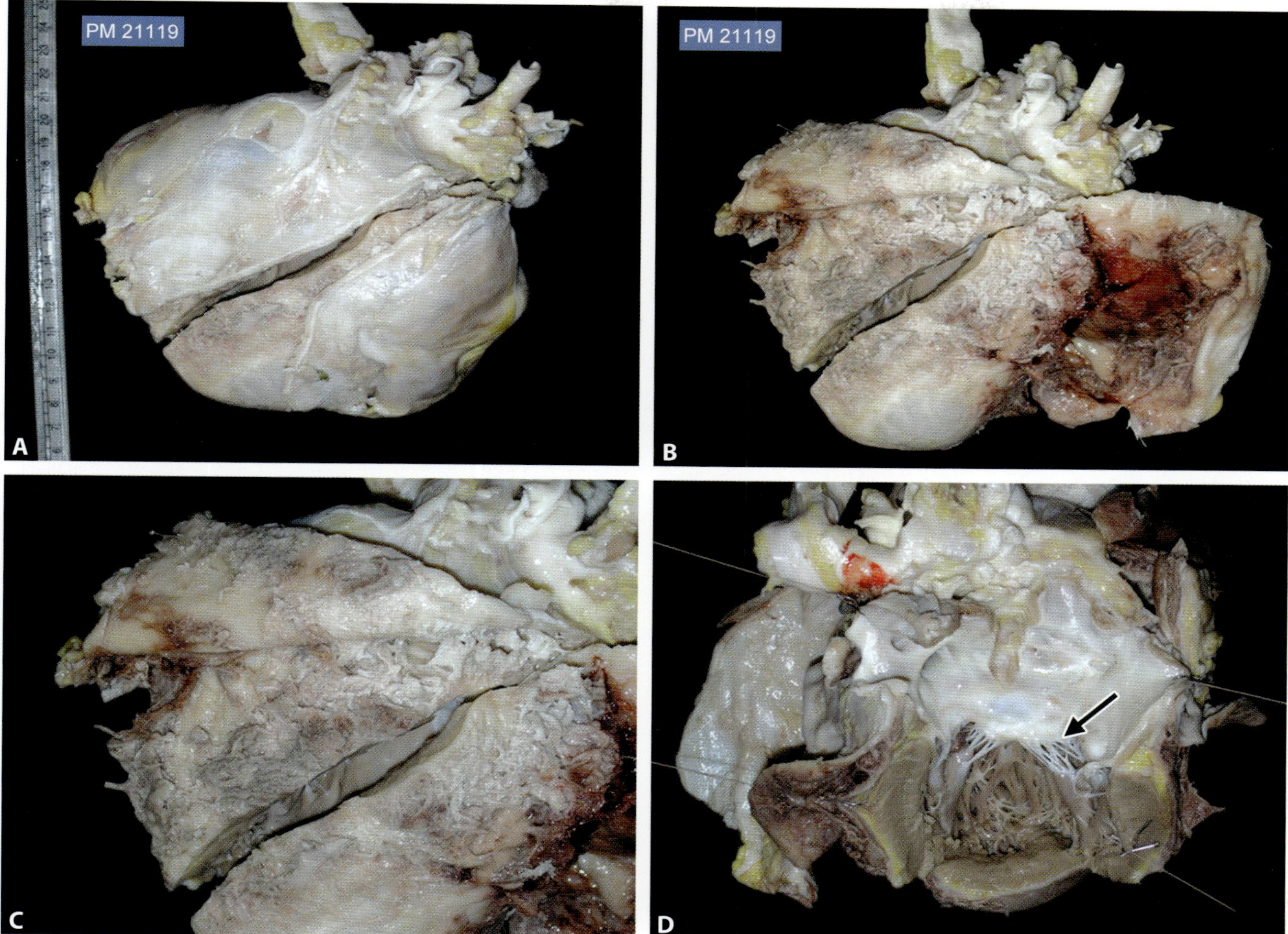

Figs 1A–D: (A) Gross picture of the dilated and enlarged heart; (B and C) The thickened parietal pericardium is reflected, shows the classic bread and butter, acute-on-chronic fibrinous pericarditis; (D) Mitral valve shows thickening of the free margin, commissural fusion, short and thick chordae tendineae and hypertrophied papillary muscles.

occurs after an episode of group A streptococcal throat infection. Rarely, it may follow streptococcal infections at other sites, particularly that of the skin. ARF is a disease of the developing countries (poor sanitation, crowded living) and is rare in the developed countries. It affects the joints, tendons, fascia, muscles, subcutaneous tissue, serous membranes, connective tissue, arteries, heart, brain and the lungs. The primary sequelae of ARF consist of arthritis, chorea and carditis which can occur together or in isolation. ARF is diagnosed by the Jones criteria. Presence of two major criteria (migratory polyarthritis of the large joints, subcutaneous nodules, erythema marginatum, pancarditis, Sydenham's chorea) or one major and two minor criteria (fever, arthralgia, laboratory parameters, i.e. elevated C-reactive protein and erythrocyte sedimentation rate, prolonged PR interval on electrocardiograph) with evidence of preceding group A streptococcal infection, i.e. positive throat culture/rapid streptococcal antigen test positivity/elevated or rising antistreptolysin titer. ARF affects children (5–15 years) but at times can occur later in life. It is immune-mediated, occurs 2–6 weeks after a group A streptococcal infection in about 3% of patients. The antibodies and CD4+ T cells produced against the group A streptococcal antigens (streptococcal M proteins), cross reacts with the host proteins, i.e. can recognize the cardiac antigens as self. The antigen–antibody reaction thus, activates complement, recruits neutrophils, macrophages and activates T cells to produce cytokines which thereby activate the macrophages. Cardiac damage thus occurs as a result of both antibody and T cell-mediated reactions. The throat swab cultures are generally negative by

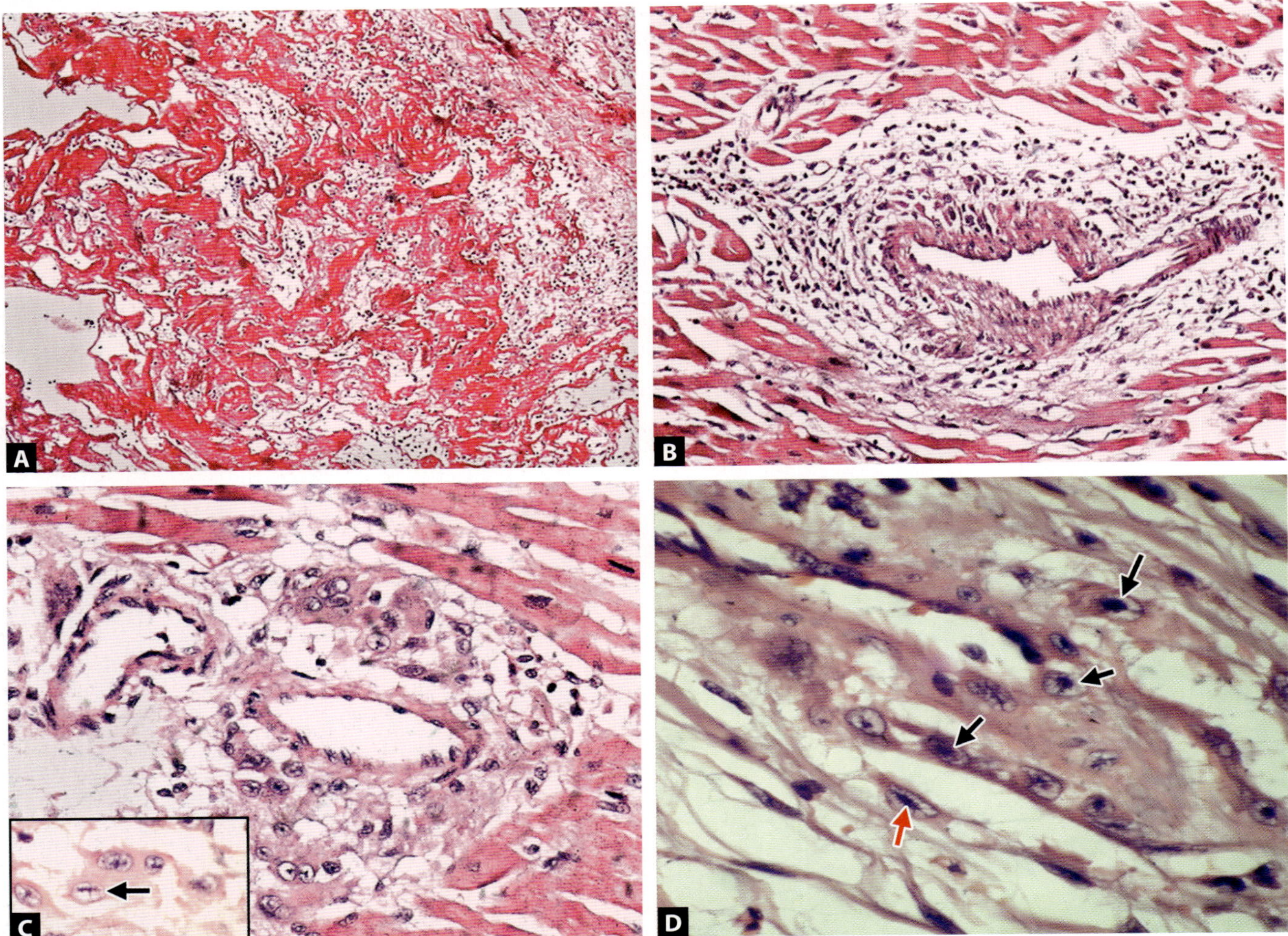

Figs 2A–D: (A) Fibrinous pericarditis; (B and C) Classic perivascular Aschoff bodies in the interstitial connective tissue of the myocardium. Inset in "C"shows the characteristic caterpillar type (arrow) of Anitschkow cell; (D) Aschoff body showing the owl eyed (black arrows) and caterpillar type (red arrow) of Anitschkow cells.

the time ARF begins, but the antibodies to the streptococcal antigen (streptolysin O, DNase B) can be found in the sera of most patients. Extracardiac manifestations of ARF vary in severity, but do not result in any permanent deformity. In contrast, the cardiac damage in ARF, grouped under the umbrella of RHD are the most destructive and devastating lesions. This is the primary cause of acquired valvular heart disease in the world. In approximately 50% cases of ARF, there is involvement of either the pericardium, myocardium, endocardium or there could be pancarditis. Myocarditis is the most common, but endocarditis is more serious. Valvulitis is the most devastating of all lesions and leads to chronic RHD. Mitral valve is most commonly involved with isolated involvement occurring in approximately 75% cases. Both mitral and aortic valves being involved in another 25% cases. Involvement of the tricuspid valve is very infrequent and if at all, occurs as part of a multivalvular involvement. Pulmonary valve is rarely ever affected. Recurrent attacks occur as there is increased predisposition to reactivation of the disease and this leads to cumulative damage to the heart valves. Clinical manifestations of valvular disease may occur years after the attack of ARF. Chronic RHD causes murmurs, cardiac dilatation and hypertrophy, arrhythmias, thromboembolic complications, heart failure and infective endocarditis.

Pathology*:** Acute rheumatic fever may show ***pancarditis with diffuse inflammation in all the three layers of the heart, along with the characteristic ***Aschoff bodies***. These are found in the interstitial connective tissue of the myocardium, in the

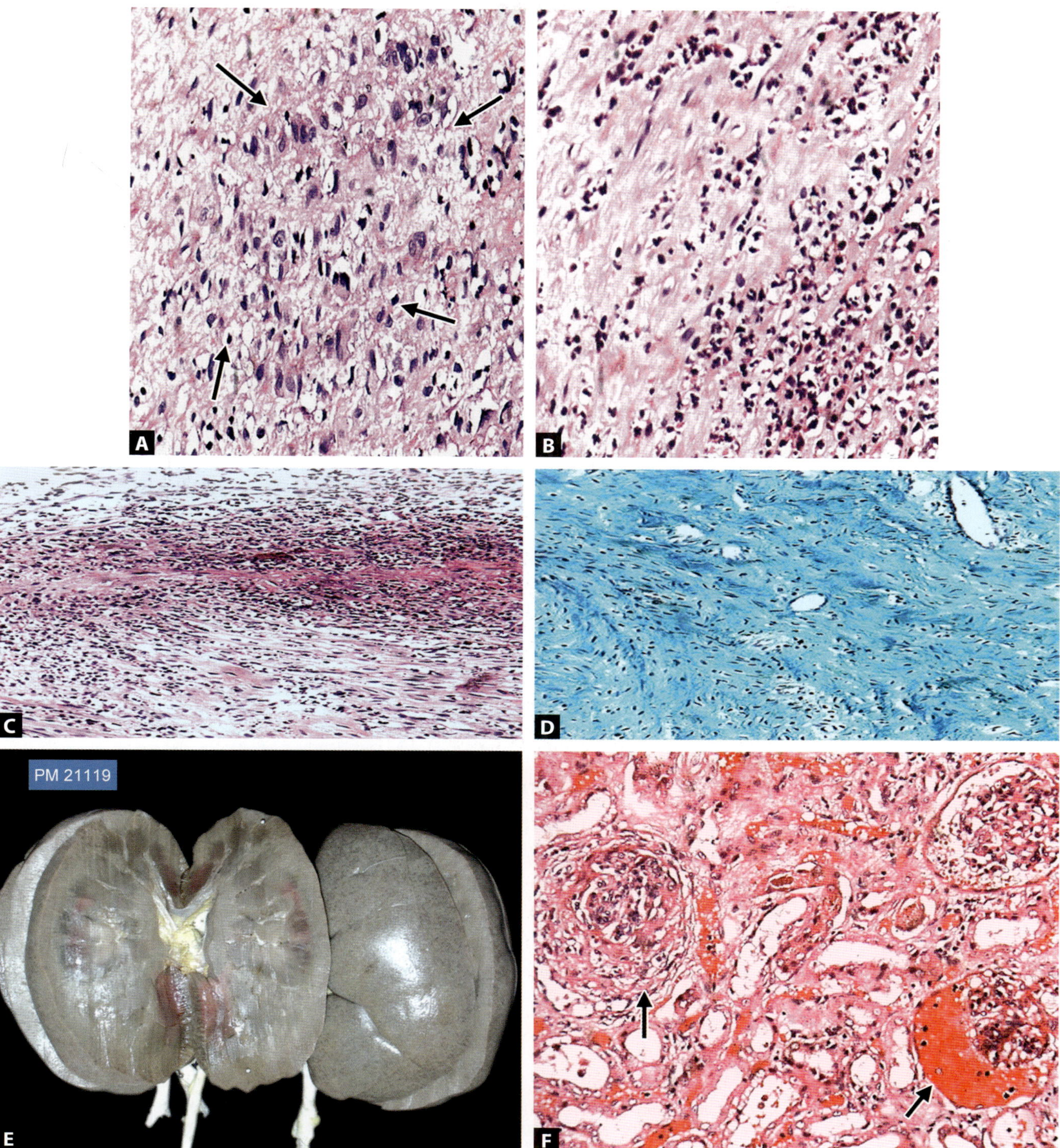

Figs 3A–F: (A) Aschoff nodule noted in the endocardium (in between the four arrows); (B) Dense acute inflammation in the endocardium; (C) Dense inflammation in mitral valve; (D) Mitral valve (Massons trichrome stain) showing changes of chronic rheumatic valvulitis, i.e. hyalinization, fibrosis, and neovascularization; (E) Enlarged and flea bitten kidneys; (F) Photomicrograph showing crescent (arrow) and blood in the Bowman's space (Lower arrow).

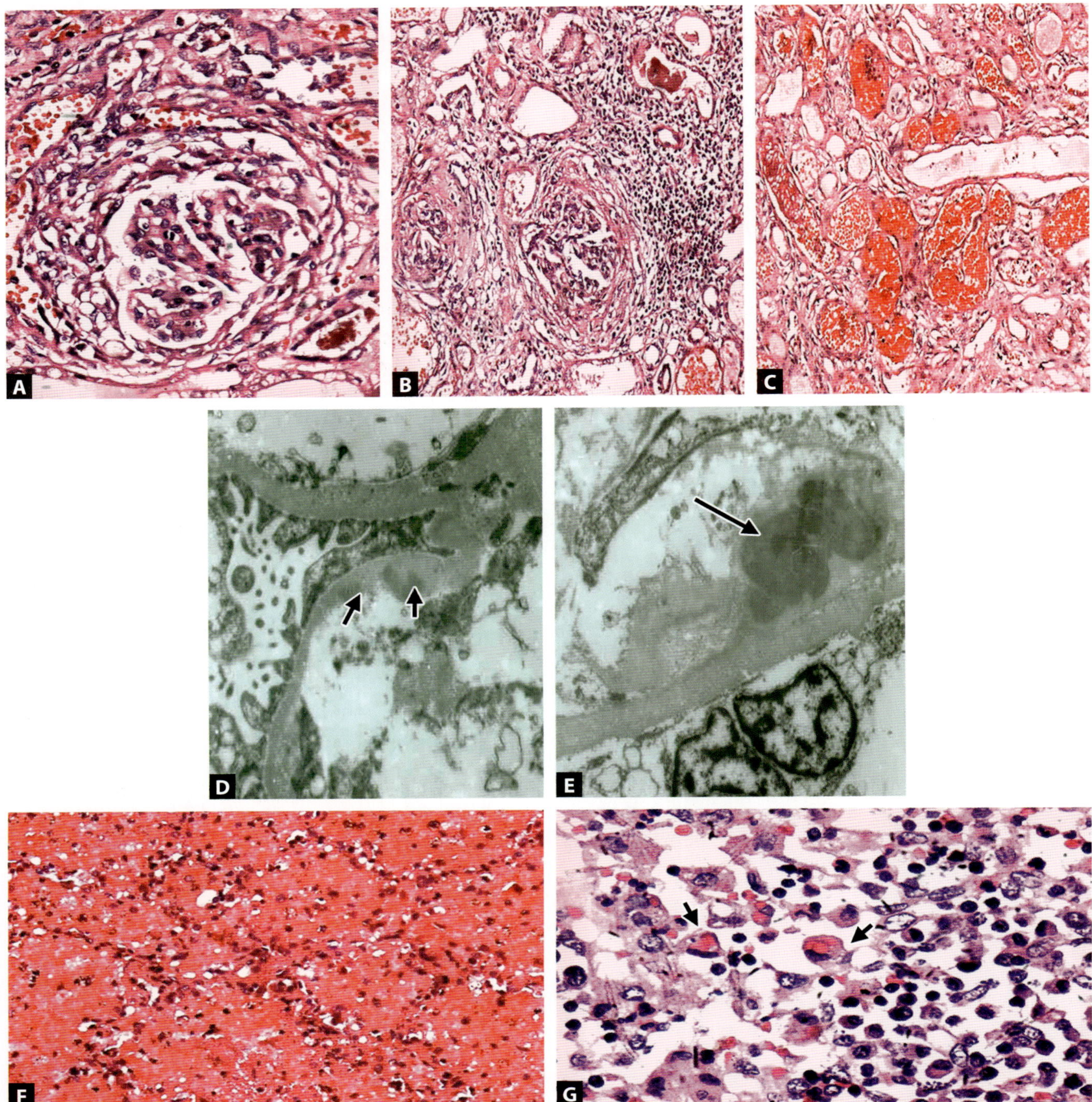

Figs 4A–G: (A) Cellular crescent. (B) Interstitium showing inflammation. (C) Dilated tubules with red blood cells. Electron microscopy showing (D) subendothelial and (E) subepithelial electron dense deposits (arrow). (F) Lung showing extensive pulmonary hemorrhage. (G) Lymph node showing hemophagocytosis (arrows).

perivascular location, may also be prominent in the subendocardial connective tissue, but rarely occur in the valves. In ARF, pericarditis is of the typical acute fibrinous, bread and butter type, composed of fibrin, polymorphs, lymphocytes, macrophages, plasma cells and at times Aschoff bodies. In recurrent attacks, it displays dense shaggy exudates with adhesions, the so called "cor villosum" or the shaggy heart, which leads to chronic pericarditis. In acute rheumatic ***myocarditis***, dense inflammation and Aschoff bodies are seen. They are composed of T lymphocytes, plasma cells and activated macrophages known as the Anitschkow cells which are pathognomic of rheumatic fever. These macrophages may have a round to ovoid nucleus with an owl eyed prominent nucleoli or may have the chromatin condensed into a central, slender wavy ribbon reminiscent of a caterpillar. Aschoff bodies are most eye-catching in their granulomatous state, which is reached 3–4 weeks after the onset of ARF. They are seen more in the sections from the ventricular septum, left ventricular free wall and left atrial free wall. Severe myocarditis leads to a globular heart and ventricular cavity enlargement. In chronic RHD, small scars are visible in the myocardium, which are the burnt out areas of Aschoff nodules and inflammation. Rheumatic valvulitis is the most serious form of rheumatic endocarditis, as it leads to chronic rheumatic valvulitis. It involves primarily the mitral valve followed by the aortic valve. Inflammation leads to fibrinoid necrosis in the cusps and in the chordae tendineae. Along the lines of closure of the valves and over the necrotic foci, small vegetations, 1–2 mm, called verrucae are formed. MacCallum patch, an area of irregular thickening is seen in the left atrium and occurs due to subendocardial lesions, further exacerbated by regurgitant jets. In chronic RHD, the valve leaflets are thick, commissural fusion occurs, chordae tendineae are thick, short and the papillary muscle is hypertrophied. Mitral valve involvement shows the characteristic "fish mouth" appearance, that results from fibrous bridging and calcification over the valvular commissures. Mitral stenosis leads to left atrial dilatation and mural thrombi develop which can embolize. Back pressure congestive changes occur in the lungs leading to pulmonary arterial hypertension, chronic passive venous congestion and over time lead to right ventricular hypertrophy. Microscopically in chronic RHD, the distorted valves show hyalinization, neovascularization, calcification and transmural fibrosis that obliterates the architecture of the leaflet.

ACUTE POSTSTREPTOCOCCAL GLOMERULONEPHRITIS[5]

This is an immune-mediated disorder, occurs 1–4 weeks after a throat or skin infection with certain so called nephritogenic strains (>90% occur due to 12, 4 and 1) of beta-hemolytic streptococci and occurs most frequently in young children (5–10 years, but no age is exempted). The immunologic basis of the disease is supported by many facts:

- The latent period between the onset of nephritis and the preceding infection is compatible with the time needed for the production of antibodies and the immune complexes.
- Antibodies against one or more streptococcal antigens are raised, two principal antigens being pyogenic exotoxin B (SpeB)[6] and nephritis-associated plasmin receptor (NAPlr),[7] identified as glyceraldehyde-3-phosphate dehydrogenase.
- Serum complement levels are low due to consumption.
- Electron microscopy shows subepithelial and subendothelial immune deposits.

Signs and symptoms generally appear after a bout of sore throat. These include fever, malaise, oliguria, hematuria, hypertension and periorbital edema. Urine examination shows dysmorphic red cells, casts and proteinuria less than 1 g/day. Atypical presentation can occur, wherein subclinical nephritis is present and diagnosis is suspected by the presence of microscopic hematuria. Other important laboratory investigations which further help in the diagnosis are elevated ASO titers and a decline in the serum levels of C3 and other components of the complement cascade. Conservative therapy leads to recovery in 95% of children. But less than 1% (with prolonged proteinuria and abnormal GFR) develop rapidly progressive glomerulonephritis, a few of which progress to chronic glomerulonephritis. Microscopic examination of the kidney shows enlarged, hypercellular glomeruli, a change which is global and diffuse. The hypercellularity is due to infiltration by neutrophils or monocytes, proliferation of endothelial or mesangial cells and due to crescent formation. Interstitium shows inflammation, edema and tubules show red cell casts. Electron microscopy shows discrete, amorphous electron dense deposits (antigen antibody complexes) in the subepithelial and subendothelial location. Immunofluorescence microscopy shows granular IgG and C3 (at times IgM) in the mesangium and along the GBM.

COEXISTENCE OF ACUTE-ON-CHRONIC RHEUMATIC HEART DISEASE AND ACUTE POSTSTREPTOCOCCAL GLOMERULONEPHRITIS

Epidemiological surveys in 1970s[8] suggested that "nephritogenic strains" of Streptococci do not cause acute rheumatic fever and "rheumatogenic" strains do not lead to glomerulonephritis. This was ingrained in our minds. But, simultaneous occurrence of acute rheumatic fever and acute poststreptococcal glomerulonephritis has been reported in literature. The concept that rheumatogenicity and nephritogenicity are distinct properties of group A

Streptococcus, does not negate the possibility that some strains possess both capabilities. Literature says that 51% patients with rheumatic fever will have clinical evidence[9] and up to 39% may have histologic evidence[10] of kidney disease. Epidemiological data is soft, but two serotypes 1 and 3 are associated with both sequelae. Presence of gross or microscopic hematuria, hypertension, low C3 levels and oliguria in a patient with acute rheumatic fever, should alert the physician to suspect a coexistent acute poststreptococcal glomerulonephritis. Literature is replete[11-21] and incidence of ARF coexisting with APSGN has been found to vary from 0.7–1.3%. In most reported cases, ARF was generally the presenting feature which was followed by APSGN. Only in an occasional case,[22] the ARF followed APSGN.

COMMENTARY INDEX CASE: PM 21119

A 15-year-old male, known case of chronic RHD on penicillin prophylaxis, came with swelling of face/feet, gross hematuria, oliguria, shortness of breath, progressive pallor and easy fatigability since 1 month. He was emaciated, anemic, JVP was raised and pulse rate was 110/min. Bilateral diffuse crepitations, pansystolic murmur, renal parenchymal disease, cardiomegaly and pulmonary arterial hypertension were present. Investigations revealed a Hb of 3.4 g/dL, markedly deranged renal function tests and coagulogram, raised ESR, positive CRP, raised ASO titers, prolonged PR interval and albumin 3+ with RBCs full field on urine examination. Clinical diagnosis considered was chronic RHD, MR/AR/PAH, rapidly progressive renal failure, ? infective endocarditis, hematuria, ? DIC and sepsis. Autopsy revealed a coexistence of acute-on-chronic RHD and crescentic poststreptococcal glomerulonephritis with electron microscopy showing subepithelial and subendothelial deposits. The patient fulfilled the Jones criteria of acute rheumatic fever—one major (pancarditis—found at autopsy) and two minor (raised ESR, positive CRP, prolonged PR interval) along with evidence of preceding group A streptococcal infection, i.e. raised ASO titer. At autopsy, there was acute-on-chronic RHD, with the characteristic Aschoff bodies (containing both caterpillar and owl eyed Anitschkow cells) found in the myocardium and the endocardium. Dense acute inflammation was noted in the endocardium and in the mitral valve. The mitral valve showed all changes of chronic rheumatic valvulitis along with acute inflammation. Coexisting immune complex-mediated crescentic glomerulonephritis with subendothelial and subepithelial electron dense deposits was seen. This association is well-known in literature and indicates that some strains (especially serotypes 1 and 3) of group A ***Streptococcus*** have both rheumatogenic and nephritogenic properties.

TAKE HOME MESSAGE

- Coexistence of acute rheumatic heart disease and acute poststreptococcal glomerulonephritis is well-documented in literature.
- Some strains (especially serotypes 1 and 3) of group A ***Streptococcus*** have both rheumatogenic and nephritogenic properties.
  Presence of gross or microscopic hematuria, hypertension, low C3 levels and oliguria in a patient with acute rheumatic fever, should alert the physician to suspect a coexistent acute poststreptococcal glomerulonephritis.

ACKNOWLEDGEMENT

This autopsy case has been published as a 'Clinicopathological conference' as—Kakkar N et al. A case of rheumatic heart disease with gross hematuria and RPGN. Indian J Nephrol. 2006;16:36-42.

REFERENCES

1. Carapetis J, Steer A, Mulholland E, et al. The global burden of group A streptococcal diseases. Lancet Infect Dis. 2005; 5(11):685-94.
2. Carapetis J, McDonald M, Wilson N. Acute rheumatic fever. Lancet. 2005;366(9480):155-68.
3. Steer A, Carapetis JR. Acute rheumatic fever and rheumatic heart disease in indigenous populations. Pediatr Clin North Am. 2009;56(6):1410-9.
4. Kumar RK, Tandon R. Rheumatic fever and rheumatic heart disease: The last 50 years. Indian J Med Res. 2013;137:643-58.
5. Rodriguez-Iturbe B, Musser JM. The current state of poststreptococcal glomerulonephritis. J Am Soc Nephrol. 2008; 19:1855-64.
6. Parra G, Rodríguez-Iturbe B, Batsford S, et al. Antibody to streptococcal zymogen in the serum of patients with acute glomerulonephritis: a multicentric study. Kidney Int. 1998; 54:509-17.
7. Oda T, Yamakami K, Omasu F, et al. Glomerular plasmin-like activity in relation to nephritis-associated plasmin receptor in acute poststreptococcal glomerulonephritis. J Am Soc Nephrol. 2005;16:247-54.
8. Stollerman GH. Rheumatogenic and nephritogenic streptococci. Circulation. 1971;43:915-21.
9. Gibney R, Reineck H, Bannayan G, et al. Renal lesions in acute rheumatic fever. Ann Intern Med. 1981;94(3):322-6.
10. Grishman E, Cohen S, Salomon MD, et al. Renal lesions in acute rheumatic fever. Am J Pathol. 1967;51:1045-61.

11. Bisno AL. The coexistence of acute rheumatic fever and acute post streptococcal glomerulonephritis. Arthritis Rheumatism. 1989;32:230-2.
12. Narula AS, Mishra A, Anand AC, et al. Poststreptococcal glomerulonephritis coexisting with acute rheumatic fever—a case report. J Assoc Physicians India. 1992;40:685.
13. Ben-Dov I, Berry EM, Kopolovic J. Poststreptococcal nephritis and acute rheumatic fever in two adults. Arch Intern Med. 1985;145(2):338-9.
14. Matsell DG, Baldree LA, DiSessa TG, et al. Acute post-streptococcal glomerulonephritis and acute rheumatic fever: occurrence in the same patient. Child Nephrol Urol. 1990;10(2):112-4.
15. Castillejos G, Padilla L, Lerma A, et al. Coincidence of acute rheumatic fever and acute post streptococcal glomerulonephritis. J Rheumatol. 1985;12(3):587-9.
16. Kujala GA, Doshi H, Brick JE. Rheumatic fever and post-streptococcal glomerulonephritis: a case report. Arthritis Rheum. 1989;32(2):236-9.
17. Imanaka H, Eto S, Takei S, et al. Acute rheumatic fever and poststreptococcal acute glomerulonephritis caused by T serotype 12 Streptococcus. Acta Paediatr Jpn. 1995;37(3):381-3.
18. Said R, Hussein M, Hassan A. Simultaneous occurrence of acute poststreptococcal glomerulonephritis and acute rheumatic fever. Am J Nephrol. 1986;6(2):146-8.
19. Kakkera DR, Khan AJ, Bastawros MN, et al. Acute rheumatic pancarditis associated with poststreptococcal acute glomerulonephritis: a patient report. Clin Pediatr (Phila). 1998;37(9):569-72.
20. Sinha R, Al-Alsheikh K, Prediville J, et al. Acute rheumatic fever with concomitant poststreptococcal glomerulonephritis. Am J Kidney Dis. 2007;50(10):A33-5.
21. Lin W, Lo W, Ou T, et al. Haematuria, transient proteinuria, serpiginous border skin rash and cardiomegaly in a 10-year-old girl. Eur J Pediatrics. 2003;162(9):655-7.
22. Kwong YL, Chan KW, Chan MK. Acute poststreptococcal glomerulonephritis followed shortly by acute rheumatic fever. Postgrad Med J. 1987;63(737):209-10.

CONTRIBUTIONS BY:

1. Dr Navneet Sharma, Professor, Department of Internal Medicine (Clinician In-Charge)
Post Graduate Institute of Medical Education and Research, Chandigarh, India.

CASE 32

A Classical Case of Marfan Syndrome with Aortic Root Dilatation, Aneurysm of the Ascending Aorta and Acute Aortic Dissection: PM 22554

Nandita Bharadwaj Kakkar

HIGHLIGHTS OF THE CASE

A young male came with sudden onset severe lacerating epigastric pain, radiating to the upper chest and neck. He was a diagnosed case of Marfan syndrome on follow-up. There was a strong family history of sudden cardiac deaths following severe chest and abdominal pain. His mother and two brothers (one with Marfanoid features) had died under similar circumstances. Echocardiography of the index case revealed massive dilatation of the aortic root and ascending aorta, with aortic dissection, moderate to severe aortic regurgitation (AR) and left ventricular systolic dysfunction. Autopsy revealed a cystic medial degeneration of the ascending aorta, (florid changes), brachiocephalic, right and left common carotids/subclavians, abdominal aorta (milder changes) leading to marked aortic root dilatation, aneurysm of the ascending aorta, acute dissection of the ascending and arch of aorta—DeBakey type 2, chronic dissection, i.e. double lumen of the left subclavian artery, myxomatous degeneration of the mitral valve, left ventricular dilatation and right ventricular hypertrophy.

Keywords: Marfan syndrome, aortic dissection, cystic medial degeneration, aortic root dilatation, autopsy.

CLINICAL DETAILS

Date of Admission: 16.04.2008, Date of Death: 17.04.2008, Duration of Hospital Stay: 34 Hours.

A 24-year-old male came to our institute emergency services with a 3-day history of pain abdomen and vomiting. The pain was severe, sudden in onset, epigastric in location, lacerating in nature, radiating to the upper chest and neck and had no relation to posture. This was associated with recurrent vomiting, which was non-bilious. There was no hematemesis. He was a diagnosed case of Marfan syndrome on follow-up. There was a strong family history of sudden cardiac deaths in the family. Mother had died of sudden abdominal pain, ? valvular heart disease, younger brother died of sudden onset chest and abdominal pain at the age of 20 years and was suspected to have a valvular heart disease and his elder brother, who had Marfanoid features, too died of sudden onset chest and abdominal pain due to aortic dissection. The index case was a nondiabetic, nonhypertensive and a nonsmoker. On examination, he was very uncomfortable and restless. The pulse was—96/min regular and bounding, BP: right upper limb—110/70 mm Hg, left upper limb—110/64 mm Hg, bilateral lower limbs—180/40 mm Hg. He had a Marfanoid habitus, was tall (height 192 cm), thin built, had a high arched palate, arachnodactyly and an arm span of 213 cm. The cardiovascular system examination revealed normal S1/S2, early diastolic murmur in left third space radiating all over the precordium and a short ejection systolic murmur heard in the right second space. Chest auscultation revealed bilateral vesicular breath sounds. The abdomen was soft, tender with no organomegaly. The central nervous system examination was normal. ***Investigations*** revealed a normal hemogram, coagulogarm and blood biochemistry. Electrocardiogram done demonstrated a left ventricular hypertrophy. The chest X-ray showed cardiomegaly with right lower zone haziness. Two-dimensional echocardiography revealed a massively dilated aortic root and ascending aorta with aortic annulus—35 mm, aortic sinus—66 mm and sinotubular junction—72 mm. The aortic valve had a poor coaptation of leaflets, moderate to severe AR and jet filling the left ventricular outflow tract. The dissection flap was seen originating 34 mm from the aortic valve annulus, extending from ascending aorta, arch of aorta, descending aorta and going up to abdominal aorta. Flow was present in both the true and false lumen. Branches of aortic arch, i.e. the brachiocephalic, left common carotid and left subclavian artery seemed to be supplied by the false lumen. Left ventricle was globally dilated with mild hypokinesia and visual ejection fraction of 40%. Diastolic mitral regurgitation (MR) and trivial tricuspid regurgitation (TR) were present. The impression was—massive dilatation of the aortic root and ascending aorta with aortic dissection (Type I, Type A), moderate to severe aortic regurgitation and left ventricular systolic dysfunction. Patient was planned for urgent surgery, but he sustained a cardiac arrest and succumbed to his illness. The units final clinical diagnosis was Marfan syndrome with acute aortic dissection, moderate to severe aortic regurgitation and left ventricular systolic dysfunction.

AUTOPSY FINDINGS: PM 22554

A partial autopsy was performed. The body was tall and thin built with arachnodactyly. The heart (Fig 1A) was massively enlarged and weighed 708 g (normal—250–350 g). The right atrium was normal. Tricuspid valve circumference was 12 cm (n—11.2–11.8 cm). The right ventricular wall thickness was 0.5 cm and the interventricular septa was bulging into the right ventricle. Pulmonary valve circumference was 6 cm (n—6.1–7.5 cm). The left atrium (Fig 1B) was dilated; mitral valve annulus was dilated, with the valve circumference being 11 cm (n—9.2–9.9 cm). The mitral valve leaflets (Fig 1B—arrows) were myxomatous, chordae tendineae and papillary muscles were thinned out and no vegetation was noted. The left ventricle was markedly dilated and thinned

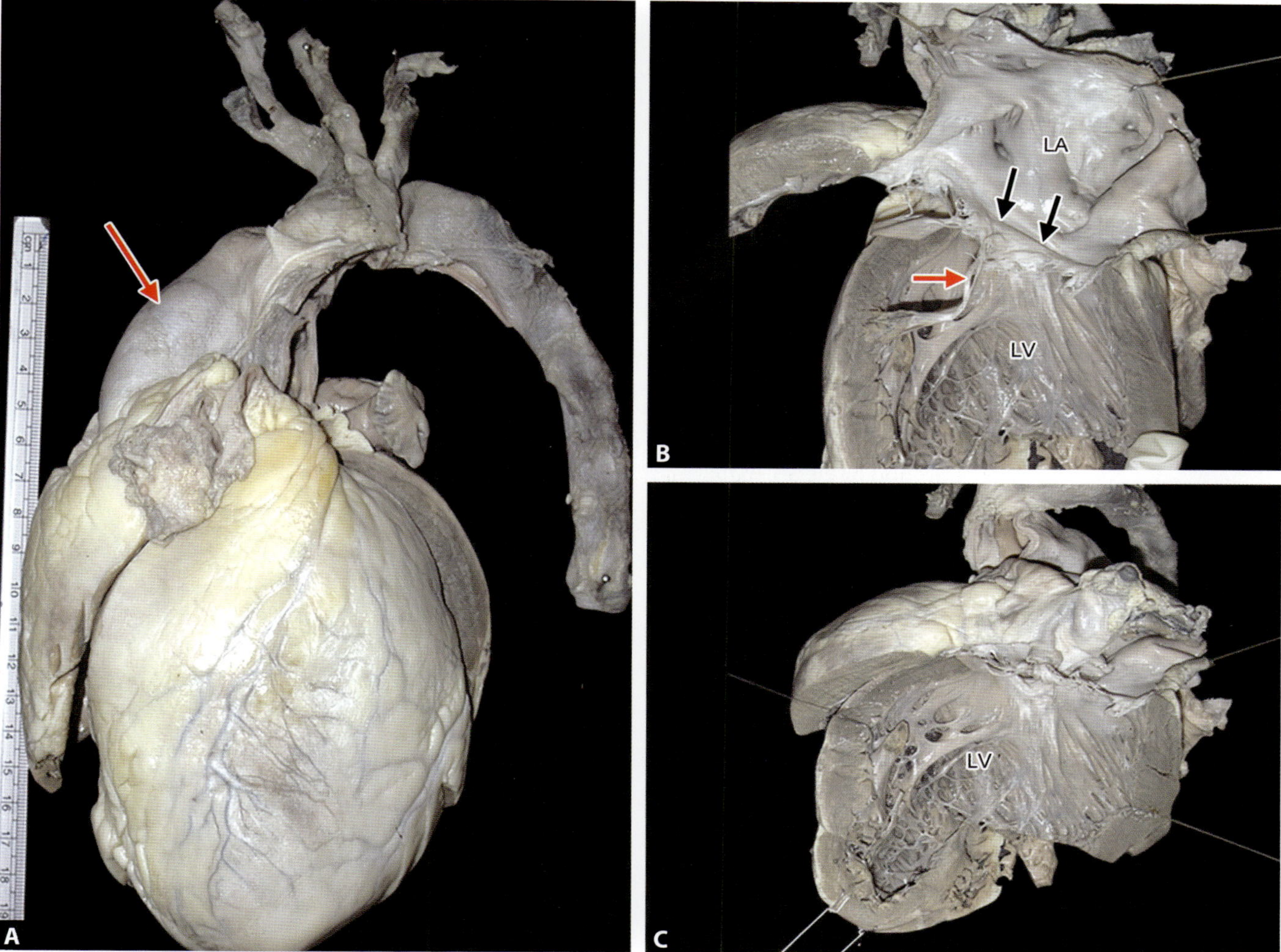

Figs 1A–C: (A) Massively enlarged heart showing marked dilatation of the ascending aorta (arrow); (B) Left inflow tract showing left atrial (LA) and left ventricular (LV) dilatation. The mitral valve leaflets are myxomatous (arrows), chordae tendineae (red arrow) and papillary muscles are thinned out; (C) Markedly enlarged left ventricle with the septum pushed to the right side.

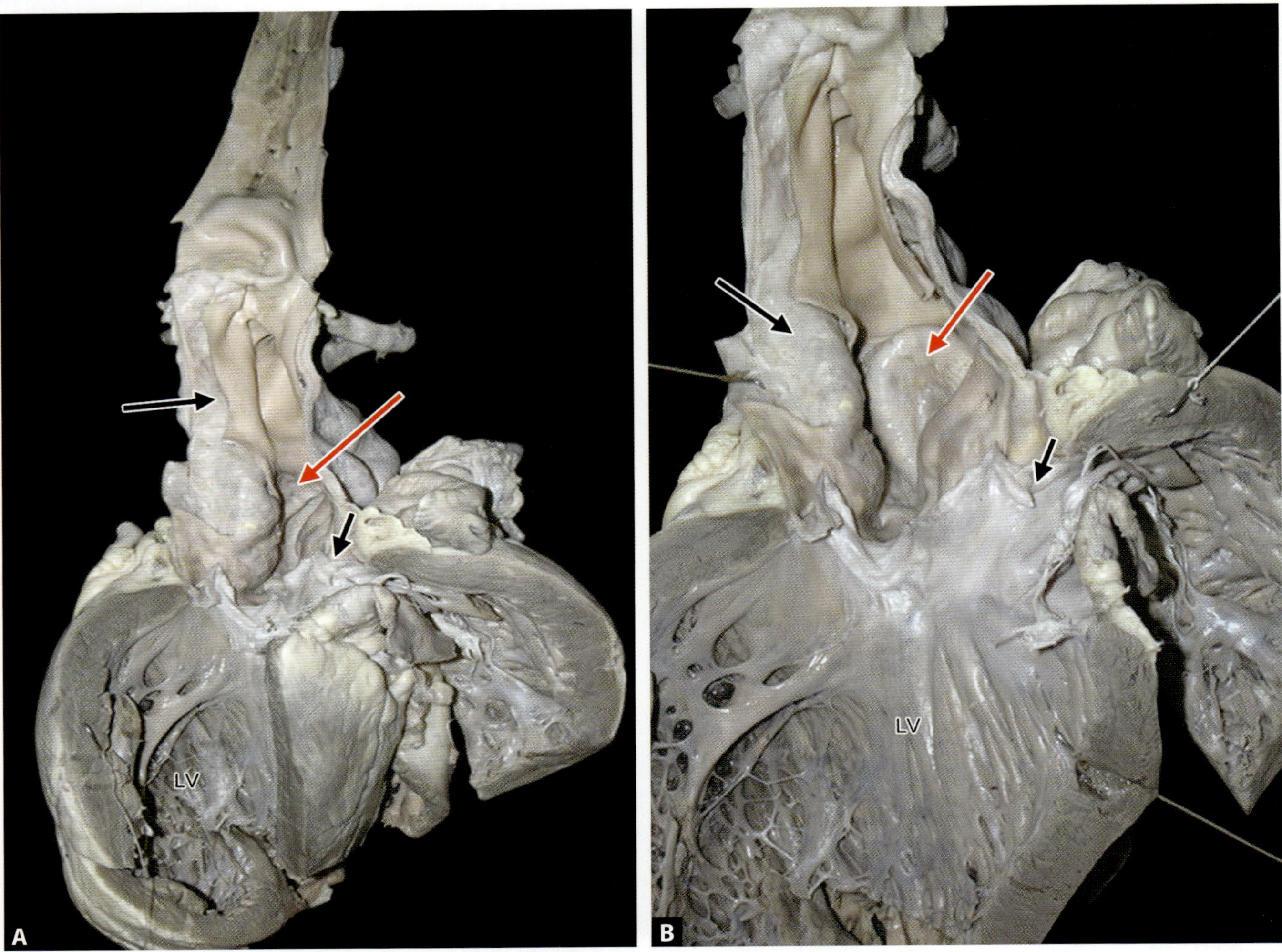

Figs 2A and B: Left outflow tract showing aortic valve (lowest arrows) with dilated annulus, leaflets are redundant and rolled back. There is aneurysmal dilatation of the ascending aorta (red arrows) along with aortic dissection (black upper arrows).

out, the interventricular septa was bulging into the right ventricle (Fig 1C). Left ventricular wall thickness was 1.5 cm. The aortic valve was tricuspid, circumference at annulus was 4 cm, leaflets were redundant and rolled back. The aortic sinus measured 7 cm. The aortic root was markedly dilated, with an aneurysmal dilatation of the ascending aorta (max width—8 cm) (Figs 1A, 2A and B, Fig 3A). Aortic dissection was seen 1 cm above the origin of the aorta till 4 mm beyond the origin of left subclavian artery (Fig 3B). Grossly the origin of the three main arteries was normal, coronaries and descending/abdominal aorta was normal. On microscopic examination, sections studied from the ascending aorta showed features characteristic of cystic medial degeneration (Figs 4A–F), i.e. extensive loss and fragmentation of the elastic fibers of the media, separation of the elastic and fibromuscular components of the media by small cleft-like spaces and laying down of amorphous extracellular connective tissue matrix. No inflammation was seen. Microphotograph from a normal age matched aorta is seen in Figs 5A and B. Sections from the left subclavian artery (Fig 6A) showed a chronic dissection in the form of a double lumen. Sections from the major arteries at the arch, i.e. brachiocephalic, right and left common carotids and subclavians (Figs 6B and C) showed milder changes of cystic medial degeneration. However the descending aorta (Fig 6D) and abdominal aorta (Figs 6E and F) showed moderate to severe changes. Sections from the mitral valve (Figs 7A–C) showed degeneration of the connective tissue core with marked loss of elastic fibers and increase in mucopolysaccharide ground substance and fibrous tissue better known as myxomatous degeneration.

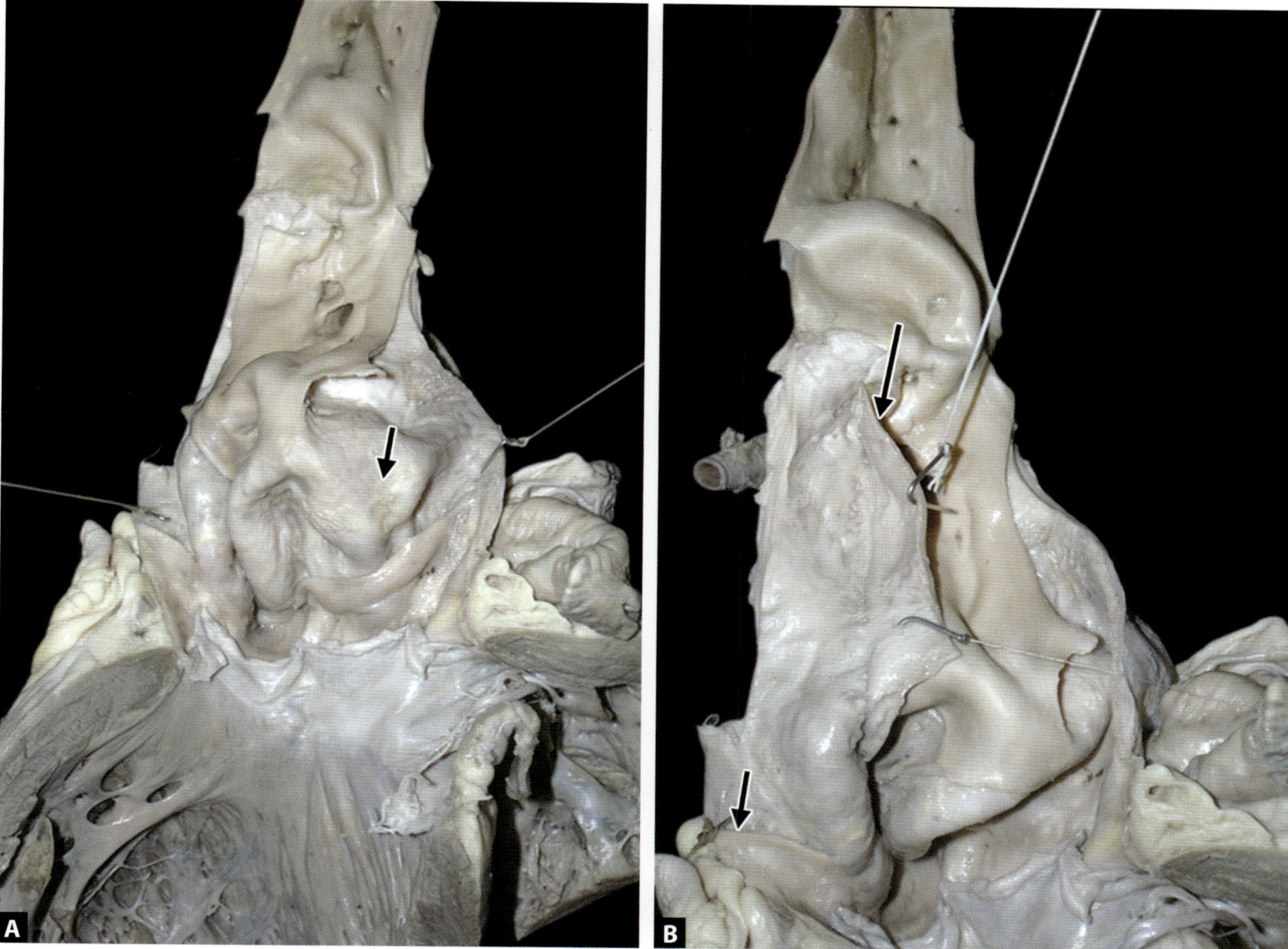

Figs 3A and B: (A) Ascending aorta showing aneurysmal dilatation (arrow); (B) Aortic dissection seen, 1 cm (lower arrow) above the origin of the aorta till 4 mm beyond the origin of left subclavian artery (upper arrow).

Microscopic sections from the lungs showed focal pulmonary hemorrhage, organizing pneumonia and grade 1 pulmonary arterial hypertension.

FINAL AUTOPSY DIAGNOSIS: PM 22554

22 Year Old Male—In A Known Case of Marfan Syndrome with Affected Mother and Two Sibling Deaths

- Cystic medial degeneration of the ascending aorta (florid changes), brachiocephalic, right and left common carotids/subclavians, abdominal aorta (milder changes) leading to:
  - Marked aortic root dilatation
  - Aneurysm of the ascending aorta
  - Acute dissection of the ascending and arch of aorta—DeBakey type 2
  - Chronic dissection, i.e. double lumen—left subclavian artery
  - Myxomatous degeneration—mitral valve
  - Left ventricular dilatation and right ventricular hypertrophy.
- Organizing pneumonia, pulmonary hemorrhage and pulmonary arterial hypertension Grade 1.

MARFAN SYNDROME AND CYSTIC MEDIAL DEGENERATION

Marfan syndrome[1-6] is a disorder of connective tissue and can affect many organ systems, principle being eyes, skeletal and the cardiovascular system. Prevalence is 1 in 5,000 and can affect men, women and children. About 80% cases are familial and have an autosomal dominant transmission. Some new mutations give rise to the rest of the cases. Microfibrils

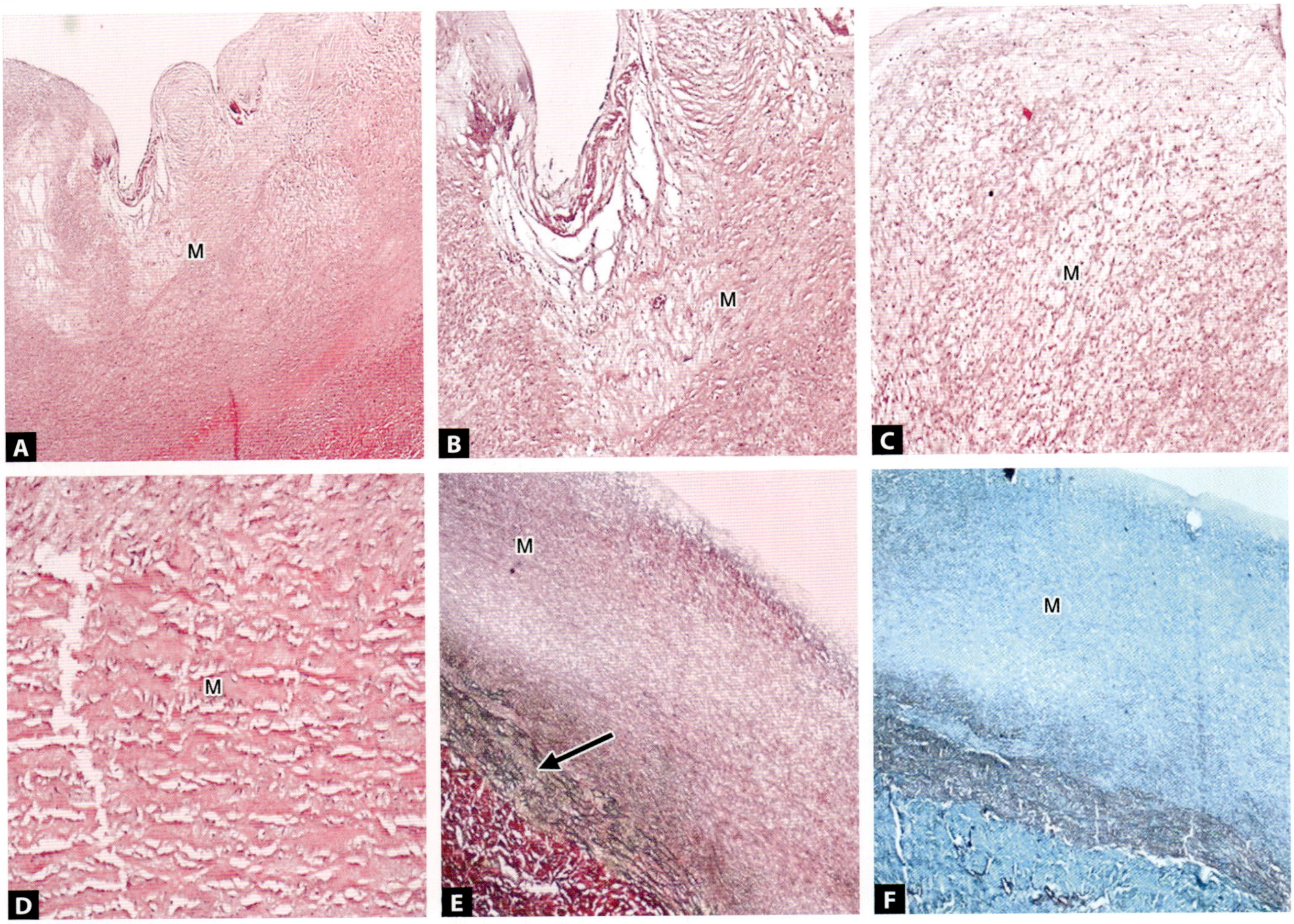

Figs 4A–F: (A) Photomicrographs from the ascending aorta showing cystic medial degeneration, i.e. extensive loss and fragmentation of the elastic fibers of the media (M); (B and C) Separation of the elastic and fibromuscular elements of the media (M) by small cleft-like spaces; (D) Laying down of amorphous extracellular connective tissue matrix in the media (M); (E) Elastic van Gieson stain shows extensive loss of elastic tissue in the media. Some black colored elastic fibers are seen in the outer layer of the media (arrow); (F) Masson trichrome stain shows increased collagen laying down in the media (M).

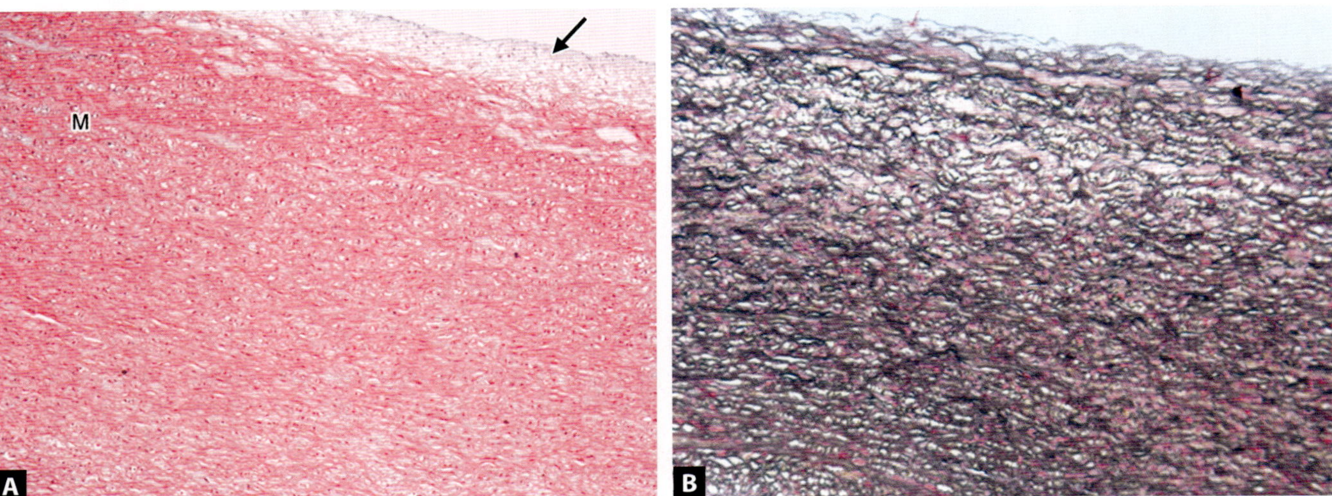

Figs 5A and B: Normal age matched aorta (A) H&E stained section of aorta showing intima (arrow) and media (M). Note the pink elastic fibers arranged uniformly; (B) Elastic van Gieson stain stains the elastic fibers black.

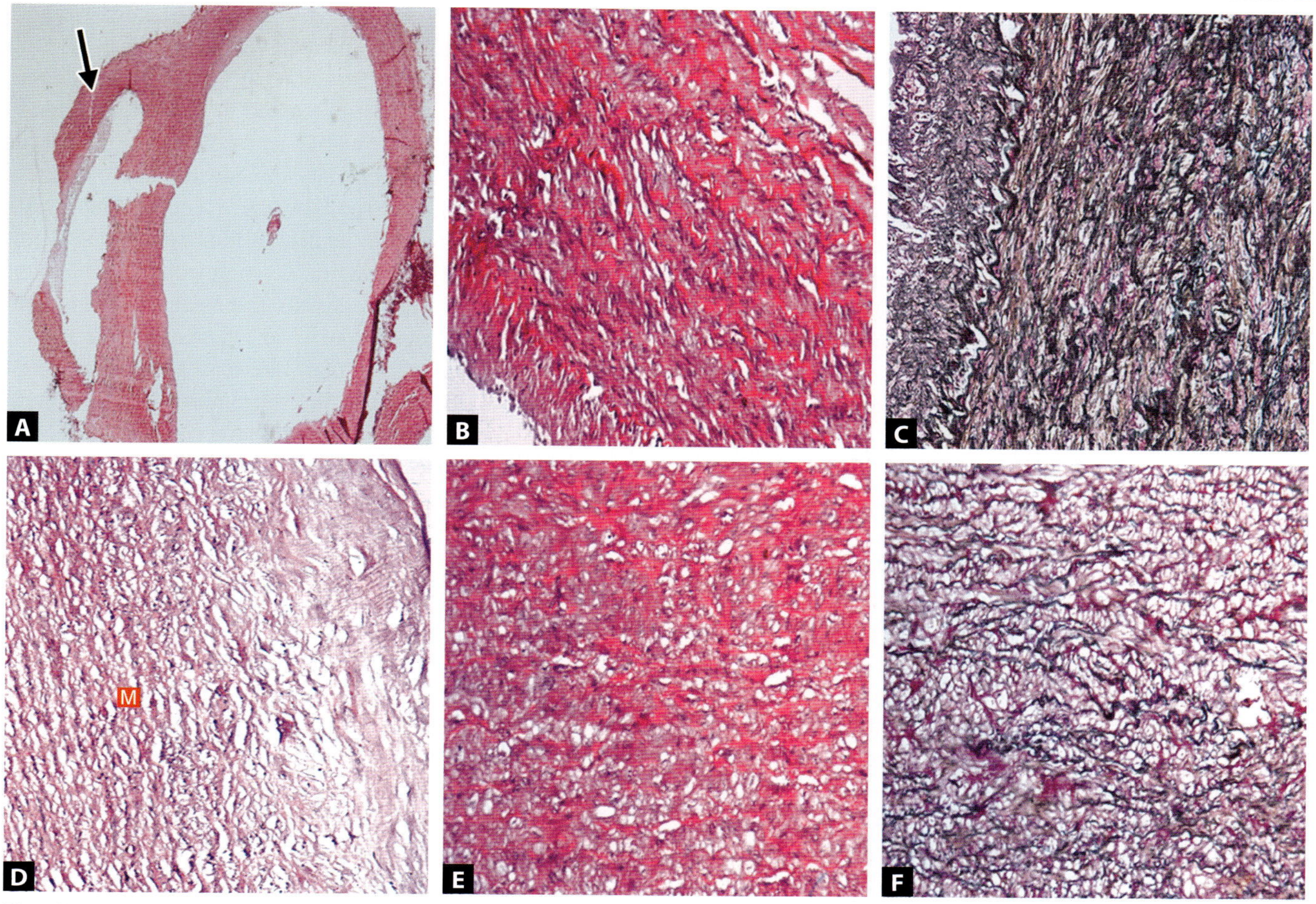

Figs 6A–F: Left subclavian artery showing (A) chronic dissection in the form of a double lumen (arrow); (B and C) Elastic tissue fragmentation in the media—H&E and EVG stains; (D) Descending thoracic aorta showing cystic medial degeneration in the media (M); (E and F) Abdominal aorta showing elastic tissue fragmentation in the media—H&E and EVG stains.

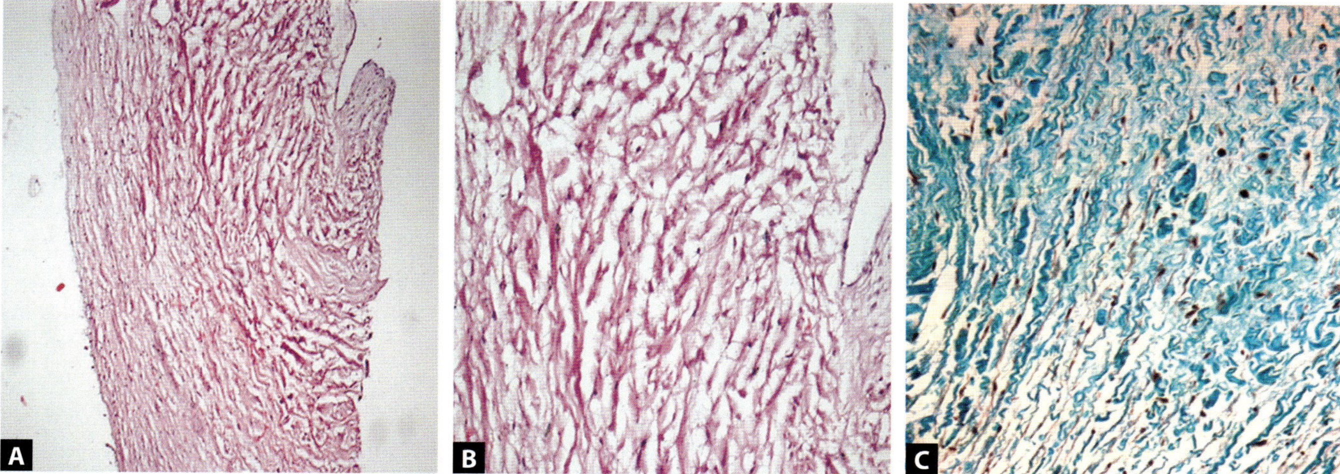

Figs 7A–C: H&E and Masson trichrome stains on the mitral valve show changes of myxomatous degeneration with marked loss of elastic fibers and increase in mucopolysaccharide ground substance and fibrous tissue.

with their important component fibrillin-1 (an important extracellular glycoprotein) are the scaffold on which the tropoelastin is deposited to form elastic fibers. These microfibrils are present in large quantities in the suspensory ligaments of the lens, ligaments and aorta. In Marfan syndrome[7,8] there is an inherited defect in fibrillin-1→ leading to defective microfibrils on which the tropoelastin cannot be deposited and thus the elastic fibers are defective. This leads to fatal complications in the above mentioned organs. There are two homologous forms of fibrillin (FBN 1 and FBN 2) encoded by two separate genes on chromosome 15q21 and 5q3, respectively. This syndrome is associated with more than 500 distinct mutations in ***FBN1*** gene, majority of which being missense mutations giving rise to abnormal fibrillin-1.

Patients with Marfan syndrome are abnormally tall, have disproportionately long limbs (span> height), reduced upper to lower segment ratio and long tapering fingers (arachnodactyly) and toes. The ligaments of the joints of the hand and feet are lax and give an impression of double joints. A characteristic finding is the hyperextension of the thumb, back to the wrist. These patients have long heads, prominent frontal eminences or supraorbital ridges. Chest shows a depressed sternum, i.e. pectus excavatum or a pigeon chest deformity. Kyphosis, scoliosis and slipping of the lumbar vertebrae can be seen. High arched palate and crowding of the teeth is present. The hallmark of Marfan syndrome is bilateral subluxation of the lens which is symmetrical and upward, known as ectopia lentis. This is present in 60–80% of patients. Cardiovascular abnormalities are fatal. The most important and life-threatening are the dilatation of the aortic root leading to aortic regurgitation, dilatation/aneurysm of the ascending aorta and aortic dissection. The other common lesion is the mitral valve prolapse. Other salient features are skin striae and dural ectasia. Presentation of the disease varies greatly even among members of the same family. Some have mild effects, whereas others have severe life-threatening problems.

Cystic medial degeneration[9] leads to elastic degeneration of the tunica media of the ascending aorta, as a result of which the major support is lost, leading to progressive dilatation and aneurysm formation. The aortic valve ring and the root of the aorta show dilatation, thereby giving rise to a significant AR. A weak tunica media is the biggest risk factor for an intimal tear, leading to an intramural hematoma that can separate the layers of the aorta, leading to an aortic dissection which is generally fatal. Here, there is dissection of blood through the wall of the aorta, usually between the middle and outer thirds, producing a blood-filled channel, which can rupture outward leading to massive hemorrhage. This blood-filled channel can at times re-rupture into the lumen of the aorta producing a distal tear, leading to the formation of a double barreled aorta. In due course of time the double barrel can get endothelialized leading to chronic dissection. In aortic dissection, the intimal tear occurs within 10 cm of the aortic valve, are generally oblique and approximately 3 cm in length with sharp, but jagged edges. This aortic dissection can go down till the iliac or femoral arteries or can go back to the root of the aorta. Cystic medial degeneration is characterized by elastic tissue fragmentation which on microscopic examination looks very haphazard on Elastic Van Gieson staining. Small cleft like spaces appear between the lost elastic tissue and the fibromuscular component of the media. The cleft like spaces are not true cysts, but are spaces filled with amorphous extracellular matrix of connective tissue. The term "cystic medial degeneration" is a misnomer, as there are no cysts or any necrosis, but the pathology is due to the lack of the proper elastic support due to the absence of the microfibrils, on which the tropoelastin is laid down to form the elastic fibers of the media. In 90% of the cases, the cause of aortic dissection is hypertension which occurs in middle-aged and older individuals. Causes of aortic dissection are Marfan syndrome, iatrogenic as a complication of arterial cannulation and rarely for unknown reasons following pregnancy. Hypertensive patients who have aortic dissection generally show mild fragmentation of the elastic tissue of the media, but can even show medial degeneration.

Myxomatous degeneration of the mitral valve or mitral valve prolapse is a common form of valvular heart disease, usually an incidental finding, but can lead to serious complications. The affected leaflets are thick, enlarged, rubbery and show ballooning or hooding. The chordae tendineae are thinned out, elongated and at times are ruptured but show no commissural fusion. Annular dilatation is present. There may at times be involvement of other valves as well. On microscopic examination, there is destruction of the fibrosa layer of the valve on which the integrity depends, deposition of myxomatous material and focal thickening of the spongiosa layer. The mitral valve undergoes secondary changes due to the stress and injury. Pathogenesis of this condition favors the theory of underlying developmental defect of connective tissue. Thus, it is seen in Marfan syndrome and some other hereditary disorders of connective tissues. In patients without any syndromes, there are features like the presence of scoliosis and high arched palate present in the patient, that favors structural abnormalities of connective tissue.

Marfan syndrome is heterogeneous as there is a great variation in the clinical picture, even within families. Patients with prominent cardiovascular and eye changes may have few skeletal system changes. Others with prominent Marfanoid habitus, may have no eye changes. Due to these variations, a diagnosis of Marfan syndrome is acceptable when there is a significant defect in two of the four organ systems which include the cardiovascular system, skeletal system, eye and skin along with a minor involvement of others. The clinical expression is thus variable and this is due to the allelic mutations within the same locus.

COMMENTARY INDEX CASE: PM 22554

A young male came with sudden onset, severe lacerating epigastric pain, radiating to the upper chest and neck. He was a diagnosed case of Marfan syndrome on follow-up. There was a strong family history of sudden cardiac deaths following severe chest and abdominal pain. His mother and two brothers (one with Marfanoid features) had died under similar circumstances. Echocardiography of the index case revealed massive dilatation of the aortic root and ascending aorta with aortic dissection, moderate to severe AR and left ventricular systolic dysfunction. Autopsy revealed a cystic medial degeneration of the ascending aorta (florid changes), brachiocephalic, right and left common carotids/subclavians, abdominal aorta (milder changes), leading to marked aortic root dilatation, aneurysm of the ascending aorta, acute dissection of the ascending and arch of aorta—DeBakey type 2, chronic dissection, i.e. double lumen of the left subclavian artery, myxomatous degeneration of the mitral valve, left ventricular dilatation and right ventricular hypertrophy.

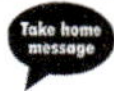

TAKE HOME MESSAGE

- Marfan syndrome is a disorder of connective tissue and mainly affects the eyes, skeletal and cardiovascular systems.
- Eighty percent cases are familial and have an autosomal dominant transmission.
- There is an inherited defect in fibrillin-1, an important extracellular glycoprotein, which is an important component of the microfibrils, present in large quantities in the ciliary zonules, ligaments and aorta.
- These microfibrils form the scaffold on which the tropoelastin is deposited to form elastic fibers.
- In Marfan syndrome, the basic foundation for the formation of the elastic fibers is defective and the above said organs are maximally affected, leading to fatal complications.
- Marfan syndrome is associated with more than 500 distinct mutations in *FBN1* gene. Most of these are missense mutations that give rise to an abnormal fibrillin-1.
- In Marfan syndrome, cystic medial degeneration leads to elastic degeneration of the tunica media of the ascending aorta, leading to various complications as seen above.

REFERENCES

1. Ramirez F, Dietz HC. Marfan syndrome: from molecular pathogenesis to clinical treatment. Curr Opin Genet Dev. 2007;17(3):252-8.
2. Loeys BL, Chen J, Neptune ER, et al. A syndrome of altered cardiovascular, craniofacial, neurocognitive and skeletal development caused by mutations in TGFBR1 or TGFBR2. Nat Genet. 2005;37:275.
3. De Paepe A, Devereux RB, Dietz HC, et al. Revised diagnostic criteria for the Marfan syndrome. Am J Med Genet. 1996;62:417.
4. Radonic T, de Witte P, Groenink M, et al. Critical appraisal of the revised Ghent criteria for diagnosis of Marfan syndrome. Clin Genet. 2011;80:346.
5. Dean JC. Marfan syndrome: clinical diagnosis and management. Eur J Hum Genet. 2007;15:724-33.
6. Adams JN, Trent RJ. Aortic complications of Marfan syndrome. Lancet. 1998;352:1722.
7. Dietz HC, McIntosh I, Sakai LY, et al. Four novel FBN1 mutations: significance for mutant transcript level and EGF-like domain calcium binding in the pathogenesis of Marfan syndrome. Genomics. 1993;17:468.
8. Singh KK, Rommel K, Mishra A, et al. TGFBR1 and TGFBR2 mutations in patients with features of Marfan syndrome and Loeys-Dietz syndrome. Hum Mutat. 2006;27(8):770-7.
9. Trotter SE, Olsen EG. Marfan's disease and Erdheim's cystic medionecrosis. A study of their pathology. Eur Heart J. 1991;12:83.

CONTRIBUTIONS BY:

1. Dr Rajesh Vijayvergiya, Professor, Department of Cardiology (Clinician In-Charge)
2. Dr S Reddy, Additional Professor, Department of Cardiology (Compilation of Clinical Details)

Post Graduate Institute of Medical Education and Research, Chandigarh, India.

CASE 33

Adult Tetralogy of Fallot with Tricuspid Valve Infective Endocarditis and Thromboembolic Botryomycotic Cerebral Abscess: PM 26941

Nandita Bharadwaj Kakkar

HIGHLIGHTS OF THE CASE

A 28-year-old male, a known epileptic since the past 15 years was incidentally detected to be a case of tetralogy of Fallot (TOF) at the age of 13 years. At that point of time, he was doing routine physical activities with ease. He started having dyspnea on exertion at the age of 20 years and was put on a low dose of diuretic. Presently, he came with history of fever and headache of one day duration, had two episodes of generalized tonic-clonic seizures (GTCS), after which there was loss of consciousness. He was gasping and SpO_2 was 74% on room air. There was neck rigidity and decreased movements in the left upper limb. Angiogram was suggestive of TOF. Contrast-enhanced computed tomography (CECT) brain showed a single ring enhancing lesion in right parieto-occipital region ? brain abscess ? glioblastoma multiforme. Echocardiography did not reveal any vegetation. Autopsy revealed a classical TOF with infective endocarditis of the tricuspid valve and thromboembolic cerebral abscess (botryomycotic).

Keywords: Tetralogy of Fallot, infective endocarditis, tricuspid valve, cerebral abscess, botryomycosis, autopsy.

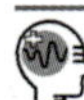

CLINICAL DETAILS

Date of Admission: 29.09.2015, Date of Death: 30.09.2015, Duration of Hospital Stay: 38 Hours

A 28-year-old male presented with history of fever and headache of one day duration. He had two episodes of (GTCS) after which there was loss of consciousness. His past medical history dates back to 15 years, when he presented to the emergency in PGIMER, with the first episode of GTCS in the year 2000. At that point of time, at the age of 13, he was incidentally detected to be a case of TOF, but he was doing routine physical activities with ease. He was recommended antiepileptic drugs (AEDs) for 3 years, to which he complied well. After this, he remained apparently asymptomatic until January 2013, when he again had two episodes of GTCS and was restarted on AED. Since then he was on irregular treatment. In February 2013, he was admitted to the cardiology ward with complaints of dyspnea on exertion for 4–5 years and history of one episode of GTCS, 7 days before admission. Cardiac catheterization was done at this time and it was suggestive of TOF. He was hemodynamically stable and afebrile, was put on low dose diuretic, advised to continue antiepileptics and discharged. Thereafter, he was on irregular follow-up. Family history revealed that his parents are alive and healthy. He had two brothers and two sisters, of which the eldest brother had sudden cardiac death at the age of 34 years. The patient was educated until the eighth standard. He was married and has two healthy children, 5 and 3 years old. He was a laborer by occupation. ***Examination***: BP—140/100 mm Hg, Pulse—70/min. Respiration—gasping at presentation, afebrile, SpO_2 = 74% on room air, height 172 cm; S1 and ? S2 normal, ejection systolic murmur heard in pulmonary area, bilateral air entry normal with no added sounds. ***CNS***: E2 V1 M4, neck rigidity present, pupils—bilateral nonsymmetric and nonreactive, he was moving all four limbs but decreased movements were noted in the left upper limb, DTR bilateral ++, Planters—bilateral up going, fundus examination could not be done as the patient was irritable and not cooperative.

Investigations and Course of Management

Hemogram: Hb—21 g/dL; TLC—10,600/μL, platelets—80,000/μL, random blood sugar—113 mg%, Na^+—136 mEq/L, K^+—6.8 mEq/L, LFT/RFT—WNL, PT—16' (N: 14'), PTI—87%, INR—1.16 and aPTT—43'.

Echocardiography: PGI (06.08.2012); Tetralogy of Fallot physiology with small-sized pulmonary arteries, No AR, 50% aortic override, valvular and infundibular pulmonary stenosis, peak systolic gradient 80 mm Hg and main pulmonary artery (MPA)—7 mm. ***Cardiac catheterization report (11.02.2013)***: Hemodynamic data—pressures (mm Hg): Aorta (s/d/m) = 105/04/42; LV = 113/10; RV 109/10. Oxymetry: ascending aorta 54.6%. ***Angiogram***: Large ventricular septal defect (VSD), 40% aortic override; no aortomitral discontinuity, normal origin and course of coronaries, large major aortopulmonary collateral arteries (MAPCAs) on right side, pulmonary artery (PA) is anterior to aorta, infundibular and valvular; right ventricular outflow tract obstruction (RVOTO), small-sized confluent PAs, MPA = 9 mm, LPA and RPA = 7 mm each. McGoon index: 0.77. Suggestive of TOF with small confluent PAs and was advised medical therapy. ***Echocardiography***: (29.09.2015–present admission): Bedside echo emergency outpatient department (EMOPD)—no obvious vegetation seen. Septae tricuspid valve—thickened. Moderate tricuspid regurgitation, right ventricular systolic pressure (RVSP) = RAP + 50 mm Hg. Transesophageal echo not done as patient was unstable. ***CECT brain***: (24.10.2014) Normal study, 29.09.2015 (present admission) Single ring enhancing lesion in right parieto-occipital region, ? brain abscess ? and glioblastoma multiforme.

This 28-year-old male presented with long standing history of TOF and seizure disorder for last 15 years. He had recurrent episodes of GTCS for last 2 years and was on irregular treatment for the same. He was advised medical therapy for his cardiac problem. Presently, he had fever and headache associated with recurrence of GTCS followed by loss of consciousness. At admission, patient was E2V1M4, BP was 140/100 mm Hg, HR 70/min, afebrile and gasping for breath. He was appropriately treated but developed cardiorespiratory arrest from which he could not be revived. ***Units final diagnosis***: A known case of cyanotic congenital heart disease—adult TOF, NYHA II, reactive polycythemia and seizure disorder—epilepsy. ***Current presentation***: Intracranial space occupying lesions (ICSOL) ? cerebral abscess associated with meningismus/meningitis ? glioblastoma multiforme, raised intracranial tension (ICT), infective endocarditis—cannot be ruled out. ***Cause of death***: Possibly cardiac arrhythmias, ? status epilepticus/raised ICT.

AUTOPSY FINDINGS: PM 26941

A complete autopsy was performed. The prosector found that the patient was emaciated. All serous cavities were within normal limits.

The ***heart*** weighed 280 g. The external look was boot-shaped with dextroposition of the aorta (Fig 1A). The tricuspid valve showed multiple vegetations (Fig 1B), which were friable, ranging in size from 0.5 to 0.8 cm, present on the atrial surface of the cusps. Abnormalities detected were (Figs 1C–E): (1) Large VSD (2.3 cm) was present. The size of the VSD was equivalent to 60–70% of the aortic ring. The margins of the VSD were free of any scar and free of any attachment of chordae tendineae. Falciparum membrane on the posterior border of the defect was present, which represented a remnant of membranous ventricular septum. The right anterior aortic leaflet and a portion of the posterior aortic leaflet arose from a part of the aortic ring that extended across the septum and got inserted in the right ventricular myocardium, where it formed the superior border of the right outflow tract. (2) Pulmonic stenosis was severe and present in the middle part of the infundibulum. Calcification was noted and no post-stenotic dilatation was present. Due to the severe infundibular stenosis was difficult to open the hypoplastic pulmonary artery (PA) via the right ventricle. Hence, a probe was inserted from the PA, into the right ventricle to ascertain the connection. (3) There was hypoplasia of the pulmonary valve ring and pulmonary arteries (main, right, left), but no pulmonary valve leaflet deformity was noted. This would behave as a functional stenosis. (4) Dextroposition of the aorta, i.e. overriding of aorta over the VSD was 60–70%. (5) Right ventricular hypertrophy (RVH) (2.3 cm). Features were consistent with a diagnosis of classical TOF. Microscopic examination of the vegetations (Figs 2A–C) revealed organization and calcification at the base, fibrin and acute inflammatory cells with an occasional cluster of bacteria. Coronary arteries were within normal limits.

The ***brain*** weighed 1,205 g. The meninges were markedly congested and showed a prominent exudate (Figs 3A–C) more so on the superolateral surfaces, which was also seen on the cerebellar surfaces and at the base of the brain. There was a prominent bulge of the parietal lobe on the right side (Fig 3A). Tonsillar herniation was seen on the right side. Bilateral uncal (right > left) herniation were also noted. The blood vessels at the circle of Willis were normal. Coronal slicing revealed a hemorrhagic, well-defined abscess, measuring 6 × 4 × 3 cm, which was extending over six coronal slices of the brain (Figs 3D and E). Anteriorly it was seen in the white matter and at the level of the splenium of the corpus callosum, it had ruptured into the right ventricle, due to which the right lateral and third ventricles were distended. Posteriorly it was very close to the surface. The brain stem and the cerebellum did not show any lesion, but were covered by thick exudate. Sections studied

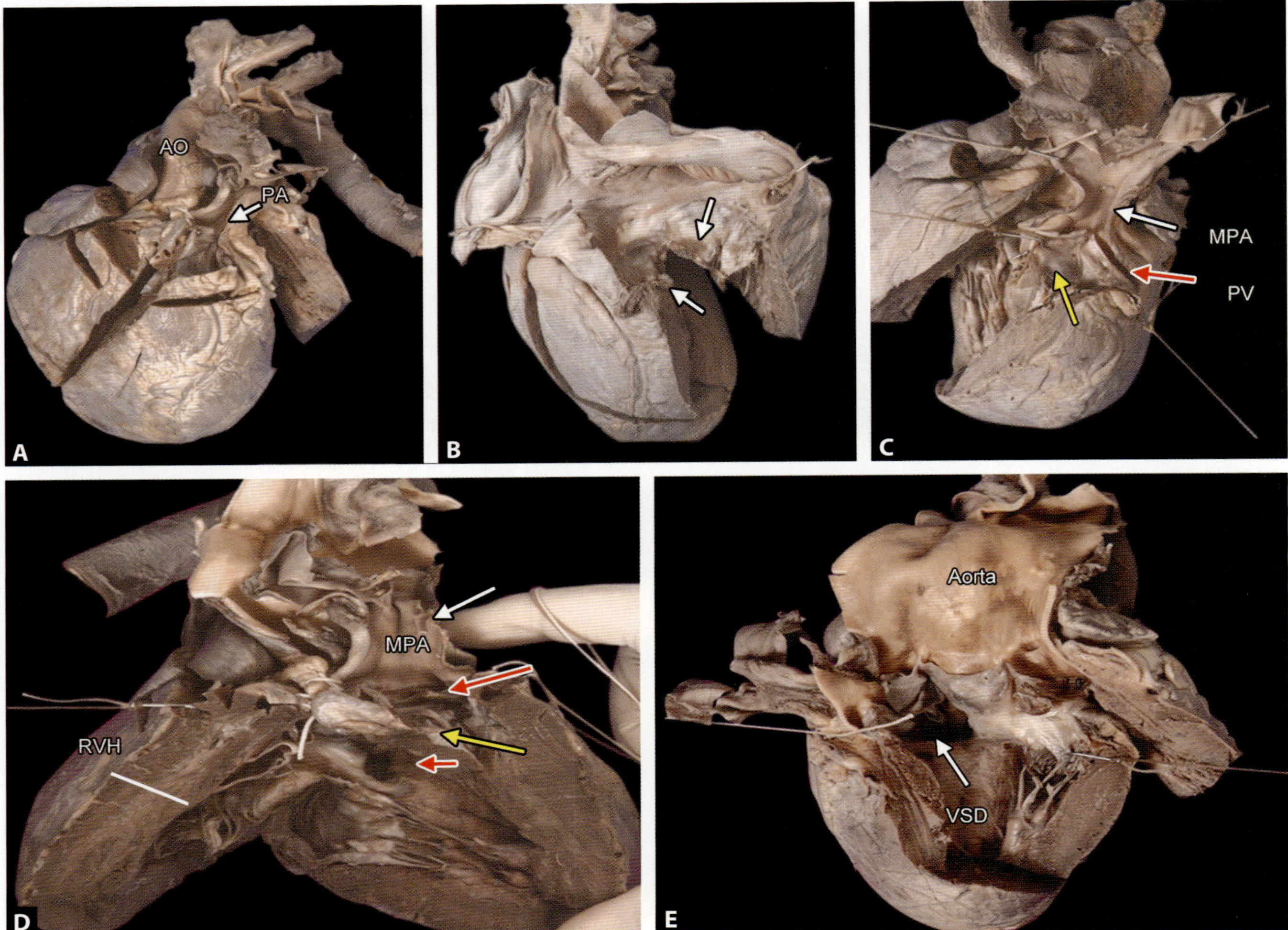

Figs 1A–E: (A) Gross photograph of the heart which is boot-shaped with dextroposition of the aorta. Opened up hypoplastic pulmonary artery (PA) is seen to the right (arrow); (B) Opened up right atrium. Tricuspid leaflets show vegetations (arrows); (C and D) Right outflow tract showing hypoplastic main PA (white arrow), pulmonary valve cusps (red arrow), and subpulmonic stenosis (yellow arrow). Figure "D" in addition shows the ventricular septum defect (VSD) (red small arrow) and marked right ventricular hypertrophy (white line); (E) Left outflow tract showing the large VSD (arrow).
(AO: Aorta; MPA: Main pulmonary artery; PA: Pulmonary artery; PV: Pulmonary vein; RVH: Right ventricular hypertrophy; VSD: Ventricular septum defect.)

from the abscess (Figs 3F and 4A–C) revealed a purulent exudate composed of polymorphs with nuclear debris in the central areas and organization going on at the periphery. Densely packed clusters or conglomerates of hematoxyphilic bacteria known as granules (strongly Gram positive) were seen embedded in a pink hyaline eosinophilic material (Figs 4B and C). This unique characteristic pattern is known as Splendore–Hoeppli phenomenon and is very characteristic of a botryomycotic abscess. The abscess had ruptured into the ventricles (Figs 4D–F and 5A–C) leading on to ventriculitis, ependymitis, choroid plexitis, border zone encephalitis, early infarcts and meningitis (Figs 5D and E). A large vessel at the base of the brain, caught up in the meningeal exudate revealed vasculitis. Surrounding the abscess there was gliosis, perivascular lymphomononuclear cell infiltrate and edema. Overall features were those of thromboembolic cerebral abscess (botryomycotic)—right parietal lobe with rupture into the ventricle causing ventriculitis, ependymitis, choroid plexitis, border zone encephalitis and meningitis. There was right tonsillar and uncal herniation.

Lungs showed hemorrhage and pulmonary arteriopathy. Extensive extramedullary hematopoiesis was seen in the ***liver, spleen and lymph nodes***. The ***bone marrow*** showed marked erythroid hyperplasia.

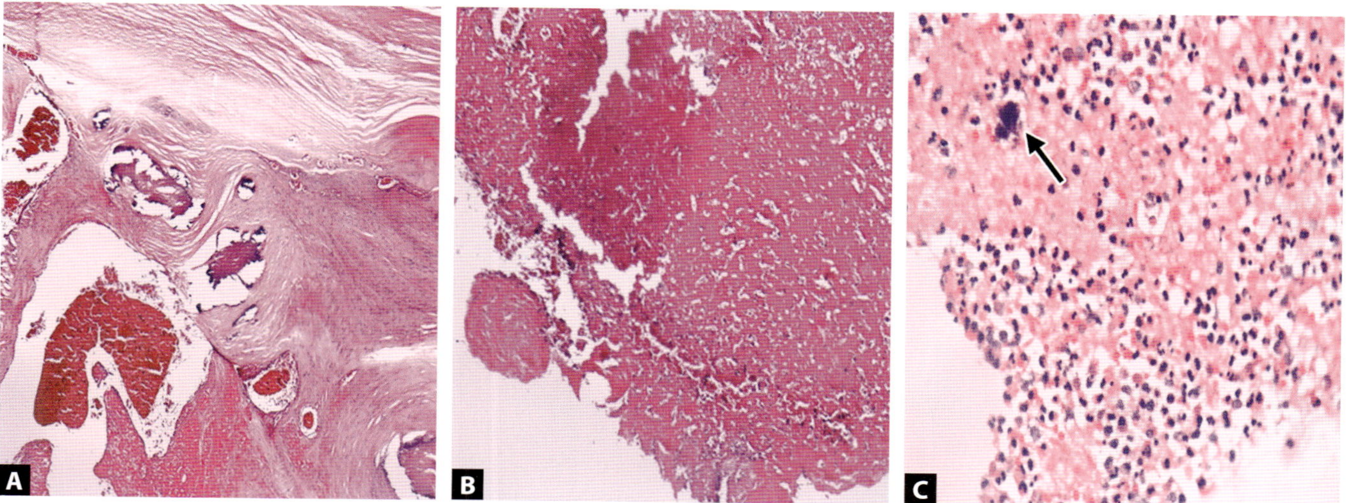

Figs 2A–C: Photomicrographs from the vegetations showing (A) Hyalinization at the base; (B) Fibrin; (C) Polymorphs with nuclear debris and cluster of bacteria (arrow).

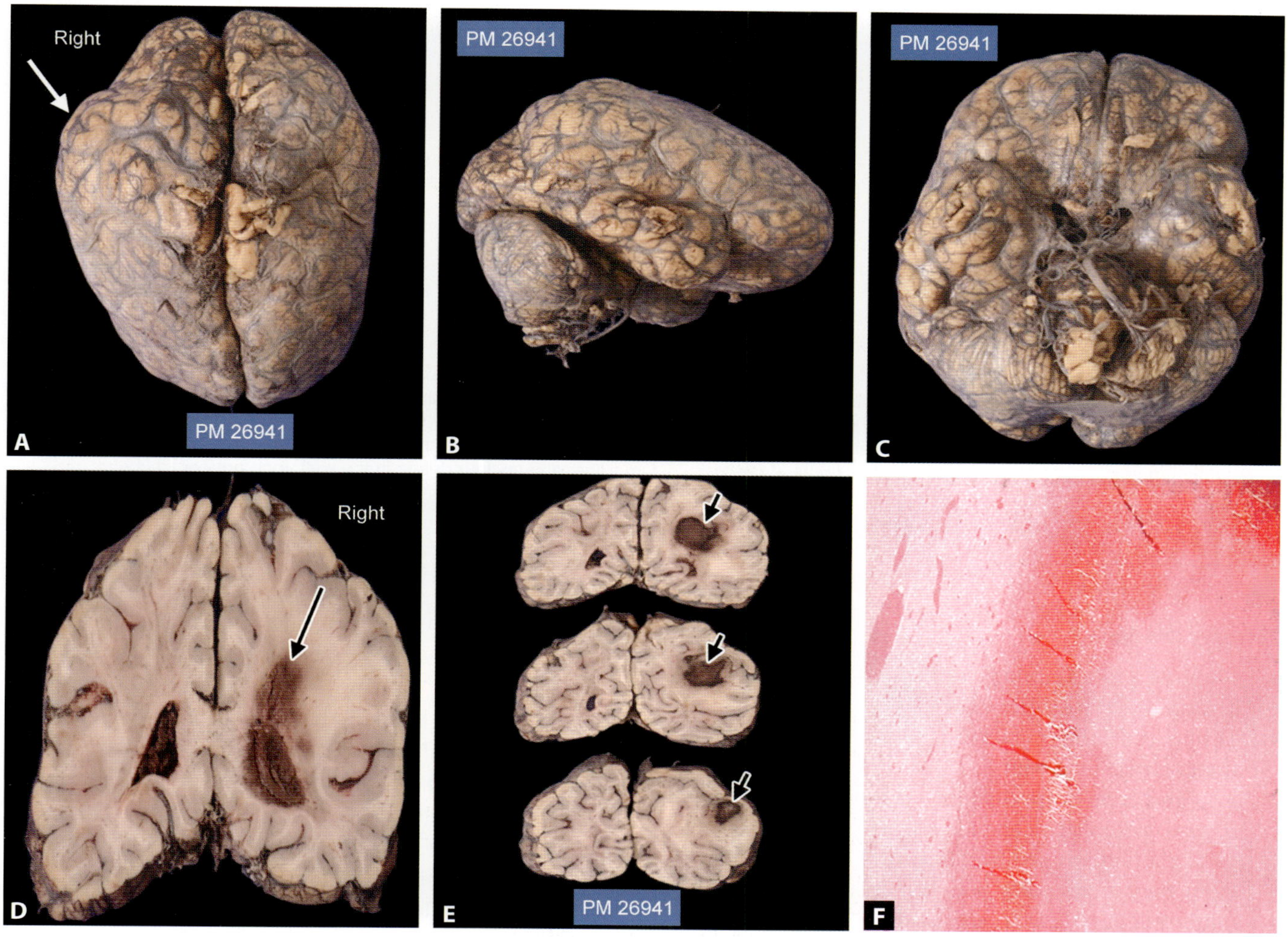

Figs 3A–F: Gross photographs of the brain showing thick exudate over the superior surfaces. (A) Here a bulge (arrow) is noted in the right parietal lobe; (B) Thick exudate seen over the right lateral surface of the brain and cerebellum; (C) Thick exudate seen over the base of the brain; (D) Coronal slice of the brain showing an abscess (arrow) rupturing into the right ventricle; (E) Coronal slices of the brain showing the extent of the well-defined abscess (arrows); (F) Photomicrograph taken from the edge of the brain abscess showing a band of hemorrhage.

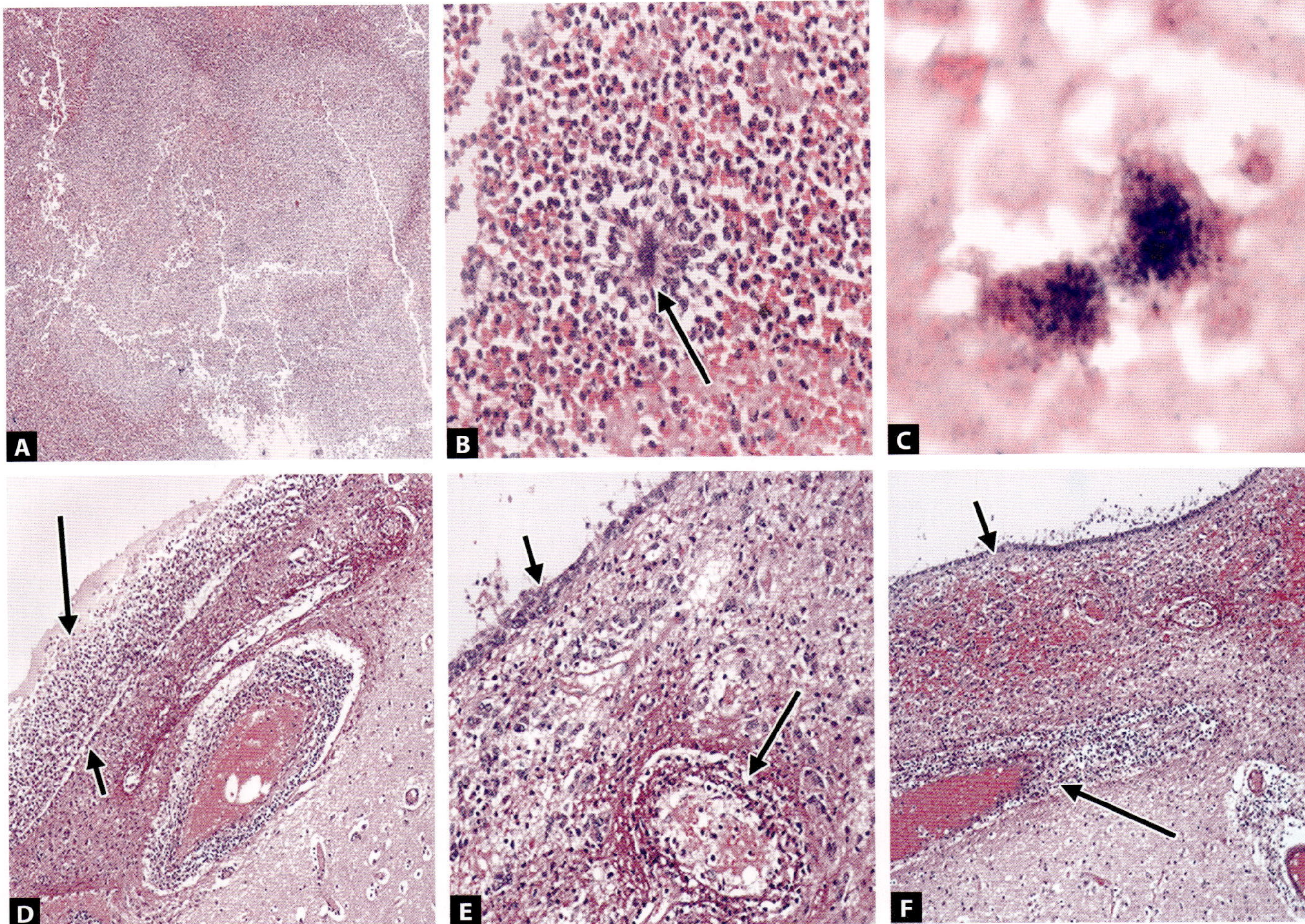

Figs 4A–F: Photomicrographs from the center of the abscess shows (A) Polymorphs and nuclear debris; (B) Polymorphs along with conglomerates of hematoxyphilic bacteria together known as granules, seen embedded in a pink hyaline eosinophilic material, known as Splendore–Hoeppli phenomenon; (C) Splendore–Hoeppli phenomenon showing Gram positive granules (Grams stain); (D) Exudate within the ventricle (long arrow), ventricular lining appreciated (small arrow); (E and F) Photomicrographs show ventricular lining (small arrows), periventricular area shows inflammation, vessels show vasculitis, i.e. fibrinoid necrosis, polymorphs, and nuclear debris in the wall (long arrows).

FINAL AUTOPSY DIAGNOSIS: PM 26941

28 Years Old Male

- Classical adult Tetralogy of Fallot with infective endocarditis of the tricuspid valve
- Thromboembolic cerebral abscess (botryomycotic)—right parietal lobe with:
  - Ventriculitis, ependymitis, choroid plexitis, border zone encephalitis and meningitis
  - Right tonsillar and bilateral uncal herniation
- Pulmonary arteriopathy with hemorrhage
- Extramedullary hematopoiesis—liver, spleen and lymph nodes
- Marked erythroid hyperplasia—bone marrow.

TETRALOGY OF FALLOT

Tetralogy of Fallot is the most widely known of the congenital heart diseases and comes under the group of "right to left shunts". The term "tetralogy" in some ways is superfluous as all components of the tetrad are not equally important. It is more justified to call this entity as a "deuterology" comprising of VSD and the pulmonic stenosis. Variations in the four components lead to a wide spectrum of congenital heart disease, that resembles "Tetralogy of Fallot". All these features occur embryologically due to anterosuperior displacement of the infundibular septum: (1) ***Classical TOF*** has a large VSD of a characteristic type and a severe pulmonic stenosis to cause a right to left shunt via the

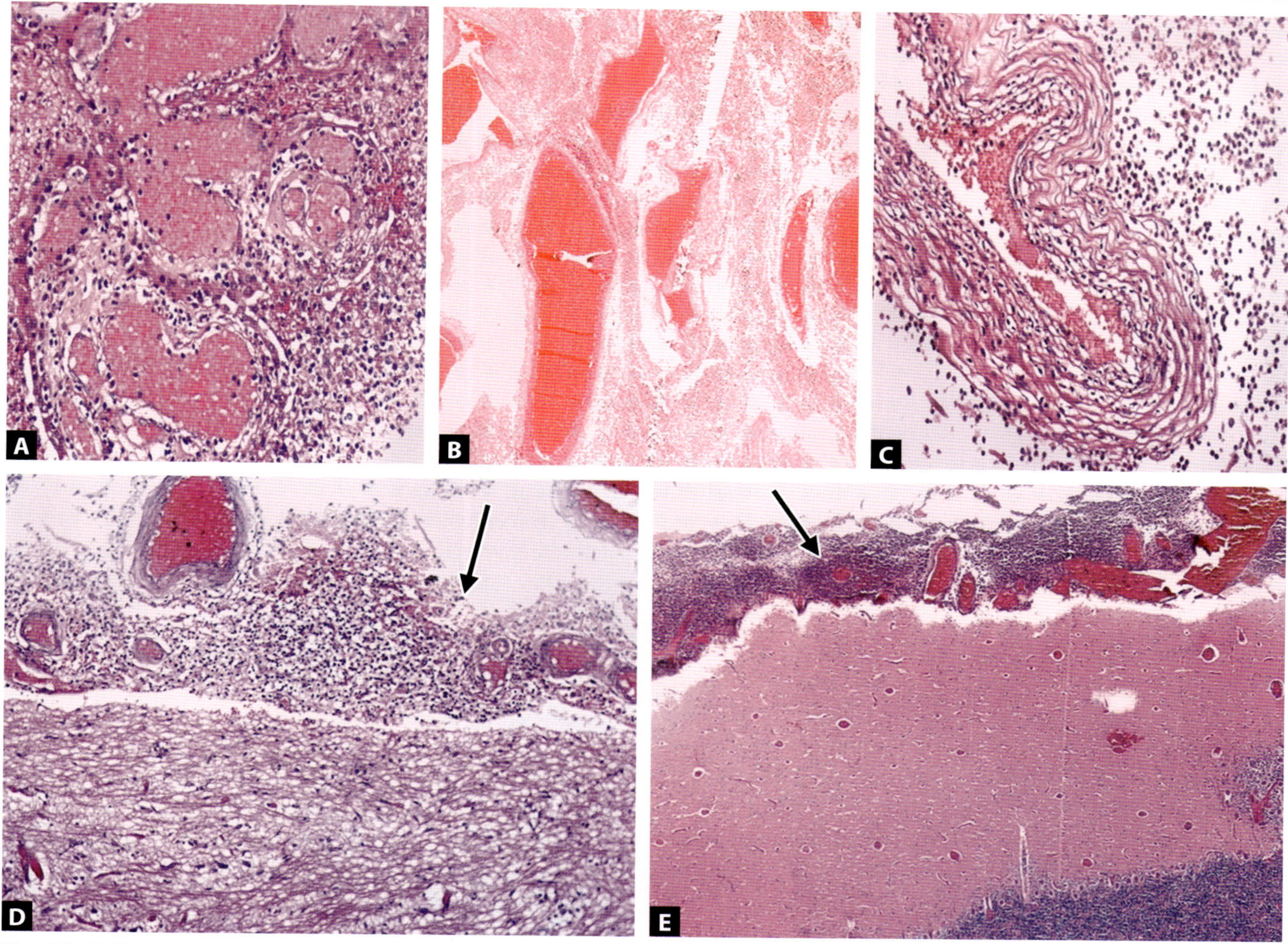

Figs 5A–E: Photomicrographs from the brain showing (A) Choroid plexitis; (B) Vessels at the base of the brain caught up in the thick exudate; (C) A large vessel at the base of the brain showing vasculitis; (D and E) Acute meningeal exudate (arrows) in the cerebral cortex (D) and cere-

VSD. (2) ***Atypical tetralogy***: Here either the VSD is not characteristic or other complicating lesions may be present. If the VSD is small and no shunt occurs, then the defect functions like a pure pulmonic stenosis. If the VSD is large and pulmonic stenosis is slight, it functions as an isolated VSD. There may be little resistance to pulmonary blood flow and left to right shunt occurs, as in an isolated VSD. (3) ***Balanced tetralogy***: Here the degree of pulmonic stenosis is just appropriate to allow an adequate pulmonary flow, which protects the pulmonary vasculature from acquiring secondary hypertensive changes. This is the most favorable functional situation in Fallot tetralogy. (4) ***Pseudotruncus arteriosus***: The pulmonic stenosis may be complete and here the term "pseudotruncus arteriosus" applies. This is the most severe form of tetralogy. The pulmonary trunk is atretic or severely hypoplastic. It may be a thin fibrous cord leading to the major pulmonary arteries, which are supplied by a patent ductus arteriosus or dilated bronchial arteries or both. The obliterated pulmonary trunk may be hidden in the epicardial fat.

The various components of ***classical TOF*** are: (1) ***VSD***, which is very large and includes the entire or part of the membranous septum. The view of the left ventricular structures can be seen through the VSD. (2) ***Pulmonic stenosis***: This can be infundibular, valvular or both. The most common is the infundibular stenosis, which can be seen in any portion of the conus, but is mostly subvalvular. Middle or low infundibular stenosis leads to dilatation of the infundibulum distal to the stenosis, thus forming a conus chamber. With subpulmonic stenosis, the pulmonary valve ring and PA are hypoplastic, thus functionally stenotic, even though there may be no leaflet deformity. A severe subpulmonic stenosis leads to severely hypoplastic pulmonary arteries (main right and left) which are smaller and thin-walled and also cause a greater degree of overriding of aorta. In classical TOF, isolated pulmonary valve stenosis is rare. In valvular stenosis, there is fusion of the cusps along the commissures, forming a membrane with a central orifice or slit. (3) ***Dextroposition of the aorta***: This feature is determined by examination of the left outflow tract. (4) ***RVH***: This is a secondary change due to hypertension in the right ventricle, which is largely due to the VSD, which equalizes the right and left pressures. The "boot shape" of the heart is due to marked RVH. (5) ***Other findings***: The ascending aorta undergoes compensatory enlargement and the ring of the aortic valve is also enlarged, due to the increased flow of blood as a result of the right to left shunt. To maintain competency, the aortic cusps are widened and as they are poorly supported in the portion where they overlie the VSD, they become redundant and eversion may occur. The coronary artery may have a single orifice. Their first portions may be distorted due to the muscle changes at the conus, due to the myocardial hypertrophy and due to the position of the aorta. The ductus arteriosus in TOF is mostly hypoplastic and may be absent. If present, it tends to obliterate after birth and this may be responsible for death in the neonatal period, as the neonate may be totally dependent on this structure for his pulmonary blood flow. In TOF, the ductus is a useless structure as, pulmonic stenosis makes the pulmonary blood flow so scanty, that the only way for the blood to escape to the systemic circulation is via the VSD. Thus, the ductus has no demand in the fetal state and undergoes resolution.

Patients with TOF, even if untreated, can survive into adult life. Ten percent of untreated patients are alive at 20 years and approximately 3% at 40 years. Bertranou et al, in their study highlighted that 86% of persons with TOF, not treated surgically live to age 1 year, 49% to age 3 years and 24% to age 10 years. Thereafter, the instantaneous risk of death remains constant. The chance of survival is significantly less with pulmonary atresia, rather than stenosis. Survival depends upon the degree of subpulmonic stenosis. If mild it resembles an isolated VSD, shunt is left to right without cyanosis and known as "pink tetralogy". In severe subpulmonic obstruction, right sided pressure is more and leads to right to left shunt, producing cyanosis, i.e. "blue or the classic tetralogy". Untreated children with TOF who survive into adult life, have a moderate degree of subpulmonic stenosis, i.e. have a balanced tetralogy. As the child grows, size of the heart increases, but the pulmonary orifice does not expand as it normally should. This makes the obstruction worse progressively and these patients manifest later in life (as did the patient in the index case). Patients with TOF do not have right ventricular failure, because the subpulmonic stenosis decompresses the right ventricle by shunting the blood via the VSD into the left ventricle and protects the pulmonary vasculature from pressure overload.

Complications of TOF are those of cyanotic heart disease. Polycythemia leads to increased viscosity of blood and this may cause thrombosis especially in the dural sinuses and in the peripheral pulmonary vessels, due to reduced and slow blood flow. Cyanosis occurs as a result of the decreased pulmonary blood flow and proper oxygenation does not occur. The right to left shunt further increases the cyanosis. Cyanosis further leads to more susceptibility to infections. Pneumonia is difficult to treat due to the reduced pulmonary blood flow. The right to left shunt provides a route for paradoxical embolus, so that any localized phlebitis or right-sided infective endocarditis can disseminate via the systemic circulation. This was the pathogenesis of brain abscess in the index case.

BOTRYOMYCOSIS

Botryomycosis is an unusual chronic suppurative bacterial infection of the skin and viscera, which clinically and histologically mimics infection by ***Actinomyces*** species. It shows the presence of granules or "grains" and may be associated with a granulomatous component. The "grains" show non-branching bacteria by appropriate stains and this is the most specific feature for the diagnosis of botryomycosis. The term botryomycosis comes from botrys (Greek), which means a bunch of grapes. The disease was first reported in 1870 in a horse who underwent castration. It occurs in two forms—cutaneous and visceral. Lung is the main site of visceral involvement, but it has been reported in the liver, kidney, trachea, heart, oral cavity, conjunctiva, orbit, bowel and the brain. Most patients have no apparent predisposing factors. In the integumentary type, trauma and foreign body may precede the development of botryomycosis. Cystic fibrosis, diabetes, HIV infection, post-surgery and steroid intake have been implicated as the predisposing factors. The essential factor is the development of a symbiotic relationship as a result of a delicate balance between the low virulence of the infecting agent and the tissue resistance of the host. Since, there is a symbiosis struck between the intruder and the host, it is a chronic disease and generally detected, years after acquisition. The most frequent causative organism is ***Staphylococcus aureus***. The other organisms implicated are ***Pseudomonas***, ***Actinobacillus***, ***E. coli***, ***Proteus vulgaris***, alpha hemolytic and nonhemolytic ***Strepto-***

coccus, gram negative ***Coccobacillus***, ***Propionibacterium acnes*** and other anaerobic organisms. Histopathology shows the characteristic Splendore–Hoeppli phenomenon, wherein clusters of bacteria known as granules, embedded in a pink hyaline matrix, are found lying in foci of acute inflammatory infiltrate. Surrounding area may show giant cells and epithelioid cells, i.e a granulomatous reaction. The granules are brightly periodic acid-Schiff (PAS) positive and the bacteria in the center of the grains are positive for Gram stain. This phenomenon is particularly striking in actinomycosis, mycetoma and botryomycosis. Pus should be sent from the lesion for culture and sensitivity. Surgical resection, drainage and appropriate antibiotics are needed for a permanent cure.

COMMENTARY INDEX CASE: PM 26941

A 28-year-old male, a known epileptic, on treatment since the past 15 years, was incidentally detected to be a case of TOF at the age of 13 years. At this point of time, he was doing routine physical activities with ease. He started having dyspnea on exertion, for the first time, at the age of 20 years and was put on a low dose of diuretic. In the present admission, he came with history of fever and headache of one day duration, had two episodes of GTCS after which there was loss of consciousness. He was gasping and SpO_2 was 74% on room air. There was neck rigidity and decreased movements in the left upper limb. Angiogram was suggestive of TOF. CECT brain showed a single ring enhancing lesion in right parieto-occipital region ? brain abscess ? glioblastoma multiforme. Echocardiography did not reveal any vegetation. Polycythemia was present. Autopsy revealed a classical TOF with infective endocarditis of the tricuspid valve and thromboembolic cerebral abscess (botryomycotic). The heart showed a very large VSD, with an aortic override of 60–70%. The pulmonic stenosis was very severe and present in the middle part of the infundibulum. Calcification was present, but no poststenotic dilatation was noted. There was hypoplasia of the pulmonary valve ring and pulmonary arteries (main, right, left), but no pulmonary valve leaflet deformity was noted. This would behave as a functional stenosis. Overriding of aorta over the VSD was to the tune of 60–70% and marked RVH was present. Complications of TOF, i.e. tricuspid valve vegetations which had dislodged and via the VSD went into the systemic circulation, to produce the abscess in the right parietal lobe of the brain and polycythemia with extensive extramedullary hematopoiesis were present. The brain abscess had ruptured into the ventricle producing ventriculitis, ependymitis, choroid plexitis, border zone encephalitis and meningitis. There was raised intracranial tension leading on to right tonsillar and bilateral uncal herniation. The abscess showed the characteristic Splendore–Hoeppli phenomenon seen in botryomycotic abscess. This young male had presented for the first time with dyspnea on exertion, at the age of 20 years. So he had the most favorable functional situation in Fallot tetralogy, i.e. a balanced tetralogy to begin with, where the degree of pulmonic stenosis is just appropriate to allow an adequate pulmonary flow, which protects the pulmonary vasculature from acquiring secondary hypertensive changes. With time, as the child grows, size of the heart increases, but the pulmonary orifice does not expand, as it normally should, this makes the pulmonic obstruction worse and these patients manifest later in life, as the index case did.

TAKE HOME MESSAGE

- Tetralogy of Fallot is a cyanotic congenital heart disease with a right to left shunt. The cardinal features of classical TOF are VSD, pulmonic stenosis (infundibular, valvular or both), dextroposition or overriding of aorta and RVH.
- Patients with TOF, even untreated can survive into adult life. Ten percent of untreated patients are alive at 20 years and approximately 4% at 40 years
- Complications include polycythemia, thrombosis, infections, infective endocarditis and paradoxical embolus.

SUGGESTED READING

1. Bertranou EG, Eugene H, Blackstone EH, et al. Life expectancy without surgery in tetralogy of Fallot. Am J Cardiology. 1978;42:458-66.
2. Defraigne JO, Demoulin JC, Pierard GE, et al. Fatal mural endocarditis and cutaneous botryomycosis after heart transplantation. Am J Dermatopathol. 1997;19(6):602-5.
3. Gillock CB, Sahni KS, Mumaw VR, et al. Cerebral Botryomycosis: Case Report. J Infectious Dis. 1990;162:765-7.
4. Richmond I, Mene A. Renal Botryomycosis. Histopathol. 1992;20(1):67-9.
5. Schlossberg D, Pandey M, Reddy R. The Splendore–Hoeppli phenomenon in hepatic botryomycosis. J Clin Pathol. 1998; 51:399-400.
6. Sherman FE. Ventricular septal defect with pulmonary stenosis or atresia, Tetralogy of Fallot. In: Sherman FE (Ed). An Atlas of Congenital Heart Disease (compiled from the

museum of Congenital Heart Disease at Childrens Hospital of Pittsburgh). Philadelphia: Lea and Febiger; 1963. pp. 187-95.

7. Toth IR, Kazal HL. Botryomycosis in acquired immunodeficiency syndrome. Arch Path Lab Med. 1987;111:246-9.
8. Vasishta RK, Gupta N, Kakkar N. Botryomycosis- a series of integumentary and visceral forms with review of literature. Ann Trop Med Parasit. 2004;98(6):623-9.

CONTRIBUTIONS BY:

1. Dr Parminder S Otaal, Associate Professor, Department of Cardiology (Compilation of Clinical Details)
2. Dr SC Varma, Ex-Professor and Head, Department of Internal Medicine (Clinician In-Charge)

Post Graduate Institute of Medical Education and Research, Chandigarh, India.

CASE 34

Cocaine-induced Vasculopathy Leading to Cardiomyopathy, Renal Infarcts, Gangrene of Digits with Autoamputation: PM 23445

Nandita Bharadwaj Kakkar

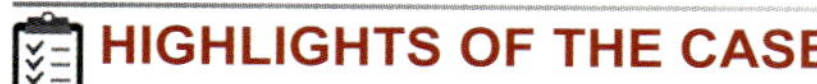

HIGHLIGHTS OF THE CASE

This 26-year-old male, a polysubstance abuser, presented to medical emergency with history of Raynaud's phenomenon, upper/lower limb digital gangrene since 4 years and a short febrile illness, associated with cough, progressive dyspnea of recent onset, along with altered sensorium, 3 days prior to admission. Echocardiography exhibited dilated cardiomyopathy. The clinical diagnosis was—multiple drug abuser, multiple digital gangrene with Raynaud's phenomenon ? vasculitis, bronchopneumonia, cardiomyopathy ? infective endocarditis. Autopsy revealed cocaine-induced florid small vessel arterial vasculopathy leading to dilated cardiomyopathy, renal infarcts and digital gangrene along with infective endocarditis of aortic valve with ring abscess.

Keywords: Cocaine, vasculopathy, cardiomyopathy, gangrene, autopsy, toes, autoamputation.

CLINICAL DETAILS

Date of Admission: 01.12.2009, Date of Death: 04.12.2009, Duration of Hospital Stay: 4 Days

A 26-year-old male came with presenting complaints of multiple episodes (with winter exacerbations) of bluish discoloration and ulceration of toes and fingers, since 4 years. Both his little toes had undergone autoamputation. For the past 15 days, there was fever (102°F), cough with mucoid expectoration, not associated with hemoptysis or chest pain and shortness of breath that was gradually worsening leading to orthopnea. There was altered sensorium since 3 days with marked restlessness, incoherent speech and he was verbally abusive. There was a history of skin rash and skin tightness. There was no past history of photosensitivity, oral ulcers, joint pains, hematuria, preceding flu-like illness, bleeding from any site, dyspnea, limb claudication, presyncope/syncope, diabetes mellitus, hypertension or pulmonary tuberculosis. There was history of polysubstance abuse—alcohol, smoking, opioids and cocaine. On examination he was conscious, with incoherent speech. He was febrile, pulse rate was 100/min, regular with no radio femoral delay, BP was 110/60 mm Hg and RR 32/min. There was pallor, mild icterus, pedal edema, jugular venous pressure (JVP) was raised and blackish discoloration of bilateral toes and finger tips was noted. The respiratory system revealed bilateral basal crepitation (right > left). Cardiovascular system was within normal limits with normal S1/S2 and no added sound or murmur was heard. No signs of meningeal irritation were seen. The liver and spleen were not palpable and the bowel sounds were present.

Investigations

***Hematological*:** Hb 7.8 g/dL, TLC—9800/μL with normal differential and adequate platelets. The ESR 48 mm first hour. Coagulogram—PT: 22', PTI: 54%, APTT: 29', fibrinogen: 5.4 g/L, D-dimer test (qualitative)—negative.

Blood Biochemistry and Microbiology*:** S.urea—220 mg%, S.creatinine—5.5 mg%, S.bilirubin— 1.76 mg%, SGOT—557 U/L, SGPT—484 U/L, alkaline phosphatase—213 U/L; total serum proteins/albumin—6.1/3.0 gm, Serum electrolytes: Ca^{2+}—7.9 mg%, K^{+}—6.5 mEq/L, Routine urine examination—within normal limits, Blood/urine cultures sterile, Endotracheal tube aspirate culture grew ***Klebsiella pneumoniae.

***Serology*:** Antinuclear antibody (ANA), antineutrophil cytoplasmic antibody (ANCA), C-reactive protein (CRP)—negative. C3, C4—normal, anti-HCV, HBsAg, anti-HBc, IgM anti-HAV—negative, anticardiolipin antibodies and

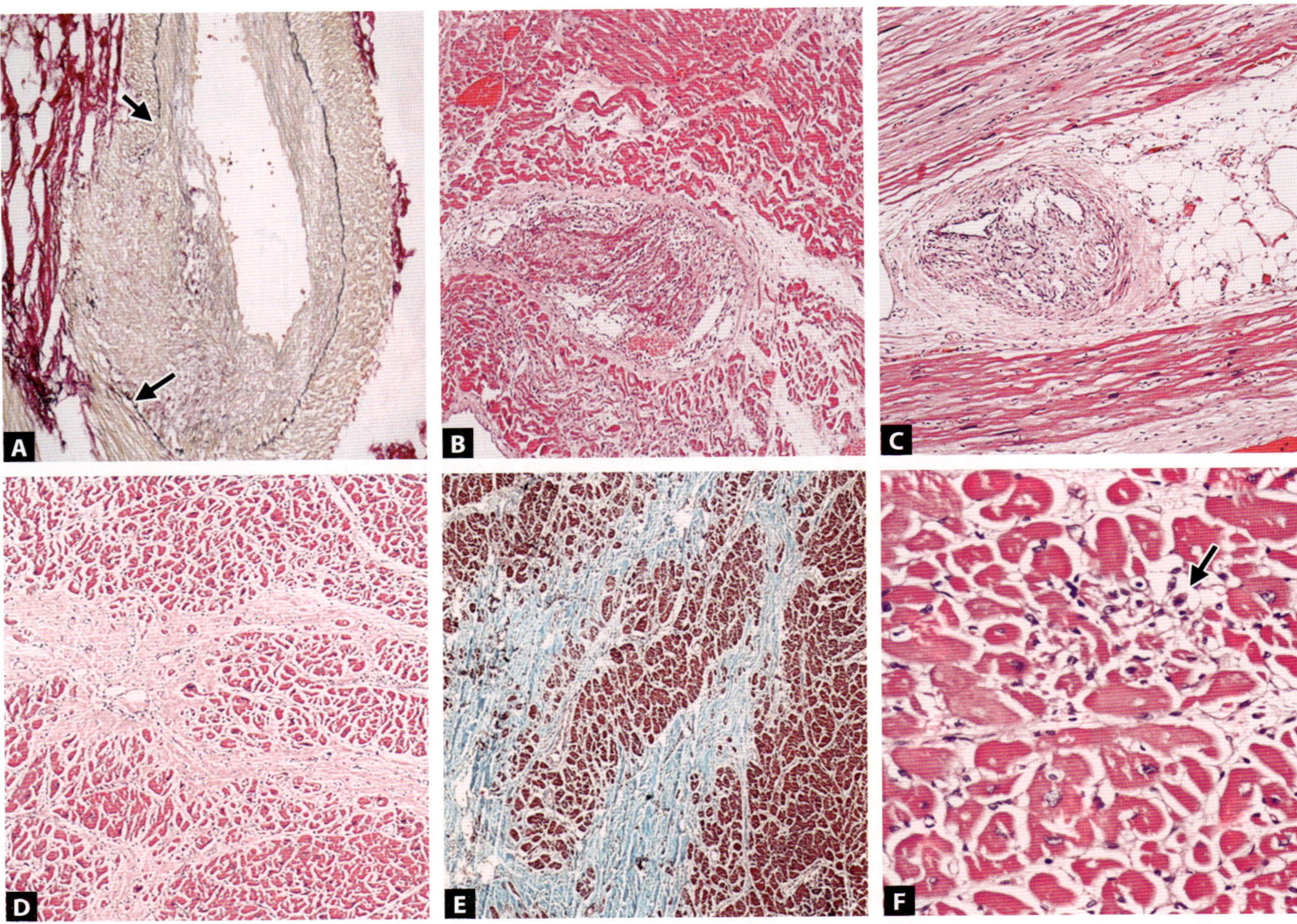

Figs 2A–F: (A) Pericardial artery showing break of the internal elastic lamina (EVG stain, arrows); (B) Myocardial vessel showing fibrin thrombi; (C) Myocardial vessel showing chronic thrombotic vasculopathy; (D and E) Myocardium showing interstitial fibrosis, better highlighted by the Masson trichrome in "E"; (F) Myocardium showing contraction band necrosis with invasion by macrophages (arrow).

can lead to sudden death. Cocaine is responsible for more hospital admissions than any other illicit drug.

Cocaine causes angina and myocardial ischemia due to coronary artery thrombosis or spasm. It leads to increased myocardial oxygen demand as a result of tachycardia or increased arterial pressure, ventricular fibrillation due to the local anesthetic action of cocaine and direct toxicity. Other adverse effects of cocaine include early atherosclerosis, apoptosis of the myocyte, arrhythmias and cardiomyopathy (hypertrophic or dilated). On microscopic examination of the heart at autopsy (in cocaine users) there is focal myocyte necrosis, patchy fibrosis, bland inflammatory infiltrates, myocarditis (could be eosinophilic), cardinal signs of myocardial dysfunction, i.e. the contraction band necrosis, myocyte hypertrophy, interstitial fibrosis, platelet thrombosis of the coronaries, myocardial infarction and features of dilated cardiomyopathy. Myocyte necrosis is a frequent finding, involves single cells interspersed among normal myocytes and is multifocal in nature. The necrotic cells show a hypereosinophilic sarcoplasm, with loss of striations and vacuolization. Tazelaar et al reported a 93% incidence of contraction band necrosis in the myocardium of cocaine-associated deaths in comparison to an incidence of 45% in control deaths due to sedative-hypnotic overdose. They attributed the presence of contraction bands to cocaine-induced catecholamine myocardial damage. Virmani et al noted a 20% incidence of myocarditis in cocaine users. Although the foci of myocarditis were small and usually sparse, these areas of cell death and inflammation may have induced ventricular fibrillation and sudden death. The features described above in cocaine users can be seen with excessive sympathoexcitation, epinephrine, norepinephrine, or isoproterenol

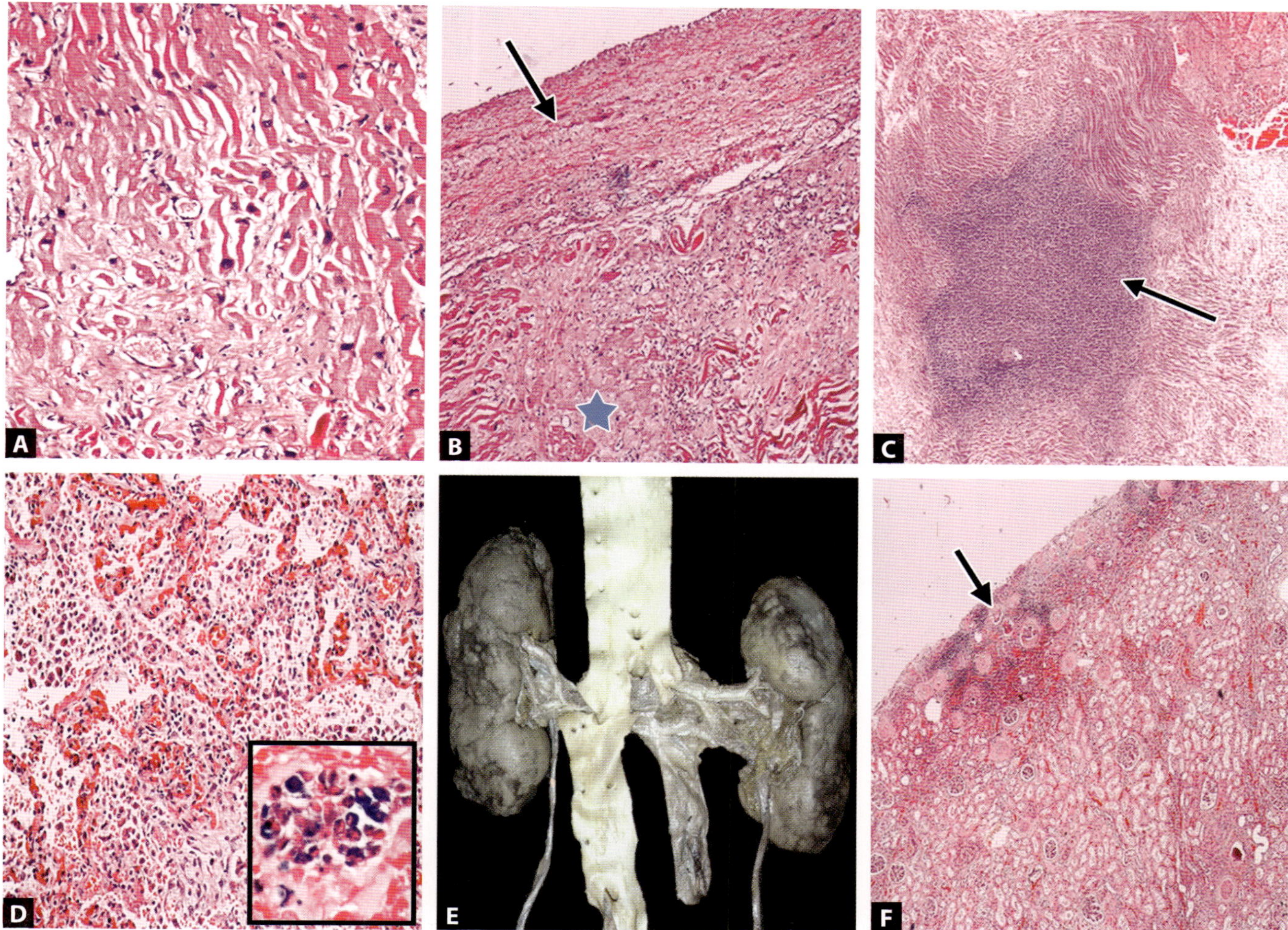

Figs 3A–F: Microphotographs of the myocardium showing (A) Attenuated myocytes; (B) Endocardial sclerosis (arrow) with subendocardial ischemic fibrosis (star); (C) Ring abscess in the myocardium (arrow); (D) Alveolar spaces packed with hemosiderin-laden macrophages—heart failure cells. Inset shows Perls' positivity in the macrophages; (E) Capsular aspect of both kidneys showing coarse scars; (F) Microphotograph of the kidney showing subcapsular infarct (arrow).

administration and adrenal medullary tumors. There is a much higher incidence of myocardial infarction in cocaine users as compared to the normal population. Extracardiac complications of cocaine use include hemorrhagic or thromboembolic brain strokes, seizures, excited delirium, rhabdomyolysis and renal failure.

Lately, there is a lot of talk on cocaine-induced vasculitis. Berman et al described two distinct vasculitic syndromes. The first one is a cocaine-induced midline destructive lesion which mimics granulomatosis with polyangiitis. The second one is ANCA-associated vasculitis, which occurs due to adulteration by levamisole, which has been used previously as a chemotherapeutic and immunomodulator for many conditions. The contamination by levamisole occurs in 70% of cocaine which is in use.

COMMENTARY—INDEX CASE: PM 23445

The index case was a young, polysubstance abuser of alcohol, nicotine, opioids and cocaine. Clinically he was diagnosed to have multiple digital gangrene, autoamputation of both little toes, Raynaud's phenomenon, vasculitis, cardiomyopathy, moderate LV systolic dysfunction, infective endocarditis, deranged renal and liver function tests, coagulopathy and septic shock. Autopsy revealed a florid cocaine-induced, acute/chronic vasculopathy involving the pericardial/myocardial small arteries (leading to cardiomyopathy) and the intralobular/arcuate arteries of the kidneys (leading to renal infarcts and ischemic damage). The main coronary arteries (LAD, LCA, RCA) were however normal. Microscopic sections from the heart revealed changes of cocaine-induced damage,

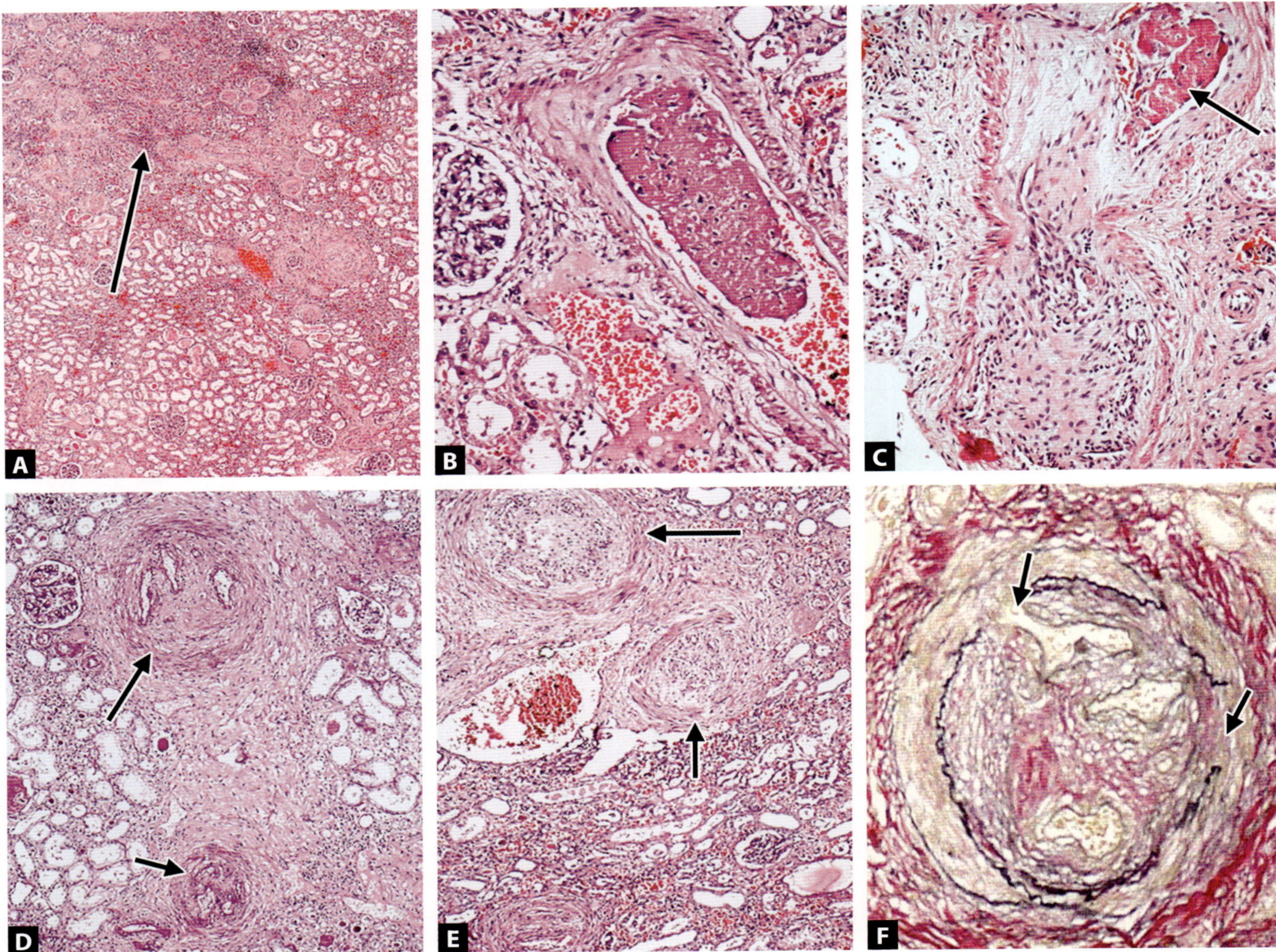

Figs 4A–F: (A) Microphotograph of the kidney showing infarct (arrow); (B) Arcuate artery showing acute fibrin thrombi; (C) Intralobular artery showing chronic thrombotic occlusion with recanalization. One end of the artery (arrow) still shows fresh fibrin; (D and E) Kidney showing chronic thrombotic vasculopathy with arcuate/intralobular arteries (arrows) showing occlusion with recanalization. "D" is Periodic acid–Schiff stain; (F) Elastic van Gieson stain showing break of the internal elastic lamina (arrows).

i.e. focal myocyte necrosis, bland inflammatory infiltrates, myocarditis, cardinal sign of myocardial dysfunction, i.e. the contraction band necrosis, myocyte hypertrophy, interstitial fibrosis, acute/chronic thrombotic vasculopathy of small arteries and dilated cardiomyopathy. The kidneys were small in size with coarse scars, showing florid acute/chronic vasculopathy, leading to infarcts and ischemic damage. The multiple episodes of bluish discoloration, ulceration of toes and fingers and the autoamputation of both little toes are also due to the thrombotic vasculopathy, although the leg vessels could not be sampled due to lack of consent from the patient's relatives. The brain could not be sampled as this was a partial autopsy.

TAKE HOME MESSAGE

- Cocaine use is associated with pathological alterations in the heart which includes focal myocyte necrosis, bland inflammatory infiltrates, myocarditis (could be eosinophilic), cardinal sign of myocardial dysfunction, i.e. the contraction band necrosis, myocyte hypertrophy, interstitial fibrosis, acute/chronic thrombotic vasculopathy, myocardial infarction and dilated cardiomyopathy
- Cocaine can cause thrombotic vasculopathy in any organ as seen in the heart, kidneys and leg vessels in the index case.

SUGGESTED READING

1. Berman M, Paran D, Elkayam O. Cocaine-induced vasculitis. Rambam Maimonides Med J. 2016;7(4):e0036.
2. Cruz AS, Marrero S, Betancourt J, et al. Cocaine-induced vasculitis: have we found a culprit? Case Reports in Rheumatology. 2012;2012.
3. Hogya PT, Wolfson AB. Chronic cocaine abuse associated with dilated cardiomyopathy. Am J Emerg Med. 1990;8:203-4.
4. Karch SB, Billingham ME. The pathology and etiology of cocaine induced heart disease. Arch Pathol Lab Med. 1988;112:225-30.
5. Knuepfer MM. Cardiovascular disorders associated with cocaine use: myths and truths. Pharmacol Ther. 2003;97:181-222.
6. Morcos NC, Fairhurs A, Henry WL. Direct myocardial effects of cocaine. Cardiovasc Res. 1993;27:269-73.
7. Peng SK, French WJ, Pelikan PCD. Direct cocaine cardiotoxicity demonstrated by endomyocardial biopsy. Arch Pathol Lab Med. 1989;113:842-5.
8. Tazelaar HD, Karch SB, Stephens BG, et al. Cocaine and the heart. Hum Pathol. 1987;18:195-9.
9. Virmani R. Cardiovascular complications of chronic cocaine abuse. Adv Bioscience. 1991;80:199-210.
10. Virmani R, Robinowitz M, Smialek JE, et al. Cardiovascular effects of cocaine: an autopsy study of 40 patients. Am Heart J. 1988;115:1068-76.
11. Zimmerman FH, Gustafson GM, Kemp HG. Recurrent MI associated with cocaine abuse in a young man with normal coronary arteries: evidence for coronary artery vasospasm culminating in thrombosis. J Am Coll Cardiol. 1987;9(4):964-8.

CONTRIBUTIONS BY:

1. Dr Shiv Bagga, Additional Professor, Department of Cardiology (Compilation of Clinical Details)
2. Dr Kartar Singh, Ex-Professor and Head, Department of Gastroenterology (Clinician In-Charge)

Post Graduate Institute of Medical Education and Research, Chandigarh, India.

CASE 35

Aftermath of Hypertension in a Middle-aged Male—Intraparenchymal Brain Hemorrhage, Pontine and Thalamic: PM 26485

Nandita Bharadwaj Kakkar

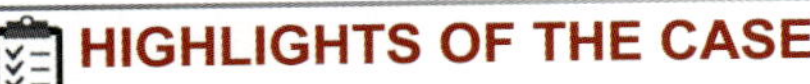

HIGHLIGHTS OF THE CASE

A 50-year-old male patient, a known hypertensive, had acute onset headache with sudden loss of consciousness and slipped from the bicycle that he was riding on. He however did not suffer from any head injury. At admission the blood pressure was 220/110 mm Hg, the pupils were pinpoint initially and later asymmetric and nonreacting. The doll's eye reflex was absent and bilateral plantars were extensor. Noncontrast CT (NCCT) revealed thalamic and brainstem bleed with extension into the fourth ventricle. Autopsy revealed intracranial hemorrhage—pontine and thalamic with intraventricular extension, left ventricular hypertrophy, coronary artery disease with old healed myocardial infarction and arterionephrosclerosis.

Keywords: Hypertension, pontine, thalamic, hemorrhage, coronary artery disease, hyaline arteriolosclerosis, arterionephrosclerosis, autopsy.

CLINICAL DETAILS

Date of Admission: 20.02.2015, Date of Death: 20.02.2015, Duration of Stay: 6 Hours.

A 50-year-old male was referred from an outside facility with sudden onset headache followed by loss of consciousness since 1 day. This episode occurred while he was riding a bicycle, from which he slipped on to soft grass without a head injury. There was no history of similar illness in the past. He was a known hypertensive but the duration or control of the disease, drugs taken and compliance was not known. There was no history of diabetes mellitus, tuberculosis or seizure disorder. On examination there was no fever, pallor, icterus, cyanosis, clubbing, edema or any lymphadenopathy. The blood pressure at admission was 220/110 mm Hg; Pulse rate: 110/min, he was on intermittent positive pressure respiration (IPPR) and the SpO_2 was 98%. CNS examination: E1VTM2, pupils pinpoint at the time of presentation—left 3 mm, right 5 mm, both nonreacting to light after few hours, Doll's eye reflex absent, bilateral plantars were extensor, decreased movement on the right side. Other systems were within normal limits. There was no murmur, air entry present on both sides, no added sounds were present and the abdomen was soft with no organomegaly.

Investigations and Course of Management

Investgations revealed a normal hemogram, normal serum electrolytes, liver/renal function tests and normal coagulogram. The random blood sugar was high, i.e. 456 mg%. NCCT head revealed hyperdensity in the right thalamus and brainstem with extension to right middle cerebellar peduncle, right cerebellar hemisphere and fourth ventricle with mild hydrocephalus.

He was managed with antihypertensives, Lasix and mannitol. The blood sugars were high, so was given insulin infusion and continued on Ambu Bag ventilation. Neurology consultation was taken and advised conservative measures in view of poor Glasgow Coma Scale (GCS) status. He soon went into cardiac arrest from which he could not be revived. Units final clinical diagnosis was—Cerebrovascular accident, intracranial bleed involving brainstem Etiology—hypertension.

AUTOPSY FINDINGS: PM 26485

A complete autopsy was performed. The prosector found that he was moderately built and there were burn scars over the chest and shoulders. All serous cavities were within normal limits. The brain weighed 1,450 g. The leptomeninges over the convexities were dull and the cortical veins were not thrombosed. The left internal carotid artery and posterior communicating artery showed small atheromas. On slicing (Fig 1A) a large hemorrhage occupying 40% area was seen in the dorsal half of the pons measuring 3 × 3.5 cm with extension into the fourth ventricle. The cerebellum was however spared. Apart from this, there was an area of hemorrhage seen in the right thalamus extending into the right hypothalamic area measuring 2 × 1 × 1 cm (Fig 1B). Bilateral tonsillar herniation was noted. On microscopic examination of the pons, the hemorrhage was fresh (Fig 1C). The adjacent brain (Figs 1D and E) showed focal hemorrhage, edema, ischemic neurons and diffuse axonal injury with presence of axonal balls. The heart (Figs 2A–D) was enlarged and weighed 380 g (Fig 2A). On cutting, mild right atrial dilatation was noted. There was left ventricular hypertrophy (2.1 cm), grade 3 atherosclerosis at the root of aorta and a dense fibrotic scar in free wall of left ventricle which was confirmed microscopically. The scarred area (Figs 2E and F) showed replacement fibrosis which was better appreciated in the Masson trichrome stain. The valves were normal. The coronary arteries (Figs 3A–E), i.e. the left anterior descending (LAD), left circumflex (LCX), left marginal (LMA) and the right coronary artery (RCA) were dissected out. They were stiff, gritty to cut and showed

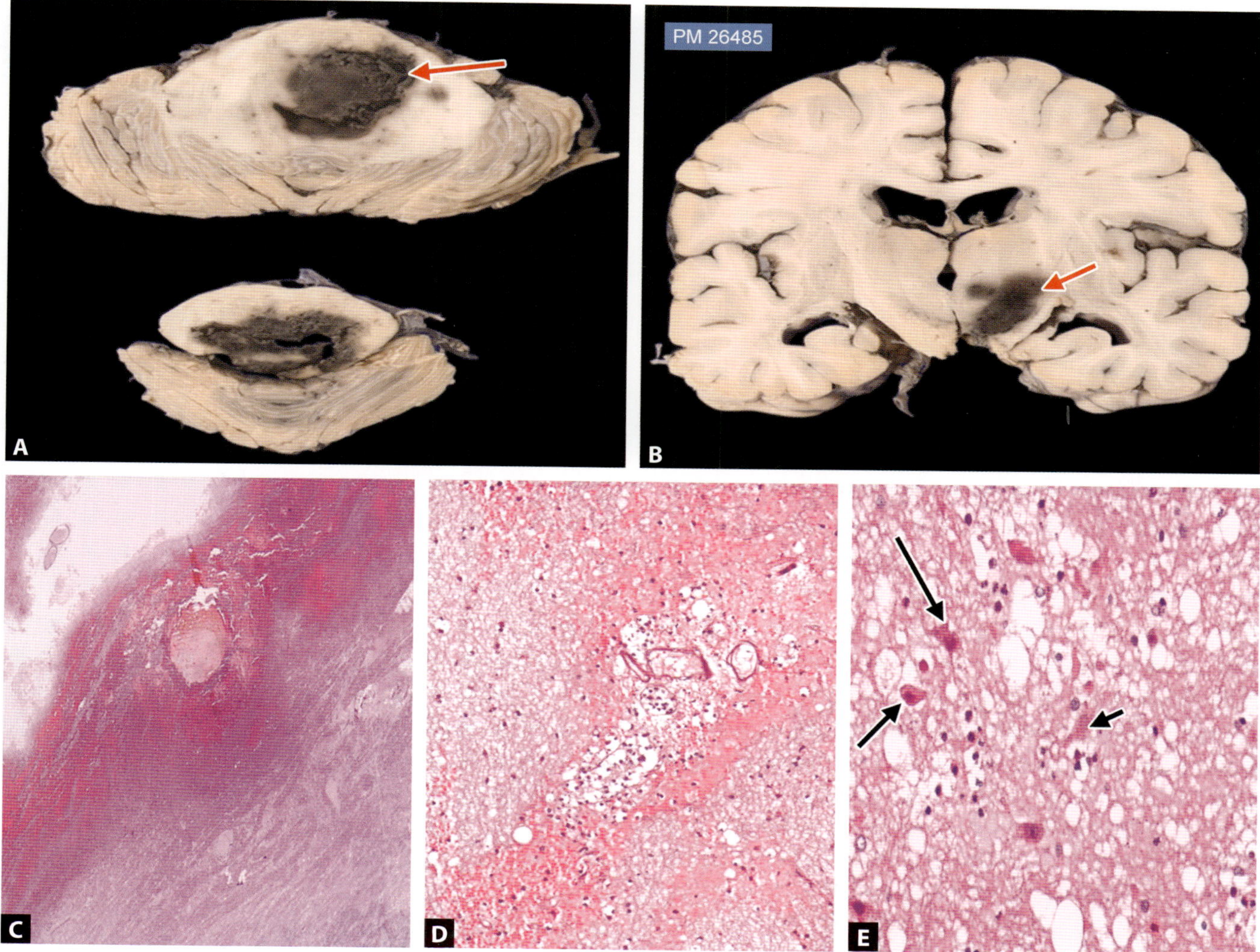

Figs 1A–E: (A) Cut slices of the pons with cerebellum. The pons shows a large area of acute hemorrhage occupying 40% of the area. No hemorrhage is seen in the cerebellum; (B) Coronal slice of the brain showing a large well-circumscribed area of acute hemorrhage in the right thalamus (arrow); (C) Photomicrograph of the pons showing fresh hemorrhage; (D) Adjacent brain parenchyma shows edema and foci of perivascular hemorrhage. (E) Adjacent brain parenchyma shows edema, ischemic neurons (long arrows), and axonal retraction balls (short arrow).

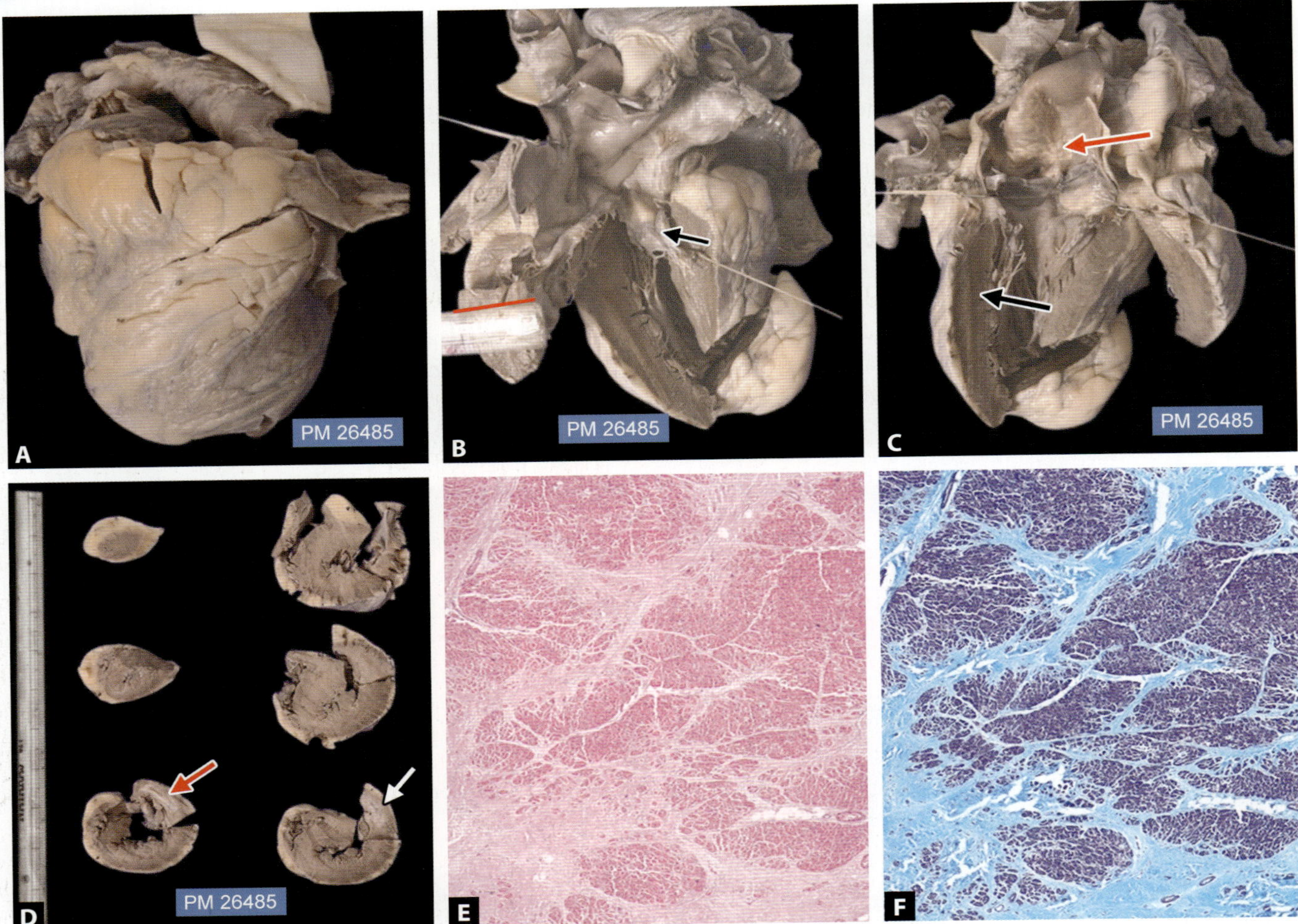

Figs 2A–F: (A) Gross photograph of the enlarged heart; (B) Opened up left inflow tract showing the mitral valve (black arrow) and left ventricular hypertrophy (redline); (C) Left outflow tract shows Grade 3 atherosclerosis at the root of the aorta (arrow) and thick left ventricular wall (black arrow); (D) Coronal slices of the left ventricle showing areas of infarct (arrows) in the free wall of left ventricle; (E) Section from the infarct shows replacement fibrosis (H&E); (F) Masson trichrome stain better highlights the myocardial fibrosis.

varying degrees of atherosclerotic narrowing (40–60%) which was confirmed on microscopy, by the presence of calcified plaques with luminal occlusion. The ***lungs*** revealed diffuse pulmonary edema and patchy hemorrhage. The ***kidneys*** (Fig 4A) were slightly shrunken and the capsular aspect revealed fine scars. The ***abdominal aorta*** was atherosclerotic (grade 3). Microscopic examination of the kidneys (Figs 4B–D) revealed hyaline arteriolosclerosis and focal nodular hyalinosis in afferent and efferent arterioles along with hyperplasia of the juxtaglomerular apparatus (JGA). The intralobular and the arcuate arteries showed changes of hypertension in the form of reduplication of the internal elastic lamina (Fig 4E). Tubular atrophy and interstitial fibrosis was noted (Fig 4F). Overall features in the kidney reflected changes of both hypertension, i.e. arterionephrosclerosis and diabetes. The ***liver*** was pale and greasy and showed centrizonal macrovesicular steatosis. A few ***pancreatic islets*** showed the presence of amyloid (Fig 5A) which was positive for Congo red stain (Fig 5B) and showed green birefringence with polarized light (Fig 5C).

FINAL AUTOPSY DIAGNOSIS: PM 26485

50-Year-Male, a known Hypertensive

- Intraparenchymal, i.e. pontine and thalamic hemorrhage with ventricular extension and bilateral tonsillar herniation

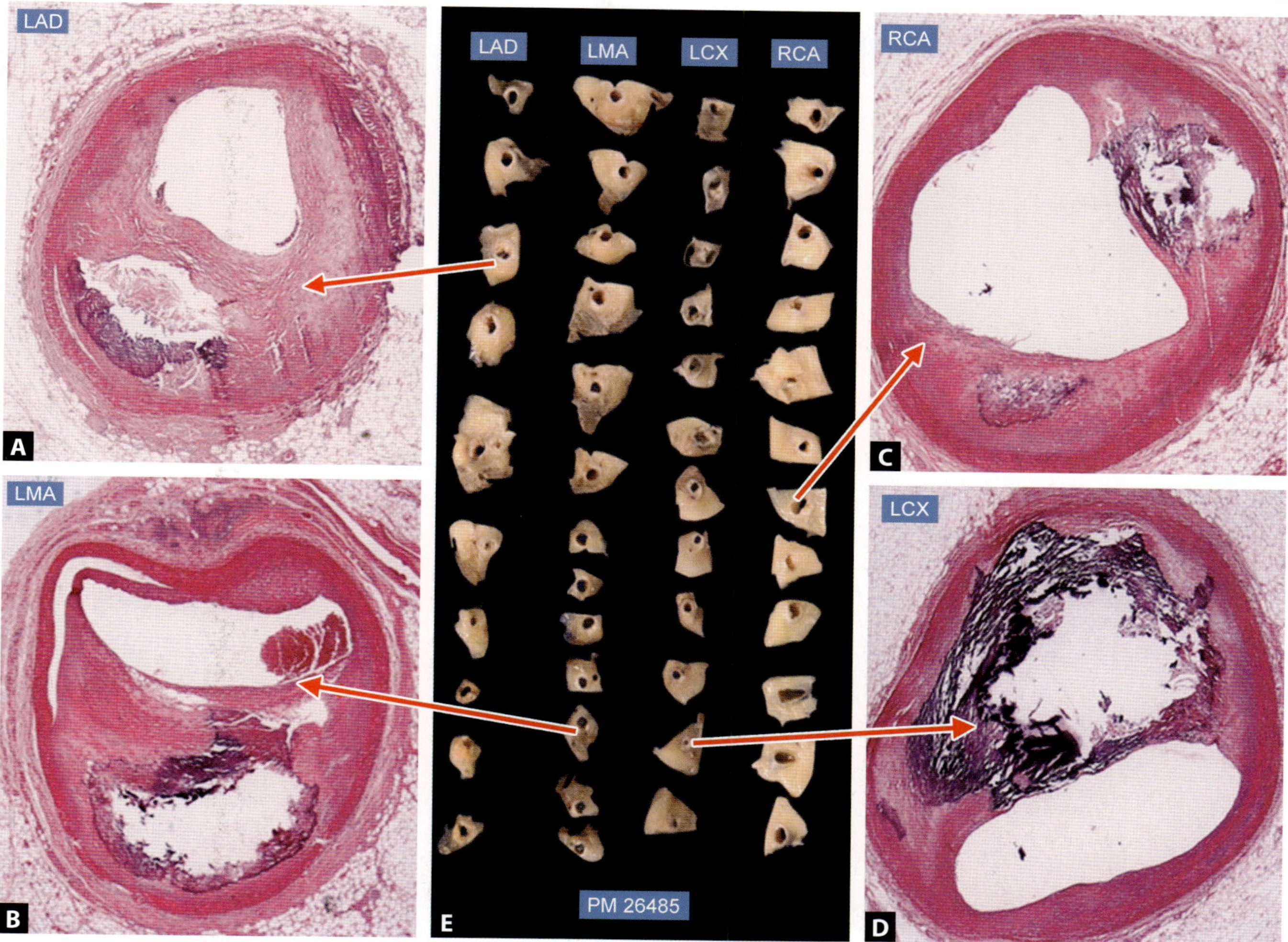

Figs 3A–E: (A–D) Photomicrographs of the left anterior descending (LAD), right coronary (RCA), left marginal (LMA), and left circumflex (LCX) arteries showing varying degrees of atheromatous narrowing with calcification; (E) Gross picture of the serial sections of the LAD, LMA, LCX, and RCA, which are stiff and show atheromatous plaques.

- Left ventricular hypertrophy, triple vessel coronary artery disease and old healed myocardial infarction (LAD territory)
- Grade 3 atherosclerosis
- Pulmonary edema
- Arterionephrosclerosis and diabetes related changes
- Pancreatic islet amyloid
- Macrovesicular steatosis in liver.

HYPERTENSIVE CEREBROVASCULAR DISEASE

Hypertension can lead to a variety of changes in the brain, i.e. lacunar infarcts, slit hemorrhages, hypertensive encephalopathy and intracranial hemorrhage. Traumatic hemorrhage generally occurs in the epidural or subdural space. Hypertensive cerebrovascular disease is the most common cause of intraparenchymal hemorrhage which leads to stroke, a medical emergency with a very poor prognosis and high morbidity/mortality. It occurs due to rupture of a small vessel. Other causes of intraparenchymal nontraumatic hemorrhages are amyloid angiopathy, hemorrhagic transformation, i.e. reperfusion injury of an ischemic infarct, arteriovenous malformation, rupture of an aneurysm, Moyamoya disease, intracranial neoplasm, coagulopathy, cerebral venous thrombosis, sympathomimetic drug abuse, sickle cell disease, eclampsia/postpartum vasculopathy, infection and vasculitis. Intraparenchymal hemorrhage leads to displacement of brain parenchyma, increased intracranial pressure and fatal herniations. Hypertensive intraparenchymal

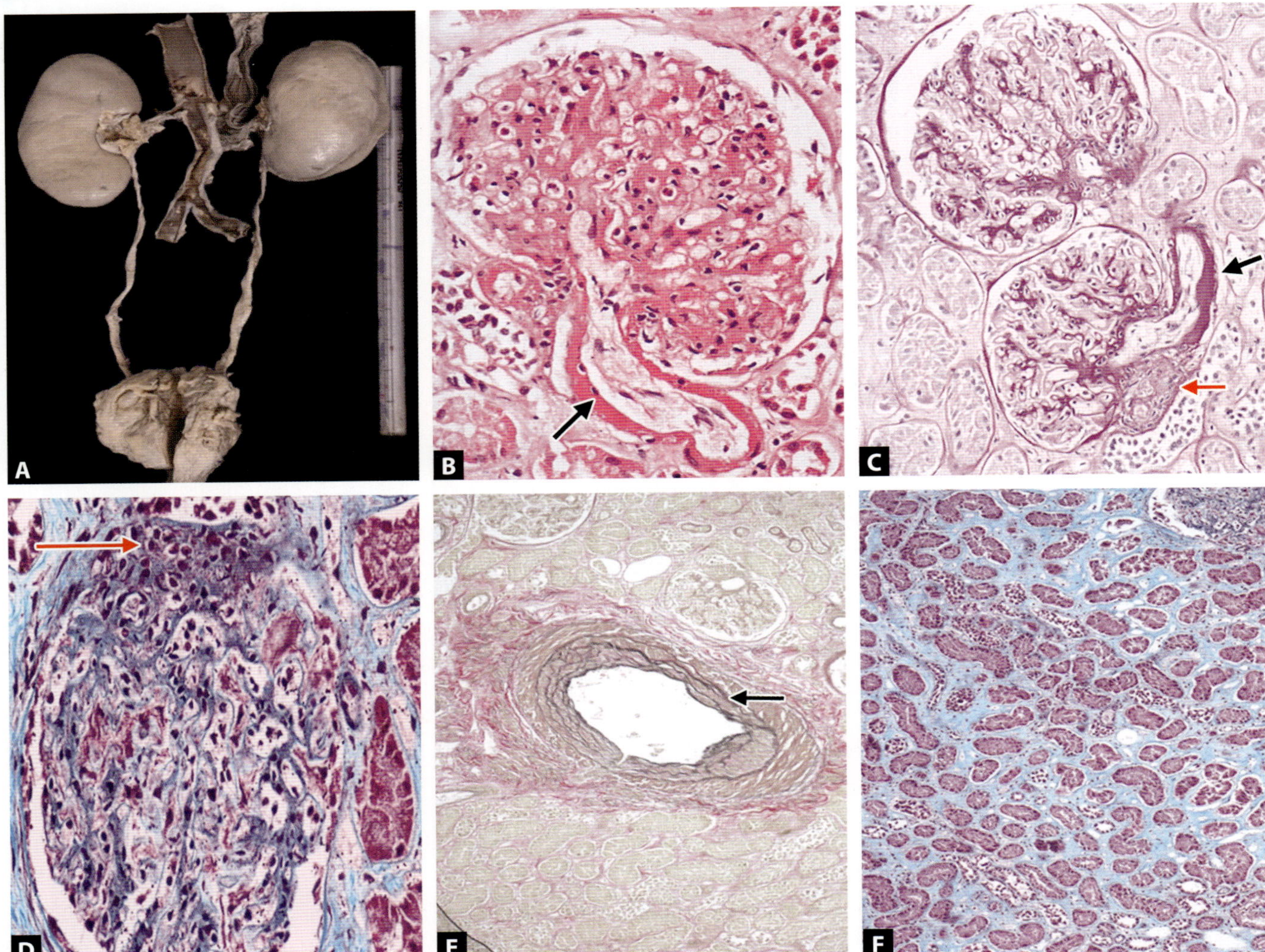

Figs 4A–F: (A) Gross picture of the kidneys which are shrunken with fine scars; (B) Photomicrograph of the kidney shows hyaline arteriolosclerosis (arrow); (C) Periodic acid–Schiff stain shows hyaline/nodular arteriolosclerosis (black arrow), and juxtaglomerular apparatus (JGA) hyperplasia (red arrow); (D) Masson trichrome stain shows JGA hyperplasia (red arrow); (E) Arcuate artery shows reduplication of the internal elastic lamina (Elastic van Gieson stain); (F) Masson trichrome stain shows interstitial fibrosis.

hemorrhages occurs in the putamen (50% cases), thalamus, pons, deep white matter and occasionally in the cerebellum. Hypertension leads to accelerated atherosclerosis in the larger arteries and hyaline arteriolosclerosis in the smaller arteries, which leads to a weakening of the walls and subsequent rupture. Acute hemorrhages show clotted blood with the adjacent brain showing edema and anoxic neuronal damage. Old hemorrhages show cavitation with a rim of brownish-yellow discoloration. Microscopy shows lipid laden macrophages and reactive astrocytosis.

COMMENTARY—INDEX CASE: PM 26485

This is a classical case of intracranial hemorrhage involving the pons and thalamus with ventricular extension, along with bilateral tonsillar herniation. The patient presented with acute onset headache with sudden loss of consciousness and slipped from the bicycle that he was riding, but without head injury. At admission the blood pressure was 220/110 mm Hg, pupils were pinpoint and later became asymmetric and nonreactive to light. The doll's eye reflex was absent and

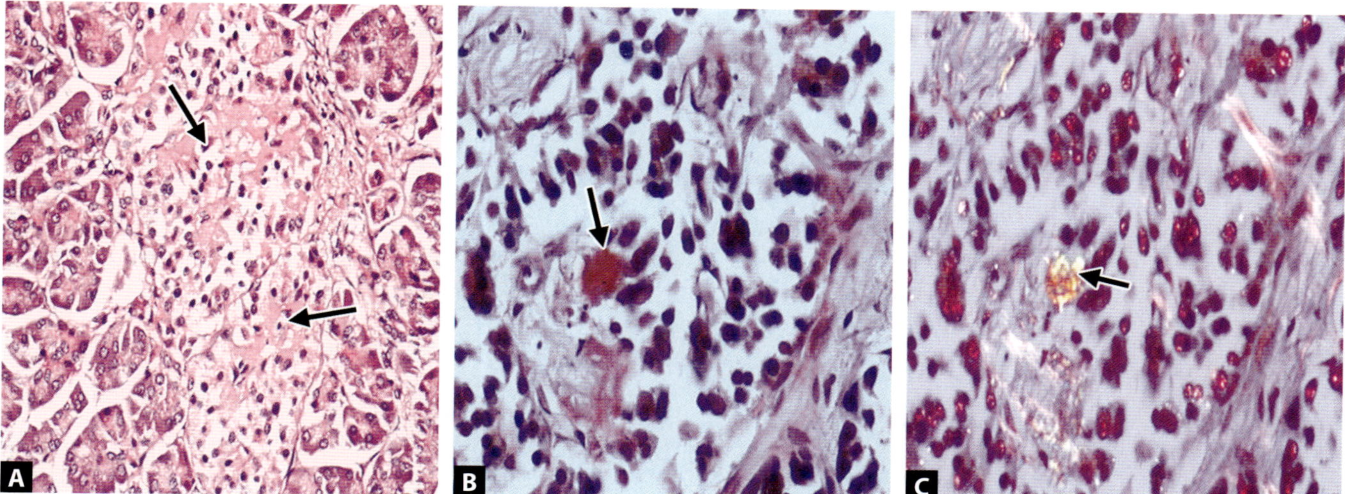

Figs 5A–C: (A) Amyloid deposition in the pancreatic islets (arrows); (B and C) Pancreatic amyloid stains orange with Congo red stain and shows green birefringence with polarized light (arrows).

bilateral plantars were extensor. NCCT revealed thalamic and brainstem bleed.

Autopsy Revealed

- Acute intraparenchymal hemorrhage—pontine and thalamic with ventricular extension along with raised intracranial pressure leading to bilateral tonsillar herniation. The surrounding brain parenchyma showed edema and ischemic neuronal damage and axonal retraction balls. Atheromas were seen in the left internal carotid artery and posterior communicating artery
- The hypertension had its effect on the heart in the form of left ventricular hypertrophy, the wall thickness being 2.1 cm. The hypertension also led to accelerated atherosclerosis, leading to triple vessel coronary artery disease with old healed myocardial infarction in the territory of the left anterior descending artery
- The kidneys were small in size with fine scars. It showed hyaline arteriolosclerosis and JGA hyperplasia, which could be attributed both by hypertension and diabetes. The kidneys showed interstitial fibrosis, tubular atrophy and reduplication of internal elastic lamina and so were consistent with a diagnosis of arterionephrosclerosis
- Although the relatives did not give history of diabetes, the patient's blood sugar levels were high. The pancreatic islets revealed amyloid, positive for Congo red, showing green birefringence with polarized light, which further indicated the presence of diabetes in this patient. The kidneys however did not show any diffuse mesangial sclerosis/nodular lesions, i.e. Kimmelstiel-Wilson disease/fibrin caps/capsular drops. Diabetes along with hypertension had contributed to coronary atherosclerosis.

TAKE HOME MESSAGE

- The most common cause of intraparenchymal brain hemorrhage is hypertension. It has high morbidity and mortality
- Hemorrhage occurs in the putamen (50% cases), thalamus, pons, deep white matter and occasionally in the cerebellum. It leads to raised intracranial pressure and subsequent herniations.

CONTRIBUTIONS BY:

1. Dr Saumya Gupta, Senior Resident, Department of Pathology (In working up the case)
2. Dr R Nithiyanandan, Junior Resident, Department of Internal Medicine (Compilation of Clinical Details)
3. Dr Parimal Agrawal, Senior Resident, Department of Pathology (In working up the case)
4. Dr Navneet Sharma, Professor, Department of Internal Medicine (Clinician In-Charge)
5. Dr BD Radotra, Professor, Department of Histopathology (Consultation)

Post Graduate Institute of Medical Education and Research, Chandigarh, India.

SECTION 6

Systemic Vasculitides Adult and Pediatric Cases

Systemic Vasculitides—Introduction

Nandita Bharadwaj Kakkar

INTRODUCTION AND REVIEW OF CLASSIFICATIONS

Systemic vasculitides[1,2] are defined as inflammation of the walls of the blood vessels with varying degrees of inflammatory infiltrate (predominantly neutrophilic and at times granulomatous), with structural injury like disruption of the elastic lamina with or without fibrinoid necrosis, leading to tissue or end organ injury. The diagnosis of vasculitides is a constant challenge, due to its protean manifestations and overlapping clinical and pathologic features. But, broadly it is divided into either primary or secondary vasculitides. There are conflicting approaches to diagnostic categorizations. Various classification criteria/nomenclature systems have come up over time with their own refinements and controversies. The important development has been the recognition of dominant blood vessel size, distinction between primary and secondary vasculitis and the incorporation of surrogate markers such as antineutrophil cytoplasmic antibodies (ANCA). The American college of Rheumatology (ACR) criteria[3] came up in 1990. The Chapel Hill Consensus Conference (CHCC) nomenclature system was proposed in 1994 and revised in 2012.

American College of Rheumatology Criteria[3]

This came up in 1990 and laid down criteria for the diagnosis of seven types of established vasculitides which included polyarteritis nodosa (PAN), Churg–Strauss syndrome (CSS), Wegener's granulomatosis (WG), hypersensitivity vasculitis, Henoch–Schönlein purpura (HSP), giant cell arteritis and Takayasu arteritis. It was based on the analysis of a pooled data from 48 centers and 807 patients. These criteria were accepted and it led to advancements in the field of vasculitic research. But there were important limitations[4] which soon became a major hindrance to clinical research and practice. The problem pertained to ANCA-associated small vessel vasculitis, as ANCA started to play a pivotal role in their diagnosis and the ACR criteria were laid down before the introduction of ANCA testing. The term "Microscopic polyangiitis" was not used in the ACR classification and this entity came under the common umbrella of PAN. Moreover, the patients did not fit well into the various divisions and there were considerable overlaps, especially amongst the small vessel vasculitides.

Chapel Hill Consensus Conference[5] (CHCC 1994)

This was a major milestone, convened in Chapel Hill, North Carolina in 1994 and is a nomenclature of systemic vasculitides, based on the size of the vessels involved. The large vessels were designated as the aorta and its largest branches which go toward the major body regions, i.e. the extremities (subclavians) and the head and neck (carotids). The medium vessels were designated as the main visceral vessels, i.e. the renal, hepatic, coronary and mesenteric arteries. The small vessels referred to the venules, capillaries, arterioles and the intraparenchymal distal arterial radicals that connect with the arterioles. They further went on to say that some small and large vessel vasculitides can involve medium-sized arteries, but large and medium-sized vessel vasculitides do not involve vessels smaller than arteries. The main drawback was that, although the importance of ANCA was stressed upon, its role was not fully appreciated. Vasculitis secondary to systemic disease was not included. Microscopic polyangiitis and classic PAN became distinct entities, but there were considerable overlaps and these shortcomings in classification, diagnosis and definitions, affected both the practicing clinicians and researchers. Sorensen et al[6] tested the usefulness of this nomenclature and concluded that it failed to act as diagnostic criteria for WG and MPA. The CHCC 1994 nomenclature did well, but as always happens with time and with better understanding of the etiopathogenesis, a change in nomenclature has to come in. Thus a revised and a better system of classification was needed which obviously needed a major international effort.[7]

International Chapel Hill Consensus Conference Nomenclature of Vasculitides 2012[8] (CHCC 2012)

CHCC 2012, took up the task of improving the CHCC 1994 nomenclature, changing the names and definitions as needed and added important categories of vasculitis that were not included in CHCC 1994. It is based (as before) on the predominant size of vessel involved:

- ***Large vessel*** vasculitis involves predominantly the aorta and its major branches and the analogous veins
- ***Medium vessel*** vasculitis involves predominantly the main visceral arteries and veins, e.g. renal artery or veins and their initial branches, i.e. interlobar artery. The latter, i.e. "the initial branches" was the new addition. Small vessels, i.e. the arterioles, capillaries and venules are spared
- ***Small vessel*** vasculitis involves predominantly the intraparenchymal arteries, arterioles, capillaries, venules and veins.

But all three categories can affect any sized artery with certain exceptions, i.e. large and medium vessel vasculitis do not involve the arterioles, capillaries and venules. This is true, because if classic PAN involves vessels smaller than arteries, i.e. the arterioles, capillaries and venules, glomerulonephritis would occur and then the case would be labeled as microscopic polyangiitis. CHCC 2012 replaced the term "Wegener's granulomatosis" with "Granulomatosis with polyangiitis (Wegener's)" and "Churg–Strauss disease" with Eosinophilic granulomatosis with polyangiitis, i.e. "EGPA". Please read the rest of the definitions etc. from the main article.[8]

REFERENCES

1. Parums DV. The arteritides. Invited review. Histopathology. 1994;25:1-20.
2. Weidner N. Introduction. Vasculitis. Semin Diagn Pathol. 2001;18(1):1-2.
3. Hunder GG, Arend WP, Bloch DA, et al. The American College of Rheumatology 1990 criteria for the classification of vasculitis: Introduction. Arthritis Rheumatism. 1990;33: 1065-7.
4. Rao JK, Allen NB, Pincus T. Limitations of the 1990 American College of Rheumatology classification criteria in the diagnosis of vasculitis. Ann Intern Med. 1998;129: 345-52.
5. Jennette JC, Falk RJ, Andrassy K, et al. Nomenclature of systemic vasculitides. Proposal of an international consensus conference. Arthritis Rheum. 1994;37:187-92.
6. Sorensen SF, Slot O, Tvede N, et al. A prospective study of vasculitis patients collected in a five year period: evaluation of the Chapel Hill nomenclature. Ann Rheum Dis. 2000; 59(6):478-82.
7. Watts RA, Suppiah R, Merkel PA, et al. Systemic vasculitis–is it time to reclassify? Rheumatology (Oxford). 2011;50(4): 643-5.
8. Jennette JC, Falk RJ, Bacon PA, e al. 2012 Revised International Chapel Hill Consensus Conference Nomenclature of Vasculitides. Arthritis Rheum. 2013;65(1):1-11.

Small Vessel Vasculitides

Nandita Bharadwaj Kakkar

INTRODUCTION

Small vessel vasculitis (SVV)[1] predominantly affects the small vessels, defined as intraparenchymal arteries, arterioles, capillaries, venules and veins. By definition, all intraparenchymal vessels are small vessels with the exception of the initial penetrating branch, which is a medium artery. Medium arteries and veins may also be affected. Under this broad umbrella, there are two major entities—antineutrophil cytoplasmic antibodies (ANCA)-associated vasculitis (AAV) and immune complex vasculitis. ANCA-associated small vessel systemic vasculitides harbors three entities, i.e. microscopic polyangiitis (MPA), granulomatosis with polyangiitis (GPA) and eosinophilic granulomatosis with polyangiitis (EGPA). They show involvement of various organ systems in different frequencies (Table 1).

Renal involvement is maximally seen in MPA followed by GPA and EGPA. Renal lesions in all three are indistinguishable with some minor differences. They show a pauci-immune necrotizing crescentic glomerulonephritis and present with rapidly progressive glomerulonephritis, hematuria, proteinuria and deranged renal function tests. They show ANCA positivity in 85–95% cases. Granulomatous glomerulonephritis can be seen in all three entities. Pulmonary and upper respiratory tract involvement occurs maximally in GPA and each entity has specific pathology. Likewise cutaneous and neurologic involvement is maximally seen in EGPA.

CLINICAL FEATURES OF ANCA-ASSOCIATED VASCULITIS

Microscopic Polyangiitis

Microscopic polyangiitis had its birth at the Chapel Hill Consensus Conference in 1994,[3] where it was universally accepted and considered a distinct entity. Before this, it was a part of polyarteritis nodosa (PAN). CHCC 2012[1] defines MPA as a necrotizing vasculitis with few or no immune deposits, predominantly affecting the small vessels, i.e. arteries, arterioles, capillaries, venules and veins. Medium arteries and veins may be affected. It shows necrotizing glomerulonephritis and often pulmonary capillaritis. Extravascular inflammation, i.e. inflammation not centered on vessels, including granulomatous inflammation is absent. MPA[4,5] predominantly affects the kidneys, lungs and skin. It has an incidence of 1–8/1000,000 in the US and Europe and 15/1000,000 in the Asian and Arab countries. Any age can be affected, but average age of onset is 50 years. Clinical manifestation[5] is extremely variable. Nephritis, rapidly

Table 1: Frequency[2] of organ involvement in microscopic polyangiitis (MPA), granulomatosis with polyangiitis (GPA) and eosinophilic granulomatosis with polyangiitis (EGPA).

Organ systems	*MPA- %*	*GPA (WG) %*	*EGPA (CSS) %*
Renal	90	80	45
Pulmonary	50	90	70
ENT	35	90	50
Cutaneous	40	40	60
Musculoskeletal	60	60	50
Neurologic	30	50	70
Gastrointestinal	50	50	50

(WG: Wegener's granulomatosis; CSS: Churg–Strauss syndrome)

Source: Jennette JC, Falk RJ. Small vessel vasculitis. NEJM. 1997;337:1512.

progressive renal failure, pulmonary hemorrhage, purpura, ulcers, digital gangrene, mononeuritis multiplex, abdominal pain due to ischemia, gastrointestinal bleed/perforation, myalgias, arthralgias, mouth/genital ulcers, retinal vasculitis, scleritis, blepharitis, conjunctivitis, keratitis, uveitis, fever and weight loss can occur. Rarely heart involvement occurs in the form of pericarditis, myocardial infarction and congestive cardiac failure. Renal involvement occurs in 90%, pulmonary in 50%, musculoskeletal in 60%, gastrointestinal (GI) tract in 50%, cutaneous in 40%, upper respiratory 35% and neurologic in 30% (Table 1). Rapidly progressive or oliguric acute renal failure and pulmonary hemorrhage are the major causes of mortality. Anti-myeloperoxidase, i.e. p-ANCA positivity is seen in 50% cases, anti-PR3 positivity, i.e. c-ANCA in 40% cases and rest are ANCA-negative.

Granulomatosis with Polyangiitis (GPA, Wegener's)

CHCC 2012[1] replaced the term "Wegener's granulomatosis (WG)" with "Granulomatosis with polyangiitis (Wegener's)". GPA[1] shows the triad of necrotizing or granulomatous vasculitis of small (small intraparenchymal arteries, arterioles, capillaries, venules and veins) to medium-sized vessels, necrotizing granulomatous inflammation involving the upper and lower respiratory tract and pauci-immune necrotizing crescentic glomerulonephritis. Vasculitis involving the eye and pulmonary capillaritis with hemorrhage is frequent. Granulomatous and non-granulomatous extravascular inflammation is common. Limited GPA[6] can occur which involves either the lower or upper respiratory tract or the eye, without systemic vasculitis. If such cases are ANCA positive and show clinicopathological changes of GPA, they should be labeled as such. GPA[7] predominantly affects the upper or lower respiratory tract, followed by the kidneys, eyes, musculoskeletal system, skin, GI tract and CNS. Multisystem involvement with inflammation in the upper airways, lung nodules and glomerulonephritis is highly suggestive of GPA. Diagnosis of GPA at an early stage is a challenge, because the initial manifestations are protean and the diagnostic triad is not present.

Clinical manifestations as such are diverse, from lung limited disease to a florid systemic necrotizing vasculitis. Involvement of the nose and paranasal sinuses leads to nasal congestion or obstruction, pain over the dorsum of the nose, epistaxis, rhinorrhea, anosmia and chronic sinusitis which leads to headache, chronic cough, nasal drip, nasal crusting which does not respond to treatment. Ulceration of the nasal mucosa, crusting and septal perforation occurs. Granulomatous inflammation leads to a saddle nose deformity, seen in 10–25% of patients.[8] Upper airway (trachea and larynx) involvement occurs more in females and in patients less than 30 years of age. It leads to ulceration, pseudomembrane formation, granulomas, cobblestone mucosa which causes recurrent cough, hemoptysis, change in voice and breathing difficulty. Subglottic stenosis is a rare complication of systemic GPA. Pulmonary involvement occurs in 90% cases of GPA. Lung nodules, which could be asymptomatic and life-threatening pulmonary hemorrhage occurs. The nodules can be single/multiple or cavitary/solid and mimic lung abscess, tuberculosis and even carcinoma. Pulmonary hemorrhage occurs due to capillaritis and leads to hemoptysis and lung infiltrates. Renal involvement occurs in 80% of cases, as a rapidly progressive renal failure with oliguria, microscopic hematuria, red cell casts and with markedly deranged renal function tests. Renal biopsy reveals a pauci-immune and crescentic necrotizing glomerulonephritis with small vessel vasculitis. Oral cavity is involved in approximately 5% cases leading to strawberry gingivitis associated with pain and bleeding gums, ulcers over the tongue/mucosa and cobblestone appearance of the palate and oroantral fistula. Eyes show necrotizing scleritis, keratitis, orbital pseudotumor, proptosis; skin shows palpable purpura/nodules, ulcers and digital infarcts; and nervous system shows mononeuritis multiplex, distal sensorimotor neuropathy, rarely cranial neuropathies or mass lesions. Unusual manifestations[9] include pituitary involvement leading to diabetes insipidus, prostatic vasculitis and mass lesions in the muscles, breast and anterior mediastinum. In GPA, conventional X-rays show significant pulmonary involvement and computed tomography provides better definitions of the lesions. The best seen radiographic patterns of GPA are multiple nodules, 50% showing cavitation and opacities in the adjacent pulmonary parenchyma.

Several clinical syndromes are recognized in GPA, which can facilitate in making an early diagnosis. These are: (1) Classic GPA,[10] i.e. involving the upper/lower respiratory tract and kidneys, occurs only in 21% of patients. (2) Limited pulmonary or renal GPA which can progress to classic form. (3) Protracted superficial variant of GPA,[11] that involves the nasal and sinus mucosa with chronic inflammation/ulceration, at times for many years. They may also have involvement of trachea, larynx and may progress to classic GPA. (4) Diffuse alveolar hemorrhage,[12,13] requires aggressive treatment and is an unusual variant with a poor prognosis.

Eosinophilic Granulomatosis with Polyangiitis (EGPA, Churg–Strauss)

CHCC 2012[1] replaced the eponym "Churg–Strauss" by "Eosinophilic granulomatosis with polyangiitis". This is the rarest of the major vasculitides. According to the CHCC 2012 definition, EGPA shows eosinophil-rich necrotizing granulomatous inflammation of the respiratory tract, necrotizing vasculitis of predominantly the small to medium-sized vessels, asthma and eosinophilia. In the presence of renal disease, ANCA[14] is positive in more than two-thirds cases and in the absence of renal disease, in one-fourth cases. Limited expression of EGPA, confined to the upper and lower respiratory tract, may occur. Clinical manifestations include constitutional symptoms like fever, weight loss, arthralgias and myalgia. Upper and lower respiratory tract manifestations include allergic rhinitis, sinonasal polyps, asthma, pleural effusion and bronchoalveolar lavage fluid shows eosinophils. Skin is involved in 60% cases and show palpable purpura and maculopapular lesions. Allergic rhinitis is the most common initial manifestation of EGPA, seen in approximately 80% of cases and is generally accompanied by nasal polyposis. Others reported are cutaneous nodules, erythema multiforme, livedo reticularis, bullae, vesicles, ulcers, digital ischemia and panniculitis. Peripheral nerve (most affected are the peroneal and tibial branches of the sciatic, ulnar and median nerves) involvement leads to mononeuritis multiplex with asymmetric motor and or sensory signs. Cardiac involvement[15,16] occurs in 15–50% cases. There may be eosinophilic and or granulomatous infiltration of the myocardium, fibrosis, coronary artery and myocardial small vessel vasculitis leading to ischemic events. Cardiomyopathy, eosinophilic pericardial effusion, conduction defects and supraventricular arrhythmias can occur. Kidneys when involved show a pauci-immune focal segmental glomerulonephritis. Gastrointestinal manifestations include vomiting, diarrhea, eosinophilic granulomatous colitis, abdominal pain and mesenteric artery vasculitis leading to bowel infarction and perforation. Uveitis, episcleritis, retinal vasculitis, thromboembolic events and later in the course of the disease, intracranial hemorrhage and cerebral infarction may occur.

ANTINEUTROPHIL CYTOPLASMIC ANTIBODIES SEROLOGY[10,17,18]

Neutrophils play the key role in causing acute injury, i.e. endothelial damage in ANCA-associated small vessel vasculitis. ANCA targets two main antigens in the cytoplasm which are the neutrophil azurophil granules—proteinase 3 (PR3) and myeloperoxidase (MPO). These are two distinct proteins and differ in structure and function. Both PR3 and MPO are proinflammatory and modulate the inflammatory response, wherein they have synergistic activities. Active untreated pauci-immune crescentic glomerulonephritis shows ANCA positivity in 85–95% cases. Serologic detection of ANCA is a useful diagnostic marker for GPA, MPA, EGPA and renal limited pauci-immune crescentic glomerulonephritis. Active untreated GPA and MPA shows ANCA positivity in 90–95% cases and EGPA is positive in 45% cases. ANCA testing is done by indirect immunofluorescence technique, using alcohol-fixed neutrophils as substrate, which makes use of the distinct biochemical properties of PR3 and MPO. There are two staining patterns, cytoplasmic (c-ANCA) and perinuclear (p-ANCA) seen in patients with pauci-immune crescentic glomerulonephritis and small vessel vasculitis. The most common c-ANCA specificity is for PR3 (PR3ANCA) and the most common p-ANCA specificity is for MPO (MPO-ANCA). In systemic GPA, 85% cases have c-ANCA and less than 10% show p-ANCA positivity. However, p-ANCA positivity is seen in 60–70% patients of systemic MPA and in 30–38% cases of EGPA. ANCA serology is least specific for EGPA, but is seen in 75% cases of EGPA with glomerulonephritis. The strongest ANCA association is seen between PR3–ANCA and GPA. The specificity of ANCA testing in GPA has been reported to be more than 95%. Sensitivity is variable and depends on the phase or type of GPA. In active classic GPA, sensitivity ranges between 90% and 98%. In inactive disease or limited GPA, the sensitivity is much lower (65–70%) and in remission it is less than 35%. A positive ANCA is a surrogate marker and should not be used as a sole criterion for making a diagnosis of small vessel vasculitis. Clinical and biopsy findings are mandatory. Some inflammatory disorders like ulcerative colitis, sclerosing cholangitis, rheumatoid arthritis, autoimmune hepatitis and Felty syndrome show p-ANCA positivity, which however does not show specificity for MPO. This is considered a false positive result as far as the small vessel vasculitis is concerned, but is a true positive result for inflammatory bowel disease. c-ANCA positivity can be seen in tuberculosis.[19] Because of these discrepancies, it is recommended[20] that both indirect immunofluorescence assay for c-ANCA/p-ANCA and ELISA for PR3–ANCA/MPO–ANCA should be performed. ANCA, although far more frequently seen in pauci-immune crescentic necrotizing small vessel vasculitides, is also seen in 30–40% cases of anti-GBM disease. This is not a cross reaction, but the result of two different antibodies.

PATHOLOGY OF ANCA-ASSOCIATED SMALL VESSEL VASCULITIS—MPA, GPA, EGPA

Renal Pathology in ANCA-associated Vasculitis[21]

The renal lesions in MPA, GPA and EGPA are indistinguishable. The hallmark terminology used is ANCA positive/negative, pauci-immune, necrotizing and crescentic glomerulonephritis. Extraglomerular vasculitis is however

- Parenchymal necrosis—microabscesses and geographic necrosis
- Granulomatous inflammation accompanied by mixed inflammatory infiltrate—microabscess surrounded by granulomatous inflammation, palisading histiocytes, scattered giant cells, poorly formed granulomas and rarely sarcoid like granulomas.

The ***minor pathologic manifestations*** of GPA included:

- Parenchymal—nodular interstitial fibrosis, endogenous lipoid pneumonia, pulmonary hemorrhage, organizing intraluminal fibrosis, lymphoid aggregates, tissue eosinophils, xanthogranulomatous lesions and alveolar macrophage accumulation
- Bronchial/bronchiolar—chronic bronchiolitis, acute bronchiolitis/bronchopneumonia, bronchiolitis obliterans or a BOOP-like picture, bronchocentric granulomatosis, follicular bronchiolitis and bronchial stenosis.

Travis et al found vasculitis in 96% of the surgical specimens, mostly within the nodules and arteries/veins (size <5 mm)/capillaries were affected. On histopathology the vasculitic changes could vary from chronic to acute inflammation with fibrinoid necrosis and necrotizing/non-necrotizing granulomatous inflammation. Cicatricial vascular changes were medial thickening along with intimal proliferation and could be the effect of treatment. Capillaritis, i.e. neutrophilic infiltration of the alveolar septa was seen in 43% of cases, most often in the presence of pulmonary hemorrhage. Travis et al concluded that arteritis and venulitis may be absent in 10% of open lung biopsies and especially those showing predominantly nodular interstitial fibrosis or diffuse pulmonary hemorrhage associated with capillaritis. Parenchymal changes are characteristic and show geographic areas of necrosis with basophilic material at the center, having a serpentine border, lined by palisading histiocytes and multinucleated giant cells with the periphery showing dense mixed inflammation. There could be neutrophilic microabscesses (represent foci of early parenchymal necrosis) alone or surrounded by granulomatous inflammation. Poorly formed granulomas composed of loose clusters of histiocytes, scattered giant cells and palisading histiocytes arranged in a cartwheel pattern can be seen. ***Minor histopathologic features*** of GPA as listed above, are usually inconspicuous and seen at the periphery of typical nodules of GPA that show vasculitis, necrosis and granulomas. Awareness about these nonspecific changes is very important, as at times (18%) they may predominate the picture in open lung biopsies. Thus, the absence of the major diagnostic features of GPA does not exclude its diagnosis on a lung biopsy. Amongst these, dense interstitial fibrosis and diffuse pulmonary hemorrhage are most common. Diffuse pulmonary hemorrhage is now considered a well-known and life-threatening complication of GPA. Travis et al in their series of 34 cases of diffuse pulmonary hemorrhage confirmed on open lung biopsies, found GPA or probable GPA in 33% of their cases. In most of these cases of GPA, pulmonary hemorrhage was a minor associated finding and major histologic features were also present. In cases where the hemorrhage was extensive, capillaritis was a frequent finding and in a few of these cases, no typical features of GPA could be identified. Few studies have however shown that lung biopsies showing only hemorrhage and capillaritis may either precede or follow the classic pathologic features of GPA. Interstitial fibrosis can be seen as loose intraluminal fibrosis indicating organizing pneumonia or as dense fibrosis which can be localized or diffuse. Cases reported as BOOP-like variant of GPA are those where organizing pneumonia is a prominent feature. GPA has been classified as angiocentric rather than bronchocentric. In about 1% cases of GPA, inflammation is centered on bronchi and bronchioles. Thus, it is very important to keep in mind while interpreting lung biopsies with atypical histologic features, limited GPA or a solitary pulmonary lesion, that GPA is a clinicopathologic diagnosis. So, a diagnosis of GPA is made after clinical and laboratory correlation and exclusion of infections with special stains and cultures.

Differential Diagnosis of GPA

GPA has many mimics and the situation is further complicated by ANCA positivity in a number of other conditions:

- ***Infections***: Tuberculosis is the most important differential diagnosis of GPA. Tuberculosis can at times show c-ANCA positivity. Nonreactive tuberculosis can produce geographic areas of necrosis with surrounding giant cells and epithelioid cells. Small vessel vasculitis may be seen in uninvolved areas of lung and other organs. Thus the picture mimics GPA. The only way to distinguish is to demonstrate acid-fast bacilli (AFB) positivity. An autopsy case of c-ANCA positive nonreactive tuberculosis with pulmonary and mesenteric vasculitis mimicking GPA is published in this book (Case 48). In this case, the Ziehl–Neelsen stain for AFB was strongly positive and it clinched the diagnosis. Fungal infections can be diagnosed on hematoxylin and eosin stained sections and special stains can demonstrate the fungal profiles
- *Other ANCA positive small vessel vasculitis*:
    - *Microscopic polyangiitis* mimics GPA. Renal lesions are indistinguishable in both. The only way to

diagnosis is, if typical lesions of GPA are seen in upper and lower respiratory tract. The most common lung biopsy finding in MPA is pulmonary hemorrhage with capillaritis. As discussed above, this can be seen in a few cases of suspected GPA without the major histologic features. But at autopsy, where both the lungs are there for evaluation and after multiple sections have been studied, if only pulmonary hemorrhage with capillaritis is noted, a diagnosis of MPA rather than GPA should be made (our experience)
- *EGPA or Churg–Strauss* can mimic GPA. The renal lesions are the same, but there is a history of asthma and peripheral eosinophilia, apart from the systemic vasculitis. Striking tissue eosinophilia in lung biopsy raises the possibility of EGPA and fungal/parasitic infections.

- *Necrotizing sarcoid granulomatosis (NSG)* or nodular sarcoid is characterized by confluent granulomatous nodules of sarcoid (nodular sarcoid) with prominent necrosis. The large areas of coalescent, sarcoid type granulomas seen in NSG are virtually absent in GPA. Granulomatous vasculitis in NSG is often more exuberant than in GPA. ANCA is negative and they have a more indolent clinical course
- *Diffuse pulmonary hemorrhage syndrome:* GPA may be associated with alveolar hemorrhage that is indistinguishable from other causes of diffuse alveolar hemorrhage such as collagen vascular disorder [systemic lupus erythematosus (SLE)], Goodpasture syndrome, MPA and others
- *Lymphomatoid granulomatosis (LYG):* This is a T-cell rich B cell lymphoma, is EBV related and shows prominent vascular infiltration. It consists of vasocentric and vasodestructive infiltrate, composed of a polymorphous population of atypical lymphoid cells in an inflammatory background of T lymphocytes. LYG may form nodules with central necrosis. It involves the lung, kidney, skin and upper respiratory tract. Distinction between the two conditions is aided by the immunophenotyping of the lymphoid infiltrates. Cytologic atypia and paucity of granulomatous necrosis are typical of LYG.
- *Classic PAN*: Does not involve arterioles, venules and capillaries but affects small and medium-sized arteries. It shows lesions of varying age with fibrinoid necrosis in acute lesions and involvement of abdominal viscera along with GIT is typical. It does not show any granulomatous inflammation, glomerulonephritis and lung involvement.

Lung Pathology in Microscopic Polyangiitis

Lung is affected in 50% cases of MPA. Chest CT scans show diffuse bilateral opacities with absence of nodules in the upper and lower lobes. At times ground glass opacities, consolidation and dense small nodules can be seen. The most common lung finding is pulmonary hemorrhage and neutrophilic capillaritis. The alveolar septa are thickened with neutrophils and nuclear debris and at times they spill into the surrounding alveolar spaces, mimicking acute pneumonia. Healing leads to a picture of organizing pneumonia. Hemosiderin may be seen with chronic hemorrhage. At times, hyaline membranes may be seen, mimicking diffuse alveolar damage. Differential diagnosis includes GPA and other causes of diffuse pulmonary hemorrhage. GPA is ruled out by lack of necrosis, granulomatous inflammation and vasculitis in the small arteries and venules. Capillaritis can however occur in both entities. Goodpasture syndrome and SLE show the typical immune profile.

Lung Pathology in Churg–Strauss Syndrome or EGPA

The lungs are involved in 70% of cases. The major pathologic features of EGPA are necrotizing vasculitis affecting the small to medium-sized arteries and veins, eosinophilic tissue infiltration and extravascular granulomas. On microscopic examination, there is asthmatic bronchitis wherein the submucosal glands and smooth muscle of the airways show hypertrophy, subepithelial basement membrane is thickened, edema is present and eosinophilic inflammation of the wall along with mucous plugs are seen. Apart from this, eosinophilic pneumonia with organizing intraluminal fibrosis, vasculitis and extravascular granulomas are seen. The extravascular granulomas show a central area of necrotic eosinophils with palisading histiocytes and multinucleated giant cells. These granulomas can be fibrotic or calcified. Vasculitis affects predominantly the small-sized muscular arteries or veins which show transmural eosinophil rich inflammation with epithelioid cells, giant cells and may also show fibrinoid necrosis. Allergic granulomas, occasionally, can be centered on the vessels. The vasculitis can subsequently heal leading to cicatricial changes. The differential diagnosis includes GPA, allergic bronchopulmonary fungal disease, parasitic infection, drug-induced vasculitis, eosinophilic pneumonia and necrotizing sarcoid.

REFERENCES

1. Jennette JC, Falk RJ, Bacon PA, et al. 2012 Revised International Chapel Hill Consensus Conference Nomenclature of Vasculitides. Arthritis Rheum. 2013;65(1):1-11.

2. Jennette JC, Falk RJ. Small vessel vasculitis. NEJM. 1997; 337:1512-23.
3. Jennette JC, Falk RJ, Andrassy K, et al. Nomenclature of systemic vasculitides. Proposal of an international consensus conference. Arthritis Rheum. 1994;37:187-92.
4. Savage CO, Winearls CG, Evans DJ, et al. Microscopic polyarteritis: Presentation, pathology and prognosis. QJM. 1985;56:467-83.
5. Guillevin L, Durand-Gasselin B, Cevallos R, et al. Microscopic polyangiitis: clinical and laboratory findings in eighty-five patients. Arthritis Rheum. 1999;42:421-30.
6. Holle JU, Gross WL, Holl-Ulrich, et al. Prospective long term follow up of patients with localized Wegener's granulomatosis: does it occur as persistent disease stage? Ann Rheum Dis. 2010;69:1934-9.
7. Eunhee S Yi, Thomas V Colby. Wegener's granulomatosis. Semin Diagn Pathol. 2001;18(1):34-46.
8. Martinez Del Pero M, Walsh M, Luqmani R, et al. Long term damage to the ENT system in Wegener's granulomatosis. Eur Arch Otorhinolaryngol. 2011;268:733-9.
9. Sharma A, Gopalakrishan D, Nada R, et al. Uncommon presentations of primary systemic necrotizing vasculitides: the Great Masquerades. Int J Rheum Dis. 2014;17(5):562-72.
10. DeRemee RA. ANCA-associated diseases: A pulmonologist's perspective. Am J Kidney Dis. 1991;28:180-5.
11. Fienberg R. The protracted superficial phenomenon in pathergic Wegeners granulomatosis. Hum Pathol. 1981;12: 112-25.
12. Travis WD, Colby TV, Lommbard C, et al. A clinicopathologic study of 34 cases of diffuse pulmonary hemorrhage with lung biopsy confirmation. Am J Surg Pathol. 1996;14:112-25.
13. Myers JL, Katzenstein ALA. Wegener's granulomatosis presenting massive pulmonary hemorrhage and capillaritis. Am J Surg Pathol. 1987;11:895-8.
14. Sinico RA, Di Toma L, Maggiore U, et al. Renal involvement in Churg–Strauss syndrome. Am J Kid Dis. 2006;47:770-9.
15. Lanham JG, Cooke S, Davies J, et al. Endomyocardial complications of Churg–Strauss syndrome. Postgrad Med J. 1985;61:341-4.
16. Marmursztejn J, Guillevin L, Trebossen R, et al. Churg-Strauss syndrome cardiac involvement evaluated by cardiac MRI and PET: a prospective study on 20 patients. Rheumatology (oxford). 2013;52:642-50.
17. Savige J, Davies D, Falk RJ, et al. Antineutrophil cytoplasmic antibodies (ANCA) and associated disease. Kidney Int. 2000;57:846-62.
18. Harper L, Savage COS. Pathogenesis of ANCA-associated systemic vasculitis. J Pathol. 2000;190:349-59.
19. Vasishta RK, Kakkar N, BR Thapa. c-ANCA positive non-reactive tuberculosis with mesenteric and pulmonary vasculitis. Bull PGI. 1995;29(2):82-90.
20. Savige J, Gillis D, Beason E, et al. International consensus statement on testing and reporting of ANCA. Am J Clin Pathol. 1999;111:507-13.
21. Jennette JC, Thomas DB. Pauci-immune and ANCA mediated crescentic glomerulonephritis and vasculitis. In: Jennette JC, Olson JL, Silva FG, D' Agati VD (Eds). Heptinstall's Pathology of the kidney, 7th edition. Philadelphia: Lippincott Williams and Wilkins; 2015. pp. 685-713.
22. Yoshikawa Y, Watanabe T. Granulomatous glomerulonephritis in Wegeners granulomatosis. Virchows Arch [A]. 1984;402: 361.
23. D'Agatti V, Chander P, Nash M, et al. Idiopathic microscopic polyarteritis nodosa: Ultrastructural observations on the renal vascular and glomerular lesions. Am J Kidney Dis. 1986;7:95.
24. Bhathena DB, Migdal SD, Julian BA, et al. Morphologic and immunohistochemical observations in granulomatous glomerulonephritis. Am J Pathol. 1987;126:581.
25. Travis WD. Vasculitis. In: Tomashefski JF, JR, Cagle PT, Farver CF, Fraire AE (Eds). Dail and Hammer's Pulmonary Pathology, Volume 1: Nonneoplastic Lung Disease. New York: Springer; 2008. pp. 1088-1137.
26. Travis WD, Hoffman GS, Leavitt RY, et al. Surgical pathology of the lung in Wegener's granulomatosis. Review of 87 open lung biopsies from 67 patients. Am J Surg Pathol. 1991;15:315-33.
27. Travis WD, Carpenter HC, Lie JT. Diffuse pulmonary hemorrhage: An uncommon presentation of Wegeners granulomatosis. Am J Surg Pathol. 1987;11:701-8.
28. Travis WD, Colby TV, Lombard C, et al. A clinicopathologic study of 34 cases of diffuse pulmonary hemorrhage with lung biopsy confirmation. Am J Surg Pathol. 1990;14:112-25.

CASE 36

Renal Limited Microscopic Polyangiitis: PM 13127

Nandita Bharadwaj Kakkar

 HIGHLIGHTS OF THE CASE

A 70 years old male was admitted with swelling of large/small joints, hematuria, hemoptysis, anasarca, dyspnea, orthopnea, hypertension, oliguria followed by anuria and acute renal failure. A clinical diagnosis of rapidly progressive glomerulonephritis? Polyarteritis nodosa? Henoch-Schonlein purpura was rendered. Autopsy revealed renal limited microscopic polyangiitis with pulmonary hemorrhage. Postmortem serum sample was positive for perinuclear antineutrophil cytoplasmic antibody (pANCA).

Keywords: Small vessel vasculitis, microscopic polyangiitis, renal limited, pauci-immune, crescentic, necrotizing, focal glomerulonephritis and autopsy.

 CLINICAL DETAILS

Date of Admission: 09.10.92, Date of Death: 10.10.92, Duration of Hospital Stay: One Day

A 70 years old male was admitted to the indoor services of PGIMER Chandigarh. A month and a half prior to this, he developed swelling of large and small joints. Fifteen-days later he developed smoky urine and hemoptysis for which he was admitted at the local Medical College. Soon after that he developed, anasarca, dyspnea, oliguria followed by anuria for a day with rise in blood urea and serum creatinine. He was then referred to our institute for further management. There was history of decreased appetite, cough with expectoration and progressive breathlessness. He was an alcoholic, a smoker, was nonhypertensive and a nondiabetic. On ***examination*** he was obese, temp: 37.2°C, pulse: 96/min, BP: 150/90 mm Hg. There was anasarca, orthopnea, raised JVP and pallor. The liver was palpable 4 cm below the right costal margin. CVS: WNL, CNS: Drowsy, flaps +, no localizing sign, Chest: Bilateral crepts noted.

Investigations and Course of Management

Investigations: Hb: 6.75 g/dL, TLC: 4,800/uL, P65, L32, M02, E01, platelets normal, blood urea: 110 mg%, serum creatinine: 5.2 mg%, random blood sugar: 126 mg%, K+ 6.4 mEq/L, Rheumatoid factor/antistreptolysin O/C-reactive protein/HBsAg: Negative, 24-hour urinary protein: 800 mg/day, Routine urine –full of RBC's.

Patient had hyperkalemia, fluid overload, metabolic acidosis, anuria and was taken up for urgent peritoneal dialysis. He received 2-units of blood, during the dialysis. A day after admission he had copious frothy expectoration followed by cardiopulmonary arrest. Unit clinical diagnosis was – Rapidly progressive glomerulonephritis ? polyarteritis nodosa ? Henoch-Schönlein purpura.

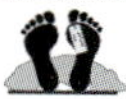 AUTOPSY FINDINGS: PM 13127

A complete autopsy was performed on this 70-years old male. The serous cavities were within normal limits. The kidneys (Figs 1A and B) weighed 260 g and were normal in size. Capsular surface showed blotchy congestion and petechial hemorrhages. Microscopy (Figs 1C–F and 2A) revealed a focal segmental/diffuse necrotizing glomerulonephritis. An occasional crescent was noted. Florid acute vasculitis with fibrinoid necrosis and transmural inflammation was seen, involving the arterioles, interlobular and arcuate arteries (Figs 2B, C and E). A few vessels showed break of internal elastic lamina (Fig 2D). No granulomatous glomerulonephritis or granulomatous arteritis was noted. Interstitial inflammation, fibrosis, RBC casts, tubular destruction and atrophy were noted. Immunofluorescence: IgG – no linear staining, IgA:

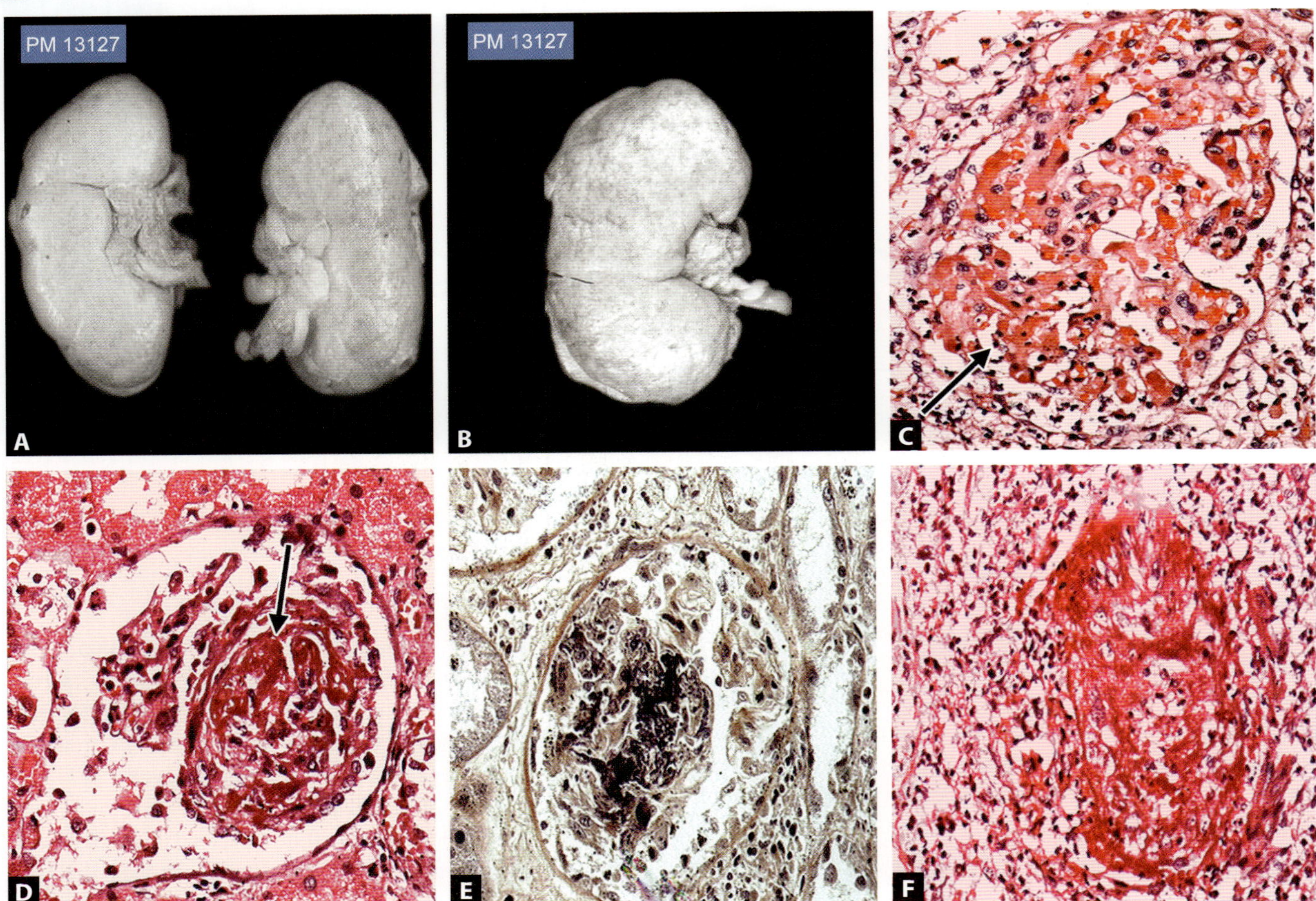

Figs 1A to F: (A and B) Capsular aspect of the kidneys showing blotchy congestion. No infarct is noted; (C and D) Glomerulus showing segmental necrotizing lesions (arrows) with polymorphs, nuclear debris and fibrin; (E) Phosphotungstic Acid-Hematoxylin (PTAH) stains the fibrin black in the glomerulus; (F) Acute glomerulitis wherein the glomerulus is destroyed by acute inflammation and replaced by fibrin.

Traces in glomeruli and casts, IgM - negative, C3+ in few casts, fibrinogen +ve in the crescents. Overall features were those of a pauci-immune, necrotizing glomerulonephritis with florid extraglomerular acute vasculitis of the arterioles, interlobular and arcuate (occasional) arteries consistent with a diagnosis of a small vessel vasculitis. Postmortem sample was positive for pANCA. The lungs (Figs 3A and B) weighed 1,250 g and were subcrepitant with areas of consolidation. Microscopic examination (Fig 3C) revealed alveolar hemorrhage, bronchopneumonia and pleuritis. No vasculitis, capillaritis, necrosis or any granulomatous inflammation was noted. Multiple sections from the tracheobronchial tree were studied, which were normal. The heart weighed 380 g, left ventricular hypertrophy was noted and all the three main coronaries (LAD, LCA and RCA) revealed approximately 50% atherosclerotic narrowing. Aorta showed grade IV atherosclerosis. No vasculitis was noted in any organ, i.e. the lungs, heart, liver, spleen, skin, GI tract, mesentery, testis, pancreas, adrenals and brain. The vasculitis (small vessel) was limited to the kidneys only. The lungs were meticulously sampled and it did not show any necrosis, granulomatous inflammation or capillaritis. There was no tissue eosinophilia, history of asthma or peripheral blood eosinophilia, hence eosinophilic granulomatosis with polyangiitis, i.e. Churg-Strauss is negated. Thus, this case fits into a renal limited form of microscopic polyangiitis.

FINAL AUTOPSY DIAGNOSIS: PM 13127

70 Years Male

- Renal limited Microscopic Polyangiitis. Postmortem sample positive for pANCA

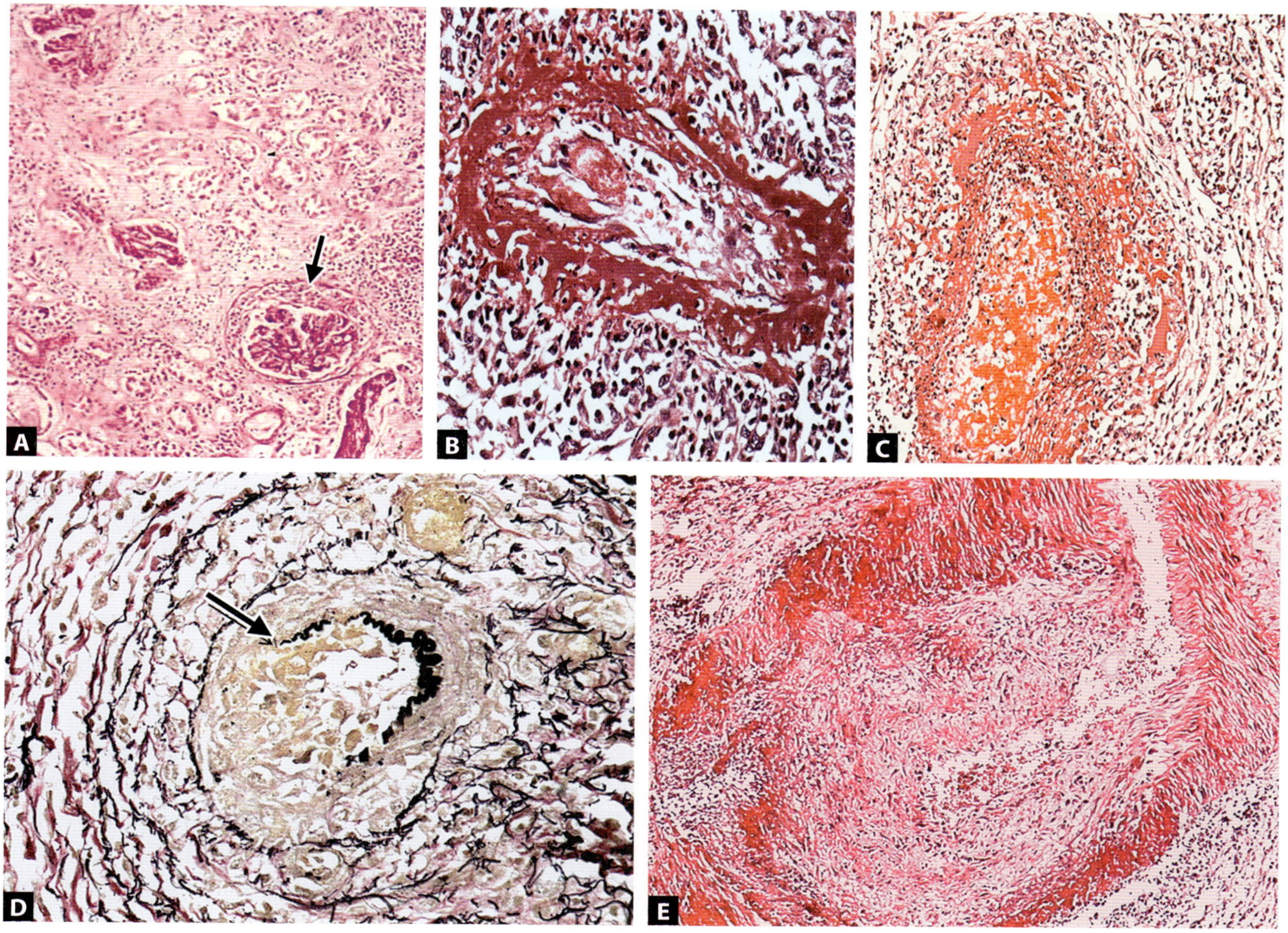

Figs 2A to E: (A) Periodic acid-Schiff stain of the kidney showing a crescent (arrow); (B and C) Interlobular arteries showing acute vasculitis with transmural fibrinoid necrosis and acute inflammation; (D) Elastic Verhoeff-Van Gieson stain showing break of the internal elastic lamina (arrow); (E) Arcuate artery showing acute vasculitis with fibrinoid necrosis and transmural inflammation.

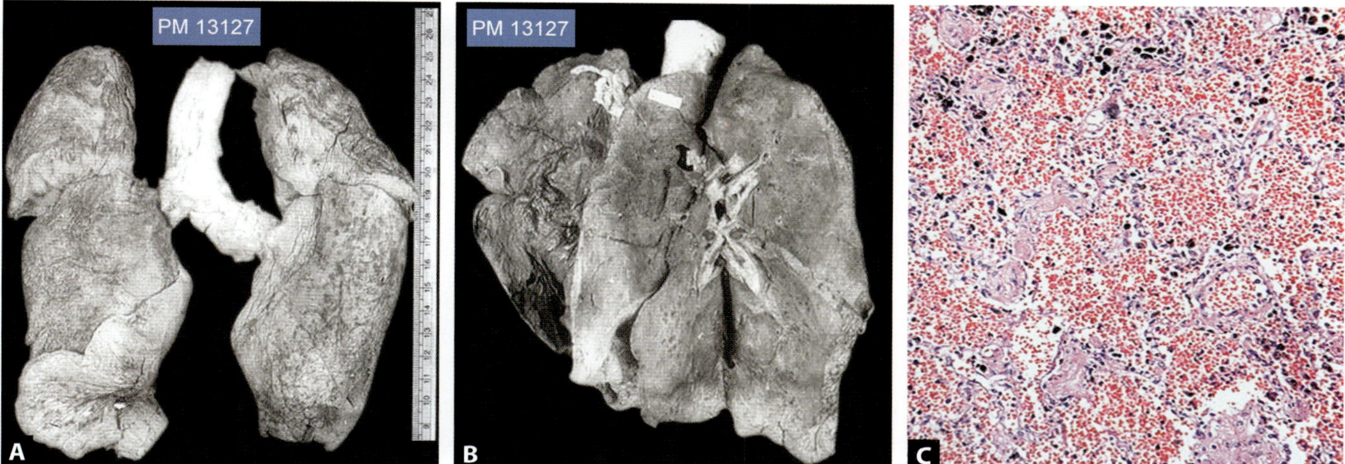

Figs 3A–C: (A) Pleural aspect of the lungs appears normal; (B) Cut section of the lungs showing areas of hemorrhagic consolidation; (C) Photomicrograph of the lung showing alveolar hemorrhage. No capillaritis is noted.

- Pauci-immune necrotizing, focal, segmental/diffuse, glomerulonephritis, with occasional crescent, with extra-glomerular acute vasculitis of the arterioles, interlobular and arcuate arteries
- *Lungs*: Hemorrhage, bronchopneumonia and pleuritis
- Left ventricular hypertrophy, coronary atherosclerosis
- Grade 4 atherosclerosis of the ascending aorta.

For Microscopic Polyangiitis: See "Small Vessel Vasculitis"

RENAL-LIMITED MICROSCOPIC POLYANGIITIS

The characteristic renal histopathologic manifestation of ANCA associated small vessel vasculitides is a pauci-immune, necrotizing crescentic glomerulonephritis (NCGN). More than three-fourths of patients with pauci-immune, ANCA-associated NCGN present with systemic small-vessel vasculitis. However, in a small number of these patients, there is no evidence of extra-renal vasculitis and hence are labeled as "renal limited vasculitis" as it is pathologically identical to the glomerulonephritis in patients with concurrent vasculitis elsewhere. In most of these cases ANCA is positive and directed against MPO. Patients present with the telltale findings of NCGN, i.e. rapidly progressive glomerulonephritis with hematuria, cellular casts, mild proteinuria and renal insufficiency. In addition general malaise, arthralgias and myalgias may be seen. Majority of these patients do not develop systemic vasculitis, but a small number does, later in the course of the disease. The histopathologic findings are indistinguishable from those seen in patients with MPA and hence can be labeled as a "***renal-limited form of MPA***". Limited expression of GPA can also occur, with the disease confined to the upper and lower respiratory tract. The author has seen a consult case of a young male with severe chronic sinusitis, who had had three biopsies over a period of 18 months, each time diagnosed on histopathology as ***chronic inflammation*** at an outside facility. The third biopsy from the maxillary sinus was sent for consultation and it revealed acute/chronic inflammation and areas of necrosis. Stain for acid-fast bacilli (AFB) and PAS stain for fungus were negative. Elastic Verhoeff-Van Gieson stain however revealed an artery with break of the internal elastic lamina. A diagnosis of "Granulomatosis with polyangiitis" was rendered with the note to look for systemic vasculitis and ANCA status. The ANCA done was positive for c-ANCA, but at that time no systemic vasculitis was detected, after thorough investigations. He was started on steroids. However, three-months later he presented with cough with expectoration and a rapidly progressive renal failure. Hence, this case was limited to begin with and later changed into a systemic vasculitis.

COMMENTARY—INDEX CASE: PM 13127

This 70-year old male had a short history (one month) and was admitted with swelling of large/small joints, hematuria, hemoptysis, anasarca, dyspnea, orthopnea, hypertension, oliguria followed by anuria and acute renal failure. A clinical diagnosis of Rapidly progressive glomerulonephritis ? Polyarteritis nodosa ? Henoch-Schonlein purpura was kept. Autopsy revealed renal limited MPA with pulmonary hemorrhage. There was a pauci-immune, necrotizing, focal glomerulonephritis with occasional crescent along with extra-glomerular acute vasculitis of the arterioles, interlobular and arcuate arteries. No extra-renal vasculitis was noted in multiple sections, meticulously studied from all the extra-renal organs. Postmortem serum sample was positive for pANCA. The lungs were graciously sampled and meticulously examined. It revealed pulmonary hemorrhage, but no vasculitis, capillaritis, areas of necrosis or granulomatous inflammation. Thus the vasculitis was renal limited. A small number of cases of renal limited small vessel vasculitis can develop systemic vasculitis, later in the course of the disease. This patient did have hemoptysis, joint pains, hematuria and acute renal failure and so clinically one cannot go away from a diagnosis of systemic vasculitis. But with no capillaritis in approximately 20 sections, meticulously studied from the lungs and no vasculitis in any other organ except for the kidneys, one can safely label this case as renal-limited microscopic polyangiitis.

TAKE HOME MESSAGE

- Characteristic renal histopathologic manifestation of ANCA associated small vessel vasculitides is a pauci-immune, necrotizing (focal segmental/diffuse), crescentic glomerulonephritis
- A small number of patients with ANCA associated, pauci-immune, necrotizing glomerulonephritis present with disease limited to the kidneys only. They have no evidence of extra-renal vasculitis and hence are labeled as renal-limited vasculitis
- A small number of cases of renal limited small vessel vasculitis can develop systemic vasculitis, later in the course of the disease.

SUGGESTED READING

1. Falk RJ, Jennette JC. Anti-neutrophil cytoplasmic autoantibodies with specificity for myeloperoxidase in patients with systemic vasculitis and idiopathic necrotizing and crescentic glomerulonephritis. N Engl J Med. 1988;318(25):1651-7.
2. Hernandez- Rodriguez J, Hoffman GS. Updating single organ vasculitis. Curr Opin Rheumatol. 2012;24(1):38-45.
3. Holle JU, Gross WL, Holl-Ulrich K, et al prospective long term follow up of patients with localized Wegener's granulomatosis: does it occur as persistent disease stage? Ann Rheum Dis. 2010;69(11):1934-9.

CONTRIBUTIONS BY:

1. Dr Savita Kumari, Professor and Head, Department of Internal Medicine (Compilation of Clinical Details)
2. Dr Ranjana Minz, Professor and Head, Department of Immunopathology (ANCA Testing)
3. Dr SK Mehta, Ex-Professor and Head, Department of Gastroenterology (Clinician In-Charge)

Post Graduate Institute of Medical Education and Research, Chandigarh, India.

CASE 37

Microscopic Polyangiitis, ANCA Negative, with Florid Glomerulitis and Granulomatous Glomerulonephritis: PM 15649

Nandita Bharadwaj Kakkar

HIGHLIGHTS OF THE CASE

A 30-year old male was admitted with a three months history of fever, joint pains followed by rash, palpable purpura, bilateral pedal edema, dyspnea, cough with expectoration, pleuritic chest pain, generalized weakness and weight loss. There was anemia, abnormal coagulogram, deranged renal function tests, proteinurea, hematuria and ultrasonography revealed bilateral enlarged kidneys with altered echotexture, iliofemoral/popliteal vein thrombosis. The clinical diagnosis was pulmonary-renal syndrome, antineutrophil cytoplasmic antibody (ACNA) negative ? Wegener's granulomatosis ? Goodpasture syndrome and left-sided iliofemoral deep vein thrombosis (DVT) with pulmonary thromboembolism. Autopsy however revealed features of small vessel vasculitis consistent with microscopic polyangiitis along with pulmonary hemorrhage and thromboembolism.

Keywords: Small vessel vasculitis, microscopic polyangiitis, granulomatous glomerulonephritis, glomerulitis, ANCA negative, autopsy.

CLINICAL DETAILS

Date of Admission: 26.05.1997, Date of Death: 01.06.1997, Duration of Hospital Stay: 7 Days

A 30-years old male, working as a truck-cleaner was admitted to our institute with history of low to moderate grade fever for 3 months. Five-days after the onset of fever he had developed joint pains initially involving the left knee and later other joints. The joint pain subsided after 15 days. He also noticed a transient rash ? Palpable purpura over the legs and developed bilateral pedal edema with progressive swelling of the left lower limb, persisting for 2-months before admission. He was having exertional dyspnea for the same duration, but the respiratory symptoms had worsened a week ago, when he developed increasing dyspnea, cough and expectoration as well as pleuritic chest pain on right side. He had been admitted at an outside facility where he had received antitubercular treatment, steroids and antibiotics for 2½ months, without any improvement. There was generalized weakness and weight loss of 15 kg during the last 2 months. There was no history of diabetes, hypertension, tuberculosis or any significant renal disease in the past.

Examination: At admission the patient was conscious, sick-looking, having marked pallor, facial swelling, bilateral pedal edema and swelling of left lower limb with calf tenderness. A palpable lymph node was noted in the left axilla. There was no icterus, clubbing, cyanosis or any rash. The pulse was 106/min, BP: 120/80 mm Hg, RR: 36/min, JVP was normal. Chest revealed dullness and bronchial breathing over the right inframammary and infra-axillary areas, as well as bilateral crepitation (right > left) and occasional rhonchi at the bases. Pleural rub was present on the right side, the liver was palpable 4 cm below the right costal margin and the spleen was just palpable. There was evidence of free fluid. CVS and CNS examination were normal.

Investigations and Course of Management

Investigations done outside: Hb—6.5 g/dL, TLC—23,000/μL, DLC P85 L12, M02, E01, ESR 72 mm, urea 67 mg%, creatinine 3.4 mg%, urine albumin 2–3+, rheumatoid factor positive, anti-nuclear factor and human immunodeficiency virus negative.

Investigations at PGIMER

Hematological: Hb—7.5 g/dL; TLC – 23,100/ uL; Platelets — 5,50,000/uL; retic count 4%; PBF: severe anisopoikilocytosis with few tear-drop cells, ovalocytes and fragmented

RBCs; ESR: 80 mm 1st hour; Coagulogram —PT/PTI—22'/59%, INR: 3.5, PTTK: 65', fibrinogen 240 mg%, FDP negative.

***Blood Biochemistry/Microbiology*:** S urea—136 mg%; S creatinine—6.6 mg%; Na^+/K^+—130/4, mEq/L; uric acid: 14 mg%; cholesterol: 124 mg%; RBS: 108 mg%; S.bilirubin: 0.7 mg%, SGOT/SGPT: 11/6 IU; alkaline phosphatase: 5 U/L; total protein 6.4 g, albumin/globulin—2.5/3.9 gm; calcium: 7.7 mg%; amylase: 133 U/L; blood culture done three times sterile; urine examination—albumin 3–4+, sugar: Nil, pus cells: 2–3/hpf, RBC: 8–10/hpf, no casts; Urine culture sterile.

***Serology*:** Antinuclear factor negative; human immunodeficiency virus negative; ANCA negative; candida serology: 1:512; aspergillus niger serology ++.

Radiology/Cardiac—Chest X-ray: Enlarged cardiac silhouette, bilateral homogeneous opacities in parahilar region. ***USG abdomen***: Bilateral enlarged kidneys, right 14.1 cm, left 13.2 cm with altered echotexture and accentuated corticomedullary distinction. Hepatomegaly with minimal free fluid in abdomen and pelvis. ***Compression ultrasonography*** of venous system: Left iliofemoral and popliteal vein thrombosis noted. No obstruction in inferior vena cava and renal veins. ***Echocardiography***: Pulmonary artery hypertension, moderate tricuspid regurgitation, mild pericardial effusion. No tamponade. ***ECG***: Showed normal sinus rhythm.

At the time of admission a diagnosis of DVT and pulmonary thromboembolism was considered and he was given heparin infusion and oxygen inhalation and later acitrom was also added. In view of the persistent fever and possible chest infection, patient received parenteral antibiotics. Administration of thrombolytic therapy was later withheld since patient had streaky hemoptysis and alveolar hemorrhage was suspected. Renal parameters showed evidence of rapidly progressive renal failure with reduced urine output (400–700 mL/day), proteinuria and rising serum urea/creatinine. Patient's condition continued to deteriorate with persistence of fever, progressive breathlessness, cough, hemoptysis and worsening of lung shadows. He was given intravenous methylprednisolone pulse and blood transfusions. He developed epistaxis and hemoptysis. Later on there was malena. Patient had refractory hypoxemia for which he was put on mechanical ventilation. Despite 100% FiO_2 there was no improvement. He was also given injection endoxan pulse. At this time his urine output had fallen to 120 mL/day and he developed severe acidosis, not responding to intravenous sodium bicarbonate. He developed a tension pneumothorax on right side. Despite the treatment, he developed cardiorespiratory arrest and could not be resuscitated. The ***Unit clinical diagnosis*** was pulmonary renal syndrome ? Wegener's granulomatosis ? Goodpasture syndrome, left-sided ileofemoral DVT ? pulmonary thromboembolism.

AUTOPSY FINDINGS: PM 15649

A complete autopsy was performed and the prosector found all serous cavities within normal limits. The kidneys (Figs 1A and B) were enlarged and together weighed 700 g. External surface and cut surface showed blotchy congestion. No infarcts were seen. On microscopic examination the glomeruli were diffusely involved and revealed a variety of lesions. Some glomeruli were discernable and showed fibrinoid necrosis with scant nuclear debris (Fig 1C). Some showed crescents with compressed glomerular tufts and florid attack by polymorphonuclear infiltrate i.e. glomerulitis, along with break of the Bowman's capsule and mergence with the interstitium (Figs 1D and E). Many glomeruli (Figs 2A–D) were not discernable due to florid glomerulitis with total destruction and replacement by polymorphs, nuclear debris and fibrin. The Bowman's capsule was totally destroyed and they in fact looked like small abscesses. Others showed a very prominent granulomatous glomerulonephritis (Figs 3A–C) wherein a destroyed glomerulus showing fibrinoid necrosis/sclerosis was surrounded by a mantle of epithelioid cells and giant cells. Some glomeruli were in the healing phase with sparse inflammation and others were totally sclerotic (Fig 3D) and appeared as virtual graveyard/tomb stones of once existing glomeruli. The arcuate and interlobular arteries (Figs 4A–C) showed acute vasculitis with transmural fibrinoid necrosis and inflammation. An occasional vessel showed thrombosis (Fig 4D). The interstitium showed dense inflammation and there was tubular atrophy. Immunoperoxidase stain showed fibrin/fibrinogen deposition in the glomeruli which correlated with the necrotizing glomerulitis. However, stains for IgA, immunoglobulin A (IgA), IgM and C3 were negative. Postmortem ANCA could not be done. Overall features were of a diffuse necrotizing crescentic glomerulonephritis with florid glomerulitis, granulomatous glomerulonephritis and acute vasculitis of the interlobular and arcuate arteries, consistent with a diagnosis of small vessel vasculitis. Renal lesions of granulomatosis with polyangiitis (GPA) and microscopic polyangiitis (MPA) are indistinguishable. The deciding factor is the status of the upper and lower respiratory tract. The lungs (Fig 5A) were heavy and weighed 2.1 Kg. The pleural aspect was normal and the cut section revealed hemorrhagic consolidation. Grossly, no focal lesion or any area of necrosis was seen. Thromboembolism was noted in

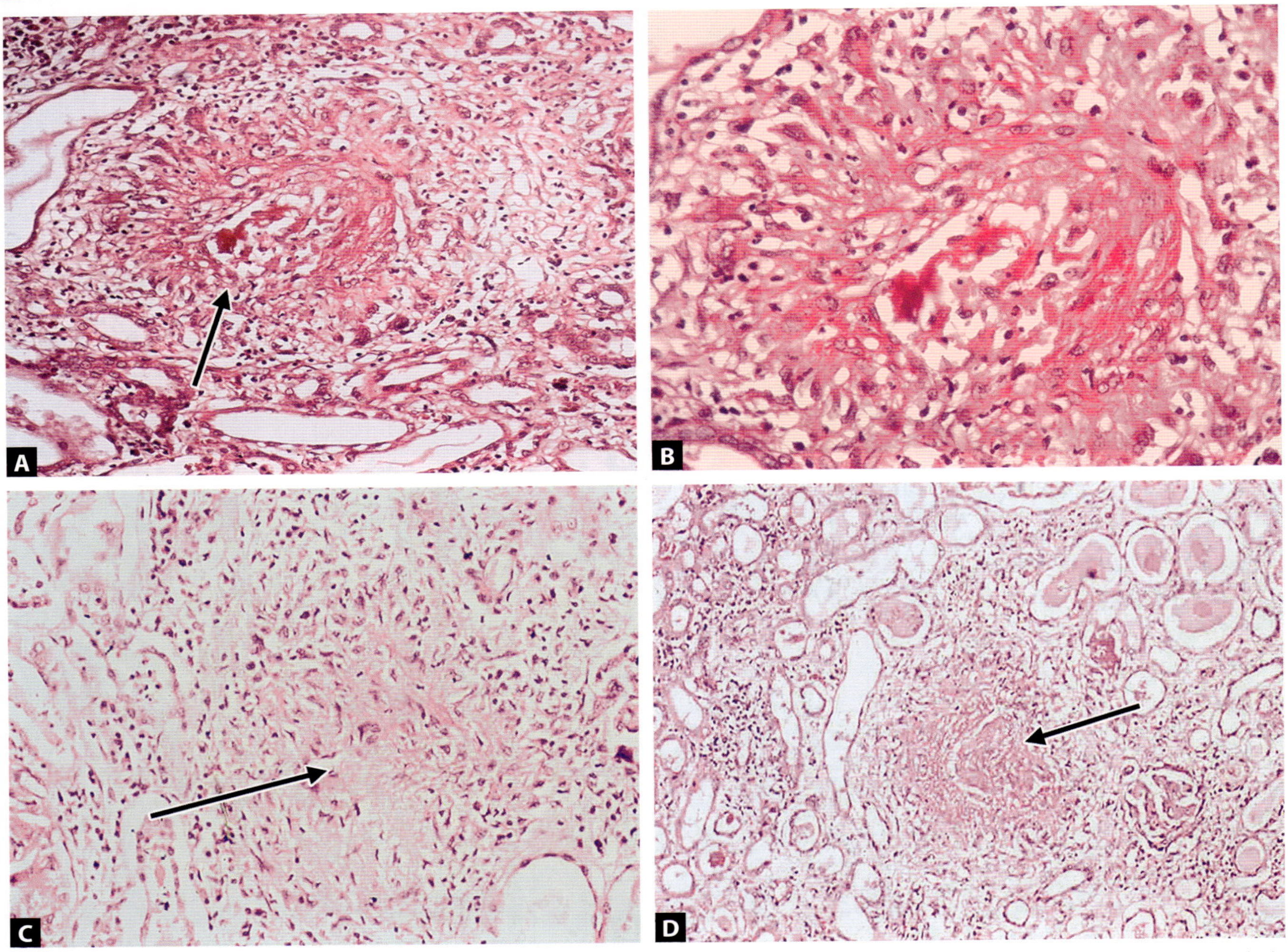

Figs 3A–D: (A–C) Granulomatous glomerulonephritis wherein a destroyed glomerulus (arrows) showing fibrinoid necrosis or sclerosis is surrounded by a mantle of epithelioid cells and giant cells; (D) A sclerotic glomerulus (arrow) that appears as a tomb stone.

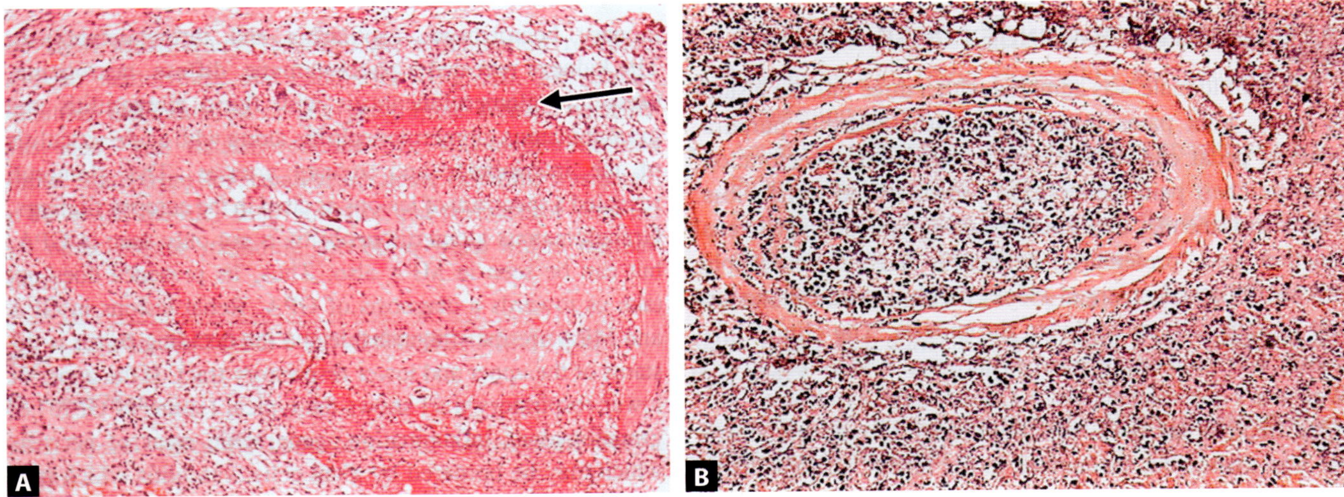

Figs 4A and B:

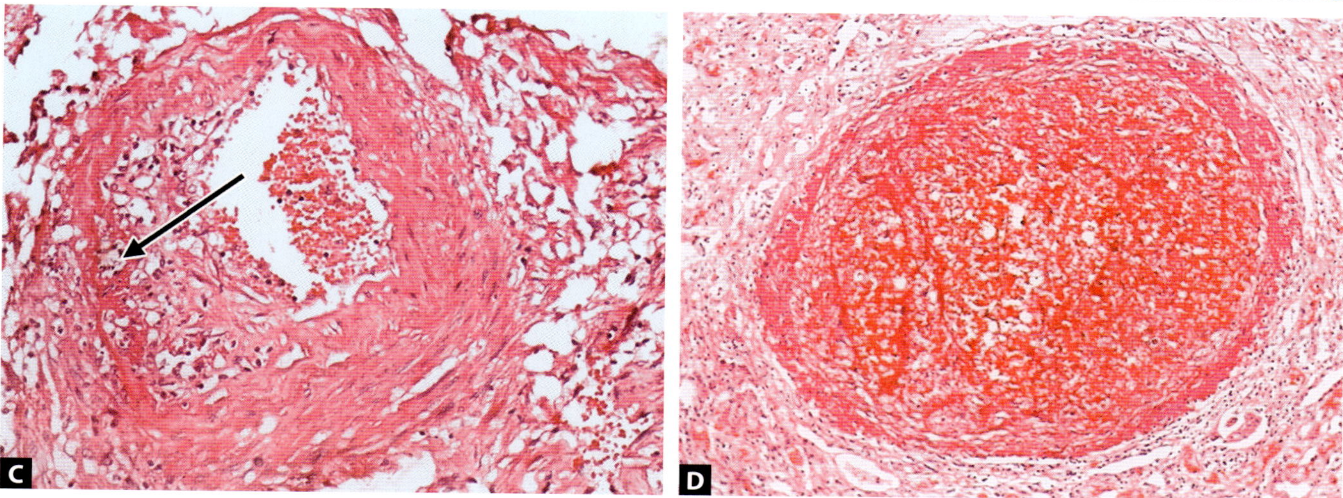

Figs 4A–D: (A) An arcuate artery showing fibrinoid necrosis (arrow), transmural inflammation and intimal proliferation with occluded lumina; (B) An interlobular artery showing acute vasculitis; (C) An interlobular artery showing acute vasculitis in one half of the vessel (arrow); (D) Artery showing thrombosis.

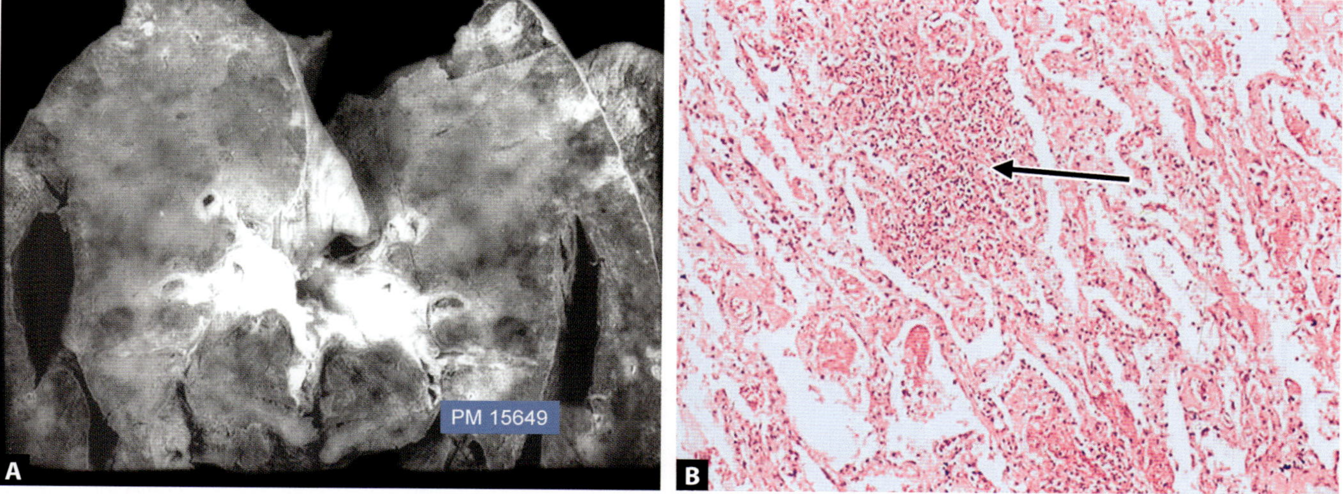

Figs 5A and B: (A) Cut-section of the lungs showing hemorrhagic consolidation; (B) Foci of capillaritis in the lungs (arrow).

the case should be labeled as MPA. The odd point in this case was that the patient was ANCA negative (done once) despite the florid acute glomerulitis and acute vasculitis.

TAKE HOME MESSAGE

- Renal lesions in granulomatosis with polyangiitis and microscopic polyangiitis are indistinguishable and the deciding factor is the status of the upper and lower respiratory tract
- Granulomatous glomerulonephritis is not only seen in GPA, but can be seen in MPA also
- Antineutrophil cytoplasmic antibody can be negative in florid cases of small vessel vasculitis and repeat ANCA is advisable.

CONTRIBUTIONS BY:

1. Dr KL Gupta, Professor and Head, Department of Nephrology (Compilation of Clinical Details)
2. Dr Shobha Sehgal, Ex-Professor and Head, Department of Immunopathology (ANCA Testing)
3. Late SD Deodhar, Professor, Department of Internal Medicine (Clinician In-Charge)

Post Graduate Institute of Medical Education and Research, Chandigarh, India.

CASE 38

Microscopic Polyangiitis in a Child: PM 16450

Nandita Bharadwaj Kakkar

HIGHLIGHTS OF THE CASE

An 8-year old child came with a 1-month history of edema, decreased urine output and on and off hematuria. Respiratory distress was there since 1 day. Investigations revealed deranged renal function tests with albumin urea and hematuria. X-ray chest revealed bilateral patchy opacities. Units clinical diagnosis was immunoglobulin A (IgA) nephropathy, antiglomerular basement membrane disease or collagen vascular disease, nephrotic/nephritic syndrome with renal vein thrombosis. At autopsy a diagnosis of microscopic polyangiitis with extensive pulmonary hemorrhage and capillaritis was made. Small vessel vasculitis in childhood is very rare.

Keywords: Childhood vasculitis, microscopic polyangiitis, necrotizing crescentic glomerulonephritis, pauci-immune, autopsy.

CLINICAL DETAILS

Date of Admission: 17.12.1998, Date of Death: 18.12.1998, Duration of Hospital Stay: 30 Hours

An 8-year-old female child came with generalized edema, decreased urine output, pain abdomen (epigastric, lumbar, periumbilical and of varying intensity) and hematuria off and on, since 30 days. Prior to this she had fever for a day, which had subsided with antipyretics. There was rapid breathing for the last 1 day. There was no history of pyoderma, intake of nephrotoxic drugs, photosensitivity, rash, altered sensorium, seizures, wheezing, chest pain, hemoptysis, Raynaud's phenomenon or deafness. On examination she weighed 23 Kg, with a height of 124 cm. She was conscious, oriented and there was no rash, pallor, lymphadenopathy, raised JVP, jaundice or clubbing. Vitals were within normal limits, bilateral basal crepts were present, liver was palpable 2.5 cm below right costal margin and there was minimal ascites. CNS and CVS were within normal limits. ***Investigations*** revealed Hb of 5.2 g/dL, TLC 14000/uL with normal platelet count. Renal function tests—serum creatinine: 6.1 mg%, serum urea: 168 mg%, Na^+—157 mEq/L and K^+—5.7 mEq/L. ANCA and ANA were not done. Routine urine examination—pH: 6.5, specific gravity: 1.025, albumin: 4+, WBC: Nil, RBC's: Full field, no casts and occasional epithelial cell. X-ray chest revealed bilateral patchy opacities with obliteration of the right costophrenic angle. Clinical impression was acute renal failure/rapidly progressive glomerulonephritis, severe anemia and pulmonary edema. She was started on restricted IV fluids, injection Lasix, one dose of nifedipine, antibiotics, peritoneal dialysis with blood transfusions. She had pulmonary hemorrhage and died after a hospital stay of one day. Units clinical diagnosis was IgA nephropathy, anti-GBM disease or collagen vascular disease, nephrotic/nephritic syndrome with renal vein thrombosis.

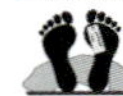

AUTOPSY FINDINGS: PM 16450

A partial autopsy was performed on this 8-year-old female child. The peritoneal cavity yielded 150 mL of straw-colored fluid. The ***kidneys*** together weighed 250 g and the external surface was flea bitten (Figs 1A–C). On microscopic examination most of the glomeruli contained cellular crescents (Figs 2A–C—arrows) and many showed necrosis of the tuft with fibrin and nuclear debris, better known as necrotizing lesions or acute glomerulitis (Figs 2D, 3A and B). Break of Bowman's capsule and mergence of the glomerulus with the interstitium was also seen (Figs 2B and C). Fibrinoid necrosis of the afferent arterioles was noted which was propagating into the glomerular tuft (Fig 2D). Phosphotungstic acid hematoxylin stain (PTAH), stained the fibrin blue

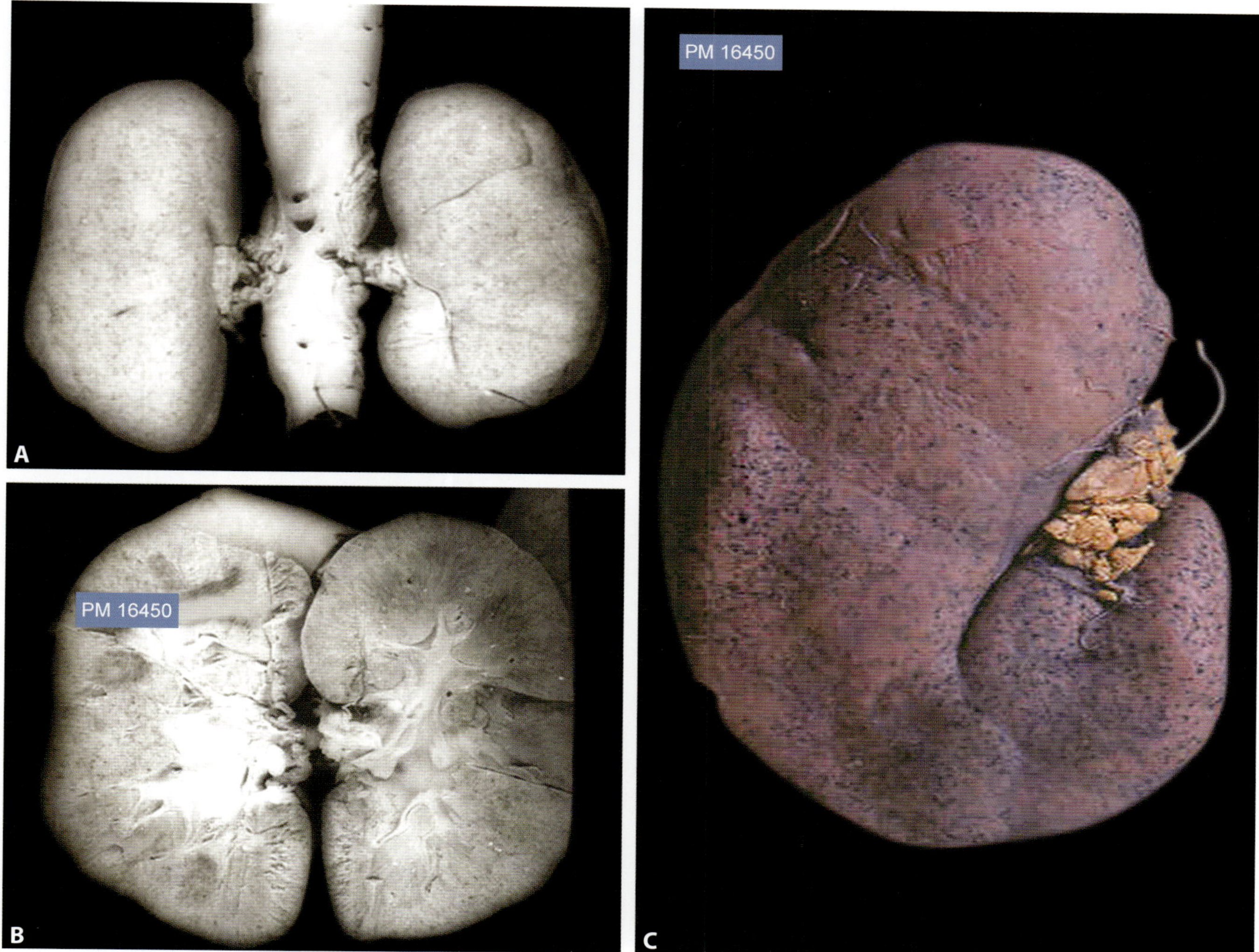

Figs 1A–C: (A) Gross photograph of both the kidneys which are normal in size and show petechial hemorrhages; (B) Cut section of the kidney showing medullary congestion; (C) Close view of the capsular aspect of the kidney showing petechial hemorrhages i.e. flea bitten appearance.

(Fig 2E). Tubules showed hyaline and RBC casts and the interstitium showed dense inflammation (Fig 3C). Apart from the afferent arterioles no other vessel showed vasculitis. Immunoperoxidase stain for IgG (Fig 3D), IgM, IgA and C3 were negative and electron microscopy (Fig 3E) did not show any electron dense immune deposits. Diagnosis was that of a pauci-immune necrotizing crescentic glomerulonephritis with acute vasculitis of the afferent arterioles. The ***spleen*** weighed 60 g and microscopy revealed florid acute vasculitis (Figs 4A and B) with fibrinoid necrosis of the central arterioles. Lesions were of the same age. A medium-sized vein in the spleen showed acute intimitis (Fig 4C). The ***heart*** weighed 220 g, valves and chambers were unremarkable and on microscopy there was acute vasculitis of the small vessels in the myocardium. The ***lungs*** (Fig 4D) weighed 500 g, pleural aspect and cut section showed hemorrhages. Microscopy (Figs 4E and F) showed extensive alveolar hemorrhage, capillaritis with nuclear debris and fibrinoid necrosis present in the septal capillaries. The differential diagnosis in this case was between microscopic polyangiitis and granulomatosis with polyangiitis (Wegener's). Glomerular lesions of MPA and GPA are indistinguishable. Absence of granulomatous inflammation, typical necrosis and vasculitis in arteries and veins, in the upper and lower respiratory tract rules out GPA.

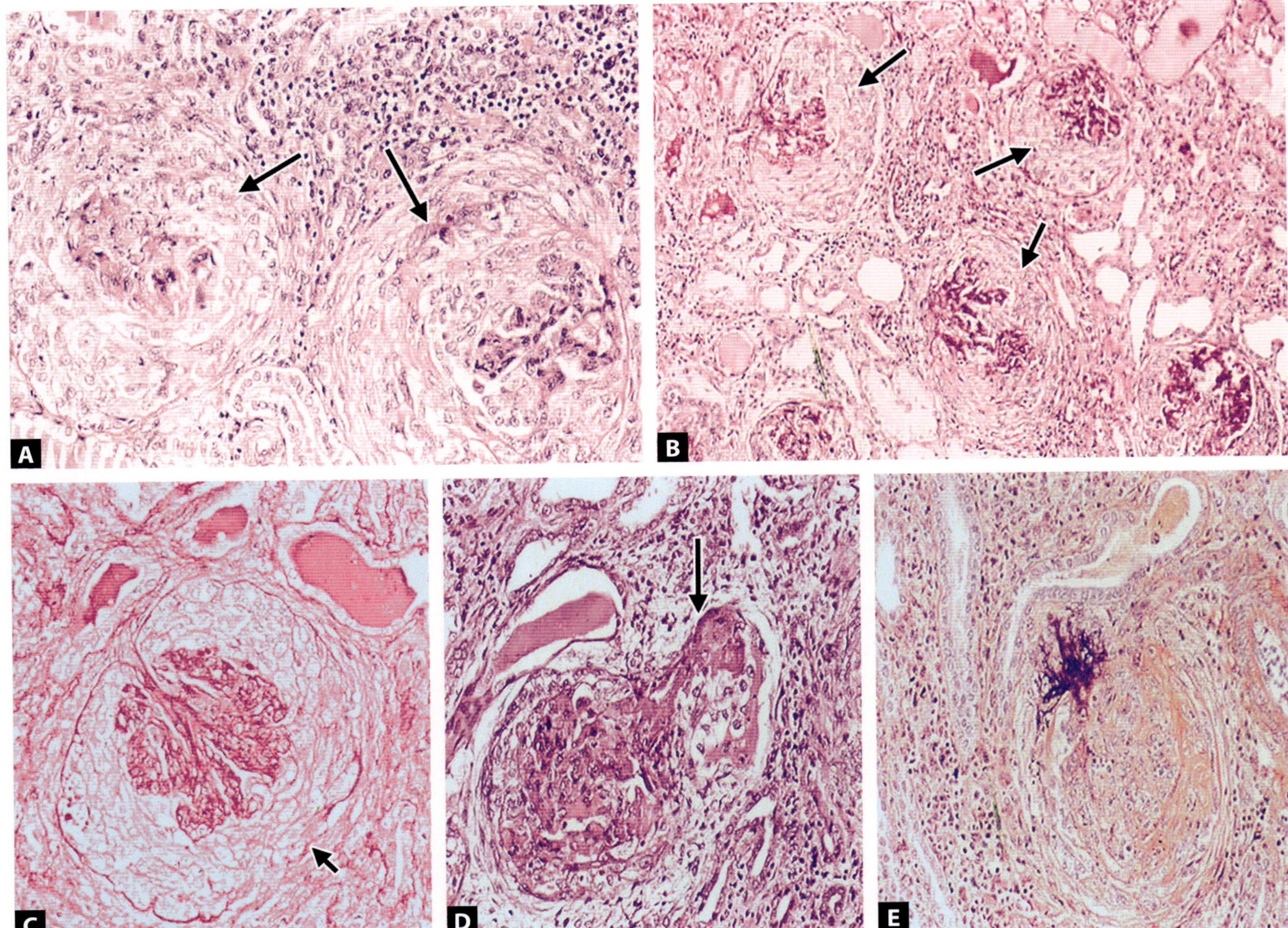

Figs 2A–E: (A) Photomicrograph from the kidney showing cellular crescents (arrows) and interstitial inflammation; (B and C) PAS-stain highlights the shrunken glomerular tufts, cellular crescents (arrows) and the break of Bowman's capsule (arrow in C); (D) Glomerulus wherein the afferent arteriole (arrow) shows fibrinoid necrosis which is propagating into the glomerular tuft, which shows necrotizing lesion with fibrin and nuclear debris; (E) Phosphotungstic acid-hematoxylin stain shows fibrinoid necrosis of the afferent arteriole, wherein it stains the fibrin blue.

FINAL AUTOPSY DIAGNOSIS: PM 16450

8 Years Female Child

- Consistent with Microscopic Polyangiitis (ANCA status unknown).
  - Pauci-immune, necrotizing, crescentic, glomerulonephritis with acute vasculitis of afferent arterioles
  - Small vessel vasculitis in spleen and myocardium
  - Extensive pulmonary hemorrhage with capillaritis.

CHILDHOOD VASCULITIS

Vasculitis is less common in childhood,[1] but Kawasaki disease occurs exclusively in children. Other vasculitides like Takayasu's aortoarteritis and Henoch-Schönlein purpura are common in children. Polyarteritis nodosa and small vessel vasculitis are rare and giant cell arteritis does not occur in children. The most common of the ANCA-associated small vessel vasculitides in children is granulomatosis with polyangiitis (Wegener's), but microscopic polyangiitis and eosinophilic granulomatosis with polyangiitis (Churg-Strauss syndrome) can also be seen in children. Ankara 2008 classification[2] defines GPA in children and stresses on 3 of the 6 criteria to be present which include—histopathology i.e. vascular and extravascular granulomas, upper airway involvement, subglottic/tracheal/bronchial stenosis, pulmonary involvement, presence of ANCA and renal disease

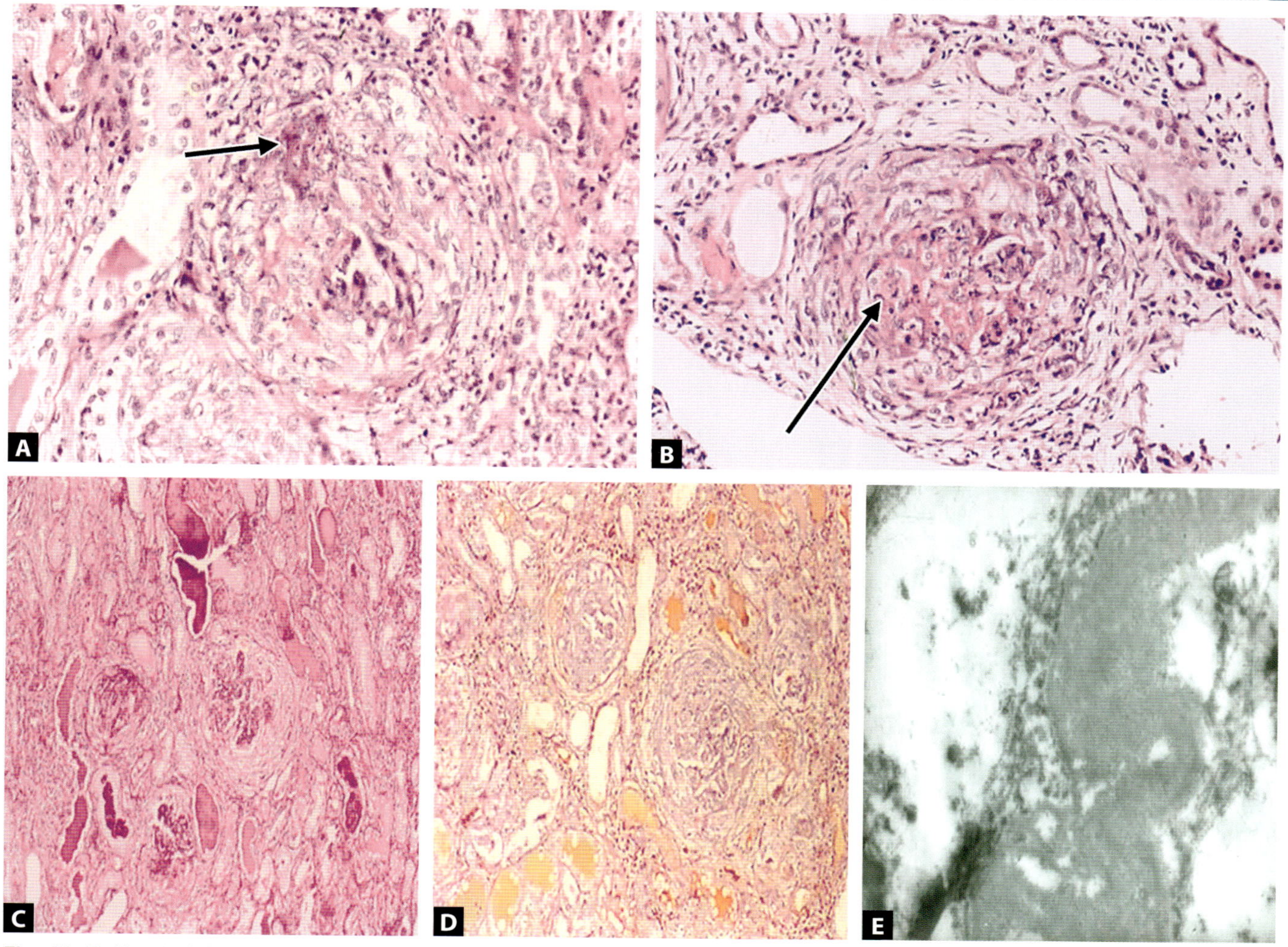

Figs 3A–E: (A and B) Glomeruli showing tuft necrosis (arrows) with polymorphs, nuclear debris and fibrin; (C) Kidney showing RBC and hyaline casts along with interstitial inflammation; (D) Immunoperoxidase stain for IgG is negative; (E) Electron microscopy showing absent immune complexes.

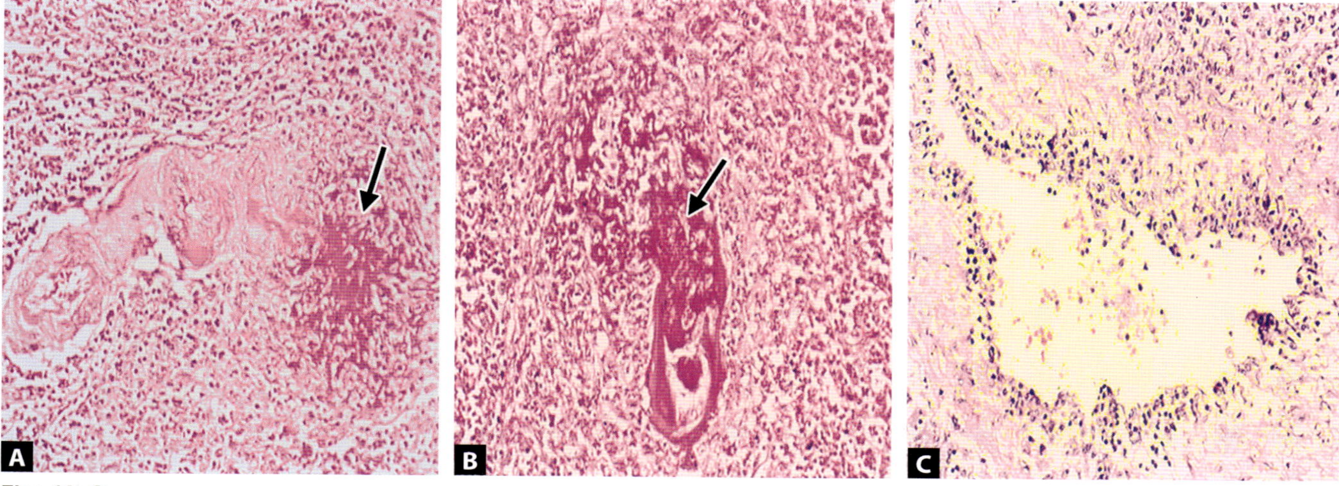

Figs 4A–C

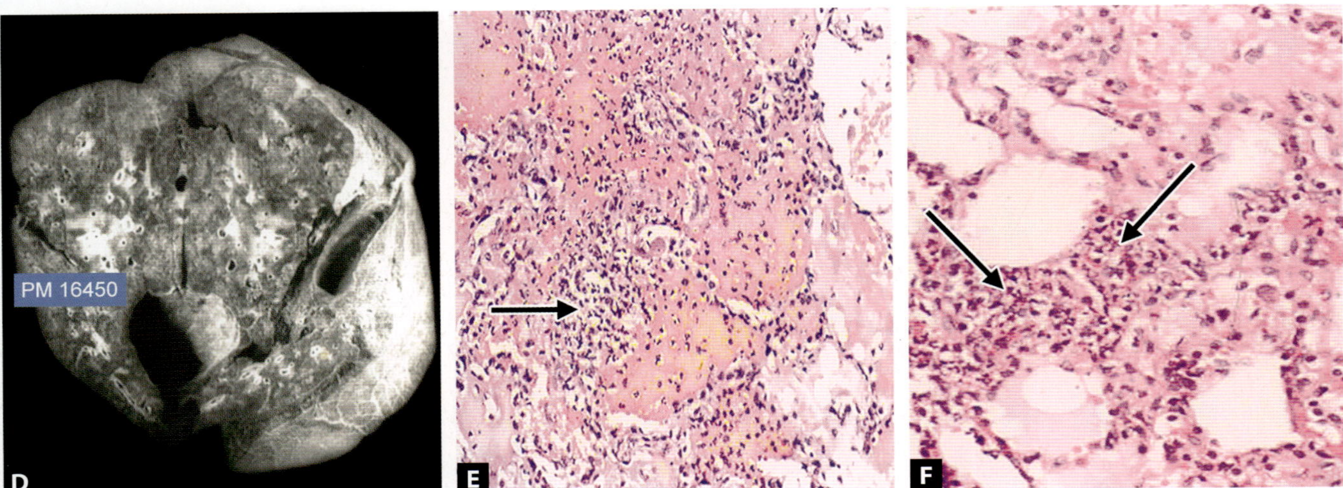

Figs 4A–F: (A and B) Acute vasculitis with fibrinoid necrosis of the small vessels of the spleen (arrow); (C) A medium-sized vein in the spleen showing acute intimitis; (D) Cut section of lungs, showing hemorrhages; (E and F) Alveolar septa shows acute capillaritis with polymorphs and nuclear debris (arrows). Alveolar hemorrhage is seen in *E*.

(proteinuria, hematuria, RBC casts or pauci-immune glomerulonephritis). Children with MPA[3] present with acute onset of symptoms involving the lung and kidney.

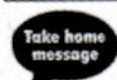

TAKE HOME MESSAGE

- Although rare, small vessel vasculitides are seen in children
- Kawasaki disease occurs exclusively in children
- Takayasu's aortoarteritis and Henoch–Schönlein purpura are commonly seen in children.

REFERENCES

1. Dolezalova P, Telekesova P, Nemcova D, et al. Incidence of vasculitis in children in the Czech Republic: 2-year prospective epidemiologic survey. J Rheumatol. 2004;31(11):2295-9.
2. Ozen S, Pistorio A, Lusan SM, et al. EULAR/PRINTO/PRES criteria for HSP, childhood PAN, childhood Wegener's garnulomatosis and Takayasu arteritis Ankara 2008: Part 11: Final classification criteria. Ann Rheum Dis. 2010;69(5):798-806.
3. Peco-Antic, Bonaci-Nikolic B, Basta-Jovanovic G, et al. Childhood microscopic polyangiitis associated with MPO-ANCA. Pediatr Nephrol. 2006;21(1):46-53.

CONTRIBUTIONS BY:

1. Dr Bhavneet Bharti, Professor, Department of Pediatrics (Clinician In-Charge)
Post Graduate Institute of Medical Education and Research, Chandigarh, India.

CASE 39

Microscopic Polyangiitis, ANCA Negative, Clinically Mimicking Granulomatosis with Polyangiitis (Wegener's Granulomatosis) and Presenting with a Breast Mass: PM 18473

Nandita Bharadwaj Kakkar

HIGHLIGHTS OF THE CASE

A 50-year old female presented with a history of symptoms going on for a year. She had fever, nasal blockage, arthralgias, joint pains, red eye, cough with expectoration, dyspnea, oliguria, vaginal bleeding, rapidly developing breast mass and renal failure. CT revealed multiple splenic infarcts, normal-sized kidneys and extensive consolidation in both lungs. A clinical diagnosis of Wegener's granulomatosis (WG) i.e granulomatosis with polyangiitis (GPA) was entertained. At autopsy, a diagnosis consistent with microscopic polyangiitis was made. The lungs and the upper respiratory tract did not show the typical lesions of GPA/WG. The worth stressing points in this case are clinical signs and symptoms of an upper/lower respiratory tract involvement, suggesting GPA/WG, vasculitis in the breast leading to a large hemorrhagic mass, granulomatous glomerulonephritis, occasional granulomatous arteritis/extravascular granulomatous lesions (area of necrosis with palisading of epithelioid histiocytes and giant cells) in the spleen and a negative ANCA, in the presence of florid untreated disease.

Keywords: Microscopic polyangiitis, mimicking, granulomatosis with polyangiitis, granulomatous glomerulonephritis, total splenic necrosis, splenic granulomatous arteritis, splenic extravascular granulomatous lesion, ANCA negative, active disease, breast mass, autopsy.

CLINICAL DETAILS

Date of Admission: 12.05.2002, Date of Death: 23.05.2002, Duration of Hospital Stay: 11 Days

This 50-years female presented with high grade fever, loss of appetite and weight, cough with minimal expectoration, breathlessness, oliguria and a right breast mass which developed spontaneously and was rapidly enlarging. She had been symptomatic since one year with history of nasal blockage, nasal discharge, otitis media, red eye, arthralgias and joint pains involving the wrist, hands and ankle. Two-months prior to admission she had hearing loss which lasted for a few days and then improved. On physical examination the patient was drowsy, restless, there was pallor, anasarca, raised JVP, normal BP, an indurated swelling in the right breast (6 x 8 cm), an ejection systolic murmur and normal liver/spleen. CNS examination revealed a drowsy patient, responding to few oral commands and to painful stimuli.

Investigations

Investigations revealed a Hb of 6.5 g/dL; TLC: 25,000/uL with a differential count, showing a slight shift to the left and 10/100 nucleated RBC's; platelet count of 4,95,000/uL; ESR of 76 mm and a normal coagulogram. Serum biochemistry revealed raised urea (210 mg%) and creatinine (13.5 mg%); albumin/globulin of 2.1/3.9 gm; total bilirubin of 1.4 mg% with a conjugated fraction of 0.7; normal transaminases and blood sugar. Routine urine examination showed albuminuria, 50–100 RBC/hpf and 10–20 WBC/hpf. Antinuclear factor, anti-nuclear antibodies, HIV and HbsAg were negative. ***X-ray chest*** showed diffuse opacification of both lungs with lymphadenopathy. ***Plain computerized tomography (CT) of the abdomen*** showed low attenuation in the spleen suggestive of infarcts/abscess; liver/pancreas/ lymph nodes were normal; both kidneys were normal in size but showed small cysts on the surface. The uterus was enlarged, but no mass was identified. ***A contrast-enhanced CT***, confirmed the splenic infarct, extensive bilateral consolidation of both lungs, absence of thromboembolism and an enlarged right atrium ? pulmonary arterial hypertension. ***Echocardiograph***y revealed pulmonary arterial hypertension, severe tricuspid regurgitation, right and left ventricular ejection fraction of 50% and 60% respectively, no clot, vegetations or effusion. A ***clinical diagnosis*** of multi-organ dysfunction: Systemic vasculitis ? Wegener's granulomatosis with glomerulonephritis, sepsis, bronchopneumonia, dysfunctional uterine bleed and ?? infective endocarditis was made.

AUTOPSY FINDINGS: PM 18473

A partial autopsy was performed (brain was not examined). The serous cavities were within normal limits.

The ***kidneys*** were normal sized, weighed 450 g together, showed blotchy congestion (Fig 1A) and occasional small cyst (0.5–1 cm) on the surface. Cut section (Fig 1B) showed congestion, but no infarcts were noted. On microscopy, glomeruli revealed a variable morphology from acute to chronic lesions, indicating thereby that the disease process had been operating for some time. Segmental (Fig 1C) and diffuse (Fig 1D) necrotizing (showing fibrinoid necrosis and leukocytoclasia i.e. nuclear debris) glomerulonephritis was seen with many glomeruli showing crescents (Fig 1D). Break of the Bowman's capsule with mergence of the glomeruli with the interstitium and abundant polymorphs infiltrating and destroying the glomeruli i.e. acute glomerulitis (Fig 2A) was prominent. Granulomatous glomerulonephritis (Fig 2B) where a glomerulus showing acute necrotizing or chronic fibrotic lesion is palisaded by epithelioid histiocytes, giant cells and lymphocytes was also seen. Chronic glomerular lesions showing fibrosis with palisading histiocytes/giant cells/lymphocytes (Fig 2C) and totally burnt-out lesions, many appearing as granulomatous glomerular tomb stones

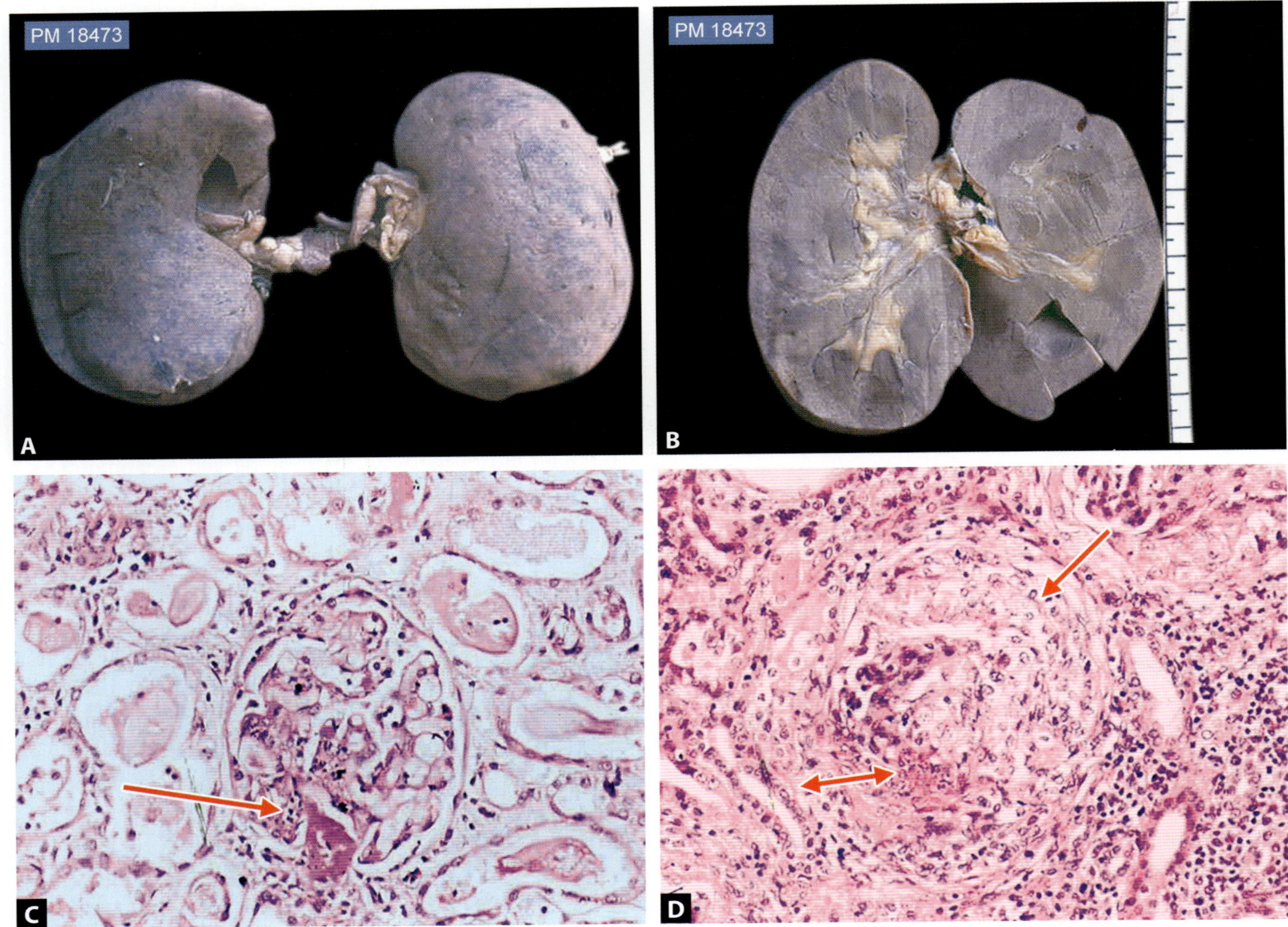

Figs 1A–D: (A) Capsular aspect of the kidney shows blotchy congestion; (B) Cut section of the kidney shows medullary congestion, but no infarcts; (C) Glomerulus showing a segmental necrotizing lesion (arrow) with fibrinoid necrosis, polymorphs and nuclear debris; (D) Diffuse lesion wherein the glomerulus shows a cellular crescent (arrow) and the glomerular tuft showing polymorphs, nuclear debris and fibrinoid necrosis is compressed to the left side (double arrow).

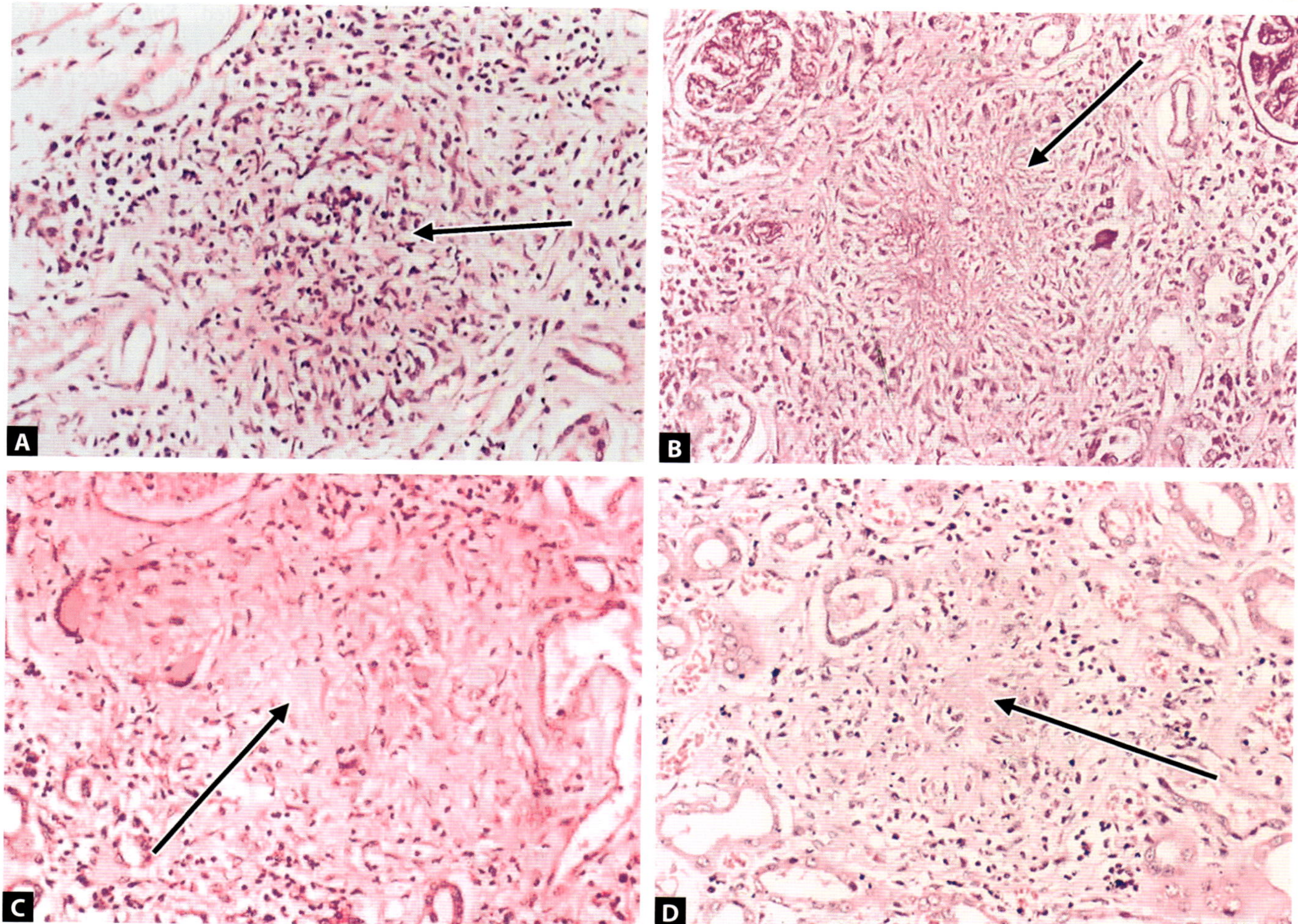

Figs 2A–D: (A) Acute glomerulitis (arrow) wherein the glomerulus is totally destroyed by infiltrating polymorphs; (B) Granulomatous glomerulonephritis (arrow) where the glomerulus shows a chronic fibrotic lesion palisaded by epithelioid histiocytes, giant cells and lymphocytes; (C) Chronic glomerular lesions (arrow) showing fibrosis with palisading histiocytes and giant cells; (D) Burnt-out glomerular lesion (arrow) i.e. a virtual tomb stone of a glomerulus.

were present (Fig 2D). Interlobular arteries showed florid acute vasculitis, showing fibrinoid necrosis and transmural inflammation along with nuclear debris (Fig 3A). Some interlobular arteries showed early vasculitis in the form of acute intimitis (Fig 3B). Vasculitis was also seen in the afferent arterioles and glomerular capillaries. The arcuate and interlobar arteries were however spared of the vasculitic process. The interstitium showed dense interstitial inflammation without eosinophils and interstitial granulomatous inflammation (typically seen in GPA and EGPA) was absent. Tubules contained hyaline and RBC casts. Immunoperoxidase staining performed on the kidney for IgG, IgM, IgA and C3 was negative and hence the glomerulonephritis was of the pauci- immune type. The renal artery and veins were normal. A diagnosis of pauci-immune crescentic necrotizing glomerulonephritis with granulomatous glomerular lesions and extraglomerular florid acute vasculitis, involving the interlobular vessels, consistent with an ANCA negative small vessel vasculitis was made. Differential diagnosis considered at this point of time was:

- Microscopic polyangiitis
- Granulomatosis with polyangiitis i.e. Wegener's granulomatosis.

Eosinophilic granulomatosis with angiitis was ruled out as eosinophils were not seen in the inflammatory lesions in the kidney or peripheral blood and there was no history of asthma. Idiopathic pauci-immune crescentic glomerulonephritis, not associated with ANCA, was ruled out as extraglomerular

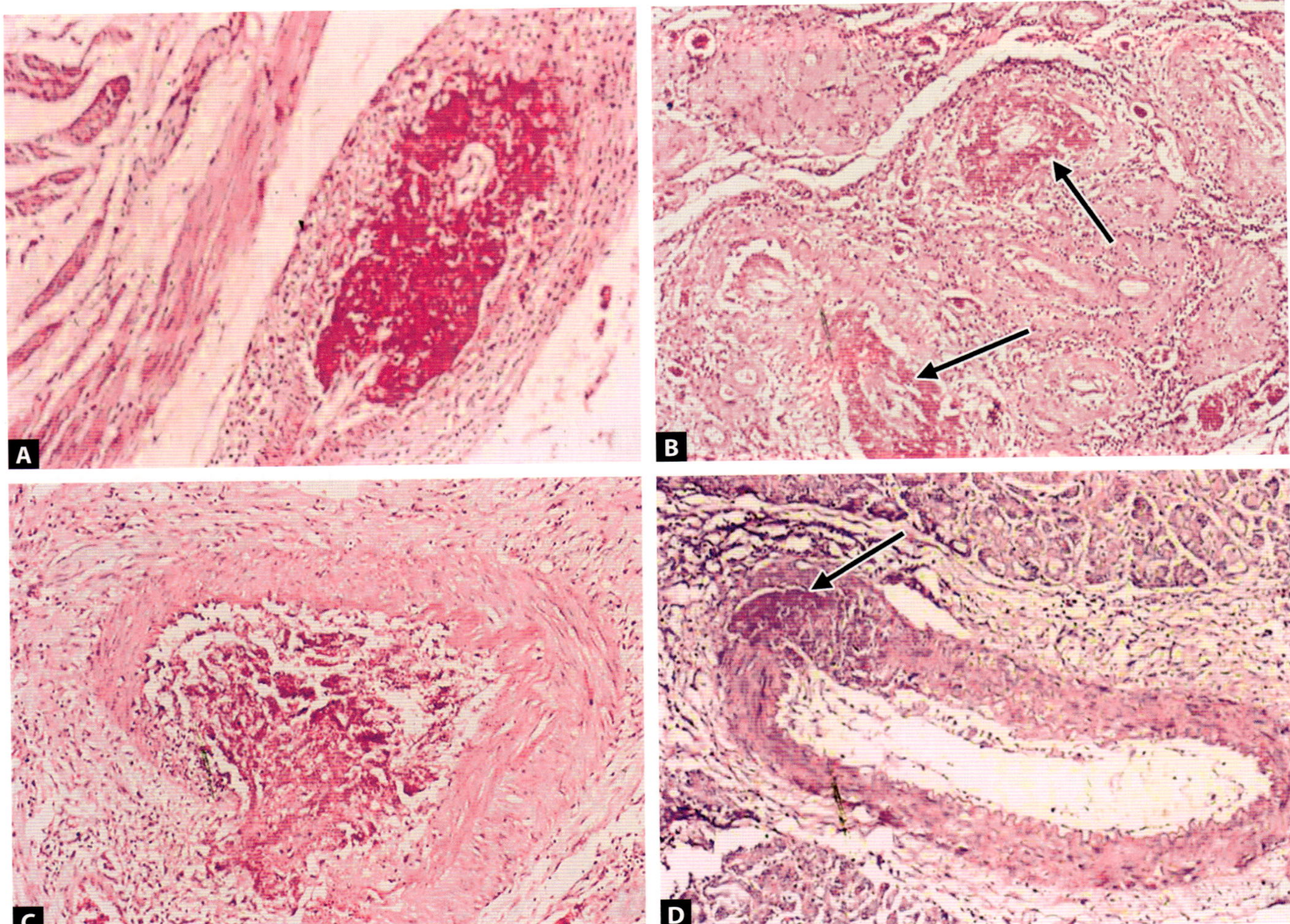

Figs 5A–D: Acute vasculitis seen in (A) Serosa of the stomach; (B) Ovary; (C) Periadrenal tissue; (D) Pancreas. Normal pancreatic acini can be seen in the vicinity.

- Adenomyosis and fibroid—Uterus.
- Pulmonary arterial hypertension grade 1.
- Mild right ventricular hypertrophy and right atrial dilatation.

For Microscopic Polyangiitis: See chapter on ***"Small Vessel Vasculitides"***.

COMMENTARY—INDEX CASE: PM 18473

This case of MPA was unique in a number of ways:

- Clinically the patient presented with upper and lower respiratory tract symptoms with diffuse consolidation of the lungs, a red eye and renal failure, so the clinicians could not go away from a diagnosis of GPA. At autopsy (after studying multiple sections) the lungs and upper respiratory tract did not show any diagnostic feature i.e. granulomatous vasculitis, necrosis and granulomatous inflammation to suggest a GPA (Wegener's). The presence of only capillaritis and hemorrhage seen in the lungs, in this case was more in favor of MPA. In MPA, upper respiratory tract disease and pulmonary involvement occurs in 33% and 50% of cases respectively and is caused by vasculitis alone and not by granulomatous inflammation.
- Travis et al in 1991[1] proposed the major and minor histopathologic features of GPA, which was based on 75 open lung biopsies, 11 lobectomies and one pneumonectomy in a cohort of 67 patients. Awareness about these non-specific changes is very important, as at times (18%) they may predominate the picture in open lung biopsies. Thus, the absence of the major diagnostic features of GPA does not exclude its diagnosis on a lung biopsy.

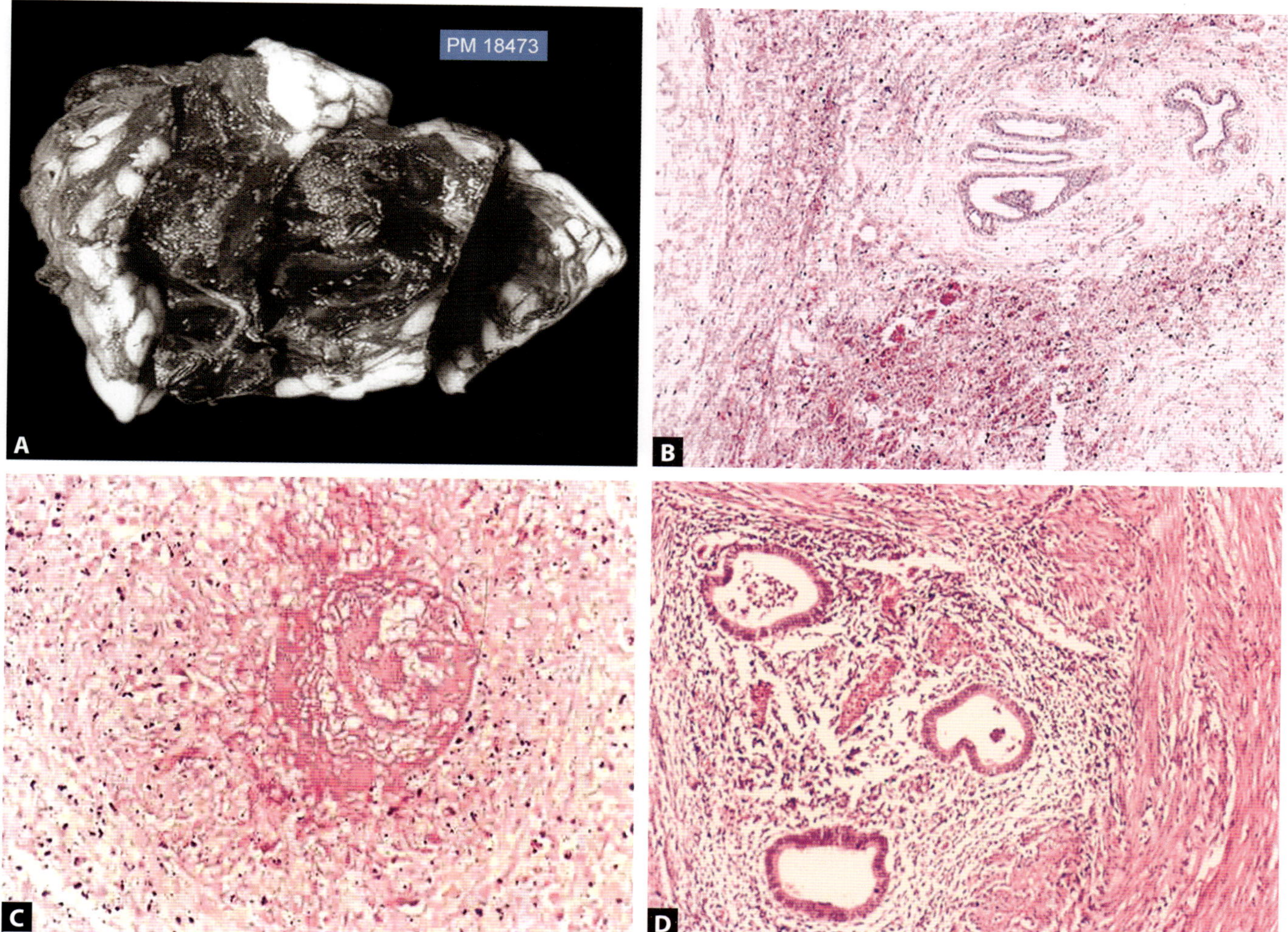

Figs 6A–D: (A) Breast mass showing extensive hemorrhagic; (B) Microphotograph from the breast mass shows hemorrhage and ducts; (C) Acute vasculitis seen in the breast; (D) Microphotograph from the uterus showing adenomyosis.

- Diffuse pulmonary hemorrhage is now considered a well-known and life-threatening complication of GPA. Travis et al[1] in their series of 34 cases of diffuse pulmonary hemorrhage confirmed on open lung biopsies, found GPA or probable GPA in 33% of their cases. In most of these cases of GPA, pulmonary hemorrhage was a minor associated finding but the major histologic features were also present. In cases where the hemorrhage was extensive, capillaritis was a frequent finding and in a few of these cases, no typical features of GPA could be identified. Few studies on lung biopsies have however shown that lung biopsies showing only hemorrhage and capillaritis, may either precede or follow the classic pathologic features of GPA.
- Going by the above statements, the index case can be labeled as a case of GPA (Wegener's). But it is important to keep in mind that the statement "Awareness about these non-specific changes is very important, as at times (18%) they may dominate the picture in open lung biopsies". Thus, the absence of the major diagnostic features of GPA does not exclude its diagnosis on a lung biopsy. It can be argued that the cases labeled as "GPA" by Travis et al[2] where only pulmonary hemorrhage with capillaritis was seen, assessment of the rest of the lung was not done as they were biopsies. Autopsy studies are few, but they bring out the picture of the entire lung as multiple sections are studied. So, the index autopsy case, where multiple sections were studied from the lung and only diffuse pulmonary hemorrhage with capillaritis was

noted, where no necrosis or granulomatous inflammation or granulomatous vasculitis was noted, would definitely fall more into the category of MPA, rather than GPA.

- Kidneys in the index case revealed a pauci-immune crescentic necrotizing glomerulonephritis (with segmental and diffuse lesions), granulomatous glomerular lesions (of all ages) and extraglomerular florid acute vasculitis, involving the interlobular arteries and afferent arterioles. The arcuate and interlobar arteries were not involved. Hence, according to the Chapel Hill Consensus Conference (CHCC 2012) this case fits very well with an ANCA negative, small vessel systemic vasculitis (SVV) and along with the pathological findings in the upper and lower respiratory tract, of capillaritis with absent granulomatous inflammation, seems consistent with a diagnosis of MPA.
- Granulomatous glomerulonephritis (of all ages) was noted in this case and this can be seen in cases of MPA as discussed in case 37.
- The spleen in the index case was converted into a bag of necrotic tissue. It showed florid vasculitis (acute, granulomatous and burnt out) of the small central arterioles and of the intraparenchymal arteries. Granulomatous arteritis was noted. The single extravascular granulomatous lesion seen in the spleen, cannot be confirmed to be truly extravascular. CHCC 2012 however mentions under MPA, in context with the lungs that "Inflammation that is not centered on vessels, including granulomatous inflammation is absent". There is however no mention about such a finding in extrapulmonary organ like spleen. Autopsy studies on vasculitides are few and splenic findings can only be picked up at autopsy.
- Approximately 90–95% cases with untreated active MPA are ANCA positive. ANCA can be negative in small vessel, systemic vasculitides, but negative ANCA in the index case with florid active disease is rather odd.
- MPA presenting as a breast mass has not been documented before.

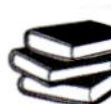

TAKE HOME MESSAGE

- Clinical mimicry of MPA and GPA is very common. In MPA, upper and lower respiratory tract involvement occurs in 33% and 50% of cases respectively and is caused by vasculitis alone and not by granulomatous inflammation.
- Diffuse pulmonary hemorrhage with capillaritis, if seen at autopsy with no evidence of any major histopathologic feature of GPA, should be considered more in favor of MPA.
- Granulomatous glomerulonephritis occurs in MPA.
- Granulomatous arteritis and extravascular granulomatous lesions seen in the spleen is odd. But literature does not speak on splenic lesions, as there is a paucity of autopsy studies.

REFERENCES

1. Travis WD, Hoffman GS, Leavitt RY, et al. Surgical pathology of the lung in Wegener's granulomatosis. Review of 87 open lung biopsies from 67 patients. Am J Surg Pathol. 1991;15(4):315-33.
2. Travis WD, Carpenter HC, Lie JT. Diffuse pulmonary hemorrhage: an uncommon presentation of Wegener's granulomatosis. Am J Surg Pathol 1987;11(9):701-8.

CONTRIBUTIONS BY:

1. Dr Ashish Bhalla, Professor, Department of Internal Medicine (Compilation of Clinical Details)
2. Dr Ranjana Minz, Professor and Head, Department of Immunopathology (ANCA testing)
3. Dr Vinay Sakhuja, Ex-Professor and Head, Department of Nephrology (Clinician In-Charge)

Post Graduate Institute of Medical Education and Research, Chandigarh, India

CASE 40

Microscopic Polyangiitis—Chronic Phase: PM 18987

Nandita Bharadwaj Kakkar

HIGHLIGHTS OF THE CASE

An 18-year-old male was admitted for nearly 3 months in our institute. He presented with renal failure, nephritic/ nephrotic picture, was antineutrophil cytoplasmic antibody (ANCA)/ antinuclear antibody (ANA) negative and kidney biopsy revealed a diffuse proliferative glomerulonephritis with no basement membrane thickening, crescents or vasculitis. A diagnosis of poststreptococcal glomerulonephritis was made. The patient deteriorated. Second renal biopsy showed a necrotizing glomerulonephritis with crescents, but with no extraglomerular vasculitis. He was then put on methylprednisolone followed by oral prednisolone and cyclophosphamide. At autopsy, a pauci-immune, focal proliferative, sclerosing glomerulonephritis with crescents and healed vasculitis (interlobular/arcuate arteries) was noted. Extrarenal healed vasculitis was seen in the heart, tunica and periadrenal arteries and acute vasculitis in the heart and lungs (capillaritis). Thus, renal lesions of small vessel vasculitis evolve with time and sequential biopsies may be needed to clinch the diagnosis.

Keywords: Microscopic polyangiitis, chronic phase, autopsy.

CLINICAL DETAILS

Date of Admission: 23.01.2003, Date of Death: 28.01.2003 and Duration of Hospital Stay: 5 days

An 18-year-old male had three admissions in PGIMER, Chandigarh.

First Admission

It was for a month in November 2002 (30-10-2002 to 30-11-2002). He was admitted with history of fever and sore throat which was there since 11 days. There was facial puffiness, pedal edema and decreased urinary output. The blood pressure (BP) was 170/90 mm Hg.

Investigations Hemogram: Revealed a Hb of 11.2 g/dL which later came down to 6.3 g/dL, TLC—15000/uL, DLC - P90,L6,M3,E1, peripheral blood film revealed a normocytic normochromic picture with hypersegmented polymorphs and toxic granules. Coagulation profile was normal. ***Blood biochemistry***: Renal functions tests: Serum creatinine was 4.5 mg% and later came down to 2.7 mg%, total proteins 6.6 gm, albumin being 3.1 gm. Complement levels were 47.4 mg/dL (N-50-90), ASO <200 (x2), CRP positive (x2), HBsAg, ANA, ANCA negative. ***Routine urine examination***—albumin 2+ with 12–15 RBC's, 24-hour urinary proteins 5 gm. ***Ultrasonography***—Right kidney 13.5 cm, Left kidney 12.7 cm, loss of corticomedullary distinction, ascites and bilateral pleural effusion. ***Kidney biopsy*** (s-13661/02) revealed a picture of diffuse proliferative glomerulonephritis with no basement membrane thickening, crescents or vasculitis. Immunofluorescence revealed IgG/fibrinogen in traces and IgM/IgA negative, C3 was 2+ along capillary loops with lobular accentuation. These findings were considered to be suggestive of poststreptococcal glomerulonephritis or membranoproliferative glomerulonephritis. He was treated with NSAIDS, antibiotics and was put on antitubercular therapy. He continued to be febrile and was further investigated. The ***urine/blood culture*** (x2) were sterile; ***Widal*** negative; ***Ascitic fluid***—150 cells/mm^3 with 70% polymorphs, proteins 1 gm/dL, Gram stain negative, culture sterile, proteins—1 gm/dL; ***Pleural fluid***—30 cells/mm^3 with 90% polymorphs, proteins 5 g/dl, sugar 77 mg/dL, ADA 7 IU/L, AFB negative on smear and culture; ***Echocardiography***—no vegetations, EKG – normal; ***Chest X-ray***—within normal limits; ***Mantoux***—negative; ***FNAC*** axillary lymph node—reactive hyperplasia; Bone marrow aspiration—mildly hypocellular, rest within normal limits; ***CT chest/abdomen***—enlarged kidneys, hepatomegaly, retroperitoneal lymph nodes (aorto-caval, para-aortic) 1–1.5 cms, bilateral pleural effusion seen. Edema and BP was controlled with amlodipine and diuretics, antitubercular therapy was started emperically and he was discharged on request.

Second Admission

The second admission (7-12-2002 to 14-01-2003, duration 5 weeks) was a week later when he came back with malaise, anorexia, nausea, vomiting, slurred speech and decreased urinary output. On examination he was conscious, flaps, myoclonic jerks, edema, ascites was seen and the BP was 150/100 mm Hg. ***Investigations*** revealed Hb of 7.8 g/dL, TLC of 14,000/uL (P86, L10, M2, E2), adequate platelets, serum creatinine 8.9 mg%, urea 300 mg%, total proteins/albumin 7.6/3 g, normal liver function tests, routine urine examination showed albumin 1+, 3–4 RBCs, few granular casts and 24-hour urinary proteins: 2.4 g. ***Kidney biopsy*** (s–15003/02) was repeated which revealed three glomeruli with a necrotizing glomerulonephritis and crescents. Rest of the glomeruli showed increased cellularity and infiltration with polymorphs. No vasculitis was seen. Repeat ANA and ANCA were negative. Antitubercular treatment was stopped, he was put on hemodialysis, antibiotics, antihypertensives were increased and blood transfusions were administered. He was given pulse Methylprednisolone followed by oral prednisolone and cyclophosphamide (on 26-12-2002).

Third Admission

In the third admission (23-01-2003 to 28-01-2003), he had low-grade fever, holocranial headache, cough with expectoration, two episodes of right focal seizures with secondary generalization associated with transient loss of consciousness for a day, orthopnea and hemoptysis. On examination, there was drowsiness, flaps, pallor, edema, raised jugular venous pressure (JVP), icterus, BP 150/90 mm Hg, orthopnea, purpuric and ecchymotic lesions, bilateral coarse crepitations and liver palpable 3 cm below the right costal margin. The renal function tests were markedly deranged, coagulopathy was present, D-dimers were positive, SGOT/SGPT were 99/86 U/L and X-ray chest showed bilateral lower/mid-zone alveolar shadows with cardiomegaly. He suffered a cardiorespiratory arrest and could not be revived. Final clinical diagnosis was Crescentic glomerulonephritis, bilateral bronchopneumonia, ? tuberculosis with ATT induced hepatitis, seizures ? accelerated hypertension. Cause of death–Sepsis.

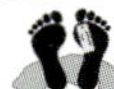 AUTOPSY FINDINGS: PM 18987

Two antemortem kidney biopsies had been done on this patient. The first (S-13661/02) one revealed diffuse proliferative glomerulonephritis with immunofluorescence (pathologists interpretation) indicating a pauci-immune nature with traces of IgG, IgA, IgM and fibrinogen. The second one (S–15003/02) showed a necrotizing crescentic glomerulonephritis. The ANCA (done both by immunofluorescence and ELISA) and ANA were negative. The patient succumbed to his illness. A complete autopsy was performed. All serous cavities were within normal limits. The ***kidneys*** together weighed 295 g and the external surface showed blotchy congestion with coarse scars (Figs 1A and B). The capsule was removed with difficulty. On cut section, the medulla was congested, a few arteries showed thrombosis and early infarcts were noted (Figs 1C and D). Both renal arteries and veins were normal. On microscopic examination the glomeruli (Figs 2A–F) showed proliferative lesions, synechiae formation, segmental sclerosis, fibrous (Figs 3A and B) and tubularized crescents (Fig 3C). No acute necrotizing lesion was seen. The interlobular and arcuate arteries showed evidence of healed vasculitis i.e. break of the internal elastic lamina, intimal fibroplasia, compromised lumen and recanalized thrombi (Figs 4A–F). Fresh thrombi were noted (Fig 3D). An occasional acute vasculitic lesion was seen in a small artery. Chronic interstitial inflammation, tubular atrophy and infarcts were seen (Fig 3E). ***Electron microscopy*** did not show any immune deposits (Fig 3F) and immunohistochemistry done for IgG, IgM, IgA, compliment and fibrinogen were negative. The diagnosis in the kidney was a pauci-immune focal proliferative, sclerosing glomerulonephritis with crescents, no necrotizing glomerular lesion, healed (an occasional fresh) vasculitis of the small sized arteries (interlobular and arcuate) with infarcts. The ***lungs*** weighed 1,350 g and the cut section showed hemorrhagic consolidation (Fig 5A). Microscopy (Figs 5B and C) revealed capillaritis with alveolar hemorrhages. There was no evidence of any tubercular focus. No necrosis, vasculitis or granulomatous inflammation was seen, thus negating granulomatosis with polyangiitis (GPA—Wegener's). The ***heart*** was normal grossly. Microscopically two foci of acute necrosis with nuclear debris and a small vessel showing fibrinoid necrosis were noted (Fig 5D). Occasional healed vasculitis was noted in the heart (Fig 5E). ***Periadrenal arteries*** and arteries in the tunica of the testes show healed vasculitis. The liver revealed feature of shock in the form of centrizonal hemorrhagic necrosis. The ***brain*** weighed 1,280 g, bilateral tonsillar herniation with mild uncal notching and edema was noted. There was no demyelination, lacunar infarcts or any vasculitis.

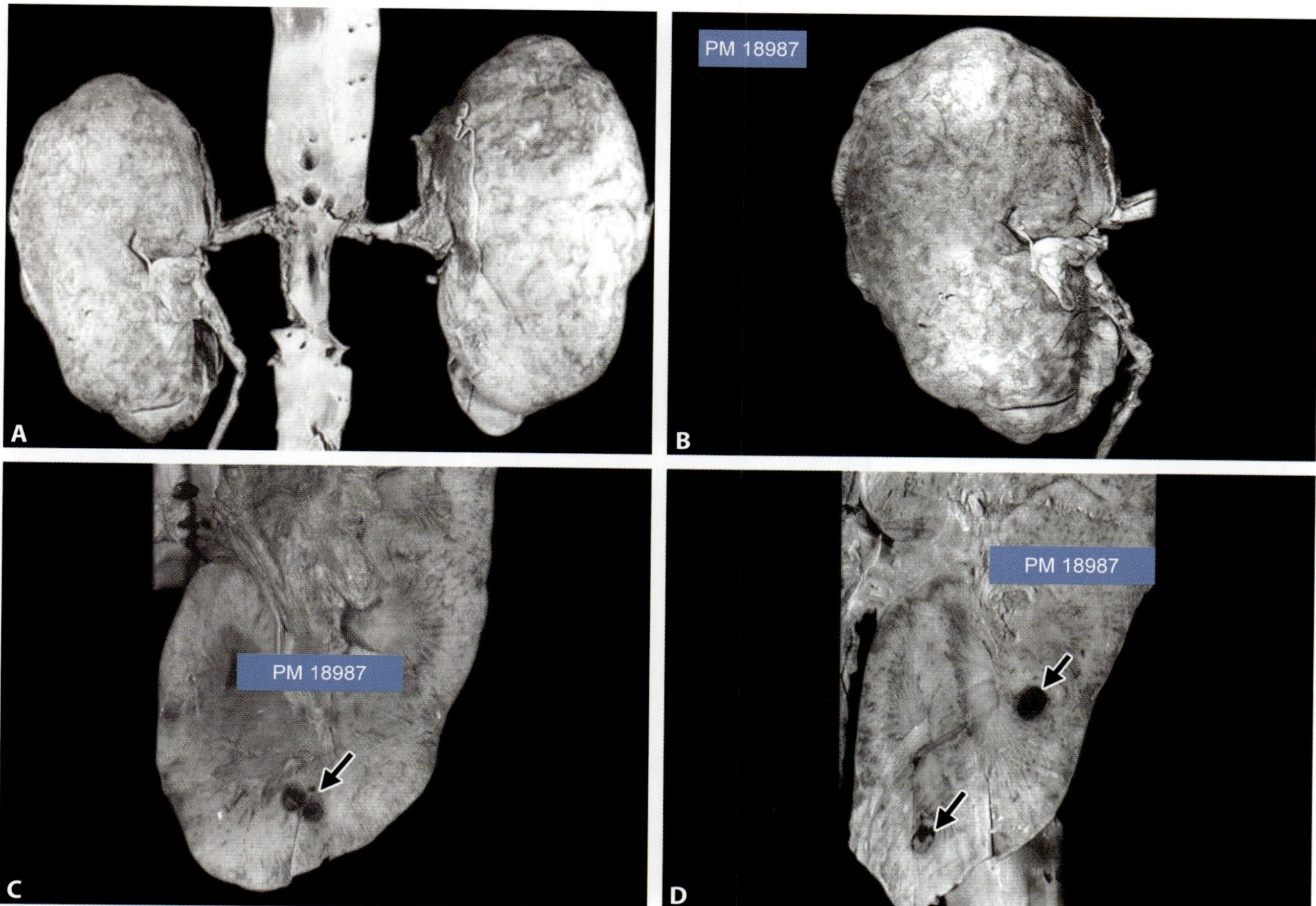

Figs 1A–D: (A and B) Gross picture of the kidneys showing blotchy congestion with coarse scars; (C and D) Cut section of the kidneys showing thrombosis (arrows) and infarcts.

FINAL AUTOPSY DIAGNOSIS: PM 18987

18 Years Male with Renal Failure

Microscopic polyangiitis: Chronic phase (ANCA negative):

- ***Kidneys***: Pauci-immune, focal proliferative sclerosing glomerulonephritis with crescents, predominantly healed (an occasional fresh) vasculitis of the small sized arteries (interlobular and arcuate) with infarcts
- ***Vasculitis***: Heart (acute and chronic), tunica and periadrenal arteries (healed)
- Pulmonary hemorrhages with capillaritis.

Shock: Liver, Cerebral edema.

For microscopic polyangiitis: See chapter on Small Vessel Vasculitis.

COMMENTARY—INDEX CASE: PM 18987

This was a young-male who had three admissions in our institute. In the first admission (duration—1 month), he came with history of fever and sore throat since 11 days and investigations revealed deranged renal function tests, hematuria, albuminuria with a nephrotic range proteinuria (5 g/24 hours), normal sized kidneys and negative ANCA/ANA. Kidney biopsy revealed a focal proliferative glomerulonephritis with no basement membrane thickening, crescents or vasculitis. Immunofluorescence revealed a pauci-immune nature of the disease. He was treated on lines of poststreptococcal glomerulonephritis. A week after discharge, he came back with worsening of symptoms and markedly deranged renal function tests. Repeat kidney biopsy showed a necrotiz-

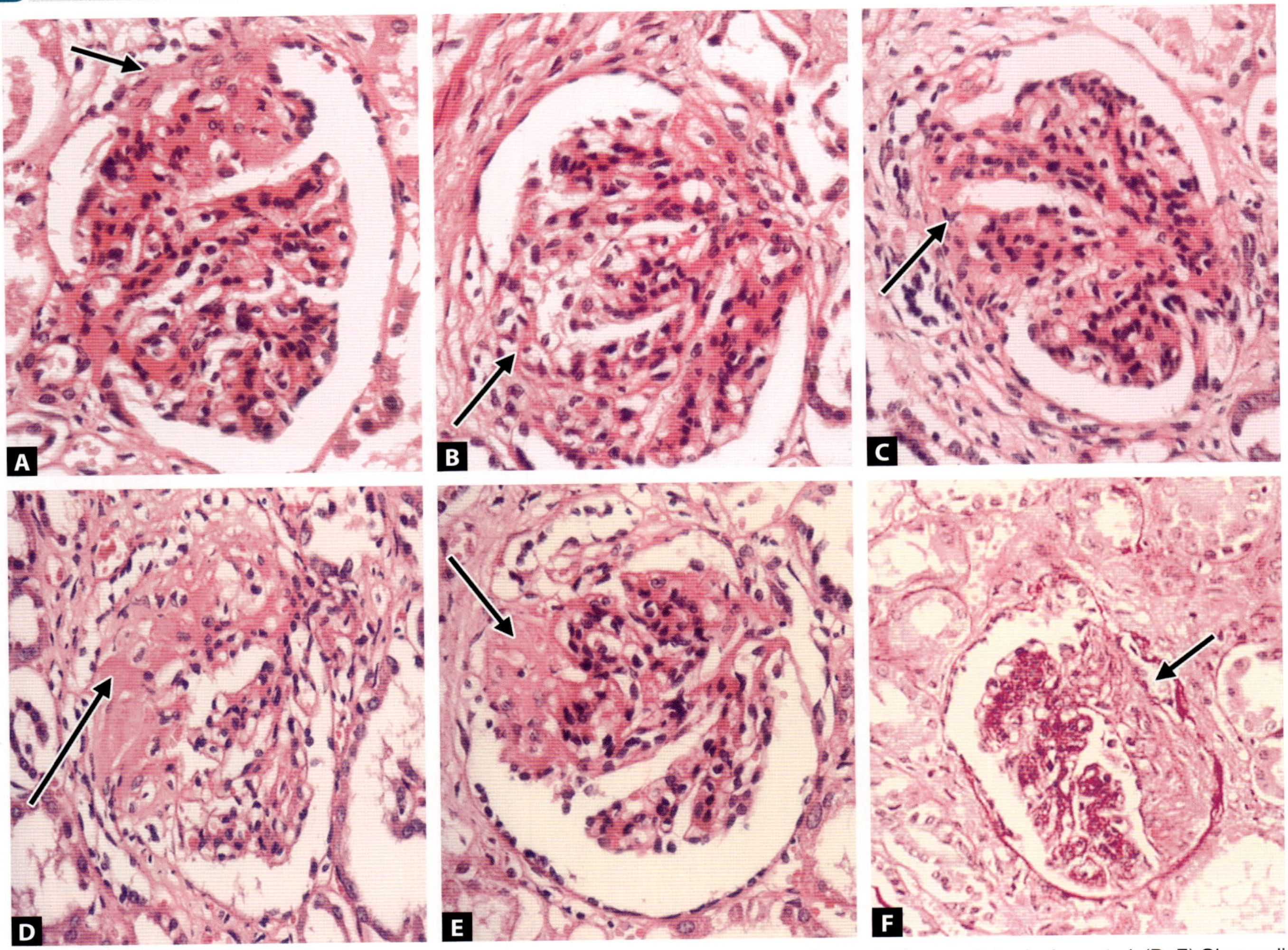

Figs 2A–F: (A–C) Glomeruli showing diffuse proliferative lesions with synechiae formation (arrows). No necrotizing lesion noted; (D–F) Glomeruli showing varying degrees of segmental sclerosis of the glomerular tuft (arrows).

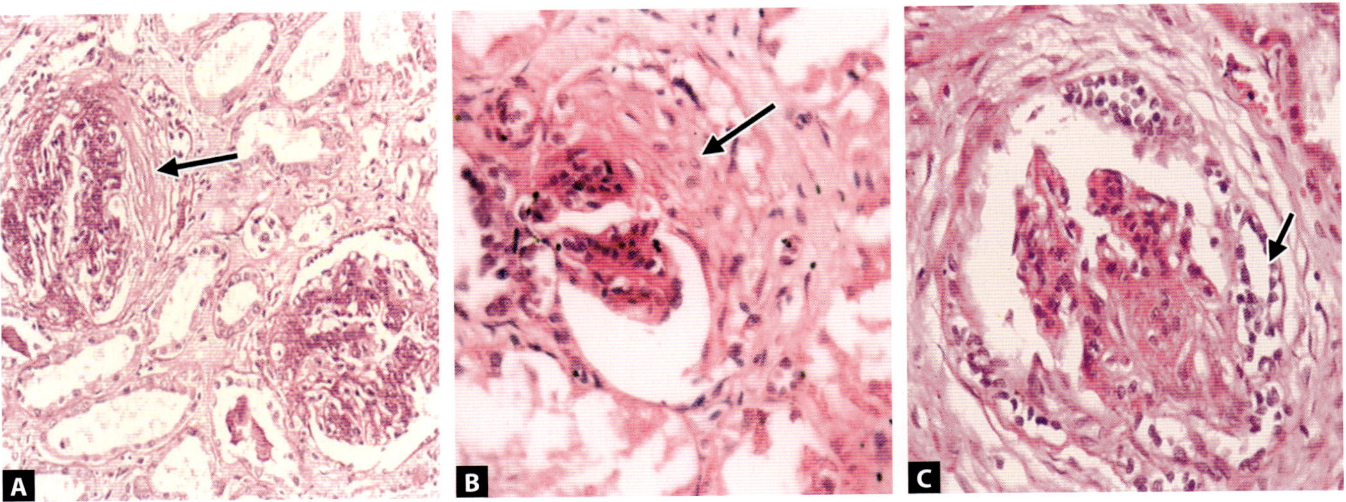

Figs 3A–C

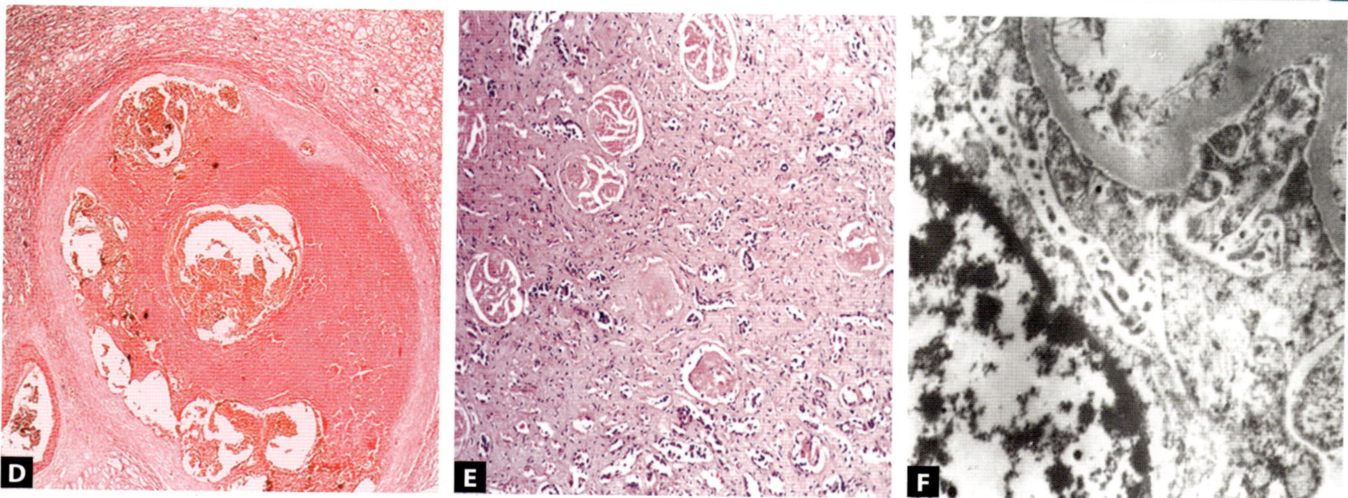

Figs 3A–F: Glomeruli showing (A and B) Fibrous crescents (arrows); (C) Tubularized crescent (arrow); (D) Arcuate artery showing thrombosis; (E) Photomicrograph of the kidney showing infarct; (F) Electron microscopy does not show any immune deposits.

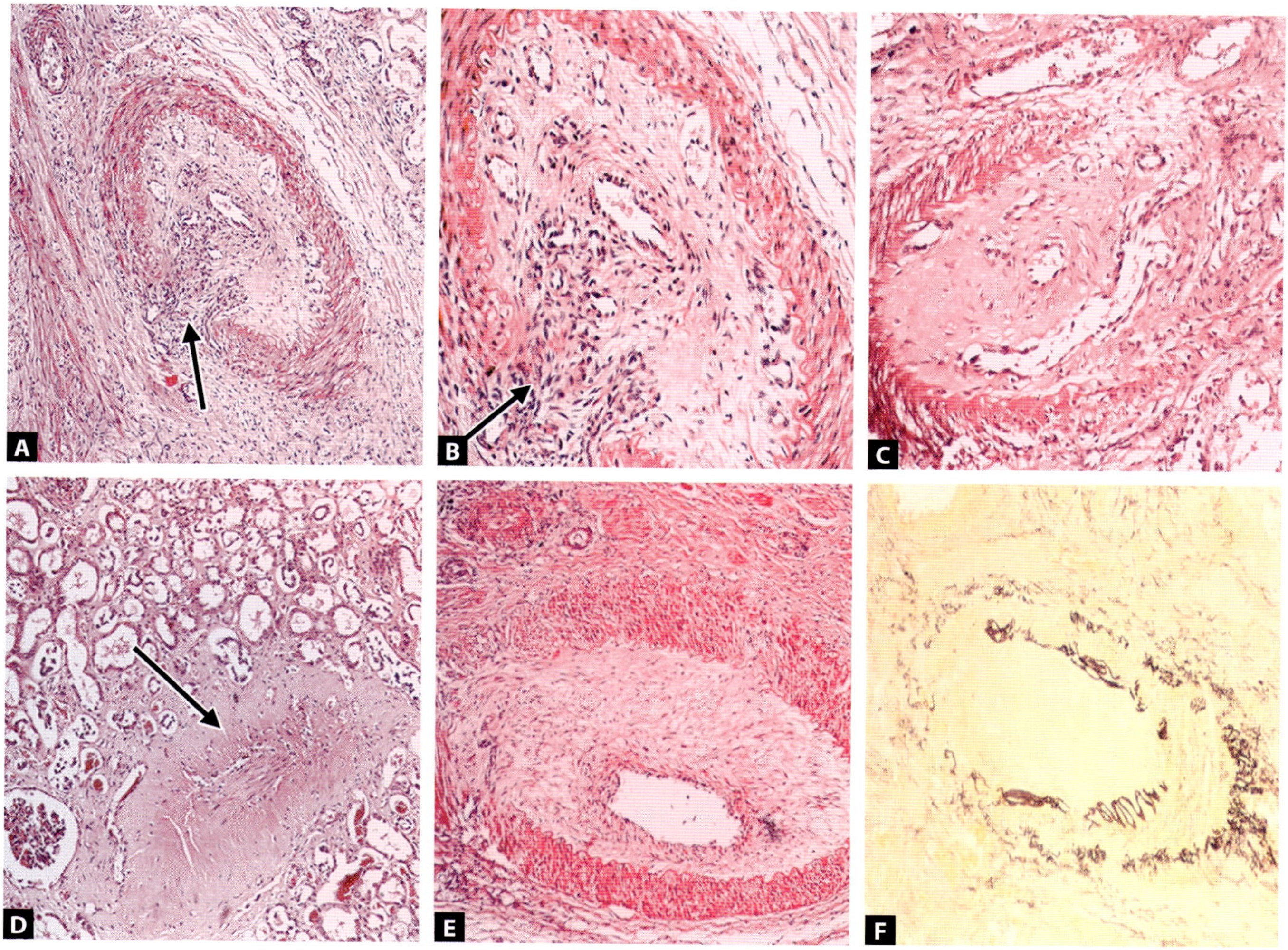

Figs 4A–F: Photomicrographs of the kidney. (A–C) Arcuate arteries showing healed vasculitis with break of the internal elastic lamina (arrows) and recanalization; (D and E) Healed vasculitis with near total occlusion of the lumina; (F) Elastic Verhoeff-Van Gieson stain showing break of the internal elastic lamina.

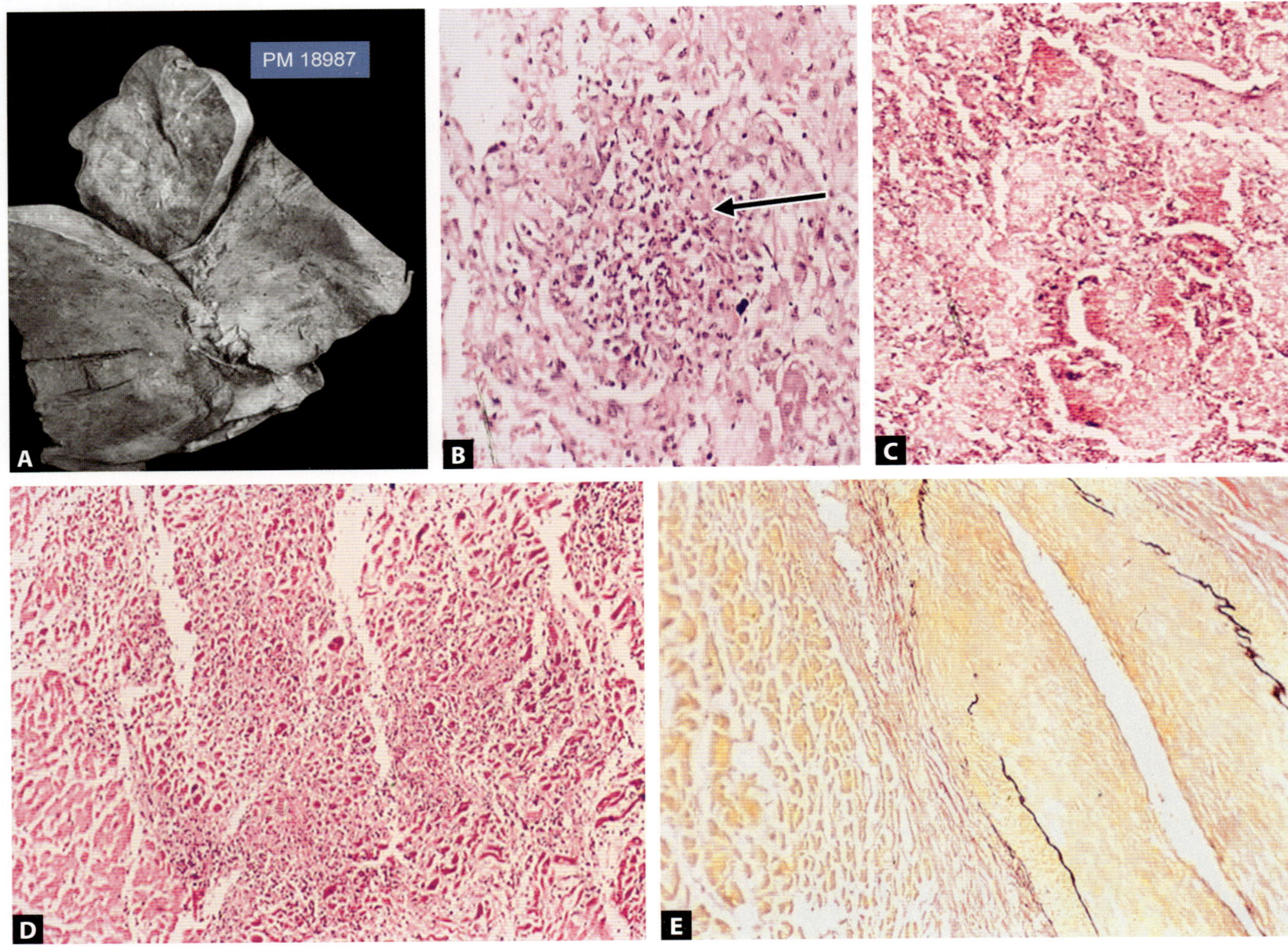

Figs 5A–E: (A) Cut section of the lung showing areas of hemorrhagic consolidation; (B) Photomicrograph of the lung showing a focus of capillaritis (arrow); (C) Lung showing alveolar hemorrhage; (D) Photomicrograph of the heart showing focus of acute vasculitis with polymorphs and nuclear debris; (E) Healed vasculitis in the heart showing break of the internal elastic lamina (Elastic Verhoeff-Van Gieson).

ing glomerulonephritis and crescents. No vasculitis was however seen. Repeat ANA and ANCA were negative. This time he underwent hemodialysis and was put on methylprednisolone followed by oral prednisolone and cyclophosphamide. In the third admission, 10 day later, he came with worsening symptoms, was hospitalized for a week, but succumbed to his illness. He had methylprednisolone followed by prednisolone and cyclophosphamide for 1 month before demise. At autopsy, a pauci-immune, focal proliferative, sclerosing glomerulonephritis with crescents and healed (occasional acute) vasculitis (interlobular/arcuate arteries) was noted. Extrarenal vasculitis, mostly healed was seen in the heart, tunica and periadrenal arteries. Capillaritis was seen in the lungs along with pulmonary hemorrhage. The kidney lesions, both glomerular and those seen in the small arteries were in the chronic phase. This was due to the effect of treatment and the patient seemed to have responded well to it. But there was evidence of acute vasculitis in the heart and capillaritis in the lungs led to pulmonary hemorrhage, which took away the patient. This case highlights the fact that two antemortem renal biopsies were done and vasculitis could not be demonstrated, although at autopsy healed extraglomerular vasculitis was prominent in the kidneys, which at the time of the biopsy must have been acute. In the first biopsy, glomeruli showed diffuse proliferative changes with no necrotizing lesion or crescents. But in the second biopsy, necrotizing lesion and crescents were noted. ANCA or ANA were negative throughout. Thus, renal lesions of small vessel vasculitis evolve with time and sequential biopsies may be needed to clinch the diagnosis.

TAKE HOME MESSAGE

- Renal lesions of small vessel vasculitis, evolve with time and sequential biopsies may be needed to clinch the diagnosis
- Diagnosis of small vessel vasculitis is an enigma.

CONTRIBUTIONS BY:

1. Dr Ranjana Minz, Professor and Head, Department of Immunopathology (ANCA testing)
2. Dr Vinay Sakhuja, Ex-Professor and Head, Department of Nephrology (Clinician In-Charge)

Post Graduate Institute of Medical Education and Research, Chandigarh, India.

CASE 41

Microscopic Polyangiitis with Acute Vasculitis of Small, Medium and Large-sized Arteries: PM 20415

Nandita Bharadwaj Kakkar

HIGHLIGHTS OF THE CASE

A 52-year-old female was hospitalized with fever, vomiting, reduced urinary output, altered sensorium and joint pains. She had a right mid zone opacity in the lung, deranged renal function tests with microscopic hematuria and respiratory distress. During the hospital stay she developed purpuric rashes on the palms and soles along with non-tender papules on the pulp of the fingers and toes. Antemortem anti-neutrophil cytoplasmic antibody (ANCA) testing was not done. A clinical diagnosis of bronchopneumonia ? tubercular ? pyogenic; acute renal failure ? acute cortical necrosis ? rapidly progressive glomerulonephritis (RPGN); encephalopathy ? metabolic ? sepsis was made. At autopsy, the case was labeled as cANCA positive microscopic polyangiitis (MPA) showing a pauci immune, necrotizing crescentic glomerulonephritis with granulomatous glomerulonephritis, occasional granulomatous arteritis with systemic acute vasculitides affecting the small, medium and large-sized arteries. Worth stressing point in this case was—arteries of all sizes were involved by the vasculitic process—large (abdominal aorta, right common carotid, left anterior descending), medium (spleen, mesenteric, interlobar artery of the kidney) and small including arterioles and capillaries (kidney, spleen, skin, colon, ovary, liver, bone marrow, lymph node, pericardium and periadrenal tissue).

Keywords: microscopic polyangiitis, granulomatous glomerulonephritis, granulomatous arteritis, involvement of large, medium and small-sized arteries, autopsy.

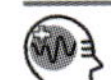

CLINICAL DETAILS

Date of Admission: 03.01.2005, Date of Death: 08.01.2005 and Duration of Hospital Stay: 5 Days.

A 52-year-old female came with fever (low to moderate grade, intermittent, up to 102°F) of 2 months duration, vomiting and reduced urinary output since 1 month, joint pains involving large/small joints since 2–3 weeks and altered sensorium since 1 week. Chest X-ray done outside showed right mid zone consolidation and she was put on anti-tubercular therapy, following which she developed vomiting. Rifampicin was stopped, but the vomiting continued and she also developed loss of appetite. There was no history of pain abdomen, bowel alteration or weight loss. A month before admission, she developed decreased urine output, 150–300 mL/day and was found to have raised serum creatinine. She received four hemodialysis and seven units of blood transfusion. On ***examination*** she was drowsy, incoherent, afebrile, pulse 88/min, blood pressure (BP) 130/70 mm Hg and respiratory rate 24/min. There was no pallor, cyanosis, jaundice, clubbing, lymphadenopathy and the jugular venous pressure was not raised. Edema feet was present. On chest auscultation, bronchial breathing was present in the right inter/infrascapular regions along with bilateral basal crepitations along with decreased air entry and occasional wheeze. Flow murmur and pericardial rub was identified. She was not oriented to time, place and person. There was debatable neck rigidity, no focal deficit, plantars were mute and she was moving all four limbs. ***Investigations*** revealed a hemoglobin (Hb) of 8.7 g/dL, TLC of 11,800/uL, DLC P67, L30, M2, E1, platelets: 1,13000/uL, ESR: 135 mm first hour, random blood sugar: 72 mg%, serum bilirubin: 3.5 mg% and later 0.7 mg%, aspartate transaminase/ alanine transaminase (SGOT/SGPT): 67/112 U/L, alkaline phosphatase: 27 U/L, total proteins: 5.8 g, albumin: 2.9 g, globulins: 3 g, serum urea: 120 mg% and serum creatinine: 6.3 mg%. HBsAg, serum electrophoresis of urine for Bence–Jones proteins, HIV, antinuclear antibody (ANA) and blood/urine culture were negative. X-ray chest showed a right mid zone consolidation. On ultrasonography, both kidneys revealed increased echogenicity with accentuated corticomedullary distinction and left pleural effusion. Routine urine examination showed 8–10 pus cells, RBCs were full-field and there were no eosinophils. CSF examination showed proteins: 1.6 g%, sugar: 12 mg% (RBS 120), WBCs nil, RBCs ++ and adenosine deaminase (ADA) of 11. ANCA was not done. ***Course in hospital***: Patient was given hemodialysis and antibiotics, anti-tubercular therapy was stopped due to rise in serum bilirubin which later came down to normal, patient was mostly afebrile and the urinary output ranged from nil to 150 mL/day. Four days after admission she developed rash on the palms and soles. On dermatology consultation a crusted ulcer was noticed on the left little finger along with purpuric nontender papules on the pulp of the fingers and toes. She soon developed sudden onset shortness of breath and a possibility of pulmonary hemorrhage was kept. The respiratory distress worsened to which she succumbed. Units final diagnosis was bronchopneumonia ? tubercular ? pyogenic; acute renal failure ? acute cortical necrosis ? RPGN ; encephalopathy ? metabolic ? sepsis.

AUTOPSY FINDINGS: PM 20415

A complete autopsy was performed. The peritoneal cavity yielded 500 mL of straw-colored fluid. The ***kidneys*** weighed 240 g. The external surface and cut section showed multiple infarcts and blotchy congestion (Figs 1A–C). The renal arteries were within normal limits. On microscopic examination, the glomeruli revealed few crescents (Fig 1D) and a florid necrotizing glomerulonephritis with few segmental (Figs 1E and 2A) and predominantly diffuse lesions. Florid acute glomerulitis (Figs 2B–D) with complete destruction of the glomerulus by an acute necrotizing inflammation (polymorphs and nuclear debris) was a prominent feature. Granulomatous glomerulonephritis (Figs 2E and F) wherein epithelioid cells and giant cells are seen surrounding a glomerulus, which shows diffuse necrotizing lesion along with break in the Bowman's capsule were noted. Acute florid transmural acute inflammation with nuclear debris and fibrinoid necrosis was seen affecting the interlobar, arcuate and interlobular arteries as well as afferent arterioles (Figs 3A–F and 4A). Occasional granulomatous arteritis (Fig 4B) was seen, where an artery showing inflammatory changes in the wall, was surrounded by epithelioid cells and giant cells. Elastic stains showed extensive destruction of the internal elastic lamina (Fig 4C). Multiple infarcts and dense interstitial inflammation was also seen. Immunohistochemistry done for IgG, IgM, IgA, C3 and fibrinogen was negative, hence indicating the pauci-immune nature of the glomerulonephritis. cANCA (on the postmortem serum) was strongly positive by both indirect immunofluorescence and by ELISA technique. Thus, the diagnosis in the kidney was a cANCA positive, pauci immune, necrotizing crescentic glomerulonephritis with granulomatous glomerulonephritis with extraglomerular acute vasculitis affecting the interlobar (medium sized), arcuate, interlobular, small intraparenchymal arteries, arterioles, capillaries and venules with occasional granulomatous arteritis. The differential diagnosis at this point was a small vessel vasculitides (since glomerular capillaries are affected) either GPA or MPA. To decide upon this, pathology in the upper and lower respiratory tract gives the answer as renal lesions in both entities are indistinguishable. The ***lungs*** (Fig 5A) weighed 520 g and grossly were subcrepitant to feel, but did not show any area of necrosis, infarcts or hemorrhage. Microscopic examination (Figs 5B and C) revealed an occasional area of capillaritis but no hemorrhage was noted. No lesions of granulomatosis with polyangiitis (GPA), i.e. Wegener's granulomatous were seen in the lungs or in the lower respiratory tract. The ***spleen*** weighed 200g and its capsular aspect and cut section showed multiple geographic areas of infarction converting it into a bag of necrotic tissue (Fig 5D). Microscopy (Figs 5E and F) revealed acute vasculitis with fibrinoid necrosis of the small and medium-sized arteries. The ***heart*** weighed 290 g, parietal and visceral pericardium (Fig 6A) was thickened with fibrinous tags but the valves and chambers were normal. The arch of the aorta and its branches were normal (Fig 6B). Microscopy showed acute fibrinous pericarditis (Fig 6C) and acute vasculitis of the small vessels of the pericardium (Fig 6D). Left anterior descending artery (Fig 6E) showed acute vasculitis with transmural inflammatory infiltrate. Sections studied from the arch of aorta were normal but the right common carotid artery showed florid intimitis (Fig. 6F). Sections studied from the abdominal aorta also showed florid intimitis (Figs 7A and B). Discrete small ulcers were present diffusely in the ***colon*** (Fig 7C), which revealed acute vasculitis with fibrinoid necrosis of the mucosal and

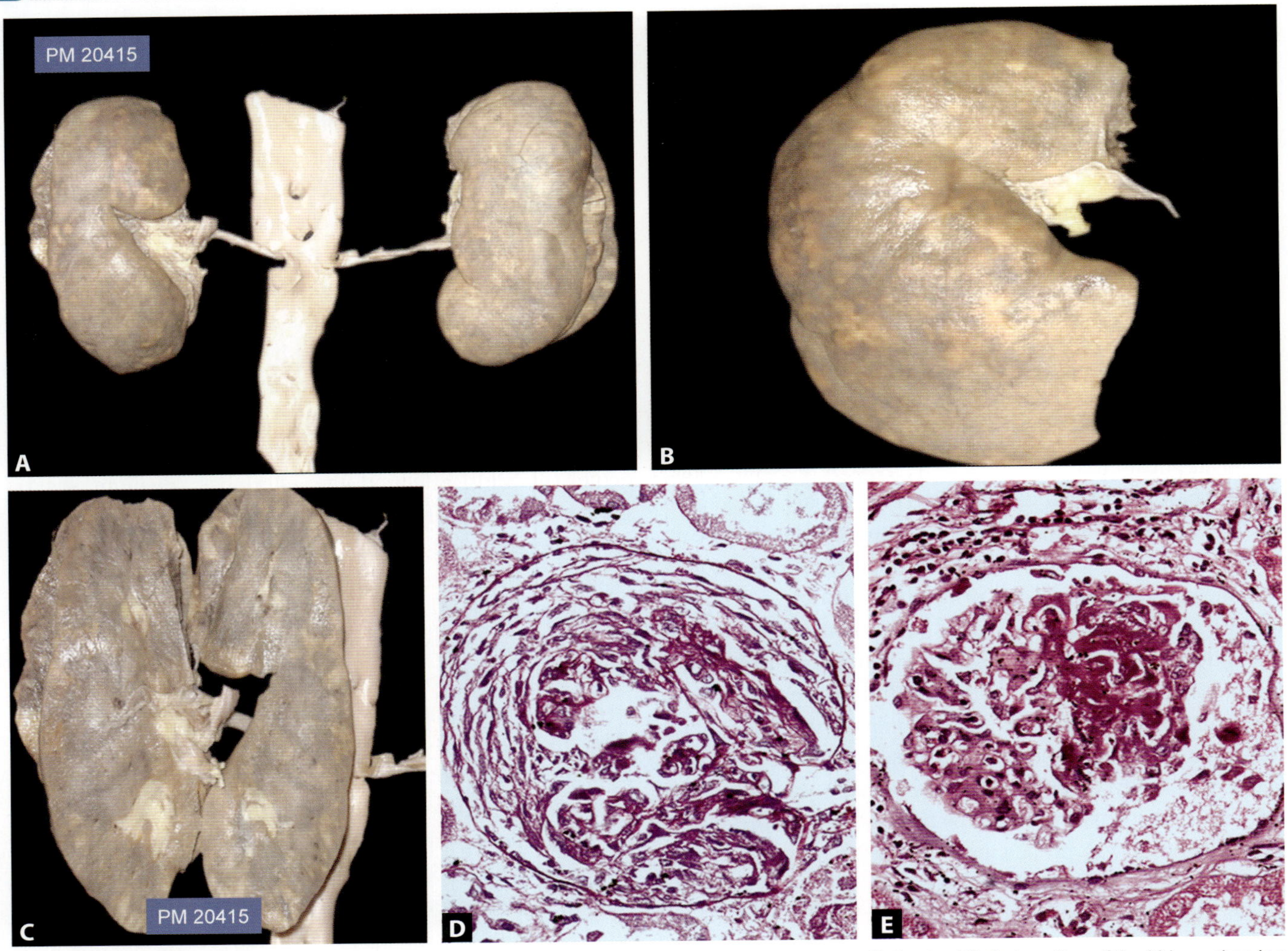

Figs 1A–E: (A and B) External aspect of the kidneys, showing multiple pale and irregular areas of infarcts; (C) Cut section of the kidney showing pale infarcts, many in the subcortical area. Photomicrographs of the kidney (PAS stain) showing; (D) A crescent; and (E) Segmental fibrinoid necrosis.

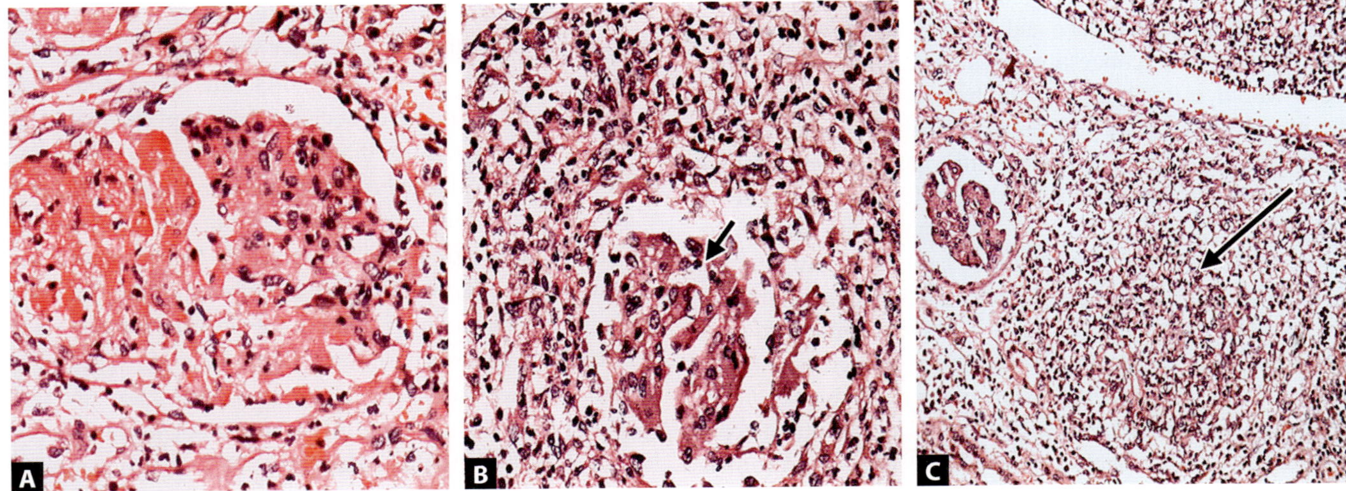

Figs 2A–C:

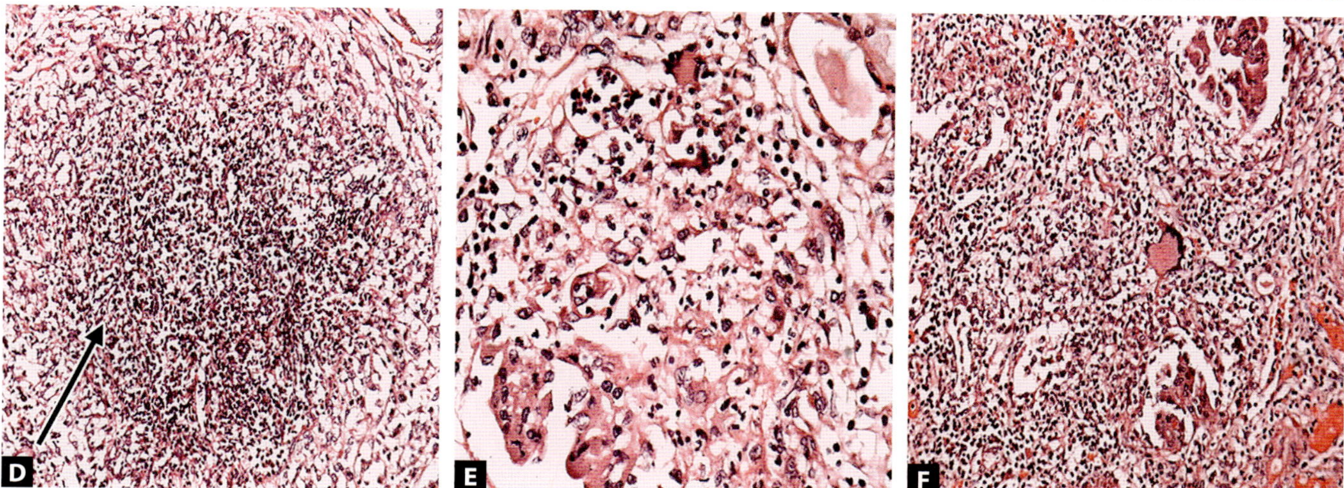

Figs 2A–F: Glomeruli showing (A) Segmental necrosis; (B) Acute glomerulitis where part of the glomerulus (arrow) is visible; (C) Acute glomerulitis where a vague impression of a glomerulus is visible at low power (arrow); (D) Acute glomerulitis where the glomerulus is totally destroyed by acute inflammation, mimicking an abscess (arrow); (E and F) Glomeruli in the process of destruction with surrounding giant cells, i.e. granulomatous reaction.

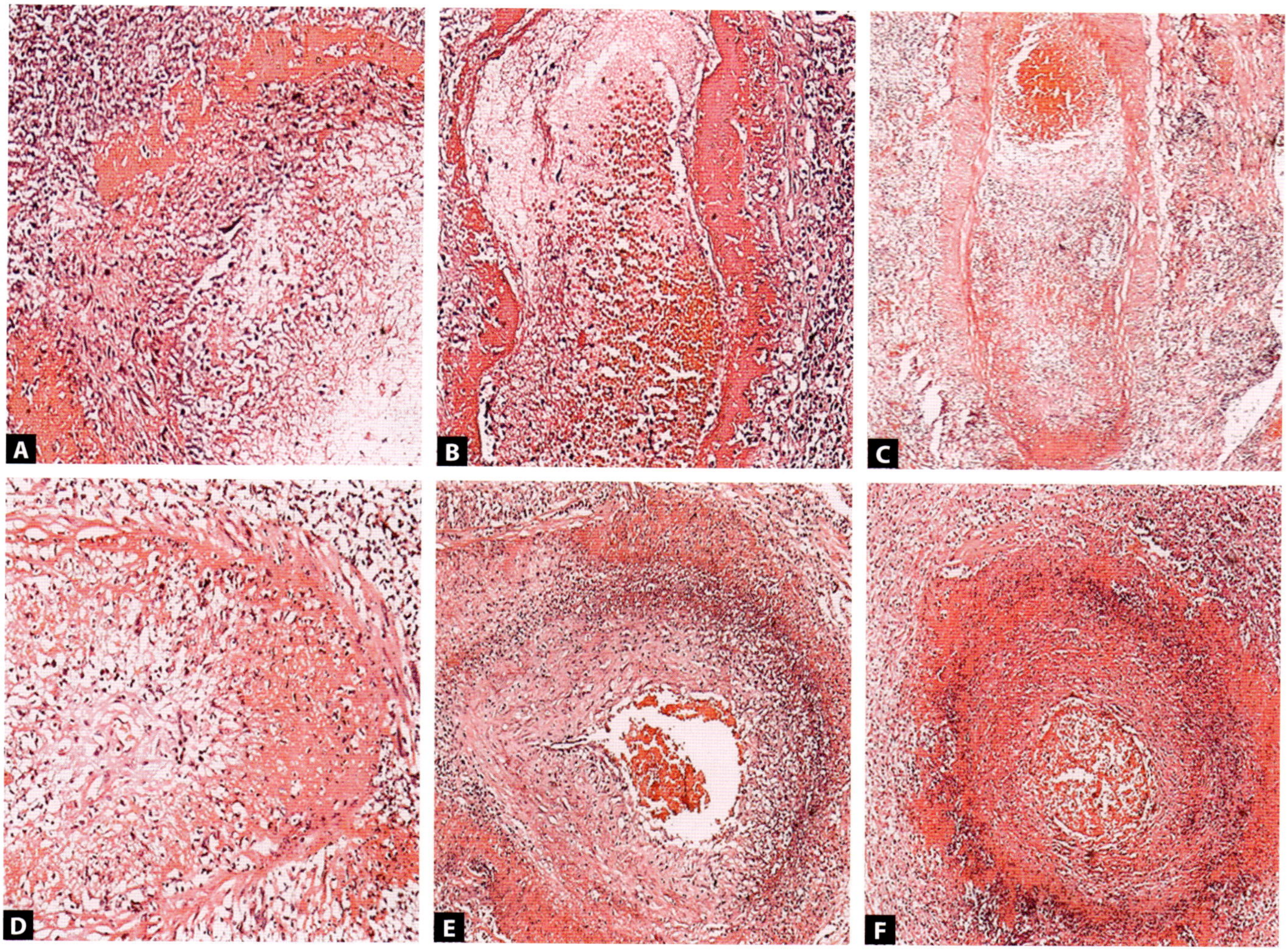

Figs 3A–F: Renal acute vasculitis with transmural necrotizing inflammation, nuclear debris and fibrinoid necrosis in (A and B) Interlobar arteries; (C and D) Arcuate artery; (E and F) Interlobular arteries.

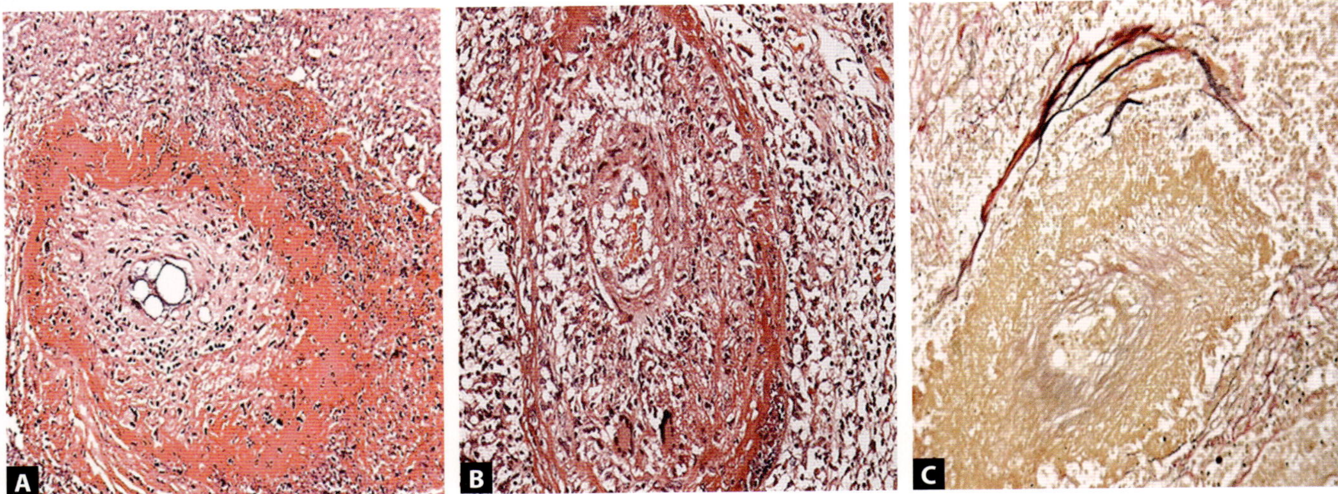

Figs 4A–C: Renal vasculitis. (A) Acute vasculitis in interlobular artery; (B) Granulomatous arteritis with palisading epithelioid cells and giant cells; (C) Elastic Van Gieson stain showing break of the internal elastic lamina.

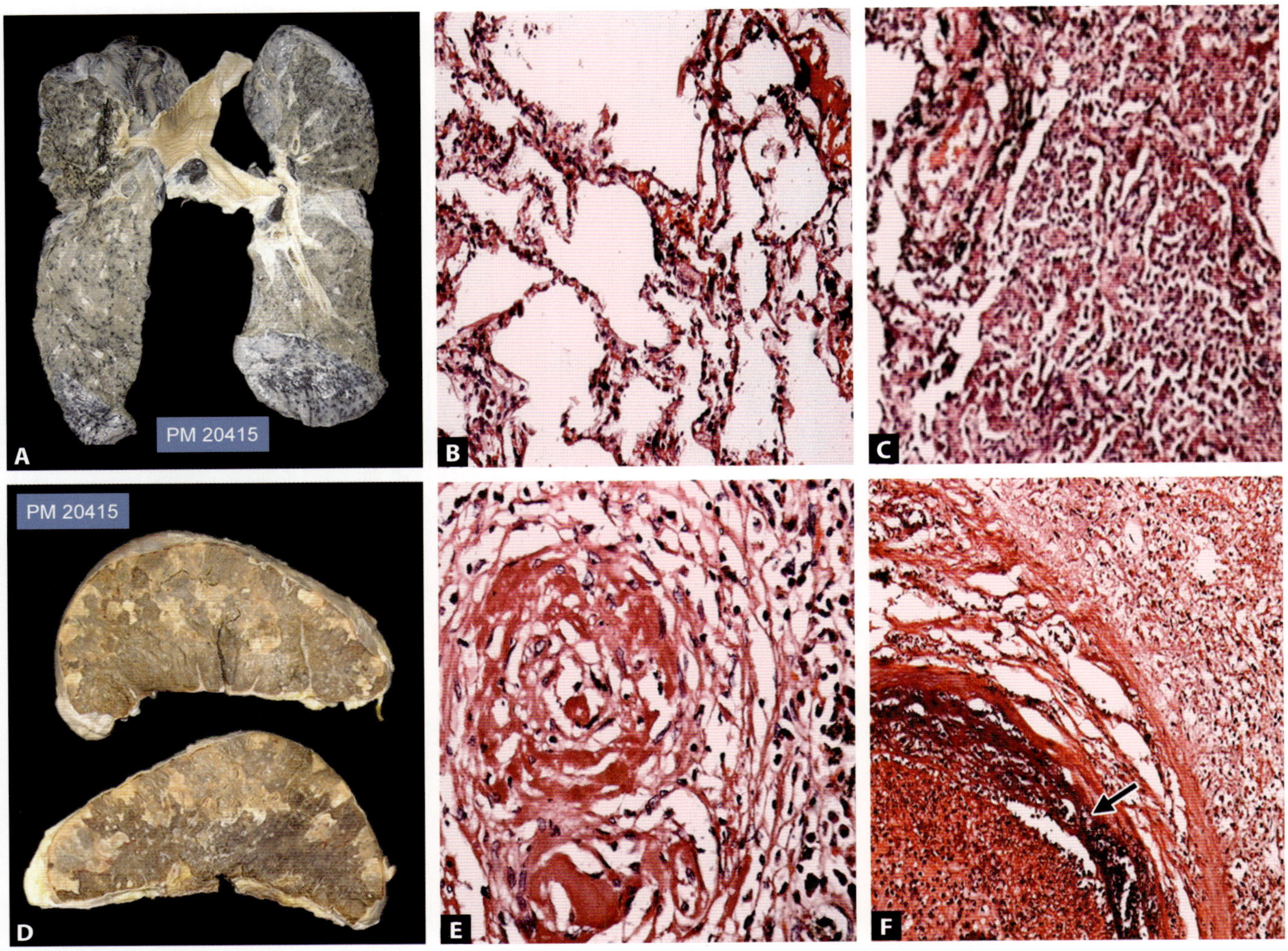

Figs 5A–F: (A) Gross picture of the lungs (cut section) which does not show any hemorrhage, necrosis or nodule; (B) Lung showing normal alveolar spaces. No hemorrhage is seen; (C) Lung showing focal capillaritis; (D) Coronal slices of the spleen showing multiple geographic areas of infarction; (E) Acute vasculitis of the central arteriole of the spleen; (F) Acute vasculitis of the medium-sized artery of the spleen (arrow). Only a part of the artery is in the photograph.

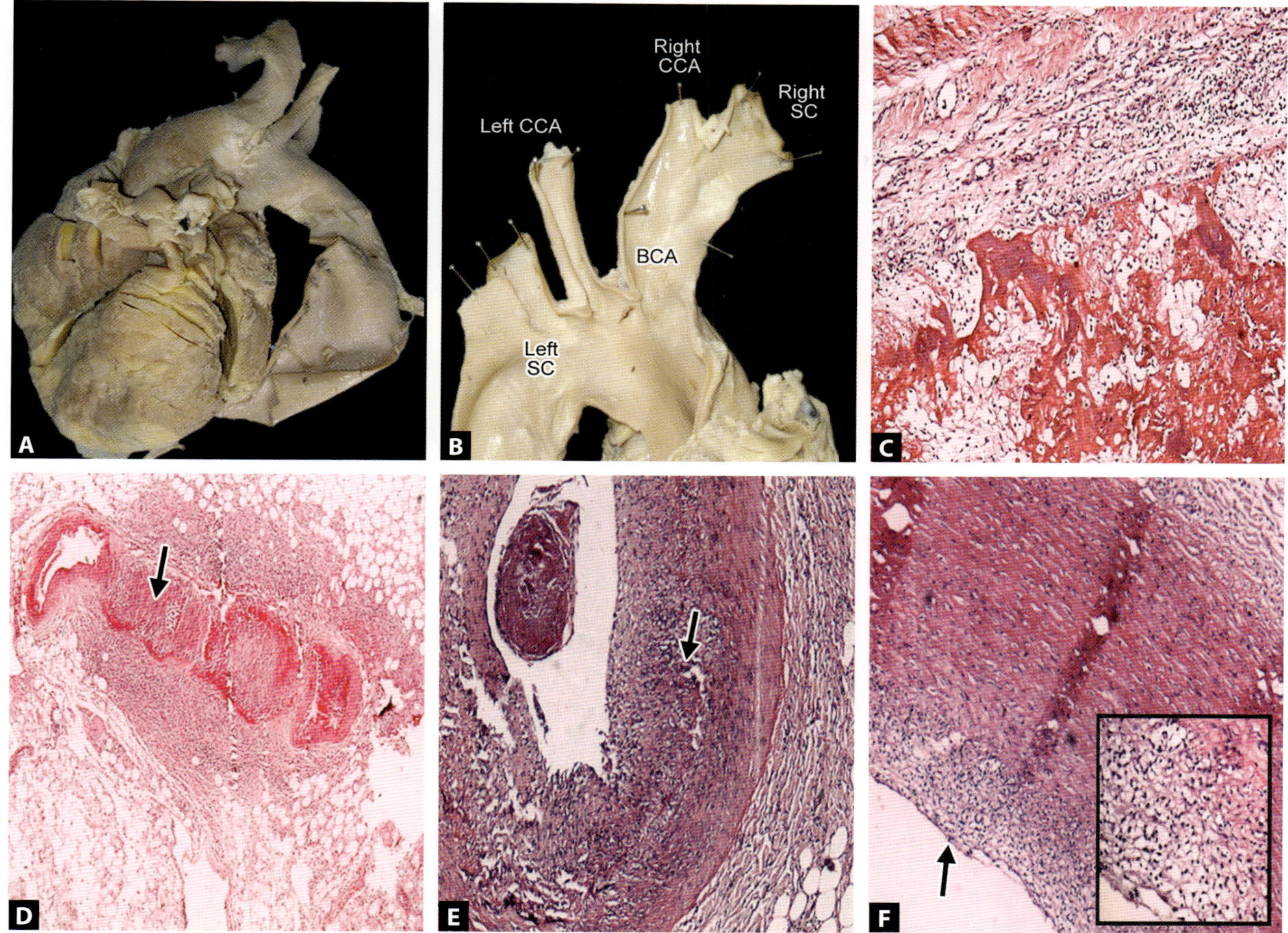

Figs 6A–F: (A) Gross picture of the heart showing pericarditis; (B) Arch of the aorta is normal. Photomicrographs of the heart showing; (C) Acute fibrinous pericarditis; (D) Acute vasculitis seen in the pericardial vessels (arrow); (E) Left anterior descending artery showing acute inflammatory cells in the intima and media (arrow); (F) Right common carotid artery showing acute intimitis (arrow) with polymorphs and nuclear debris (inset).

submucosal small vessels (Figs 7D and E). Acute vasculitis (Figs 8A–E) was also seen in the peradrenal arteries, small arteries of the lymph nodes, ovary, liver and few medium-sized arteries of the mesentery. Skin (Fig 8F) biopsies taken from the lesional areas showed acute vasculitis. In the brain (Figs 9A and B), there was subarachnoid hemorrhage over the cerebellum and at the base. The left vertebral artery was rudimentary. Sections examined did not show any vasculitis, but however it cannot be ruled out.

FINAL AUTOPSY DIAGNOSIS: PM 20415

52 Years Old Female, c-ANCA Positive

- Cytoplasmic anti-neutrophil cytoplasmic antibody (c-ANCA) positive microscopic polyangiitis (MPA)
- Pauci-immune necrotizing glomerulonephritis with crescents, lorid acute glomerulitis and granulomatous glomerulonephritis.
- Acute vasculitis of the small arteries, including arterioles and capillaries (kidney, spleen, skin, colon, ovary, liver, bone marrow, lymph node, pericardium and periadrenal tissue), medium arteries (spleen, mesenteric, interlobar artery of the kidney) and large arteries (abdominal Aorta/right common carotid/left anterior descending). Occasional granulomatous arteritis seen in the kidney.
- Fibrinous pericarditis
- Focal resolving bronchopneumonia
- Subarachnoid hemorrhage—base of the brain.

For microscopic polyangiitis: See chapter on 'Small Vessel Vasculitis'.

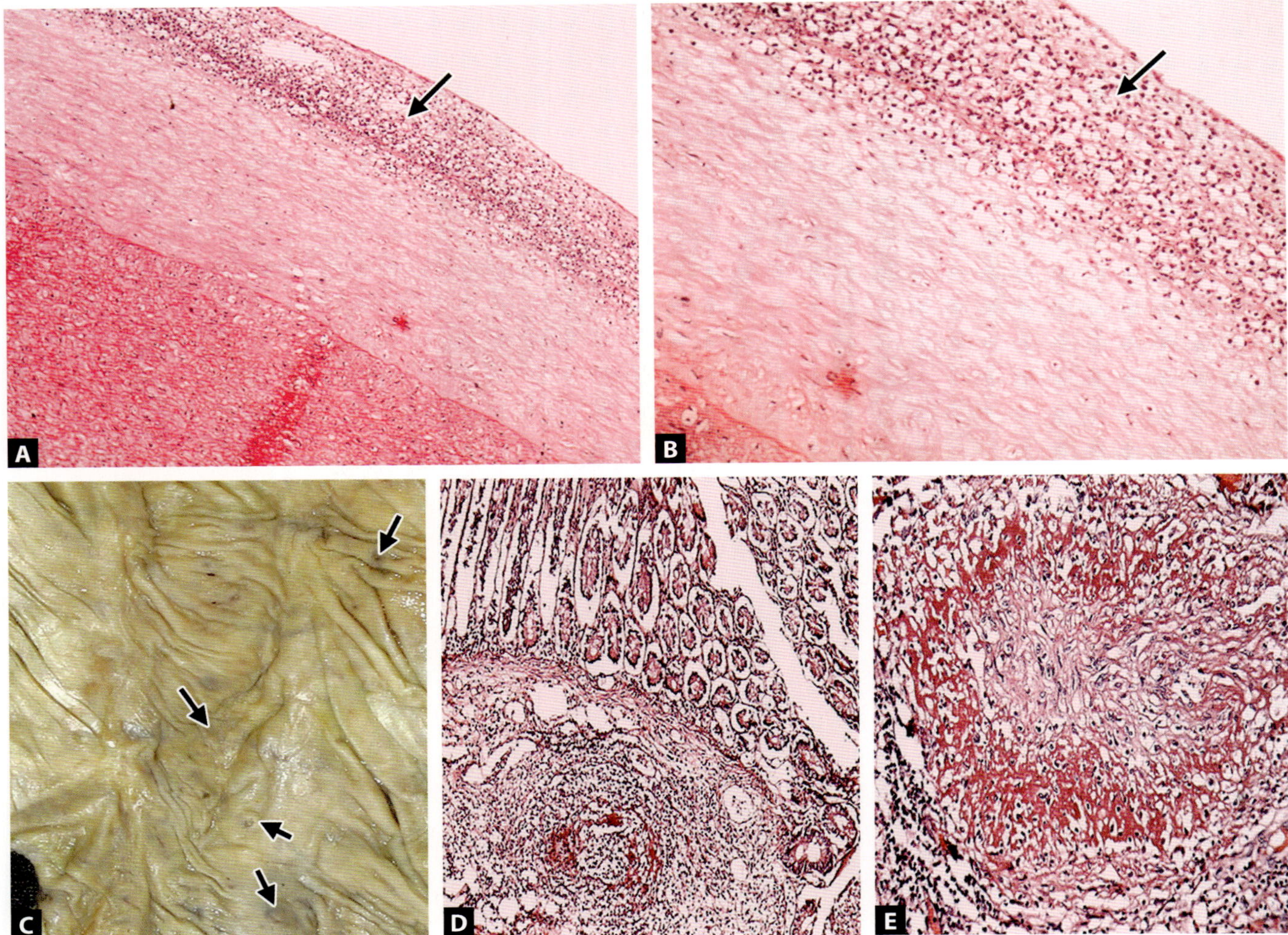

Figs 7A–E: (A and B) Abdominal aorta showing acute intimitis with polymorphs and nuclear debris in the intima (arrows); (C) Large intestine showing small ulcers (arrows); (D and E) Large intestine showing acute vasculitis with fibrinoid necrosis in the submucosa.

COMMENTARY—INDEX CASE: PM 20415

In 2005, when this case was discussed in the clinicopathological conference, it was an enigma, as it showed vasculitis of the small, medium and large-sized arteries along with glomerulonephritis. It was labeled as "cANCA positive MPA with involvement of small, medium and large sized arteries." There were no lesions to suggest GPA (necrosis, vasculitis, granulomatous inflammation) in the upper and lower respiratory tract and presence of glomerulonephritis ruled out classic polyarteritis nodosa (PAN). The lungs did not reveal any hemorrhage, but only an occasional focus of capillaritis.

But now the CHCC2012[1] consensus nomenclature answers all queries. It is based (as before) on the predominant type of vessel involved, i.e. large vessels (aorta and its major branches and the analogous veins), medium vessels (main visceral arteries and veins, i.e. renal, hepatic, coronary and mesenteric and veins and their initial branches, i.e. interlobar artery in the kidney, right and left hepatic arteries. The latter. i.e. "the initial branches" is the new addition) and small vessels (intraparenchymal arteries, arterioles, capillaries, venules and veins). CHCC2012[1] highlights that large vessel vasculitis affects the large arteries more often than medium or small vessel vasculitis, the medium vessel vasculitis affects predominantly the medium arteries and the small vessel vasculitis affects predominantly small arteries and other small vessels (arterioles, capillaries and venules). *But the key concept is that the vasculitis of all three major categories can affect any sized artery*.[1] CHCC2012[1] also says that—"It is important to realize that medium vessel vasculitis and even large vessel vasculitis can affect small arteries".

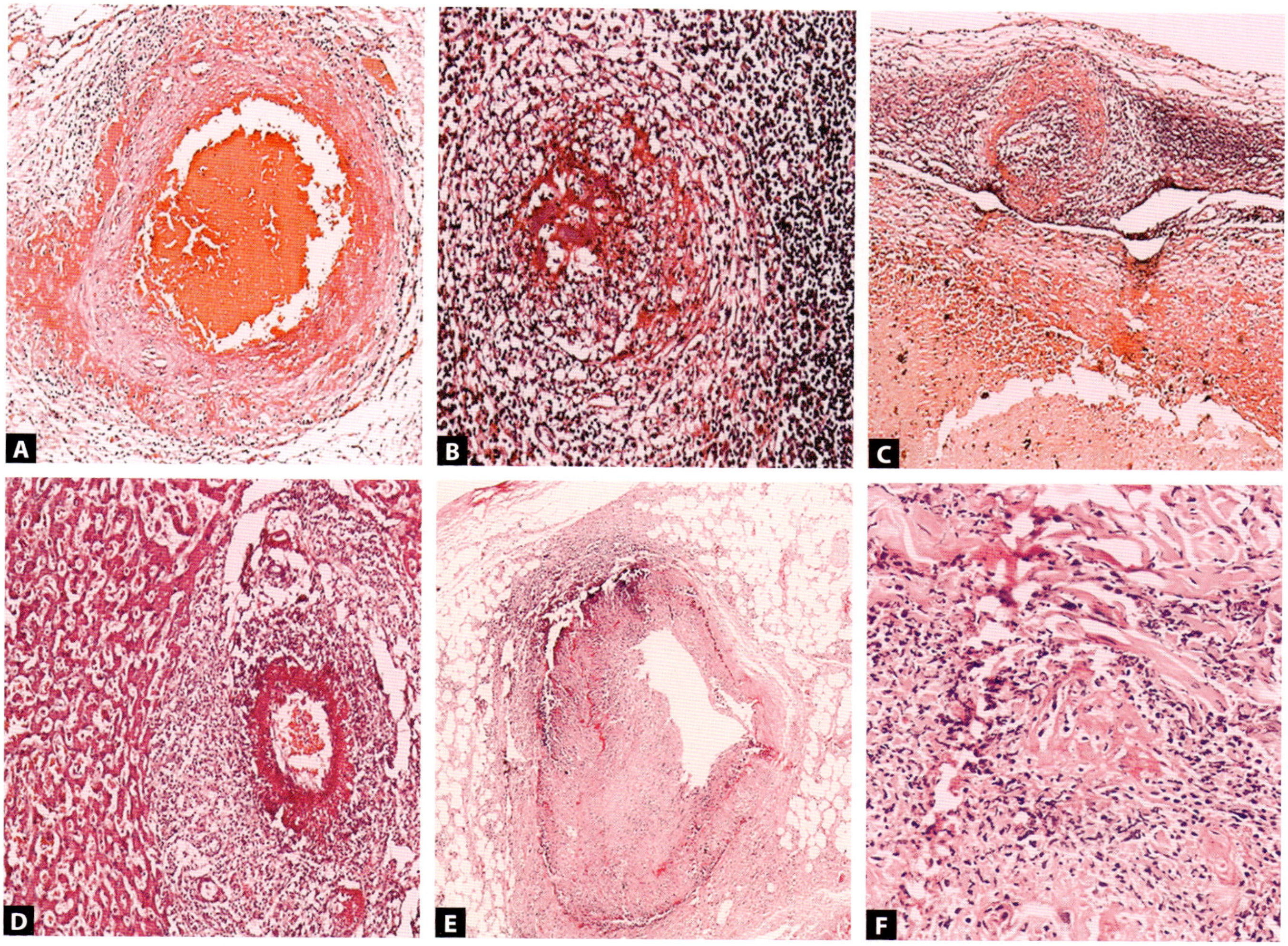

Figs 8A–F: Acute vasculitis seen in the (A) Periadrenal arteries; (B) Lymph node; (C) Ovary; (D) Liver; (E) Medium-sized artery of the mesentery; (F) Skin.

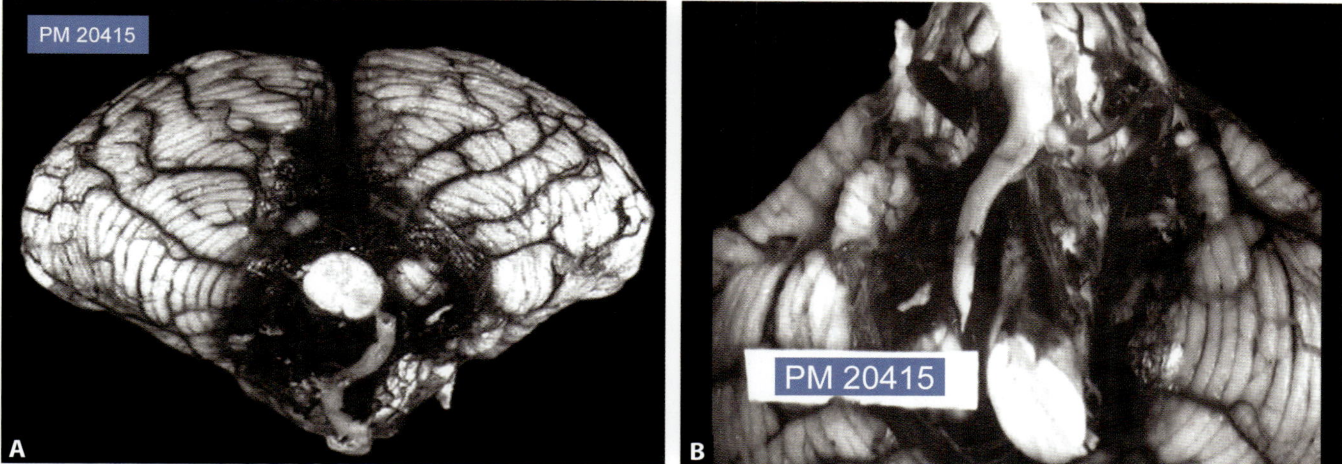

Figs 9A and B: Gross pictures of the brain showing hemorrhage (A) Cerebellar surface; (B) At the base of the brain.

So, according to this concept, the large and medium vessel vasculitis can affect small arteries but not the arterioles, capillaries and venules. This is true, because if classic PAN involves vessels smaller than arteries, i.e. the arterioles, capillaries and venules, glomerulonephritis would occur and then the case would be labeled as MPA.

The index case very well endorses the above key concept of CHCC2012. The kidneys on gross examination showed multiple infarcts as extraglomerular acute vasculitis was affecting the medium-sized arteries (interlobar) along with small-sized arteries (arcuate and interlobular). The index case also showed florid acute glomerulitis and granulomatous glomerulonephritis which can be seen in cases of MPA. In granulomatous glomerulonephritis, epithelioid cells and giant cells are seen surrounding a glomerulus, which shows diffuse necrotizing lesion along with break in the Bowman's capsule. Thus, cases of MPA where florid acute glomerulitis is seen will also show granulomatous glomerular lesions which develop subsequent to the acute glomerular destruction. Similarly, granulomatous arteritis can be seen in the kidneys subsequent to the florid acute vasculitis. The pericarditis in the index case was due to uremia. The brain showed subarachnoid hemorrhage at the base, but no evidence of vasculitis was noted. This however cannot be ruled out.

TAKE HOME MESSAGE

- CHCC2012 highlights that the vasculitis of all three major categories, i.e. large, medium and small size, can affect any sized artery.
- CHCC2012 also says that "It is important to understand that medium vessel vasculitis and even large vessel vasculitis can affect small arteries." So, according to this concept, the large and medium vessel vasculitis can affect small arteries but not the arterioles, capillaries and venules.
- This case of MPA highlights the above facts, as here acute vasculitis was seen in large, medium and small arteries along with arterioles, capillaries and venules.
- Granulomatous glomerulonephritis can be seen in cases of MPA.

Acknowledgement

This case was published as a Clinicopathological conference in our hospital bulletin. Das A, Kakkar N, Khurana D, kalra N, Sakhuja V. A case of ANCA associated systemic vasculitis. Bulletin PGI. 2005;39:84-96. (Nonindexed)

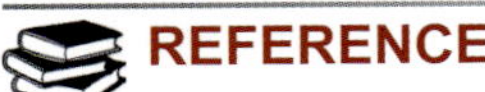

REFERENCE

1. Jennette JC, Falk RJ, Bacon PA, et al. 2012 Revised International Chapel Hill Consensus Conference Nomenclature of Vasculitides. Arthritis & Rheumatism, 2013; 65 (1):1–11

CONTRIBUTIONS BY:

1. Dr Dhiraj Khurana, Professor, Department of Neurology (Compilation of the Clinical Details)
2. Dr Ranjana Minz, Professor and Head, Department of Immunopathology (ANCA testing)
3. Dr Surjit Singh, Ex-Professor, Department of Internal Medicine (Clinician In-Charge)
4. Dr Kusum Joshi, Ex-Professor and Head, Department of Histopathology (Consultation)

Post Graduate Institute of Medical Education and Research, Chandigarh, India

CASE 42

p-ANCA Positive Classic Polyarteritis Nodosa: PM 24277

Nandita Bharadwaj Kakkar

HIGHLIGHTS OF THE CASE

A 62-year-old male presented with fever, progressive weakness of both limbs which was subacute, asymmetrical in onset and painful, mononeuritis multiplex, myalgias, weight loss, malaise, melena, oliguria, generalized edema, deranged renal function tests, hematuria and altered sensorium with left basal ganglia infarct. The perinuclear antineutrophil cytoplasmic antibodies (p-ANCA) was strongly positive by immunofluorescence and ELISA. This led to a clinical diagnosis of a small vessel vasculitis, i.e. microscopic polyangiitis (MPA). The autopsy however revealed this to be a case of classic polyarteritis nodosa (PAN). The point is whether p-ANCA can be positive in classic PAN.

Keywords: Polyarteritis nodosa, p-ANCA positive, mononeuritis multiplex, autopsy.

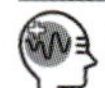

CLINICAL DETAILS

Date of Admission: 09.05.2011, Date of Death: 23.06.2011, Duration of Hospital Stay: 15 days

A 62-year-old male, presented with progressive weakness of upper limbs (UL) and lower limbs (LL) since 3 months. This was subacute, asymmetrical in onset and painful. It began on the right side and went over to the left (Right UL → Right LL → Left UL and Left LL) but there was no bladder involvement. He had associated low grade fever off and on, severe myalgia, weight loss and general malaise. He received intravenous steroids (alternate day dexamethasone injection) followed by transient improvement. There were 6–7 episodes of melena and the steroids were stopped. There was oliguria since 1 month, associated with vomiting, generalized edema and he subsequently lapsed into altered sensorium. He was unable to recognize his relatives and would talk incoherently. There was history of bronchial asthma since 10 years. There was no history of cranial nerve palsies, headache, seizures or hemiplegia. No history of cough, expectoration, hematuria, jaundice, joint pains, rash, oral ulcers and photosensitivity. He was a reformed smoker and an occasional alcohol consumer. On ***examination*** he was drowsy, disoriented and afebrile, pulse was 86/min, BP was 120/80 mm Hg and respiratory rate was 18/min. There was pallor, pitting edema, clubbing, bilateral basal crepts and CNS examination revealed a status of E3-4 V5M6. There was left lateral rectus palsy, right upper motor neuron (UMN) 7th nerve palsy, wasting of bilateral intrinsic hand muscles, hypotonia of all four limbs, power grade 0/5 in right UL/LL and grade 3/5 in left UL/LL, bilateral wrist drop along with generalized areflexia with mute planters.

Investigations

Hemogram: Hb – 7.5 g/dL; TLC – 29,400/uL with polymorphonuclear leucocytosis; platelets—220,000/uL; ESR—60 mm in the first hour; PTI – 100%, INR – 1.01, APTT – 45 seconds; fibrinogen—4.91 g/L, D-dimer positive.

Blood Biochemistry: Serum creatinine/urea—4.81/127 mg%; serum Na^+/K^+ 136/6.32 mEq/L; serum protein/albumin–5.6/1.7 gm; serum alkaline phosphatase (ALP)—1065 U/L; Serum uric acid—10.43 mg%; TSH – 7.54; Liver function tests and lipidogram—within normal limits.

Microbiological tests: Routine urine—15–20 pus cells, RBCs 3+; blood/urine culture: Sterile × 3; fungal serology negative.

Immunological investigations: ANA negative; pANCA ++ by Immunofluorescence and ELISA; HIV nonreactive; Serum electrophoresis—no M band; Bence-Jones proteins negative; Nerve conduction study (NCS)—sensorimotor polyneuropathy predominantly axonal, Lower limb > upper limb (done outside), CSF - no WBCs, RBC ++, protein - 39 mg/L, sugar—41 mg%; Gram stain negative.

Radiology: ***NCCT Head*** - (L) basal ganglia infarct, ***MRI brain*** - acute focal infarcts in left basal ganglia and left paraventricular white matter; ***MRI Cx Spine***—NAD, no cord compression; ***CT chest (plain)***—patchy nodular opacities bilateral lower lobes (right >left, posterior segments), likely infective. Minimal right-sided pleural effusion; ***CT abdomen (plain)***—suspicious thickening of colonic wall with subtle pericolonic stranding ? Inflammatory; ***USG Abdomen***—moderate ascites, mild pericardial and bilateral pleural effusion, mild hepatomegaly, bilateral mildly increased renal cortical echogenicity; ***Compression USG***—no evidence of deep vein thrombosis.

The patient had upper gastrointestinal bleed and underwent an endoscopy, which revealed duodenal ulcer which was cauterized. He was managed on the lines of vasculitis, had renal failure (underwent peritoneal dialysis), hyperkalemia, sepsis and septic shock (antibiotics, ionotropes and peritoneal dialysis). Developed cardiac arrest on 17.5.2011 and was revived. He succumbed to the second cardiac arrest on 23.5.2011. ***Units Clinical Diagnosis***—Mononeuritis multiplex, diffuse cerebral infarctions—Vasculitis ? Microscopic polyangiitis, severe sepsis, acute kidney injury and refractory septic shock.

AUTOPSY FINDINGS: PM 24277

Antemortem sural nerve biopsy (S—7941/11) was done in this case. The sural nerve was lightly stained by H&E stain (Fig 1A, control-A1), showed total myelin loss (Fig 1B, control-B1) and immunohistochemistry with neurofilament protein (NFP) revealed total loss of axons (Fig 1C, control-C1). Overall features were those of severe demyelination with axonopathy. A complete autopsy was performed. The pleural cavity contained 2 liters of straw-colored fluid. The kidneys were small in size, distorted and (Figs 2A–C) weighed 240 gm. The capsular surface (Figs 2A and B) showed blotchy congestion and depressed scars. The cut section revealed medullary congestion and small pale infarcts. On microscopic examination, there were geographic areas of infarcts (Figs 2D and E). The interlobar, arcuate and interlobular arteries showed vasculitis in the form of a spectrum of lesions of different ages, present simultaneously. It began with fibrinoid necrosis and acute inflammation, evolved through chronic inflammation and fibroplasias and culminated in varying degrees of vascular sclerosis, i.e. acute vasculitis (Figs 2F and 3A), subacute vasculitis or healing vasculitis (Figs 3B–D) and healed tomb stone of vasculitis, where the vessel was barely discernable (Figs 3E and F). Varying degrees of luminal occlusion due to intimal hyperplasia was seen in the affected arteries. The interlobar arteries showed aneurysmal dilatation (Figs 4A and B). Elastic Van Gieson stain showed break of the internal elastic lamina of the affected arteries (Fig 4C). Glomeruli were within normal limits (Figs 4D and E). No granulomatous lesions were noted. Interstitial inflammation was present (Fig 4D). Immunofluorescence was negative for IgG, IgA, IgM, kappa, lambda, C3 and C1q. Electron microscopy did not show any immune deposits (Fig 4F). The p-ANCA was strongly positive by both immunofluorescence and ELISA [MPO ELISA—reading 2.4 (cut off of 0.4)]. Morphology was consistent with the diagnosis of classic PAN. Extrarenal vasculitis (acute/chronic) was seen in the small-sized arteries in the mesentery (Figs 5A–C), nerve (Fig 5D), muscle (Fig 5E), liver (Fig 5F), spleen (Fig 6A) and colon (Figs 6B and C). The ***brain*** weighed 1,493 g. Microscopic examination revealed small infarct in the left basal ganglia suggestive of subacute ischemia. Atherosclerotic occlusion of a small branch of middle cerebral artery was also noted. Cerebral ischemia was present, but no vasculitis was seen in the CNS. ***Lungs*** were normal grossly (Fig 6D) and showed early bronchopneumonia and pulmonary edema (Fig 6E). However, there was no capillaritis or any pulmonary hemorrhage. Testes revealed testicular atrophy. In the jejunum, an incidental well-circumscribed mass, 4 × 4 × 3 cm (Fig 6F) was seen on the serosal aspect, the microscopy of which was consistent with the diagnosis of a benign gastrointestinal stromal tumor (Fig 6F-inset). An organized thrombus was seen in the common iliac vein and grade 2 atherosclerosis was noted. Other organs were within normal limits.

FINAL AUTOPSY DIAGNOSIS: PM 24277

62 Years Old Male

- Classic polyarteritis nodosa—p-ANCA positive with vasculitis in the kidneys, mesentry, muscle, nerve, spleen, liver and intestine
- Demyelination with axonopathy—sural nerve
- Old infarct—left internal capsule (atherosclerotic) with cerebral hypoxia
- Early bronchopneumonia, pulmonary edema and bilateral pleural effusion
- Grade II atherosclerosis—aorta, testicular atrophy
- Incidental gastrointestinal stromal tumor (GIST)—jejunum
- Organized thrombus—common iliac vein.

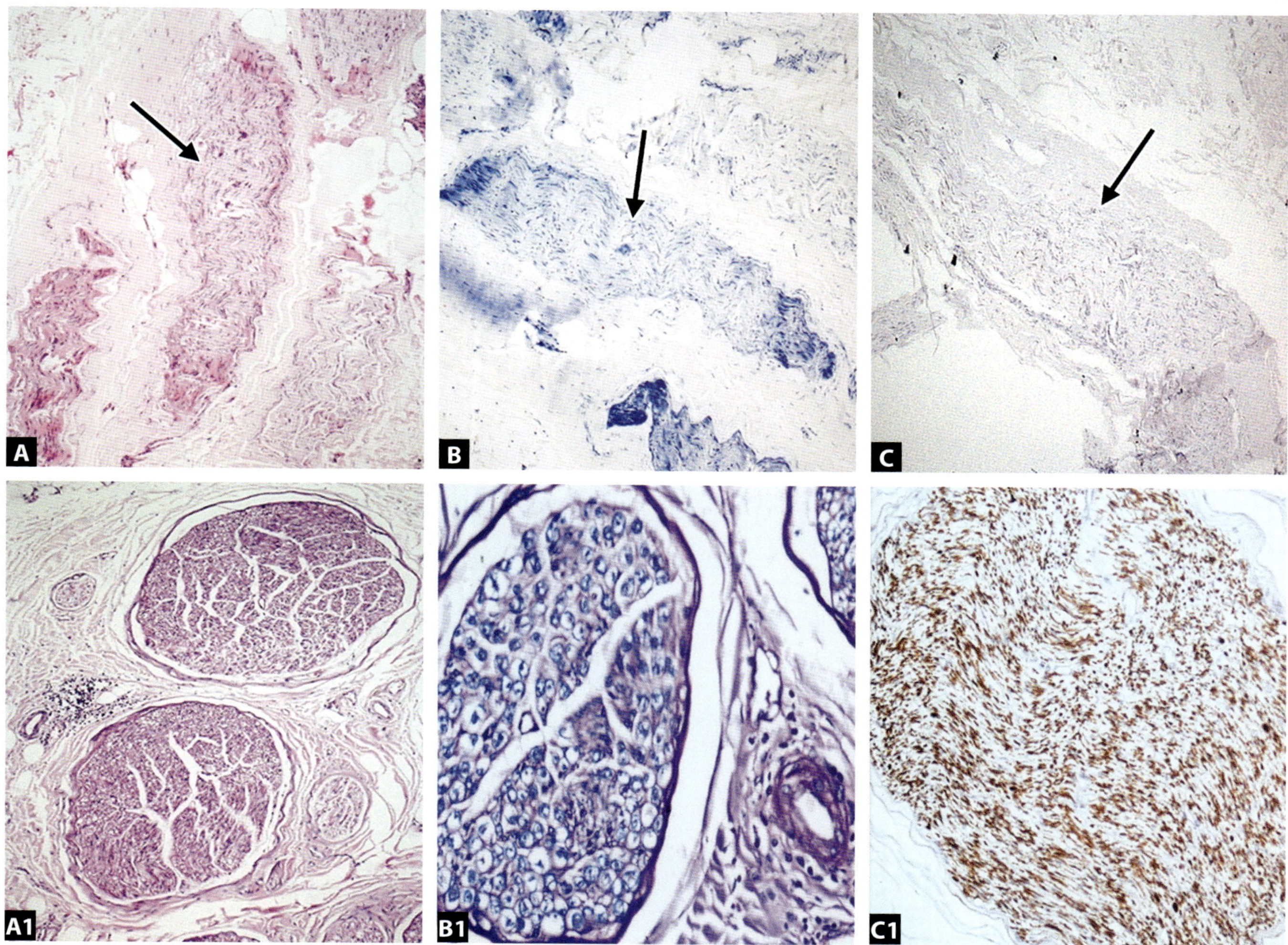

Figs 1A–C: Sural nerve shows (A) Pale staining nerve on H&E (arrow); (A1) Normal control. (B) Myelin stain shows extensive loss of myelin; (B1) Normal control. (C) Immunostain for neurofilament protein shows extensive axonal loss; (C1) Normal control.

POLYARTERITIS NODOSA

Polyarteritis nodosa comes in the category of a medium vessel vasculitis, which predominantly affects the medium vessels (defined as the main visceral arteries or veins and their initial branches). Any sized artery can however be affected. Inflammatory aneurysms and stenosis are common. PAN is a necrotizing arteritis of predominantly medium and small arteries without glomerulonephritis or vasculitis in arterioles, capillaries or venules and is not associated with ANCAs. It is a systemic disease with an incidence of 2–3 per million and has a male predominance (2:1). Any age can be affected, but it occurs mostly in adults.

Clinical Features of Polyarteritis Nodosa

Polyarteritis nodosa is a chronic disease characterized by remissions and exacerbations. Patients present with fever, weight loss, peripheral neuropathy, myalgias, arthralgias, abdominal pain, signs and symptoms of renal disease, hypertension, melena, visual disturbances, focal neurological deficits and nonspecific features of chronic inflammation such as anemia or elevated erythrocyte sedimentation rate.

- ***Neurological manifestations***: The most common indicator of vasculitis is peripheral neuropathy which occurs in 50–75% of cases, typically in the form of mononeuritis multiplex (earliest symptom in 30% of cases). It occurs acutely, but can be indolent. Usually the sensory signs (hypo/hyper/dysesthesia or pain) come before the motor deficits (which affect the lower limbs). Initially a single nerve is involved, i.e. mononeuritis followed by others, i.e. multiplex. The nerves involved in order of preference are superficial peroneal, sural, radial, cubital and median. The CNS is involved in 5% cases only.

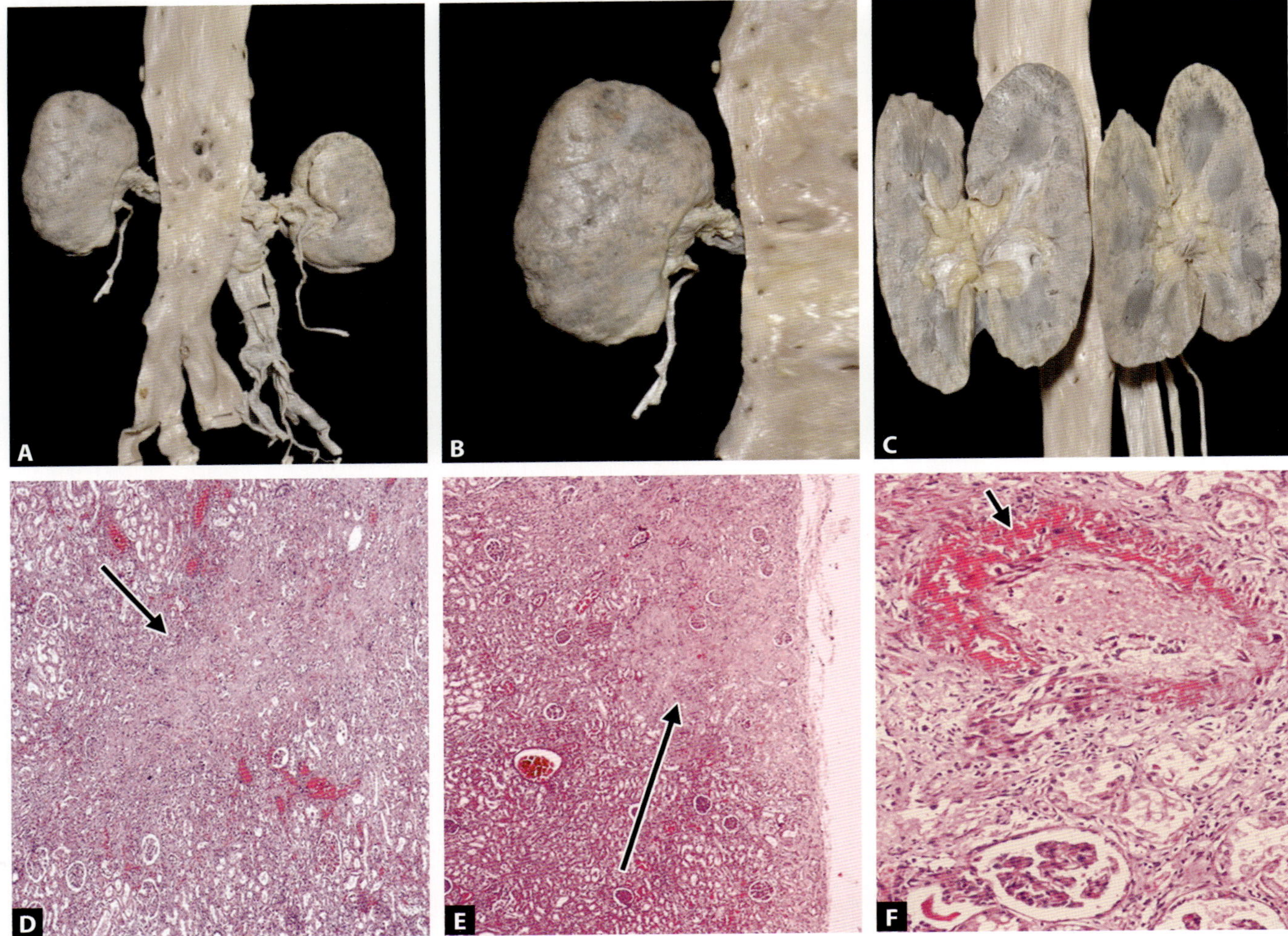

Figs 2A–F: (A and B) Kidneys with the aorta and inferior vena cava. They are smaller in size and show coarse scars; (C) Cut section of the kidneys show medullary congestion and ischemic scars; (D and E) Photomicrographs of the kidney showing areas of infarction (arrows); (F) Kidney showing acute vasculitis with fibrinoid necrosis (arrow) of the wall and inflammation.

It presents as encephalopathy, cognitive disturbances presenting as disorientation, psychosis, hallucinations, delusions or diminished consciousness. Vasculitis of a cerebral artery can lead to seizures, strokes and subarachnoid hemorrhages.

- ***Gastrointestinal*** (GI) involvement occurs in approximately one third cases, more often in those with HBV-related PAN. GI symptoms may be the first manifestation of the disease and these include abdominal pain, GI hemorrhages leading to melena and perforations. The small bowel is more affected as compared to the colon or stomach. Intraperitoneal rupture of the aneurysms can be catastrophic. Severe GI manifestations like perforation, peritonitis, bowel ischemia and intestinal occlusion have a poor prognosis.
- ***Renal*** involvement manifests as flank pain, hematuria and as hemorrhage due to rupture of an aneurysm. Renovascular hypertension occurs in up to one-third of patients. Renal biopsy is contraindicated when aneurysms are present. Acute renal failure usually occurs early during disease progression or flare.
- ***Cardiac*** involvement can present as congestive heart failure, myocardial infarction, or as cardiomyopathy. In cases with infarction, angiography can prove the coronary involvement by arteritis in 85% of cases, whereas in the other 15%, infarction is due to involvement of the smaller coronary vessels or due to spasms.
- Skin involvement occurs in approximately half of the cases of PAN as cutaneous or subcutaneous nodules. The most important cutaneous finding is a palpable purpura.

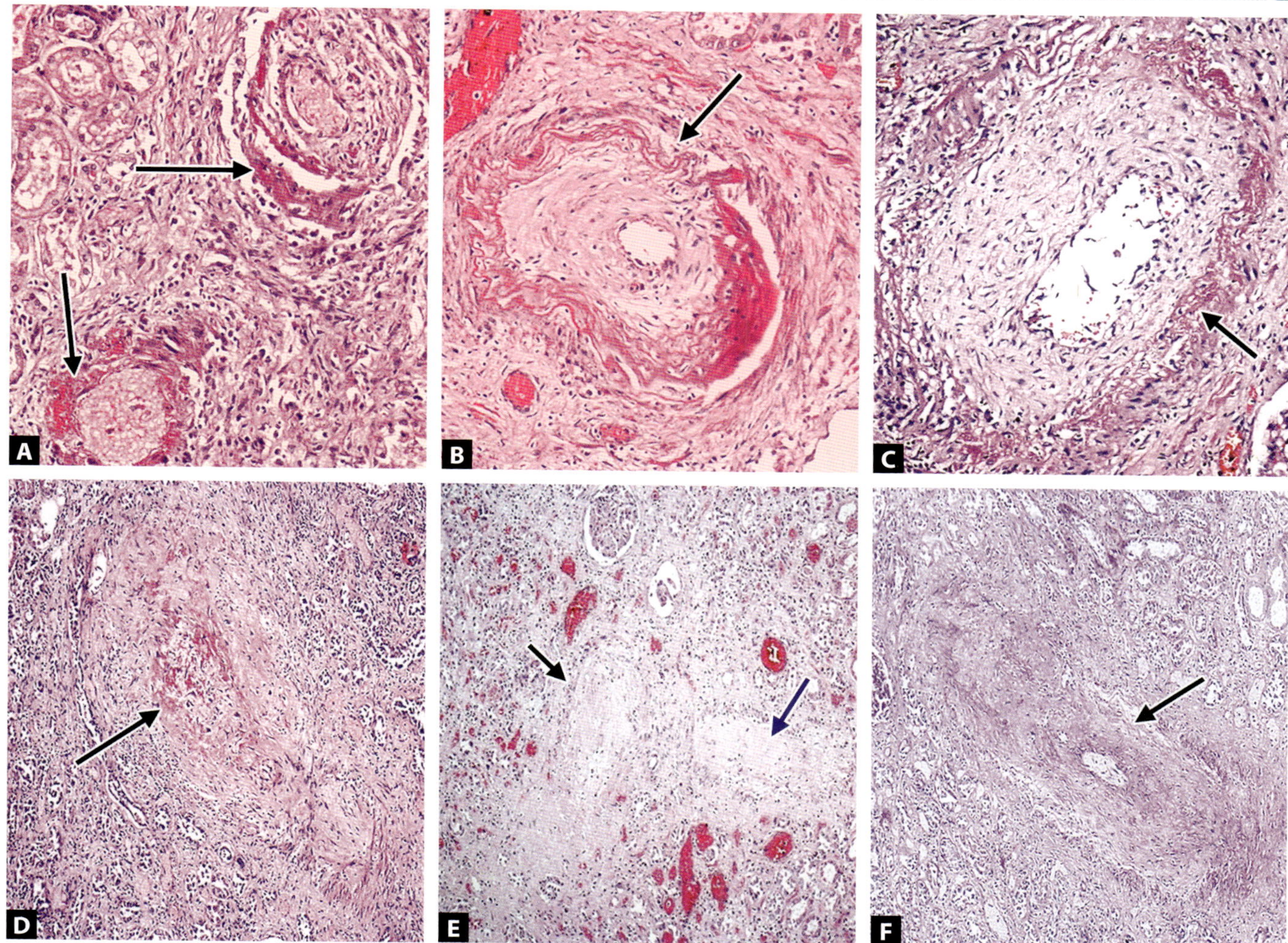

Figs 3A–F: Photomicrographs of the kidney showing. (A) Acute vasculitis in the intralobular arteries (arrows); (B–D) Subacute or healing vasculitis in the intralobular arteries showing intimal fibrosis, luminal compromise, focal fibrin deposition (in B and D), and mild inflammation; (E and F) Healed vasculitis showing tombstones of the vessels which show fibrosis and occlusion of the lumina (arrows).

This could be the first sign of a systemic disease, which occurs later in the course.

- Orchitis is one of the most characteristic manifestations of PAN and is one of the American College of Rheumatology (ACR) classification criteria. Occurs due to testicular artery ischemia and is unilateral.
- Lungs are spared in PAN, unlike MPA, GPA and EGPA.

Associated conditions include hairy cell leukemia, rheumatoid arthritis, Sjögren's syndrome, hepatitis B and cryoglobulinemia. Clinical severity of PAN depends on the location, number and caliber of arteries affected. Factors associated with a poor prognosis include age >50 years and gastrointestinal, renal, or cardiac involvement. PAN, most commonly involves the renal, coronary, hepatic and mesenteric, medium and small arteries. Rarely may involve veins or large elastic arteries such as aorta or its primary branches. Vasculitis leads to ischemia, infarction and hemorrhage in the affected organ. PAN has predilection for arterial branch points and thus produce aneurysms. Diagnostic criteria are met if the patient has three of the following symptoms (ACR 1990 criteria for PAN)—weight loss > 4 Kg; livedo reticularis; testicular pain or tenderness; myalgias or muscle weakness; mono or poly neuropathy; hypertension (diastolic > 90 mm of Hg); elevated blood urea nitrogen or creatinine; serum positivity for hepatitis B surface antigen or antibody (up to 30% cases); abnormal arteriogram; biopsy showing features suggestive of PAN or

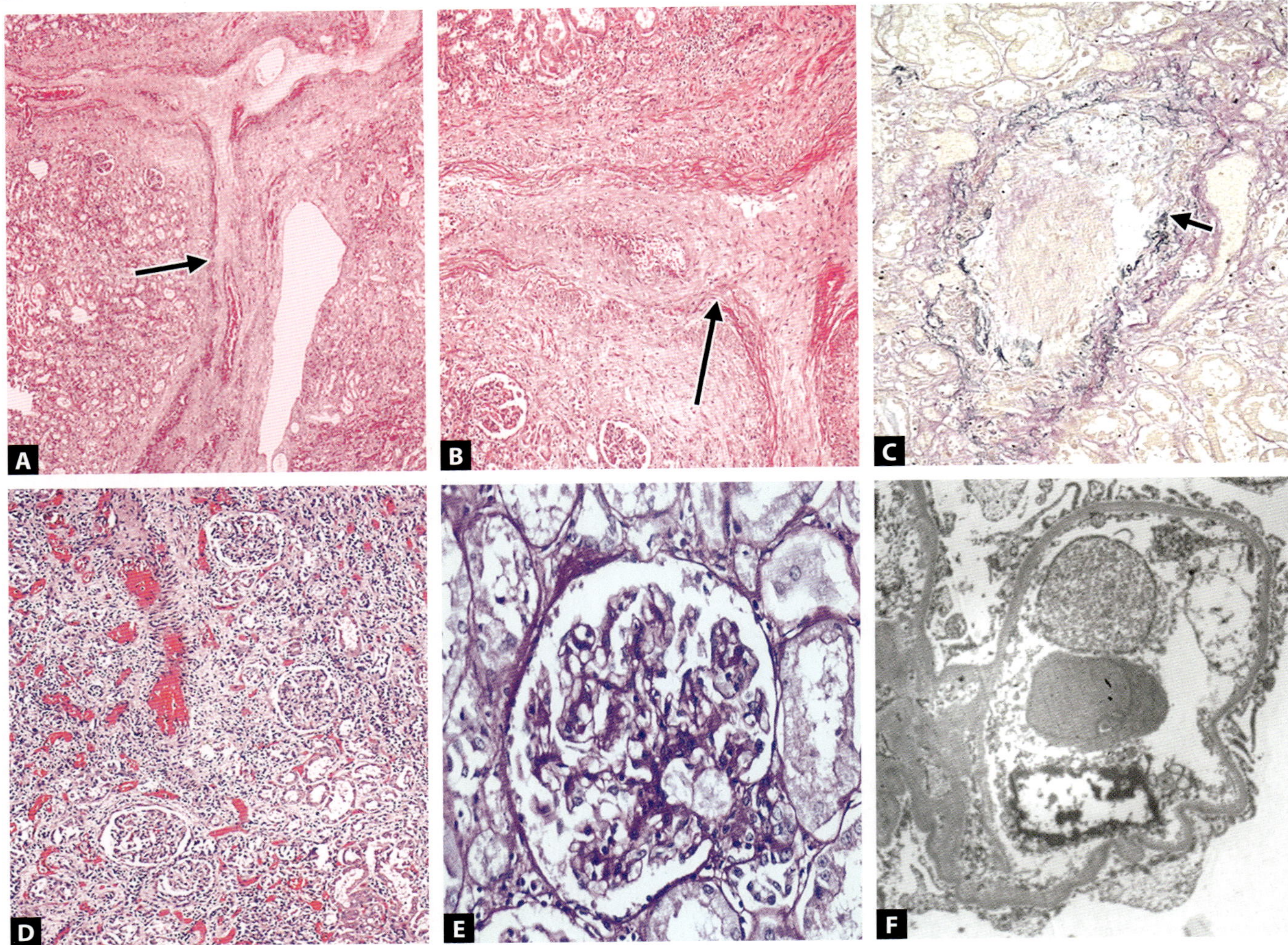

Figs 4A–F: (A and B) Interlobar artery showing aneurysm with intimal fibrosis (arrows); (C) Elastic Van Gieson stain showing break of the internal elastic lamina; (D) Section shows normal glomeruli and interstitial inflammation; (E) Periodic acid–Schiff stain shows normal glomerulus; (F) Electron microscopy shows absence of any immune deposits.

diagnostic biopsy showing fibrinoid necrosis of vessel wall. Presence of three or more of the above criteria yields an 82% sensitivity and 86 % specificity.

Pathology of Polyarteritis Nodosa

The gross abnormalities in the kidneys are the result of arterial pseudoaneurysms, thrombosis, infarction and hemorrhage. On microscopic examination, acute vasculitis is characterized by fibrinoid necrosis which destroys the endothelial and smooth muscle fibers, elastic lamina and collagen. Wall is suffused by a proteinaceous material rich in fibrin and neutrophils. The fibrinoid necrosis may be focal, segmental or circumferential. Apart from the acute necrotizing lesions, healed and healing lesions are characteristic and are seen simultaneously. So, a combination of several lesions at different stages, i.e. acute, healing and healed is the hallmark of PAN. They begin with fibrinoid necrosis and acute inflammation, evolve through chronic inflammation and fibroplasia and culminate in varying degrees of vascular sclerosis. Healing lesions show granulation tissue within the wall and healed lesions show transmural scarring. Aneurysms develop typically at branch points due to weakening of the vessel wall. Kidney shows infarcts due to involvement of interlobar and arcuate arteries. Glomerulonephritis is not seen and if seen, the case is labeled as MPA. Immunofluorescence microscopy and electron microscopy do not reveal evidence of vascular immune complex deposition. Extrarenal vasculitis involves the medium and smaller arteries. Aneurysms may be seen at the branching points. All varieties of vasculitic lesions can be appreciated, i.e. (A) Acute lesions with

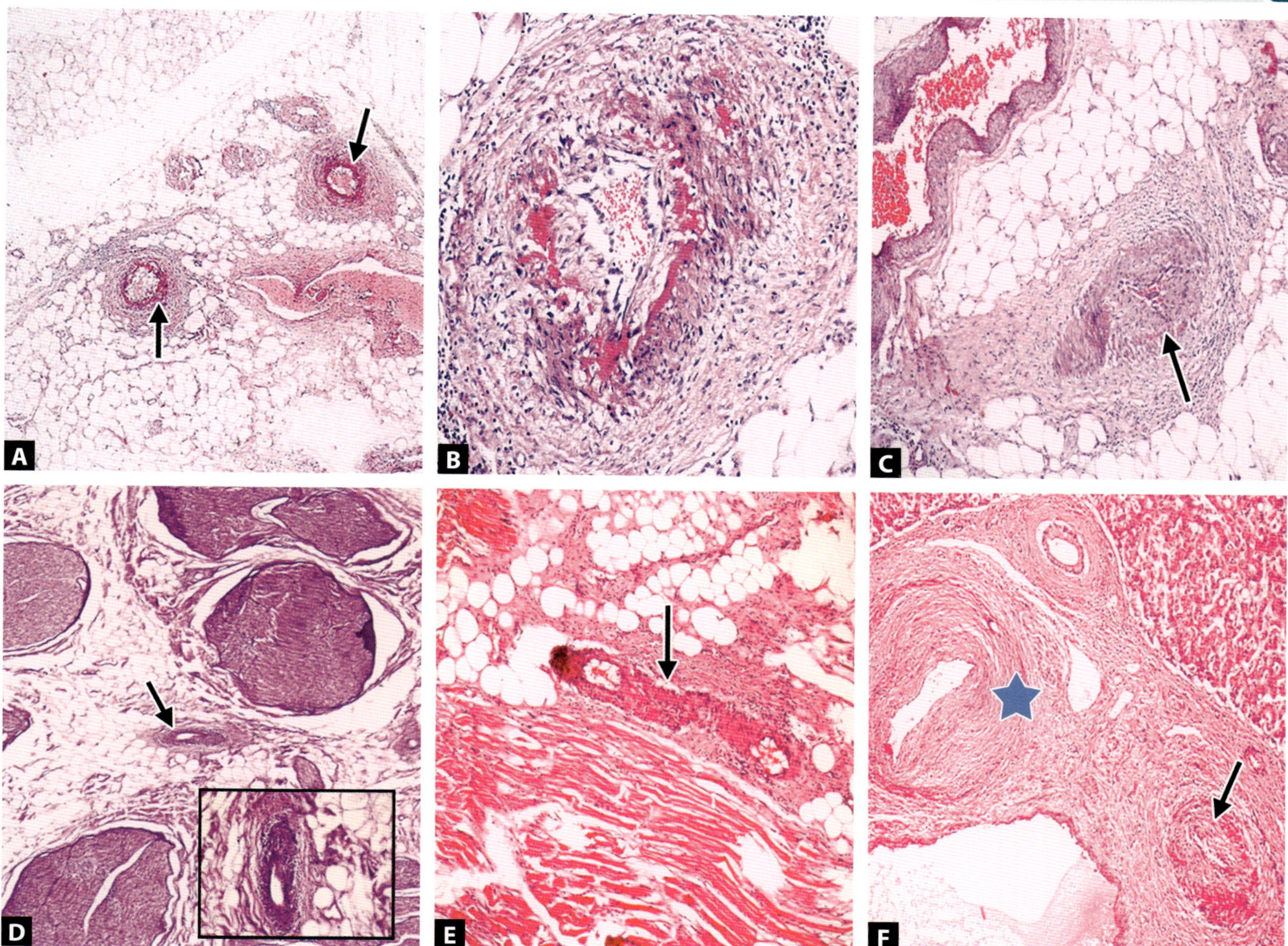

Figs 5A–F: Photomicrographs of the mesentery showing. (A and B) Acute vasculitis of small arteries; (C) Healing vasculitis. Photomicrographs showing acute vasculitis (arrows) of small arteries in the (D) Nerves; (E) Muscle, and (F) Liver. Liver in addition shows an artery showing healed vasculitis (star).

fibrinoid necrosis and transmural inflammation; (B) Healing or subacute lesions where inflammation is less, remnant of fibrinoid necrosis can still be seen and fibrosis has set in leading to intimal fibroplasia and luminal compromise and (C) Healed lesions wherein inflammation is hardly seen no fibrin is seen and scarring has led to vessels with totally occluded lumina (some may show recanalization) or as virtual tombstones where vessels are barely discernable.

Classic PAN is an incompletely understood entity. There is an association between classic PAN and hepatitis B infection. Other infections that have been rarely associated with PAN include hepatitis C, HIV and parvovirus B19. ANCA is negative in classic PAN and thus does not play a role in its pathogenesis. ANCA is however positive in small vessel vasculitides like MPA, GPA (Wegener's) and EGPA (Churg-Strauss), where inflammatory involvement of capillaries or venules is present.

COMMENTARY—INDEX CASE: PM 24277

This 62-year-old male presented with fever, progressive weakness of both limbs which was subacute, asymmetrical in onset and painful, mononeuritis multiplex, myalgia, weight loss, malaise, melena, oliguria, generalized edema, deranged renal function tests, hematuria and altered sensorium. The p-ANCA was strongly positive both by immunofluorescence and ELISA and a clinical diagnosis of a small vessel vasculitis, i.e. MPA was made. The autopsy however revealed

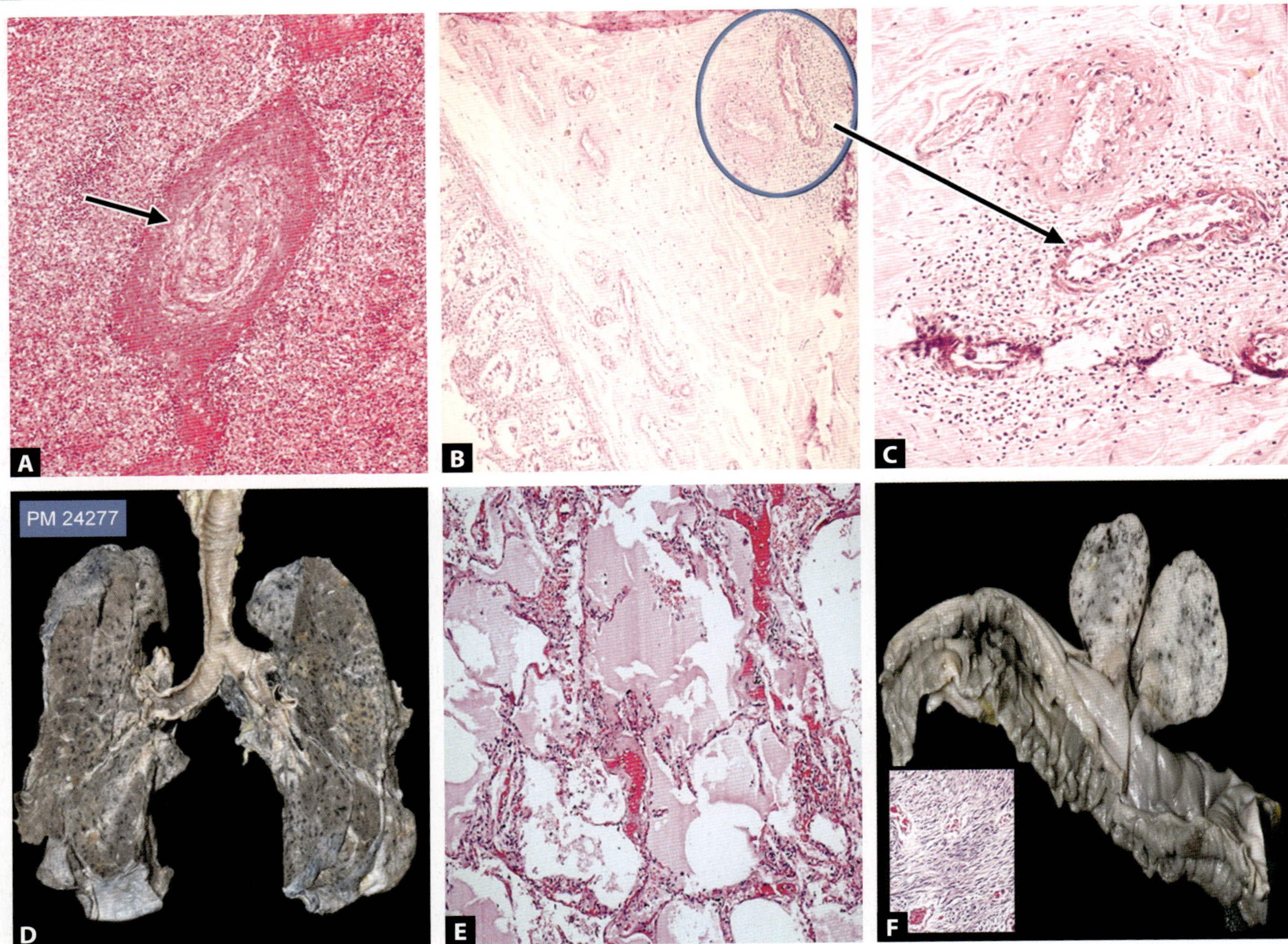

Figs 6A–F: Photomicrographs showing acute vasculitis in the (A) spleen and (B and C) submucosa of the small intestine; (D) Cut section of the subcrepitant lungs. No hemorrhage or infarct seen; (E) Lungs showing edema fluid; (F) Small intestine showing a well-circumscribed tumor on the serosal aspect which on microscopy is a gastrointestinal stromal tumor (inset).

this to be a case of classic PAN. At autopsy acute, subacute and chronic vasculitis was noted in the kidneys involving the medium and small-sized arteries. However, the extrarenal organs, i.e. the mesentery, nerve, muscle, liver, spleen and colon revealed small artery (acute to chronic) vasculitis only. Only an occasional medium-sized artery was involved in the mesentery. The brain showed atherosclerotic occlusion of a small branch of middle cerebral artery which led to a small infarct in the left basal ganglia. Cerebral ischemia was present, but no vasculitis was however noted.

Polyarteritis nodosa and MPA have to be correctly diagnosed as their treatment differs substantially. ANCA positivity is generally not seen in patients with arteritis without capillaritis or venulitis. Hence, ANCA is negative in classic PAN. But in the index case, p-ANCA was positive by both immunofluorescence and by ELISA. There are occasional case reports in literature stating the presence of p-ANCA positivity in classic PAN. They state that when a patient presents with acute renal failure, alveolar hemorrhages and MPO-ANCA but with no evidence of glomerulonephritis, classic PAN should be considered in the differential diagnosis. But it is finally the renal biopsy which will clinch the diagnosis. In the index case, the kidney showed acute, healing and healed vasculitis more so in the interlobular arteries, i.e. the smaller arteries. Vasculitis was also seen in the medium-sized arteries, i.e. the interlobar or arcuate of the kidney and multiple infarcts were noted. However, in the extrarenal locations, i.e. the muscle, nerve, liver, spleen, colon and mesentery, acute vasculitis was seen in the smaller arteries only. Could this have led to the p-ANCA positivity, is a matter of debate.

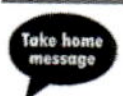

TAKE HOME MESSAGE

- Polyarteritis nodosa and MPA have to be correctly diagnosed as their treatment and prognosis differs substantially.
- There are occasional case reports in literature stating the presence of p-ANCA positivity in classic PAN.

Acknowledgement

This case was published as a CPC in the official journal of our institute—Kakkar et al pANCA positive classic polyarteritis nodosa. Journal of Post Graduate Institute of Medical Education and Research. 2012;46(4);204-11.

SUGGESTED READING

1. Guillevin L, Lhote F, Amouroux J, et al. Antineutrophil cytoplasmic antibodies, abnormal angiograms and pathological findings in polyarteritis nodosa and Churg-Strauss syndrome: indications for the classification of vasculitides of the polyarteritis nodosa group. Br J Rheumatol. 1996;35:958.
2. Guillevin L, Lhote F. Distinguishing polyarteritis nodosa from microscopic polyangiitis and implications for treatment. Curr Opin Rheum. 1995;7:20.
3. Hanegar C, Pagnoux C, Puechal X, et al. A paradigm of diagnostic criteria for PAN: analysis of a series of 949 patients with vasculitides. Arthritis Rheum. 2008;58:1528-38.
4. Jennette CJ, Singh H K. Renal involvement in polyarteritis nodosa, Kawasaki disease, Takayasu arteritis and giant cell arteritis. In: Jennette, JC, Olson JL, Schwartz MM, Silva FG (Eds). Heptinstall's Pathology of the Kidney, 6th edition. Philadelphia: Lippincott Williams & Wilkins; 2007. p. 676.
5. Lhote F, Guillevin L. Polyarteritis nodosa, microscopic polyangiitis and Churg-Strauss syndrome: clinical aspects and treatment. Rheum Dis Clin North Am. 1995;21:911.
6. Lightfoot RW Jr, Michel BA, Bloch DA, et al. The American College of Rheumatology 1990 criteria for the classification of PAN. Arthritis Rheum. 1990;33:1088-93.
7. Pagnoux C, Seror R, Henegar C, et al. Clinical features and outcomes in 348 patients with PAN: a systematic retrospective study of patients diagnosed between 1963 and 2005 and entered into the French Vasculitis Study Group Database. Arthritis Rheum. 2010;62:616-26.
8. Sakaguchi Y, Uehata T, Kawabata H, et al. An autopsy proven cases of MPO-ANCA positive polyarteritis nodosa with acute renal failure and alveolar haemorrhages. Clin Exp Nephrol. 2011;15(2):281-4.
9. Yamamoto T, Matsuda J, Kadoya H, et al. A case of MPO-ANCA- positive polyarteritis nodosa complicated by exudative otitis media, mononeuritis multiplex and acute renal failure. Clin Exp Nephrol. 2011;15(5):754-60.

CONTRIBUTIONS BY:

1. Dr RK Vasishta, Professor and Head, Department of Histopathology (Consultation)
2. Dr Vivek Lal, Professor and Head, Department of Neurology (Compilation of Clinical Details)
3. Dr Ranjana Minz, Professor and Head, Department of Immunopathology (Immunological Workup)
4. Dr Surjit Singh, Ex-Professor, Department of Internal Medicine (Clinician In-Charge)

Post Graduate Institute of Medical Education and Research, Chandigarh, India.

CASE 43

Takayasu's Aortoarteritis, Pulmonary Hypertension, and Pulmonary Capillary Hemangiomatosis: PM 14993

Nandita Bharadwaj Kakkar

HIGHLIGHTS OF THE CASE

This is a classic case of Takayasu's aortoarteritis (TA) type 3 in a 6-year-old female child affecting the ascending/arch/abdominal aorta, brachiocephalic artery, right and left subclavians and left common carotid. Takayasu's aortoarteritis is associated with pulmonary hypertension which generally occurs either due to pulmonary arterial involvement by TA or due to elevated left ventricular end diastolic pressure, or both. In the index case of TA, the cause of pulmonary hypertension was a rare lesion termed pulmonary capillary hemangiomatosis. This entity has a very distinct histopathologic picture.

Keywords: Takayasu's aortoarteritis, pulmonary arterial hypertension, pulmonary capillary hemangiomatosis, autopsy.

CLINICAL DETAILS

Date of Admission: 16.12.1995, Date of Death: 30.12.1995 and Duration of Hospital Stay: 15 Days.

A 6-year-old girl presented with fever, generalized weakness, dyspnea, increased precordial activity, orthopnea, paroxysmal nocturnal dyspnea, anorexia and weight loss since the last 4 months. On examination, the radial, brachial and subclavian pulses were absent, carotid pulses were week (right > left) and the blood pressure (BP) in the lower limbs was 150/100 mm Hg. No bruit was heard. Jugular venous pressure was raised till the angle of the mandible. Apex beat was felt in the 5th left intercostal space, 3 cm outside the midclavicular line and a left parasternal heave grade II was noted. On auscultation, the first heart sound was normal and the pulmonary component of the second heart sound was loud. Third and fourth heart sounds were heard. There was no murmur. Liver was palpable 5 cm below the left costal margin. Fundus examination disclosed copper wire arteries but no papilloedema. ***Investigation*** revealed a normal hemogram, erythrocyte sedimentation rate of 28 mm in the first hour and a normal routine biochemistry. X-ray of the chest revealed cardiomegaly with a CT ratio of 70% and right middle and upper zone infiltrates. Electrocardiography disclosed biventricular hypertrophy, left atrium 3.1 cm, aorta 2.0 cm; left ventricular end diastole/end systole (ed/es) 5.2/4.7 cm; E point septal separation 1.8 cm; left ventricular ejection fraction 16%; dilatation of the left ventricle; global hypokinesia; moderate MR (MR jet area 5.7 cm^2, left atrial area 13.9 cm^2), TR+; calculated right ventricular pressure 31+, right atrial pressure; trivial aortic regurgitation; normal endocardium and normal origin of the left coronary artery; no vegetations, thrombi, rheumatic or congenital heart disease were noted. Clinical diagnosis was TA with systemic and pulmonary hypertension and congestive cardiac failure. She died of sudden cardiorespiratory arrest before angiography could be done.

AUTOPSY FINDINGS: PM 14993

A complete autopsy was performed. The ascending aorta one cm proximal to the origin of the brachiocephalic artery, arch of aorta at and around the ostia of the three major vessels, along with 3 cm of the brachiocephalic trunk, was thickened, with a dull, ulcerated and tree bark-like intima (Fig 1A). The ostia of the left common carotid artery and the left subclavian artery were narrowed (Fig 1A) and just beyond their origin, they felt cord-like with near total origin of their lumina for a distance of 2–3 cm. The right subclavian artery (Fig 1A) right from its origin from the brachiocephalic trunk also revealed an ulcerated, dull, tree bark-like intima. Three cm of the abdominal aorta, at the level of the origin of the renal arteries was thickened with a thickened, dull and ulcerated intima. Microscopically both acute and healed changes were seen. The ascending aorta (Figs 1B–E), brachiocephalic artery (Figs 2A–E and 3A), right subclavian artery (Fig 3B) and the abdominal aorta showed a granulomatous arteritis with presence of transmural acute necrotizing inflammation, polymorphs, nuclear debris, plenty of giant cells, intimal fibrosis, total destruction and haphazardness of the elastic fibers of the media, break of the internal elastic lamina and neovascularization. The vasa vasorum showed perivascular lymphomononuclear infiltrate with endothelial proliferation and obliteration of the lumen. The left subclavian artery (Figs 3C–E) and the left common carotid artery showed healed lesions with a near total occlusion of the lumen due to marked intimal fibrosis. They also showed break and destruction of the elastic fibers of the media, break of the internal elastic lamina, neovascularization, but minimal inflammation. Macroscopically and microscopically, the renal, mesenteric, carotid and pulmonary arteries were normal. Overall features are those of a granulomatous arteritis of the large vessels, i.e. the aorta (arch and abdominal aorta) and its branches (brachiocephalic artery, right and left subclavian arteries and left common carotid artery) consistent with the diagnosis of TA. The ***lungs*** were overweight (350 g). Pleural aspect (Figs 4A and B) showed prominent lines forming

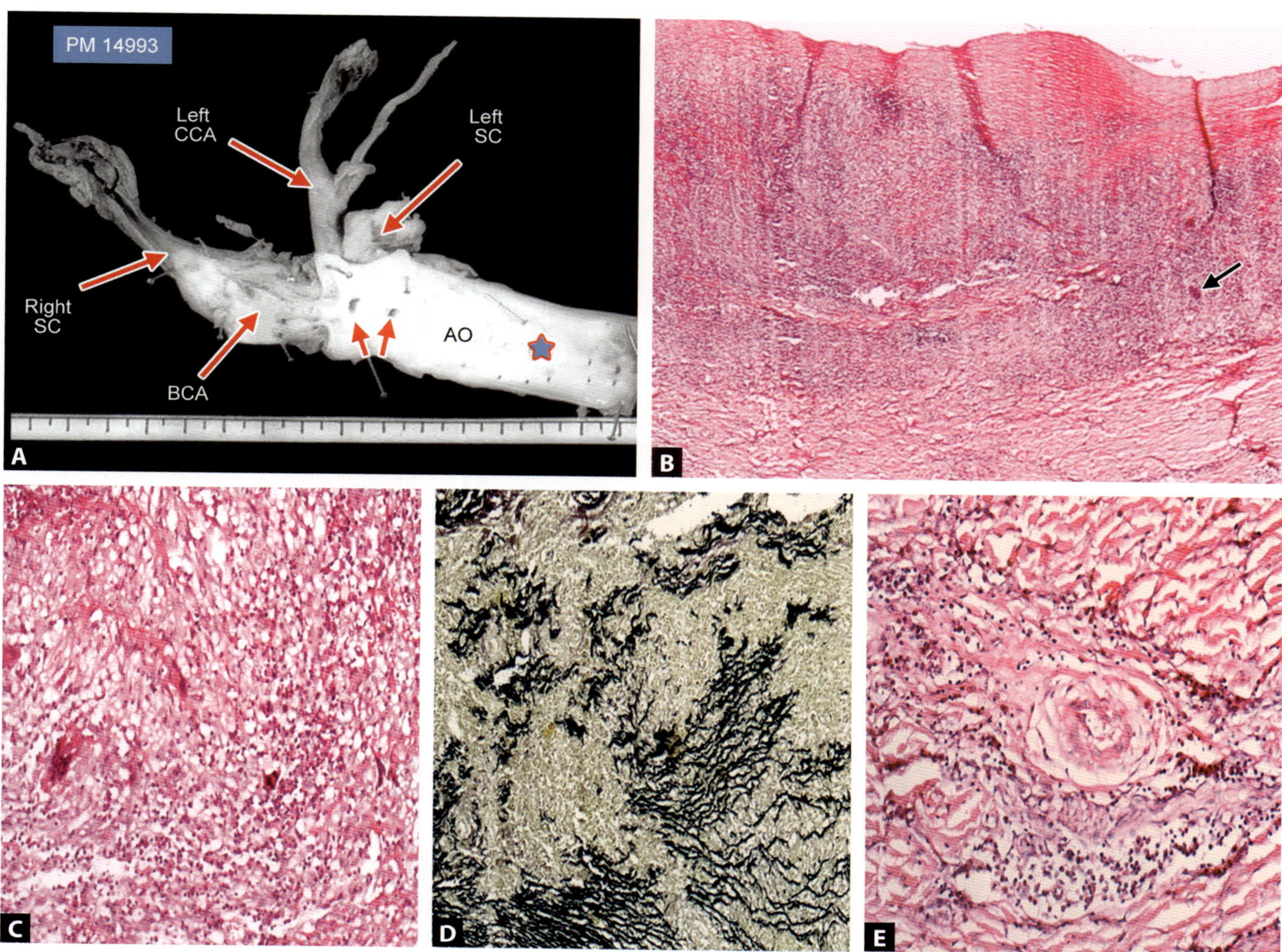

Figs 1A to E: (A) Gross photograph showing the arch of aorta with the origin of the brachiocephalic artery (BCA) which is opened up and shows ulcerated tree bark appearance (arrow). Also seen are the narrowed left common carotid (Lt CCA) and left subclavian arteries (Lt SC). The origin of the Lt CCA and Lt SC artery from the arch of aorta shows narrowing (small red arrows). The descending aorta (red star) is seen but the ascending aorta is not in the picture. Photomicrographs from the affected ascending aorta shows; (B) Transmural inflammation with giant cells (arrow); (C) Media of the aorta showing inflammation, giant cells and destruction of the elastic tissue; (D) EVG stain showing devastation of the elastic tissue of the media; (E) Inflammation seen around the vasa vasorum in the adventitia.

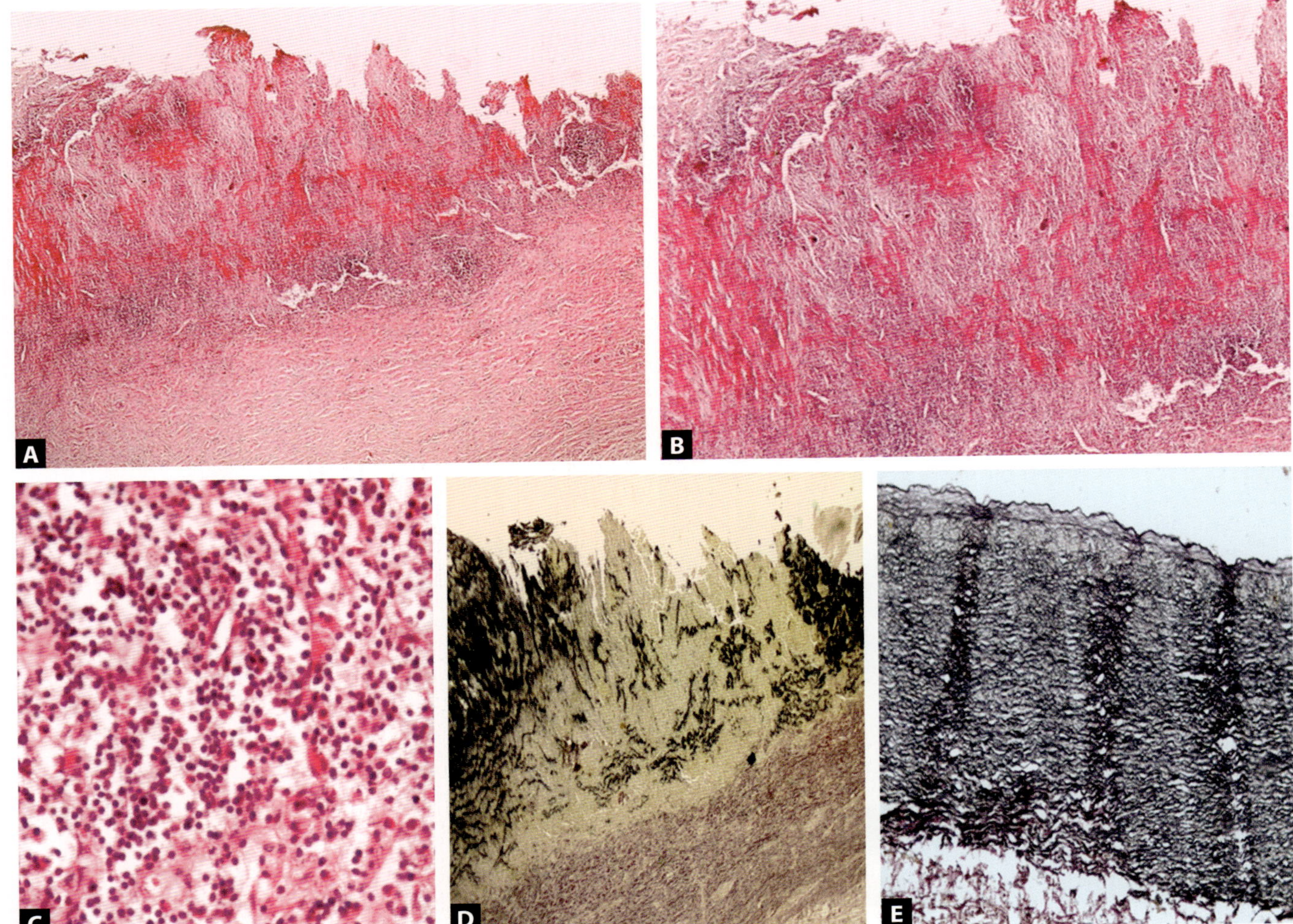

Figs 2A to E: Photomicrographs from the brachiocephalic artery shows (A) Transmural inflammation; (B) Total destruction of the elastic tissue of the media, giant cells and dense inflammation; (C) Dense collection of lymphomononuclear cells; (D) EVG stain shows destruction of the elastic tissue of the media; (E) EVG stain showing the normal organized elastic tissue of the media of a normal brachiocephalic artery.

a mosaic pattern and cut surface (Fig 4C) revealed areas of hemorrhage interrupted by prominent lines. Microscopically there was diffuse capillary proliferation (Figs 5A–C) in the lung parenchyma. This capillary proliferation was seen in the alveolar and bronchiolar walls (Fig 5D), interlobular fibrous septa and in the walls of pulmonary veins (Figs 6A–C) causing near total occlusion of their lumina. Many small muscular arteries manifested medial hypertrophy, cellular intimal proliferation and intimal fibrosis (Figs 6D and E) amounting to grade II pulmonary hypertension. Old and fresh intra-alveolar hemorrhages were present. Features in the lung are consistent with the diagnosis of pulmonary capillary hemangiomatosis. The ***heart*** weighed 190 g. There was biventricular (right 0.7 cm and left 1.2 cm) hypertrophy and the coronary arteries were normal.

FINAL AUTOPSY DIAGNOSIS: PM 14993

6 Years Female

- Takayasu's Aortoarteritis Type 3 (involving the ascending/arch/abdominal aorta, brachiocephalic, right and left subclavian and left common carotid artery)
- Pulmonary capillary hemangiomatosis
- Grade II pulmonary hypertension
- Biventricular hypertrophy—heart.

About Takayasu's Aortoarteritis: See Case 44

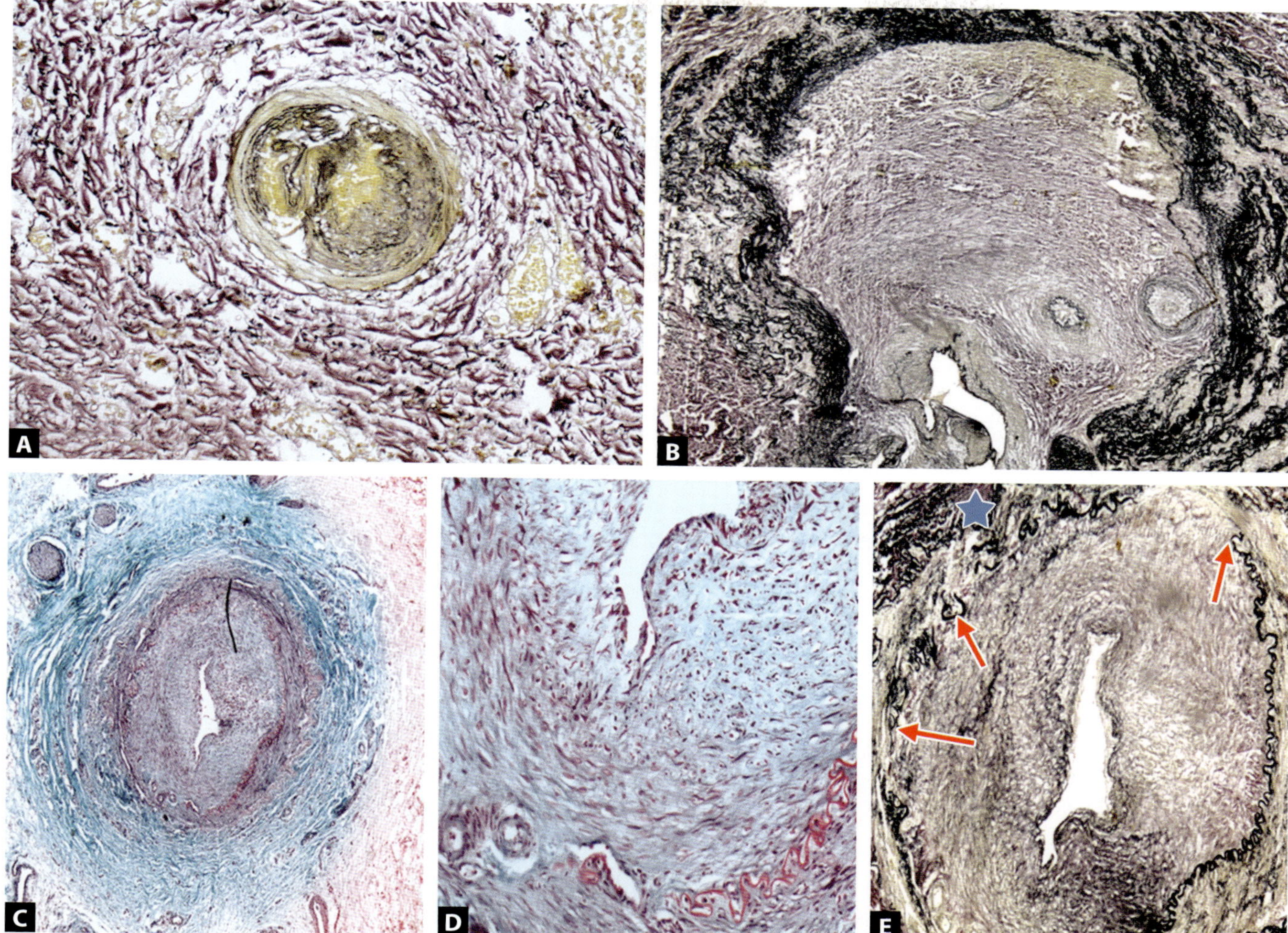

Figs 3A to E: (A) A small artery of the vasa vasorum of the brachiocephalic artery showing destruction of the internal elastic lamina and occlusion of the lumen (Elastic Van Gieson stain). (B) Elastic Van Gieson stain on the section of the right subclavian artery showing destruction of the elastic tissue of the media, marked intimal fibrosis with a chink like lumina. (C and D) Left subclavian artery shows marked intimal fibrosis, chink like lumina, destruction of the media and internal elastic lamina with minimal inflammation (Massons trichrome stain). (E) Elastic Van Gieson stain shows broken internal elastic lamina (arrows) and elastic tissue of the media (star).

PULMONARY CAPILLARY HEMANGIOMATOSIS

The entity pulmonary capillary hemangiomatosis (PCH) was discovered by Wagenvoort et al[1] in 1978, but its etiopathogenesis is still an enigma. So far, few cases have been reported in the literature.[1-7] It is a rare cause of pulmonary hypertension as the proliferation of capillaries within the walls of the pulmonary veins and venules causes a secondary veno-occlusive disease. Patients present with exertional dyspnea which progressively worsens. Chest X-rays show prominent pulmonary arteries and reticulonodular shadows, seen on both sides. On echocardiogram there is right ventricular hypertrophy, dilatation of the pulmonary arteries and high (normal 30 mm Hg) right ventricular systolic pressure. Grossly the lung on cut section shows scattered hemorrhagic areas giving a mosaic look. On microscopic examination, these patchy lesions show a diffuse proliferation of thin-walled capillary-sized blood vessels containing numerous erythrocytes. Capillary proliferation is prominently seen in the walls of pulmonary veins inducing a secondary pulmonary "veno-occlusive disease". This capillary proliferation is also demonstrable in the alveolar and bronchiolar walls, in the interlobular fibrous septa and as confluent areas in the parenchyma. The pleura, bronchial walls and pulmonary arteries may also be involved but to a lesser extent. Even though it is sometimes not possible to distinguish small pulmonary veins from arterioles, this lesion is most marked

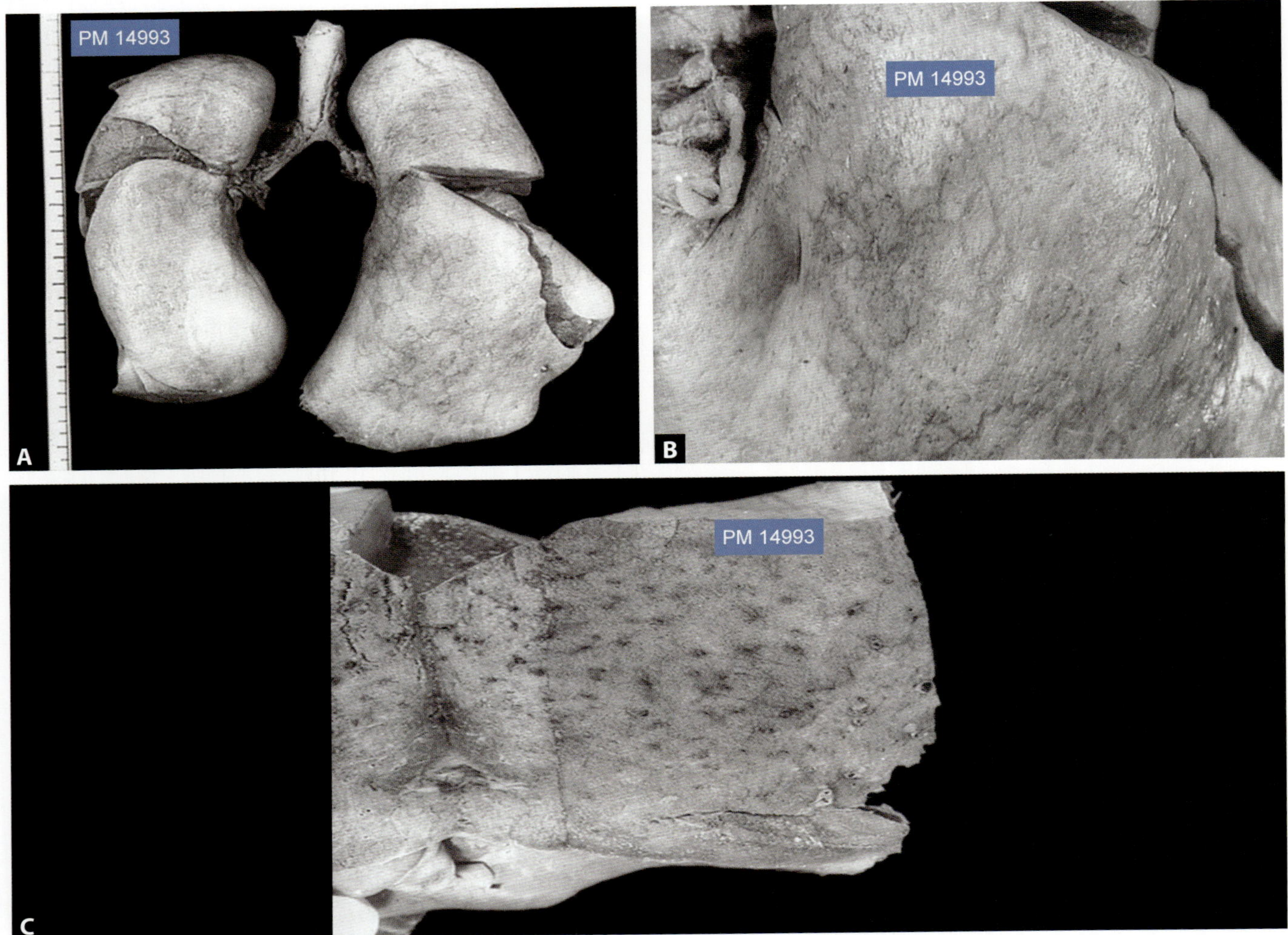

Figs 4A to C: (A and B) Lungs showing prominent lines on the pleural aspect forming a mosaic pattern; (C) Cut surface revealed areas of hemorrhage interrupted by prominent lines.

in the vessels adjacent to the venous septa, suggesting that the small vessels involved are indeed the veins. Muscular pulmonary arteries reveal changes of pulmonary hypertension. Intra-alveolar hemorrhages and hemosiderosis are frequently observed. The precise nature of this condition is debated. Wagenvoort et al[1] have considered this entity to be neoplastic but Magee et al[2] were unable to detect any pleomorphism or nuclear hyperchromatism in the endothelial cells.

COMMENTARY—INDEX CASE: PM 14993

This is a classical case of TA Type 3 in a 6 years female child affecting the ascending/arch/abdominal aorta, brachiocephalic artery, right and left subclavians and left common carotid. TA is associated with pulmonary hypertension which generally occurs either due to pulmonary arterial involvement by TA or due to elevated left ventricular end diastolic pressure, or both. In the index case of TA, the cause of pulmonary hypertension was a rare lesion termed PCH. This entity has a very distinct histopathologic picture, wherein proliferation of capillaries within the walls of the pulmonary veins and venules causes a secondary veno-occlusive disease.

TAKE HOME MESSAGE

- Takayasu's aortoarteritis is a chronic inflammatory arteriopathy of unknown etiology affecting large vessels, particularly the aorta and its main branches and to a lesser extent, the pulmonary artery.

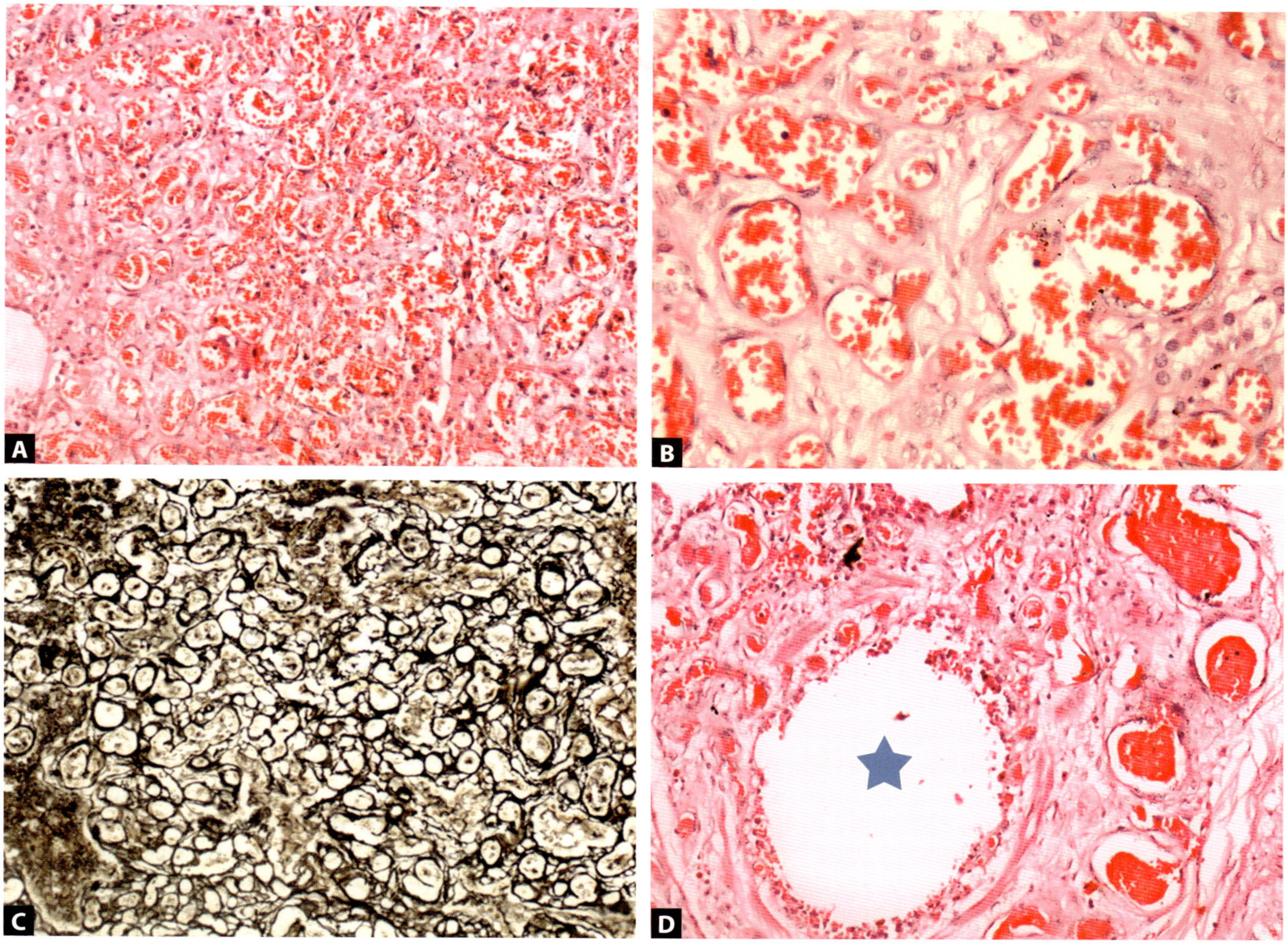

Figs 5A–D: Photomicrographs of the lung showing (A and B) Diffuse capillary proliferation; (C) Reticulin stain highlights capillary proliferation. (D) Variable-sized capillary proliferation seen in the wall of the bronchiole. The lumen of the bronchiole is marked by a star.

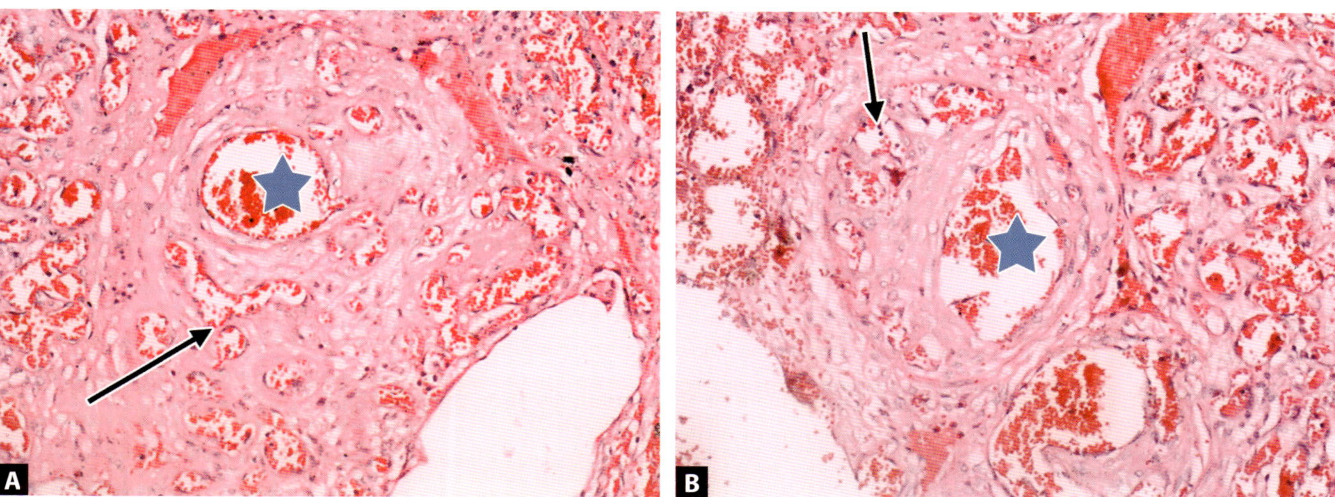

Figs 6A and B

icterus, cyanosis, edema or any lymph node enlargement. Cardiovascular (CVS) examination: precordial bulge +, left parasternal heave grade 3 with P2 loud. Liver was palpable, 3 cm below right costal margin. ***Investigations***: HIV, Mantoux, ANA, HbsAg, HCV, nitroblue tetrazolium test (NBT), dihydrorhodamine (DHR) and thyroid function tests were negative. ESR: 48, CRP: 174 mg/L and immunoglobulins (IgG/ IgD/IgM/ IgG2) were raised. ***X-ray*** revealed cardiomegaly, prominent main pulmonary artery and normal lung fields. ***HRCT and CECT*** done on 4.10.2013 revealed: RV and RA enlarged, dilated main PA (22.5 mm) and it is dilated compared to aorta, right PA (11.5 mm) and left PA (14 mm), 12 mm beyond main PA bifurcation there is abrupt severe attenuation in size of right pulmonary artery (1.2 mm) which is seen as a thin contrast opacifying line, there is evidence of mural thickening of ascending aorta, arch, descending thoracic aorta and major branches of aorta, few patchy mosaic attenuation are seen in left lower lobe of lung, likely due to vascular cause (PAH). Overall features are suggestive of aortoarteritis and with this right pulmonary artery possibility she was then transferred to pediatric immunology and rheumatology unit. A diagnosis of TA type 4 with right pulmonary artery stenosis with severe PAH was made and patient was started on tablets prednisolone, methotrexate, sildenafil and diuretics. Peripheral pulses were examined at this point and they were all present and equal. Renal Doppler done did not show evidence of renal artery stenosis. Cardiology opinion was taken for pulmonary artery stenting to ease her symptoms, which were mainly due to PAH. However, possibility of stenting was ruled out because of extensive disease and diffuse tapering of right PA. Subsequently patient was discharged in a hemodynamically stable condition.

Third Admission (24.03.2014–6 hours)

This time she presented to pediatric emergency with fever, cough and breathlessness for 2 days. Evaluation revealed left mid zone consolidation with increased TLC with severe hypoxemia and metabolic acidosis. On ***examination*** she was tachypneic, afebrile with RR of 50/min and HR of 132/min. She was irritable, peripheral pulses were feeble and blood pressure was 128/94 to 78/44 mm Hg. There was grade 1 clubbing and SaO_2 was 84% on room air and 90% on nasal prong oxygen. She was not thriving well. Respiratory system revealed respiratory distress, subcostal/intercostal/suprasternal retractions, active accessory muscles, dull percussion note below the 4th intercostal space on (L) side with adequate air entry. Cardiovascular system examination revealed left parasternal heave, loud P2 component of second heart sound and no murmur. Abdominal examination did not reveal any organomegaly. Nervous system examination revealed extreme irritability with Glasgow Coma Scale of 15/15.

Investigations

Investigations: Hb: 17 g/dL; TLC: 13,300/uL; platelets: 400,000/uL; blood urea: 40 mg%; serum creatinine: 0.7 mg%; serum Na^+: 131 mEq/L; serum K^+: 4.2 mEq/L; Chest X-ray: consolidation on left mid and lower lung regions; arterial blood gases—pH: 7.26, HCO_3^-: 9, pO_2: 74 mm Hg, pCO_2: 22 mm Hg. Blood culture was sterile. The child was treated with supplemented oxygen, fluid boluses, addition of inotropes and broad spectrum antimicrobials. She had worsening hypoxemia and metabolic acidosis requiring intubation and manual positive pressure ventilation. In spite of all measures, her condition was worsening and finally died at 6 hours of admission. ***Units clinical diagnosis***: TA type 4, severe PAH, right pulmonary artery stenosis and left lung pneumonia. Cause of death: cardiorespiratory failure with severe hypoxemia and severe metabolic acidosis due to (L) lung pneumonia.

AUTOPSY FINDINGS: PM 25988

A partial autopsy was performed. The pleural cavities contained 500 mL of serosanguinous fluid. The ***heart*** weighed 280 g. ***Left side of heart***: The left atrium was normal. Left ventricular hypertrophy was present with the wall measuring 1.6 cm (Fig 1A—black arrow). The aorta was normal for 2 cm from its origin (Fig 1A—black double arrow). Beyond that, the aorta (ascending/arch/descending thoracic) was markedly thickened (Fig 1A—blue arrow) and fibrotic (like a hose pipe) with the intima showing a dull, tree bark-like appearance (Figs 1A and B). All the three main branches (Figs 1C–F) arising from the arch of aorta, i.e. the brachiocephalic artery (BCA), left common carotid artery (LCC) and left subclavian artery (LSA) were involved by the disease process from their very origin. They were thickened, intima showed a dull, tree bark appearance and there was varying degrees of luminal occlusion. The occlusion was more at the origin with the LCC and LSA showing near total occlusion (Figs 1E and F). Microscopic sections from the aorta (Figs 2A–F) show marked intimal fibrosis and dense granulomatous inflammation in the outer part of the media, composed of lymphocytes, histiocytes and giant cells. The media showed extensive destruction of the elastic tissue (Fig 3A) and in areas total break of the media was noted (Fig 2F). The adventitia showed inflammation, more so around the vasa vaso-

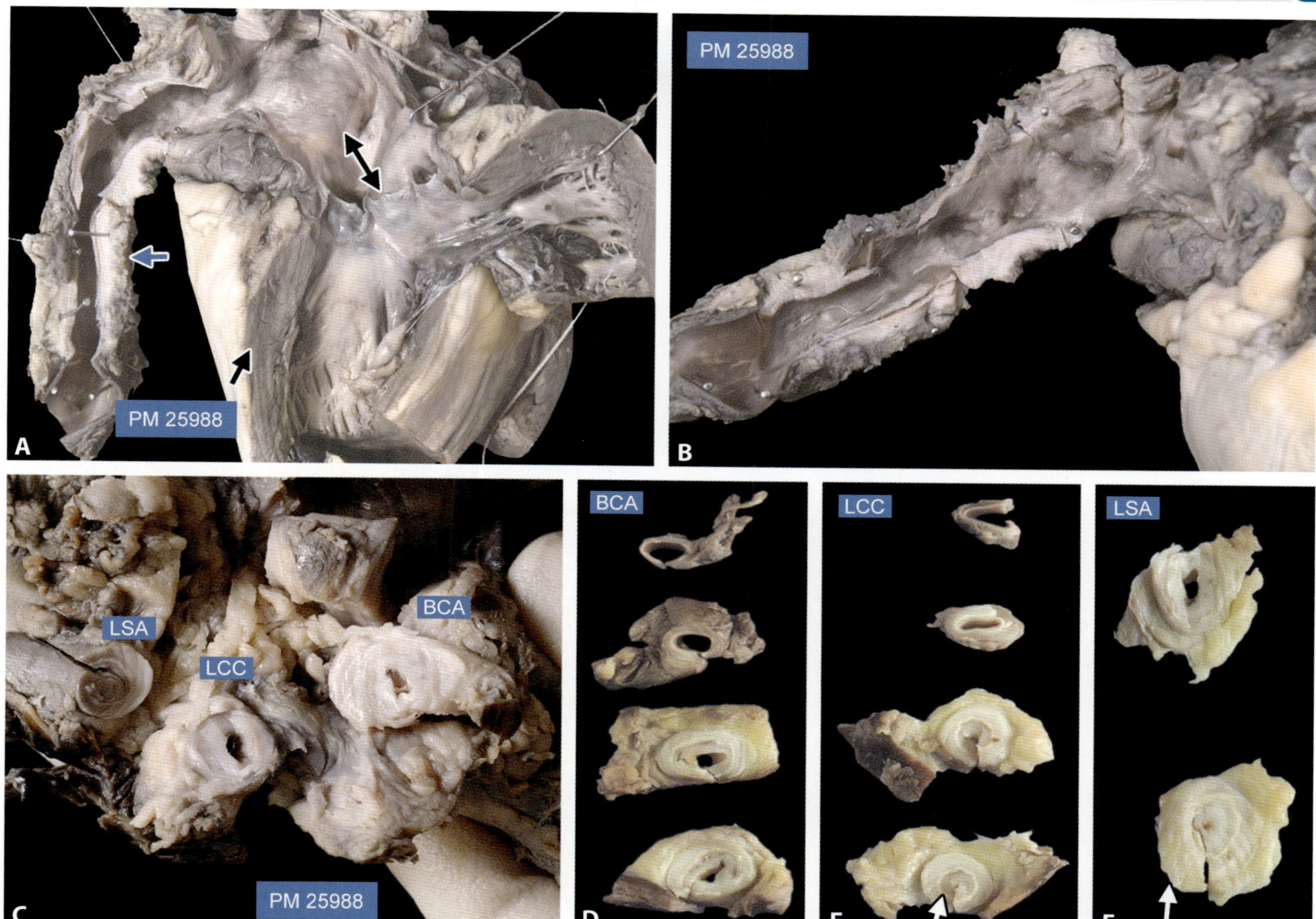

Figs 1A–F: (A) Outflow tract of the heart showing left ventricular hypertrophy (black arrow). The aorta is normal for 2 cm from its origin (double arrow). Beyond that it is thick and fibrotic like a hose pipe; (B) Opened up aorta showing a thick wall, with the intima showing a dull, tree bark like appearance; (C) Cut section of the brachiocephalic artery (BCA), left common carotid artery (LCC) and left subclavian artery (LSA) showing a thick wall and varying degrees of luminal occlusion; (D to F) Serial cuts of the BCA, LCC and LSA from their origin (below upward). The LCC and LSA show near total occlusion at the origin (arrows).

rum and vascular proliferation. Many small vessels of the vasa vasorum showed marked intimal fibrosis and near total occlusion of the lumina (Fig 3B). On immunohistochemistry, the inflammatory infiltrate was predominantly composed of T cell, (strong CD3 positivity, Fig 3C) along with few histiocytes (CD68 positive, Fig. 3C). The BCA (Figs 3D and E), LCC (Figs 4A–C) and LSA (Figs 4D–F) on microscopic examination revealed marked intimal fibrosis, dense inflammation (composed of lymphocytes, histiocytes and giant cells) in the media leading to its disruption and adventitial inflammation mostly around the vessels. ***Right side of heart***: The right atrium and right ventricle were dilated (Fig 5A), right ventricular hypertrophy (0.6 cm) was present (Fig 5A-arrow), the root of the main pulmonary artery was dilated, the ostia of the right pulmonary artery was firm and slightly narrowed with visible humps (Fig 5B-arrow) and the right branch of the pulmonary artery, 1.5 cm beyond its origin was firm and stenotic (Fig 5C-arrow). On microscopic examination, the right pulmonary artery (Figs 5D–F) showed florid intimal fibrosis leading to near total luminal occlusion and extensive inflammation of the media (Fig 5D-arrow). The elastic van Gieson (Fig 5F) stain showed disruption of the media with near total loss of elastic tissue at places. The abdominal aorta, renal arteries and mesenteric arteries were however normal. Overall features were consistent with a diagnosis of TA type 4. The ***lungs*** (Fig 6A) weighed 380 g. The pleural surface was shaggy. The cut section was firm with areas of breaking down and hemorrhage. Microscopic examination revealed confluent necrotizing pneumonia with multiple abscesses, getting confluent, composed of

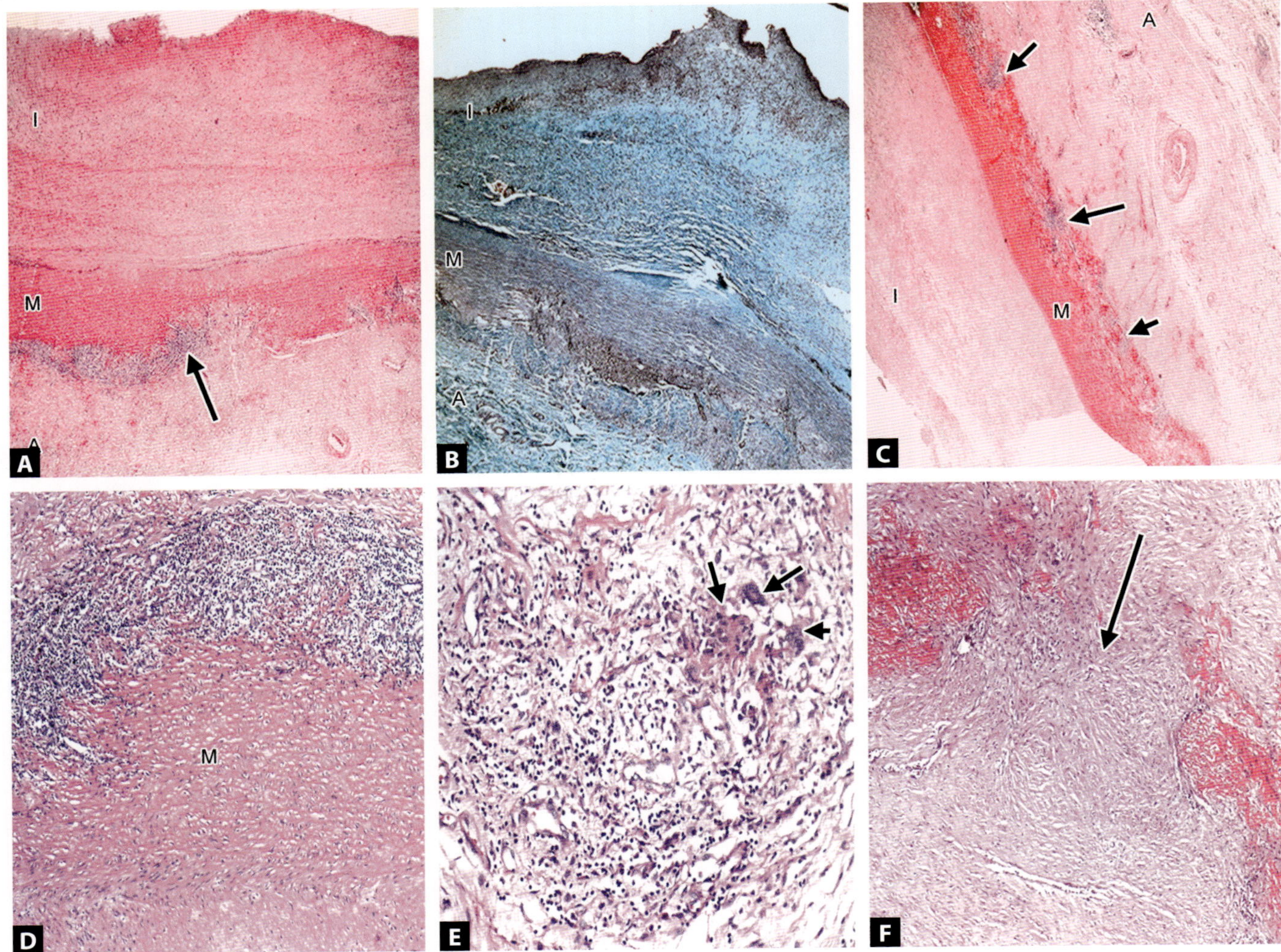

Figs 2A–F: (A–C [Trichrome stain]) Photomicrographs from the aorta showing intima (I), media (M), and adventitia (A). The intima is markedly thick with intimal fibrosis, media shows dense lymphomononuclear inflammation (arrows). (D and E) Media showing dense inflammation replete with giant cells. (F) Total break of the media (arrow).

polymorphs, nuclear debris and scattered giant cells (Figs 6B–D). Periodic acid–Schiff (PAS) stain revealed fungal profiles, ranging in size from 5–12 μm, showing prominent budding, morphology consistent with that of Cryptococcus (Fig 6E). The capsule stained pink with mucicarmine and deep blue with alcian blue (Fig 6F). The entire organism stained magenta with PAS and black with Grocott's silver stain (Fig 6G). Apart from this, alveolar hemorrhage, edema (Fig 7A), organization and lesions of pulmonary arterial hypertension (medial hypertrophy, intimal fibrosis and plexiform lesion—Figs 7B and C) were noted. The ***liver*** was enlarged and on microscopy showed passive venous congestion. Congestive splenomegaly was also seen.

FINAL AUTOPSY DIAGNOSIS: PM 25988

13-year-old Female

- Takayasu's aortoarteritis type 4—involving the:
  - Ascending aorta , arch of aorta , descending thoracic aorta
  - Brachiocephalic, left common carotid and left subclavian arteries
  - Right pulmonary artery.
- Biventricular hypertrophy, pulmonary arterial hypertension

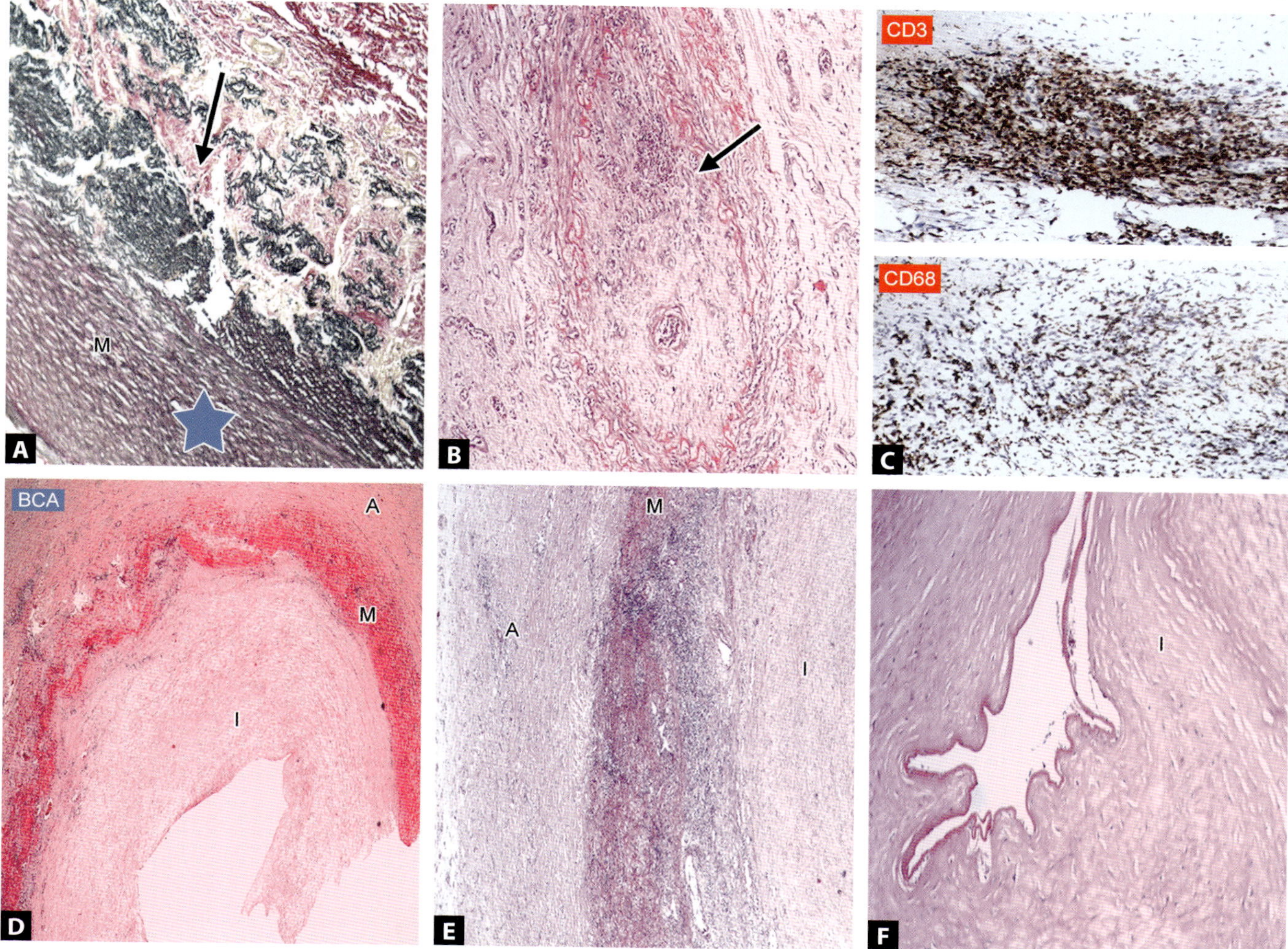

Figs 3A–F: (A) Aorta showing disruption (arrow) of the elastic fibers of the media-EVG stain. The inner part of the media is spared (star); (B) Occluded vessel (arrow) in the adventitia of the aorta; (C) Inflammatory infiltrate in the wall of the aorta showing strong positivity for CD3 along with scattered CD68 positive histiocytes; (D and E) Brachiocephalic artery with thickened intima (I) showing fibrosis and media (M) showing marked disruption due to inflammation. Adventitia (A) is thickened, shows fibrosis and sparse inflammation; (F) Near total luminal occlusion.

- Passive venous congestion—liver, congestive splenomegaly
- Confluent necrotizing pneumonia with abscesses–cryptococcal
- Pulmonary hemorrhage, edema and pleural effusion.

LARGE VESSEL VASCULITIS

Large vessel vasculitis[1] affects predominantly the large arteries, i.e. the aorta and its major branches. It consists of two entities, TA and giant cell arteritis, both of which may show granulomatous inflammation and affect the aorta and/or its major branches. Giant cell arteritis has a propensity to involve the branches of the vertebral or carotid arteries, may affect the temporal artery and often is associated with polymyalgia rheumatica. Both entities occur predominantly in females, age being the deciding factor between the two, TA occurs in younger individuals (<50 years) and giant cell arteritis in older individuals (>50 years).

TAKAYASU AORTOARTERITIS

Takayasu aortoarteritis (TA) is an inflammatory arteriopathy, often granulomatous, which involves the large vessels, i.e. the aorta and its main branches and to a lesser extent the pulmonary artery. It has varied names which include pulseless

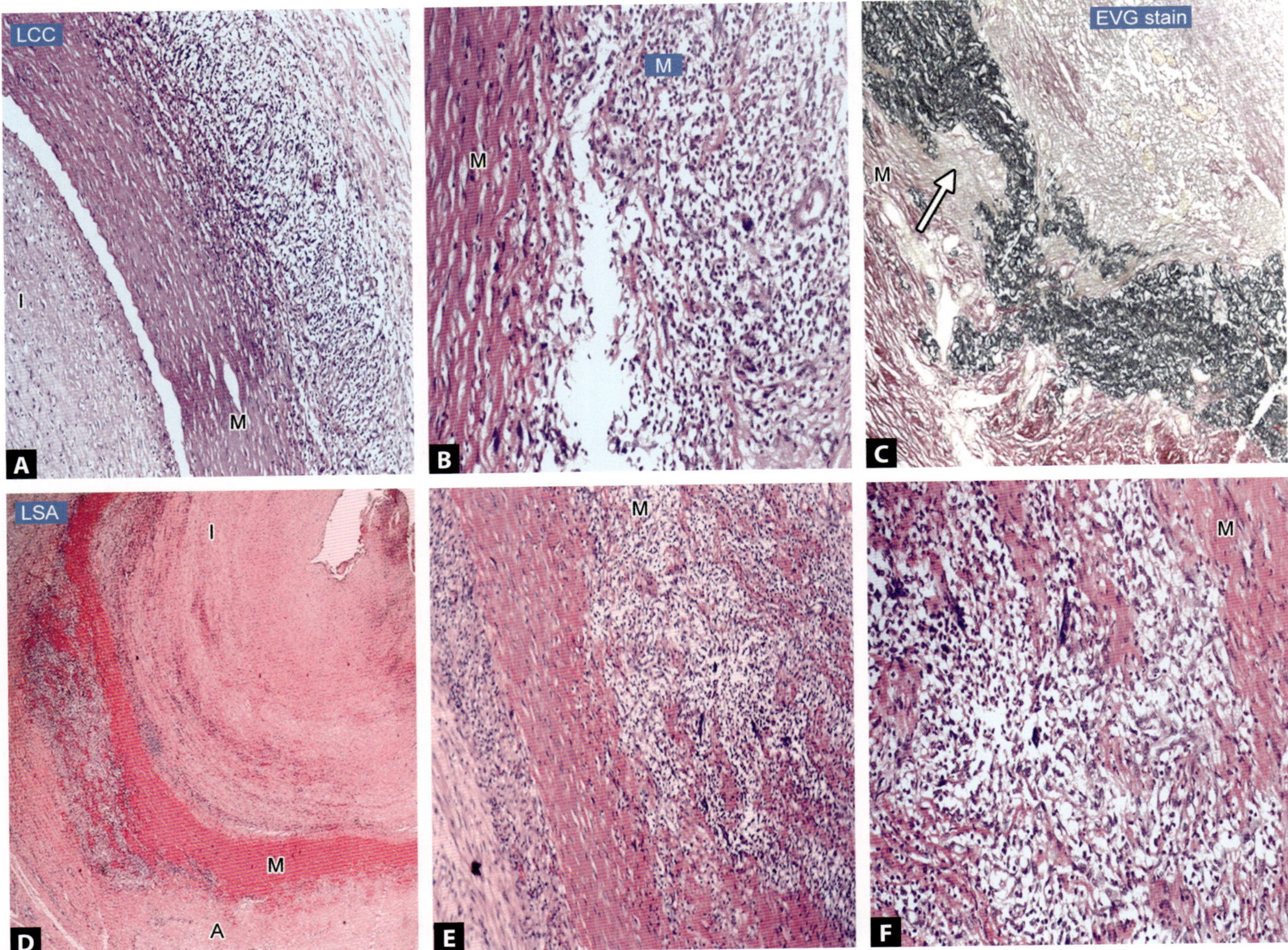

Figs 4A–F: Left common carotid artery-LCC (A–C (EVG stain)) and Left subclavian artery (LSA) (D–F) showing intimal fibrosis (I), dense inflammation in the media (M) with giant cells and disruption of the elastic tissue (arrow) along with luminal occlusion (seen in D).

disease, reverse coarctation, aortic arch syndrome, occlusive thromboaortopathy, etc. But it is referred to as Takayasu's disease after the name of the ophthalmologist who first described the characteristic retinal abnormalities in 1908. It occurs predominantly in young Asian females (less than 50 years) with female to male ratio of almost 9:1.[2] Chugh et al.[3] recorded a female to male ratio of 1.5:1 in India. The highest prevalence rate of TA has been described in Japan. TA is usually diagnosed in young women in the second or third decade but can also occur in early childhood.[4]

Natural history[5-7] is variable and divided into (A) Early pre-pulseless phase characterized by nonspecific signs and symptoms of a systemic inflammatory process like fever, fatigue, malaise, anorexia, weight loss, myalgias, night sweats and arthralgias. (B) Stage of vessel wall inflammation which is manifested by a characteristic sign such as "carotidynia". This is a pathognomonic finding which reflects inflammation of the carotid arteries and is seen in approximately 30% patients of TA. (C) Late phase characterized by signs and symptoms of vascular occlusion like claudication, angina, abdominal angina and renovascular hypertension. A mean of 8 years, with a range of months to several years may separate the early and late phases.

Absence of at least one arterial pulse (radial, ulnar, carotid) is seen in 98%; bruit in 86% and symptoms of claudication affect upper limb more than lower limb.[8] Systemic hypertension,[9,10] is seen in more than 50% of cases. The blood pressure in the lower limbs should be measured as the reading in the arm is low. Hypertension is due to renal ischemia, may be due to renal artery stenosis or else

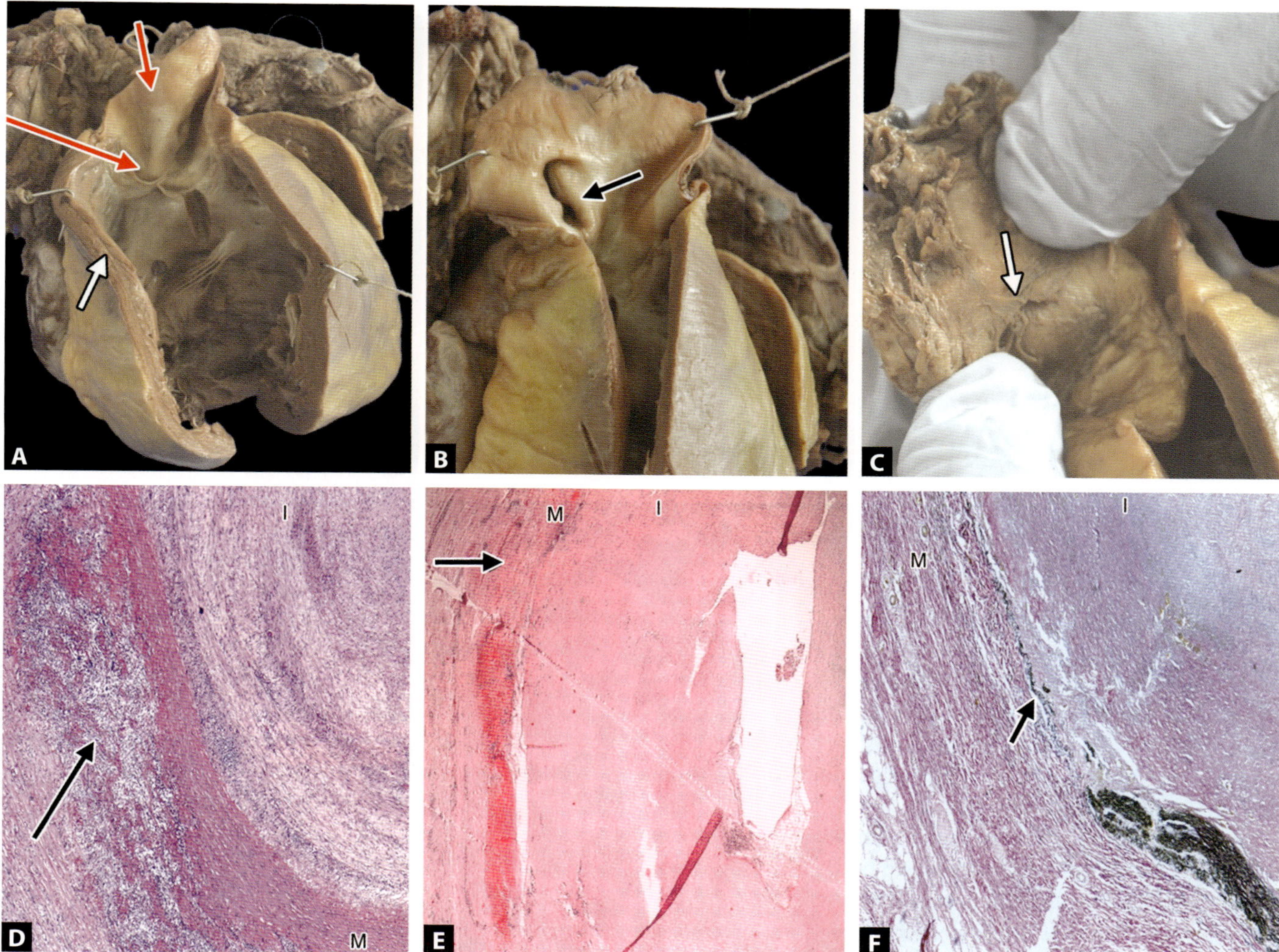

Figs 5A–F: (A) Right outflow tract showing pulmonary valve (long red arrow), dilated main pulmonary artery (upper red arrow) and right ventricular hypertrophy (white arrow); (B) Ostia (arrow) of the right pulmonary artery (RPA) showing narrowing with visible humpsl (C) Right pulmonary artery showing stenosis (arrow) 1.5 cm from its origin; (D) Right PA showing intimal (I) fibrosis and dense medial (M) inflammation (arrow); (E) RPA shows intimal (I) fibrosis, luminal narrowing and disruption of the media (M) (arrow); (F) EVG stain confirms the loss of elastic tissue of the media (arrow).

attributed to a loss of vascular compliance. Pulmonary hypertension has been observed in 27% of TA patients and may be either due to pulmonary arterial involvement or due to elevated left ventricular end diastolic pressure or both.[6] The arteries commonly involved in TA are the aorta, subclavian arteries, brachiocephalic, renal arteries at the ostia, carotids, vertebral, superior mesenteric, celiac, pulmonary and the coronaries. Inferior mesenteric artery is often spared. TA has four subtypes on the basis of arteriography: Type 1 involves the aortic arch and its branches; Type 2 involves the descending thoracic and abdominal aorta; Type 3 is a mixture of both 1 and 2 and Type 4 involves the pulmonary artery in addition to involvement of any part of aorta. Arteriography is the gold standard for evaluation.

Subclavian artery (Lt>Rt) is involved in up to 90% of cases leading to upper extremity claudication and at times Raynaud's phenomenon. Carotid artery involvement leads to transient decrease in visual acuity and narrowing of the visual fields may occur particularly with the face up position. Patients therefore tend to keep their neck flexed with a face down position. Neurological manifestations include headache, syncope, seizures, hypertensive encephalopathy, hemiplegia (7%) and subclavian steal syndrome when the subclavian artery proximal to the origin of the vertebral artery is involved. Significant aortic involvement occurs in more than 50% of patients. This causes aortic regurgitation in 5–19% due to aortic root dilatation. Congestive heart

Etiology of TA is unknown. It is said to be an outcome of interactions between genetic susceptibility, environmental trigger line infectious agents and epigenetic changes. Various postulations are infections (tuberculosis, streptococcus), immune-mediated, estrogens and genetic factors. Differential diagnosis is from giant cell arteritis (histologically they show the same features) which typically involves the temporal artery, affects females more than 50 years and is associated in 75% cases with polymyalgia rheumatica.

COMMENTARY—INDEX CASE: PM 25988

This young girl came with progressive dyspnea, cough, congestive heart failure (since 2½ years) and was initially diagnosed to have ASD with PAH. On follow up, a repeat echocardiography ruled out ASD and contrast echo showed no evidence of shunt and the right pulmonary artery could not be seen beyond its origin. This finding was however not investigated further. In the second admission, a year and nine months later, she came with complaints of cough, breathlessness and occasional hemoptysis. The peripheral pulses were normal, clubbing was present, she was emaciated, liver was palpable, cardiomegaly and prominent main pulmonary artery were noted. There was hypergammaglobulinemia and CRP/ESR were raised. HRCT and CECT clinched the diagnosis of TA type 4. Peripheral pulses at this point were re-examined and were all present and equal. Stenting was not possible as angiography revealed extensive involvement of right PA with diffuse tapering. She was started on tablets prednisolone, methotrexate, sildenafil and diuretics. In her final admission, she came with pneumonia, severe hypoxemia and metabolic acidosis. She succumbed to a florid cryptococcal infection of the lungs which was acquired, as she was emaciated and was on immunosuppressive therapy. The unique feature in this case of TA, was the initial presentation with PAH secondary to pulmonary artery involvement and peripheral pulses were present and equal, when on HRCT and CECT, significant disease was detected. This patient was diagnosed as TA, one year and nine months after the initial presentation and hence significant time was lost in initiating the correct treatment. Diagnosis of TA can be a diagnostic problem, especially in the pre-pulseless stage and in the stage of vessel wall inflammation, due to the nonspecific signs and symptoms. This period is a reversible phase of the disease, which should not be lost at any cost. Large vessel vasculitides contribute to 17% cases of pyrexia of unknown origin (PUO).[22] Noninvasive modalities like positron emission tomography (PET) imaging can be useful in detecting vessel wall inflammation in the early phase of TA, which present with nonspecific manifestations and pyrexia of unknown origin (PUO). Delay in diagnosis is common in TA and younger patients have four times higher diagnostic delay than their adult counterparts.[23] Thus, with a high degree of clinical suspicion and PET imaging, it would be possible to salvage patients in the early phases, so as to prevent life threatening interventions later on.

TAKE HOME MESSAGE

- Pulmonary artery involvement is fairly well seen in TA, but the initial presentation with severe pulmonary hypertension is uncommon.
- Diagnosis of TA can be a diagnostic problem, but with a high degree of clinical suspicion and PET imaging, it would be possible to salvage patients in the early phases, so as to prevent life threatening interventions later on.

REFERENCES

1. Jennette JC, Falk RJ, Bacon PA, et al. 2012 Revised International Chapel Hill Consensus Conference Nomenclature of Vasculitides. Arthritis & Rheumatism. 2013;65(1):1-11.
2. Cupps TR, Fauci AS. The Vasculitides. Philadelphia: Saunders; 1981. pp. 107-15.
3. Chugh KS, Sakhuja V, Malik N, et al. Nonspecific aortoarteritis is a major cause of renovascular hypertension in Asian countries. Proc Asian Pacific Congr Nephrol, Beijing. 1990;450-6.
4. Hass A, Stiehm ER. Takayasu's arteritis presenting as pulmonary hypertension. Am J Dis Child. 1986;140:372-4.
5. Lupi HE, Sanchez IG, Marcushamer J, et al. Takayasu's arteritis: clinical study of 107 cases. Am Heart J. 1977;93:94-103.
6. Chugh KS, Sakhuja V. Takayasu's arteritis as a cause of renovascular hypertension in Asian countries- Editorial. Am J Nephrol. 1992;12:1-8.
7. Johnson SL, Lock RJ, Gompels MM. Takayasu arteritis: a review. J Clin Pathol. 2002;55:481-6.
8. Hall S, Barr W, Lie JT, et al. Takayasu arteritis: A study of 32 North American patients. Medicine. 1985;64:89-99.
9. Sharma BK, Sagar S, Chugh KS, et al. Spectrum of renovascular hypertension in the young in North India: a hospital based study on occurrence and clinical features. Angiology. 1985;36:370-8.
10. Chugh KS, Sakhuja V. Aortoarteritis, a common cause of renovascular hypertension in Asia. Int J Artif Organs. 1988; 11:319-21.
11. Green NB, Baughman RP, Kim CK. Takayasu's arteritis associated with intestinal lung disease and glomerulonephritis. Chest. 1986;89:605-6.
12. Lai KN, Chan KW, Ho CP. Glomerulonephritis associated with Takayasu's arteritis. Report of 3 cases and review of the literature. Am J Kidney Dis. 1986;7:197-204.

13. Yoshikawa Y, Iri H, Hata J, et al. Granulomatous aortitis associated with necrotizing angiitis and glomerulonephritis. Acta Pathol Jpn. 1973;23:129-38.
14. Yamada I, Shibuya H, Matsubara O, et al. Pulmonary artery disease in Takayasu's arteritis: angiographic findings. AJR. 1992;159:263-9.
15. Lupi E, Sánchez G, Horwitz S, et al. Pulmonary artery involvement in Takayasu's arteritis. Chest. 1997;67:69-74.
16. Elsasser S, Soler M, Bolliger CT, et al. Takayasu disease with predominant pulmonary involvement. Respiration. 2000; 67:213-5.
17. Garcia-Olivé I, Bardají MSP, Pascual SC, et al. Severe pulmonary hypertension and Takayasu arteritis. Arch Bronconeumol. 2008;44(3):170-2.
18. Zheng D, Fan D, Liu I. Takayasu arteritis in China: a report of 560 cases. Heart Vessel Suppl. 1992;7:32-6.
19. Koyabu S, Isaka N, Yada T, et al. Severe respiratory failure caused by recurrent hemorrhage in Takayasu's arteritis. Chest. 1993;104:1905-6.
20. Arend WP, Michel BA, Bloch DA, et al. The ACR 1990 criteria for the classification of Takayasu arteritis. Arthritis Rheum. 1990;33:1129-34.
21. Sharma BK, Jain S, Radotra BD. An autopsy study of Takayasu arteritis in India. Int J Cardiol. 2000;75:S21-33.
22. Vanderschueren S, Knockaert D, Adriaenssens T, et al. From prolonged febrile illness to fever of unknown origin: the challenge continues. Arch Intern Med. 2003;163:1033-41.
23. Johnson SL, Lock RJ, Gompels MM. Takayasu arteritis: a review. J Clin Pathol. 2002;55:481-46.

CONTRIBUTIONS BY:

1. Dr Suraj Khanal, Associate Professor, Department of Cardiology (Compilation of Clinical Details)
2. Dr Surjit Singh, Professor and Head, Department of Pediatrics (Clinician In-Charge)

Post Graduate Institute of Medical Education and Research, (PGIMER), Chandigarh, India

CASE 45

Granulomatosis with Polyangiitis (Wegener's Granulomatosis) with Left Foot Gangrene and Right Hemiplegia: PM 14106

Nandita Bharadwaj Kakkar

 HIGHLIGHTS OF THE CASE

A 35-year-old male came with fever, cough, streaky hemoptysis, ulcerated lesion on the tongue, conjunctival hemorrhages, joint pains, palpable purpura, loose motions with melena, absent pulse in dorsalis pedis (both) and left posterior tibial arteries, gangrene of the left foot, terminal neck rigidity with right hemiplegia and deranged renal function tests. A diagnosis of systemic vasculitis with wet gangrene of foot, sepsis, cerebrovascular accident (CVA), pulmonary tuberculosis and renal insufficiency was made. Autopsy revealed features consistent with granulomatosis with polyangiitis (GPA), i.e. Wegener's granulomatosis involving the lungs, tracheobronchial tree, kidneys, spleen, brain, skin, ilium, colon and heart.

Keywords: granulomatosis with polyangiitis, Wegener's, hemiplegia, gangrene, foot, acute vasculitis, brain, large vessel involvement, autopsy.

 CLINICAL DETAILS

Date of Admission: 02.07.1994, Date of Death: 04.07.1994 and Duration of Hospital Stay: 2 Days

A 35-year-old male, a police constable by profession came with fever along with cough and expectoration since 2 months. The fever was moderate grade without chills and rigors. Occasional streaky hemoptysis was present and he was receiving anti-tubercular treatment on the basis of chest X-ray. He started having pain and swelling in various joints like wrist, shoulder, knee and hip joints for which he was put on nonsteroidal anti-inflammatory drugs (NSAIDs). He developed bluish-black discoloration on the feet which gradually spread to other parts. A few fluid-filled vesicles giving a purulent discharge erupted 10 days before admission. There was altered sensorium since 6 days. Loose motions with blood clots and occasional vomiting with blood clots was present since 2 days. On ***examination***, he was febrile, pale, pulse was 132/min, both dorsalis pedis and left posterior tibial arteries could not be felt and right posterior tibial was weak, BP: 140/60 mm Hg and pedal edema or periorbital puffiness was present. No cyanosis, clubbing, icterus or any lymphadenopathy was noted. Ecchymoses was seen on the lower limbs, trunk and upper limbs and multiple black patches were also seen, suggestive of skin infarction. Gangrene of left foot with secondary infection and foul smelling discharge was noted. There were large vesicular bullous lesions, 3–4 in number and pale digits. Palpable purpura in the form of ulcerated dark lesions were seen over the bony prominences and joints. An ulcerated lesion was seen over the tip of the tongue. Palpebral conjunctiva showed small hemorrhagic spots. The cardiovascular system was within normal limits. Abdomen revealed guarding but no free fluid. Conducted sounds were present in both the lungs. CNS examination revealed a comatose patient, pupils were reacting to light, neck rigidity and right hemiplegia was present and the plantars were upgoing.

Investigations and Course of Management

Investigations revealed a Hb of 7.8 g/dL which later fell to 4.5 g/dL; Reticulocyte count: 1.5%; platelets 110000/uL; ESR: 70 mm first hour; TLC: 15000/uL; DLC P86 L12, M1, E1, NRBC 15/100 WBC; Routine urine examination: protein 2+; RBCs 5–6/HPF, pus cells: 1–2/HPF; Electrolytes normal; Urea/creatinine: 94/2.9 mg%; uric acid: 10.4 mg%; cholesterol: 286 mg%; bilirubin: 0.7 mg%; SGOT/SGPT: 27/35 IU; alkaline phosphate: 11 U/L; calcium: 6.4 mg%; amylase: 133 U/L; random blood sugar: 102 mg%; ANF:

negative; C3: 100 mg%; RF: 1.8; coagulation profile: PTI 70%, PTTK 49" (38"); blood culture: E. coli (?extraneous); ABG: pH: 7.52, pO2: 55, pCO2: 21, HCO3: 17.3; ECG: deep symmetrical T inversion in V3, ST depression and T inversion V4-5; X ray chest: consolidation (L) upper zone with infiltration in both lung fields; CT head: could not be done.

He was started on antibiotics, hydrocortisone 100 mg IV 6 hourly and dexamethasone 20 mg stat and then 4 mg 6 hourly. Dermatologists opinion was active vasculitis of small and medium-sized vessels (? PAN ? Septicemia). Surgeons opinion was gangrene of left foot with absence of (L) posterior tibial pulsations and superadded infection, to be managed conservatively. Neurologists opinion was ? drug-induced vasculitis, ? occlusive ? hemorrhagic stroke and septicemia. He sustained a cardiorespiratory arrest from which he could not be revived. ***Units final diagnosis*** was—Systemic necrotizing vasculitis, wet gangrene feet with secondary infection and septicemia, right hemiparesis CVA ? Infarction ? bleed, pulmonary tuberculosis and renal insufficiency.

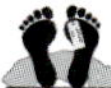

AUTOPSY FINDINGS: PM 14106

A complete autopsy was performed on this 35-year-old male. On external examination multiple (0.5–1.5 cm) ecchymotic macules, patches and plaques were present over the lower limbs, trunk and upper limbs. Skin over left foot and lower left leg was black with areas of abscess formation. Skin of the right foot was also discolored. On opening, all the serous cavities were within normal limits. Both the ***lungs*** weighed 1,600 g. Fibrinous pleuritis (Fig 1A) with adhesions were noted. Cut section (Fig 1B) showed areas of consolidation measuring 7 x 6 x 5 cm in the left upper lobe and 5 x 4 x 3 in the right lower lobe along with tracheal and bronchial ulceration. On microscopic examination (Figs 1C and D), geographic areas of necrosis bordered by granulomatous inflammation with many giant cells and histiocytes, small to medium vessel (arteries and veins) acute necrotizing (Fig 1E) and granulomatous vasculitis (Figs 2A–C), necrotizing tracheitis (Fig 1F), bronchitis, bronchiolitis and proliferative alveolitis was seen. Giant cells and histiocytes were in plenty. Elastic Van Gieson stain showed devastation of the internal elastic lamina of the arteries (Fig 2D). No organisms were identified and special stains with periodic acid–Schiff (PAS), Grocott, Gram and AFB were negative. Overall features in the lung were consistent with a diagnosis of granulomatosis with polyangiitis (Wegener's granulomatosis). The ***kidneys*** were flee bitten. Microscopy revealed focal segmental/diffuse necrotizing glomerulonephritis with the tufts showing fibrinoid necrosis and nuclear debris (Figs 3A–C). No crescent was however seen. Interlobular arteries showed acute vasculitis with transmural inflammation and fibrinoid necrosis (Figs 3D–F). No granulomatous glomerulonephritis or arteritis was seen in the kidneys. Dense interstitial inflammation was noted. Immunoperoxidase stains for IgG, IgM, IgA, fibrinogen and complement were negative. The ***spleen*** weighed 350 g and showed extensive infarction along with necrotizing vasculitis of small and medium-sized vessels. The entire ***terminal ileum, caecum and ascending colon*** were studded with small, well-defined, round ulcers, 0.3–0.5 cm in diameter with central area of necrosis (Fig 4A). Microscopic sections revealed evidence of florid small vessel acute vasculitis in the submucosa (Figs 4B and C). The ***brain*** revealed an area of discoloration in the left frontoparietal region measuring 5 x 4 x 4 cm in the domain of middle cerebral artery, but the artery itself was normal. The lesion was seen selectively in the white matter sparing the cortex. Under the microscope, it revealed extensive small vessel vasculitis with necrosis (Figs 4D and E). The ***skin*** showed acute vasculitis with fibrinoid necrosis, polymorphs and nuclear debris. The ***heart*** revealed fibrinous pericarditis and focal areas of myocarditis with polymorphs, nuclear debris and small vessel vasculitis. The dorsalis pedis and posterior tibial arteries could not be dissected out, for want of permission from the relatives. Postmortem antineutrophil cytoplasmic antibodies (ANCA) could not be done.

FINAL AUTOPSY DIAGNOSIS: PM 14106

35-Year-Old Male

Features consistent with Granulomatosis with Polyangiitis (GPA), i.e. Wegener's granulomatosis with:

- Vasculitis and granulomatous inflammation in the lungs and tracheobronchial tree.
- Pauci-immune focal segmental/diffuse necrotizing glomerulonephritis with extraglomerular acute vasculitis of the interlobular arteries.
- Acute vasculitis in the spleen, brain, skin, ileum, colon and heart.
- Fibrinous pericarditis.

Granulomatosis with polyangiitis: See Chapter 'Small vessel vasculitis'.

NEUROLOGICAL INVOLVEMENT IN GRANULOMATOSIS WITH POLYANGIITIS

Neurological manifestations are seen in GPA, more so in the peripheral nervous system where they manifest as

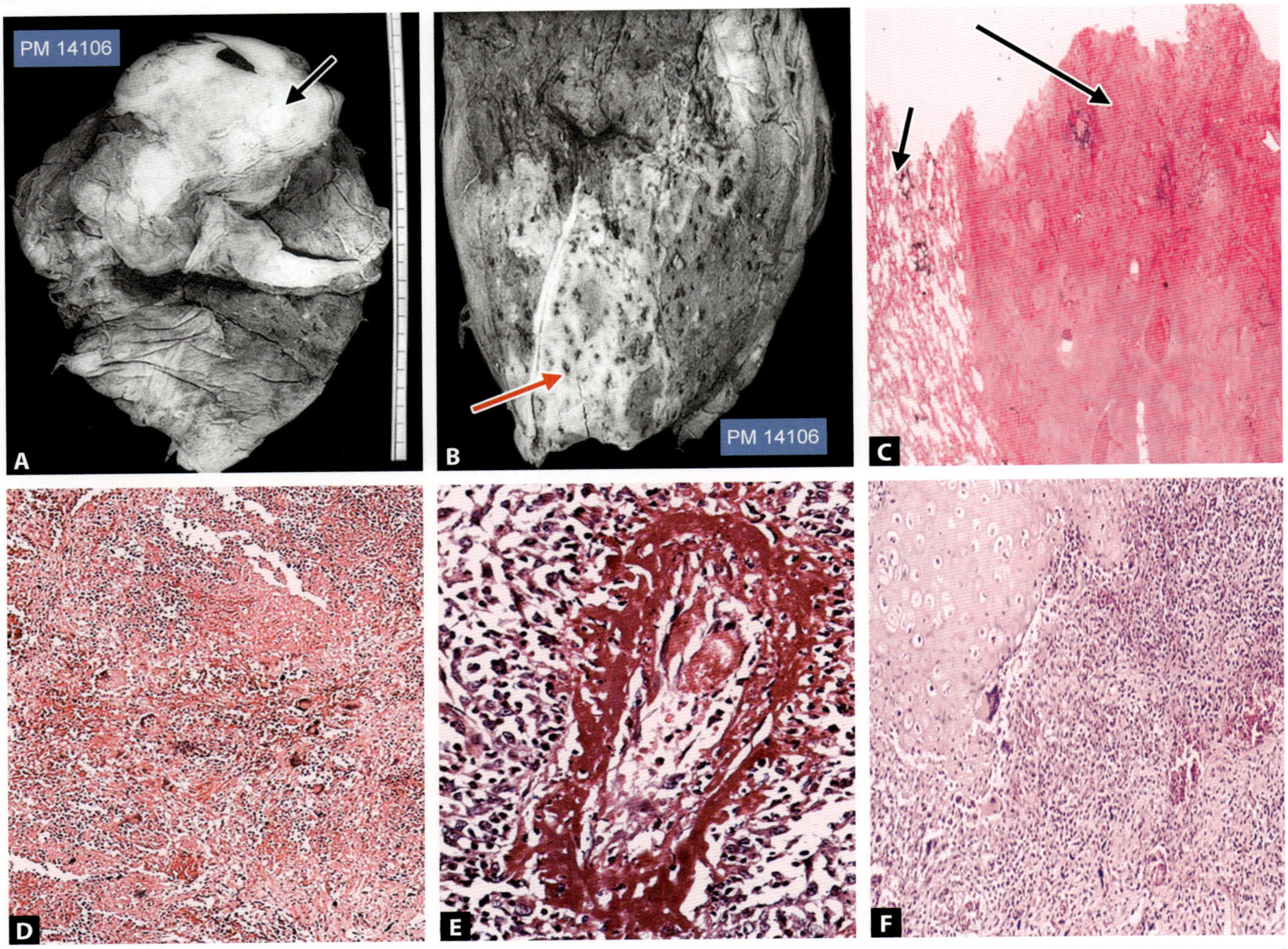

Figs 1A–F: (A) Gross picture of the lung showing thickened pleura (arrow); (B) Cut section of the lung showing well-defined whitish areas of consolidation, which shows breaking down; (C) Photomicrograph showing area of necrosis (long arrow) with adjacent normal lung parenchyma (small arrow); (D) Periphery of the necrotic area of the lung showing plenty of giant cells; (E) Lung showing acute vasculitis with fibrinoid necrosis, polymorphs and nuclear debris in the wall; (F) Trachea showing ulceration, dense inflammation with giant cells, few abutting on the cartilage.

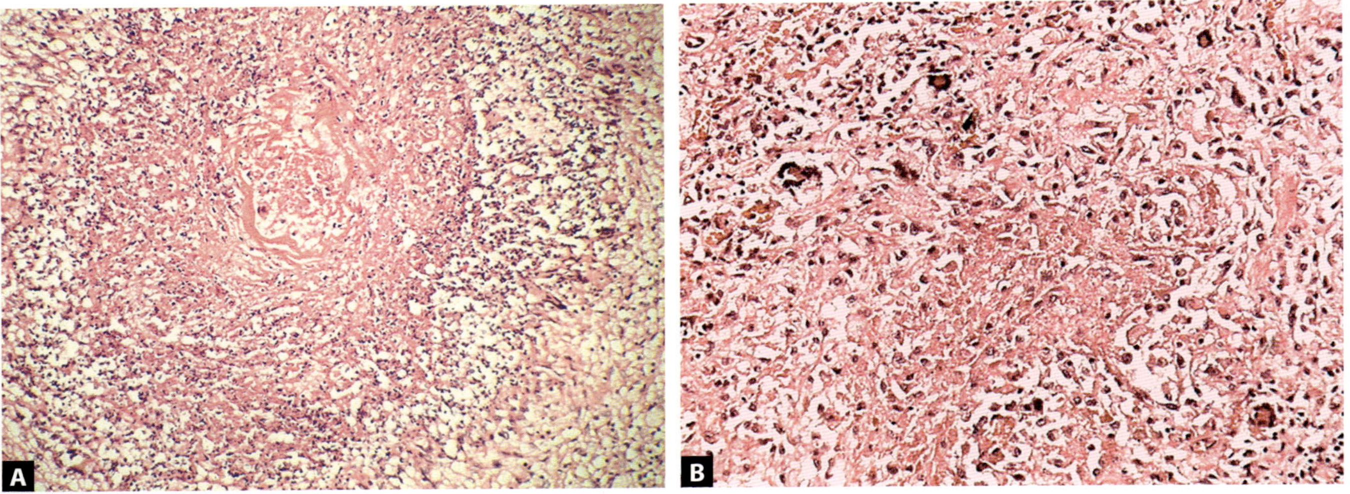

Figs 2A and B:

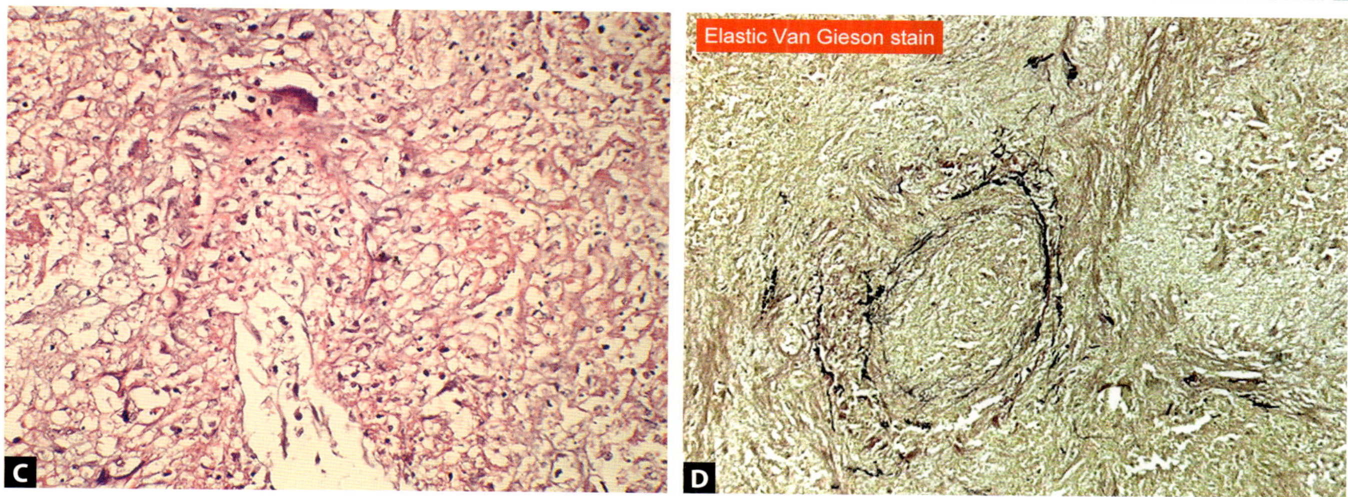

Figs 2A–D: Photomicrographs of the lung showing (A and B) Granulomatous vasculitis with fibrinoid necrosis and a collarette composed of polymorphs, nuclear debris, epithelioid histiocytes, and giant cells; (C) Vessel showing inflammation in the wall along with giant cells; (D) Elastic Van Gieson stain showing break of the internal elastic lamina.

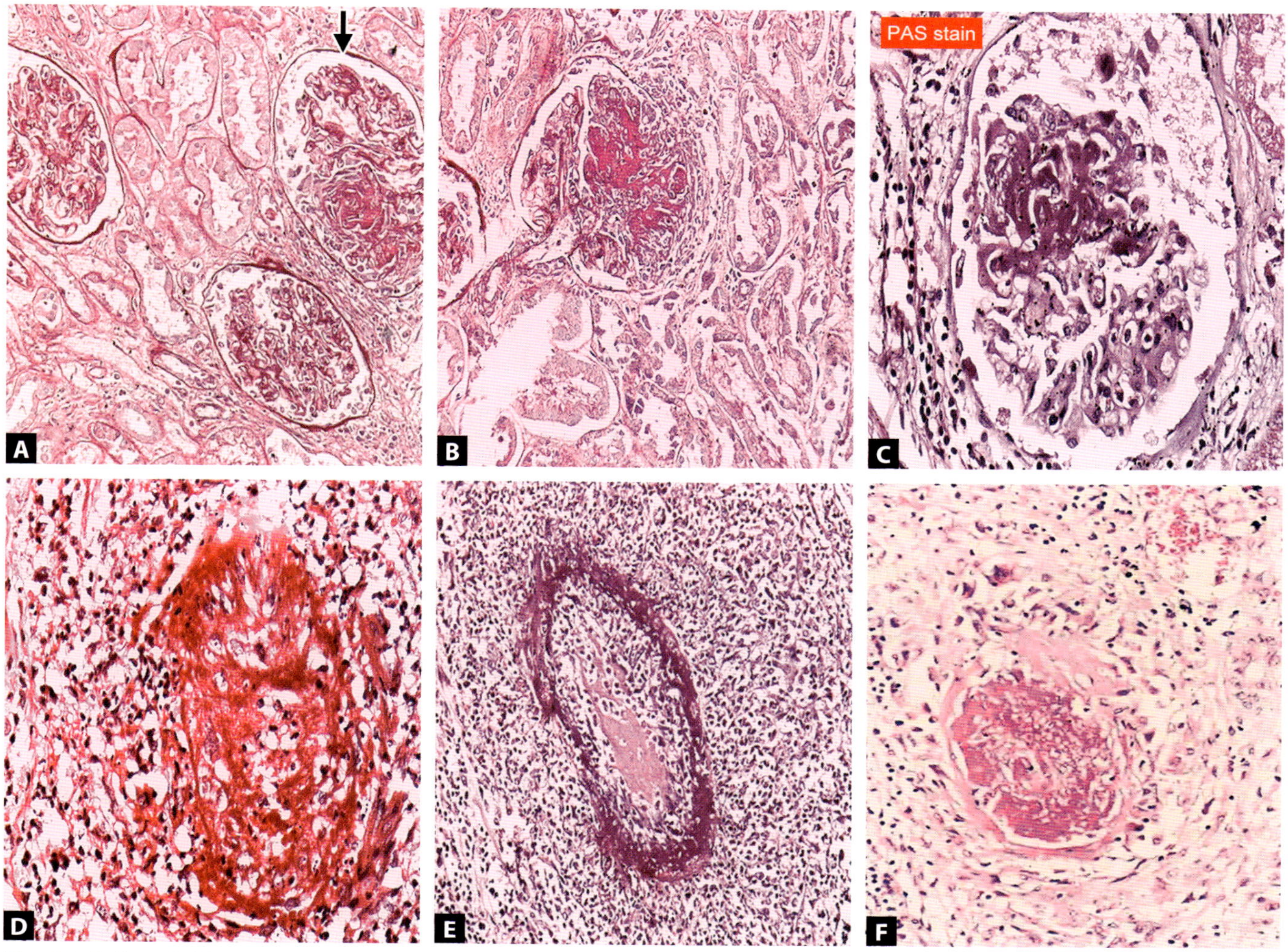

Figs 3A–F: (A to C) Photomicrographs of the kidney showing segmental to diffuse necrotizing glomerulitis with fibrinoid necrosis and nuclear debris; (D to F) Interlobular arteries showing acute vasculitis with transmural necrotizing inflammation, fibrinoid necrosis and nuclear debris.

CASE 46

Granulomatosis with Polyangiitis—Wegener's Granulomatosis, Presenting as an Anterior Mediastinal Mass: PM 18613

Nandita Bharadwaj Kakkar

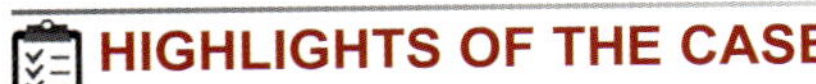

HIGHLIGHTS OF THE CASE

A young male came with fever, cough, hemoptysis and abdominal pain. Investigations revealed an anterior mediastinal mass along with pleural/pulmonary nodules. Fine needle aspiration cytology (FNAC) from the mass showed necrotic tissue, degenerated inflammatory cells, foreign body type of giant cells, with acid-fast bacilli (AFB)/fungal stains negative and a diagnosis of tuberculosis was considered. The renal function tests were mildly deranged and CT scan revealed hemorrhage in the midbrain, fourth ventricle and cerebellum along with hydrocephalus. The clinical diagnosis was anterior mediastinal mass ? tuberculosis ? lymphoma with intracerebral and cerebellar hemorrhage. Autopsy revealed a classical picture of granulomatosis with polyangiitis (GPA), i.e. Wegener's granulomatosis (WG) (cANCA 4+) presenting as a large anterior mediastinal mass with involvement of the trachea, lungs, kidneys, testes, muscle, pericardium and spleen.

Keywords: Wegener's granulomatosis, granulomatosis with polyangiitis, systemic vasculitides, mediastinal mass, uncommon presentation, autopsy.

CLINICAL DETAILS

Date of Admission: 28.06.2002, Date of Death: 19.07.2002, Duration of Hospital Stay: 22 Days

A 25-year-old male was admitted with history of high grade intermittent fever with associated malaise, headache and night sweats since 2 months. There was productive cough which was worse on lying down along with hemoptysis since the same duration and breathlessness which was progressively worsening since 15 days. The patient was in New York Heart Association class III. There was right upper quadrant abdominal pain which was severe, continuous, non-radiating and lasted for 3-4 hours at a time. There was no history of chest pain, edema, palpitations, jaundice, abdominal distension, alteration in bowel habit, joint pains, skin rash or any bleeding from any site. On examination there was pallor, pulse—30/min, BP—120/80 mm Hg and RR—24/min. There was no peripheral lymphadenopathy, icterus, clubbing or edema. The respiratory system examination revealed impaired percussion note in left upper parasternal region and the breath sounds were normal. Central nervous system examination was within normal limits.

Investigations and Course of Management

Investigations: Hb—10.6 g/dL, TLC—12000/uL, DLC P60,L35,M3,E2, platelets—3,00,000/uL, ESR—57, serum creatinine—1.1 mg%, urea 50 mg%, total proteins/albumin—6.6/3.2 gm, random blood sugar—137 mg%, liver function tests normal, CSF—hemorrhagic with 60 WBCs, 20% polymorphs, proteins—30 g%, sugar—66 mg%, culture sterile, ADA—8 U/L, Toxoplasma IgG—less than 1:40, Crypto-latex agglutination—negative, Widal—negative, HIV—non-reactive, blood cultures done thrice—negative, routine urine examination was normal, urine culture—sterile; blood film for MP x 3 negative, sputum AFB smear x 3 negative. ***USG abdomen***: 5.5 × 5.6 cm well-defined smooth-walled cystic lesion with post acoustic enhancement in segment 5 and 6 of liver; ***Chest X-ray*** shows a mass in the left upper zone, abutting the superior mediastinum with an ill-defined opacity in the retro-cardiac region; ***Contrast-enhanced CT*** chest/abdomen shows an anterior mediastinal heterogeneous hypodense mass lesion with pleural nodules and a single parenchymal nodule in left lower lobe, a single large cyst in the right lobe of liver and small ill-defined hypodense lesion in the retro-pancreatic region; ***CT head***

showed hemorrhage in the midbrain and fourth ventricle with hydrocephalus; ***FNAC*** from the mediastinal mass shows necrotic tissue, degenerated inflammatory cells, multinucleated foreign body type giant cells, AFB stain negative, fungal stain negative and no malignant cells. On the basis of the FNA, a diagnosis of tuberculosis was suggested. ***Course in hospital***: This patient was hospitalized for 22 days in our institute. The first computarized tomography of the head was done a week after his admission, which revealed hemorrhage in the midbrain and fourth ventricle along with hydrocephalus. On the 16th day of admission, the patient had severe headache with 3-4 bouts of vomiting. There was sudden profuse sweating and stiffening of the body. Sensorium improved with conservative management. He was also given broad-spectrum antibiotics and later anti-tubercular therapy. A ventriculoperitoneal shunt and digital subtraction angiography were planned. On the 19th day, he had an acute cry with clenching of mouth and tonic posturing of the body. CT head was repeated and showed a cerebellar hemorrhage. He was given anti-cerebral edema measures, remained unconscious and expired on 22nd day of admission. ***Units final diagnosis***: Anterior mediastinal mass ? tuberculosis ? lymphoma with intracerebral and cerebellar hemorrhage.

AUTOPSY FINDINGS: PM 18613

A partial autopsy was performed on this 25-year-old male. The brain was not in examined. All the serous cavities were within normal limits. The ***trachea*** showed extensive ulceration with evidence of acute vasculitis. The ***lungs along with the anterior mediastinal mass*** weighed 880 g. The mediastinal mass was present over the anterior surface of the left lung and measured 8 × 7 × 1.5 cm (Fig 1A). The mass could be separated from the lung to quite an extent (Fig 1B) but one part of it was seen to be in continuity with a mass in the middle portion of the left lung (Fig 1C). Cut section of the mass was firm with soft areas and small areas of hemorrhage (Fig 1D). On cut section, the left lung shows total consolidation of the middle portion over an area of 10 × 9 × 8 cm forming a yellowish mass with areas of breakdown. The right lung shows small yellowish nodules distributed randomly more in the lower lobes (Fig 1C). Microscopic sections from the mass within the ***lung*** showed a variety of lesions. There were large areas of necrosis bordered by hemorrhage (Fig 2A). The necrotic areas revealed dense inflammation bordered by giant cells (Fig 2B) and in some areas there were plenty of foreign body giant cells with inflammation and fibrosis (Fig 2C). The small arteries in these areas show acute vasculitis with fibrinoid necrosis and transmural inflammation of the wall (Fig 2D), granulomatous arteritis, where in an artery showing inflammatory changes in its wall was seen palisaded by histiocytes and giant cells were seen (Figs 2E and 3A). Break of internal elastic lamina was better appreciated in elastic van Gieson stain (EVG) (Fig 3B). Stains for AFB and Periodic acid-Schiff (PAS) done on multiple sections were negative. Features were consistent with granulomatosis with polyangiitis (GPA), i.e Wegener's granulomatosis (WG). The sections from the ***mediastinal mass*** showed florid acute vasculitis (Figs 3C and D, Figs 4A and B) involving the small/medium-sized arteries and veins. Apart from this, there was inflammation, areas of geographic necrosis bordered by giant cells, dense fibrosis (Fig 4C) and caught up lymph nodes and the thymus. EVG stain revealed destruction of the internal elastic lamina and an occasional artery showed marked intimal fibrosis with near total occlusion of the lumina, i.e. a healed lesion (Fig 4D). The ***kidneys*** weighed 200 g. Capsular surface exhibited a flee-bitten appearance with small infarcts (Fig 5A). Cut section (Fig 5B) shows peripheral infarcts and small hemorrhages. The renal vein and artery were normal. On microscopic examination, the glomeruli showed a variety of lesions, focal (Fig 5C) and predominantly diffuse (Fig 5D) necrotizing lesions where the glomerular tuft shows fibrinoid necrosis with polymorphs and nuclear debris. Few crescents were also noted (Fig 5E). Diffuse necrotizing lesions with break of the Bowman's capsule and emergence of the tuft with the interstitium was noted (Fig 6A). Infarcts (Fig 6B) and extraglomerular acute vasculitis involving the small (Figs 6C and D) and medium-sized arteries (Figs 6E and F) were seen. No granulomatous vasculitis or granulomatous glomerulonephritis was identified. Interstitial inflammation was prominent. Immunohistochemistry with IgG, IgM, IgA, C3 and fibrinogen were all negative, thus indicating the pauci-immune nature of the glomerulonephritis. Postmortem cANCA was strongly positive by indirect immunofluorescence and by ELISA technique. The ***heart*** weighed 210 g and the pericardium was dull. On the anterior aspect of the pulmonary artery, a hematoma 2×1×1 cm was visible. The valves and chambers were unremarkable. Microscopy shows acute small vessel vasculitis in the pericardium (Fig 7A). The pulmonary artery was microscopically normal. Apart from this, small vessel acute vasculitis with inflammation and fibrinoid necrosis was seen in the ***muscle*** (Fig 7B), ***testis*** (Fig 7C), ***epididymis*** and ***spleen***. The ***liver*** showed a simple cyst (not otherwise specified) in the right lobe measuring 4 cm in diameter. The brain was not examined due to lack of permission from the relatives, however if examined would have shown florid features of vasculitis, in view of the CT scan findings of intracranial hemorrhage (parenchymal and ventricular).

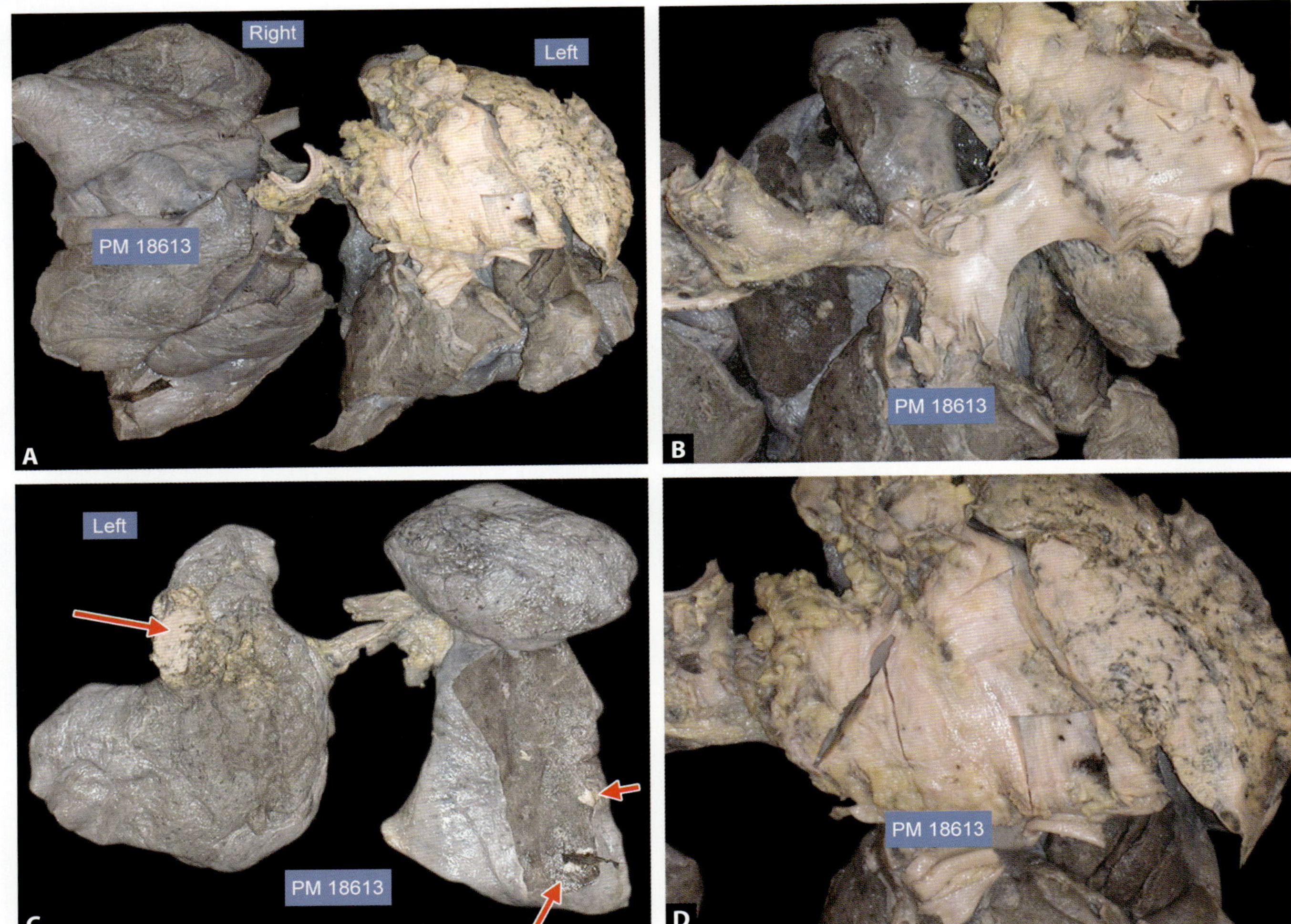

Figs 1A–D: (A) Both lungs along with the mediastinal mass present over the anterior surface of the left lung; (B) The mass could be separated from the lung to some extent; (C) Lungs viewed from the posterior aspect wherein the left lung shows a mass in the middle portion and the right lung shows small nodules (arrows); (D) Cut section of the mass was firm with soft areas and small areas of hemorrhage.

FINAL AUTOPSY DIAGNOSIS: PM 18613

25 Years Old Male

Granulomatosis with polyangiitis, i.e. WG (cANCA strongly positive) involving the:

- Anterior mediastinum in the form of a mass
- Trachea, lungs
- Kidneys
- Testes, muscle, pericardium and spleen
- Liver—simple cyst.

***Granulomatosis with polyangiitis (Wegener's)*:** See chapter on "Small Vessel Vasculitis".

COMMENTARY—INDEX CASE: PM 18613

Granulomatosis with polyangiitis (Wegener's) is a systemic, ANCA positive, predominantly small vessel vasculitis with a classical triad of—(A) Necrotizing granulomatous inflammation of the upper and lower respiratory tract; (B) Systemic/focal necrotizing vasculitis involving both arteries or veins and (C) Focal/diffuse necrotizing glomerulonephritis generally with crescents. In addition, inflammatory changes are frequently seen in the eyes, ears, joints, skin, mucous membranes, muscle, spleen, GIT, testes, etc. Hilar adenopathy and mediastinal masses are distinctly rare in patients with GPA. It has protean manifestations and this is a reason for

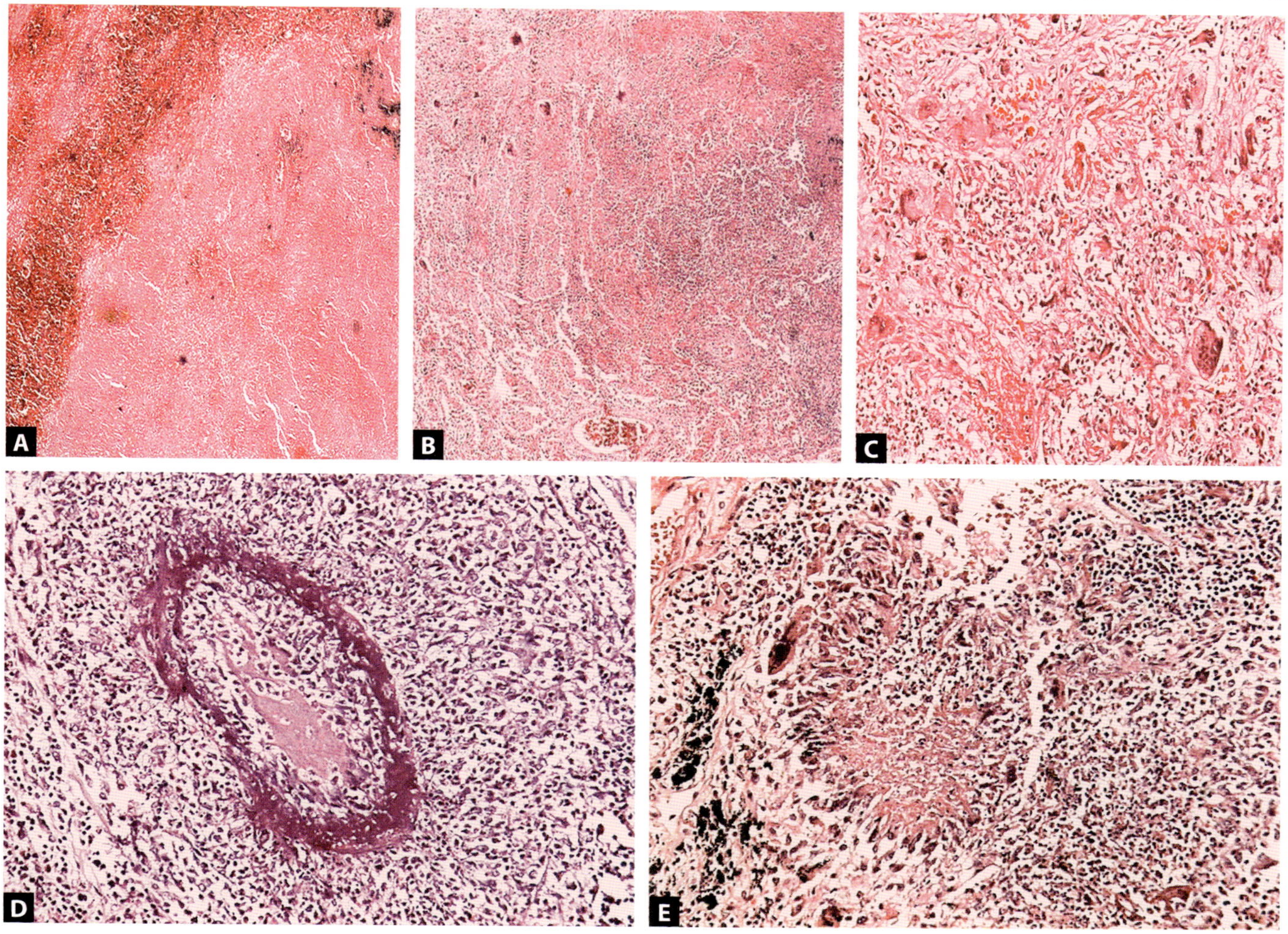

Figs. 2A to E: Photomicrographs of the lung mass showing (A) Areas of necrosis bordered by hemorrhage; (B) Dense inflammation bordered by giant cells; (C) Areas replete with foreign body giant cells, inflammation, and fibrosis; (D) Acute vasculitis with fibrinoid necrosis and transmural inflammation; (E) Granulomatous arteritis, where in the artery showing inflammatory changes in its wall is palisaded by histiocytes and giant cells.

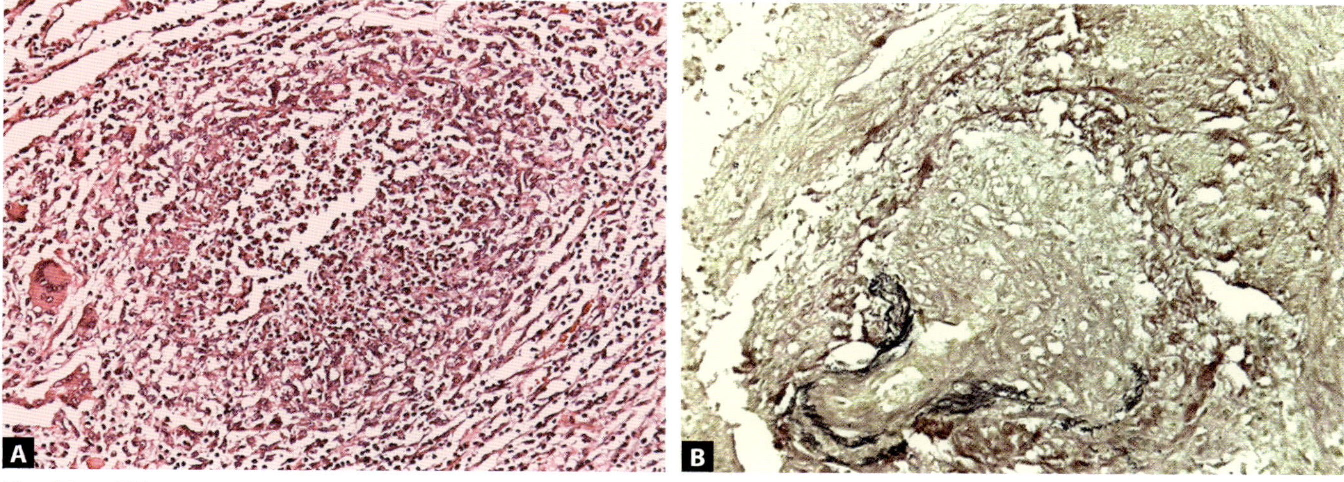

Figs 3A and B

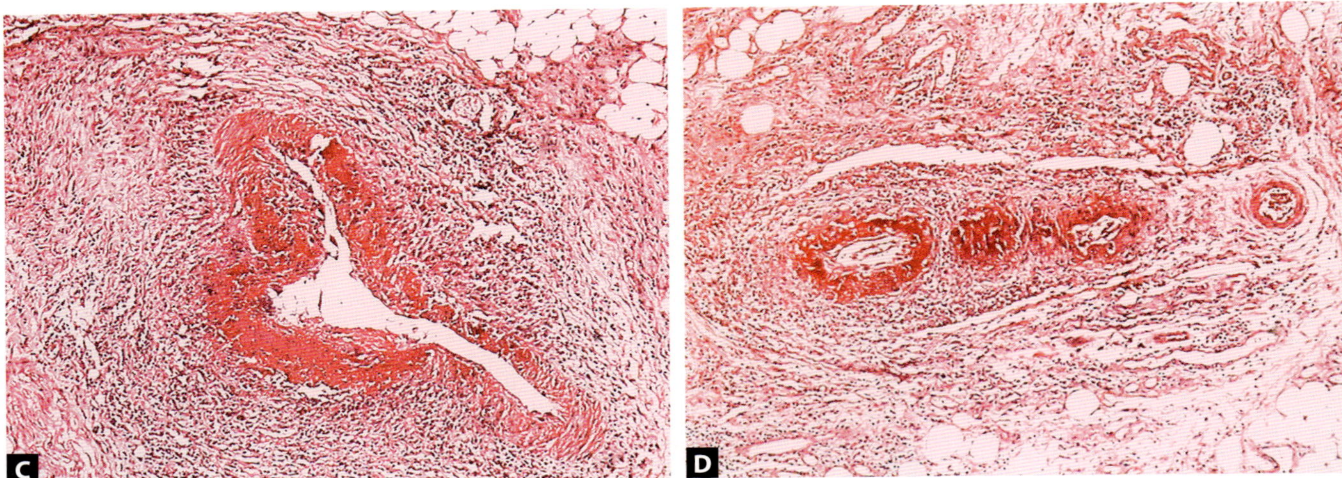

Figs. 3A–D: (A) Lung mass showing granulomatous arteritis; (B) Lung—EVG stain shows an artery with destruction of the internal elastic lamina; (C and D) Mediastinal mass showing florid acute vasculitis of small arteries.

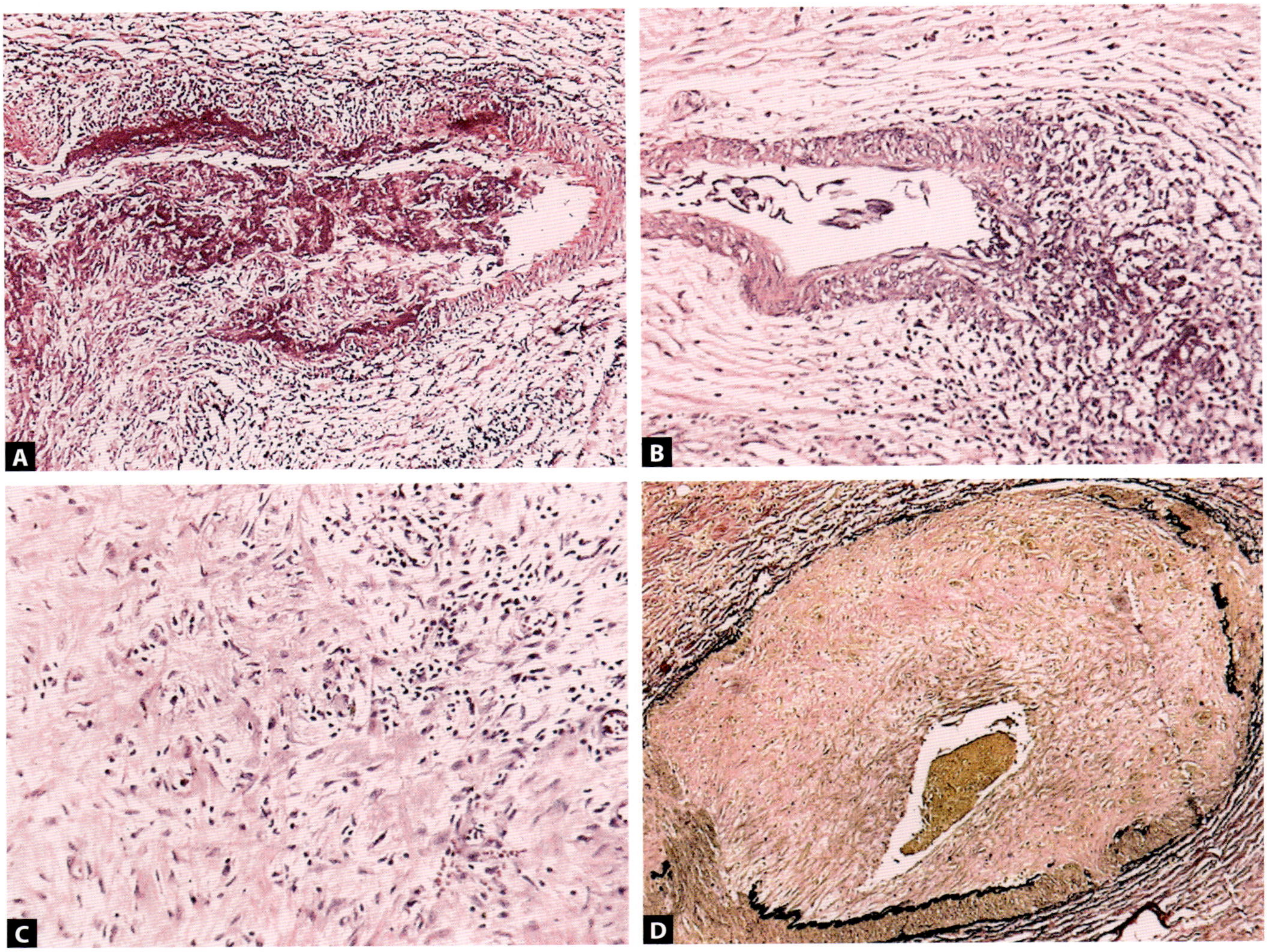

Figs 4A–D: Photomicrographs from the mediastinal mass showing (A and B) Florid acute vasculitis of medium-sized arteries; (C) Marked fibrosis with inflammatory cells; (D) Healing arteritis with intimal fibrosis, luminal occlusion, break of internal elastic lamina and sparse inflammation.

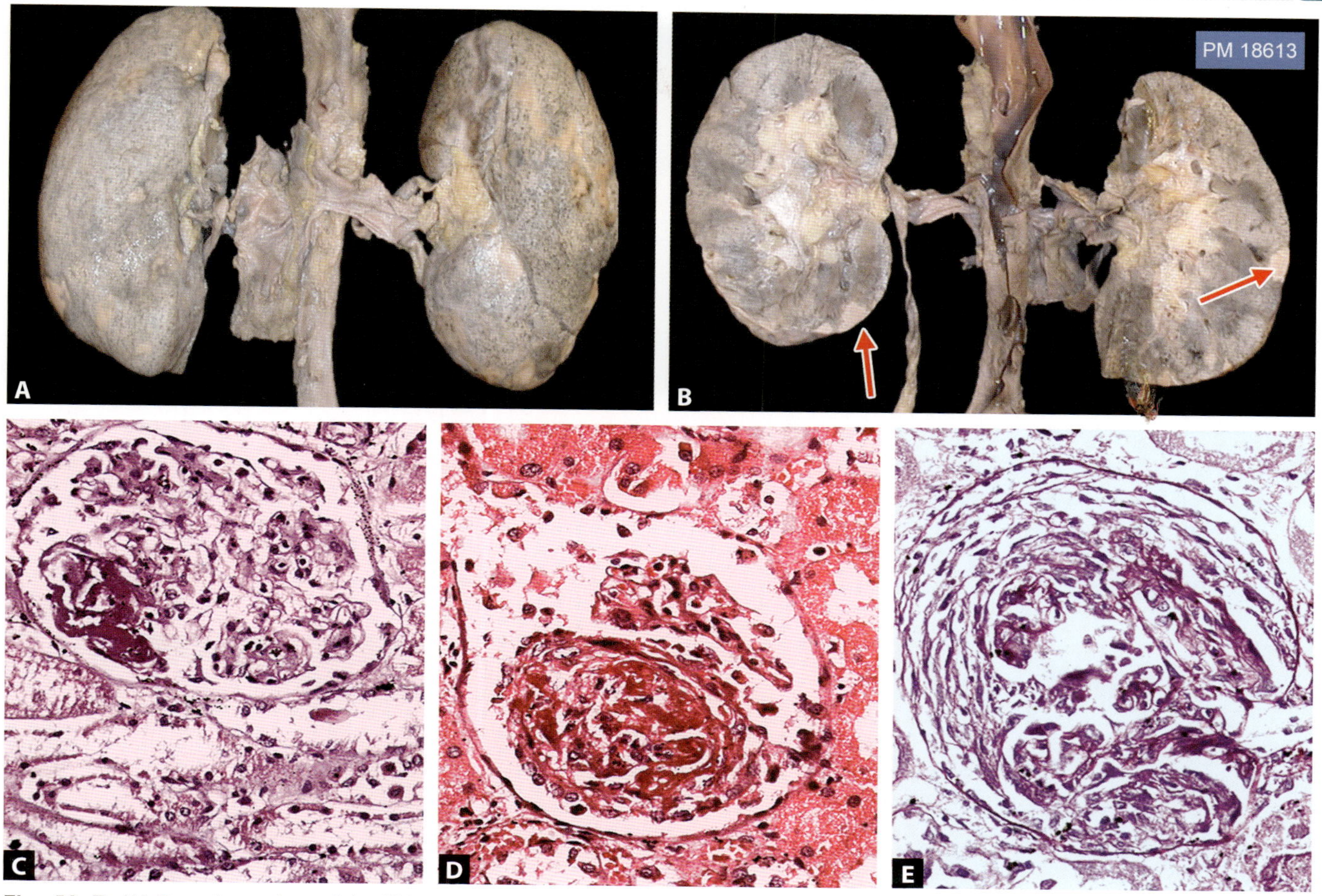

Figs 5A–E: (A) Capsular surface of the kidneys shows a flee-bitten appearance with small infarcts; (B) Cut section of the kidneys showing medullary congestion and infarcts (arrows). Glomeruli showing (C) Segmental necrotizing lesion; (D) Diffuse necrotizing lesion; (E) Crescent in PAS stain.

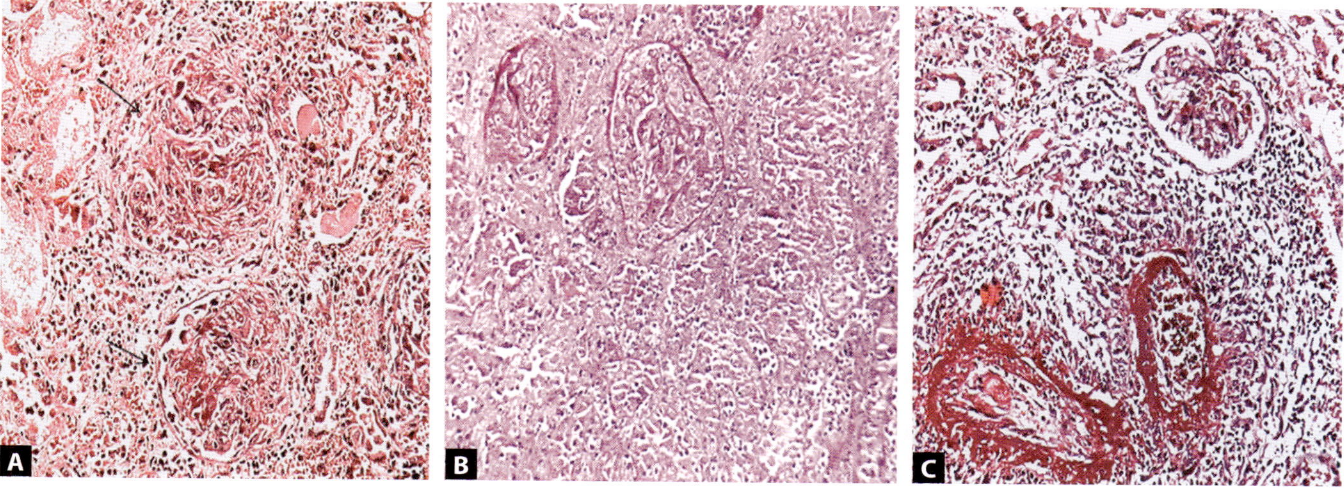

Figs 6A–C

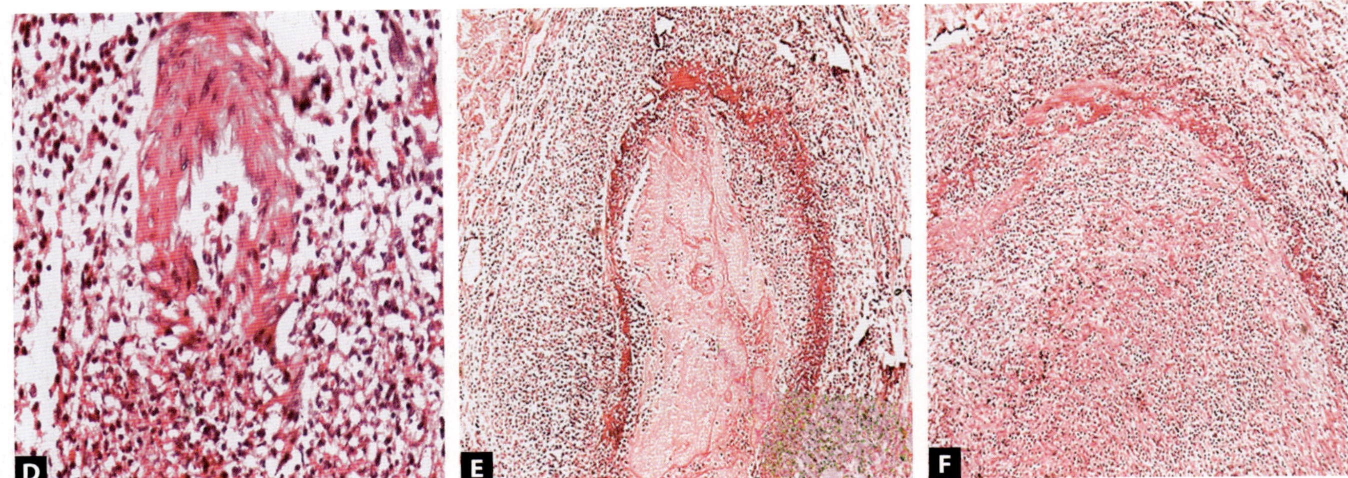

Figs 6A–F: Photomicrographs of the kidney showing: (A) Two glomeruli showing break of the Bowman's capsule and mergence of the tuft with the interstitium (B) Area of infarct. Acute necrotizing vasculitis of the (C and D) Interlobular arteries; (E) Arcuate artery; (F) Interlobar artery.

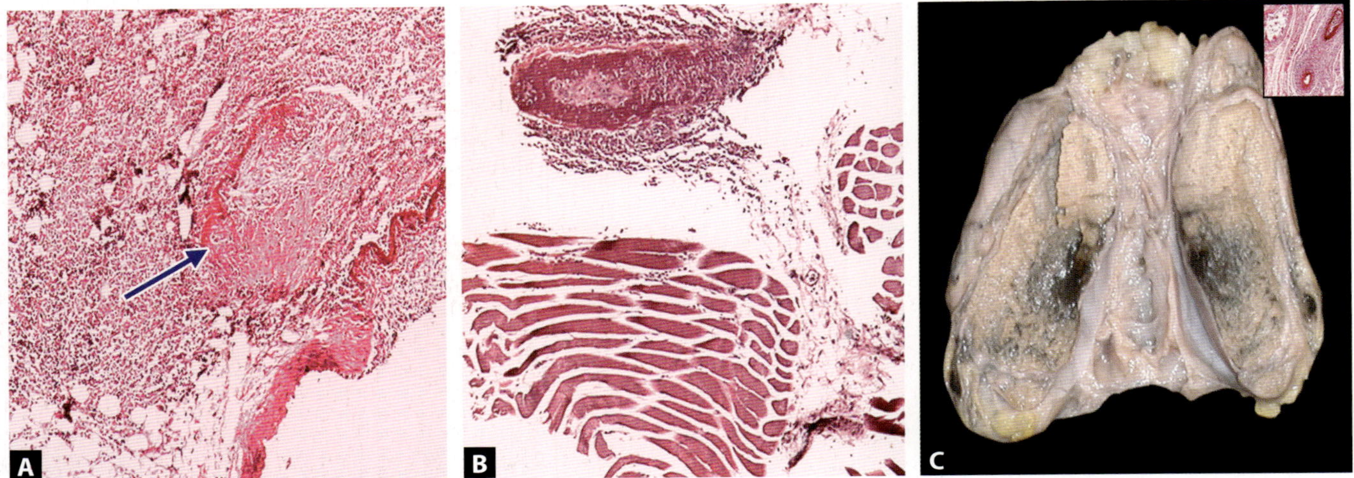

Figs 7A–C: Acute vasculitis in the (A) Pericardium; (B) Muscle and (C) Testis showing hemorrhage and inset shows acute vasculitis.

delay in diagnosis and hence the treatment. The index case is an example of this, where the primary presentation was with an anterior mediastinal mass leading to a mistaken diagnosis of tuberculosis/malignancy. When present, the mediastinal involvement is usually associated with lung parenchymal changes, as in the index case. These masses could be either lymph nodal masses showing granulomatous inflammation, geographic areas of necrosis and vasculitis or true mediastinal masses where the disease process involves the soft tissue of the mediastinum leading to the formation of a mass.

George et al[1] evaluated 302 cases from two large cohorts of patients with GPA (104 from Cleveland Clinic patients and 198 from NIH database) and found three patients (i.e. 1%) each with mediastinal masses and hilar lymphadenopathy. In all these patients, there was a suggestion of mediastinal widening and/or hilar abnormalities seen on chest X-rays. Boudes[2] reported a 42-year-old man who developed a constrictive left thoracic chest pain and a chest X-ray revealed a left mediastinal mass. A physical examination did not show any upper/lower respiratory tract, cutaneous, bony or any CNS symptoms. Left anterior thoracotomy was performed and the tumor was removed, which on microscopy revealed necrosis and granulomas with no vasculitis and a diagnosis of tuberculosis was considered. Stain for AFB and fungus were negative. A few months later this patient was readmitted with rapidly progressing renal failure, markedly abnormal renal function tests, hematuria and on a renal biopsy, a diagnosis of focal segmental necrotizing glomerulonephritis with crescents in 75% glomeruli and acute vasculitis in an afferent arteriole was made. At this time, right tonsil ulceration and a lesion on the epiglottis were noted which on a biopsy showed necrotizing granulomatous lesions without vasculitis. GPA was suspected and the slides of the mediastinal mass were reviewed where in fibrinoid necrosis was noted and granulomas without caseation necrosis were seen within and outside the arterial wall, confirming a diagnosis of GPA. Hence in GPA, granuloma formation can get tumorous as we normally see in the lungs in the form of nodules and large white areas of consolidation. Other places where we can find such tumors are the upper airways,[3] orbit,[4,5] salivary glands,[6] kidney and the mediastinum.[1,2,7,8]

The index case of GPA presented with an anterior mediastinal mass and on FNA a diagnosis of tuberculosis was made, although the stain for AFB was negative. The renal function tests were mildly deranged, although at autopsy the kidney involvement was florid. Routine urine examination was unremarkable which is very odd, taking into consideration the presence of a florid necrotizing glomerulonephritis with crescents. During life a diagnosis of GPA was not considered. cANCA done on the postmortem serum sample was strongly positive. Mediastinal tumor may be an unusual presenting manifestation of GPA, i.e. WG. This should be kept in mind to prevent delay in the institution of cyclophosphamide therapy.[9]

This patient was hospitalized for 22 days in our institute. The first computerized tomography of the head was done a week after his admission, which revealed hemorrhage in the midbrain and fourth ventricle along with hydrocephalus. On the 16th day of admission, the patient had severe headache with 3-4 bouts of vomiting. There was sudden profuse sweating and stiffening of the body. Sensorium improved with conservative management. He was also given broad-spectrum antibiotics and later anti-tubercular therapy. A ventriculoperitoneal shunt and digital subtraction angiography were planned. On the 19th day he had an acute cry with clenching of mouth and tonic posturing of the body. CT head was repeated and showed a cerebellar hemorrhage. He was given anticerebral edema measures, remained unconscious and expired on 22nd day of admission. Central nervous system involvement occurs in GPA, but intracranial hemorrhage is rare.[10,11]

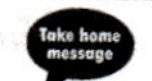

TAKE HOME MESSAGE

- Mediastinal masses and hilar adenopathy are distinctly rare in patients with granulomatosis with polyangiitis.
- On fine needle aspiration, if we find necrotic tissue, degenerated inflammatory cells and multinucleated foreign body giant cells with negative AFB and fungal stains, the first possibility still remains tuberculosis (In India) followed by granulomatosis with polyangiitis.
- Tumorous presentation of granulomatosis with polyangiitis is well-known in literature and apart from the lungs it can be seen in the upper respiratory tract, orbit, kidney, salivary glands and mediastinum.
- Central nervous system involvement occurs in granulomatosis with polyangiitis, but intracranial hemorrhage is rare.

REFERENCES

1. George TM, Cash JM, Farver C, et al. Mediastinal mass and hilar adenopathy–rare thoracic manifestation of Wegener's granulomatosis. Arthritis and Rheumatism. 1997;40(11):1992-7.
2. Boudes P. Mediastinal tumor as the presenting manifestation of Wegener's granulomatosis. J Internal Med. 1990;227(3):215-7.
3. Fauci AS, Wolff SM. Wegener's granulomatosis: studies in 18 patients and a review of literature. Medicine. 1973;52:535-61.
4. Diamond RD, Fienberg R. Case 43-1981—A 54-year-old man with an 11-year history of chronic inflammation of the orbit and paranasal sinuses. NEJM. 1981;305:999-1008.
5. Haynes BF, Fishman ML, Fauci AS, et al. The ocular manifestation of Wegener's granulomatosis: fifteen year experience and review of literature. Am J Med. 1977;63:131-41.
6. Kavanaugh AF, Huston DP. Wegener's granulomatosis presenting with unilateral parotid enlargement. Am J Med. 1988;85:741-2.
7. Song YH, Kim TH, Lee IH, et al. Wegener's granulomatosis presenting as mediastinal soft tissue mass invading the tracheal tree. Clin Rheumatol. 2000;19(6):495-8.
8. Maguire R, Fauci AS, Doppman JL, et al. Unusual radiographic presentation of Wegener's granulomatosis. 1978; 130:233-8.
9. Sharma A, Gopalakrishnan D, Nada R, et al. Uncommon presentation of primary systemic vasculitides: The great masquerades. Int J Rheum Dis. 2014;17(5):562-72.
10. Memet B, Rudinskaya A, Krebs T, et al. Wegener granulomatosis with massive intracerebral hemorrhage: Remission of disease in response to rituximab. J Clin Rheumatol. 2005; 11(6):314-8.
11. Ceri M, Ortabozkoyun L, Unverdi S, et al. Massive intracerebral hemorrhage associated with Wegener granulomatosis. Rheumatol Int. 2012;32(6):1813-14.

CONTRIBUTIONS BY:

1. Dr Ranjana Minz, Professor and Head, Department of Immunopathology
2. Dr SC Varma, Ex-Professor and Head, Department of Internal Medicine (Clinician In-Charge)

Post Graduate Institute of Medical Education and Research, Chandigarh, India

CASE 47

Granulomatosis with Polyangiitis, i.e. Wegener's with Multiple Pulmonary Nodules and Total Splenic Necrosis: PM 21594

Nandita Bharadwaj Kakkar

HIGHLIGHTS OF THE CASE

This middle-aged female had fever, generalized pustular skin rash, swelling of the limbs, breathlessness, deranged renal function tests, microhematuria, large abscess in the spleen, bilateral cavitating lung lesions and c-ANCA was negative. A diagnosis of bilateral cavitating pneumonia, acute renal failure, ? disseminated Staphylococcus or fungal infection with a possibility of vasculitis was made. At autopsy the classical triad of granulomatosis with polyangiitis (GPA), i.e. Wegener's granulomatosis (WG) was seen, along with total splenic necrosis converting it into a bag of necrotic tissue. Postmortem c-ANCA (done 2 weeks later) was strongly positive. This case highlights the importance of repeating an ANCA test, if it is negative and the clinical suspicion of GPA is strong.

Keywords: Granulomatosis with polyangiitis, Wegener's, triad, total splenic necrosis, autopsy.

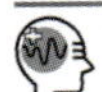

CLINICAL DETAILS

Date of Admission: 26.09.2006, Date of Death: 07.10.2006, Duration of Hospital Stay: 12 Days.

A 40-year-old lady presented with fever since 25 days for which she was given antibiotics. Five days after the start of fever she developed nonpruritic skin rash over both upper and lower limbs, associated with swelling of the limbs. For the last 5 days she was having breathlessness. There was no history of facial puffiness, oliguria, hematuria, hemoptysis, nasal bleed or stuffiness. ***On examination***, the patient was sick and toxic looking, afebrile, pulse—120/min, regular, BP—130/100 mm Hg and RR—45/ min. There was pallor, pedal edema and generalized pustular rashes present on both upper and lower limbs. No icterus, cyanosis or clubbing was present and the jugular venous pressure was normal. On auscultation there were decreased breath sounds in bilateral infrascapular areas and crepitations were audible. The liver and spleen were palpable 3 cm and 4 cm below their respective costal margins. No free fluid was present. The patient was conscious, oriented with no meningeal signs.

Investigations and Course of Management

Hematological: Hb—7.2 to 5.3 g/dL; TLC 14000/uL; DLC P82 L16, M2, E2; platelets 112000/uL; coagulogram mildly deranged; c-ANCA: negative, ANA-ve. ***Blood biochemistry/microbiology***: S creatinine 6.7 mg%; S urea 135 mg%; Total proteins/albumin—6/2.8 gm; 24 hour urinary protein 1.8 gm/day; Liver function tests within normal limits; Routine urine examination—albumin 1+, pus cells 10–15/HPF, epithelial cells 5–6/HPF, RBC 35–40/HPF; Cultures for blood, urine and aspirate from skin lesion were sterile; HBsAg -ve. ***Radiological***: Ultrasonography of the abdomen showed mild hepatomegaly, space occupying lesion measuring 7 x 5 x 4 cms in the spleen ? Abscess, bilateral pleural effusion (Left > Right); X-ray chest revealed bilateral cavitating lung lesions. ***Cytology/Biopsy***: Splenic aspirate showed polymorphs and degenerated cells in a necrotic back ground with no malignant cells; Pleural fluid—negative for malignancy. Skin biopsy showed necrotic epidermis with separation from the underlying dermis, extensive neutrophilic exudates, fibrin, nuclear debris, acantholytic cells, dermal perivascular inflammation, occasional vessel showed neutrophilic infiltrate within the wall but with no fibrinoid necrosis. Overall features consistent with vasculitis.

Echocardiography: Mild pericardial effusion with no vegetations; ECG: Sinus tachycardia; ***Coarse and management***: Possibility of staphylococcal sepsis with vasculitis was kept.

The splenic space occupying lesion was drained under guidance. She was managed with antibiotics, lasix, mechanical ventilation, blood transfusion, empirical methylpredisolone, antifungals and peritoneal dialysis. She continued to deteriorate and suffered a cardiorespiratory arrest.

Unit's Final Diagnosis: Bilateral cavitating pneumonia, acute renal failure ? disseminated staphlococcus/fungal infection, ?? systemic vasculitis with multi organ dysfunction and septicemia.

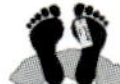 AUTOPSY FINDINGS: PM 21594

A partial autopsy was performed on this 49-year-old female with a clinical diagnosis of bilateral cavitary pneumonia with acute renal failure. The pleural cavity yielded 150 mL of straw-colored fluid (left > right) and the pericardial cavity contained minimal fluid. The antemortem skin biopsy (s-11262/06) was consistent with a diagnosis of vasculitis. The ***lungs*** (Fig 1A) were heavy and weighed 1,325 g. The pleurae were thickened over both lower lobes and tracheobronchial ulceration was noted. On cut section the left lung (Fig 1B) showed multiple well-circumscribed white necrotic nodules varying in size from 0.5 cm to 5 cm in diameter scattered in both lobes. The right lung (Fig 1C) showed fewer nodules, the largest measuring 6 cm in diameter. On microscopic examination, granulomatous inflammation, i.e. geographic areas of bland necrosis with nuclear debris, bordered by giant cells and histiocytes was noted (Figs 1D–F). There was florid small vessel vasculitis (acute and chronic) with prominent granulomatous arteritis where

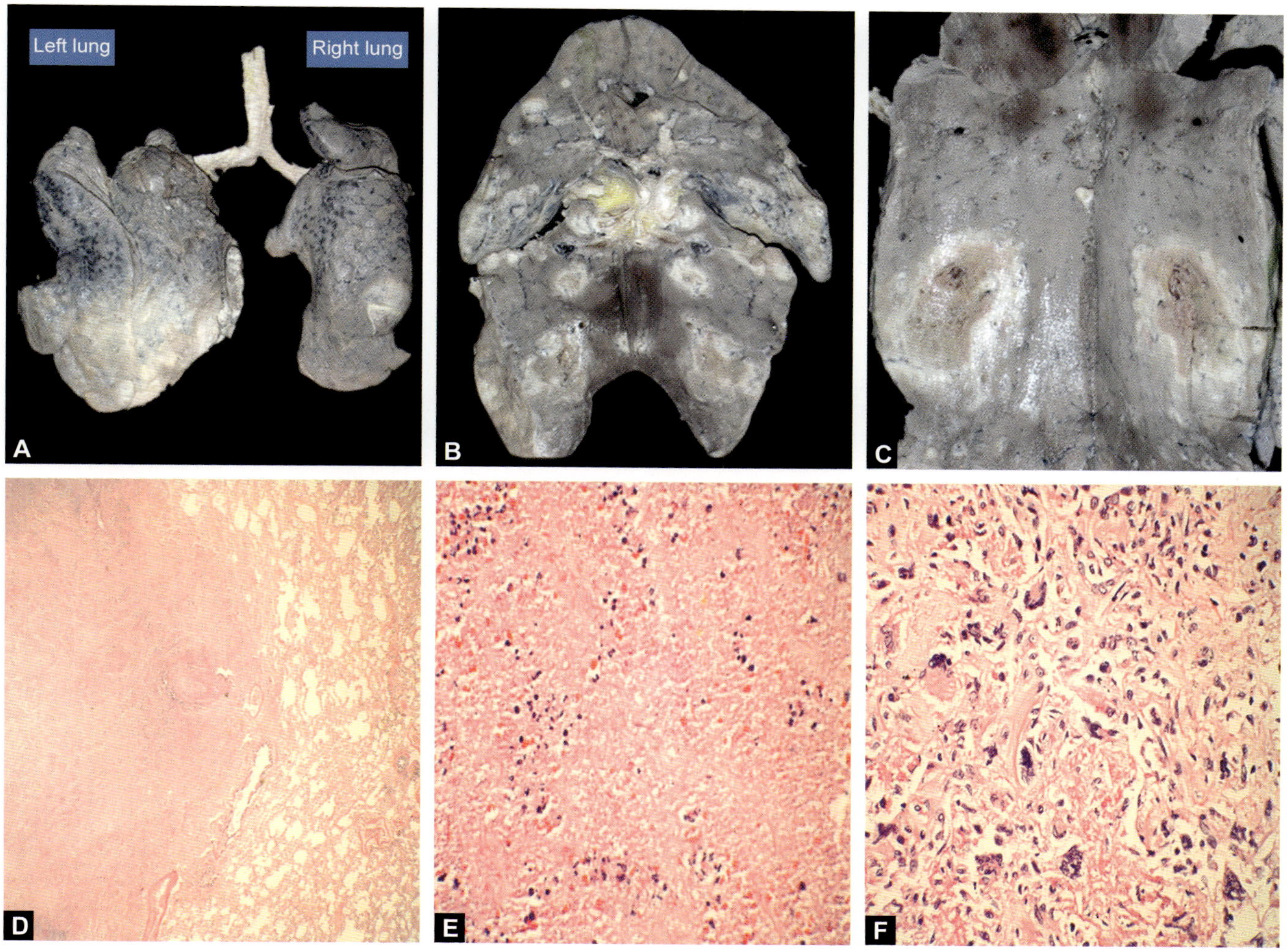

Figs 1A–F: (A) Pleural aspect of the lungs showing thickened pleura (left > right); (B and C) Cut section of the lungs showing multiple, well-circumscribed, breaking down nodules; (D) Low power of a nodule showing necrosis with adjacent normal lung parenchyma; (E) Nodule showing bland necrosis with nuclear debris; (F) Periphery of the nodule, replete with giant cells.

in a perivascular, well-defined collar of palisading epithelioid macrophages with giant cells was noted (Figs 2A–D). Acute fibrinous and chronic pleuritis, bronchopneumonia, thromboembolism, bronchial and tracheal ulcerations were also seen. No organism was identified and stains for AFB, PAS and Gram were negative on multiple sections. Overall features were consistent with granulomatosis with polyangiitis (GPA). The ***kidneys*** (Figs 3A and B) were swollen and weighed 340 g. The surface showed coarse scars with petechial hemorrhage and the renal arteries were normal. On microscopic examination the glomeruli showed cellular crescents (Fig 3C), focal and segmental necrotizing glomerulitis, where in a part of the glomerular tuft showed fibrinoid necrosis and nuclear debris (Fig 3D). Extraglomerular small vessels showed acute vasculitis with inflammation and fibrinoid necrosis of the wall (Figs 3E and F). RBC casts and interstitial inflammation was noted. No granulomatous glomerulonephritis/arteritis was seen. Immunohistochemistry for IgG, IgA, IgM, C3 and fibrinogen were negative indicating the pauci-immune nature of the glomerulonephritis. Electron microscopy did not reveal any immune deposits. Thus, kidney showed a pauci-immune necrotizing crescentic glomerulonephritis with extraglomerular small vessel vasculitis. The ***spleen*** weighed 260 g. The capsule was markedly thickened and on cut section practically the entire spleen was converted into a bag of necrotic tissue (Fig 4A). Microscopic examination showed necrosis, replete with giant cells and florid acute and chronic vasculitis along with gran-

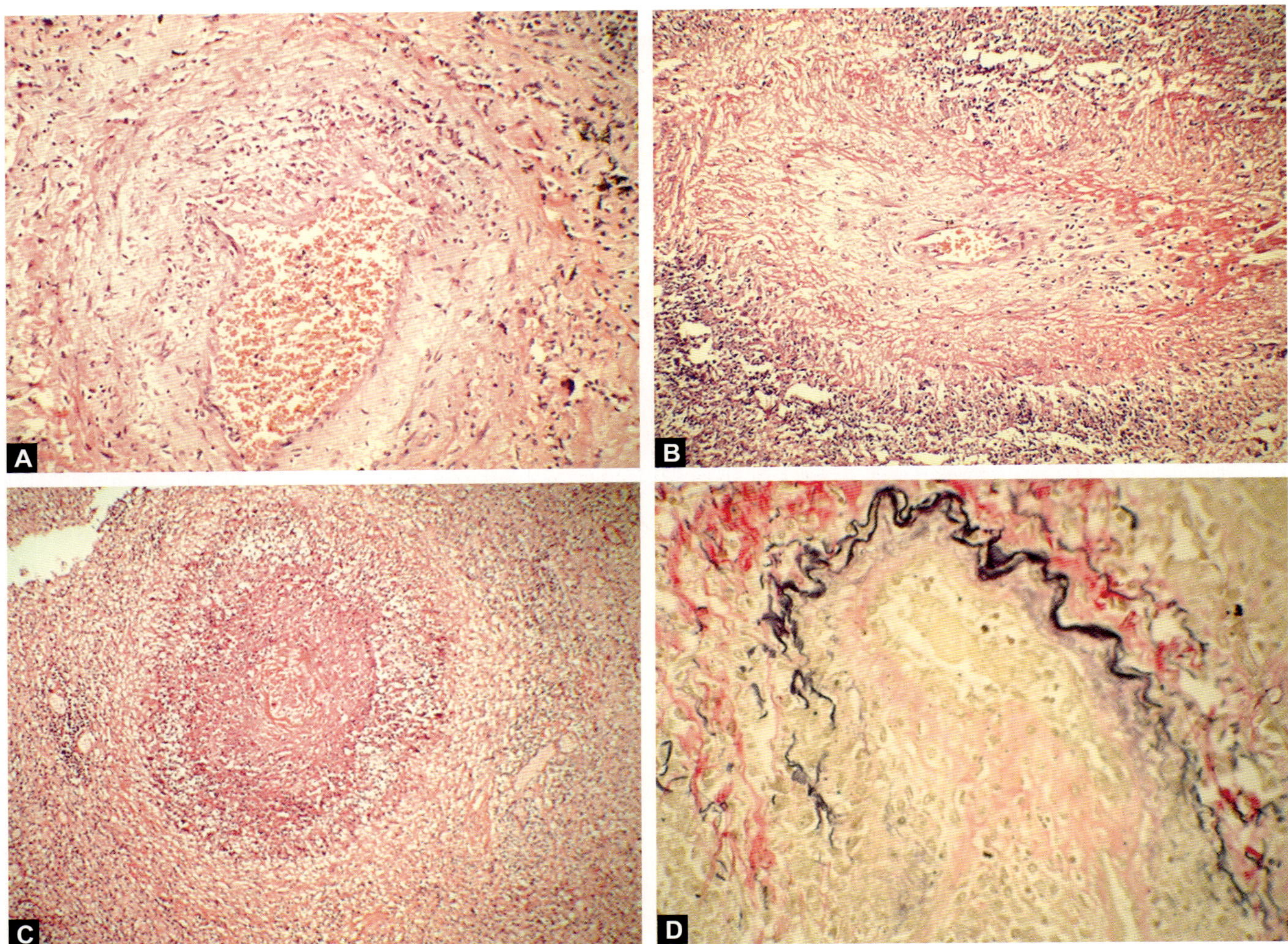

Figs 2A–D: Photomicrographs of the lung. (A) Small artery showing acute vasculitis; (B) Subacute vasculitis with inflammation in the wall, break of the internal elastic lamina, intimal fibrosis with luminal compromise; (C) Granulomatous arteritis with fibrinoid necrosis in the center surrounded by a collar composed of polymorphs, epithelioid histiocytes, and giant cells; (D) Elastic van Gieson stain showing break of the internal elastic lamina of a small artery.

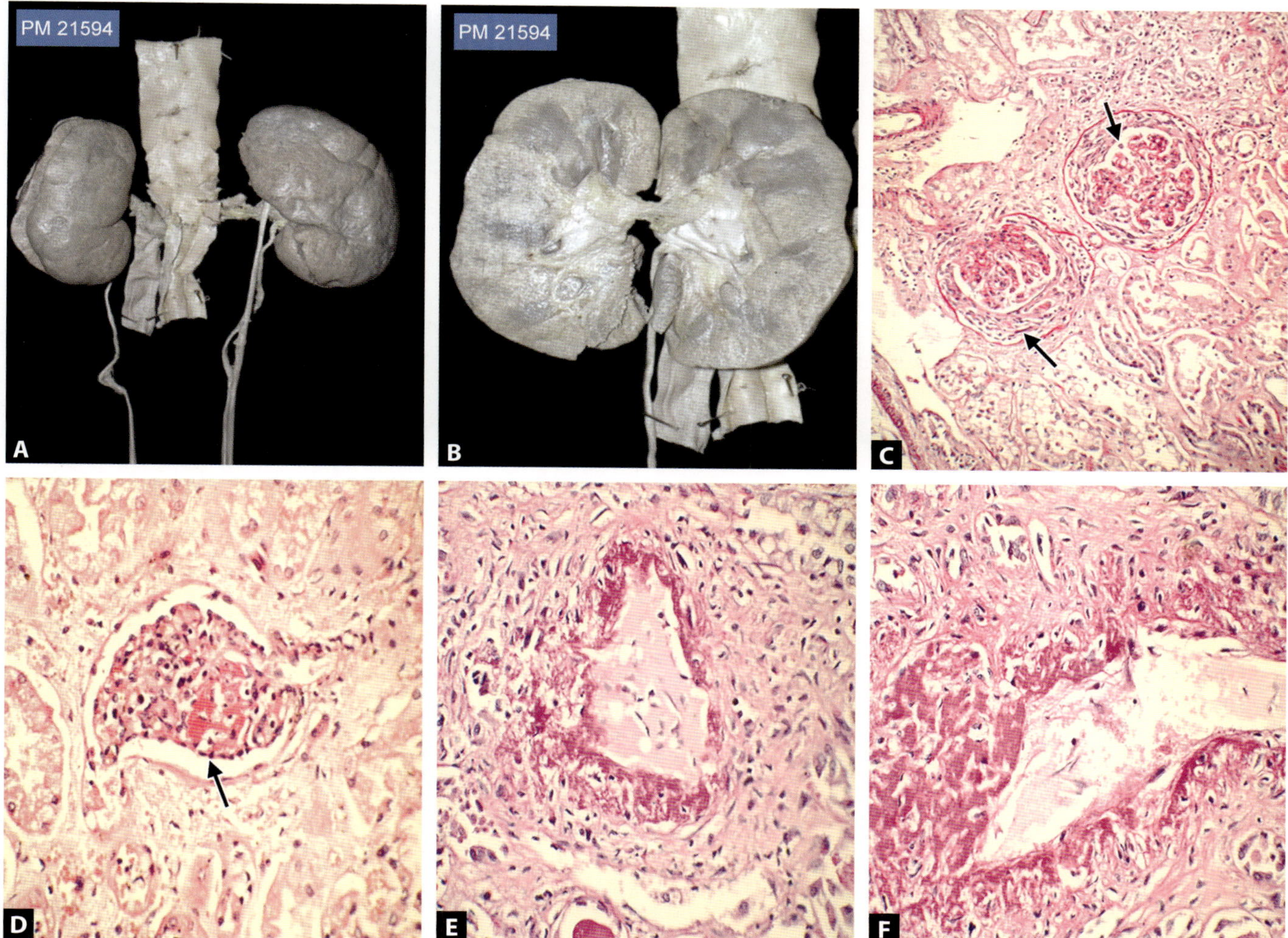

Figs 3A–F: Kidneys. (A) Capsular aspect showing petechial spots; (B) Cut section shows medullary congestion. No infarcts were seen. Photomicrograph of the kidney; (C) Showing cellular crescents (arrows); (D) Glomerulus showing segmental necrotizing lesion with fibrinoid necrosis and nuclear debris (arrow); (E and F) Interlobular arteries showing acute vasculitis.

ulomatous vasculitis (Figs 4B–D). The ***liver*** showed an occasional focus of acute small vessel vasculitis (Fig 5A). The skin revealed acute vasculitis in the superficial dermis leading to separation of the epidermis (Fig 5B). The ***heart*** was normal grossly and microscopically and there was minimal pericardial effusion. Other organs were within normal limits. ***c-ANCA*** done on the postmortem sample (2 weeks after the antemortem testing) was strongly positive.

FINAL AUTOPSY DIAGNOSIS: PM 21594

49 Years Old Female

Granulomatosis with polyangiitis, i.e. Wegener's, (c ANCA 4+) involving the lungs, skin, kidneys, spleen and liver.

Granulomatosis with polyangiitis (Wegener's)—See chapter on "***Small vessel Vasculitis***".

COMMENTARY—INDEX CASE: PM 21594

This middle-aged female presented with fever, generalized pustular skin rash, swelling of the limbs, breathlessness, deranged renal function tests, microhematuria, large abscess in the spleen, bilateral cavitating lung lesions and c-ANCA was negative. A clinical diagnosis of bilateral cavitating pneumonia, acute renal failure, ? disseminated Staphylococcus/fungal infection with a possibility of vasculitis was made. Worth stressing points in this case of GPA are:

1. At autopsy the classical triad of GPA ie necrotizing/granulomatous vasculitis of small to medium sized

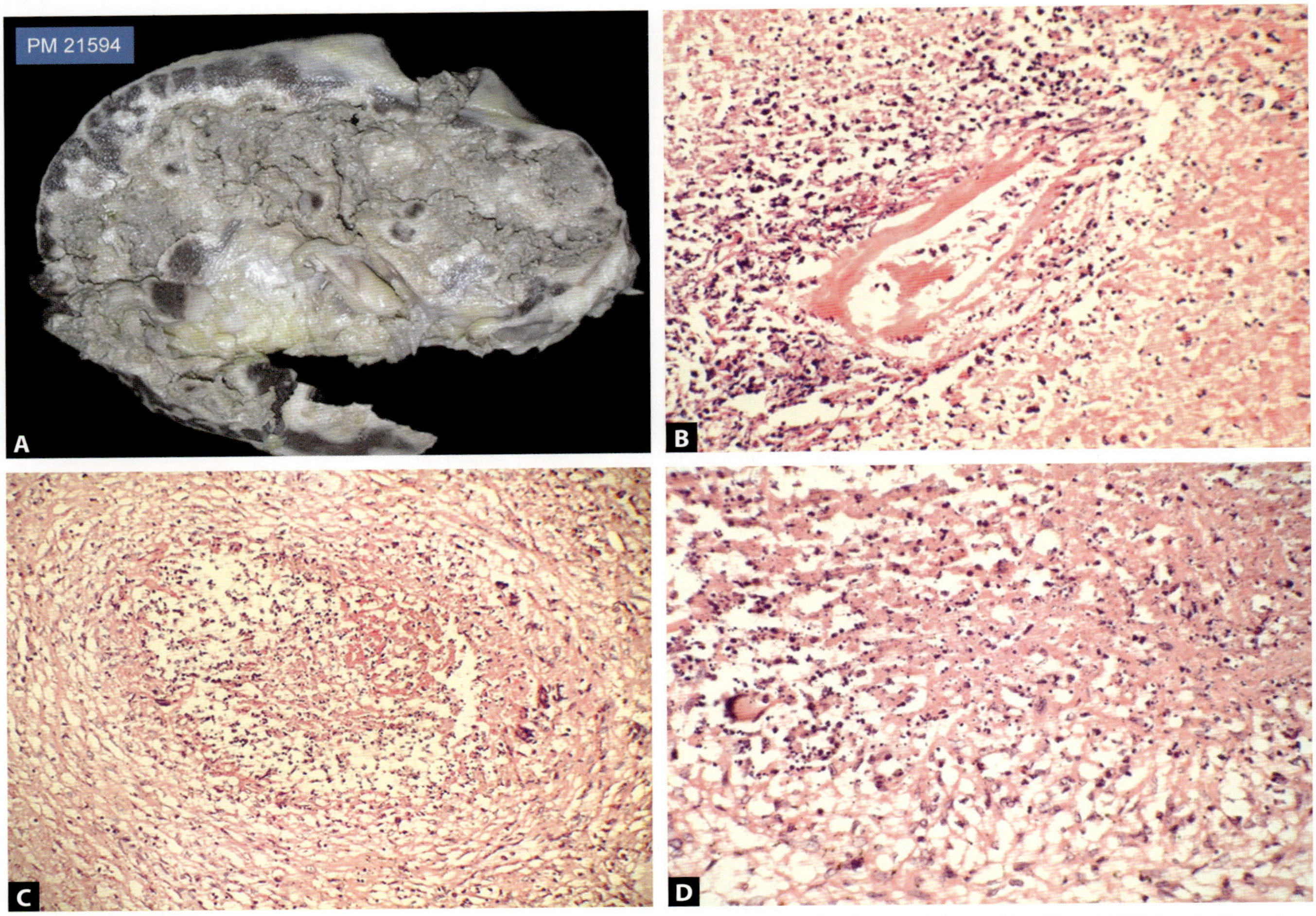

Figs 4A–D: (A) Coronal slice of the spleen showing total necrosis; (B) Central arteriole showing acute vasculitis; (C and D) Artery in the spleen showing granulomatous arteritis with palisading histiocytes and giant cells.

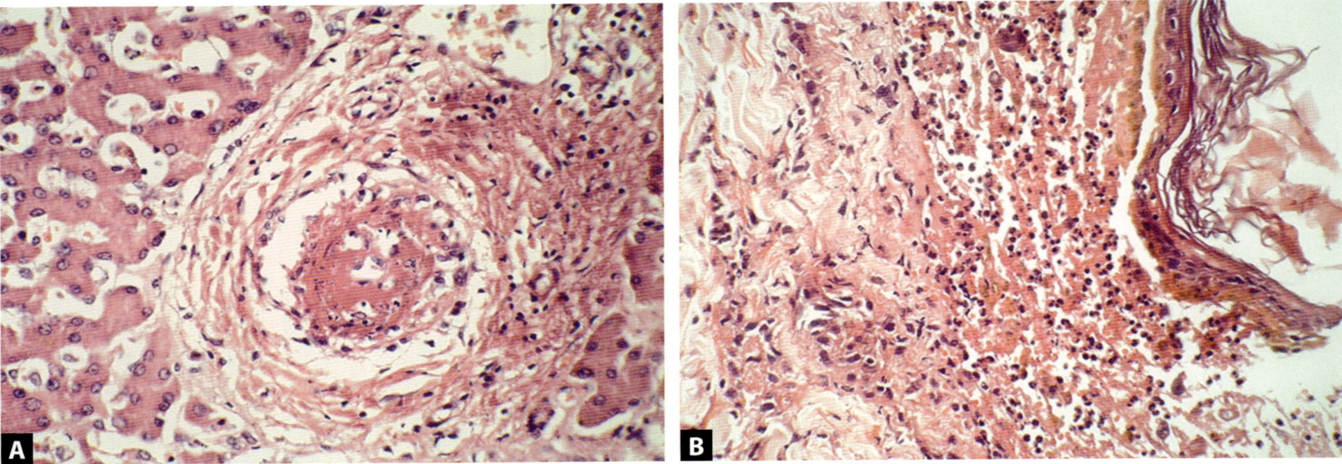

Figs 5A and B: (A) Acute vasculitis in the liver; (B) Section of the skin showing acute vasculitis in the superficial dermis with separation of the epidermis.

vessels, necrotizing granulomatous inflammation involving the upper and lower respiratory tract and pauci-immune necrotizing crescentic glomerulonephritis was seen.

2. There was extensive vasculitis in the spleen leading to total splenic necrosis, converting it into a bag of necrotic tissue. The ultrasonography revealed a space occupying lesion in the spleen measuring 7 × 5 × 4 cms and a possibility of abscess was thought of. A splenic aspirate was done which revealed polymorphs and degenerated cells in a necrotic back ground with no malignant cells. Splenic involvement[1,2] in GPA is quite prevalent than believed and leads to pain in the left upper quadrant radiating to the left shoulder. Many patients however are asymptomatic. Infarction occurs due to the occlusion of the splenic artery or its branches. Splenic infarction may be massive as seen in the index case, where the entire spleen is converted into a bag of necrotic tissue.
3. The antemortem ANCA was negative. The postmortem cANCA (done 2 weeks later) was strongly positive. So if the clinical suspicion of GPA is strong, a repeat ANCA testing should be done if found negative in the first instance.

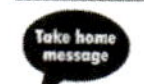

TAKE HOME MESSAGE

- This case highlights the importance of repeating an ANCA test if it is negative and the clinical suspicion of GPA is strong.
- Classic GPA i.e involving the upper/lower respiratory tract and kidneys, occurs in 21% of patients.
- Splenic involvement in GPA is quite prevalent than believed. Total splenic necrosis leading to its conversion into a bag of necrotic tissue can be seen as seen in the index case.

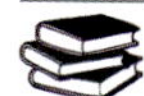

REFERENCES

1. Gal AA, Masor JJ. Splenic involvement in Wegener's granulomatosis. Arch Pathol Lab Med. 1996;120(10):974-7.
2. Rentsch J, McColl G. Splenic infarction in Wegener's granulomatosis. J Rheumatol 2000;27:1554-55.

CONTRIBUTIONS BY:

1. Dr Ranjana Minz, Professor and Head, Department of Immunopathology (ANCA Testing)
2. Dr SK Jindal, Ex-Professor and Head, Department of Pulmonary Medicine (Clinician In-Charge)

Post Graduate Institute of Medical Education and Research, Chandigarh, India

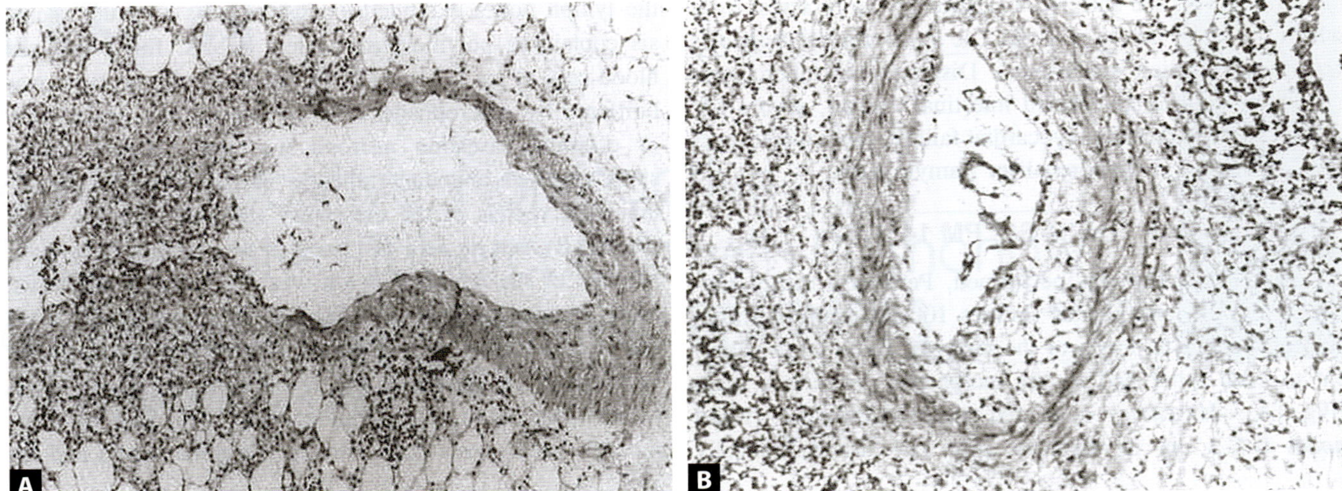

Figs 2A and B: Medium-sized mesenteric vessels showed vasculitis with transmural necrotizing inflammation and nuclear debris.

section of the ***liver*** (Figs 3B and C) showed small white lesions measuring 0.5 cm. Microscopically the liver showed features of malnutrition, i.e. diffuse periportal macrovesicular steatosis, portal tract widening with bridging, but no increase in reticulin fibers. The white lesions seen on gross examination consisted of acute necrosis bordered by Langhans giant cells and macrophages (Fig 3D). An occasional compact epithelioid cell granuloma was seen. A large number of acid-fast tubercle bacilli were demonstrated by Ziehl–Neelsen stain. Grossly the ***spleen*** showed few white nodules measuring 0.5 cm (Fig 3C). Microscopically it showed areas of acute necrosis, but no granulomas. Ziehl–Neelsen stain showed an occasional bacillus. Cut surface of both the upper lobes of the ***lung*** showed extensive areas of whitish consolidation with breaking down, measuring 4 × 3 × 2 cm (Figs 4A and B). Microscopically (Figs 5A–D) there were large areas of acute necrosis with the adjacent vessels showing changes of endarteritis obliterans. These areas of necrosis were at places bordered by Langhans giant cells and macrophages. An occasional ill-formed epithelioid cell granuloma was present (Fig 5D). Ziehl–Neelsen stain showed plenty of tubercle bacilli in the areas of necrosis. The small vessels away from the areas of necrosis, in the viable portions of the lung revealed a prominent acute vasculitis, with transmural necrotizing inflammation replete with nuclear debris (Fig 6A). No acid-fast bacillus was seen in the walls of these vessels. ***Heart*** weighed 137 g, was small and atrophic. There were multiple foci of myofiber necrosis and infiltration by lymphomononuclear cells and macrophages. In areas, the myofibers were thin, wavy and showed loss of striations, interstitial edema and vacuolization. These features were consistent with histology of a heart in malnutrition. Postmortem investigations revealed a negative HIV serology and serum for c-ANCA was strongly positive (Fig 6B).

FINAL AUTOPSY DIAGNOSIS: PM 14513

- Disseminated nonreactive tuberculosis (heavy bacillary load) involving the terminal ileum, lymph nodes (mesenteric, hilar, cervical and peripancreatic), lungs, liver and spleen. Postmortem c-ANCA strongly positive case.
- Mesenteric and pulmonary vasculitis.
- Features of malnutrition in heart and liver.

ANTINEUTROPHIL CYTOPLASMIC ANTIBODY

The past decade has seen an explosion of data on ANCA. ANCA are specific for granule proteins of granulocytes and monocytes and induce distinct fluorescence patterns, e.g. the cytoplasmic (classic) c-ANCA, perinuclear p-ANCA and atypical ANCA. c-ANCA is induced by antibodies directed against proteinase 3 in about 90% of all ANCA-positive sera and p-ANCA is induced by antibodies against myeloperoxidase in about 40%. Atypical ANCA does not have a clear cut association with a distinct granule protein. The diagnostic value of ANCA and its pathogenic implications proved to be particularly important in systemic vasculitides such as Granulomatosis with polyangiitis (GPA), microscopic polyangiitis and the closely related pauci-immune necrotizing and crescentic glomerulonephritis.[1-3] As soon as, ANCA testing became widely available, it became clear that diseases[4] other

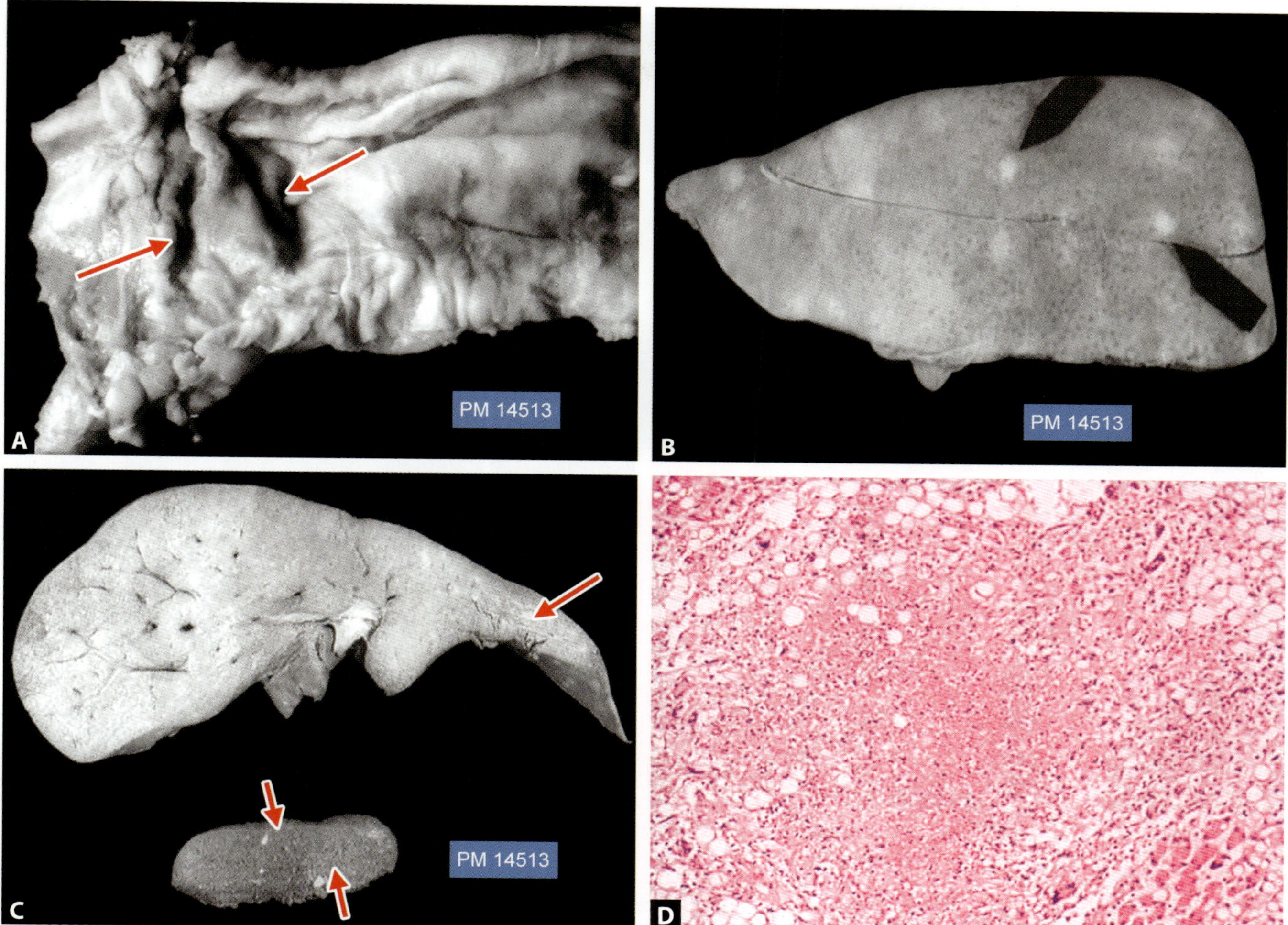

Figs 3A–D: (A) Terminal ileum shows oval ulcers located transversely (arrows); (B) Capsular aspect of the liver showing tiny white miliary nodules; (C) Coronal slices of the liver and spleen showing tiny white miliary nodules (arrows); (D) Photomicrograph of the liver showing an area of acute necrosis bordered by giant cells.

than vasculitides-like infections[5,6] were found to give positive results. Amongst the infections, HIV,[7] tuberculosis,[8,9] bacterial endocarditis, amoebiasis,[10] and malaria,[9] gave positive results. In the study by Adebajo[9] et al. 3/20 patients with tuberculosis were positive for c-ANCA, but there was no clinical evidence of vasculitis in these patients. ANCA in infections probably represent a secondary response indicating neutrophil activation as may also occur in classical ANCA associated disease.[11] Other diseases like rheumatoid arthritis,[12,13] inflammatory bowel disease,[14,15] and autoimmune hepatitis revealed ANCA positive. A number of tumors, like atrial myxoma, small cell lung cancer, non-Hodgkin's lymphoma and colon carcinomas turned out to be ANCA positive.

NONREACTIVE TUBERCULOSIS

This is tuberculosis in which there is acute necrosis, no granuloma formation and a heavy bacillary load. This is seen in immunocompromized states like HIV, primary immunodeficiencies, posttransplantation, malnutrition, etc. At times, one encounters only acute necrosis (as was seen in the index case) and here the Ziehl–Neelsen stain clinches the diagnosis.

VASCULITIS AND TUBERCULOSIS[16-18]

Any inflammation can involve the arteries, veins, or small vessels like capillaries, arterioles and venules. The inflammatory vascular lesions may be as follows: (1) Local nonspecific vasculitis in direct vicinity of the inflammatory

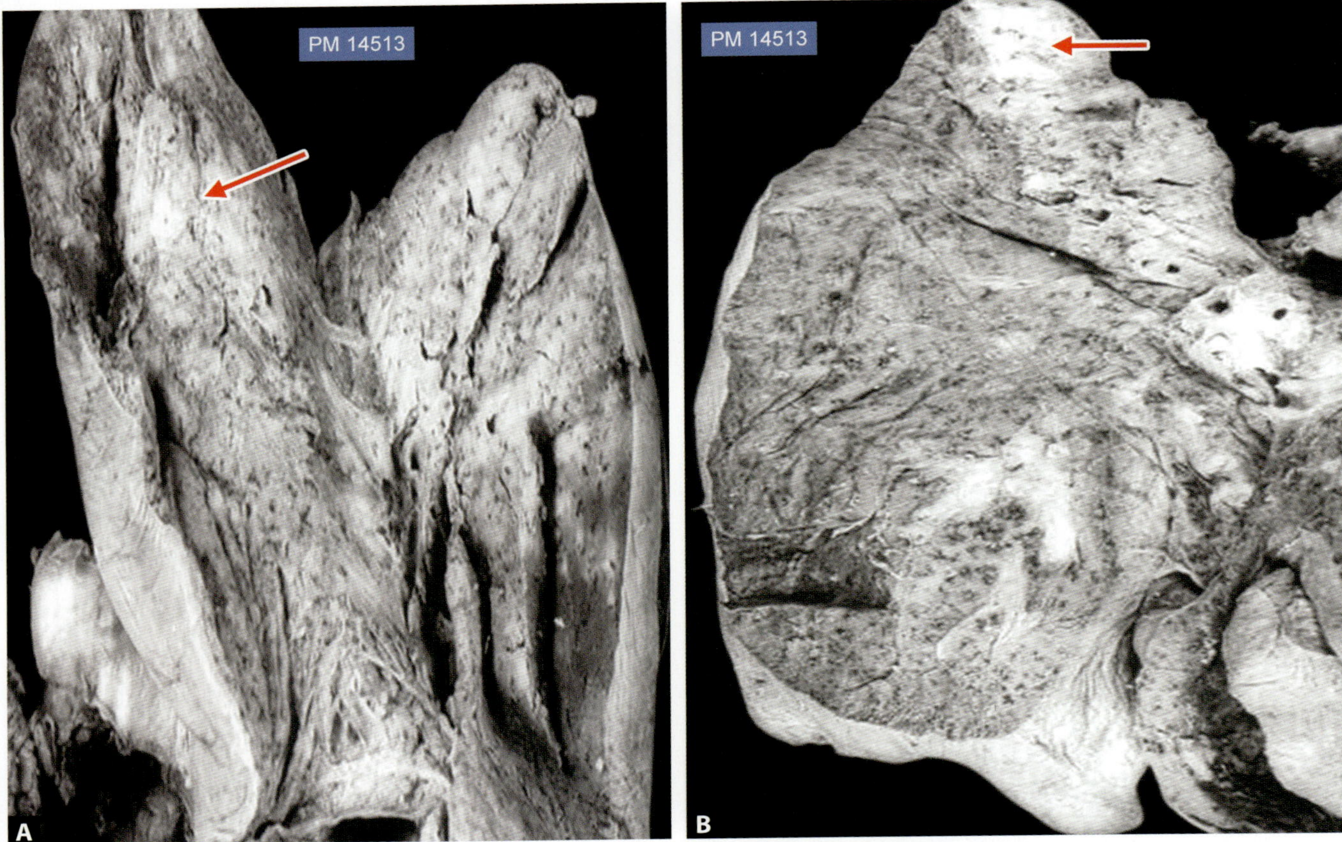

Figs 4A and B: Upper lobes of the lung showed extensive areas of whitish consolidation with breaking down (arrows).

exudates, i.e. endarteritis obliterans type of lesion seen in tuberculosis. (2) Local specific vasculitis due to direct damage to vessels by the offending agent like fungi destroying the wall or acid-fast bacilli seen in granulomas within the wall or otherwise. (3) Vasculitis distant from the primary site of inflammation (immune complex-mediated).

Mesenteric vasculitis[19-21] has been described in cases of ileocaecal tuberculosis. Vascular involvement constitutes an important part of tuberculous pathology in all organs, although its presence has been well-documented only in the central nervous system. Idiopathic ischemic strictures of the bowel are common in Indian patients between the ages of 20 years and 40 years.[22] Since there is a high incidence of abdominal tuberculosis in India, many of the idiopathic strictures could be the result of mesenteric small vessel occlusive disease. Shah et al.[19] from India performed superior mesenteric angiography in 20 patients with abdominal tuberculosis and demonstrated encasement, stretching, crowding and occlusion mostly involving larger arterial branches in 13 patients. Histological examination in six of their cases showed luminal narrowing, arterial occlusion due to vasculitis or extensive compression. Thus, they concluded that vascular involvement constitutes an important abnormality in abdominal tuberculosis and may explain some of the pathological and clinical manifestations of this disease. These authors however did not correlate the individual angiographic abnormalities with the type of histological lesion and thus the vascular abnormalities mentioned could be an inherent component of chronic inflammation itself, under the first category of local nonspecific inflammation. According to them, hypervascularity seen in the ulcerative phase of the disease may explain the occurrence of gastrointestinal hemorrhage in some patients. Occlusive arterial changes developing in the later stages of the disease would lead to stricture formation. Malik et al.[20] found one case of mesenteric vasculitis amongst 40 cases of abdominal tuberculosis. Apart from this there is a report of ileocaecal tuberculosis associated with granulomatous vasculitis[21] where the granuloma formation was seen in the wall of the vessel.

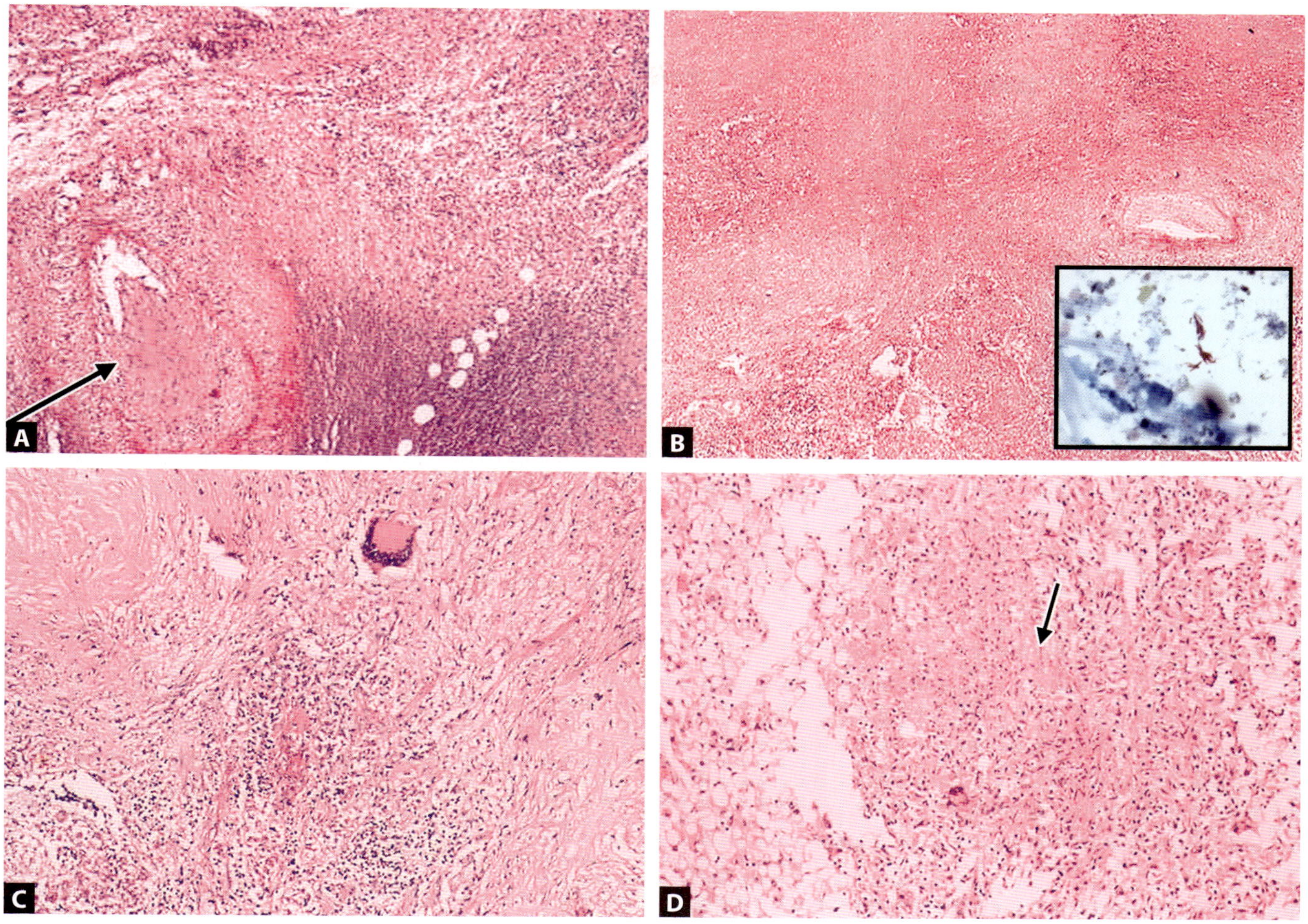

Figs 5A–D: Photomicrographs from the lung (A) Showing areas of acute necrosis and an adjacent vessel shows endarteritis obliterans (arrow); (B) Area of acute necrosis with nuclear debris. Inset in "B" shows acid-fast bacilli on ZN stain; (C) Area of cute necrosis bordered by scattered Langhans giant cells; (D) An occasional ill-formed epithelioid cell granuloma is seen (arrow).

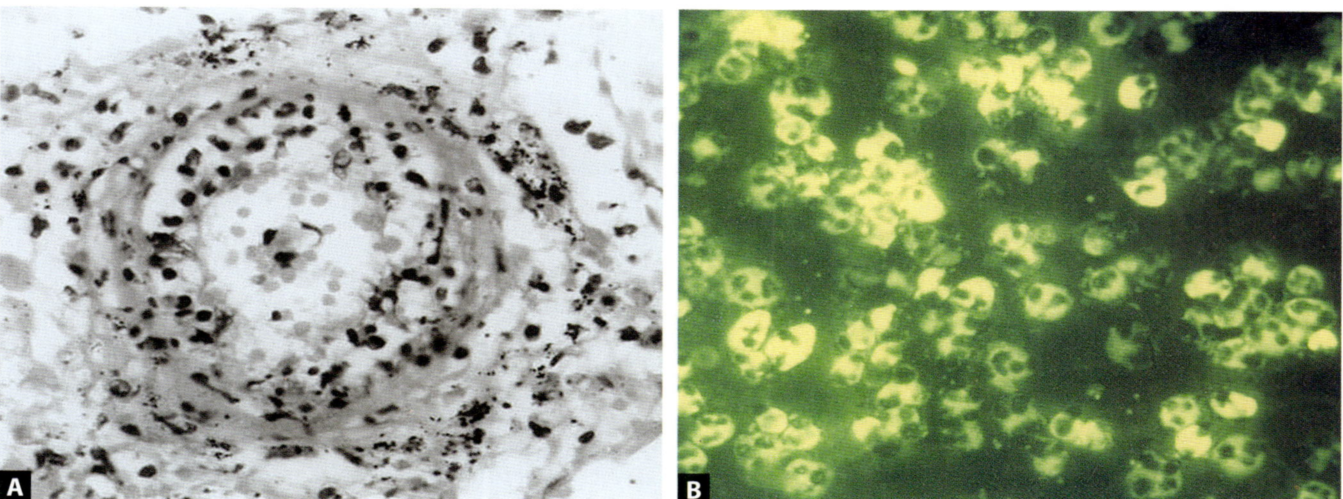

Figs 6A and B: (A) Photomicrograph from the lung showing a small vessel, away from the areas of necrosis, exhibiting acute vasculitis with transmural necrotizing inflammation replete with nuclear debris; (B) Strong c-ANCA positivity: indirect immunofluorescence performed on ethanol fixed neutrophils which demonstrate strong granular cytoplasmic fluorescence with lobular accentuation 400X.
(*Courtesy*: Dr Shobha Sehgal)

COMMENTARY—INDEX CASE: PM 14513

This 18-year-old malnourished female was admitted with complaints of acute abdominal pain, diarrhea, edema, cervical lymphadenopathy, ascites, pleural effusion and vague masses palpable in the epigastrium and the right iliac fossa. A clinical diagnosis of malabsorption syndrome, ? disseminated tuberculosis, ? immune proliferative small intestinal disease with severe left ventricular dysfunction was considered. Autopsy revealed disseminated nonreactive tuberculosis with a heavy bacillary load, postmortem c-ANCA strongly positive along with mesenteric and pulmonary vasculitis. There were changes of malnutrition in heart and liver. The important and stress worthy features in this case was:

- ***Nonreactive tuberculosis*** with widespread acute necrosis different from the usual caseation necrosis: Severe changes of malnutrition were seen in the liver and heart and it was not surprising that the patient did not evoke a granulomatous reaction. Ziehl–Neelsen stain for acid-fast bacilli was strongly positive.
- ***Strong c-ANCA positivity:*** The diagnostic value of ANCA and its pathogenic implications have proven to be very important in systemic vasculitides like GPA and microscopic polyangiitis. Now, ANCA is being found to be positive in a number of infectious conditions, autoimmune disorders, tumors, etc. How much diagnostic and pathogenic significance will be attributed to positive ANCA tests in nonvasculitic conditions remains at the time being, open for discussion and research. Patients with infectious disease such as tuberculosis can develop antiproteinase-3 antibodies resulting in c-ANCA positivity. Possibly, some of the mycobacterial antigens cross react with proteinase 3 and the antibodies so generated can evoke an immune complex-mediated vascular injury. This vasculitis may complicate and modify the clinicopathological features of the underlying disease.
- ***Pulmonary vasculitis***: There was extensive pulmonary vasculitis in the index case, notably so in the viable portions of the lung away from the areas of necrosis. This emphasized that vasculitis was not simply a consequence of tuberculosis, which this patient had. No AFB were demonstrated in the walls of these vessels and so this vasculitis was related to ANCA. Since c-ANCA was strongly positive, one could conclude that antiproteinase-3 antibodies were present and this may relate with the occurrence of vasculitis, as is seen in WG and microscopic polyangiitis. The other possibility is that some of the mycobacterial antigens may cross react with proteinase 3 and the antibodies so generated can evoke an immune complex-mediated vascular insult. Studies on a larger sample size would help substantiate this observation.
- ***Mesenteric vasculitis***: Mesenteric vasculitis as seen in this case has been described in cases of ileocaecal tuberculosis as a part and parcel of the basic disease process, i.e. local nonspecific vasculitis. It may however explain some of the pathological and clinical manifestations of this disease, like GI bleed in the early phase and strictures in the latter phase.
- ***Severe malnutrition*** had led to severe changes in the heart and the liver. The global hypokinesia and the severe left ventricular dysfunction were due to the morphological changes of malnutrition in the heart, i.e. multiple foci of myofiber necrosis and infiltration by lymphomononuclear cells and macrophages leading to severe myocardial damage.

TAKE HOME MESSAGE

- Acute necrosis (different from the usual caseation necrosis) occurs in nonreactive tuberculosis and a simple Ziehl–Neelsen stain clinches the diagnosis. At times, this stain has to be performed on multiple sections.
- Classic antinuclear cytoplasmic antibodies can be positive in conditions other than vasculitides like infections, tumors, etc. It can be positive in tuberculosis and this is a big diagnostic pitfall.
- The presence of bland acute necrosis with surrounding giant cells, vasculitis in the lungs and c-ANCA positivity takes us toward a diagnosis of Granulomatosis with polyangiitis (GPA). A positive Ziehl–Neelsen stain for AFB clinches the diagnosis. Thus, in every case of WG, tuberculosis should be ruled out and vice versa.
- Mesenteric vascular involvement constitutes an important abnormality in abdominal tuberculosis and may explain some of the pathological and clinical manifestations of this disease.

REFERENCES

1. Nolle B, Specks U, Ludemann J, et al. Anticytoplasmic autoantibodies: their immunodiagnostic value in Wegener granulomatosis. Ann Int Med. 1989;111:28-40.
2. Falk RJ, Jennette JC. Anti-neutrophil cytoplasmic autoantibodies with specificity for myeloperoxidase in patients with systemic vasculitis and idiopathic necrotising and crescentic glomerulonephritis. N Engl J Med. 1988;318:1651-7.
3. Gross WL, Schmitt HS, Csernok E. ANCA and associated diseases: immunodiagnostic and pathogenic aspects. Clin Exp Immunol. 1993;91:1-12.

4. Peter HH, Metzger D, Rump A, et al. ANCA in diseases other than systemic vasculitis. 5th International ANCA Workshop. Clinical Exp Immunol. 1993;93 (Suppl 1):12-3.
5. Efthimiou J, Spickett G, Lane D, et al. Antineutrophil cytoplasmic antibodies, cystic fibrosis and infection. Lancet. 1991;337:1037-8.
6. Schmitt WH, Csernok E, Gross WL. ANCA and infection. Lancet. 1991;337:1416-7.
7. Klaassen RJL, Goldschmeding R, Dolman K, et al. Antineutrophil cytoplasmic autonatibodies in patients with symptomatic HIV infection. Clin Exp Immunol. 1992;84:24-30.
8. De Clerk LS, Van Offel JF, Smolders WA, et al. Pitfalls with ANCA. Clin Rheumatol. 1989;8:512-6.
9. Adebajo AO, Charles P, Maini RN, et al. Autoantibodies in malaria, tuberculosis and hepatitis B in a West African population. Clin Exp Immunol. 1993;92:73-6.
10. Pudifin DJ, Duursma J, Gathiram V, et al. Serum from patients with invasive amoebiasis has anti-neutrophil cytoplasmic antibody activity. Clinical Exp Immunol. 1993;93 (Suppl 1): S33.
11. Falk RJ, Terrel RS, Charles LA, et al. ANCA induce neutrophils to degranulate in vitro. Proc Natl Acad Sci USA. 1989;87:4115-9.
12. Savige JA, Gallicchio MC, Stockman A, et al. Anti-neutrophil cytoplasm antibodies in rheumatoid arthritis. Clin Exp Immunol. 1991;86:92-8.
13. Braun MG, Csernok E, Schmitt WH, et al. Incidence and specificity of p-ANCA in rheumatic diseases. Proceedings of the 4th International Workshop on ANCA. Lubeck, Germany. 1992.
14. Saxon A, Shanahan F, Landers C, et al. A distinct subset of antineutrophil cytoplasmic antibodies is associated with inflammatory bowel disease. J Allergy Clin Immunol. 1990; 86:202-10.
15. Rump JA, Scholmerich J, Gross V, et al. A new type of perinuclear anti-neutrophil cytoplasmic antibody (po+ ANCA) in active ulcerative colitis but not in Crohn's disease. Immunobiology. 1990;181:406-13.
16. Strauss L, Liebermann KV, Churg J. Pulmonary vasculitis. In: Fishman AP (Ed). Pulmonary disease and disorders, 2nd edition. New York: McGraw-Hill Book Company; 1988. pp. 1127.
17. Bambery P, Bharti B, Datta BN. Pulmonary vasculitis: an Indian perspective. Seminars in Respiratory Medicine. 1991; 12:115-23.
18. Menon NK, Malaviya AN, Ahuja MMS. Progress in tuberculosis. In: Ahuja MMS (Ed). Progress in Clinical Medicine in India. New Delhi: Arnold Heinemann; 1976. p.480.
19. Shah P, Ramakantan R. Role of vasculitis in the natural history of abdominal tuberculosis-evaluation by mesenteric angiography. Indian J Gastroenterol. 1991;10(4):127-30.
20. Malik AK, Bhasin DK, Pal L, et al. Does vasculitis occur in abdominal tuberculosis? J Clin Gastroenterol. 1992;15(4): 355-6.
21. Mapstone NP, Dixon MF. Vasculitis in ileocaecal tuberculosis: similarities to Crohn's disease. Histopathology. 1992;21: 477-9.
22. Bapat RD, Aiyer PM, Relekar RG, et al. Ischemic bowel disease. Indian J Gastroenterol. 1990;9:19-22.

CONTRIBUTIONS BY:

1. Dr Deepak Bhasin, Ex-Professor and Head, Department of Gastroenterology (Clinician In-Charge)
2. Dr Shobha Sehgal, Ex-Professor and Head, Department of Immunopathology (ANCA workup and Fig 6B)
3. Dr BR Thapa, Professor and Head, Department of Gastroenterology, Hepatology and Nutrition (Compilation of Clinical Details)

Post Graduate Institute of Medical Education and Research, Chandigarh, India

SECTION 7

Primary Renal Mucormycosis Adult and Pediatric Cases

CASE 49

Isolated Bilateral Renal Mucormycosis with Contiguous Spread to the Adrenals, Mesentery, Pancreas and Colon in an Apparently Immunocompetent Adult: PM 27250

Nandita Bharadwaj Kakkar

 HIGHLIGHTS OF THE CASE

This 45-year-old male came with a short history of intermittent fever, abdominal pain, vomiting, cough and a rapidly progressive renal failure. Investigations revealed leukocytosis with neutrophilia, deranged renal function tests, hypoproteinemia, hypoalbuminemia, hematuria, pus cells in urine with 2+ albumin, nephrolithiasis and bulky kidneys with swollen cortical parenchyma with significant perinephric fat stranding on non-contrast computerized tomography (NCCT). A clinical diagnosis of acute on chronic kidney disease with bilateral nephrolithiasis, hypertension, acute pulmonary edema and Type 1 respiratory failure was made. Autopsy revealed isolated bilateral renal mucormycosis with contiguous spread to the adrenals, mesentery, pancreas and colon, nephrolithiasis with acute pyelonephritis. There was no evidence of any fungus in the lungs.

Keywords: Primary renal mucormycosis, contiguous spread, angioinvasion.

 CLINICAL DETAILS

Date of Admission: 28.02.2016 at 05:41 pm, Date of Death: 28.02.2016 at 06:25 pm, Duration of Hospital Stay: 45 minutes.

A 45-year-old male was being treated at an outside facility with complaints of intermittent fever, abdominal pain, vomiting and cough for last 10 days. He was diagnosed to have urinary tract infection and chronic kidney disease. He received intravenous antibiotics (imipenem and levofloxacin) and anti-hypertensives (amlodipine and arkamin). The patient did not respond to the treatment and was referred to PGIMER. On reaching the institute he was found to be in an unresponsive state with unrecordable pulse and blood pressure. Cardiopulmonary resuscitation was done but the patient could not be revived.

Investigations (Done at the Outside Facility)

Hemogram: Hb—11 g/dL, TLC—21,800/uL, DLC—P92, L4M4 and platelets—1,50,000/uL.

Blood biochemistry: Na^+—132 mEq/L, K^+—4.77 mEq/L, blood urea—141 mg%, serum creatinine—7.21 mg%, total proteins—4.75 g, albumin—2.05 g; random blood sugar—105 mg%. ***Urine examination:*** albumin—2+, sugar—nil, 8–10 pus cells/HPF, 25–30 RBC/HPF. ***Serology***: HBsAg—negative, anti-HCV—negative and HIV—nonreactive. ***Radiology:*** USG abdomen: kidneys—normal sized with normal pelvicalyceal system, 4.4 mm stone in right kidney, 4.9 mm stone in left kidney and other abdominal organs are normal. NCCT KUB—both kidneys bulky with swollen cortical parenchyma and significant perinephric fat stranding, left lung shows basal consolidation and bilateral minimal pleural effusion. ***Units final diagnosis***—chronic kidney disease with bilateral nephrolithiasis, hypertension, acute pulmonary edema and type 1 respiratory failure.

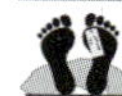 AUTOPSY FINDINGS: PM 27250

A partial autopsy was performed. The peritoneal cavity contained 1.5 liters of straw-colored fluid. Both ***kidneys*** (Figs 1A–C) were encased in a mass to which the intestines were also entangled. The kidneys weighed 600 g. The capsule was thickened with a yellowish material plastered on the outer aspect. The para-aortic nodes, aorta and the inferior vena cava were all entangled in this mass. The capsule was removed with difficulty. Capsular aspect of the kidneys showed uniform blackish discoloration. Cut section showed total infarction of both kidneys. The hilar vessels were thrombosed. Multiple small stones were present in the pelvicalyceal system on both sides. Microscopic sections from the kidney (Figs 2A–D) revealed bland infarction replete with fungal hyphae of mucormycosis (broad, aseptate, empty looking and foldable), areas of dense acute necrotizing inflammation in the medullary areas and vessels (all sizes) showed thromboses, replete with hyphae of mucormycosis. The pelvicalyceal system (Figs 3A and B) was mildly dilated and contained necrotic pultaceous material which on microscopy revealed necrotic tissue replete with fungal profiles of mucor. The inflammation was going into the perirenal fat which was also replete with the fungus. Upper parts of both ureters were caught up in the inflammatory process (Fig 3C). ***Adrenals*** were caught up in the inflammation leading to their necrosis (Fig 3D). Fungal profiles of mucormycosis were exuberant in the periadrenal tissue and also invading the adrenal gland. ***Urinary bladder*** appeared normal and microscopic sections did not reveal any ulcer or fungus. The ***mesentry*** (Figs 4A–D, 5A and B) was thick, discolored and showed thrombosed vessels. Microscopy revealed fat necrosis, exuberant proliferation of fungal hyphae of mucormycosis with thrombosis of vessels containing similar hyphae. The tail of the ***pancreas*** (Figs 5C–E) in close approximation to the mass, was discoloured and showed acute necrosis replete with mucormycosis hyphae. ***Colon*** (Figs 6A–D): A part of the descending colon was attached to the mass and this area, 8 cm in length showed thickening and transmural blackish discoloration. Microscopy showed dense inflammation on the

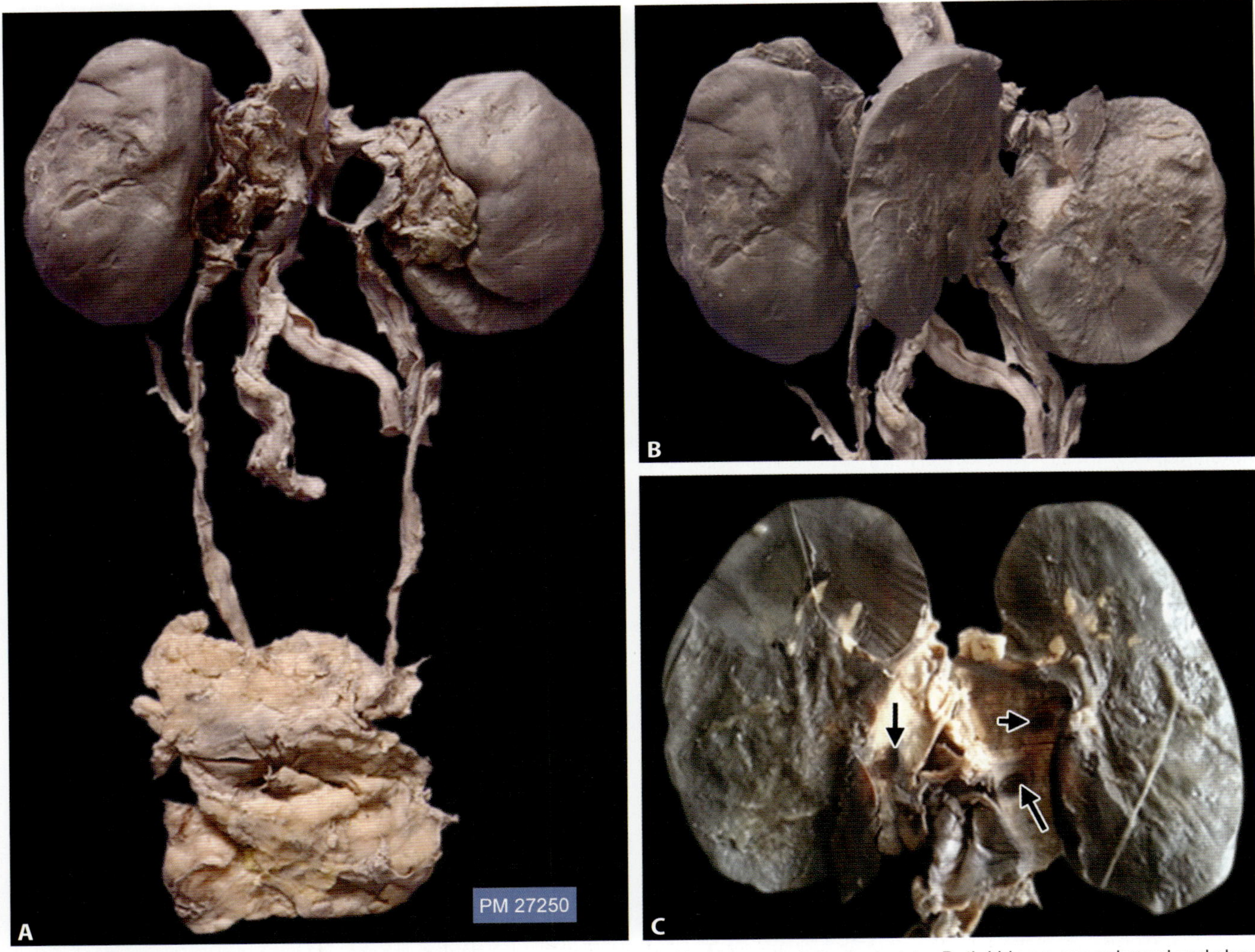

Figs 1A–C: (A) Organ complex comprising of both kidneys, ureters, urinary bladder, and abdominal aorta. Both kidneys are enlarged and show diffuse black discoloration; (B) Kidneys showing diffuse dusky discoloration and cut section shows total infarction; (C) Infarcted kidneys showing thrombosed vessels (arrows) in the hilar fat.

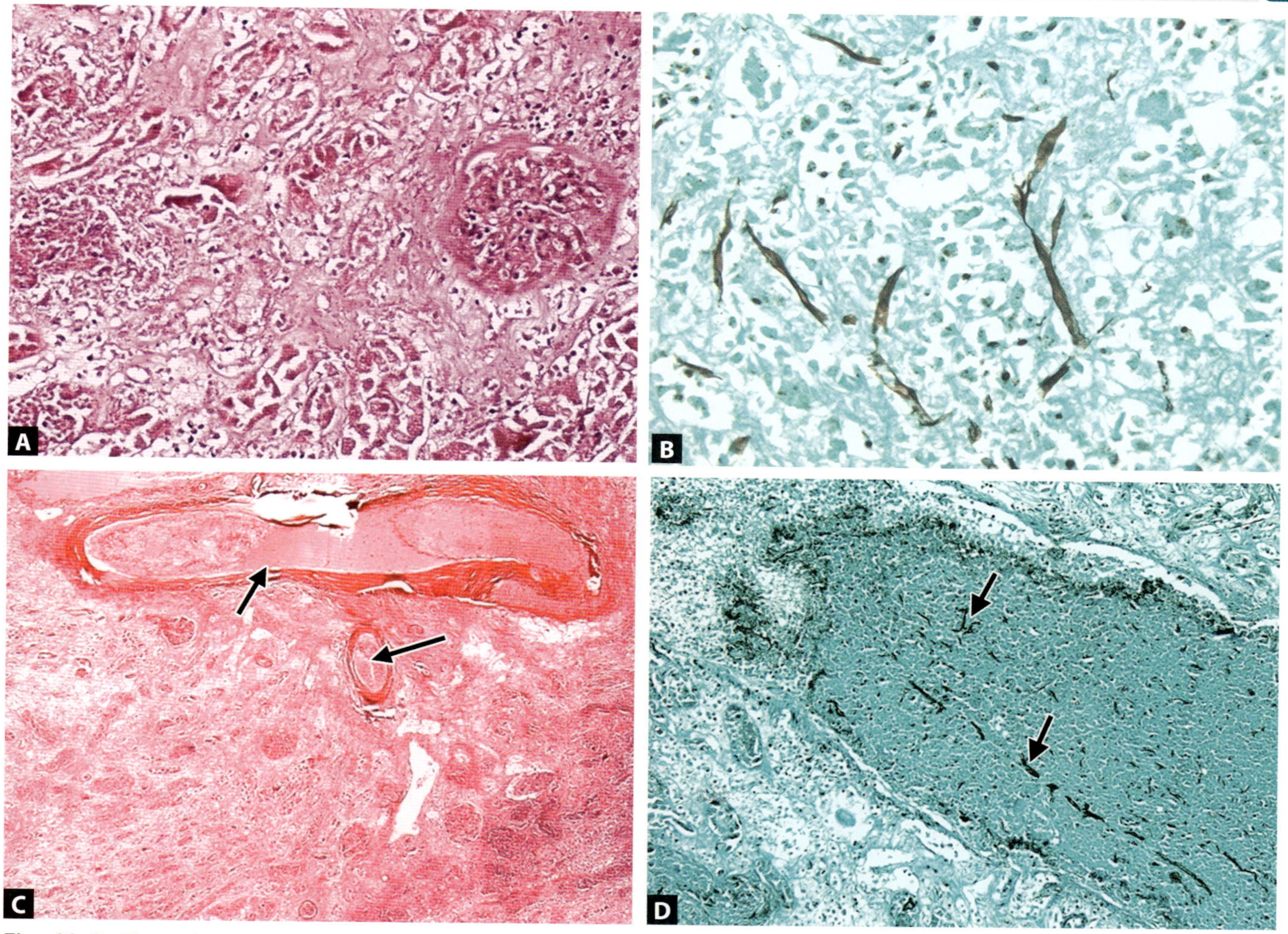

Figs 2A–D: Photomicrographs of the kidney showing (A) Total coagulative necrosis; (B) Areas of necrosis replete with fungal profiles of mucormycosis (Grocott stain); (C) Vessels of all caliber show thrombosis (arrows); (D) Grocott stain shows fungal profiles (arrows) of mucormycosis within the thrombosed vessel.

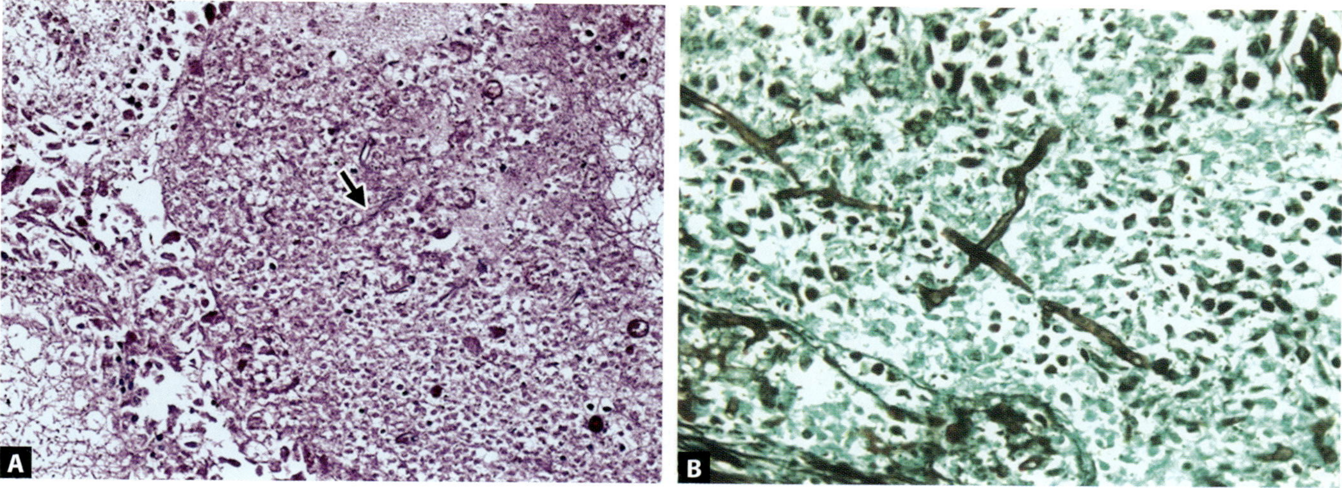

Figs 3A and B:

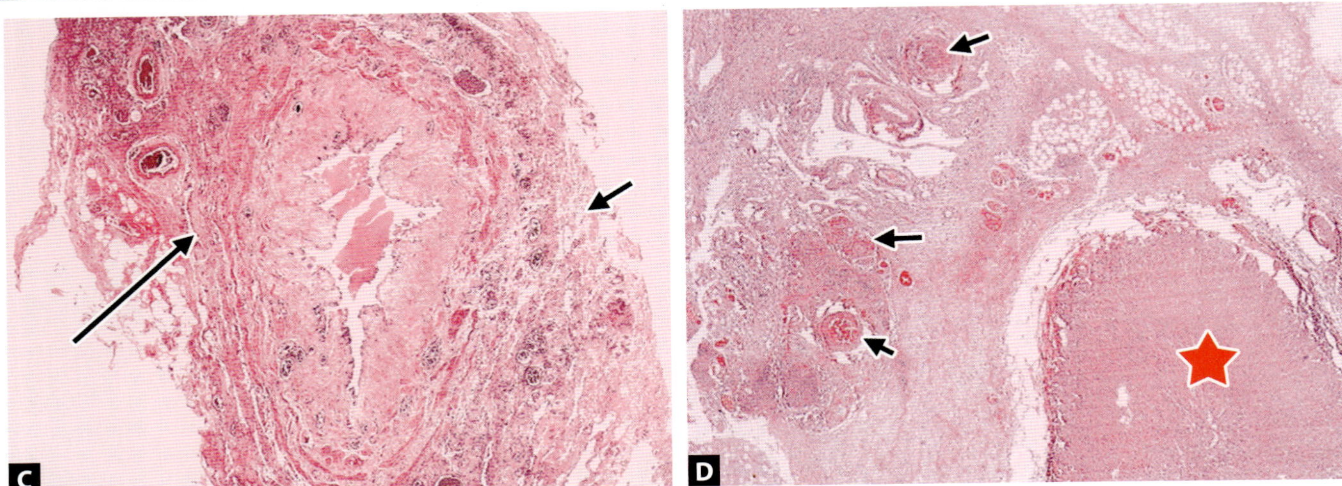

Figs 3A–D: (A and B) Pelvicalyceal system showing necrotic debris replete with fungal profiles of mucormycosis B-(Grocotts stain); (C) Section from the upper part of the ureter shows periureteral inflammation (arrows); (D) Adrenal (star) showing necrosis with extensive periadrenal inflammation showing thrombosed vessels (arrows).

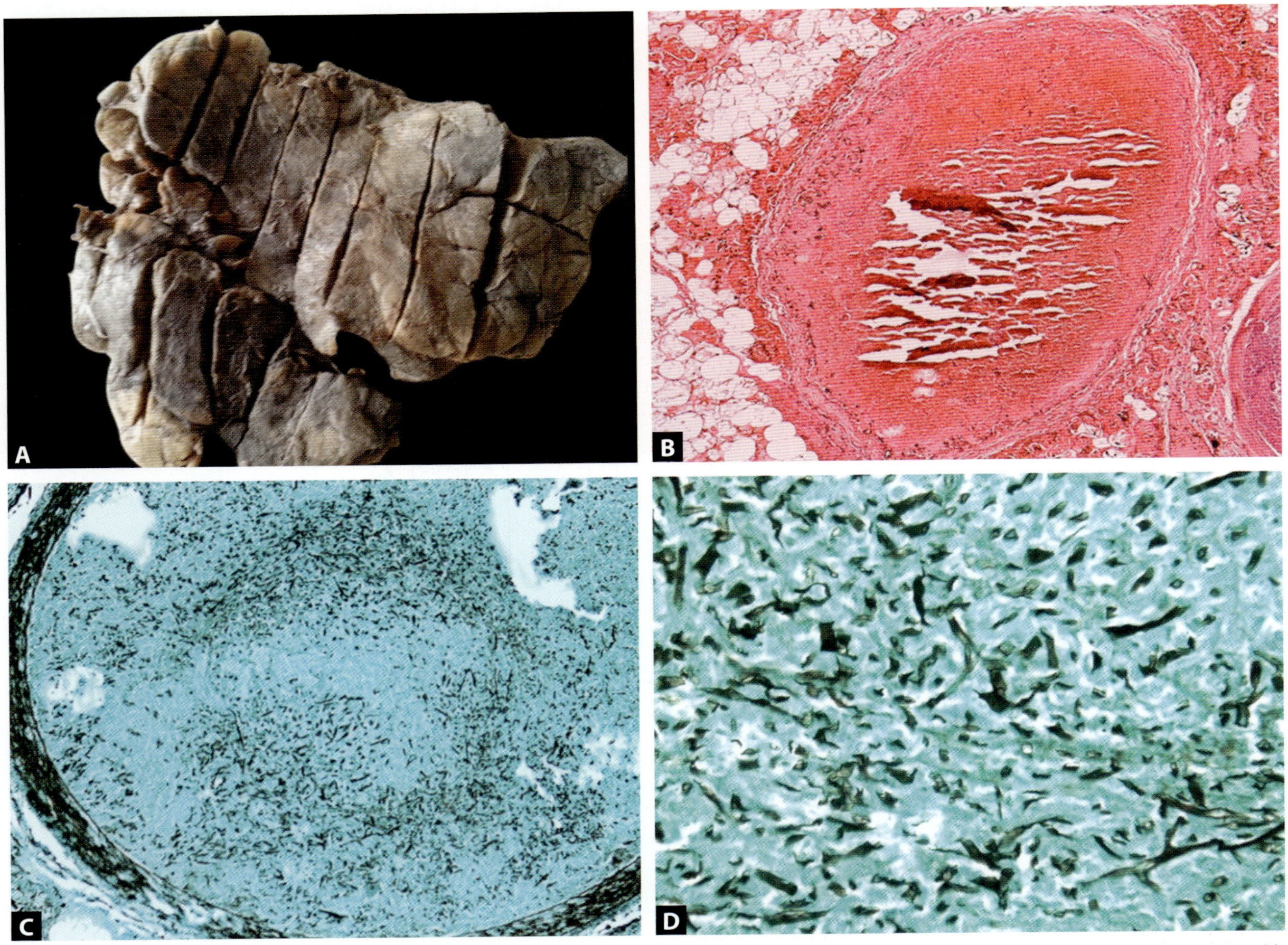

Figs 4A–D: (A) Thickened and discolored mesentery; (B) Mesenteric vessels showing thrombosis; (C and D) Mesenteric vessels replete with fungal hyphae of mucormycosis (Grocott stain).

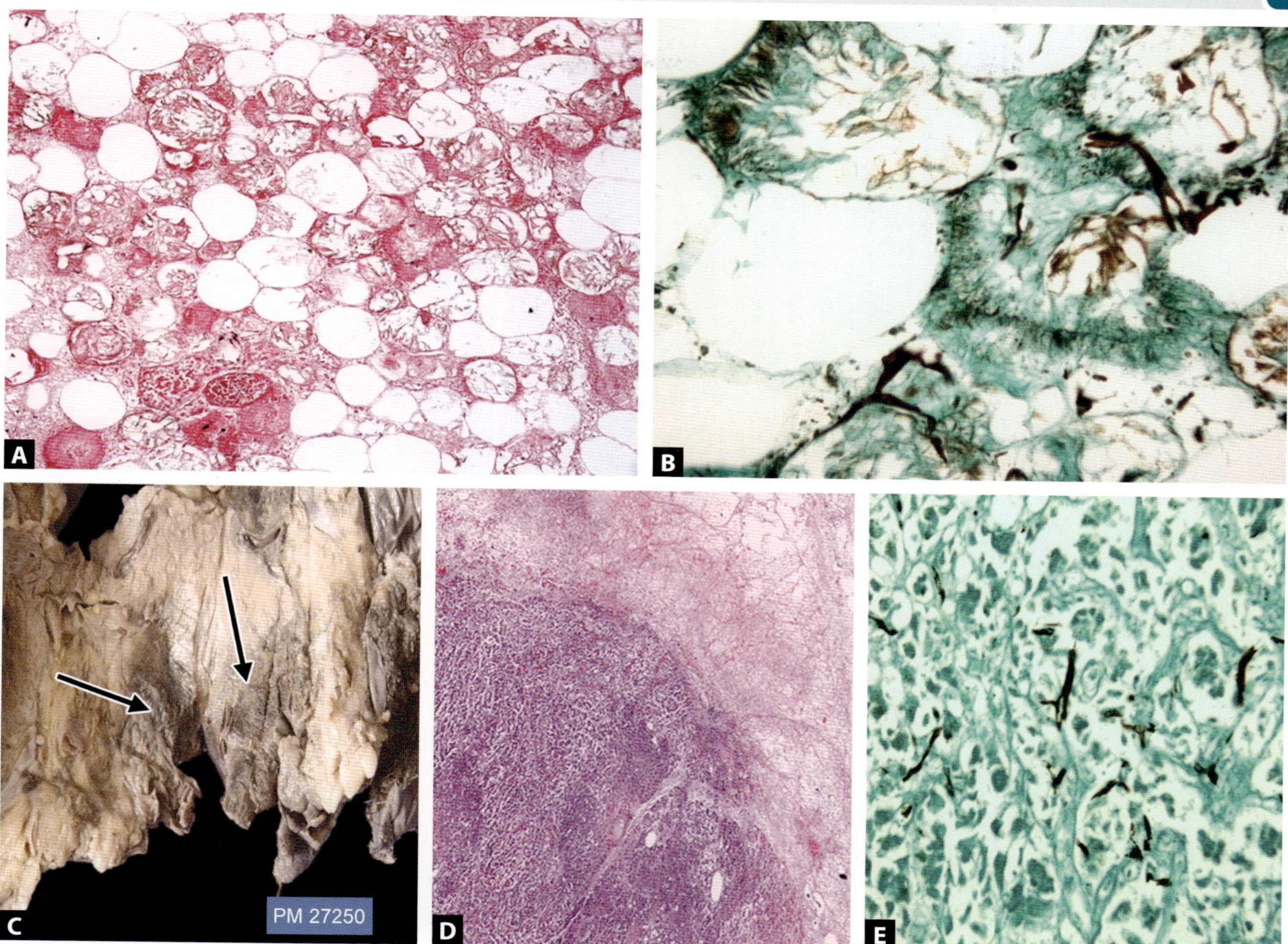

Figs 5A–E: (A and B) Photomicrograph of the mesentery showing fat necrosis and replete with fungal hyphae of mucormycosis B-(Grocott stain); (C) Cut section of the pancreas showing areas of discoloration (arrows); (D and E) Pancreas showing necrosis along with fungal profiles of mucormycosis (Grocott stain).

serosal aspect replete with fungal profiles of mucormycosis. In areas, the serosal inflammation along with the fungal hyphae was extending into the wall of the large gut leading to inflammation, hemorrhage and areas of ischemic necrosis in the muscularis propria, submucosa and mucosa. Fungal profiles of mucor were seen in the muscularis propria but not in the mucosa and submucosa. ***Lungs*** (Fig 7A) weighed 1,100 g and the pleura appeared normal. Cut section showed diffuse consolidation. Lungs (Figs 7B–F) were meticulously sampled and sections revealed organizing pneumonia with Masson bodies, prominent adenomatoid change along with silicotic nodules. No fungus was seen in the lungs in the multiple sections studied. Periodic acid–Schiff and Grocott stain were done which were negative. ***Heart*** revealed mild left ventricular hypertrophy (wall thickness 1.6 cm). The valves, chambers and coronaries were normal. ***Liver and spleen*** on microscopic examination showed septicemic changes.

FINAL AUTOPSY DIAGNOSIS: PM 27250

45 Years Old Male

- Isolated/primary bilateral renal mucormycosis with contiguous spread to the adrenals, mesentery, pancreas and colon.
- Nephrolithiasis with acute pyelonephritis.
- Lungs: organizing pneumonia with silicotic nodules.
- Septicemic changes—liver and spleen.

Primary Renal Mucormycosis—See Case No 50, PM 22863.

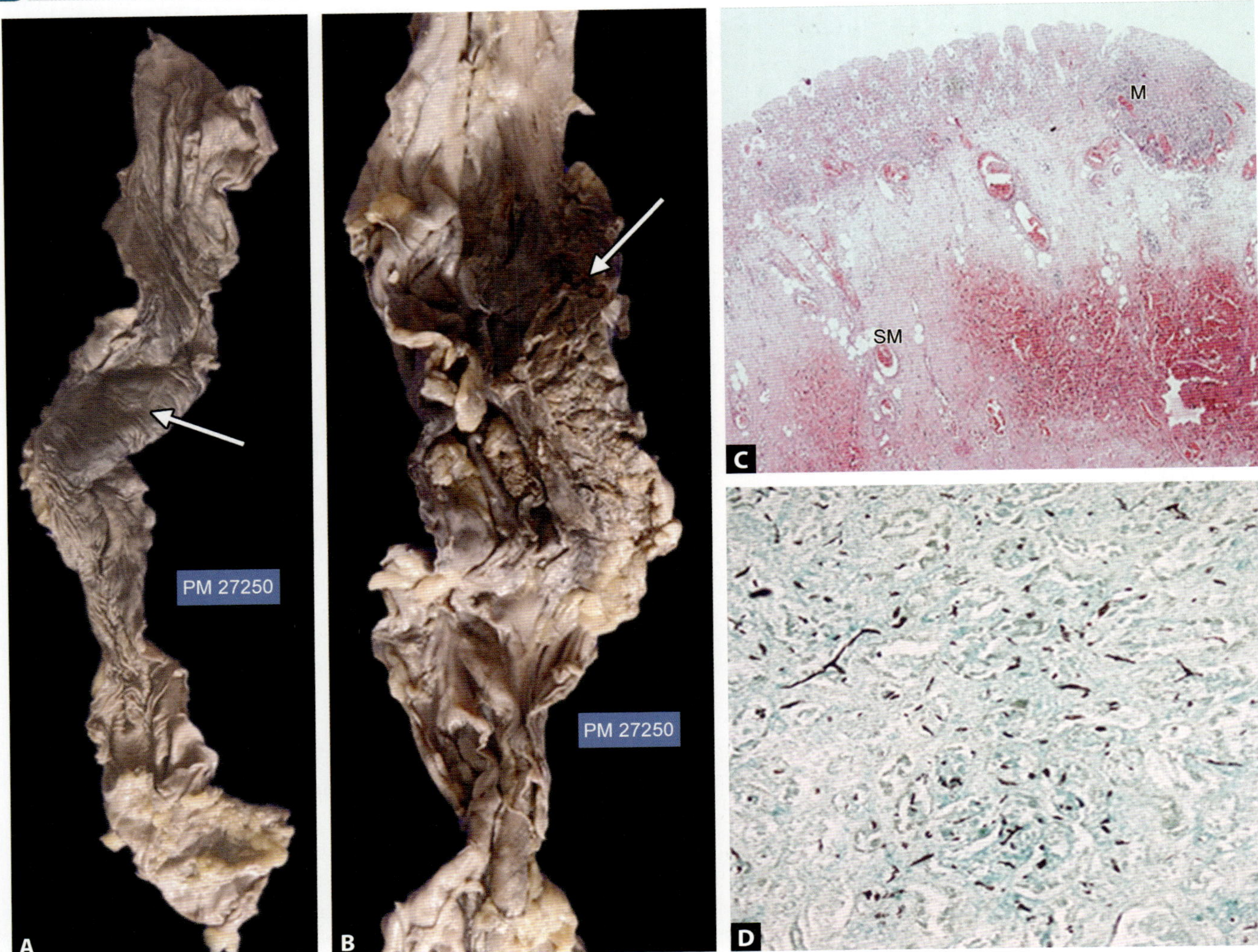

Figs 6A–D: (A and B) Mucosal and serosal aspect of the colon that was entangled in the mass, showing discoloration; (C) Photomicrograph of the colon showing transmural coagulative necrosis of the mucosa (M) with hemorrhage in submucosa (SM); (D) Colon show abundant fungal hyphae of mucormycosis in the areas of necrosis.

COMMENTARY—INDEX CASE: PM 27250

This 45-year-old male came with a short history of intermittent fever, abdominal pain, vomiting, cough and a rapidly progressive renal failure. Investigations revealed leukocytosis with neutrophilia, deranged renal function tests, hypoproteinemia, hypoalbuminemia and hematuria; pus cells in urine with 2+ albumin, hypocalcemia, hyperphosphatemia, nephrolithiasis and bulky kidneys with swollen cortical parenchyma with significant perinephric fat stranding on NCCT. Serum creatinine increased from 1.6 mg% to 7.21 mg% over 5 days, i.e. there was rapidly progressive renal failure. A clinical diagnosis of acute-on-chronic kidney disease with bilateral nephrolithiasis, hypertension, acute pulmonary edema and type 1 respiratory failure was made. Autopsy revealed isolated/primary bilateral renal mucormycosis with contiguous spread to the adrenals, mesentery, pancreas and colon and nephrolithiasis with acute pyelonephritis. There was no evidence of any fungus in the lungs. in this middle aged male, there was no apparent predisposing factor for acquiring a primary renal mucormycosis. He was thus labelled as immunocompetent.

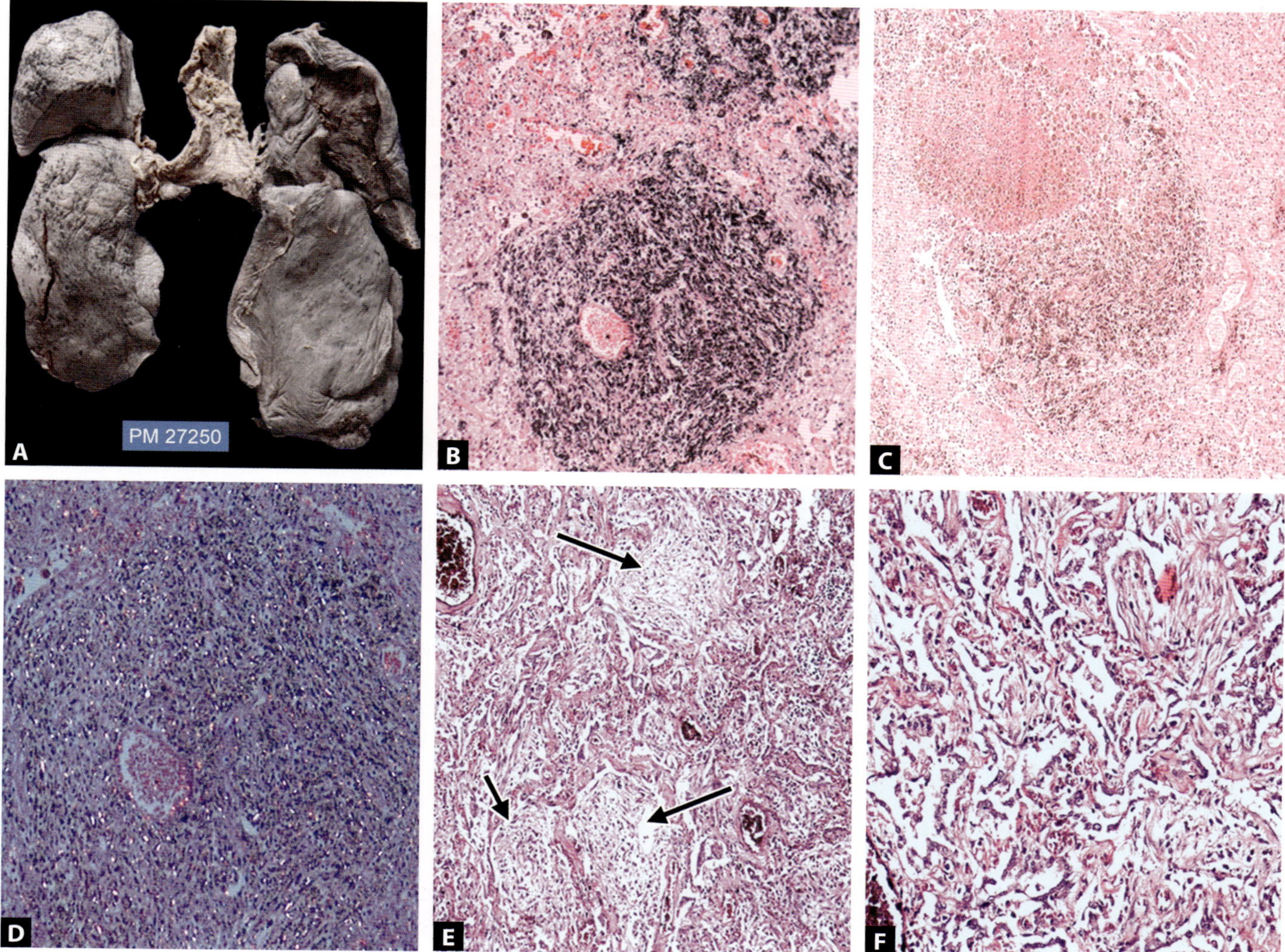

Figs 7A–F: (A) Gross photograph of both lungs. Photomicrographs of the lungs showing; (B) Silicotic nodules; (C) Silicotic nodule showing central necrosis; (D) Birefringent particles of silica under polarized light; (E) Formation of Masson bodies (arrows) in the alveolar spaces; (F) Prominent adenomatoid change.

TAKE HOME MESSAGE

- Isolated/primary renal mucormycosis is a distinct clinical entity, can occur in apparently immunocompetent hosts, is seen mostly in India and the diagnosis is frequently missed.
- Rapidly progressive renal failure with NCCT showing bulky kidneys with significant perinephric fat stranding, should alert the clinician.
- There is a rapid development of renal failure due to widespread thrombosis of renal vasculature secondary to angioinvasion.
- Bland coagulative necrosis of the kidneys replete with broad aseptate hyphae of mucormycosis, extensive angioinvasion and contiguous perinephric spread with entanglement of adjacent organs is diagnostic.

CONTRIBUTIONS BY:

1. Dr Vivek Kumar, Assistant Professor, Department of Nephrology (Compilation of Clinical Details)
2. Dr Ashish Bhalla, Professor, Department of Internal Medicine (Clinician In-Charge)

Post Graduate Institute of Medical Education and Research, Chandigarh, India.

CASE 50

Primary Bilateral Renal Mucormycosis in an Apparently Immunocompetent Child: PM 22863

Nandita Bharadwaj Kakkar

 **HIGHLIGHTS OF THE CASE**

This is a 2½-year, apparently immunocompetent, male child who presented with sudden onset fever of 20 days duration, followed by complete anuria, anasarca, altered sensorium and rapid breathing. On investigating, the renal function tests were deranged. Clinical diagnosis was sepsis, DIC, meningitis, acute renal failure ? Acute tubular necrosis ? Hemolytic uremic syndrome ? uremic encephalopathy. Autopsy revealed isolated bilateral renal mucormycosis with contiguous spread to the adrenals, mesentery and descending colon. There were multiple ulcers, replete with fungal hyphae of mucormycosis in the urinary bladder. No mucor was found in lungs and in any other organ. The kidneys were infected by ascending infection from the urinary bladder.

Keywords: Isolated renal mucormycosis, bilateral, fungal cystitis, ascending infection, immunocompetent, child, autopsy.

 **CLINICAL DETAILS**

Date of Admission: 3.10.2008, Date of Death: 18.10.2008, Duration of Hospital Stay: 15 Days.

A 2½ years old male child presented with sudden onset fever since 20 days, followed by anuria, anasarca, altered sensorium and rapid breathing since 3 days. The child was apparently well 20 days prior to admission, when he started to have intermittent high grade fever, accompanied with rigors and which came down with antipyretics. Three days prior to admission, he had anuria followed by swelling of face, abdomen and feet. He had one episode of generalized tonic–clonic seizure, 4 days back which lasted for 2 minutes. There was respiratory distress since 4 days with a high respiratory rate and in-drawing of chest. There was one episode of melena, but there was no history of diarrhea. He was born to parents with a nonconsanguineous marriage, has three older siblings who are doing well and was developmentally normal with adequate immunization. He was treated at an outside facility, but he deteriorated, was intubated and referred to PGIMER, Chandigarh. ***On examination*** he was on manual intermittent positive pressure respiration (IPPR) with SpO_2 of 98%; pulse was 140/min; temperature—37° C, BP—100/60 mm Hg, weight—12 kg (89% of expected) and length—88 cm (92% of expected). There was pallor, no icterus, cyanosis or lymphadenopathy. Periorbital puffiness and pedal edema were present. Respiratory system revealed equal air entry and bilateral crepitations. Cardiovascular system was normal. Abdomen was distended, liver and spleen were not palpable, there was a mass felt in the left hypochondrium, hard with a smooth surface and ballotable ? kidney. Central nervous system—E1 M4-5 VT, hypotonia +, deep tendon reflexes present, plantars upgoing and there were no meningeal signs.

Investigations

Hematological: Hb 11.7—7.1 g/dL; TLC—12600-39000/uL; DLC N86, L6, M6, E2; platelets—75000/uL, PBF—moderate anisocytosis, mild poikilocytosis with microcytes/macrocytes, fragmented RBC's +, low platelets, reticulocyte count—0.09%, ESR—72 mm 1st hour, Coagulogarm—PT -18', PTI 72%, aPTT-29' (c 25'-32'), Fibrinogen—7.02 g/L (N- 2–4 gm/L), D dimer—positive. Malarial parasite smear: Negative (thrice) and Card test: Negative. ANA: negative.

Blood biochemistry: Na^+—139-146 mEq/L; K^+ 5.5 mEq/L; Cl^- 96–111 mEq/L; S urea—106 mg%; S creatinine—4.1–6.9 mg%; S calcium—7.1mg%; S bilirubin—0.7 mg%; AST 90 U/L; ALT—63 U/L; ALP 363 U/L; S proteins 4.4 gm; albumin—0.9 gm; globulins—3.5 gm. Urine examination could not be done as patient was anuric throughout.

Microbiology: Blood culture: sterile; Peritoneal fluid: proteins: 0.6 g/dL, glucose: 237 mg/dL, predominantly neutrophils, Gram stain negative, culture sterile; EBV (VCA) IgM antibody positive; Parvo B19 IgM antibody negative; HIV negative, Fungal serology: Negative for aspergillus and candida; C3: 65 mg/dL (N-50-150 mg/dL), C4: 28 mg/dL (N-20-50 mg/dL).

Radiology: Chest X ray – right pneumothorax with bilateral infiltrates; NCCT head normal; USG abdomen (portable): Rt Kidney 8.6; Lt kidney 8.3 cms (Normal: 7.6+-1.3). B/l raised renal cortical echogenicity with maintained corticomedullary differentiation, pelvicalyceal system compact, upper ureters not visualized, urinary bladder empty. Mild left pleural effusion present with minimal interloop fluid. Liver, spleen and pancreas normal.

Course in hospital: Baby was on manual ventilation and anuric at admission. He received fluid bolus and Lasix, but remained anuric throughout. Renal parameters were deranged, there was acidosis and hyperkalemia. Peritoneal dialysis was done five times. On the 8th day, he had pneumothorax and cardiac arrest, but was revived with inotropes. The pneumothorax was drained. There was thrombocytopenia, coagulopathy and low albumin for which he was given fresh frozen plasma, Vitamin K and blood transfusion. Antimicrobials (vancomycin, piptaz and meropenem) were given for sepsis or meningitis. Fluconazole was added in view of prolonged hospital stay. He remained intermittently febrile, sensorium improved transiently, there was no recurrence of seizures (dilantized) but on the 14th day he went into shock and could not be revived. Units clinical diagnosis was sepsis, disseminated intravascular coagulopathy, meningitis, acute renal failure, ? acute tubular necrosis ? hemolytic uremic syndrome, ? uremic encephalopathy.

AUTOPSY FINDINGS: PM 22863

A complete autopsy was performed on this 2-year and 6-month-old male child. The peritoneal cavity yielded 1.2 liters of straw-colored fluid. Both ***kidneys*** were encased in a mass in which the para-aortic nodes, abdominal aorta, inferior vena cava and the intestines were entangled. After dissection, the kidneys (Fig 1A) were found to be enlarged and together weighed 400 g (normal 220 g). The capsule was markedly thickened with a yellowish material plastered on the outer aspect and was removed with difficulty (Figs. 1B and C). The outer surface of the kidneys revealed a mosaic pattern of hemorrhage and necrosis (Fig 1D). On cut section both the kidneys were infarcted and showed dusky discoloration (Figs 1E and F). Microscopy of the kidney (Figs 2A and B) revealed bland coagulative necrosis surrounded by areas of dense inflammation. The areas of necrosis were replete with broad, aseptate, foldable, right-angled branching fungal hyphae, consistent with morphology of mucormycosis (Figs 2C and D). Plenty of giant cells could be seen, some of them having ingested the fungal hyphae (Fig 2E). Vessels of all sizes showed florid vasculitis, with the wall and the lumen replete with fungal hyphae (Fig 2F and Figs 3A and B). The lining of the pelvicalyceal system (Fig 3C) was ulcerated and showed necrosis, giant cells and fungal hyphae. The inflammation from the renal parenchyma was contiguously spreading into the thickened capsule and into the perirenal fat, which was also replete with the fungus (Figs 3D–F). The ***urinary bladder*** (Figs 4A–C) showed deep ulcers replete with fungal profiles of mucormycosis. ***Adrenals*** were caught up in the exuberant spreading inflammation and showed bland necrosis, replete with fungal hyphae (Figs 4D–F). A part of the ***descending colon*** (8 cm) was attached to the mass and showed thickening, exudates on the serosal aspect, mucosal ulceration and discoloration (Fig 5A). On microscopy it showed transmural necrosis (Fig 5B), serosal aspect showed dense inflammation and attached mesentery showed fat necrosis which was full of fungal profiles of mucormycosis (Fig 5C). The muscularis propria in these areas showed necroinflammation and few fungal profiles. The submucosa and mucosa showed inflammation, hemorrhage and areas of ischemic necrosis. An occasional fungal profile was seen in the mucosa and submucosa. Hence, the spread of necroinflammation was contiguous from the serosa to the mucosa. The ***lungs*** weighed 200 g. The pleura was normal. Cut section revealed diffuse consolidation and on microscopy there was bronchopneumonia with focal alveolar hemorrhage (Figs 5D and E). Lungs were meticulously sampled and no fungus was detected. Bone marrow revealed adequate representation of all three haemopoietic elements along with secondary hemophagocytosis (Fig 5F). Thymus, spleen, lymph nodes, terminal ileum and appendix showed adequate lymphoid tissue and this ruled out the presence of immunodeficiency (Figs 6A–C). All other organs, including brain were within normal limits. No meningitis was seen.

FINAL AUTOPSY DIAGNOSIS: PM 22863

A 2½ years, apparently immunocompetent male with sudden onset acute renal failure:

- Isolated/primary bilateral renal mucormycosis with contiguous spread to the adrenals, mesentery and descending colon.
- Mucormycotic cystitis.

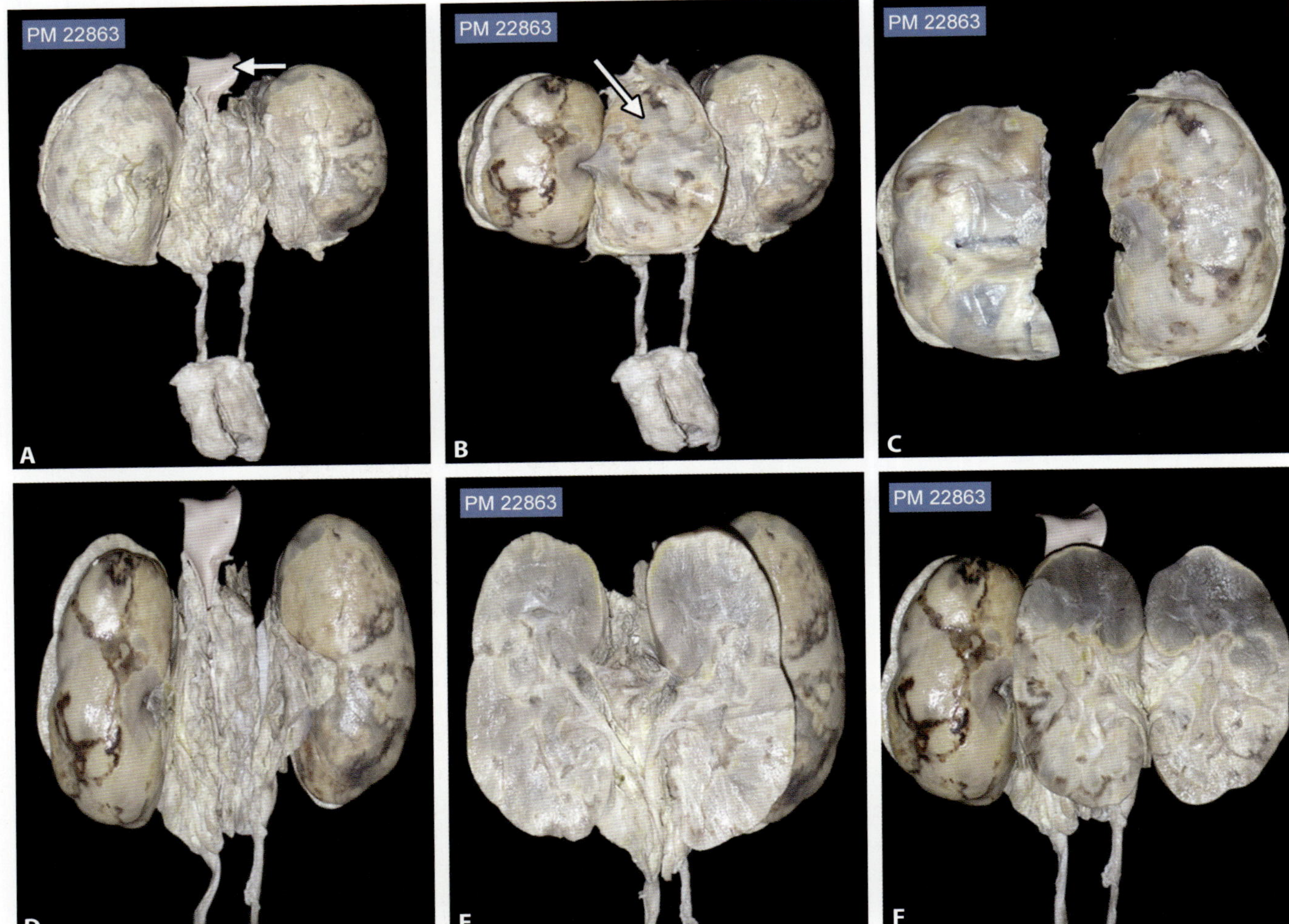

Figs 1A–F: (A) Both kidneys are enlarged, covered by a thick capsule with exudates on the surface. Necrotic material encasing the para-aortic lymph nodes, inferior vena cava (IVC), and part of aorta (arrow) is seen in-between; (B) The right renal capsule is reflected (arrow); (C) Gross picture of both the thickened capsules, showing necrosis, exudate, and hemorrhage; (D) Both kidneys after removal of the capsule show infarction and a mosaic pattern; (E and F) Cut section of both kidneys showing infarction and dusky discoloration.

- Bronchopneumonia with focal alveolar hemorrhage.
- Florid hemophagocytosis in the bone marrow.

ISOLATED/PRIMARY RENAL MUCORMYCOSIS

Mucormycosis formerly known as zygomycosis, is caused by fungi belonging to the family ***Mucoraceae*** and most often caused by species of the genera ***Rhizopus/Rhizomucor/Mucor*** and occasionally by other species under the genera ***Lichtheimia, Cunninghamella*** or ***Saksenaea***. Mucormycetaneous fungi are now members of phylum Glomeromycota and subphylum Mucormycotina. They are widely distributed in nature and in majority of the cases occur as an opportunistic infection in the immunosuppressed individuals, i.e. neutropenic individuals, those on corticosteroid therapy/chemotherapy, diabetics, post-transplantation patients on routine immunosuppressant therapy, iron overload, HIV infected individuals, intravenous drug abusers and patients with burns, trauma or surgical wounds. Mucormycotina are transmitted by airborne asexual spores, are inhaled and harbor in the sinuses or the lungs. Apart from this, infection can enter via the skin or by ingestion. Once they gain entry in the body, they are phagocytosed by the macrophages and the sporangiospores are killed. The components of the hyphae wall are recognized by the TLR2, which ignites a proinflammatory cascade of cytokines. Neutrophils have an important role in killing the hyphae by causing direct damage to its

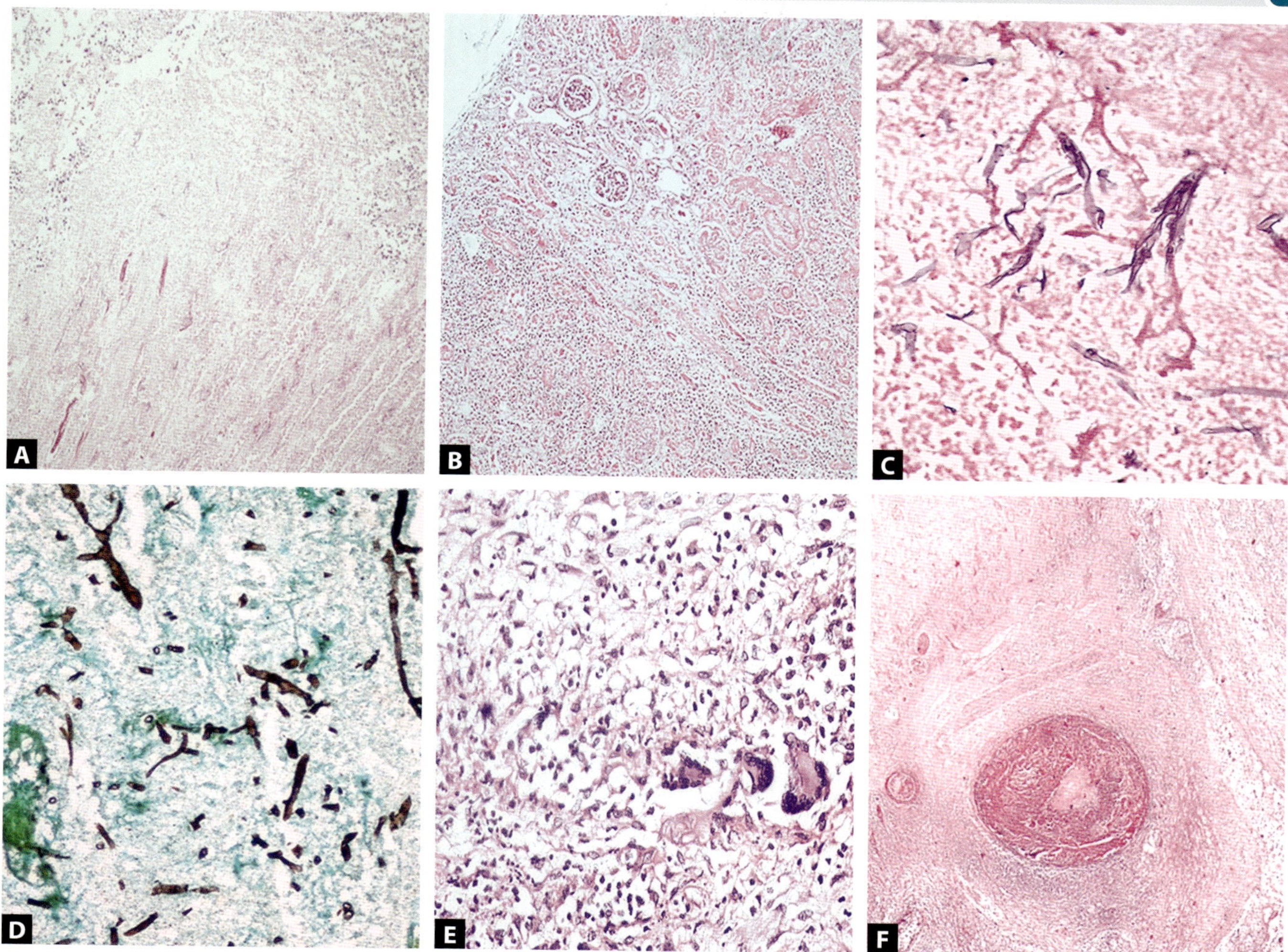

Figs 2A–F: Photomicrograph of the kidneys showing (A) Bland necrosis; (B) Bland coagulative necrosis with inflammatory infiltrate and (C) Necrosis with hyphae of mucormycosis; (D) Grocott stain better highlighting the fungal hyphae; (E) Areas of inflammation with giant cells; (F) Bland necrosis with vasculitis.

wall. Chances of invasive infection are greatly increased if the neutrophil or the macrophage number or function is compromised. Some species of mucormycotina are more aggressive and cause widespread disease. Patients with an iron overload have a higher incidence of mucormycosis, as free iron promotes its growth. In the tissue sections ***Mucormycetes*** hyphae are broad, empty looking, having variable width (5–50 μm), aseptate and show frequent right-angled branching. Inhalation or ingestion determines the primary site of inoculation, i.e. the nasal sinuses, lungs or the gastrointestinal tract. A variety of clinical forms are well-recognized which include rhinocerebral (nasal sinuses to the orbit and then the brain), pulmonary, gastrointestinal, cutaneous and disseminated. With the exception of the cutaneous form, the infection with mucor is acute and fatal due to the widespread dissemination caused by its angioinvasivness. The most commonly involved organ is the lung and from here the infection disseminates to other organs. In the tissues, the hyphae excite an acute inflammatory reaction with multinucleated macrophages, but at times the inflammatory response is poor. There is bland necrosis and a great propensity to invade the arteries, leading to thrombosis, hemorrhage, infarction and quick dissemination. Mucormycosis is an emergency as the fungus spreads very rapidly and so the diagnosis and initiation of treatment has to be very fast to save life. The mortality of different forms of mucormycosis reaches 75–100% in most series. Survival in isolated renal mucormycosis is estimated to be 65%.

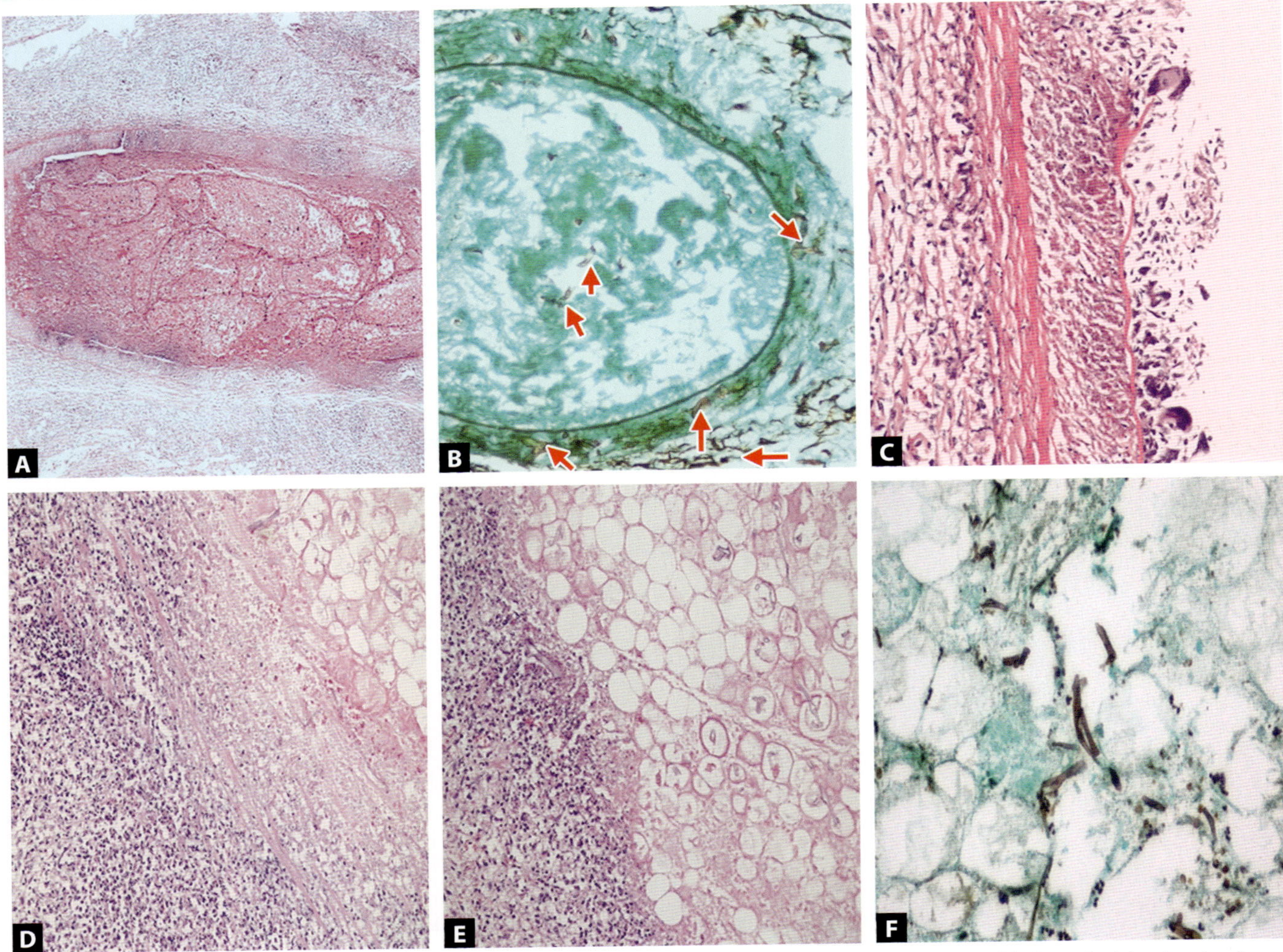

Figs 3A–F: Photomicrograph of the kidneys showing (A) Renal artery showing thrombosis and vasculitis; (B) Grocott stain showing fungal hyphae of mucor in the wall and in the lumen (arrows); (C) Lining of the pelvicalyceal system showing ulceration, necrosis, and giant cells; (D and E) Perirenal fat showing exuberant inflammation and necrosis and (F) Perirenal fat replete with fungal hyphae of mucormycosis F-(Grocott stain).

Isolated renal mucormycosis is very rare and limited to case reports. Renal involvement is frequently seen (in about 20% cases) in disseminated mucormycosis, but isolated form of infection is very occasionally seen. It is known as primary renal mucormycosis and defined as renal infection with mucor, in the absence of infection anywhere else in the body. Gupta et al. found eight isolated cases of renal mucormycosis amongst 18 cases of disseminated disease. Clinically they present with fever, flank pain, hematuria and renal enlargement. Renal failure is seen and is the result of the near total occlusion of the renal arteries and their branches. CT shows diffuse renal enlargement with multiple nonenhancing areas and perinephric collection. Pathogenesis of isolated renal mucormycosis is an enigma. Kidney involvement in disseminated mucormycosis occurs by hematogenous route. But in isolated renal involvement, retrograde spread from the lower urinary tract infection has been suggested.

COMMENTARY—INDEX CASE: PM 22863

This is a 2½-year-old, apparently immunocompetent, male child who presented with sudden onset fever of 20 days duration, followed by complete anuria, anasarca, altered sensorium and rapid breathing. On investigating, the renal function tests were deranged and he was totally anuric. Autopsy revealed isolated bilateral renal mucormycosis with contiguous spread to the adrenals, mesentery and descending colon. There were multiple ulcers, replete with fungal hyphae of mucormycosis in the urinary bladder. The lining of the

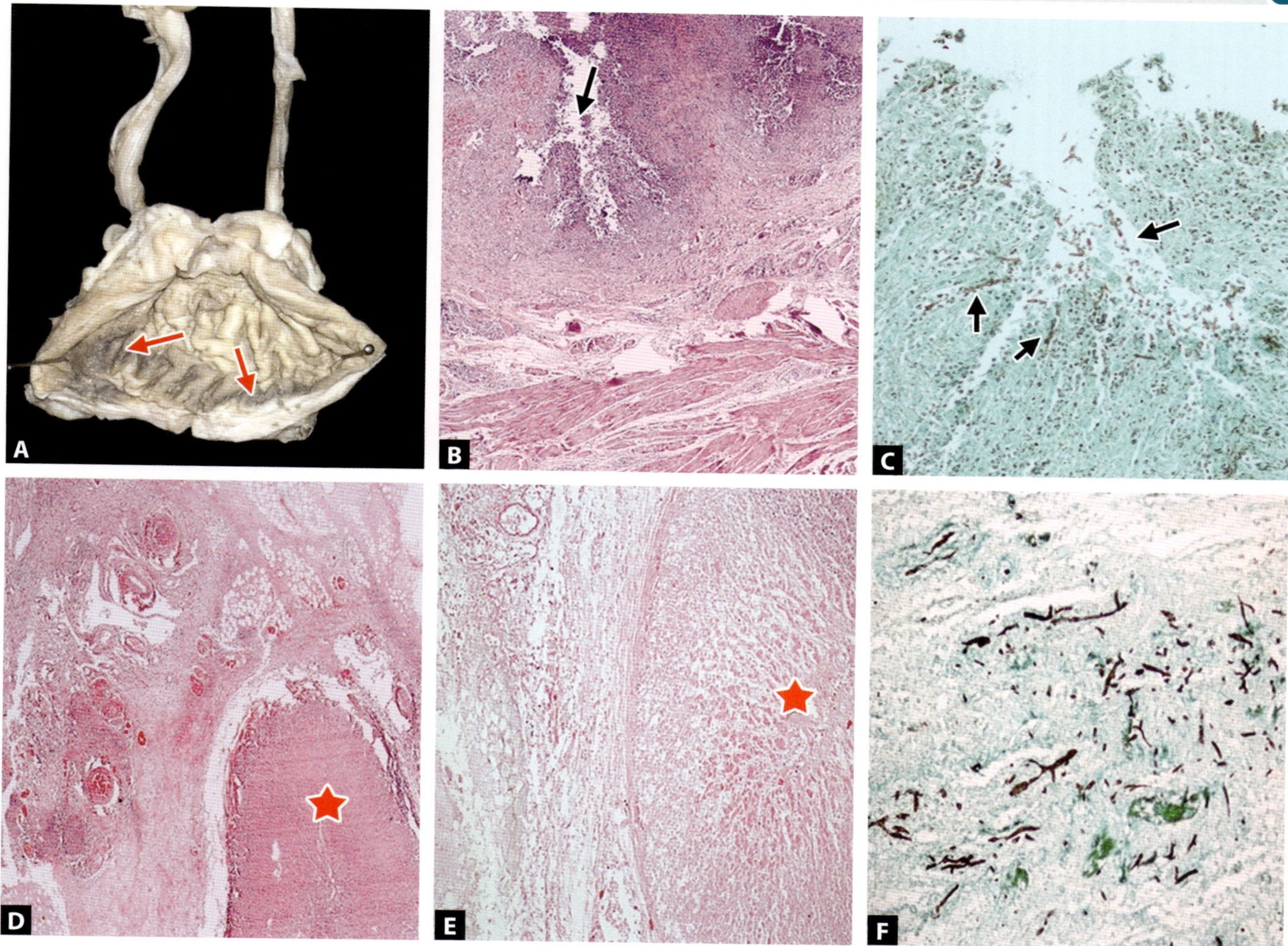

Figs 4A–F: (A) Gross picture of the urinary bladder showing ulceration (arrows). Photomicrograph of the urinary bladder showing; (B) Deep ulcer; (C) Replete with fungal hyphae (Grocott stain–arrows); (D) Adrenal gland (star) encased by necroinflammatory tissue; (E) Adrenal gland showing bland necrosis (star); (F) Adrenal gland replete with fungal hyphae (Grocott stain).

pelvicalyceal system was also ulcerated and replete with mucor. The entire parenchyma of the kidneys was necrotic and replete with fungal hyphae. The main renal arteries and all its branches were thrombosed and were teaming with fungal hyphae of mucor. No mucor was found in lungs and in any other organ. The kidneys were infected by ascending infection from the urinary bladder, thus substantiating the theory of retrograde spread of infection from the lower urinary tract. The capsule was markedly thickened and involved by mucor, which showed a contiguous spread to the adrenals and to a part of the descending colon in proximity to the kidneys. Immune workup was not done in this child and hence one cannot firmly comment upon the status of immunocompetency. All one can say is 'apparently immunocompetent'.

TAKE HOME MESSAGE

- Isolated/primary renal mucormycosis is rare and limited to case reports.
- It can occur in immunocompetent hosts.
- It is defined as renal infection with mucormycosis, in the absence of infection anywhere else in the body.
- Retrograde spread from the lower urinary tract has been suggested as the pathogenesis of isolated renal mucormycosis.

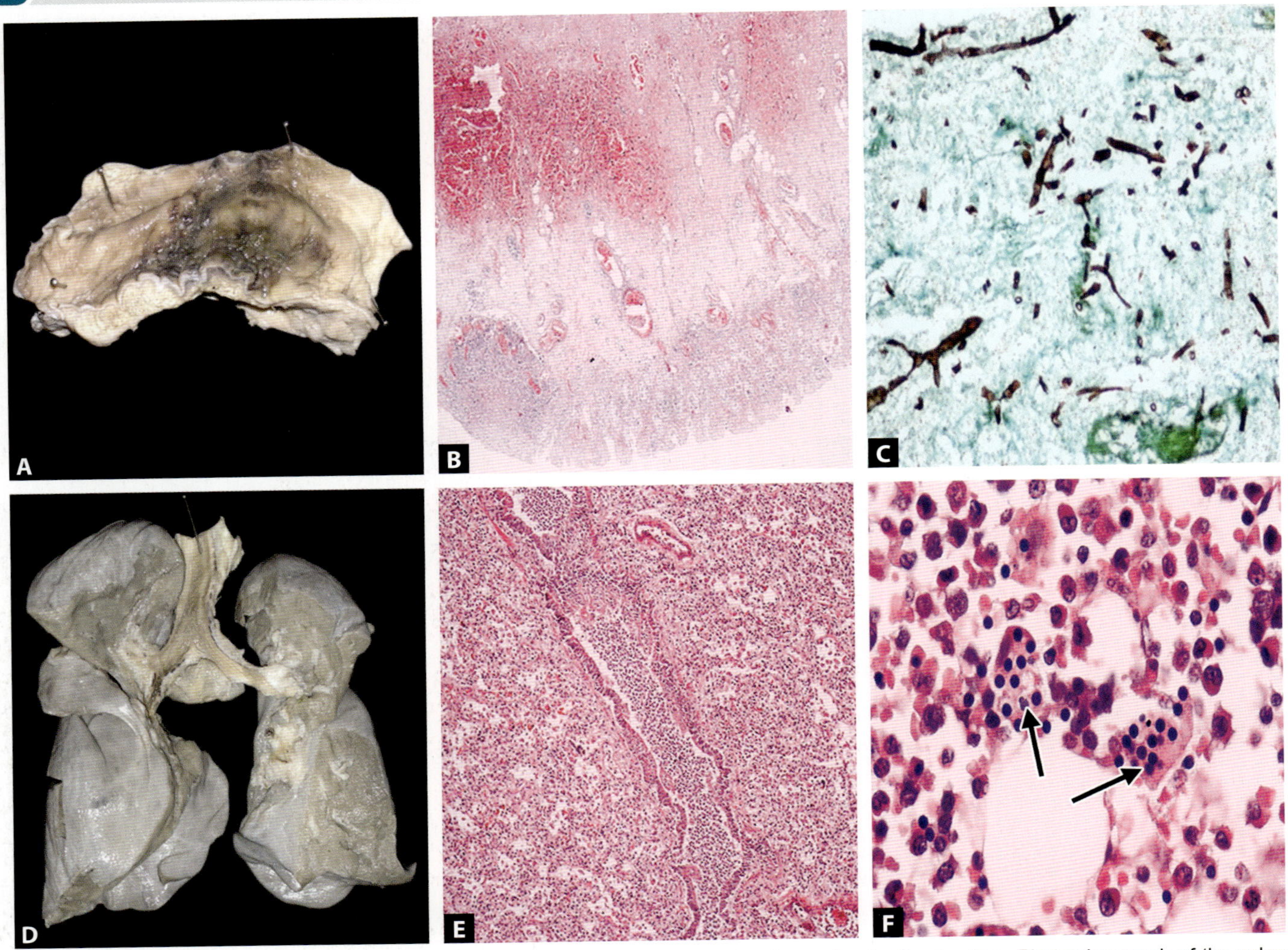

Figs 5A–F: (A) Portion of the colon that was attached to the renal mass, showing hemorrhagic discoloration. Photomicrograph of the colon showing; (B) Bland transmural necrosis with hemorrhage; (C) Serosa replete with fungal hyphae of mucor (Grocott stain); (D) Both lungs showed areas of consolidation; (E) Photomicrograph of the lung showing bronchopneumonia. No fungus seen in the lungs; (F) Photomicrograph of the bone marrow showing hemophagocytosis (arrows).

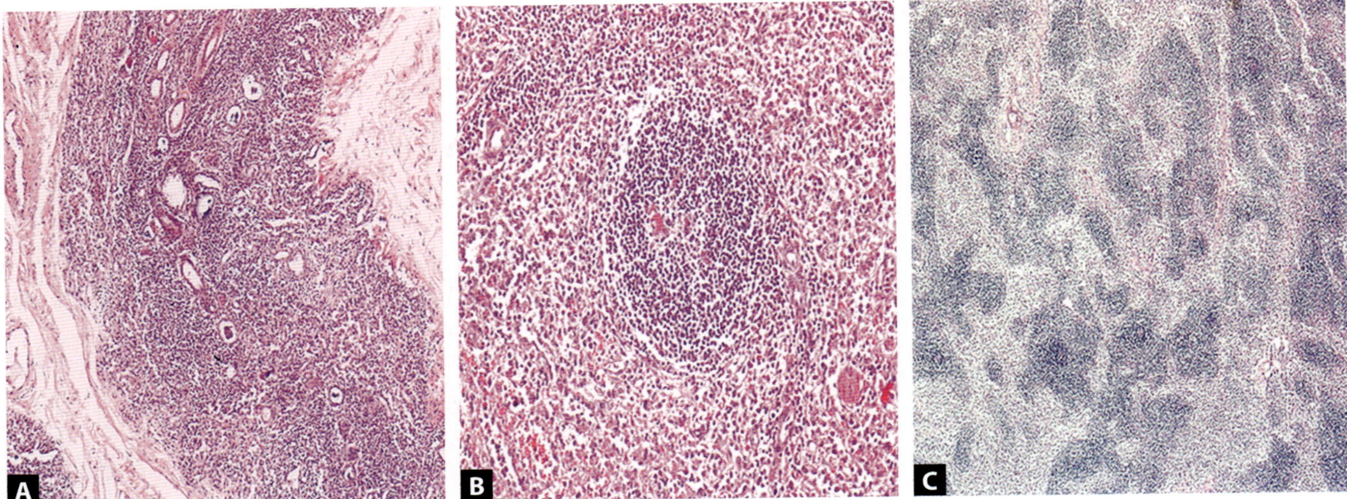

Figs 6A–C: Photomicrographs showing adequate lymphoid tissue in the (A) Thymus (B) Spleen and (C) Lymph node.

SUGGESTED READING

1. Chakrabarti A, Das A, Sharma A, et al. Ten years' experience in zygomycosis at a tertiary care centre in India. J Infect. 2001;42:261-6.
2. Chugh KS, Sakhuja V, Gupta KL et al. Renal mucormycosis: CT findings and their diagnostic significance. Am J Kid Dis. 1993;22:393.
3. Goel S, Carter JE, Culpepper M, et al. Primary renal zygomycotic infarction mimicking renal neoplasia in an immunocompetent patient. Am J Med Sci. 2009;338:330-3.
4. Gupta KL, Joshi K, Sud K, et al. Renal zygomycosis: an under-diagnosed cause of acute renal failure. Nephrol Dial Transplant. 1999;14:2720-5.
5. Jianhong LI, Xianliang HU, Xuewu J. Isolated renal mucormycosis in children. J Urol. 2004;171:387-8.
6. Singh SK, Wadhwa P, Sakhuja V. Isolated bilateral renal mucormycosis. Urology. 2004;63(5):979-80.
7. Verma R, Vij M, Agrawal V, et al. Renal mucormycosis in immunocompetent patients: report of three cases. Basic Appl Pathol. 2011;4:66-70.

CONTRIBUTIONS BY:

1. Dr Deepak Bansal, Professor, Department of Pediatrics (Compilation of Clinical Details)
2. Dr Akshay Kumar, Professor, Department of Radiodiagnosis and Imaging
3. Dr Meenu Singh, Professor, Department of Pediatrics (Clinician In-Charge)

Post Graduate Institute of Medical Education and Research, Chandigarh, India.

SECTION 8

Histiocytosis Pediatric and Adult Cases

CASE 51

Primary/Familial Hemophagocytic Lymphohistiocytosis with Extensive Involvement of the Brain: PM 20788

Nandita Bharadwaj Kakkar

HIGHLIGHTS OF THE CASE

A 2-month-old female child came with sudden onset illness of 3 days with fever, poor feeding, vomiting, altered sensorium and intractable seizures. There was no history of any consanguinity and an older sibling was normal. There was hepatosplenomegaly, bicytopenia, deranged coagulogram, low serum proteins/albumin, elevated transaminases/serum bilirubin, hyponatremia and mildly deranged renal function tests. Cerebrospinal fluid (CSF) examination exhibited lymphocytic pleocytosis with increased proteins. Autopsy revealed florid lymphohistiocytic (LH) infiltrate in the brain (Grade 3), liver, spleen, lymph nodes, bone marrow, with focal involvement of other organs, features consistent with primary/familial hemophagocytic lymphohistiocytosis (HLH).

Keywords: Hemophagocytic lymphohistiocytosis, HLH, primary or familial HLH, intractable seizures, autopsy.

CLINICAL DETAILS

Date of Admission: 11.07.2005, Date of Death: 12.07.2005, Duration of Hospital Stay: 1 Day

A 2-month-old female child came with 3 days history of fever, poor feeding, vomiting and 1-day history of altered sensorium and seizures. The baby was well 3 days prior to admission, when she developed high grade fever and nonbilious/nonprojectile vomiting. She had multiple episodes of seizures, which were initially generalized, tonic–clonic, then multifocal and later became left focal with secondary generalization. There was no history of trauma, rash, loose stools, ear discharge, hematemesis or melena. She was initially seen at her native place by a pediatrician, who diagnosed her as a case of meningitis and put her on antibiotics along with phenytoin and diazepam to control her seizures. She was then referred to PGIMER. Her neonatal period was uneventful. She was a full-term, normal vaginal delivery and cried immediately after birth. The parents had a nonconsanguineous marriage. She had an elder male sibling, 2 years old, who was doing well. The developmental history was normal for age. On ***examination*** the baby was seizuring and was cyanosed. She was given injection phenobarbitone, was intubated and put on intermittent positive pressure ventilation. The heart rate was 140/min, respiratory rate—100/min with distress, peripheral pulses were palpable, temperature was 36.7°C, weight—5 Kg (50th centile) and head circumference—38 cm (25th–50th centile). The baby was cyanosed and no icterus or pallor was detected. There was no external malformation. Neurological examination was not possible as the child was sedated, but it varied between E1M5Vt to E1M1Vt. Pupils were normal-sized and normal reacting, tone was normal and deep tendon reflexes were brisk with up going plantars. The abdomen was soft and no tenderness was elicited. The liver (5 cm) and spleen (3 cm) were enlarged.

Investigations

Investigations revealed a bicytopenia with Hb of 8 g/dL and platelets of 72,000/μL. TLC was raised to 17,300/μL with P48, L44, M5, E3. Peripheral blood film showed mild anisocytosis with microcytes/macrocytes, mild hypochromia and reduced platelets. No malarial parasite was detected. The coagulogram was deranged with PT more than 2 minutes (control 10 s) and aPTT more than 2 minutes (control 30–40 s). Blood biochemistry: serum Na^+/K^+—128/5.4 mEq/L; Ca^{2+}—8 mg%, phosphate—4.5 U/L, urea—55 mg%, creatinine—1.2 mg%, random blood sugar—117 mg%, total bilirubin—3.5 mg% with conjugated fraction of

0.7 mg%, SGOT/SGPT—82/55 U/L, total proteins/albumin—4.8/2.7 gm. VDRL and HIV by micro ELISA were non-reactive. Blood culture was sterile. X-ray chest showed bilateral infiltrates. Antemortem bone marrow could not be done due to paucity of time. The postmortem CSF examination (done by the clinicians)—60 cells/cu mm, all lymphocytes, proteins—1.3 g/dL, glucose—30 mg/dL, smear—8–10 WBC/HPF and Gram stain/culture negative. The child was treated for seizures and infection. She had bleeding from her nose, mouth, puncture sites and from the endotracheal tube. She received fresh frozen plasma, packed cells, platelet concentrates and vitamin K. She had uncontrollable seizures, went into shock and despite all measures, succumbed to her illness. ***Units clinical diagnosis*** was—Disseminated sepsis with meningitis and pneumonia, ? intrauterine infection, ? storage disorder, ? inborn error of metabolism.

AUTOPSY FINDINGS: PM 20788

A complete autopsy was performed on this 2-month-old female child. Hemorrhagic fluid was found in the pleural and peritoneal cavities. Postmortem ***bone marrow*** (Figs 1A–C) biopsy and aspirate were of normal cellularity and erythrophagocytizing histiocytes were seen in abundance, which were positive for the histiocytic marker CD68 (Fig 1D). The ***lymph nodes*** (Figs 2A–C) of the mesentery, peripancreatic area, paraaortic area and hilar showed mild enlargement. On microscopic examination, there was infiltration by a LH infiltrate, exhibiting extensive hemophagocytosis. The ***thymus*** (Figs 2D and E) was enlarged and also showed erythrophagocytizing histiocytes in abundance. The ***liver*** (Figs 3A–D) was enlarged (210 g) and there was florid centrizonal hemorrhagic necrosis indicative of shock. There was expansion of the portal tracts due to a heavy

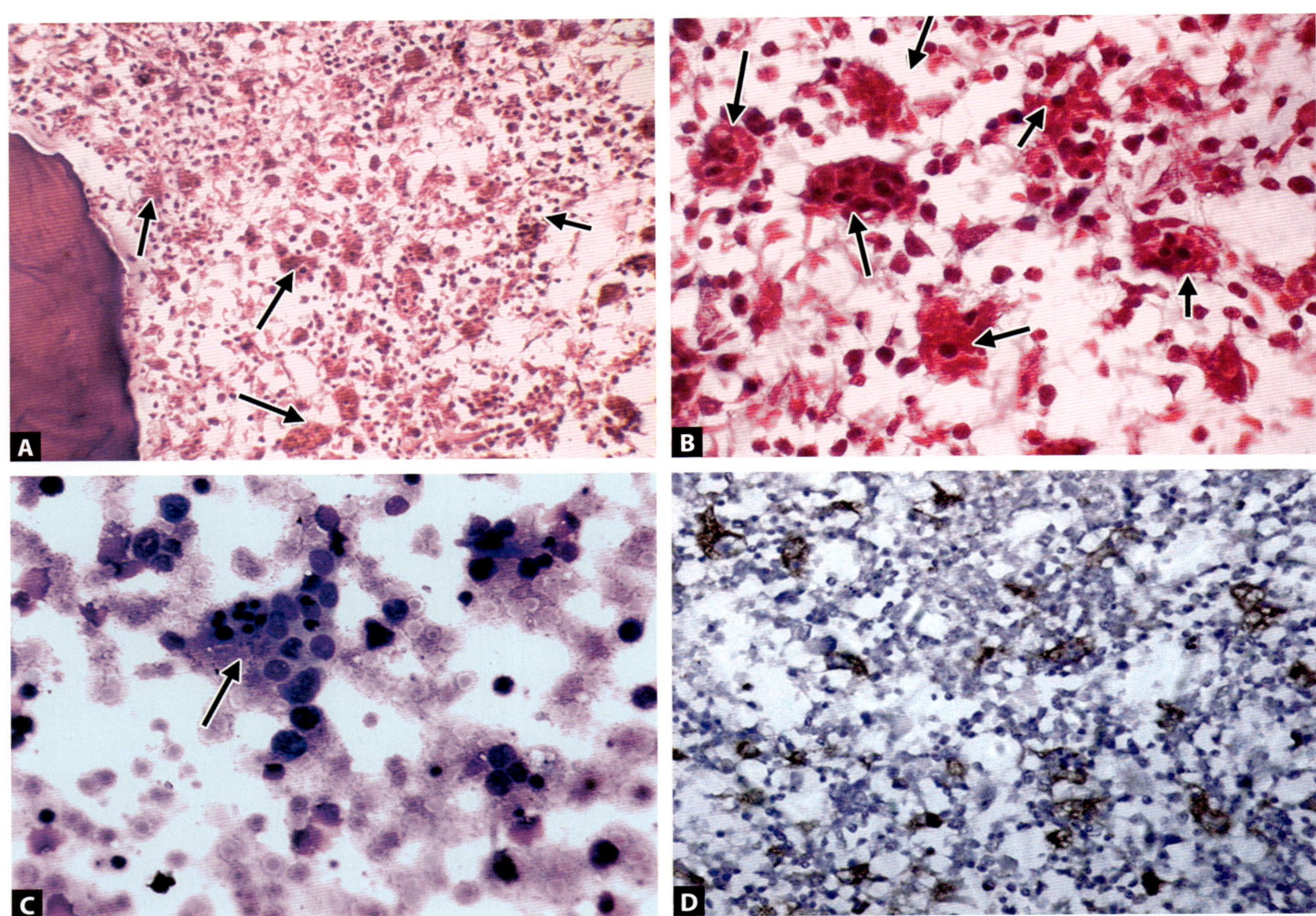

Figs 1A–D: (A and B) Section of the postmortem bone marrow replete with macrophages showing prominent hemophagocytosis (arrows); (C) Postmortem bone marrow aspirate showing a histiocyte with florid hemophagocytosis (arrow); (D) Bone marrow showing plenty of CD68 positive histiocytes showing prominent phagocytosis.

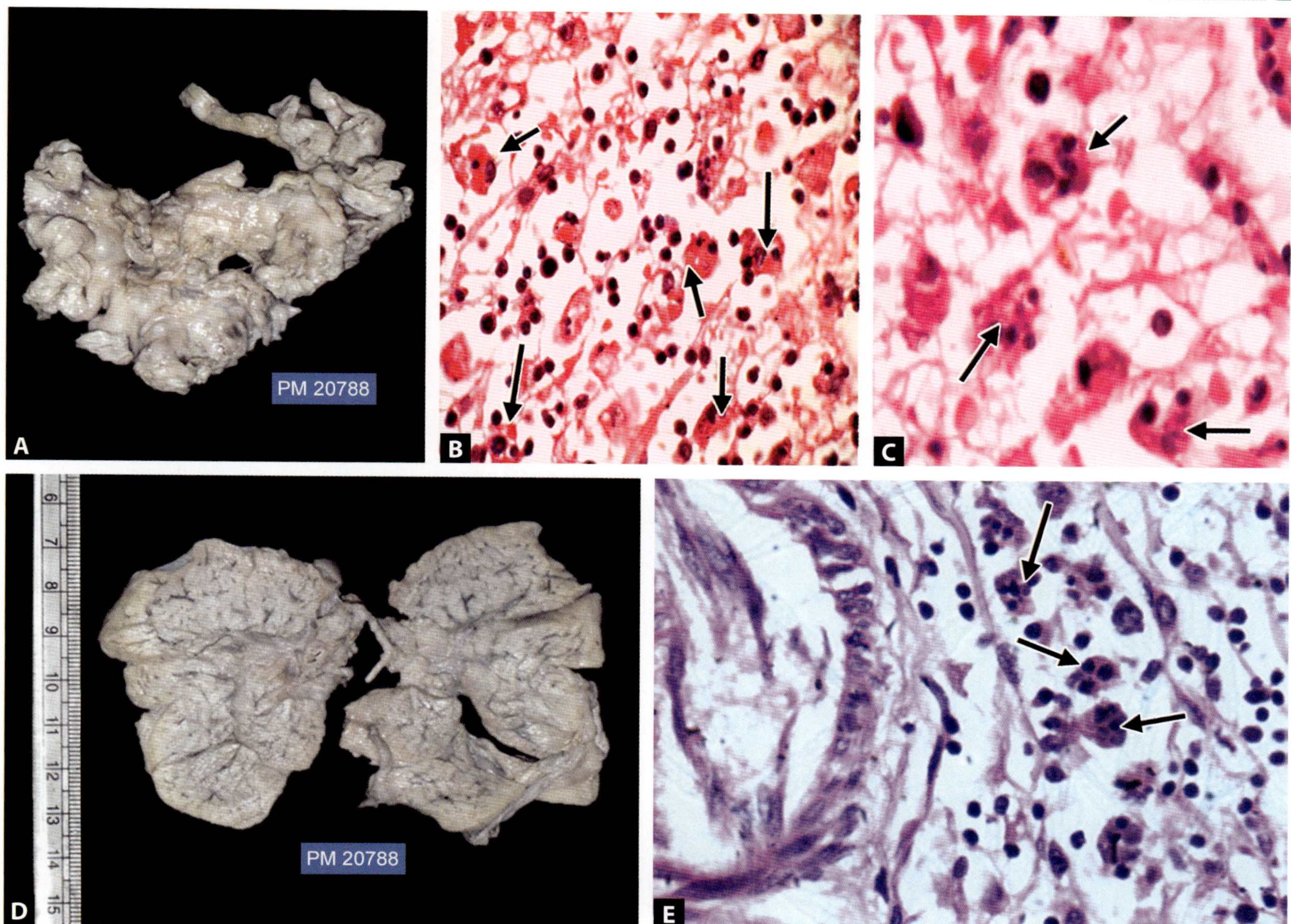

Figs 2A–E: (A) Gross photograph of the mesentery showing enlarged lymph nodes; (B and C) Photomicrograph of the lymph nodes showing plenty of histiocytes with prominent hemophagocytosis (arrows); (D) Gross photograph of the enlarged thymus; (E) Thymus showing histiocytes with prominent hemophagocytosis (arrows).

LH infiltrate showing hemophagocytosis. Phagocytizing histiocytes were also seen in the sinuses. The ***spleen*** was enlarged (93 g) and congested (Fig 3A). Microscopy revealed marked white pulp depletion. A dense LH infiltrate with hemophagocytosis was seen in the red pulp and around the penicillary arteries. The ***brain*** (Fig 4A) weighed 505 g, had a hypoxic look and coronal slices revealed central white matter softening. On microscopy, the meninges revealed a LH infiltrate (Fig 4B). There was extensive periventricular and gray/white matter perivascular LH infiltrate (Figs 4C and D, Figs 5A and B). This morphology mimicked an encephalitic process. The surrounding brain parenchyma (Figs 5C and D) revealed proliferation of astrocytes amidst the LH infiltrate. Similar infiltrates were present in the midbrain, pons, thalamus and globus pallidus. The cerebellar meninges were clogged with LH infiltrate (Fig 5E), strongly positive for CD68 (Fig 5F). Phagocytosis however was not prominent in the brain. The ***heart*** (Fig 6A) was grossly normal. Microscopic examination showed LH infiltrate, positive for CD68 in the pericardium (Figs 6B and C) and the myocardium (Figs 6D and E). The ***lungs*** (Figs 7A and B) exhibited extensive alveolar hemorrhages, bronchopneumonia and focal LH infiltrate. The ***intestine*** (small/large) showed small ulcers with a transmural LH infiltrate exhibiting hemophagocytosis. A similar LH infiltrate was seen in the ***kidneys*** (Figs 7C and D), adrenal, periadrenal fat, pancreas (Fig 7E) and skeletal muscle (Fig 7F). The LH infiltrate showed positivity for CD3 (T cell marker) and CD68 (histiocytic marker).

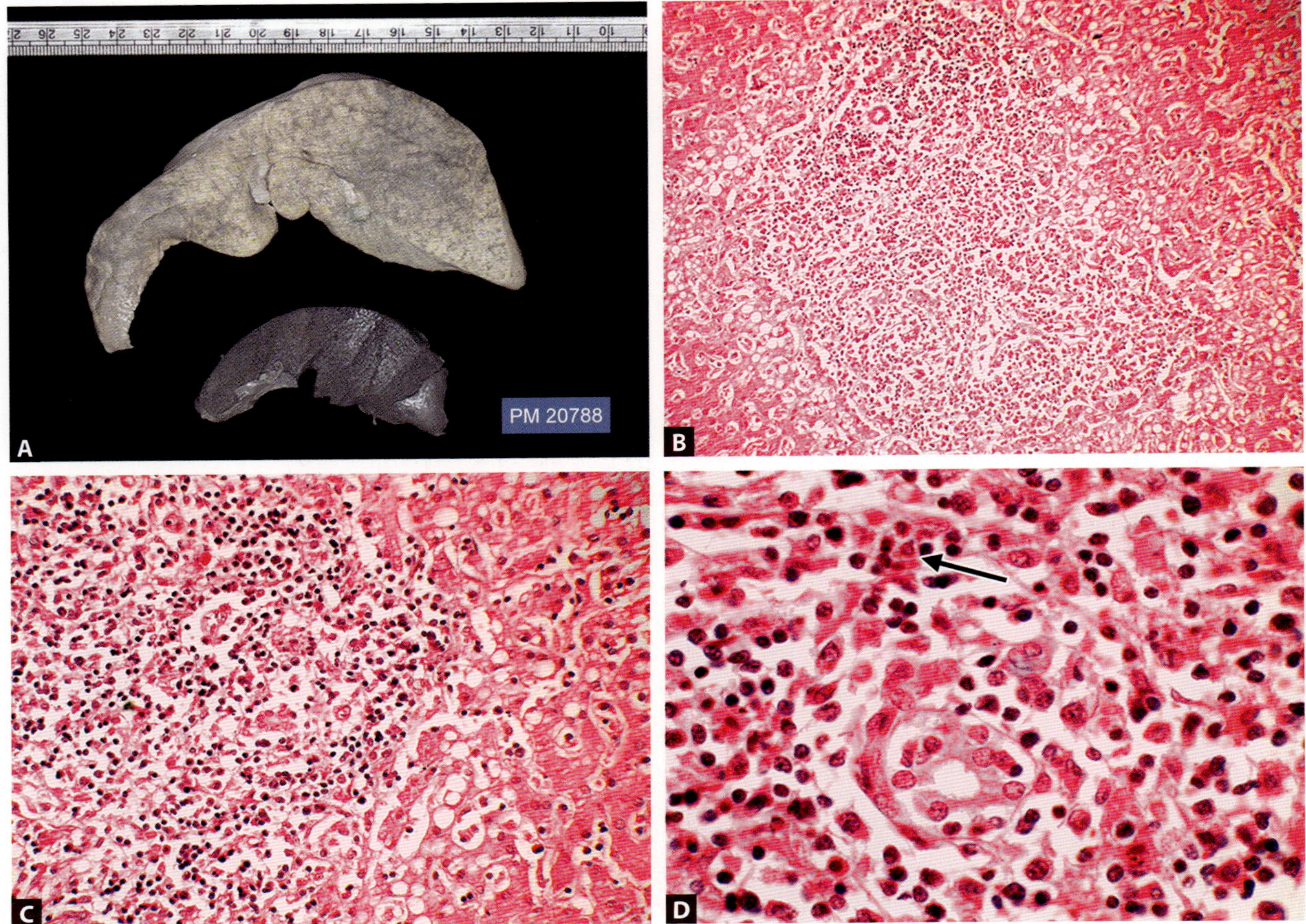

Figs 3A–D: (A) Coronal slices of the enlarged liver and spleen; (B and C) Photomicrograph of the liver showing expanded portal tracts with a florid lymphohistiocytic (LH) infiltrate; (D) Portal tract showing histiocytes exhibiting hemophagocytosis (arrow).

FINAL AUTOPSY DIAGNOSIS: PM 20788

2-Month-Old Female

Primary/familial hemophagocytic lymphohistiocytosis (HLH) with florid involvement of the brain (Grade 3), bone marrow, lymph nodes, liver, spleen and focal involvement of the lung, gastrointestinal tract (GIT), kidneys, adrenal, periadrenal fat and pancreas.

Features of shock: Extensive centrizonal hemorrhagic necrosis in the liver.

HEMOPHAGOCYTIC LYMPHOHISTIOCYTOSIS

Histiocytic disorders are rare, unfamiliar, hence a diagnostic problem and occur more commonly in the children. The two types of histiocytes are macrophages and dendritic cells, both being derived from CD34 positive hematopoietic progenitor cells in the bone marrow. ***Macrophages*** are of two basic subtypes, i.e. monocytes of the blood and macrophages of the tissue. Classical monocytes are active in innate defence against microorganisms and secrete proinflammatory cytokines. Macrophages reside in the tissues like skin, spleen, alveoli, liver (Kupffer cells), GI tract, thymic cortex, microglia of the brain, lymph nodes, etc. They have antigen processing/presenting functions, play a role in wound repair, secrete cytokines and are CD68 or alpha-1 antitrypsin positive. ***Dendritic cells*** (irregular shape with numerous processes) are the potent stimulators of primary immune response, have antigen presenting function and they interact with, stimulate, direct T cell responses and migrate selectively through tissues. The various types of dendritic cells are Langerhans cells, dermal dendrocytes, follicular

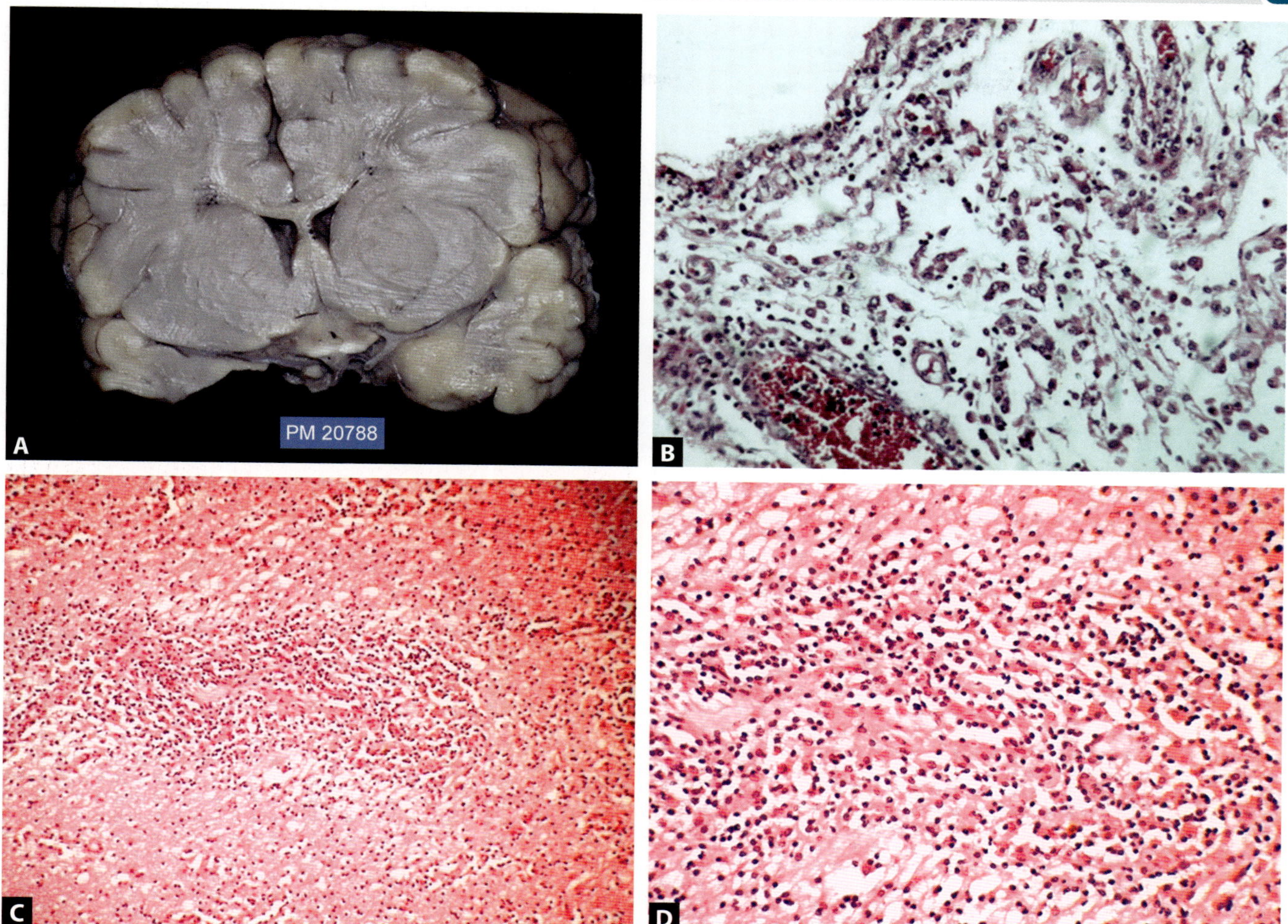

Figs 4A–D: (A) Coronal slice of the brain showing a hypoxic look and central soft matter softening; (B) Meninges showing lymphohistiocytic (LH) infiltrate; (C and D) White matter of the brain showing dense LH infiltrate.

dendritic cells of the lymph nodes, interstitial dendritic cells, etc. The ***contemporary classification of histiocytic disorders*** includes—(1) Disorders related to dendritic cells—Langerhans cell histiocytosis, juvenile xanthogranuloma and related disorders, solitary histiocytosis of various dendritic cell phenotypes. (2) Disorders related to macrophages—(a) HLH (primary/familial and secondary due to infections, malignancy and juvenile rheumatoid arthritis); (b) Rosai–Dorfman disease; (c) Solitary histiocytoma with macrophage phenotype. (3) Malignant disorders—(a) Monocyte related-leukemia, i.e. monocytic leukemia M5A/B, acute myelomonocytic leukemia M4, chronic myelomonocytic leukemia and extramedullary monocytic tumors or sarcomas; (b) Dendritic cell-related histiocytic sarcoma (localized or disseminated); (c) Macrophage-related histiocytic sarcoma (localized or disseminated).

Hemophagocytic lymphohistiocytosis is an enigmatic, underdiagnosed disease, rather a syndrome with diagnostic and therapeutic difficulties. The clinical symptoms vary widely and lack of awareness contributes greatly to the underdiagnosis. It was first reported in 1952. There is a persistent activation of natural killer (NK cell) and cytotoxic T lymphocytes which leads to a persistent macrophage activation, dissemination, organ infiltration and hemophagocytosis. HLH is of two types—(1) ***Primary or familial*** which is an autosomal recessive, fatal disease, occurs in early infancy with a survival of less than 2 months if untreated and is generally associated with consanguinity. (2) ***Secondary or acquired*** which is associated with infections (EBV, bacterial, fungal, parasitic), connective tissue diseases, malignancies and immune suppression. The genetic subtype can also be triggered by an infection. Both types of HLH have similar clinical/laboratory/morphologic

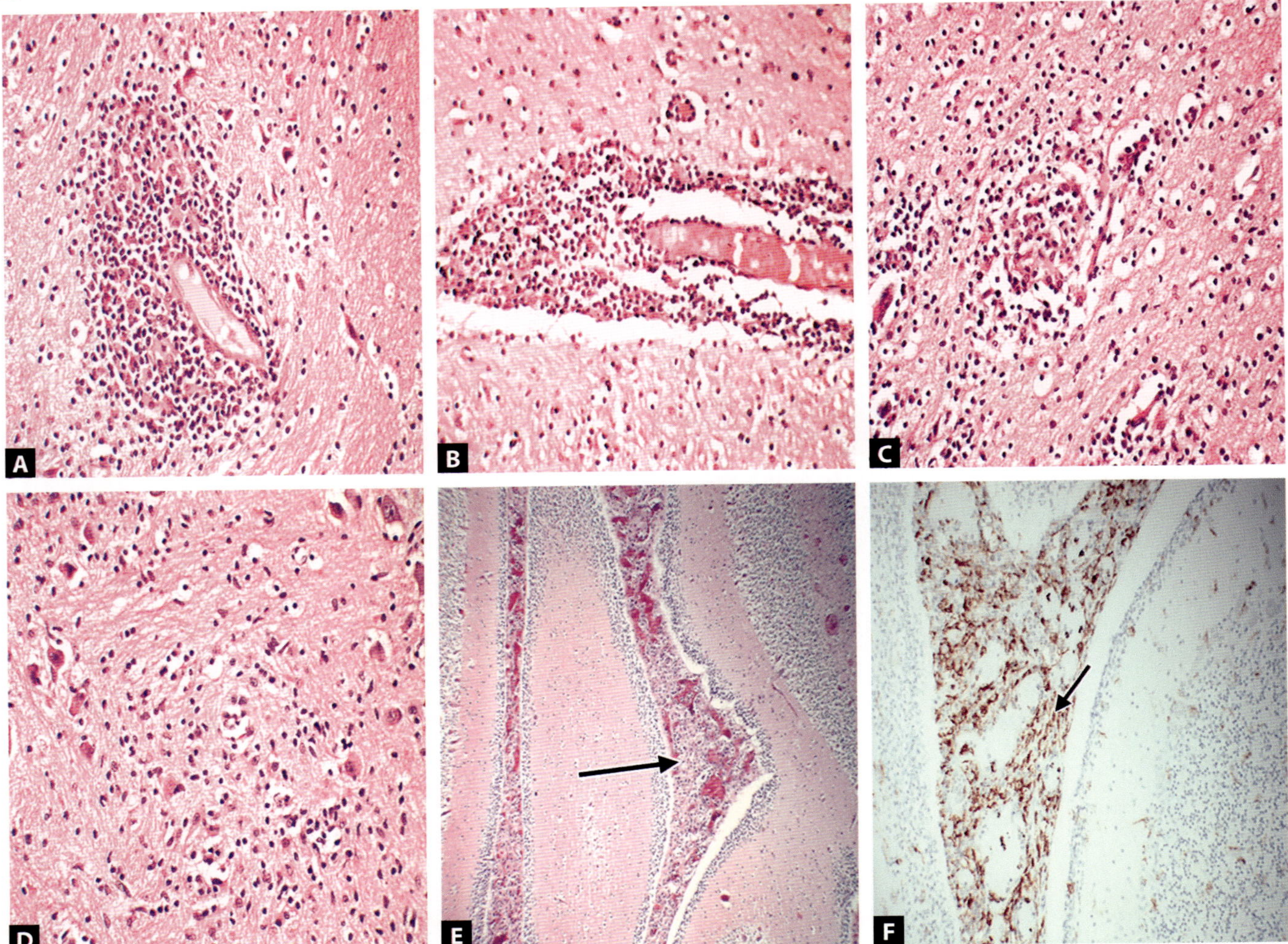

Figs 5A–F: (A and B) Photomicrographs of the brain showing dense perivascular lymphohistiocytic (LH) infiltrate; (C) The perivascular LH infiltrate is spilling into the adjacent brain parenchyma; (D) LH infiltrate amidst the neurons; (E) Cerebellum showing a dense LH infiltrate in the subarachnoid space (arrow); (F) Cerebellum showing CD68 positive histiocytes in the subarachnoid space (arrow).

features. The clinical symptoms very widely and this is the deterrent in the way of early diagnosis.

Hemophagocytic lymphohistiocytosis shows the following clinical and laboratory features—fever, hepatosplenomegaly, cytopenias particularly thrombocytopenia and anemia, hypertriglyceridemia (VLDL/LDL), coagulopathy, hypofibrinogenemia, hyperferritinemia, deranged liver function tests with hyperbilirubinemia, raised transaminases and lactate dehydrogenase, hyponatremia, hypoproteinemia, hypoalbuminemia, hypofibrinogenemia, coagulation abnormalities with prolonged activated partial thromboplastin time/prothrombin time, CSF pleocytosis with predominantly lymphocytes with increased proteins and bone marrow aspiration may show hemophagocytosis. Other abnormal laboratory findings in HLH are low NK cell activity and hypercytokinemia with elevated soluble interleukin-2 receptor (sIL-2r) levels in serum and in the CSF. Central nervous system manifestation occur in one third cases and include irritability, bulging fontanelle, neck rigidity, hypotonia, hypertonia, severe meningoencephalitis, intractable seizures, cranial nerve (6/7 nerve) palsy, ataxia, hemiplegia/tetraplegia, blindness and unconsciousness.

The ***diagnosis of HLH*** can be established if one of either "a" or "b" are fulfilled: (a) A molecular diagnosis consistent with HLH. (b) Diagnostic criteria for HLH (five out of the eight criteria needed)—fever (>7 days, >38.5°C); splenomegaly (>3 cm); cytopenia affecting at least two lineages in the peripheral blood—Hb: less than 9 g/dL

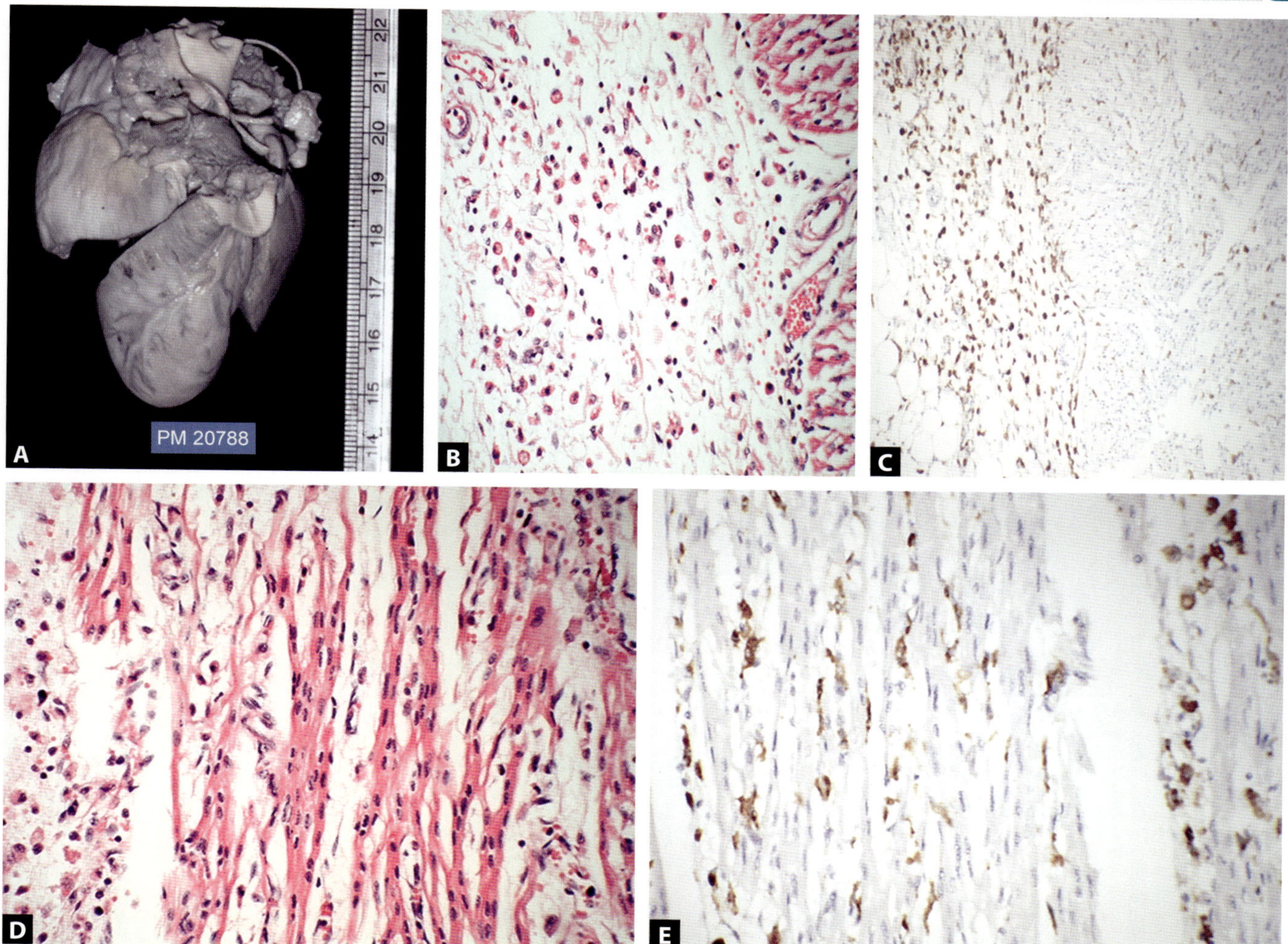

Figs 6A–E: (A) Gross photograph of the heart; (B and C) Lymphohistiocytic (LH) infiltrate in the pericardium which is positive for CD68 immunostain; (D and E) LH infiltrate in between the myocardial fibers which also shows positivity for CD68 immunostain.

(in infants <4 weeks: Hb<10 g/dL), Platelets: less than 100,000/μL, absolute neutrophil count: less than 100/μL; hypertriglyceridemia (fasting triglycerides ≥265 mg/dL) and/or hypofibrinogenemia (<1.5 g/L); and hemophagocytosis in bone marrow, spleen, or lymph nodes with no evidence of malignancy; low or absent NK-cell activity (measured by 51-Cr release assay); ferritin more than or equal to 500 μg/L; elevated soluble IL2 (CD25) levels more than or equal to 2,400 U/mL. Comments added to these criteria are—(1) first bone marrow examination may not show hemophagocytosis. Repeating bone marrow aspiration after a time may help; (2) spinal fluid pleocytosis and/or elevated spinal fluid protein and a histological picture of chronic persistent hepatitis in the liver support a diagnosis of HLH.

Pathologic hallmark of HLH is a diffuse infiltrate of lymphocytes and mature macrophages exhibiting hemophagocytosis in various organs. Hemophagocytosis should be carefully looked for in the bone marrow, it may be absent in the first sample and there should be no hesitation in taking a repeat sample after a few days. Bone marrow shows LH infiltrate with hemophagocytosis in 25–100% cases of primary HLH and is generally more florid and better appreciated in secondary HLH. Liver may show four different patterns—chronic hepatitis-like, leukemia-like, neonatal giant cell hepatitis-like and histiocytic storage disorder-like. Apart from this, there is a LH infiltrate in the portal tracts and sinusoids wherein the histiocytes may show hemophagocytosis. Performing a liver biopsy may be hazardous because of hypofibrinogenemia. The lymph nodes

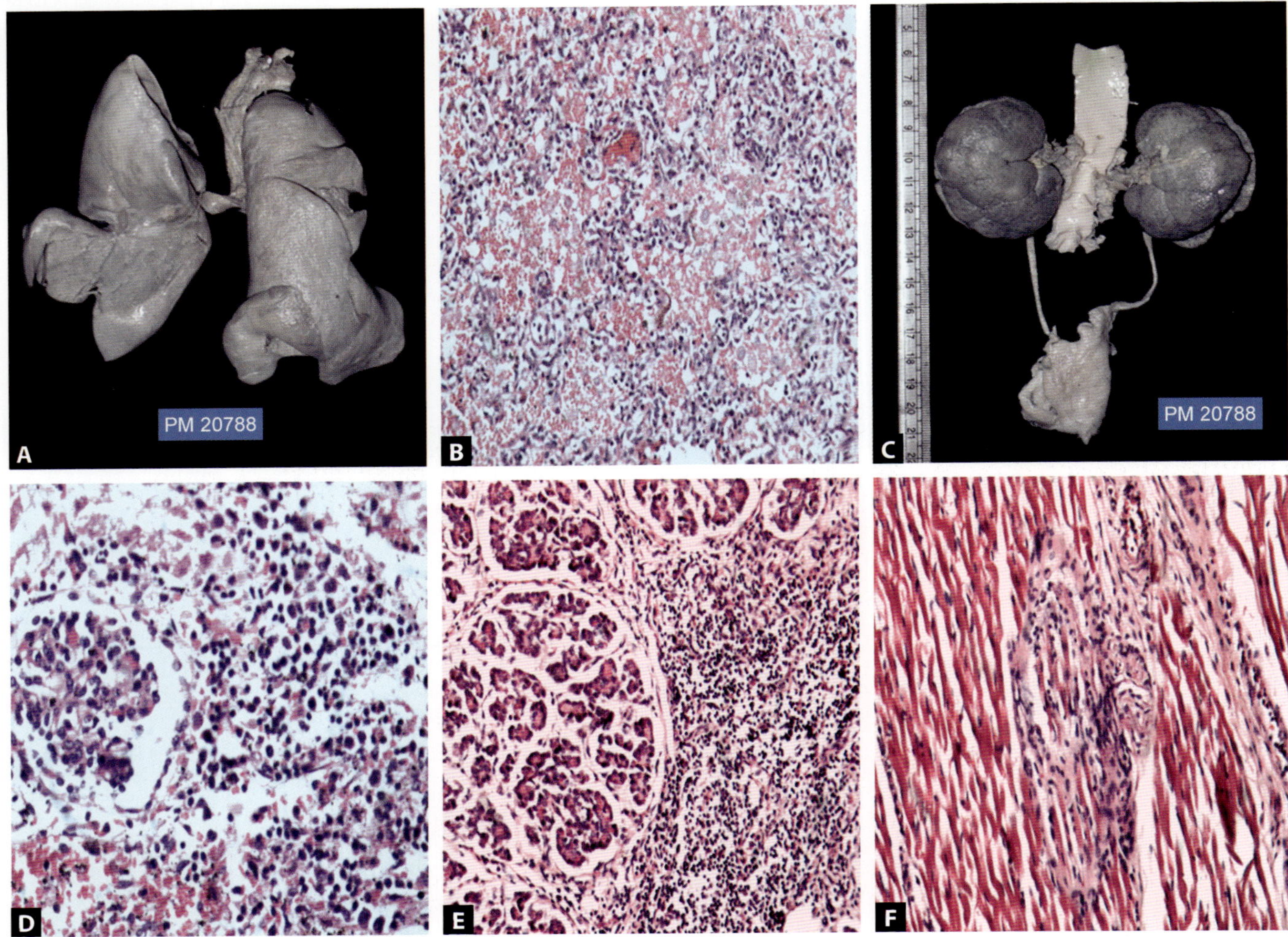

Figs 7A–F: (A) Gross photograph of the lungs; (B) Photomicrograph of the lung showing alveolar hemorrhage and lymphohistiocytic (LH) infiltrate in the thickened alveolar septae; (C) Gross photograph of the kidneys, ureters, and bladder; (D) LH in the interstitium of the kidney; (E) LH infiltrate in the pancreas; (F) LH infiltrate in the skeletal muscle.

show a progressive lymphoid depletion. CNS is involved in majority of the cases. Three grades of lesions characterized by varying degrees of infiltration by lymphocytes and macrophages have been described. Grade 1: only meningeal infiltrate, Grade 2: meningeal and perivascular infiltrate, Grade 3: diffuse meningeal, perivascular and parenchymal infiltrate of brain with or without foci of necrosis. Hemophagocytosis is most commonly seen in the meningeal infiltrate.

Pathophysiology of Familial HLH: In patients with infection there is activation of macrophages, NK cells and cytotoxic T lymphocytes (CTLs). Through receptor interaction and cytokine secretion there is continued mutual stimulation of these cells. As a result, there is lysis of the infected cells with termination of immune response. However, in HLH patients there is inability of NK cells and CTLs to cope with infection leading to persistence of activated cells which produces a cytokine storm and runaway immune system. Lymphocytes and macrophages accumulate, disseminate and infiltrate different organs. In the genetic type of HLH, there is blocking of cytotoxic activity of NK cells and CTLs. Of the five subtypes of genetic HLH, the blocking mechanism has been best elucidated in subtype 1 due to mutation of ***PRF-1*** gene. Mutation of this gene leads to deficiency of perforin. Normally perforin perforates the membrane of target cells and granzymes enter the infected cells through the pores made by perforin. This is followed by lysis and apoptosis of target cells, control of infection and termination of immune response. In the presence of perforin deficiency due to PRF 1 mutation, there is persistence of infected cells and sustained NK cells and CTL activity, macrophage activation, dissemination and organ infiltration. It is suggested that all other genetic forms of HLH and even the secondary acquired forms of HLH are due to impairment of NK cells and CTLs.

COMMENTARY—INDEX CASE: PM 20788

This 2-month-old female child had a sudden onset illness, 3 days prior to admission. She came with fever, poor feeding, vomiting, altered sensorium and intractable seizures. There was no history of consanguinity and an older sibling was doing well. On examination there was hepatosplenomegaly with no lymphadenopathy. There was bicytopenia, deranged coagulogram, low serum proteins/albumin, elevated transaminases/serum bilirubin, hyponatremia and mildly deranged renal function tests. CSF examination exhibited lymphocytosis with increased proteins. The baby had a hospital stay of only 1 day and so she could not be investigated properly. Autopsy revealed florid LH infiltrate in the brain (Grade 3—meninges, periventricular and intraparenchymal locations) and other organs consistent with the diagnosis of primary/familial HLH. Consanguinity may not be documented as many a times the parents hide this history, especially amongst the Hindus, where consanguineous marriages are not allowed. Autopsy however clinched the diagnosis. The baby fulfilled 6/8 "B" criteria, the other two however could not be done. The age of the child and such florid Grade 3 infiltrate in the brain and other organs points toward the primary/familial nature of the HLH in this case.

TAKE HOME MESSAGE

- Familial or primary HLH is a rare, fatal and autosomal recessive disorder seen in early infancy.
- The pathologic hallmark is infiltration of various organs like the bone marrow, lymph nodes, liver, spleen, etc. and most importantly the brain with a lymphohistiocytic infiltrate, where the macrophages exhibit hemophagocytosis.
- In familial HLH, there are multiple immune defects which create a "cytokine storm", thus leading to an excessive stimulation of T lymphocytes and macrophages.

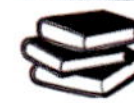

SUGGESTED READING

1. Akima M, Sumi SM. Neuropathology of familial erythrophagocytic lymphohistiocytosis. Six cases and review of the literature. Hum Pathol. 1984;15:161.
2. Arico M, Danesino C, Pende D, et al. Pathogenesis of hemophagocytic lymphohistiocytosis – Review. Br J Haematol. 2001;114:761-9.
3. Arico M, Janka G, Fischer A, et al. Hemophagocytic lymphohistiocytosis. Diagnosis, treatment and prognostic factors. Report of 122 children from the international registry. Leukemia. 1996;10:197.
4. Göransdotter EK, Fadeel B, Nilsson-Ardnor S, et al. Spectrum of perforin gene mutations in familial hemophagocytic lymphohistiocytosis. Am J Hum Genet. 2001;68:590-7.
5. Henter JI, Arico M, Elinder G, et al. Familial hemophagocytic lymphohistiocytosis. Primary hemophagocytic lymphohistiocytosis. Hematol Oncol Clin N Am. 1998;12(2):417-33.
6. Henter JI, Elinder G, Ost A. Diagnostic guidelines for hemophagocytic lymphohistiocytosis. The FHL study group of the Histiocyte Society. Semin Oncol. 1991;18:29-33.
7. Henter JI, Horne AC, Arico M, et al. HLH-2004: Diagnostic and therapeutic guidelines for hemophagocytic lymphohistiocytosis. Pediatr Blood Cancer. 2007;48(2):124-31.
8. Henter JI, Nennesmo I. Neuropathologic findings and neurologic symptoms in twenty three children with hemophagocytic lymphohistiocytosis. J Pediatr. 1997;130(3):358-65.
9. Kakkar N, Vasishta RK, Banerjee AK, et al. Familial hemophagocytic lymphohistiocytosis: An autopsy study. Pediatr Pathol Mol Med. 2003;22(3):229-42.
10. Ost A, Ardnor AN, Henter IJ. Autopsy findings in 27 children with hemophagocytic lymphohistiocytosis. Histopathology. 1998;32:310-6.
11. Sullivan KE, Delaat CA, Douglas SD, et al. Defective natural killer cell function in patients with hemophagocytic lymphohistiocytosis and in first degree relatives. Pediatr Res. 1998;44:465-8.
12. Vasishta RK, Kakkar N, Banerjee AK, et al. Neuropathology of familial hemophagocytic lymphohistiocytosis. Arch Pediatr Adolesc Med. 1999;153:546-7.

CONTRIBUTIONS BY:

1. Dr Bhavneet Bharti, Professor, Department of Pediatrics (Clinician In-Charge)
2. Dr Praveen Kumar, Professor and Head, Department of Pediatrics—Neonatology Division (Compilation of Clinical Details)
3. Dr RK Vasishta, Professor and Head, Department of Histopathology (Consultation)

Post Graduate Institute of Medical Education and Research, Chandigarh, India.

CASE 52

Langerhans Cell Histiocytosis Presenting as an Anterior Mediastinal Mass: PM 21476

Nandita Bharadwaj Kakkar

HIGHLIGHTS OF THE CASE

A 10-month-old male child presented to the emergency with abdominal distension, fever, rapid breathing, altered sensorium, loose stools and nodular lesions on the scalp. There was hepatosplenomegaly, X-ray chest exhibited mediastinal widening and ultrasonography revealed a homogenous soft tissue mass in the anterior mediastinum ? lymph nodal which was encasing the vessels of the mediastinum. Autopsy revealed multisystem Langerhans cell histiocytosis (LCH) with a mediastinal mass and extensive involvement of the lungs, lymph nodes, liver, spleen, colon and pancreas. The bone marrow and the skin could not be assessed.

Keywords: Langerhans cell histiocytosis, systemic, anterior, mediastinal mass, autopsy.

CLINICAL DETAILS

Date of Admission: 06.08.2006, Date of Death: 07.08.2006

A 10-month-old boy presented with a 4 days history of abdominal distension, fever, rapid breathing and altered sensorium. The abdominal distension was progressive. It was associated with loose stools, 4–5 per day, watery to semisolid, not blood stained and nonfrothy. Fever was low grade, continuous, not associated with chills/rigors/sweating and responded to antipyretics. There was altered sensorium and the child was not recognizing his parents or responding to commands. He was a full-term normal vaginal delivery and there was no birth asphyxia. The child was second in birth order, elder sibling being alive and healthy. There was no history of tuberculosis or any similar illness in the family. On general physical examination the heart rate was 140/min, RR 100/min, peripheral pulses were present and there was pallor. There was no cyanosis, icterus, lymphadenopathy or pedal edema. A few nodular lesions were noted on the scalp. The liver (span 15 cm) and spleen were enlarged 8 and 3 cm below the respective costal margins. There was no ascites. Respiratory system revealed tachycardia, subcostal and intercostal retractions and air entry was decreased on both sides. Bilateral crepts were present (Lt > Rt.).

Investigations

Hematological: There was bicytopenia (Hb 7.2 g/dL, TLC 20,000/uL and platelets 80000/uL). Peripheral blood film revealed moderate anisocytosis with microcytes and few macrocytes, reduced platelets and toxic granules. The coagulogram was deranged with PT 16', PTI 63%, aPTT 2'.

Blood biochemistry: Serum bilirubin 2.5 mg%, SGOT 67 U/L, SGPT 65 U/L, S creatinine 2 mg%, blood urea 100 mg%, Na^{2+} 138 mEq/L, K^{+} 5.8 mEq/L.

Radiology: ***USG abdomen*** revealed hepatosplenomegaly with bilateral increased renal cortical echogenicity. ***X ray chest*** showed mediastinal widening and ***USG chest*** showed a homogenous soft tissue density mass in the anterior mediastinum ? lymph nodal. The vessels of the mediastinum were encased by the mass. ***Course in hospital***: Child had severe respiratory distress and was intubated. At 19 hours of admission, child had endotracheal/nasal bleed and developed decompensated refractory shock and suffered a cardiac arrest.

Unit's final diagnosis: Sepsis with refractory septic shock, coagulopathy, pulmonary hemorrhage, anterior mediastinal mass with hepatosplenomegaly ? storage disorder ?? lymphoma.

AUTOPSY FINDINGS: PM 21476

A complete autopsy was performed on this 10-months-old male baby. The serous cavities were within normal limits. The ***mediastinal mass*** measured 5 × 4 × 3 cm, was firmly adherent to the lungs and was difficult to separate out (Fig 1A). It was present in the anterior mediastinum, but was extending into the superior mediastinum encasing the trachea (Fig 1B). It was seen to infiltrate the right lung (Fig 1C). On microscopic examination the mass showed a demarcation from the adjacent lung (Fig 2A). Multiple sections from the mass revealed sheets of atypical cells admixed with eosinophils, neutrophils, histiocytes and lymphocytes (Fig 2B). The atypical cells were large with a moderate amount of homogenous pink cytoplasm and reniform, lobulated or grooved nuclei (Fig 2C). Semithin section (Fig 2D) showed prominent grooving in the tumor cells. Areas of necrosis and calcification were seen. Aggregates of lymphoid cells were seen scattered within the tumor (Fig 3A). The atypical cells were strongly positive for CD1a (Fig 3B) and S100 (Fig 3C) and negative for CD68. However, few CD68 positive macrophages could be seen along with (Fig 3D). Morphology and immunohistochemistry was consistent with a diagnosis of Langerhans cell histiocytosis (LCH). The origin of LCH in the anterior mediastinum could be either the lymph nodes or the thymus. Small aggregates of lymphoid tissue were seen in the sections examined from the mass, so the origin from the mediastinal lymph node could be a possibility. Multiple mediastinal lymph nodes (Figs 4A and B) adjacent to the mass were sampled and some of them showed reactive changes, but a few showed involvement by LCH. Since the thymus or even its remnant could not be identified, despite examining multiple sections, a possibility that this mass arose in the thymus and totally replaced it, also remains a possibility. The ***lungs*** were very heavy, bulky and weighed 370 g along with the mass (normal weight of lung—110 g). Pleura showed areas of thickening and hemorrhage. Microscopic examination revealed atypical cells of LCH in the septae and in the alveolar spaces (Fig 5A). Apart from the atypical cells there was confluent necrotizing pneumonia, hyaline membrane formation indicating diffuse alveolar damage (Fig 5B) and pulmonary hemorrhage (Fig 5C). The ***liver*** was enlarged and weighed 510 g (N—300 g). Microscopically, it showed distension of sinusoids, which were packed with atypical Langerhans cells with accompanying eosinophils and macrophages (Fig 5D), at places forming nodules (Fig 5E). The infiltrate showed a strong positivity with CD1a (Fig 5F). The ***spleen*** (Fig 6A) was enlarged and weighed 52 g (N weight—24 g). The red pulp (Figs 6B and C) showed extensive infiltration by LCH. The ***pancreas*** (Fig 6D) and ***colon*** (Fig 6E) also showed focal infiltration. The ***brain*** was normal grossly but on microscopic examination revealed features of hypoxia. The bone marrow and the scalp sections were misplaced and hence could not be assessed. But both were definitely involved by the disease, as there were nodular scalp lesions and pancytopenia present in the patient.

FINAL AUTOPSY DIAGNOSIS: PM 21476

10 Months Old Male

- Multifocal, multisystem, Langerhans cell histiocytosis (LCH)—mediastinal mass (origin ? lymph node, ? thymus),

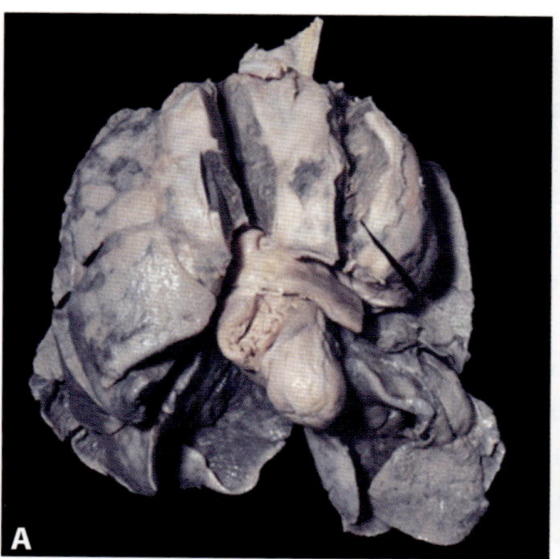

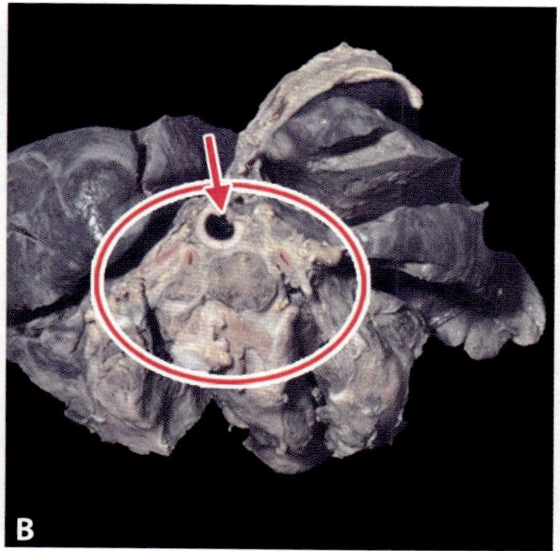

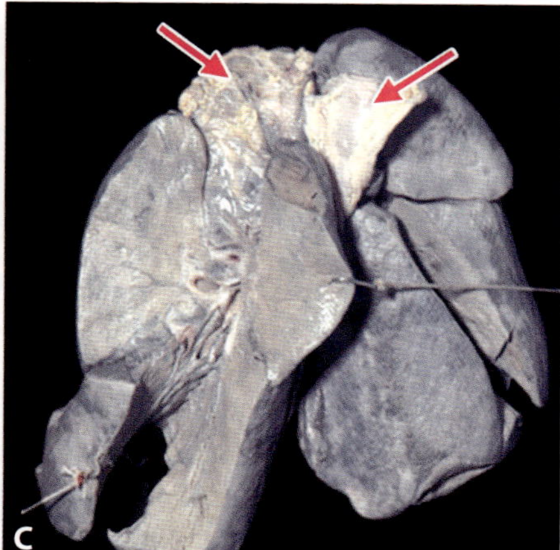

Figs 1A–C: (A) Gross picture of the heart, lung complex along with the mediastinal mass; (B) Coronal cut of the mediastinum at the level of the lower part of the trachea (arrow) showing the mass encasing the mediastinal structures; (C) Upper lobe of the right lung showing infiltration by the tumor (arrows).

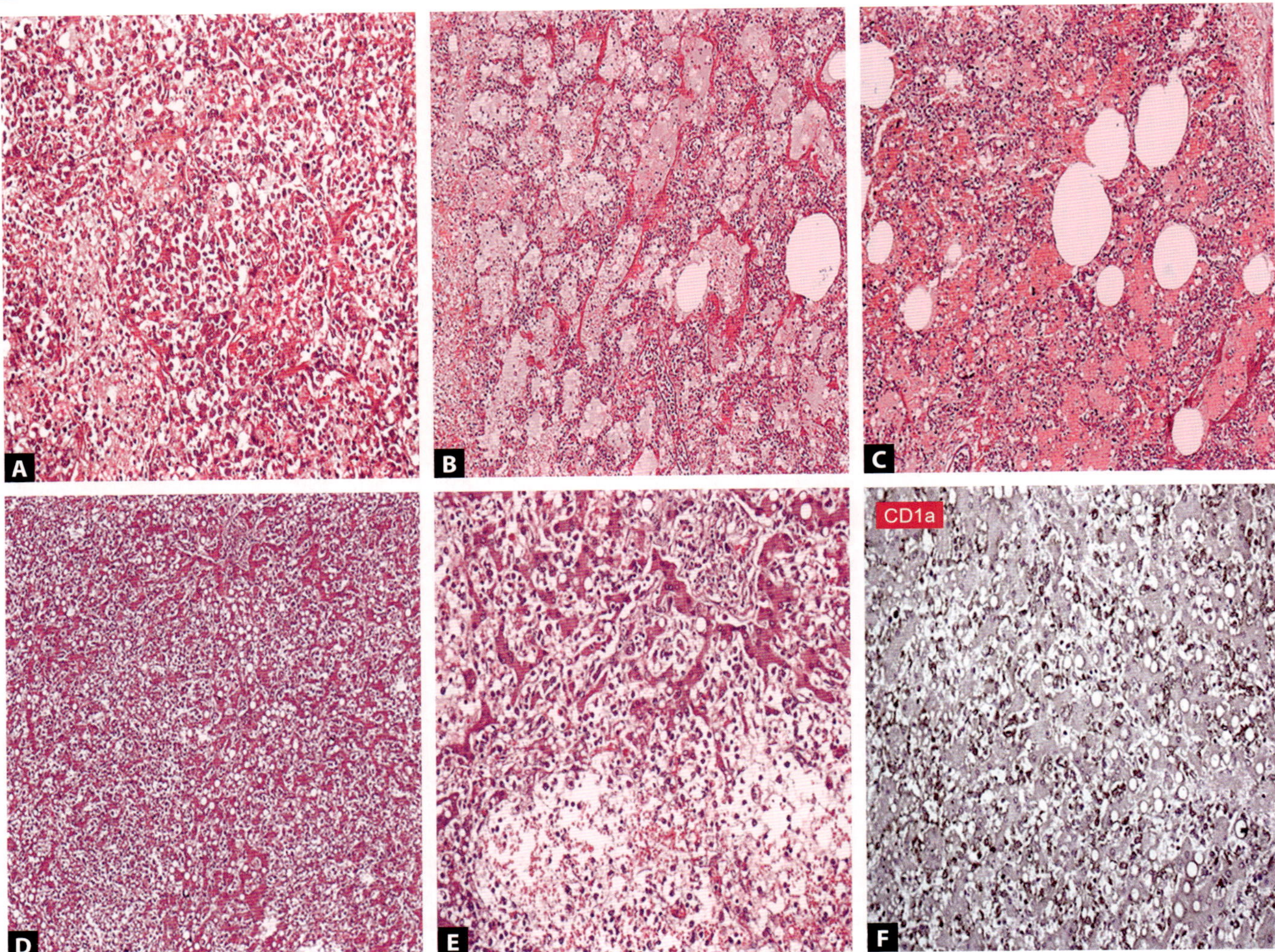

Figs 5A–F: Photomicrographs from the lung showing (A) Infiltration by Langerhans cell histiocytosis (LCH); (B) Hyaline membrane formation along with edema; (C) Alveolar hemorrhage. Photomicrographs from the liver showing; (D) Sinuses packed with atypical cells of LCH; (E) Infiltrate forming nodules; (F) Atypical cells infiltrating the sinusoids show strong CD1a positivity.

alveoli. Thymic and mediastinal lymph node involvement is rare.[8,9] LCH presenting as an anterior mediastinal mass[10-13] is restricted to case reports. In most cases, there is a coexistent pulmonary involvement. Hepatobiliary involvement occurs in multisystem LCH in 50–60% of cases, wherein they infiltrate the periportal regions, showing an affinity for the bile ducts or show sinusoidal involvement. Gastrointestinal involvement in multisystem LCH occurs in 2–6% of children and shows a characteristic rash in 86% of patients. So, in cases of LCH with skin involvement, symptoms suggestive of gastrointestinal (GI) involvement need an endoscopic biopsy. Any part of gastrointestinal tract (GIT) may be involved by the disease process. The infiltrate is initially seen in the mucosa and later becomes transmural. Multisystem LCH can involve the central nervous system (CNS) in approximately 30% cases. Affected sphenoid bone can by direct extension involve the pituitary and hypothalamus. In the CNS, perivascular histiocytic infiltrate are seen, which later form granulomatous masses at any site. The most common CNS manifestation in LCH is diabetes insipidus which is considered as a pathognomonic feature. Sites of soft-tissue involvement are the cavernous sinus, the orbit, paranasal sinuses, naso/oropharynx, the temporal region (masticator space, ear), larynx and hypopharynx, thyroid, salivary glands and the adjacent muscles.

Langerhans cell histiocytosis was first described more than a century ago when a student Paul Langerhans in 1865[14] detected the Langerhans cell in the human skin. In the past,

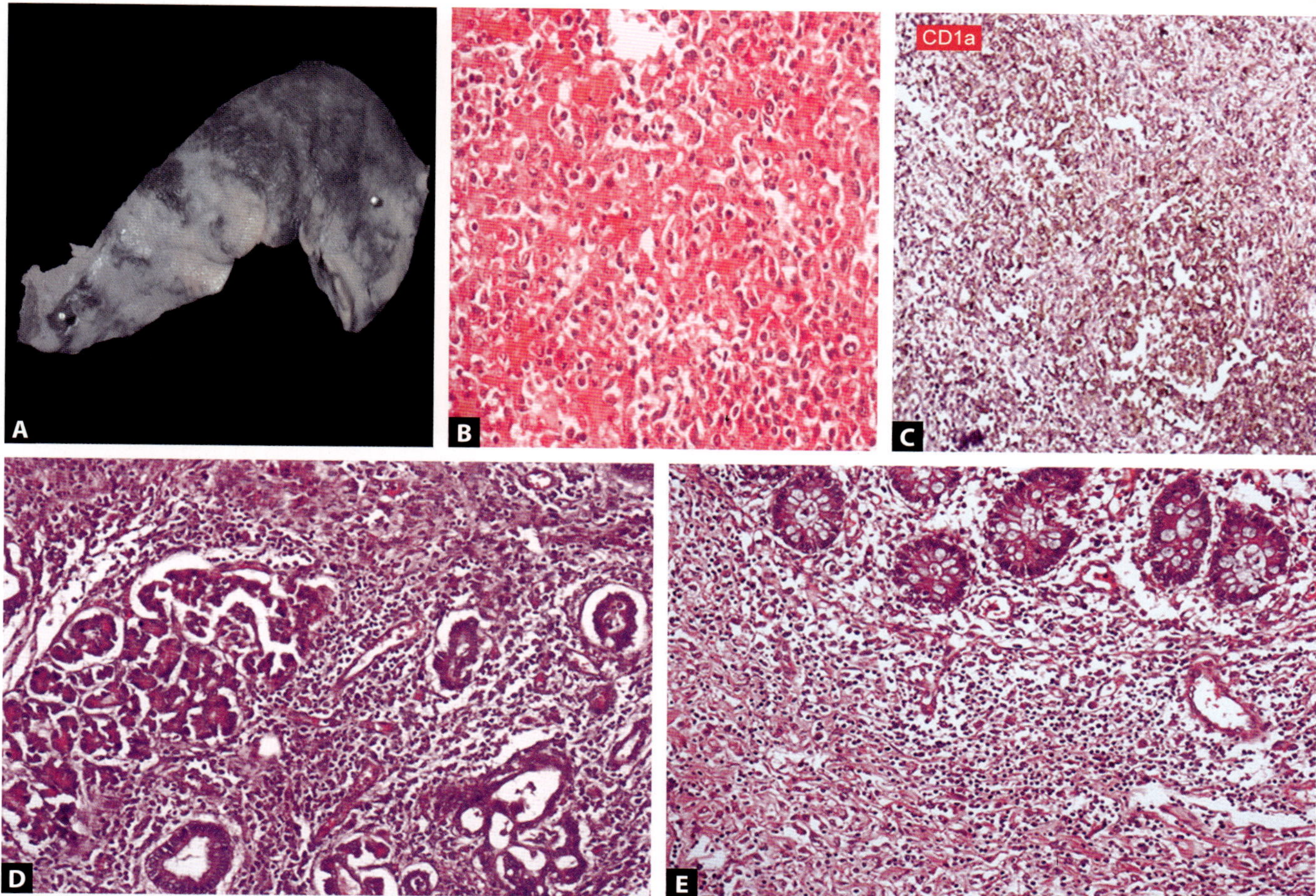

Figs 6A–E: (A) Slice of the diffusely enlarged spleen; (B) Red pulp shows extensive infiltration by Langerhans cell histiocytosis (LCH); (C) Splenic infiltrate shows strong CD1a positivity; (D) LCH infiltrate in the pancreas; (E) LCH infiltrate in the submucosa of the colon.

various terminologies have been used for LCH—Eosinophilic granuloma (solitary lesion), Hand–Schüller–Christian disease (if multiple lesions) and Letterer–Siwe disease (disseminated with visceral involvement). These three conditions are now considered to be different expression of the same basic disorder. In 1987, the histiocytosis society established a classification depicted in Table 1.[15,16] Clinically, LCH is divided into three groups: unifocal, multifocal unisystem and multifocal multisystem.

Unifocal and multifocal unisystem LCH is characterized by expanding or erosive collections of Langerhans cells within the medullary cavities of the bones. Any bone can be involved, but the common ones are calvarium, ribs and femur. Unifocal lesions are slowly progressing, affect older children or adults, can heal spontaneously or be cured by local excision or irradiation. They can be asymptomatic or painful and can occasionally lead to pathologic fracture. Multifocal unisystem LCH shows multiple bone lesions, eruptions on the scalp or auditory canals and fever. Pituitary stalk is involved in 50% cases which lead to diabetes insipidus. Many patients have spontaneous regression and others are treated successfully with chemotherapy.

Table 1: Classification of Langerhans cell histiocytosis.

Class	*Syndromes*
Class 1: Dendritic-cell related	Langerhans cell histiocytosis Juvenile Xanthogranuloma, Erdheim–Chester disease
Class 2: Macrophage related	HLH, genetic or infection associated Rosai–Dorfman (Sinus histiocytosis with massive lymphadenopathy)
Class 3: Malignant disorders	Monocyte related-monocytic leukemia Dendritic-cell related Localized or macrophage related Disseminated (malignant histiocytosis)

Multifocal multisystem LCH is seen in children < 2 years and is a fulminant disease. The prognosis is poor with a 5-year survival of 50% even with aggressive chemotherapy. Cutaneous lesions caused by infiltrates of Langerhans cells are seen over the trunk and on the scalp. These patients have hepatosplenomegaly, lymphadenopathy, pulmonary involvement and at later stage destructive osteolytic bone lesions. Marrow infiltration leads to cytopenias.

Pathogenesis of Langerhans Cell Histiocytosis

The pathogenesis[17] of LCH is ambiguous. A viral or genetic etiology has been negated and it probably seems to be a reactive, benign, immunological process. Langerhans cells are considered as specialized type of interstitial dendritic cell. These cells are located in the epidermis, oral mucosa, bronchial mucosa, tongue, tonsil, esophagus, lymph nodes and thymus. They have antigen presenting functions, stimulate and direct T cell responses and thus are said to be potent stimulators of primary immune responses. Once the Langerhans cells capture the foreign antigen or microbes, inflammatory cytokines are produced and under the cytokine influence, they migrate from the epidermis via the afferent lymphatic vessels, gain maturity on the way and reach the lymph nodes and present the antigen to the naïve T cell. The dendritic cells are originally derived from the bone marrow. The hallmark of LCH is a bizarre monoclonal proliferation of abnormal Langerhans cells that have the propensity to infiltrate any organ. This infiltration is accompanied by a variety of inflammatory cells and giant cells with occasional granuloma formation. This proliferation thus reflects an exaggerated immune response triggered by some unknown antigen which is yet to be identified.[18]

Histopathology of Langerhans Cell Histiocytosis

The histopathologic features of LCH are similar be it any site. It is composed of sheets or clusters of atypical cells admixed with macrophages, lymphocytes, numerous eosinophils and frequently multinucleated giant cells. The atypical cells are the Langerhans cells which are characterized by a moderate amount of eosinophilic cytoplasm. The nuclei are typically grooved, elongated kidney-shaped with thin nuclear membrane, delicate chromatin and inconspicuous nucleoli. Eosinophils are noted, but are not essential for the diagnosis. Large areas of necrosis and at times eosinophilic abscesses can be seen. In longstanding disease, there is a paucity of Langerhans cells and the lesion consists of fibrous tissue along with macrophages. Immunohistochemistry shows positivity with—(1) Langerin (CD207), a cell surface receptor which helps in the formation of Birbeck granules, is the best diagnostic marker with 100% positivity. It is a defining marker for LCH, is more specific than CD1a and staining is seen in the cell membrane and Golgi, in a granular pattern. (2) CD1a is another characteristic marker for Langerhans cells and shows cell membrane staining. It demarcates LCH from other dendritic cell and histiocytic proliferations. (3) S-100 is also positive in these Langerhans cells although it is not diagnostically specific. Electron microscopy shows the characteristic cytoplasmic structures known as Birbeck bodies which resemble a tennis racket. Differential diagnosis includes—(1) Rosai–Dorfman disease where there is sinusoidal distribution of histiocytes, which are larger with a round nuclei, distinct nucleoli and abundant cytoplasm. Emperipolesis is the diagnostic feature. Histiocytes are positive for S-100, CD68 but negative for CD1a and Langerin. (2) Dermatopathic lymphadenopathy shows aggregates of Langerhans and interdigitating dendritic cells, some with grooved nuclei in the paracortex admixed with melanin laden macrophages.

COMMENTARY—INDEX CASE: PM 21476

This 10-month-old male baby presented with a short history of abdominal distension, fever, rapid breathing, altered sensorium and loose stools. There was hepatosplenomegaly, lymphadenopathy and nodular lesions on the scalp. Bicytopenia was present, coagulogram, liver and renal function tests were deranged. USG of the chest revealed an anterior mediastinal mass. Autopsy revealed a systemic LCH presenting as an anterior mediastinal mass with widespread involvement of the lungs, liver, spleen, lymph nodes, pancreas and colon. Characteristic morphology was noted and the Langerhans cells were strongly positive for CD1a and S-100. The organ of origin of LCH in the anterior mediastinum could be either from the lymph nodes or the thymus. Small aggregates of lymphoid tissue were seen in the sections examined from the mass, so the origin from the mediastinal lymph node could be a possibility. Some mediastinal lymph nodes adjacent to the mass were involved by LCH. Since the thymus or even its remnants could not be identified, despite examining multiple sections, a possibility that this mass arose in the thymus and totally replaced it cannot be negated. The GIT tract was involved but the skin or bone marrow although involved, could not be assessed. LCH presenting as anterior mediastinal mass is rare and limited to case reports only.

TAKE HOME MESSAGE

- Langerhans cell histiocytosis is a rare disease that occurs mainly in the pediatric population.
- Langerhans cell histiocytosis shows a clonal accumulation of Langerhans cells in various tissues or organs.
- Fifty percent show a mutation of the B-RAF oncogene.
- Bone followed by skin is the most common organ system involved. Other organs like CNS, lungs, hepatobiliary, spleen, GIT, lymph nodes and thymus can be involved.
- Langerhans cell histiocytosis seems to be a reactive, benign, immunological process leading to an uncontrolled immune response.

REFERENCES

1. Lieberman PH, Jones CR, Steinman RM, et al. Langerhans cell (eosinophilic) granulomatosis: a clinicopathologic study encompassing 50 years. Am J Surg Pathol. 1996;20:519-52.
2. Campos MK, Viana MB, de Oliveira BM, et al. Langerhans cell histiocytosis: a 16-year experience. J Pediatr (Rio J). 2007;83:79-86.
3. Badalian-Very G, Vergilio JA, Degar BA, et al. Recurrent BRAF mutations in Langerhans cell histiocytosis. Blood. 2010;116:1919-23.
4. Nicholson HS, Egeler RM, Nesbit ME. The epidemiology of Langerhans cell histiocytosis. Hematol Oncol Clin North Am. 1998;12(2):379-84.
5. Kilpatrick SE, Wenger DE, Gilchrist GS, et al. Langerhans' cell histiocytosis (histiocytosis X) of bone: a clinicopathologic analysis of 263 pediatric and adult cases. Cancer. 1995; 76(12):2471-84.
6. Schmidt S, Eich G, Hanquinet S, et al. Extra-osseous involvement of Langerhans' cell histiocytosis in children. Pediatr Radiol. 2004;34:313-21.
7. Jubran RF, Marachelian A, Dorey F, et al. Predictors of outcome in children with Langerhans cell histiocytosis. Pediatr Blood Cancer. 2005;45(1):37-42.
8. Ducassou S, Seyrig F, Thomas C, et al. Thymus and mediastinal node involvement in childhood Langerhans Cell histiocytosis: long-term follow-up from the French National Cohort. Pediatr Blood Cancer. 2013;60:1759-65.
9. Siegal GP, Dehner LP, Rosai J. Histiocytosis X (Langerhans' cell granulomatosis) of the thymus. A clinicopathologic study of four childhood cases. Am J Surg Pathol. 1985;9:117-24.
10. Nakata H, Suzuki H, Sato Y, et al. Histiocytosis X with anterior mediastinal mass as its initial manifestation. Pediatr Radiol. 1982;12:84-5.
11. Abramson SJ, Berdon WE, Reilly BJ, et al. Cavitation of anterior mediastinal masses in children with histiocytosis-X. Report of four cases with radiographic, pathologic findings and clinical follow up. Pediatr Radiol. 1987;17:10-4.
12. Odagiri K, Nishihira K, Hatekeyama S, et al. Anterior mediastinal masses with calcifications on CT in children with histiocytosis-X (Langerhans cell histiocytosis). Report of two cases. Pediatr Radiol. 1991;21:550-1.
13. Mogul M, Hartman G, Donaldson S, et al. Langerhans' cell histiocytosis presenting with the superior vena cava syndrome: A case report. Med Pediatr Oncol. 1993;21:456-9.
14. Langerhans P. Ueber die Nerven der menschlichen Haut. Virchows Arch (Pathol Anat). 1868;44:325-37.
15. Histiocytosis syndromes in children. Writing Group of the Histiocyte Society. Lancet. 1987;1:208-9.
16. Chu T, D'Angio GJ, Favara BE, et al. Histiocytosis syndromes in children. Lancet. 1987;2(8549):41-2.
17. Nezelof C, Basset F. Langerhans cell histiocytosis research. Hematol Oncol Clin North Am. 1998;12(2):385-406.
18. The French Langerhans' Cell Histiocytosis Study Group. A multicentre retrospective survey of Langerhans' cell histiocytosis: 348 cases observed between 1983 and 1993. Arch Dis Child. 1996;75:17-24.

CONTRIBUTIONS BY:

1. Professor S Singhi, Ex-Professor and Head, Department of Pediatrics (Clinician In-Charge)
2. Dr Vipul Gupta, Assistant Professor, Department of Pediatrics (Compilation of Clinical Details)

Post Graduate Institute of Medical Education and Research, Chandigarh, India.

CASE 53

Macrophage Activation Syndrome—A Fatal Complication of Systemic Onset Juvenile Idiopathic Arthritis: PM 26202

Nandita Bharadwaj Kakkar

 HIGHLIGHTS OF THE CASE

A 2-year-old boy came with prolonged fever, arthralgia, evanescent rash, lymphadenopathy and hepatosplenomegaly. There was a progressive fall in the blood counts from the day of admission till demise (9 days). There was anemia, thrombocytopenia, elevated ESR and C-reactive protein (CRP), decreased fibrinogen levels, elevated ferritin, hypertriglyceridemia, elevated transaminases and mildly raised serum bilirubin. Bone marrow aspiration revealed only an occasional macrophage with hemophagocytosis. Clinical diagnosis was macrophage activation syndrome (MAS) complicating systemic-onset juvenile idiopathic arthritis (SoJIA). Autopsy revealed a florid hemophagocytosis in thymus, bone marrow, lymph nodes, spleen and liver, consistent with MAS along with diffuse alveolar damage and pulmonary hemorrhage.

Keywords: SoJIA, systemic-onset juvenile idiopathic arthritis, macrophage activation syndrome, type 2 histiocytosis, autopsy.

 CLINICAL DETAILS

Date of Admission: 02.08.2014, Date of Death: 10.08.2014, Duration of Hospital Stay: 8 days.

A 2-year-old male baby was admitted with complaints of fever since 3 weeks, joint pain since 2 weeks, rash and cough since 1 week. The fever was high grade, up to 104°F, intermittent with no chills and rigors. Joint pains were present in both knees and he had difficulty in walking. There was no swelling or redness. The rash was maculopapular, erythematous, nonpruritic and evanescent, involving the trunk, limbs and face. The cough was nonproductive to begin with and later became productive. There was however no hemoptysis. Past history revealed recurrent episodes of fever associated with cough since June 2014 and was treated each time with oral prednisolone (5–7 days) considering a hyperreactive airway disease. The child was developmentally normal, appropriately immunized and was first in birth order. There was no history of contact with tuberculosis. Anthropometric measurements were normal. ***On examination*** the temperature was—38.7°C, pulse rate—110/min, respiratory rate—24/min, blood pressure—96/58 mm Hg and SpO_2—99%. On systemic examination, the abdomen was soft and nontender. The liver was palpable 3.5 cm below right costal margin (span—8 cm), was soft in consistency with rounded margins and smooth surface. The spleen was palpable 2 cm below left costal margin. No free fluid was present. There was a progressive fall in the blood counts from the day of admission till demise (9 days). The Hb fell from 7.2 g/dL to 5 g/dL, TLC fell from 11,500/μL to 7,100/μL and the platelets fell from 2,07,000/μL to 15,000/μL. The ESR was 62 mm 1st hour. Electrolytes were within normal limits. Terminally the serum urea (112 mg%) was high but creatinine was 1.2 mg%, serum bilirubin was 1.7 mg% with conjugated fraction of 0.7, AST/ALT were 149/72 U/L and later went up to 218/70 U/L. Total serum proteins and coagulogram were normal. The CRP was raised, i.e. 140 mg/L. Triglycerides were elevated, i.e. 355 mg%. The blood culture was sterile, smears for malarial parasite, Widal, serology for leptospira, brucella and HIV were negative. The Weil–Felix agglutination test, Mantoux and gastric lavage for AFB (done thrice) were all negative. Fibrinogen levels were low, i.e. 2.2 g/L. Ferritin levels were 1,50,000 μg/L (N: <500). Bone marrow aspiration did not show any excess of blasts and only an occasional macrophage with hemophagocytosis was noted. ***Units final clinical diagnosis*** was MAS complicating SoJIA. Cause of death being pulmonary hemorrhage.

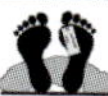

AUTOPSY FINDINGS: PM 26202

A complete autopsy was performed on this 2-year-old male baby. He was moderately built and pale. Both pleural cavities yielded 500 mL each and the peritoneal cavity yielded 1000 mL of straw-colored fluid. The pericardial cavity was within normal limits. The ***thymus*** (Fig 1A) was enlarged and weighed 30 g (N: 16.5 g). On cutting it was fleshy. Sections examined from the thymus (Fig 1B) showed marked increase in lymphoid tissue with reduction in the epithelial component. An occasional Hassall's corpuscle was seen. There was a marked increase in macrophages (confirmed by CD68 immunostain) which revealed florid hemophagocytosis (Figs 1C and D). The ***lymph nodes*** (hilar, paratracheal, carinal, paraaortic, mesenteric) (Fig 2A) were enlarged and ranged in size from 0.5 cm to 1.5 cm. On microscopic examination, there were prominent lymphoid follicles with expansion of the paracortex (Fig 2B). Macrophages were markedly increased in number and revealed prominent hemophagocytosis (Fig 2C) which was confirmed on CD68 immunostain (Fig 2D). The ***bone marrow*** was normocellular with adequate representation of all the three hematopoietic elements. However, there was marked increase in number of macrophages which exhibited prominent hemophagocytosis (Figs 3A and B). The ***liver*** (Fig 3C) was enlarged and weighed 560 g (N: 394 g). Capsular aspect was unremarkable and cut surface was pale with no focal lesion. On microscopic examination the lobular architecture was maintained and there was no increase in fibrosis. The portal tracts (Fig 3D) were expanded and showed moderate lymphohistiocytic

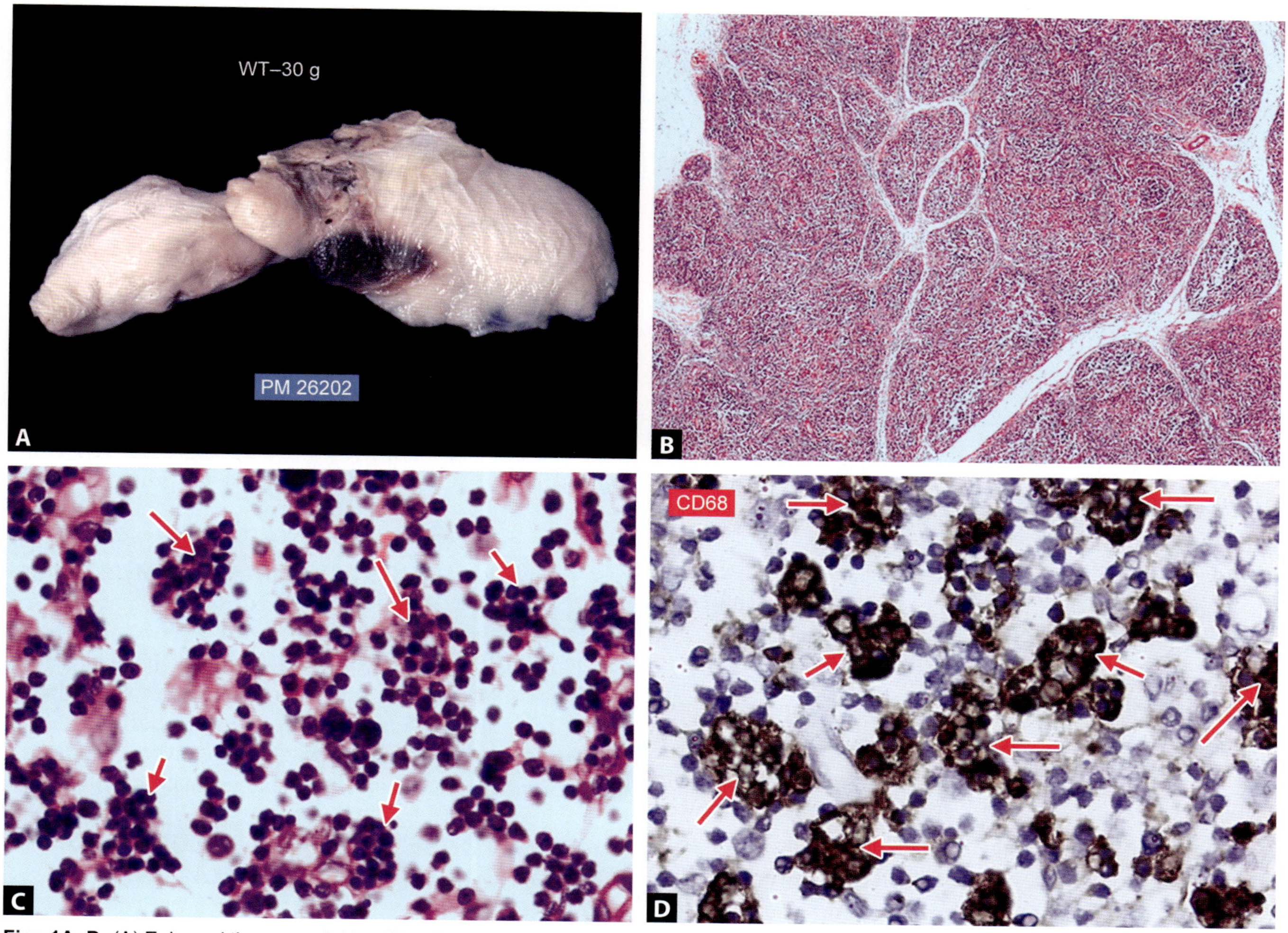

Figs 1A–D: (A) Enlarged thymus weighing 30 g; (B) Thymus shows a marked increase in lymphoid tissue, reduction in the epithelial component, and an occasional Hassall's corpuscle; (C) Macrophages are increased in number and show exuberant hemophagocytosis; (D) Macrophage marker CD68 shows strong positivity in the hemophagocytizing macrophages.

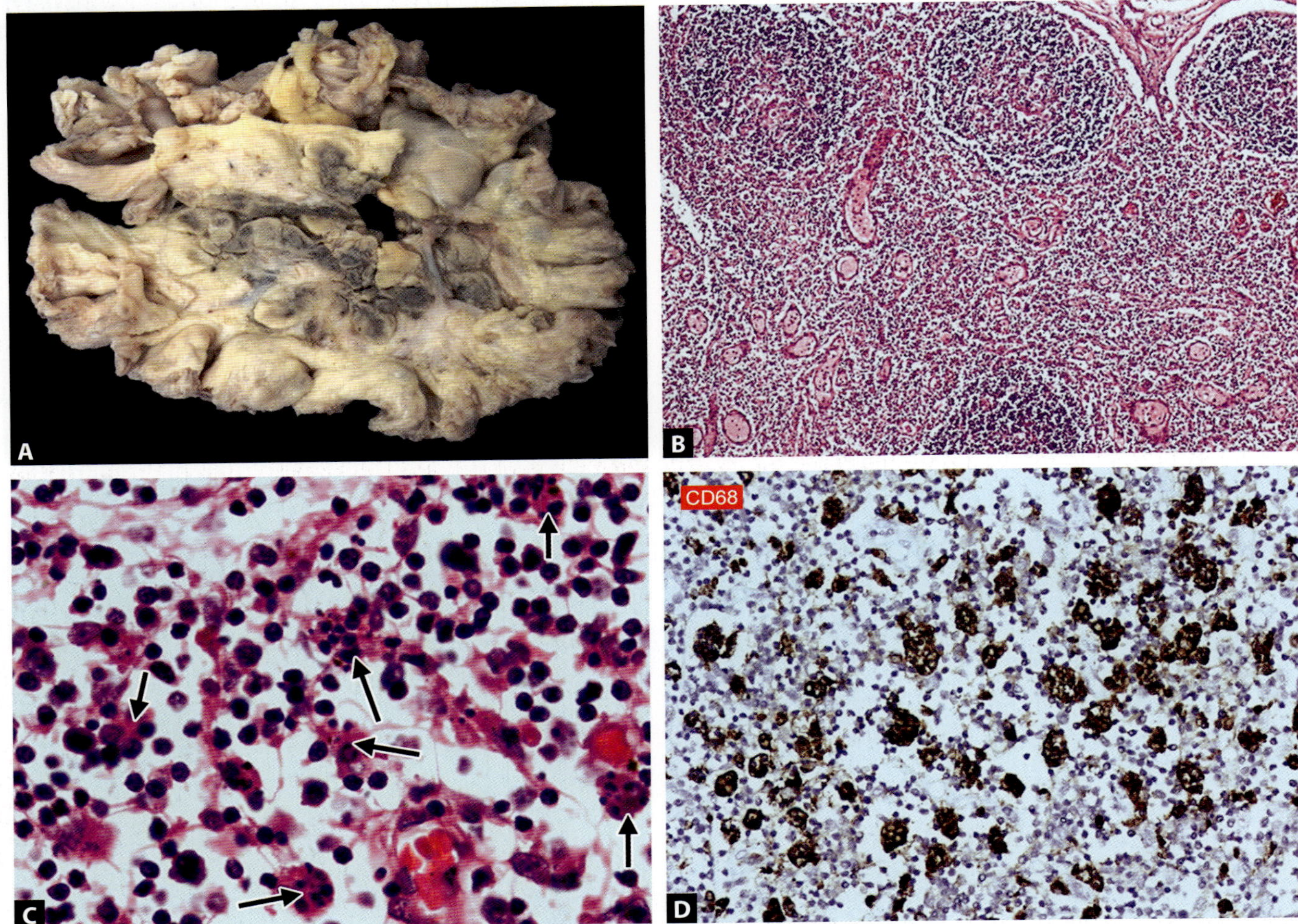

Figs 2A–D: (A) Mesentery showing enlarged lymph nodes; (B) Lymph node shows prominent lymphoid follicles with expansion of the paracortex; (C) Lymph node shows a marked increase in macrophages with hemophagocytosis (arrows); (D) CD68 immunostain confirms the marked increase in the hemophagocytizing macrophages.

infiltrate showing hemophagocytosis which were highlighted on CD68 immunostain (Fig 3E). The ***spleen*** (Fig 4A) was markedly enlarged in size and weighed 150 g (N: 33 g). The cut surface and microscopic sections showed prominence of white pulp and congested red pulp (Figs 4A and B). There was a marked increase in macrophages showing exuberant hemophagocytosis (Fig 4C). The ***lungs*** were heavy and together weighed 245 g. The pleural was dull and showed patchy areas of hemorrhage. On cut section the lungs were subcrepitant to feel and areas of hemorrhage were present. On microscopic examination hyaline membrane formation (Fig 4D), alveolar hemorrhage (Fig 4E) and edema was noted indicating diffuse alveolar damage.

FINAL AUTOPSY DIAGNOSIS: PM 26202

2 Years Old Male with SoJIA, ANA Negative

- Florid hemophagocytosis in thymus, bone marrow, lymph nodes, spleen and liver—consistent with Macrophage activation syndrome secondary to SoJIA.
- Diffuse alveolar damage with hyaline membrane formation, pulmonary hemorrhage and edema.

SYSTEMIC ONSET JUVENILE RHEUMATOID ARTHRITIS AND MACROPHAGE ACTIVATION SYNDROME

Systemic onset juvenile rheumatoid arthritis is a diagnosis of exclusion. The diagnosis can be made at presentation, but

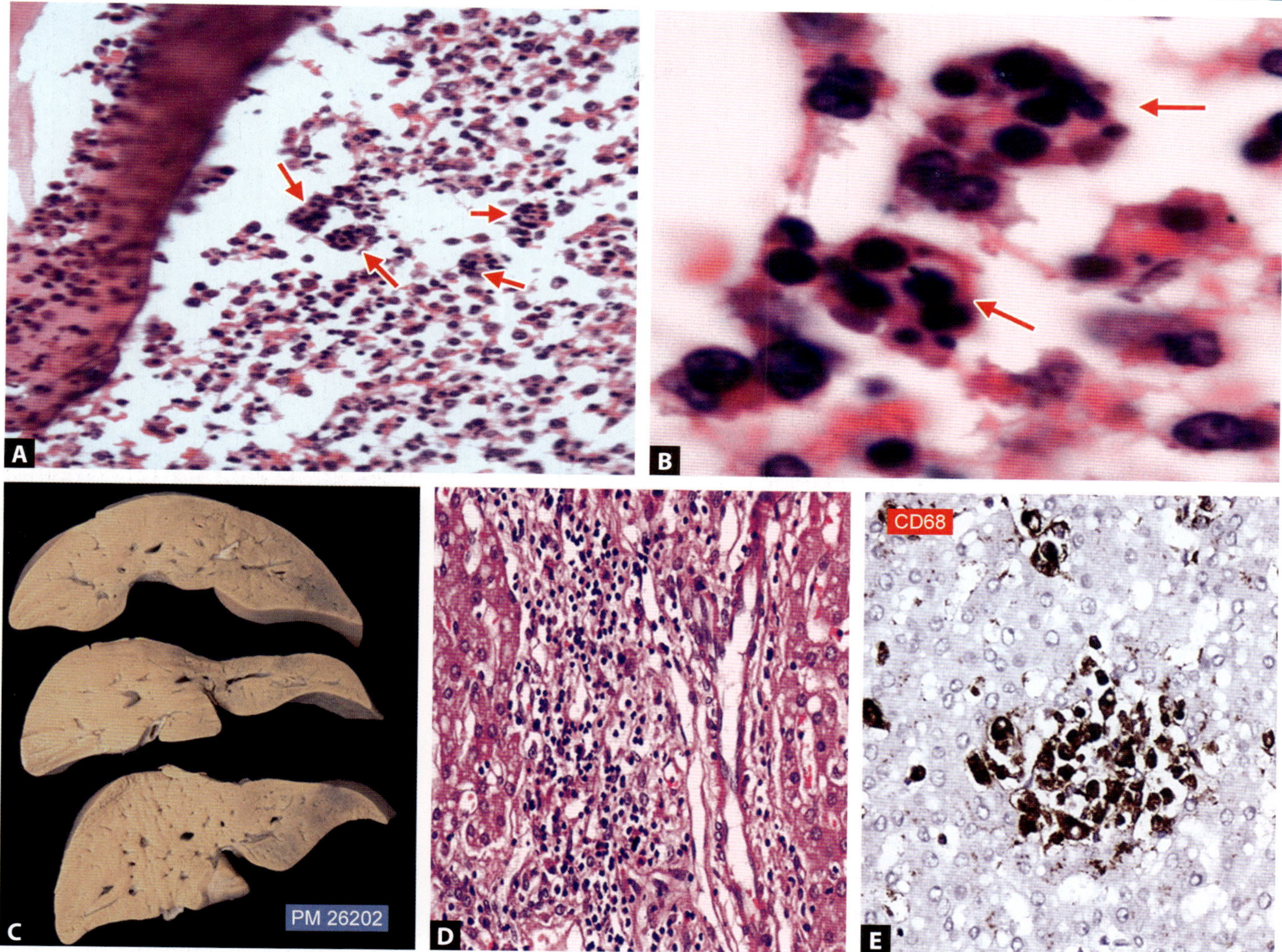

Figs 3A–E: (A) Bone marrow showing marked increase in macrophages engulfing hematopoietic elements (arrows); (B) Phagocytizing macrophages seen under oil immersion lens; (C) Coronal slices of the enlarged liver which is pale; (D) Portal tract showing a lymphohistiocytic infiltrate with phagocytizing macrophages; (E) CD68 immunostain on the liver showing a cluster of hemophagocytizing macrophages in the sinusoid.

it may be delayed for many years. International League of Associations for Rheumatology (ILAR) criteria for diagnosis of SoJIA is presence of arthritis in one or more joint with presence of fever for more than 2 weeks with one or more of the following—(A) Evanescent erythematous rash; (B) Generalized lymphadenopathy; (C) Hepatomegaly or splenomegaly or both and (D) Serositis. Laboratory profile shows anemia, thrombocytosis, neutrophilic leukocytosis and elevated ESR and CRP. SoJIA with thrombocytopenia indicates MAS which occurs in 10% cases of SoJIA. Mild or subclinical MAS occurs in one-third of patients with active systemic disease. MAS occurring as the first presenting feature in SoJIA is seen in case reports. MAS is suspected in SoJIA when there is occurrence of bleeding manifestation (occurs in 70–80% cases), CNS involvement in the form of seizures, irritability, meningeal signs, encephalopathy (occurs in 40–60% cases), hyponatremia, fall in ESR, elevation in AST, thrombocytopenia, leukopenia, decreased fibrinogen (occurs in 70–80% cases), elevated ferritin (occurs in 70–80% cases) and elevated triglycerides (occurs in 60–80% cases). Progressive fall in counts is more important than absolute values. Bone marrow examination demonstrating hemophagocytosis is seen in 67% of cases. The cut off value for serum ferritin in MAS is more than 500 µg/L and levels more than 10,000 µg/L are diagnostic. Very high levels of ferritin (>3,000 µg/L) were associated with increased mortality in a dose response fashion.

Macrophage activation syndrome in SoJIA presents with nonresponding fever, headache, jaundice, anemia, lymphadenopathy, hepatosplenomegaly, bleeding from various

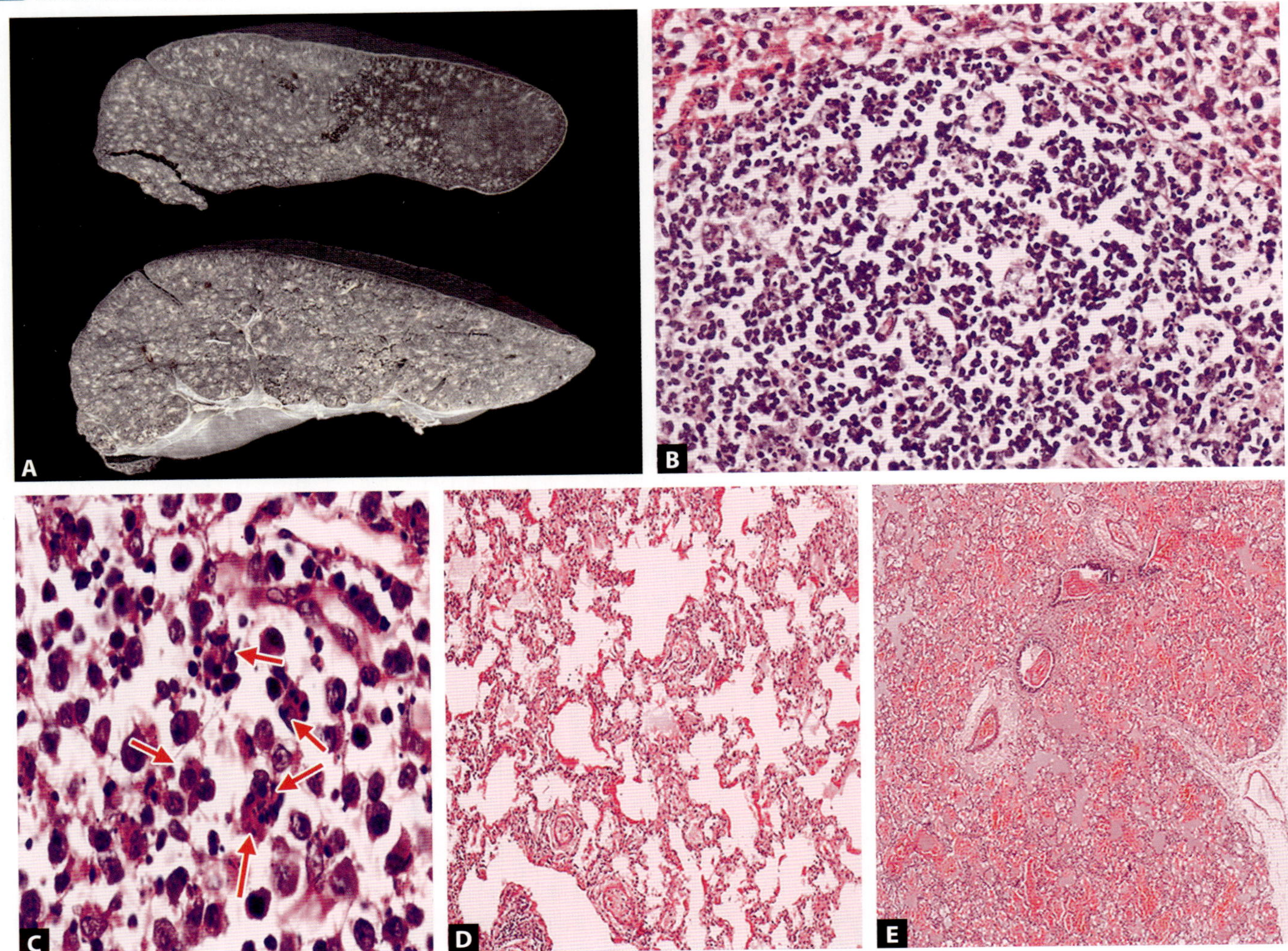

Figs 4A–E: (A) Slices of the enlarged spleen with prominence of the white pulp; (B) White pulp with lymphohistiocytic infiltrate; (C) High power showing plenty of hemophagocytizing macrophages (arrows); (D) Microphotograph of the lung showing dilated alveolar spaces lined by hyaline membranes; (E) Lung showing extensive alveolar hemorrhage.

sites, disseminated intravascular coagulation and brain dysfunction in the form of lethargy, irritability, disorientation, seizures and coma. There is radical improvement in the basic disease. Laboratory findings reveal cytopenia, abnormal coagulation profile, hypofibrinogenemia, degraded fibrin products, abnormal hepatic function tests, elevated lactate dehydrogenase levels, hypertriglyceridemia, hyperferritinemia, low Na and albumin levels and the pathognomonic feature of presence of hemophagocytizing macrophages in the bone marrow. The diagnosis of MAS needs the presence of two or more of the following clinical or two or more of the following laboratory criteria or histopathologic evidence of hemophagocytizing macrophages in the bone marrow aspirate. The clinical parameters consist of hemorrhages or mucosal bleeds, hepatomegaly at least 3 cm below the costal margin and CNS disturbances like headache, disorientation, seizures and coma. The laboratory criteria include leukopenia, thrombocytopenia, AST more than 59 U/L and hypofibrinogenemia. Differential diagnosis of MAS includes acute exacerbation of underlying juvenile rheumatoid arthritis (JRA), systemic lupus erythematosus (SLE), sepsis, visceral leishmaniasis, brucellosis and tuberculosis. The active phase of the disease is characterized by increased levels of the α-chain of the soluble interleukin-2R (sCD25). This is a valuable marker for diagnosis as well as for prognosis, since increased levels correlate with increased mortality. Macrophage activation is an ominous complication of systemic rheumatic disorders, primarily SoJIA and is associated with a bad prognosis. Early recognition and aggressive therapy with parenteral administration of high doses of methylprednisolone and cyclosporin are critical. But, despite the best of treatments, mortality is very high. In MAS, there is an uncontrolled proliferation or activation of T-cells which results in a cytokine storm with induction of IFN-γ and pro-inflammatory cytokines like IL-1, 8, 12, TNF-α, plasmin and transferrin, which triggers a pro-inflammatory response causing activation of macrophages and subsequent hemophagocytosis. Proliferation and activation of macrophages in the reticuloendothelial system thereby causes lymphadenopathy, hepatosplenomegaly and pancytopenia. This ineffective and uncontrolled immune activation finally leads to multiorgan dysfunction.

Macrophage activation syndrome is an underestimated, fatal, complication of rheumatic diseases like SoJIA and Still's disease. Other entities where it can be seen are SLE, polyarticular juvenile idiopathic arthritis and Kawasaki disease. Factors which precipitate MAS in these conditions are infections, nonsteroidal anti-inflammatory drugs—aspirin, gold salts, methotrexate, sulfasalazine therapy and autologous bone marrow transplantation. Patients with SoJIA develop MAS in about 10% cases

COMMENTARY—INDEX CASE: PM 26202

This is a classical case wherein a diagnosis of SoJIA was made along with MAS. MAS occurring as the first presenting feature in SoJIA is seen very rarely. A 2-year-old boy came with prolonged fever, arthralgia, evanescent rash, lymphadenopathy and hepatosplenomegaly. He fulfilled the ILAR criteria for diagnosis of SoJIA. There was a progressive fall in the blood counts from the day of admission till demise (9 days). There was anemia, thrombocytopenia, elevated ESR and CRP, decreased fibrinogen levels, elevated ferritin, hypertriglyceridemia, elevated transaminases and mildly raised serum bilirubin. Bone marrow aspiration revealed only an occasional macrophage with hemophagocytosis. He fulfilled the diagnostic criteria, both clinical and laboratory, for the diagnosis of MAS. Autopsy revealed a florid hemophagocytosis in thymus, bone marrow, lymph nodes, spleen and liver, consistent with MAS along with diffuse alveolar damage and pulmonary hemorrhage. There was a marked discrepancy in the number of hemophagocytizing macrophages between the antemortem and postmortem bone marrow biopsies. This discrepancy has been reported in literature, wherein the first biopsy does not show hemophagocytizing macrophages and a biopsy done a week later is replete with them.

TAKE HOME MESSAGE

- Class 2 histiocytosis is macrophage-related and comprises the primary and secondary hemophagocytic lymphohistiocytosis (HLH). Autoimmune disorders can lead to a special form of secondary HLH, termed as macrophage activation syndrome which has a prevalence of 3% and a high mortality.
- The autoimmune disorders associated with MAS are SoJIA, SLE, adult Still's disease and Sjögren syndrome.
- Approximately 10% of the patients with SoJIA develop MAS.

SUGGESTED READING

1. Haque SF. Macrophage activation syndrome. Medicine Update. 2011;446-9.
2. Kravitz MS. The hemophagocytic syndrome/ macrophage activation syndrome: A final common pathway of a cytokine storm. IMAI. 2009;11:633634.
3. Moradinejad MH, Ziaee V. The incidence of macrophage activation syndrome in children with rheumatic disorders. Minerva Pediatr. 2011;63(6):459-6.
4. Reddy VV, Myles A, Cheekatla SS, et al. Soluble CD25 in serum: a potential marker for subclinical macrophage activation syndrome in patients with active systemic onset juvenile idiopathic arthritis. Int J Rheum Dis. 2014;17(3):261-7.
5. Singh S, Chandrakasan S, Ahluwalia J, et al. Macrophage activation syndrome in children with systemic onset juvenile idiopathic arthritis: clinical experience from northwest India. Rheumatol Int. 2012;32(4):881-6.

CONTRIBUTIONS BY:

1. Dr Archana KS, Senior Resident, Department of Pathology (Working up of the Autopsy findings)
2. Dr Debasish Sahoo, Junior Resident, Department of Pediatrics (Compilation of the Clinical Details)
3. Dr Surjit Singh, Professor and Head, Department of Pediatrics (Clinician In-Charge)

Post Graduate Institute of Medical Education and Research, Chandigarh, India.

CASE 54

Epstein–Barr Virus-associated Secondary Hemophagocytic Lymphohistiocytosis—A Rare Complication: PM 21703

Nandita Bharadwaj Kakkar

 HIGHLIGHTS OF THE CASE

A 22-year-old male presented with pyrexia of unknown origin (PUO) and jaundice. On examination there was pallor, icterus, hepatosplenomegaly and ascites. Generalized lymphadenopathy was detected on ultrasonography and CECT abdomen. Investigations revealed pancytopenia with progressive fall in counts during the hospital stay, deranged liver and renal function tests, raised transaminases, hypoalbuminemia, hypertriglyceridemia, hyperferritinemia and the bone marrow revealed hemophagocytosis. The autopsy showed florid disseminated hemophagocytic lymphohistiocytosis (HLH) and the immunostains confirmed infection with Epstein–Barr virus (EBV).

Keywords: Autopsy, Epstein–Barr virus, secondary, hemophagocytic lymphohistiocytosis, pyrexia of unknown origin.

 CLINICAL DETAILS

Date of Admission: 19.11.2006, Date of Death: 26.11.2006, Duration of Hospital Stay: 7 Days

A 22-year-old male form Panchkula was admitted in the emergency with complaints of fever for 4 weeks and jaundice of one week duration. The fever was moderate-to-high grade and continuous. He was treated at an outside facility and became afebrile for a few days. However, fever recurred and he developed jaundice one week prior to admission. Jaundice was gradually progressive with no associated features of cholestasis or decompensation. He gave history of loss of appetite, weight, asthenia and myalgia. There was no history of rash, joint pains, breathlessness, chest pain, bowel alteration, decreased urine output, neurological deficit, drug intake, blood transfusion and any addiction or jaundice in the past. On ***examination,*** he was average built, conscious, temperature—39°C, pulse—100/min, BP—110/70 mm Hg, respiratory rate—20/min, pallor++, icterus++, jugular venous pressure (JVP) not raised, no edema feet, small axillary node seen on right side of neck, Chest/CVS/CNS—within normal limits (WNL), liver was palpable 3 cm below the right costal margin, spleen palpable 2 cm below the left costal margin and ascites was noted.

Investigations and Course and Management

Hematological: Hemogram—progressive fall from time of admission—Hb—fell from 8.7 gms% to 5.3 gms%, TLC—fell from 1800/uL to 500/uL, Platelets fell from 35000/uL to 12000/uL; reticulocyte count—2.6, ESR 1st hour—25; PTI-65%; fibrinogen level—1.85 g/L; plasma hemoglobin—5 mg%; G6PD—normal; urine Hb—normal; Bone marrow showed marked hemophagocytosis; S Ferrtin—7557.8 mg/dL.

Blood Biochemistry: S urea/creatinine- 130/3.6 mg%; S bilirubin/conjugated fraction—6.3/4.2 mg%; SGOT/SGPT—69/60 U/L; S alkaline phosphatase—36 U/L; S proteins—5 gm; albumin/globulin—3.1/1.9 gm; Electrolytes—Na^+/K^+—126/3.1 mEq/L; Ca^{2+}/PO_4^- 7.9/3.0 mg%; Lipidogram—total cholesterol 130 mg%; triglycerides 260 mg%; HDL 21 mg%; LDL 70 mg%.

Microbiological: Cultures—blood/bone marrow/pleural/ascitic- sterile; Hbs Ag/Hep C/HIV/Widal—negative, serology for malaria/brucella/kala-azar/fungus/ CMV- negative; serum complement—C3—29 mg/dl (N-50-90), C4—18.4 mg/dl (N-10-40); ANA/DS-DNA negative; Pleural fluid—protein 1.9, ADA 42 IU/L; Ascitic fluid—protein 1 .8, ADA 55 IU/L.

Radiology: USG abdomen—hepatosplenomegaly, peripancreatic, periportal, mesentric and retroperitoneal nodes enlarged, ascites present; Chest X-ray—WNL; CECT abdomen-narrowing at the terminal ileum with mural thickening in distal loops and at the iliocolic junction, hepatosplenomegaly present, retroperitoneal and mesenteric lymph nodes enlarged lymph nodes, mild ascites and right pleural effusion present. NCCT head—WNL.

Course and management: A young boy was admitted as a case of pyrexia of unknown origin (PUO) ? Lymphoreticular malignancy ? Tuberculosis. He was put on antibiotics and on the basis of his CT findings, pleural fluid and ascitic fluid analysis, he was put on modified anti-tubercular treatment in view of the jaundice. Since bone marrow showed hemophagocytosis with markedly elevated serum ferritin levels, he was put on cyclosporine. A day before his demise he had generalized tonic clonic seizures followed by cardio respiratory arrest. He was put on inotropic support, developed ventricular tachycardia, cardioversion was done and he attained sinus rhythm. He was put on amiodarone infusion but he again developed ventricular tachycardia and cardiac arrest from which he could not be revived. Unit's clinical diagnosis: Hemophagocytosis ? Disseminated tuberculosis, Systemic inflammatory response syndrome (SIRS) and septic shock.

AUTOPSY FINDINGS: PM 21703

A partial autopsy was performed on this 22-year-old male, a case of PUO. The peritoneal cavity contained 1,500 mL of straw-colored fluid and the pleural cavities yielded 500 mL of similar fluid. The ***bone marrow*** (Figs 1A and B) was hypocellular, erythroid series and megakaryocytes were seen but the myeloid series was depressed. There was an extensive infiltration by lymphohistiocytic (LH) infiltrate exhibiting florid hemophagocytosis (Figs 1C and D). The bone marrow

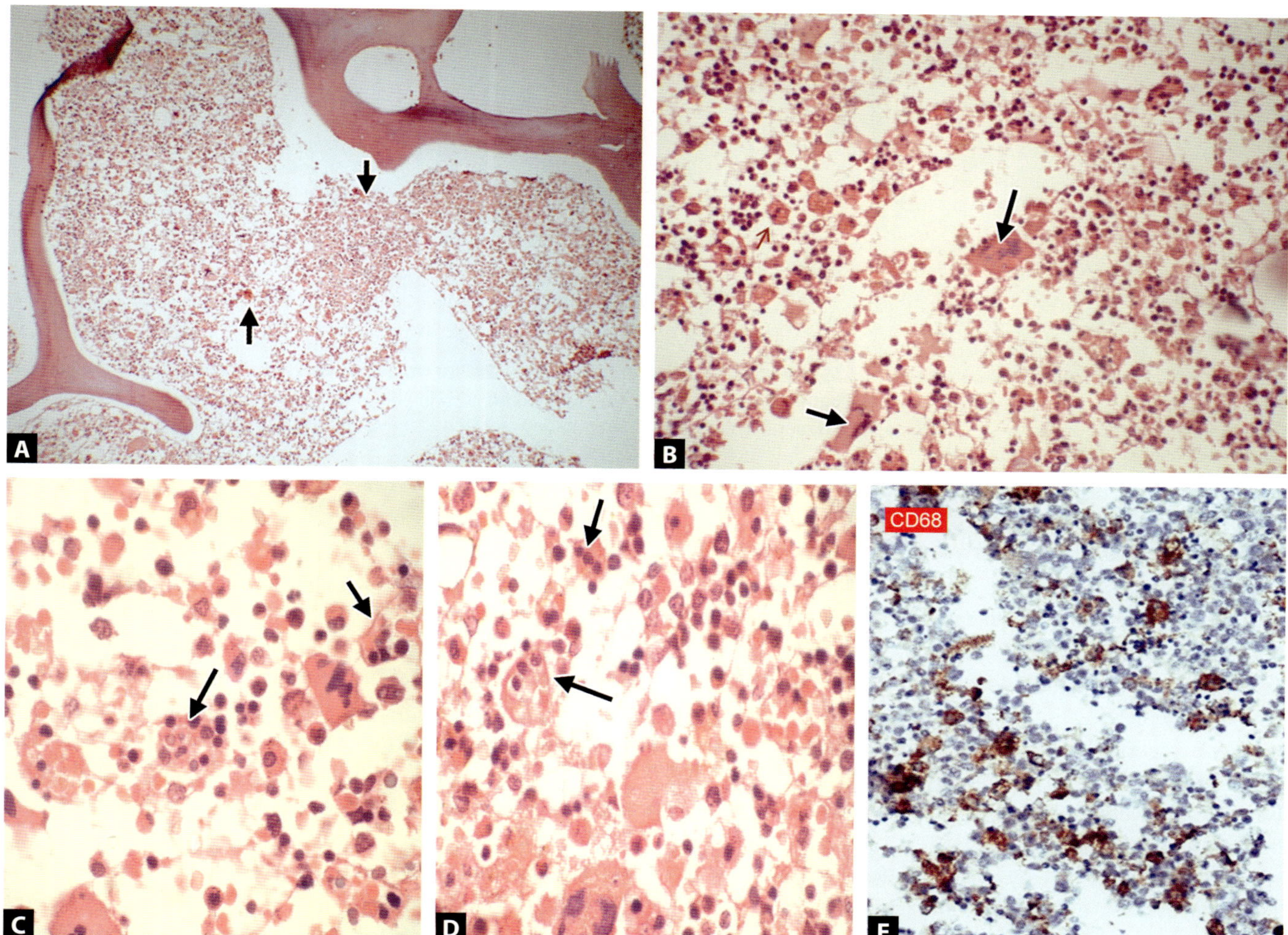

Figs 1A–E: (A and B) Bone marrow section, hypocellular showing few megakaryocytes (black arrows) and erythroid component; (C and D) Hypocellular bone marrow showing erythrophagocytizing histiocytes (arrows); (E) Bone marrow replete with CD68 positive histiocytes.

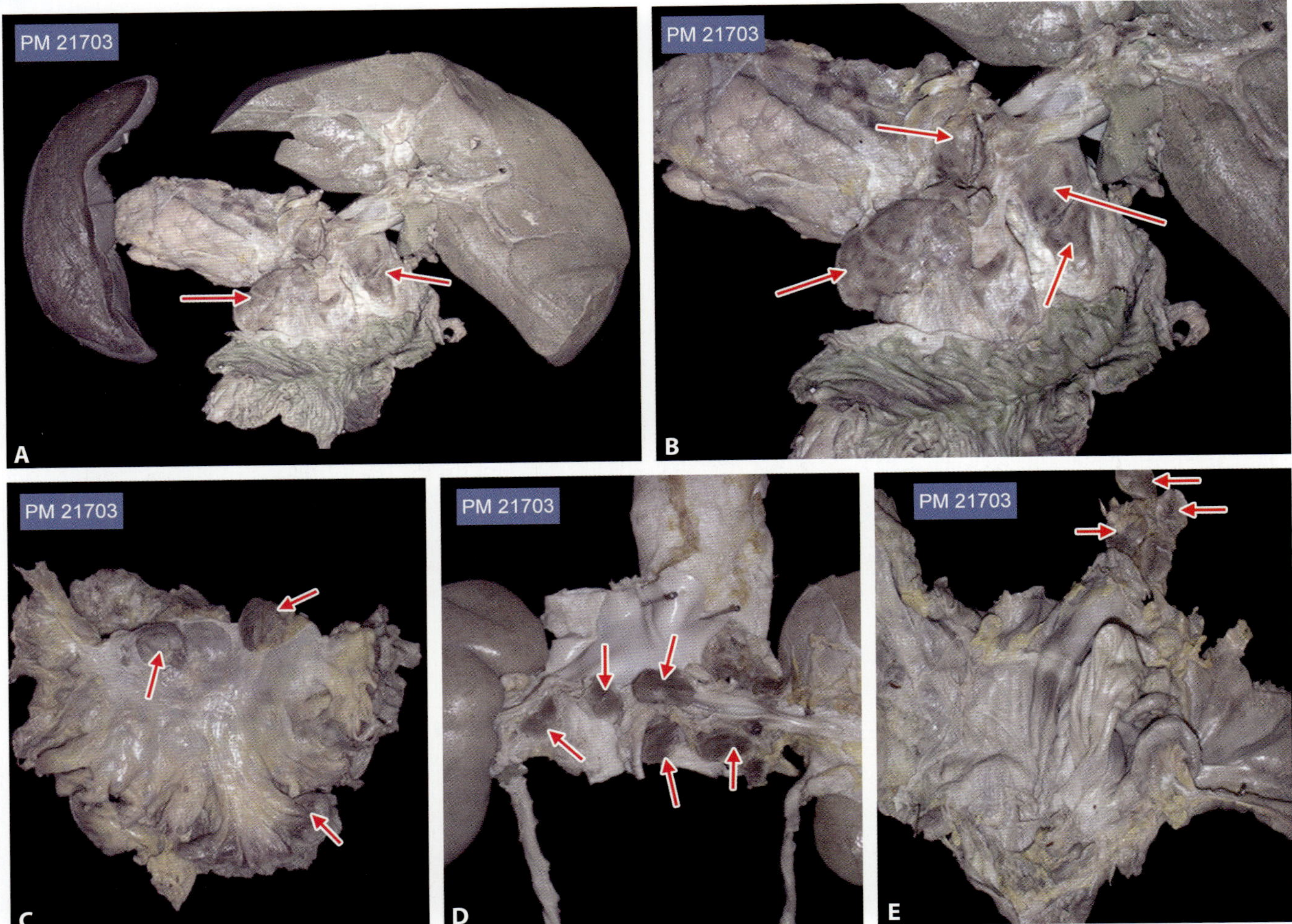

Figs 2A–E: (A and B) Complex of the liver, spleen, pancreas showing enlarged peripancreatic and periportal lymph nodes (arrows); (C) Enlarged mesenteric lymph nodes (arrows); (D) Enlarged paraaortic lymph nodes seen in between the kidneys (arrows); (E) Enlarged lymph nodes on the serosal aspect of the colon (arrows).

showed plenty of CD68 positive histiocytes (Fig 1E). There was generalized lymphadenopathy. The portal, peripancreatic, paraaortic, hilar, carinal and mesenteric ***lymph nodes*** were moderately enlarged (Figs 2A–E). On microscopy the architecture of the lymph nodes were effaced and there was lymphoid depletion (Fig 3A). No follicle could be identified on H&E sections, but a few peripherally pushed follicles could be seen on CD20 immunohistochemistry (Fig 3B). The lymph nodes were replaced by small lymphocytes which were positive for T cell marker CD3 (Fig 3C) and by histiocytes which were confirmed by positivity with CD68 (Fig 3D). These histiocytes exhibited florid hemophagocytosis (Figs 4A and B). Immunohistochemistry done on the lymph node (Figs 4C to E) with EBV ZEBRA (cytoplasmic), EBNA2 (nuclear) and LMP1 (nuclear) were positive indicating an EBV infection. The ***liver*** (Fig 5A) was enlarged and weighed 1,600 g. The portal tracts (Figs 5B and C) were expanded with a florid LH infiltrate (CD 68++, CD3 ++), but only an occasional histiocyte exhibited hemophagocytosis. The ***spleen*** (Fig. 5D) was three times enlarged and weighed 360 g. On microscopy, the sinuses were packed with a LH infiltrate showing florid hemophagocytosis (Fig. 5E). The terminal part of ***small intestine*** (Fig 6A) was thickened with a grayish discoloration. Sections examined (Fig 6B) from here showed ulceration with an extensive transmural LH infiltrate (CD68 and CD3 positive) exhibiting hemophagocytosis (Fig. 6C). The ***lungs*** showed a small focus of *Aspergillus* bronchopneumonia, focal hemorrhage and pulmonary edema. The kidneys, testis and pancreas showed LH infiltrate with occasional cell showing hemophagocytosis.

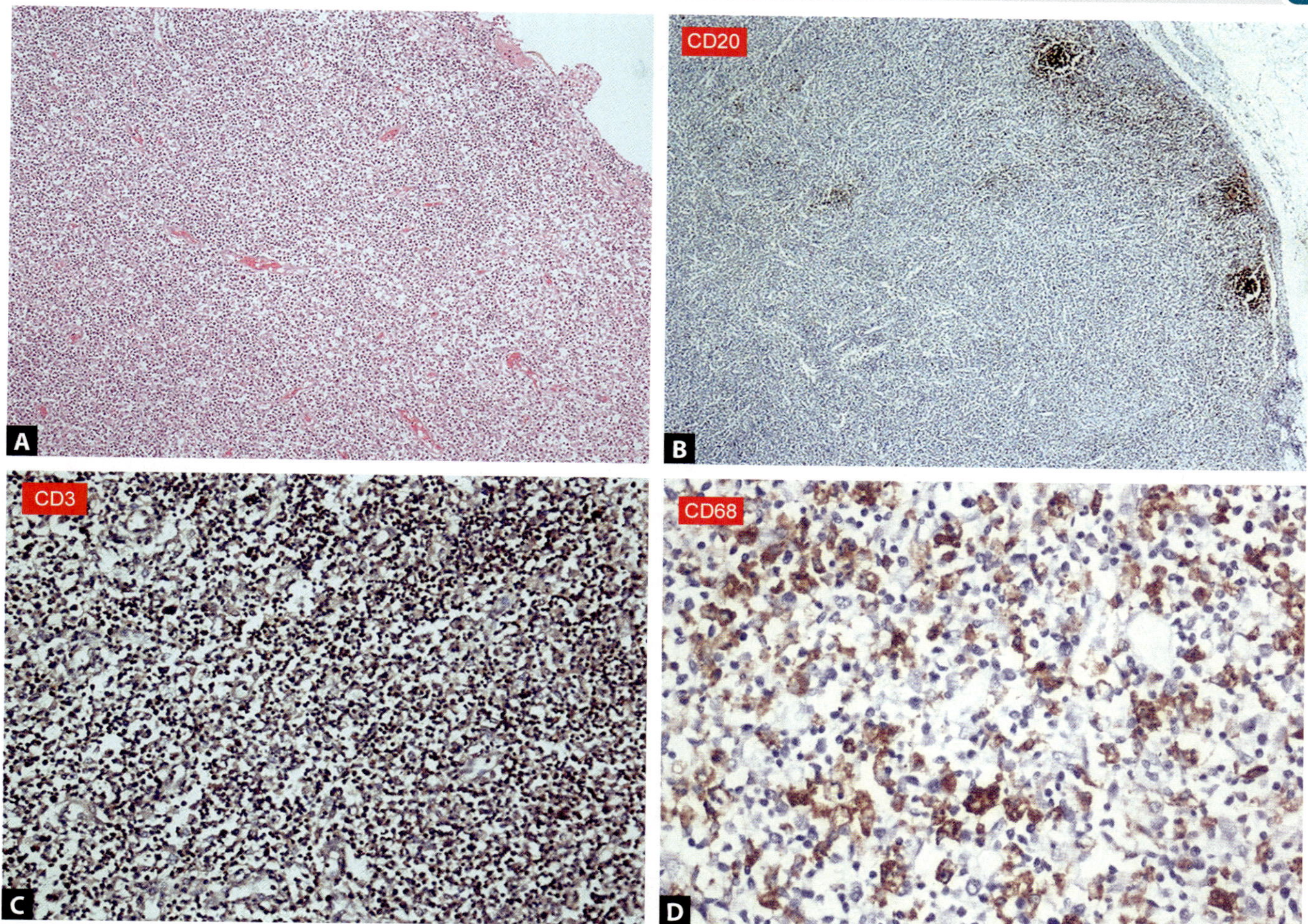

Figs 3A–D: (A) Photomicrograph of the lymph node showing effaced architecture. No lymphoid follicle is discernable. Immunostains on the same lymph node; (B) CD20 showing a few small follicles pushed to the periphery; (C) CD3 showing strong positivity; (D) CD68 showing strong positivity.

FINAL AUTOPSY DIAGNOSIS: PM 21703

22 Years Old Male with Pyrexia of Unknown Origin

Epstein–Barr virus associated Hemophagocytic lymphohistiocytosis (HLH).

Hemophagocytic lymphohistiocytosis—See case 51—PM 20778.

EPSTEIN–BARR VIRUS INFECTION

Epstein-Barr virus is a ubiquitous and predominantly B lymphotropic, gamma herpesvirus 4, which causes infectious mononucleosis, a self-limited, benign lymphoproliferative condition which is generally seen in young adults and adolescents. Infectious mononucleosis presents with fever, sore throat, generalized lymphadenopathy, splenomegaly and atypical T lymphocytes in the peripheral blood. Hepatitis, meningoencephalitis, a faint widely scattered erythematous maculopapular rash and pneumonia can be seen. EBV is also indicated in the pathogenesis of tumors like Burkitt lymphoma, B cell lymphomas in immunosuppressed individuals, a variety of Hodgkins lymphoma, some forms of T cell/NK cell lymphomas and carcinomas like nasopharyngeal carcinoma and some gastric carcinomas. It is transmitted by close contact in human beings, which are the only reservoirs of Epstein–Barr virus. The virus initially infects the epithelial cells of the oropharynx, replicates here and cell lysis leads to spread of virions to the oropharyngeal lymphoid tissues. It soon leads to viremia, with subsequent infection of the lymphoreticular system, including the liver, spleen and B lymphocytes in peripheral blood. Fifty percent

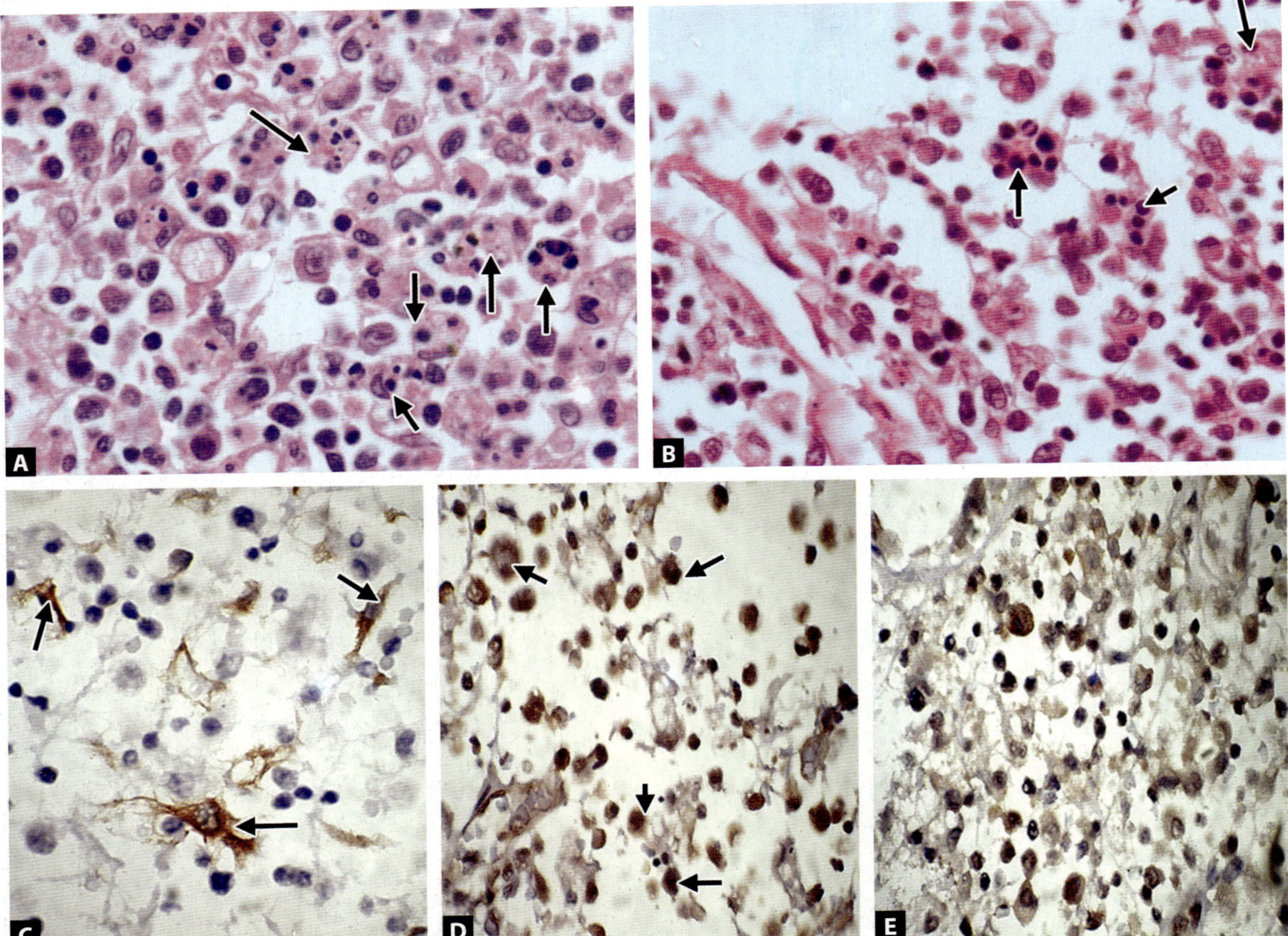

Figs 4A–E: (A and B) Photomicrograph of the lymph node showing hemophagocytizing histiocytes (arrows). Anti-Epstein–Barr virus (EBV) immunohistochemistry on the lymph nodes; (C) Anti-EBV Zebra shows positive cells; (D and E) Anti-EBV latent membrane protein and EBNA2 shows nuclear positivity.

of the population is infected by the age of 5 years and 90% by the age of 25 years. In children the primary infection may be asymptomatic or may lead to mild derangement of the liver function tests. In adolescents it may either present as a syndrome of acute infectious mononucleosis or could be totally asymptomatic. The immune response to the viral infection occurs in the form of large atypical CD8+ T lymphocytes seen in circulation, which combat the B lymphocytes infested with the EBV. Thus in the normal individuals, B cell proliferation that occurs due to EBV infestation gets controlled and the individual either remains asymptomatic or acquires a self-limited bout of infectious mononucleosis. However in the immunosuppressed individuals, reactivation of EBV leads to B cell proliferation and finally to B cell lymphomas. The B cells are infested by the EBV via the complement receptor CD21. After the primary infection, the B lymphocytes are capable of acquiring a latent infection wherein they show no viral replication, remain viable, express viral proteins as an extrachromosomal episome, which rarely integrates into the cell genome, but does replicate with cell division and are passed to subsequent generations of cells. EBV infection leads to proliferation of B cells by the process of hijacking many normal signaling pathways, thereby expanding the pool of latently infected B cells. Few EBV encoded proteins responsible for the latency, activation and proliferation of the B cells are:

- Latent membrane protein-1 (LMP-1) is an ***EBV*** gene which is oncogenic, acts like a CD40 receptor and is a key recipient of the helper T cell signals which stimulate the B cell growth. LMP-1 also activates the JAK/

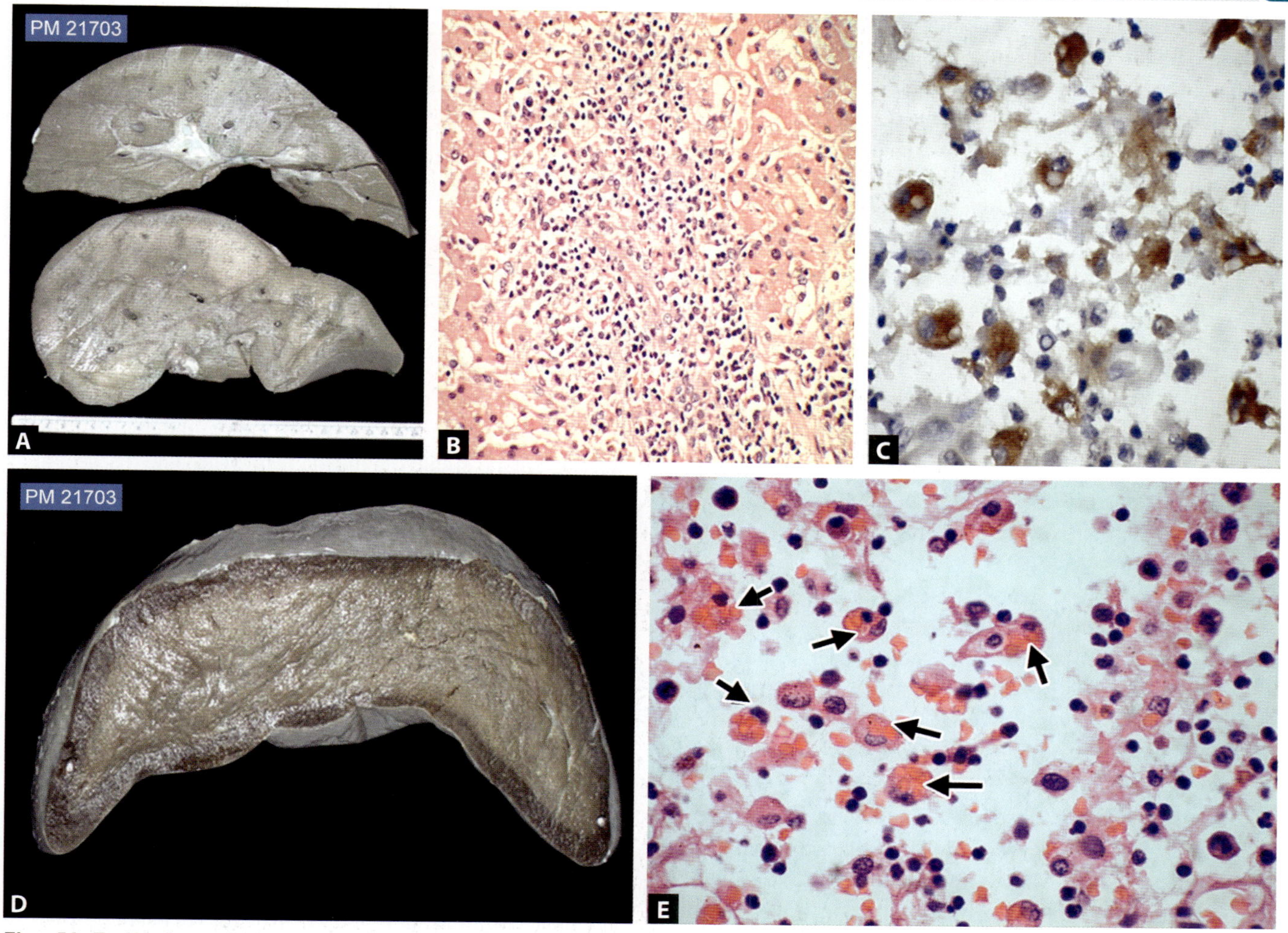

Figs 5A–E: (A) Coronal slices of the enlarged liver; (B) Photomicrograph of the liver showing dense portal lymphohistiocytic infiltrate; (C) Portal infiltrate positive for CD68 immunostain; (D) Coronal slice of the markedly enlarged spleen; (E) Photomicrograph of the spleen showing hemophagocytosis (arrows).

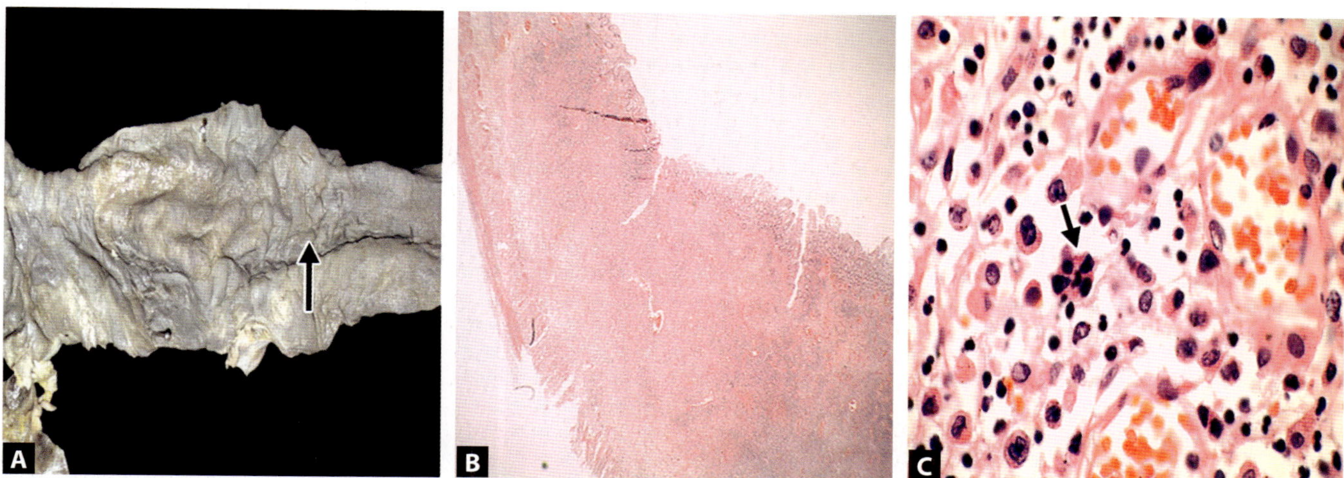

Figs 6A–C: (A) Gross picture of the mucosal aspect of the terminal ileum showing thickening and ulceration (arrow); (B) Low power photomicrograph of the thickened and ulcerated terminal ileum; (C) Terminal ileum showing dense lymphohistiocytic infiltrate showing hemophagocytosis (arrow).

STAT and the NF-kB signaling pathways, which further promote the B cell survival and proliferation by preventing apoptosis by activating ***BCL2***.

- EBNA-2 is another ***EBV*** gene that encodes a nuclear protein which mimics an active notch receptor. EBNA-2 promotes B cell activation and proliferation by activating many host genes like cyclin D and SRC family of proto-oncogenes.
- EBNA-1 binds the ***EBV*** genome to the host chromosome during mitosis, thereby ensuring that the viral episomes are present in the daughter cells, when the infected cell divides.
- EBV produces a homologue of IL-10 known as vIL10 which suppresses antiviral T cell signals and inhibit the macrophages and the dendritic cells, for the long survival of the infected B cells. The infected B cells proliferate, disseminate and secrete antibodies which form the basis of diagnostic test for mononucleosis.
- Symptoms appear when the host immune response is stimulated, which is mediated by CD8+ cytotoxic T cells and the NK cells. This reactive proliferation of the T cells leads to lymphadenopathy and splenomegaly. IgM antibodies are seen early in the course of the infection and later are replaced by IgG antibodies which persist for life. The diagnosis is based on—(A) Peripheral blood absolute lymphocytosis (>60% of WBCs are lymphocytes) with atypical activated CD8+ T lymphocytes. These are large cells, 10–16 μm in diameter with abundant cytoplasm containing multiple vacuolations, azurophilic granules and an irregular nucleus; (B) Positive heterophile antibody reaction; (C) Rising titers of viral capsid or nuclear antigens. The atypical lymphocytes are highly suggestive of the diagnosis of infectious mononucleosis. The lymph nodes are discrete, tender to palpation and enlarged throughout the body. Nodal enlargement is usually symmetric and enlarged epitrochlear nodes are highly suggestive of infectious mononucleosis. Microscopy in most instances shows an effaced architecture, due to marked paracortical expansion by the proliferating T cells. There may be a few visible follicles or they may be small and peripherally displaced or not seen at all. EBV infected B cells may resemble Reed–Sternberg like cells, thus mimicking a Hodgkin's lymphoma. Immunohistochemistry reveals B cells expressing the latency specific genes like EBNA2 and LMP1. The spleen is 2–3 times enlarged, soft, fleshy and hyperemic. The spleen can rupture from relatively minor trauma or even spontaneously. On microscopic examination it shows expanded white pulp due to the proliferation of the T cells. Liver too shows mild to moderate enlargement with atypical lymphocytes in the portal tracts and sinusoids.

Epstein–Barr Virus-associated Hemophagocytic Lymphohistiocytosis

Hemophagocytic lymphohistiocytosis is a rare, aggressive complication of EBV infection, more commonly observed in adult patients and usually encountered in the setting of primary contact with EBV. Without early and effective therapy, EBV-HLH has a high mortality due to multiorgan failure. Diagnosis of EBV-HLH is a challenge, as it is a syndrome with a combination of minor and major criteria and there is no single diagnostic test for it. The disease takes over like an avalanche and the diagnosis is generally delayed. EBV-HLH is a clinicopathological syndrome consisting of a dysregulated, hyperinflammatory, immune response leading to a cytokine storm. EBV-HLH may occur at any age and affects patients having a normal immune system, but more so in patients having immune defects. It is characterized by fever, splenomegaly, cytopenia, hypertriglyceridemia, hypofibrinogenemia, hyperferritinemia, high serum levels of lactate dehydrogenase and soluble CD25. This is accompanied by histological evidence of hemophagocytosis. The infectious agents leading to HLH are EBV, Parvovirus, Cytomegalovirus, Herpes-simplex virus, Herpes Virus 8, Varicella zoster and HIV infection alone or in combination. The most common agent associated with HLH and leading to a poor prognosis is EBV. The EBV-infested B cells stimulate cytotoxic T lymphocytes leading to hypercytokinemia. Awareness of this life-threatening syndrome is the key to early diagnosis and prompt appropriate treatment.

COMMENTARY—INDEX CASE: PM 21703

A young male presented with PUO and jaundice. On examination there was pallor, icterus, hepatosplenomegaly and ascites. Generalized lymphadenopathy was detected on ultrasonography and CECT abdomen. Investigations revealed pancytopenia with progressive fall in counts during the hospital stay, deranged liver and renal function tests, raised transaminases, hypoalbuminemia, hypofibrinogenemia, hypertriglyceridemia, hyperferritinemia and the bone marrow revealed hemophagocytosis. The autopsy exhibited florid hemophagocytic lymphohistiocytosis which was EBV associated. This case fulfills all the criteria for a secondary infection associated HLH.

TAKE HOME MESSAGE

- Hemophagocytic lymphohistiocytosis is a rare, aggressive and fatal complication of EBV infection.
- Awareness of this life-threatening syndrome is the key to early diagnosis and prompt appropriate treatment.

SUGGESTED READING

1. Fisman DN. Hemophagocytic syndromes and infection. Emerg Infect Dis. 2000;6(6):601-8.
2. Goudarzipour K, Kajiyazdi M, Mahdaviyani A. Epstein-Barr virus-induced hemophagocytic lymphohistiocytosis. Int J Hematol Oncol Stem Cell Res. 2013;7(1):42-5.
3. Henter JI, Horne A, Aricó M, et al. Diagnostic and therapeutic guidelines for hemophagocytic lymphohistiocytosis. Pediatr Blood Cancer. 2007;48(2):124-31.
4. Lay JD, Chuang SE, Rowe M, et al. Epstein-Barr virus latent membrane protein-1 mediates upregulation of tumor necrosis factor-alpha in EBV-infected T cells: implications for the pathogenesis of hemophagocytic syndrome. J Biomed Sci. 2003;10:146-55.
5. Rouphael NG, Talati NJ, Vaughan C, et al. Infections associated with haemophagocytic syndrome. Lancet Infect Dis. 2007;7(12):814-22.
6. Sadraei NH, Vejpongsa P, Baljevic M, et al. Epstein-Barr virus-related hemophagocytic lymphohistiocytosis: hematologic emergency in the critical care setting. Case Reports In Hematology. 2015;ID 491567.
7. Torti L, Larocca LM, Massini G, et al. Epstein-Barr Virus (EBV)-associated haemophagocytic syndrome. Mediterr J Hematol Infect Dis. 2012;4(1):e2012008.

CONTRIBUTIONS BY:

1. Dr Savita Kumari, Professor and Head, Department of Internal Medicine (Compilation of Clinical Details)
2. Dr Vinay Sakhuja, Ex-Professor and Head, Department of Nephrology (Clinician In-Charge)

Post Graduate Institute of Medical Education and Research, Chandigarh, India.

SECTION 9

Primary Immunodeficiency Pediatric Cases

CASE 55

Disseminated Bacillus Calmette–Guérin Infection in a Case of Severe Combined Immunodeficiency: PM 22931

Nandita Bharadwaj Kakkar

HIGHLIGHTS OF THE CASE

This was a 6½ month-old male who had recurrent chest infections since birth. There was history of three male sibling deaths due to recurrent chest infections. However, two siblings, i.e. one female (6-year-old, having recurrent urinary tract infections on prophylaxis) and one male (normal) were alive. Clinically it fitted into X-linked recessive, severe combined immunodeficiency (SCID) of T−B+ type. Autopsy revealed marked thymic atrophy with dysplasia, profound lymphoid depletion and disseminated Bacillus Calmette–Guérin (BCG) infection with a very heavy bacillary load.

Keywords: Primary immunodeficiency, severe combined immunodeficiency, SCID, T−B+ type, Bacillus Calmette–Guérin infection, disseminated, polymerase chain reaction, autopsy.

CLINICAL DETAILS

Date of Admission: 09.12.2008, Date of Death: 17.12.2008, Duration of Hospital Stay: 9 Days

This was a 6½ month-old male, who was admitted twice in the past one month to PGIMER Chandigarh, with history of recurrent chest infections since birth. He had been admitted twice outside, diagnosed as pneumonia and received antibiotics. There was history of three male sibling deaths at 5 months, 4½ months and 5½ months due to recurrent chest infections. However, two siblings, i.e. one female (6 years, was having recurrent urinary tract infections and was on prophylaxis) and one male (normal) were alive. This glaring history, however pointed toward an X-linked recessive immunodeficiency and so the index baby was referred to our institute. In the first admission in PGI, there was wet sounding paroxysmal cough, respiratory distress with retractions and oral candidiasis. Chest X-ray had shown right upper lobe (RUL) consolidation. He was again diagnosed as having pneumonia and treated with a combination of intravenous antibiotics for 10 days and discharged on oral antibiotics. Within 15 days, he was readmitted with respiratory distress, abnormal movements and an altered sensorium. On examination, the weight was 5.5 kg, length 68 cm with an occipito-frontal circumference of 38 cm. He was pale. Chest examination revealed intercostal retractions. The liver was palpable 5 cm below right costal margin, span 9 cm and was firm. The spleen was palpable 4 cm below the left costal margin. CNS examination revealed E4 M6 V.

Investigations and Course and Management

***Hemogram*:** Hb 6.5 g/dL, TLC 18800/uL, DLC P90, L5, M3, E2, platelets 11000/uL, coagulogram mildly deranged.

Other Investigations*:** Total serum proteins/ albumin—2.5/0.8 gm, total serum bilirubin/conjugated fraction—1.6/1.25 mg%, S urea/S creatinine 18/0.6 mg%, HIV ELISA non reactive, blood culture grew ***Pseudomonas aeruginosa, serology for toxoplasma, rubella and CMV negative, CSF-within normal limits and X-ray chest showed diffuse perihilar infiltrates.

Immune workup: IgG: 294 mg% (N 300-900), IgA: 49 mg % (N 15-70), IgM: 88 mg% (40–160). Absolute lymphocyte count: 940, CD3 +ve cells: absent, CD 19+ cells- 86%. Absolute B cell count 808.

The child was given oxygen, intravenous (IV) antibiotics and intravenous immunoglobulin (IVIG) 1 g/kg. On day 5, he had worsening of respiratory distress, was intubated and put on intermittent positive pressure respiration. He had two left focal seizures, was dilantinized but suffered a sudden cardiac arrest from which he could not be resuscitated. Units final clinical diagnosis was—Primary immunodeficiency, ? X-linked recessive SCID with recurrent pneumonia, ? cystic fibrosis.

AUTOPSY FINDINGS: PM 22931

A complete autopsy was performed on this 6-month-old male child, this being the fourth male sibling death with two siblings (one female and one male) being alive and doing well. The peritoneal cavity yielded 300 mL of straw-colored fluid. The entire fibrofatty tissue in the retrosternal area was processed to look for the ***thymus*** which was markedly atrophic (Fig 1A) and weighed 3 g. Microscopically, the thymus did not show any distinction between cortex and medulla, was dysplastic and was reduced to its basic epithelial structure. It was totally devoid of lymphocytes and an occasional dysplastic Hassall's corpuscle (Fig 1B) was appreciated. The entire thymus was however replaced by foamy histiocytes (Fig 1C). Immunohistochemistry for B cell marker, i.e. CD20 showed a few scattered B cells (Fig 1D) but the T cell marker, CD3 was totally negative (Fig 1E). Other ***lymphoid organs***, i.e. the appendix (Fig 2A), small intestine (Fig 2B), spleen (Fig 2C) and lymph nodes (Fig 2D), were severely depleted of lymphoid tissue. Immunohistochemistry done on the lymph node revealed an occasional small cluster of CD20 positive B cells (Fig 2E), CD3 stain did not highlight even a single T cell (Fig 2F) and the histiocyte marker CD68 (Fig 2G) was strongly positive, indicating total replacement of the lymph node by foamy histiocytes. The peripheral blood

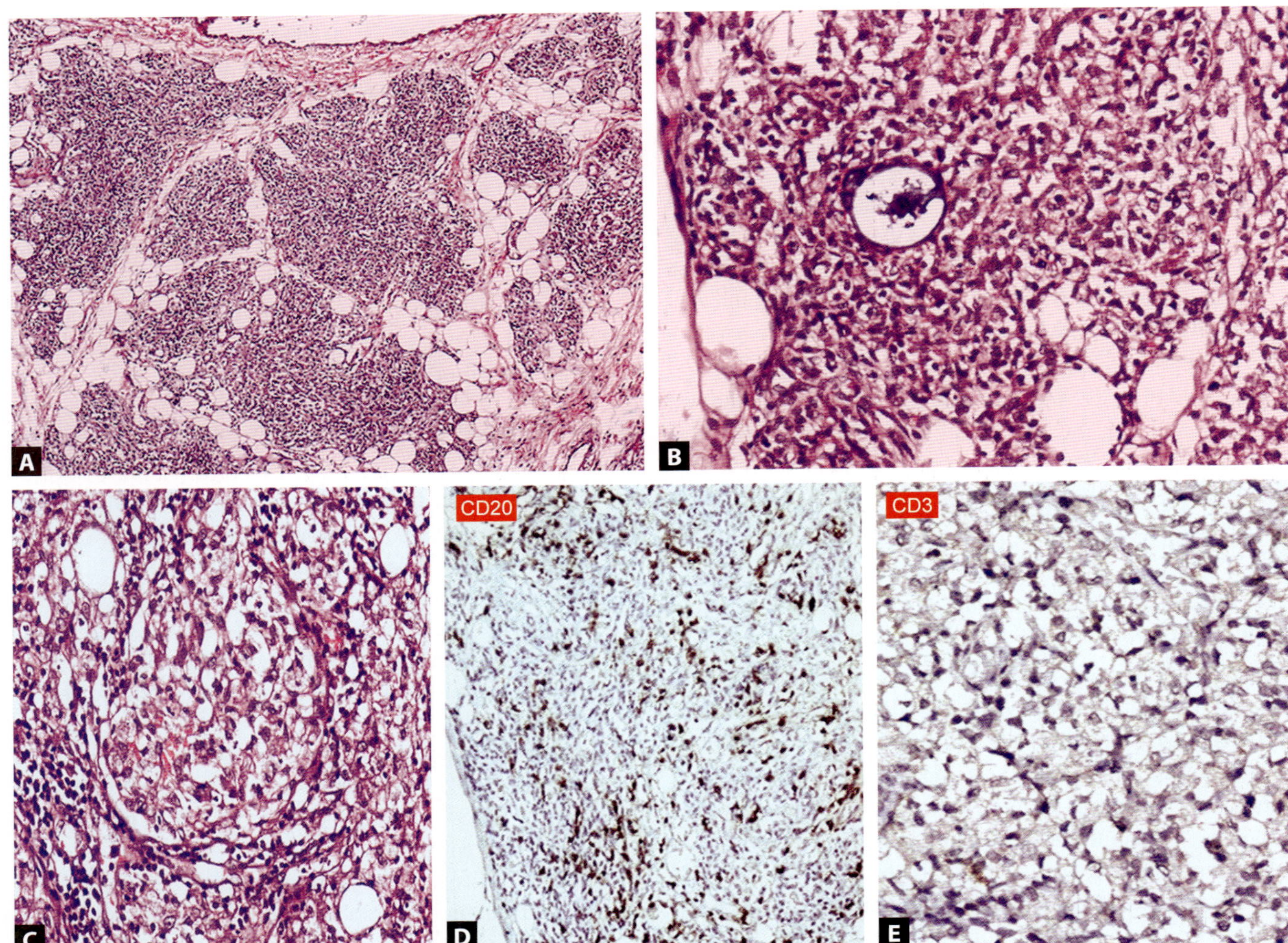

Figs 1A–E: (A) Low power view of the thymus which is markedly atrophic, devoid of lymphoid tissue, and shows no distinction into cortex and medulla; (B) Thymus showing a dysplastic Hassall corpuscle and foamy cells; (C) At a higher power, the thymus is seen depleted of lymphocytes and is replaced by foamy cells; (D) CD20 immunostain shows few scattered B lymphocytes; (E) CD3 immunostain does not show a single T cell.

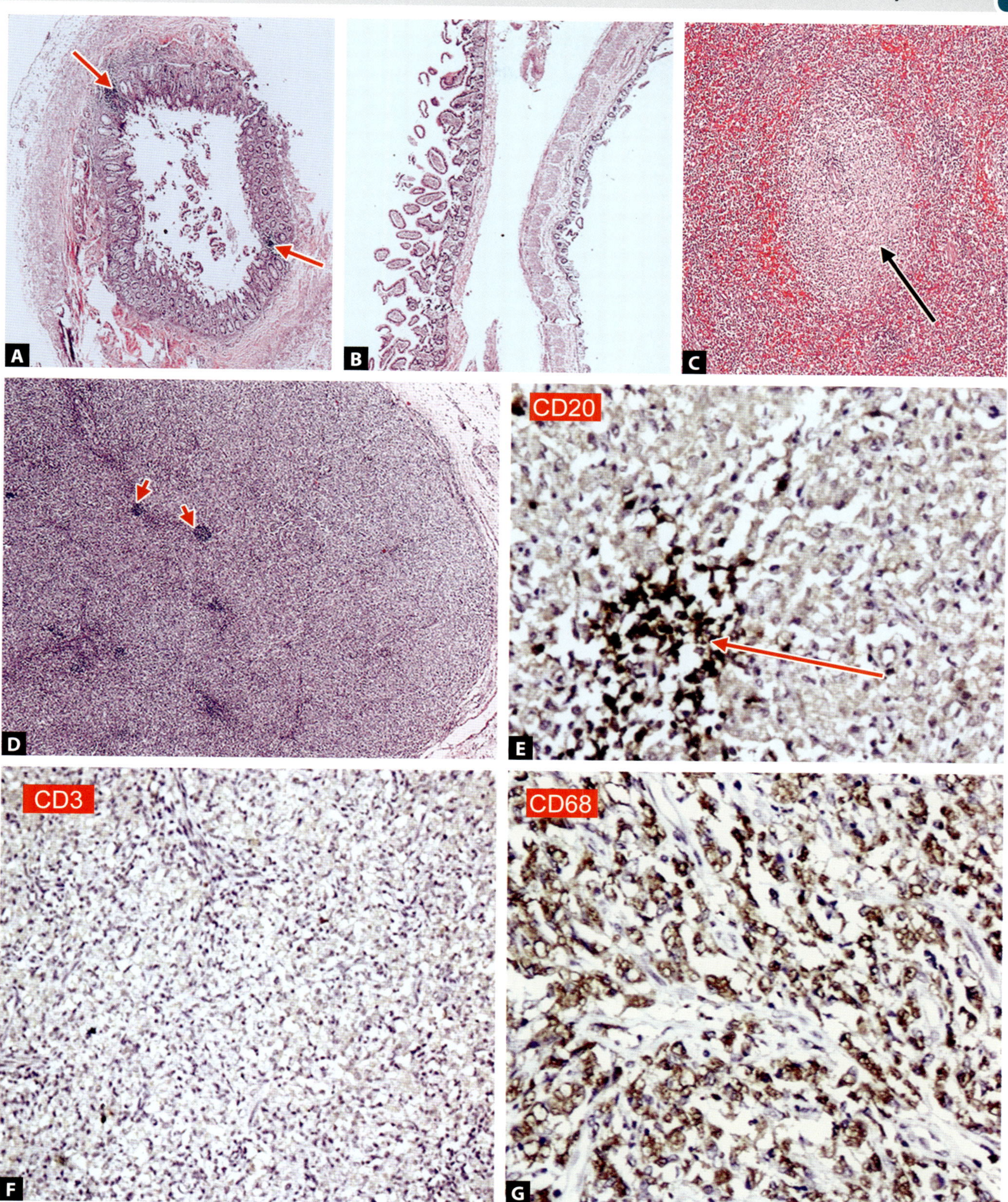

Figs 2A–G: (A to C) Section from appendix, terminal ileum and splenic white pulp show depletion of lymphoid tissue (arrows); (D) Lymph node replaced by foamy cells and shows tiny remnants of lymphocytes (arrows); (E) CD20 immunostain on the lymph node highlights the tiny cluster of B lymphocytes; (F) T cell marker CD3 on the lymph node is negative; (G) Macrophage marker CD68 on the lymph node shows strong positivity.

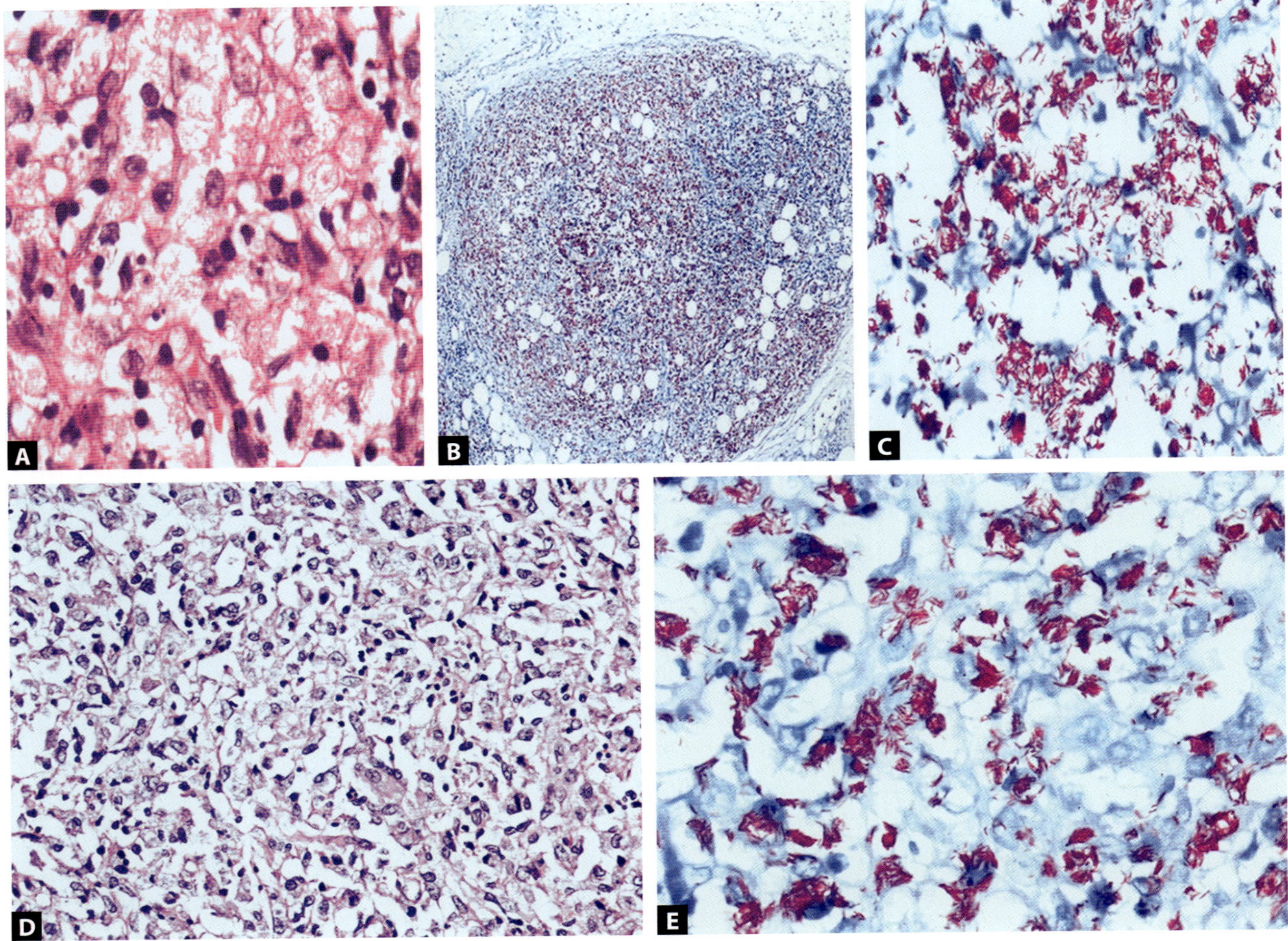

Figs 3A–E: (A) High power view of the thymus showing total replacement by foamy histiocytes; (B and C) Thymus at low and high power replete with red colored acid-fast bacilli on Ziehl–Neelsen stain; (D) Section of the lymph node at high power showing sheets of foamy histiocytes; (E) Ziehl–Neelsen stain on the lymph node, showing faggots of acid-fast bacilli.

showed a severe lymphocytopenia (TLC: 18,800/µL; P- 90, L-05, M-03, E-02), with 0% CD3 positive cells, 86% CD19 positive cells, an absolute lymphocyte count of 940, absolute T-cell count of 0 and absolute B cell count of 808. The immunoglobulins were however within normal limits [IgG 299 mg% (N: 300–900), IgA: 49 mg% (N: 15–70), IgM: 88 mg% (N: 40–160)]. Taking into consideration the above findings, the primary disorder in this case was a primary immunodeficiency, highly suggestive of SCID of the T−B+ type.

The atrophic ***thymus*** was totally replaced by foamy histiocytes (Fig 3A). Ziehl-Neelsen stain showed florid acid-fast bacilli (AFB) positivity at low power (Fig 3B) and at high power, faggots could be seen within and outside the histiocytes (Fig 3C). The ***lymph nodes*** (paraaortic, peripancreatic, hilar) were 0.5–2 cm in size. On microscopic examination there was total lymphoid depletion and replacement by foamy histiocytes (Fig 3D) loaded with acid-fast tubercle bacilli on Ziehl-Neelsen staining (Fig 3E). The ***spleen*** weighed 55 g, as against a normal weight of 23 g. On cut section tiny white nodules, 0.1–0.5 cm, were present diffusely (Fig 4A). On microscopic examination the spleen was devoid of white pulp which was replaced by leproma-like nodules (Fig 4B) composed of foamy histiocytes with granular material (Fig 4C). No epithelioid cells or lymphocytes were seen. Ziehl-Neelsen stain showed florid positivity with AFB seen diffusely at low power (Fig 4D). The liver (Fig 5A) weighed 440 g, as against a normal of

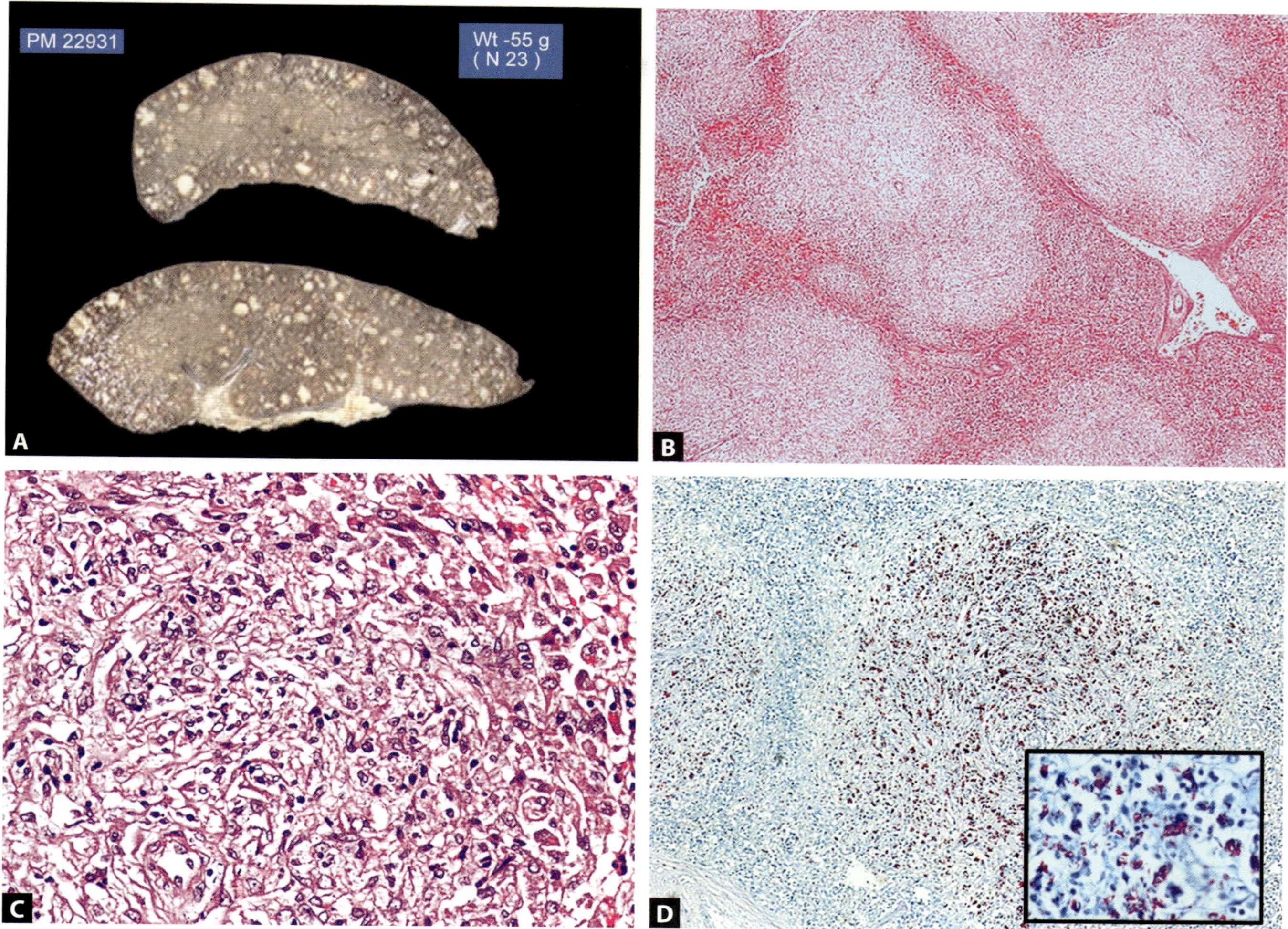

Figs 4A–D: (A) Coronal slices of the enlarged spleen showing tiny white nodules scattered diffusely; (B) Low power view of the tiny nodules which have a pale appearance; (C) Nodules at high power show leproma-like granuloma composed of foamy histiocytes; (D) Ziehl–Neelsen stain at low power and high power (inset) shows the histiocytes in the nodule packed with acid-fast bacilli.

276 g, at this age. It was pale and mildly bile stained. Cut section revealed exaggerated mottling and an occasional millet-sized nodule. On microscopic examination, diffuse macrovesicular steatosis and leproma-like granulomas (Fig 5B) composed of foamy histiocytes showing strong AFB positivity (Fig 5B inset) were seen. The lungs weighed 220 g. The pleura showed areas of hemorrhage (Fig 6A) and the cut section also revealed extensive hemorrhagic consolidation (Fig 6B). On microscopic examination alveolar spaces were seen to be packed with histiocytes and pink granular debris (Fig 7A). Confluent necrotizing giant cell pneumonia, angioinvasive and bronchoinvasive aspergillosis (Figs 7C and D), pulmonary hemorrhage and squamous metaplasia of the bronchial lining was also noted. Ziehl–Neelsen staining shows clusters of acid-fast tubercle bacilli (Fig 7B) within and outside the histiocytes. No well-formed granulomas were seen and the tuberculosis was totally nonreactive. The ***kidneys***, on gross examination, appeared congested (Fig 8A) and on microscopic examination, interstitial inflammation (Fig. 8B) with histiocytes containing acid-fast tubercle bacilli (Fig 8B inset) was seen. The ***bone marrow*** was hypocellular with increased number of plasma cells, megakaryocytes appeared dysplastic, mild erythrophagocytosis could be appreciated and scattered foamy histiocytes (Fig. 8C) were present which revealed AFB positivity (Fig. 8D). The ***brain*** weighed 650 g and was normal both grossly and microscopically. Other organs were within normal limits. The pathologist contacted the parents of the baby for the history of BCG vaccination. The parents said that the baby received BCG immunization on day 50 of life, which however did not elicit any skin reaction.

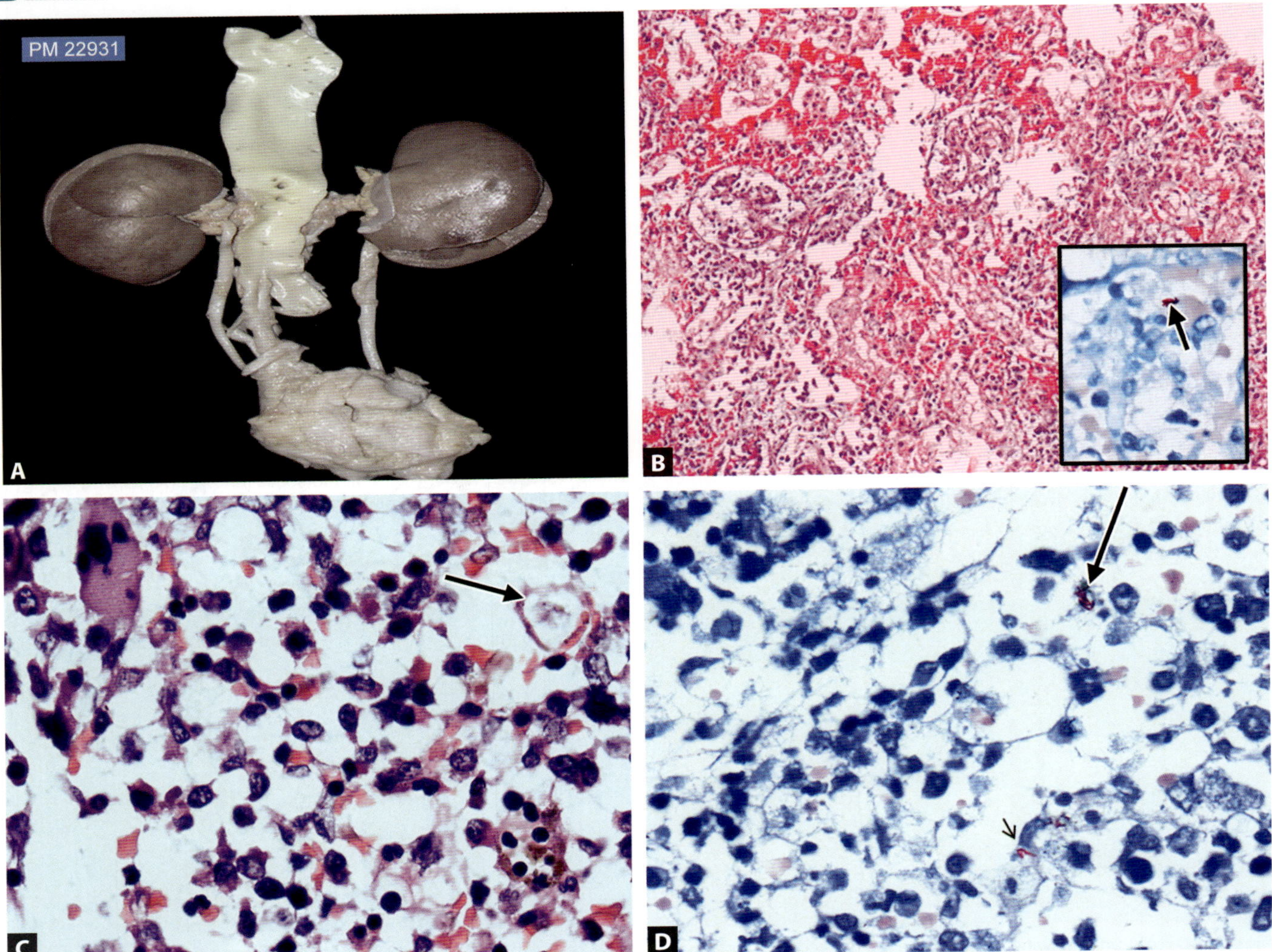

Figs 8A–D: (A) Gross photograph of both the kidneys which appear congested, ureters and urinary bladder along with the abdominal aorta; (B) Photomicrograph from the kidneys shows congestion, interstitial inflammation with foamy histiocytes wherein acid-fast bacilli are found on Ziehl–Neelsen stain (inset); (C and D) Microphotograph from the bone marrow shows interspersed foamy cells (arrow) wherein plenty of acid-fast bacilli are seen on Ziehl–Neelsen staining.

which the most common cause is the deficiency of enzyme adenosine deaminase (ADA). This leads to accumulation of deoxyadenosine and its derivatives which are toxic to the immature lymphocytes particularly of the T-cell lineage.[3] ADA deficient individuals on X-ray examination may show multiple skeletal abnormalities of chondro-osseous dysplasia, which include flaring of the costochondral junction and a bone in bone anomaly in the vertebral body. ADA deficient[4] patients have a more profound lymphopenia than other types of SCID, with mean lymphocyte count of less than 500/mm^3. Milder form of this disease is reported leading to a diagnosis being made in adulthood. Amongst the relatively rarer causes of recessive SCID are mutations of Jak 3,[2] mutations in recombination activation genes and mutations that impair the expression of the class II MHC molecules, thus preventing the development of CD4+ T cells. Infants with SCID are lymphopenic and this is the first indicator of the disease and can aid in early diagnosis. Serum immunoglobulins and antibodies are diminished to absent or can be normal. There are unique lymphocyte phenotypes for the various genetic forms of SCID as highlighted by flow cytometric studies.[4] These are T^-B^+ NK^- SCID, $T^-B^-NK^+$ SCID and T^-B^- NK^- SCID.

Patients with SCID present with thrush, diaper rash, failure to thrive, morbilliform rash (due to graft-versus-host disease as a result of transplacental transfer of maternal T cells) and are susceptible to recurrent severe infections by a wide range of pathogens. The pathogens include *Candida albicans, Pneumocystis carinii, Pseudomonas*, varicella, adenovirus, respiratory syncytial virus, parainfluenza 3, CMV, Epstein–Barr virus and BCG. These infants also lack the ability to reject allografts, leaving them at risk for fatal GVHD.[5] This condition is uniformly fatal in the first 2 years of life, unless immune reconstitution can be accomplished.

Histologic findings in SCID are variable, just as the disease shows diverse forms. The thymus is small, dysplastic, with paucity of lymphoid cells and left overs of the Hassall corpuscles reduced to their basic epithelial structures can be seen. Generally in ADA deficient SCID, left overs of the Hassall's corpuscles can be seen, whereas in X-linked SCID lobules of undifferentiated epithelial cells resembling fetal thymus is seen.[6] In most patients the lymph nodes and tonsils are rudimentary, devoid of lymphocytes and reduced to a reticular sinusoidal framework. Spleen, tonsils and gastrointestinal tract show a marked reduction of the lymphoid component in its T cell areas and most of the times in the B cell areas as well. In ADA deficiency,[7] several distinct pathologic lesions are seen. On microscopic examination, the physeal region shows disorganized chondrocyte columns, ballooned lacunae and necrotic chondrocytes, kidney may show mesangial sclerosis and adrenal gland may show cortical fibrosis. Bone marrow transplantation is the treatment of choice. Gene therapy has also been successful, but has limitations.[8]

BACILLUS CALMETTE–GUÉRIN INFECTION

Bacillus Calmette-Guérin, one of the most widely used vaccines generally given at birth, is developed from the live attenuated strain of ***Mycobacterium bovis*** and is used to prevent ***M. tuberculosis*** infection. In the majority of cases, BCG vaccine is harmless and may lead to minor complications like localized abscesses or regional lymphadenitis. But the most dreaded and fatal complication is a disseminated BCG infection[9-11] which is often associated with an underlying immunodeficiency.[12-14] This immunodeficiency could be primary like SCID, chronic granulomatous disease (CGD) of childhood, a form of specific cellular immunodeficiency (CID) or acquired like in HIV infection. In patients with immunodeficiency syndromes, BCG vaccination should not be given. Gonzalez et al.[15] highlighted nine children with immunodeficiency syndromes (2 with SCID, 2 with CGD and 4 with CID) who developed persistent or disseminated BCG infection at birth. They calculated the risk of BCG infection to be 3.4/10,00,000 vaccinated newborns, which closely reflects the incidence of severe congenital immunodeficiencies. The clinical presentations in these patients varied according to the type of underlying immunodeficiency. Gonzalez observed two siblings with SCID, who were vaccinated with BCG at birth, but in who BCG infection did not develop. It is postulated that in such patients, there is a high innate, monocyte–macrophage-mediated resistance to BCG, thereby allowing them to kill BCG in the absence of T-cell mediated immunity. Immunodeficiency, either primary or secondary should be suspected, if after giving BCG injection, no local reaction or scar is elicited. The practice of BCG revaccination, if the BCG vaccination at birth leaves no scar, should be discontinued and the child rather should be investigated for an immunodeficiency.

Casanova et al.[16] analyzed 16 cases of BCG infection with dissemination to two areas beyond the inoculation site and with no well-defined immunodeficiency condition. Of these, there were 8 boys and 8 girls and consanguinity was present in 5/16 cases. The prevalence was estimated at 0.59 cases per 1 million vaccinated children. These children presented with fever and cachexia. Of the 16 cases, BCG infection had disseminated to the lymph nodes in 15, skin in 13, soft tissues, lungs, spleen and liver in 11 each and to the bones in 9. Apart from this, 8 children had severe opportunistic infection with Salmonella enteric serotypes (7 cases) and Mycobacterium abscessus (1 case). Casanova et al.[16] concluded that BCG infection is a rare but severe complication of BCG vaccination. Why some children are prone to this, is not known. But this phenomenon could be due to a yet not determined, genetic immunodeficiency condition that affects the killing of intracellular bacteria such as BCG and ***Salmonella***.

There are other studies[17] in which no underlying immunodeficiency could be detected in cases of disseminated BCG infection. Such cases were considered as idiopathic. Tardieu et al.[18] reported two cases of BCG meningitis in children who were vaccinated previously with BCG, without any adverse symptoms. A specific or distinct mutation of the interferon-yR1 gene,[19,20] may lead to BCG infection in vaccinated children or to atypical mycobacterial infection in unvaccinated children. The former, however has a worse prognosis due to the higher virulence and higher numbers of infecting BCG organisms. Vaccination with all currently used BCG substrains is contraindicated in children with interferon-yR1 deficiency. Fatal disseminated BCG infection is due to a complete deficiency of interferon-yR1. Milder forms of the disease may however be seen. On microscopic examination, there are two distinct forms of idiopathic BCG infection. One form shows well-circumscribed tuberculoid granulomas with few AFB and is associated with a good prognosis. The other form shows ill-formed leproma-like granulomas, replete with AFB and is associated with a fatal outcome. This may be due to either different mutations of the interferon-γR1 gene or mutations of another gene.

COMMENTARY—INDEX CASE: PM 22931

This is a case of X-linked recessive, SCID of T−B+ type along with disseminated BCG infection (confirmed by PCR) in a 6½ month-old male baby. The baby had recurrent chest infections since birth. There was peripheral lymphocytopenia with an absolute lymphocyte count of 940, absolute T cell count of 0 and absolute B cell count of 808. Serum immunoglobulins, were however within normal limits due to the transplacental transfer of immunoglobulins from the mother as the child is only 6 months old. There were four male sibling deaths (index case being the fourth one), with two siblings, i.e. one female (on prophylaxis for recurrent urinary tract infection) and one male being alive and doing well. The index baby received BCG immunization on day 50 of life, which however did not elicit any skin reaction. The parents went back for revaccination, but the pediatrician asked them to wait and watch. At autopsy there was marked thymic atrophy with dysplasia and profound lymphoid depletion in the lymph nodes, spleen and gastrointestinal tract. There was disseminated BCG infection (proven by PCR) with the thymus, lymph nodes and the lung replaced by histiocytes packed with red-colored faggots of AFB. The spleen and liver however showed leproma-like granulomas replete with AFB. The bacillary load was so heavy, that the baby had virtually been converted into a culture plate of ***Mycobacterium bovis***.

TAKE HOME MESSAGE

- Severe combined immunodeficiency is a group of disorders characterized by defects in both cell- and antibody-mediated immunity.
- The most common form is the X-linked SCID, accounting for approximately 50% of the cases. This is followed by autosomal recessive SCID (30%), of which the most common cause is the deficiency of enzyme ADA.
- Various genetic forms of SCID are—T^-B^+ NK^- SCID, T^- B^- NK^+ SCID and T^- B^- NK^- SCID.
- Peripheral lymphocytopenia is the first indicator of the disease and can aid in early diagnosis.
- In SCID, the thymus is atrophic, dysplastic, devoid of lymphoid cells and remnants of Hassall's corpuscles can be found and it is reduced to its basic epithelial structure.
- In SCID, lymphoid rich organs, i.e. the lymph nodes, tonsils, appendix, small intestine and spleen show severe lymphoid depletion.
- Bacillus Calmette-Guérin, one of the most widely used vaccine, is developed from the live attenuated strain of Mycobacterium bovis and is used to prevent *M. tuberculosis* infection.
- Bacillus Calmette-Guérin vaccine is harmless and may lead to minor complications like localized abscesses or regional lymphadenitis.
- The most dreaded and fatal complication of BCG vaccination is a disseminated BCG infection, which is often associated with an underlying immunodeficiency.
- Bacillus Calmette-Guérin vaccination should be avoided in patients with underlying immunodeficiencies.
- Disseminated BCG infection can occur without an underlying immunodeficiency. This occurs in cases with interferon-γR1 deficiency.

REFERENCES

1. Rosen FS. Defects in cell mediated immunity. Clin Immunol Immunopathol. 1986;41:1-7.
2. Leonard WJ. Cytokines and immunodeficiency diseases. Nat Rev Immunol. 2001;1:200-8.
3. Resta A, Thompson LF. SCID: The role of deaminase deficiency. Immunol Today. 1997;18:371-4.
4. Buckley RH, Schiff RI, Schiff SE, et al. Human severe combined immunodeficiency: genetic, phenotypic and functional diversity in one hundred eight infants. J Pediatr. 1997;130:378-87.
5. Buckley RH, Schiff RI, Schiff SE, et al. Hematopoietic stem cell transplantation for the treatment of severe combined immunodeficiency. N Engl J Med. 1999;340:508-16.
6. Huber J, Zegers BJ, Schuurman HJ, et al. Pathology of congenital immunodeficiencies. Semin Diagn Pathol. 1992;9:31-62.
7. Ratech H, Greco MA, Gallo G, et al. Pathologic findings in ADA deficient severe combined immunodeficiency. I. Kidney, adrenal and chondro-osseous tissue alterations. Am J Pathol. 1985;120:157-69.
8. Parkman R, Weinberg K, Crooks G, et al. Gene therapy for ADA deficiency. Annu Rev Med. 2000;51:33-47.
9. Liberek A, Korzon M, Bernatowska E, et al. Vaccination-related Mycobacterium bovis BCG infection. Emerg Infect Dis. 2006;12:860-2.
10. Rezai MS, Khotaei G, Mamishi S, et al. Disseminated Bacillus Calmette-Guerin infection after BCG vaccination. J Tropical Pediatr. 2008;54(6):413-6.
11. Talbot EA, Perkins MD, Silva F, et al. Disseminated Bacillus Calmette-Guerin disease after vaccination: case report and review of literature. Clin Infect Dis. 1997;24(6):1139-46.

12. Huang LH, Shyur SD, Weng JD, et al. Disseminated cutaneous Bacillus Calmette-Guerin infection identified by PCR in a patient with X-linked severe combined immunodeficiency. Pediatr Dermatol. 2006;23(6):660-3.
13. Huang LH, Shyur SD, Weng JD, et al. Disseminated Bacillus Calmette-Guerin disease as the initial presentation of X-linked SCID: a case report. Asian Pac J Allergy Immunol. 2005;23(4):221-6.
14. Marchand I, Mahe E, Clerici T, et al. Disseminated Bacillus Calmette-Guerin infection revealing X-linked severe combined immunodeficiency. Ann Dermatol Venerol. 2008;135(8-9):587-90.
15. Gonzalez B, Moreno S, Burdach R, et al. Clinical presentation of Bacillus Calmette-Guerin infections in patients with immunodeficiency syndromes. Pediatr Infect Dis J. 1989;8(4):201-6.
16. Casanova JL, Blanche S, Emile JF, et al. Idiopathic disseminated Bacillus Calmette-Guérin infection: a French national retrospective study. Pediatrics. 1996;98:774-8.
17. Pedersen FK, Engbaek HC, Hertz H, et al. Fatal BCG infection in an immunocompetent girl. Acta Paediatr Scand. 1978;67:519-23.
18. Tardieu M, Truffot–Pernot C, Carriere JP, et al. Tuberculous meningitis due to BCG in two previously healthy children. Lancet. 1988;1:440-1.
19. Jouanguy E, Aktare F, Lamhamedi S, et al. Interferon –γ-receptor deficiency in an infant with fatal Bacillus Calmette-Guerin infection. N Engl J Med. 1996;335(26):1956-61.
20. Newport MJ, Huxley CM, Huston S, et al. A mutation in the interferon–gamma–receptor gene and susceptibility to mycobacterial infection. N Engl J Med. 1996;335:1941-9.

CONTRIBUTIONS BY:

1. Dr Kusum Sharma, Professor, Department of Medical Microbiology (Performing the PCR)
2. Dr Meenu Singh, Professor, Department of Pediatrics (Compilation of Clinical Details)
3. Dr Biman Saikia, Professor, Department of Immunopathology (Immune Workup)
4. Dr Surjit Singh, Professor and Head, Department of Pediatrics (Clinician In-Charge)

Post Graduate Institute of Medical Education and Research, Chandigarh, India.

CASE 56

Chronic Granulomatous Disease of Childhood: PM 24170

Nandita Bharadwaj Kakkar

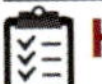

HIGHLIGHTS OF THE CASE

A 7-month-old male child with previous three male sibling deaths at the age of 3 months, 14 months and 9 months. His five female siblings are alive and normal. Maternal aunt had also lost three male babies at 6 days, 12 months and 13 months of age. Index case suffered recurrent respiratory and urinary tract infections, ischiorectal abscess and developmental delay. Splenohepatomegaly was present. There was hyperglobulinemia and the nitroblue tetrazolium (NBT) test was positive. Clinical diagnosis was 'Chronic granulomatous disease of childhood with sepsis. Autopsy was consistent with a diagnosis of chronic granulomatous disease of childhood (CGD). Florid chronic active inflammation with both histiocytic/suppurative granulomas and pigmented macrophages were seen in the lungs, lymph nodes, spleen, liver, kidneys and thymus.

Keywords: Primary immunodeficiency, chronic granulomatous disease, suppurative granulomas, inherited, X-linked, phagocyte/neutrophil dysfunction, autopsy.

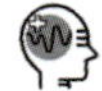

CLINICAL DETAILS

Date of Admission: 09.03.2011, Date of Death: 16.03.2011, Duration of Hospital Stay: 8 Days.

A 7-month-old male baby came with history of high grade fever since 2 months which responded partially to antipyretics. Since day 10 of life, the baby had recurrent episodes of respiratory tract infections, which were treated only to recur after sometime. About 2 months and 1 month prior to this admission, he was admitted twice, in some outside facility. There he was noted to have an ischiorectal abscess which was drained and he received multiple antibiotics. At that time, test for malaria was positive for ***Plasmodium vivax*** and he received chloroquine. Routine urine examination showed pus cells and he was treated for urinary tract infection as well. He also received RBC infusion and intravenous immunoglobulins. The fever however did not respond, his IgG/IgM levels were raised and he was referred to PGIMER, Chandigarh. The baby was born by normal vaginal delivery at 34 weeks gestation. Antenatal ultrasonography was done twice which were normal. There were no antenatal and natal problems. He was breast fed with an additional supplement of cow milk. Developmental delay was present in all sectors. There was no history of contact with tuberculosis. He was ninth in the birth order, with three previous male sibling deaths, at the age of 3 months, 14 months and 9 months. His five female siblings were alive and normal. Maternal aunt, i.e. mother's sister had also lost three male babies at 6 days, 12 months and at 13 months of age, with the reasons for mortality cited as recurrent infections. The baby was adequately immunized with BCG, DPT (3 doses) and OPV (3 doses). On ***examination***, he was afebrile, heart rate was—110/min, respiratory rate—30/min, blood pressure—86 mm Hg (systolic), weight—4.6 kg, length—62 cm and head circumference—41 cm. There was no pallor, icterus, cyanosis, clubbing, lymphadenopathy, edema, ascites the anterior fontanelle was 3 x 3 cm and was not bulging. The liver and spleen were palpable, 1 cm and 5 cm below their respective costal margins. The CNS examination was normal.

Investigations and Course of Management

***Hematological*:** Hb 9.9 g/dL which later fell to 6.5 g/dL, TLC—27000/uL, DLC—P92,L5,M2,E1, platelets were initially 152000/uL and later fell to 42000/uL. Coagulation profile was deranged with PTTK 30s, PTI 43%, fibrinogen 2.06g/dL, D—dimer positive.

Immunological work up: Nitroblue tetrazolium (NBT) test was positive ie control showed 90% neutrophils with purple blue cytoplasmic granules after reacting with a colorless solution of NBT and the neutrophils from the index case showed a total absence of the cytoplasmic reaction product; Immunoglobulins: IgG 1138 (n-54-1610), IgM 171 (n-80-280), IgE 306 (n- 50-109); HIV Elisa non-reactive; T lymphocytes—CD3 –66.7% (n-60-80%), CD19 –22.5%, CD4 -33.6% and CD8 -54.8%.

Blood Biochemistry/Microbiology/others: K^+ 2.9 mEq/l, Na^+ 141 mEq/l, S. urea-65 mg%, S. creatinine 0.9 mg%, total proteins/albumin/globulins—5.3/1.5/3.8 gm, S. bilirubin-2.6 mg%, SGOT/SGPT-491/210 U/L, alkaline phosphatase-361 U/L, Ca^{++} 5.5 mg%, blood culture grew B cepacia complex, urine/ CSF culture were sterile, CSF showed no cells, glucose 45mg%, proteins 116 mg%, grams stain negative; X ray chest was suggestive of bilateral pneumonia. ***Course and management*** – The child developed respiratory distress on the third day of admission with tachypnoea and retractions. On D4 he developed left focal seizures and was put on diazepam and phenytoin. He developed abdominal distension, sepsis, hypokalaemia, respiratory distress worsened, was intubated and ventilated manually, developed shock and cardiac arrest. ***Units clinical diagnosis*** was- Chronic granulomatous disease of childhood with sepsis ? fungal with protein energy malnutrition.

AUTOPSY FINDINGS: PM 24170

A complete autopsy was performed on this 7-month-old male child with three previous male sibling deaths. The serous cavities were within normal limits. The ***lungs*** were heavy and weighed 150 g (normal for age: 111 g). The pleural aspect showed hemorrhages (Fig 1A) and the cut section revealed hemorrhagic consolidation (Fig 1B). On microscopic examination of the lung extensive alveolar hemorrhage, confluent necrotizing pneumonia (Fig 1C), diffuse alveolar damage with prominent hyaline membranes (Fig 1D), active chronic inflammation with ill-defined histiocytic granulomas composed of epithelioid-like cells (Fig 1E) some of which contained giant cell (Fig 1F), suppurative granulomas with polymorphs and nuclear debris in the center and bordered by histiocytes and epithelioid-like cells and compact well-defined easily recognizable granulomas with giant cells (Figs 2A and B) composed of epithelioid cells and histiocytes (Fig 2C) to be appreciated. Pigmented macrophages were present in clusters surrounded by epithelioid-like cells (Fig 2D). The ***lymph nodes*** (mesenteric (Fig 3A), hilar, peripancreatic and paraaortic) were moderately enlarged. Microscopically both suppurative and histiocytic granulomas could be seen with preserved lymphoid tissue (Fig 3B). The histiocytic granulomas contained plenty of giant cells and nondescript pink amorphous material lying in clumps and also within the giant cells (Fig 3C). The pink amorphous material seems to be due to inadequate digestion of intracellular debris due to the faulty microbial killing. Suppurative granulomas were composed of polymorphs and nuclear debris, palisaded by histiocytes and epithelioid cells (Fig 3D). Granulomas with caseation like necrosis (Fig 3E) and few compact granulomas without necrosis were also seen. Pigmented macrophages were seen in plenty in the sinusoids (Fig 3F). The ***spleen*** (Fig 4A) was markedly enlarged and weighed 130 g, as against a normal of 22 g at this age. Cut section revealed tiny white millet-sized nodules present diffusely (Fig 4A). On microscopic examination, multiple suppurative granulomas (Figs 4B and C) composed of polymorphs and nuclear debris bordered by histiocytes, histiocytic granulomas replete with CD68 positive cells (Fig 4D) and pigmented macrophages were seen admixed with lymphoid tissue (Fig 4E). The ***liver*** was slightly enlarged weighing 380 g, as against a normal weight of 288 g at this age (Fig 5A). No focal lesion could be seen. On microscopic examination, it was studded with granulomas (Fig 5B), both histiocytic with pigmented macrophages (Fig 5C) and suppurative (Fig 5D), which were present both in the portal tracts and liver parenchyma. Macrovesicular steatosis was prominent. The ***kidneys*** (Fig 6A) showed multiple areas of hemorrhage on the capsular aspect and on cut section, both in the cortex and medulla. Microscopic examination showed features of acute pyelonephritis (Fig 6B) with the medullary tubules packed with polymorphs and nuclear debris. Along with this ill-formed histiocytic granulomas (Fig 6C) were also seen. Apart from this, histiocytic granulomas were seen in the ***skeletal muscle*** (Fig 6D), where they were seen to be destroying the muscle bundles. The ***brain*** revealed hemorrhages in the cerebellar folia and on microscopic examination there were histiocytic collections in the subarachnoid space (Fig 7A). The entire tissue found behind the sternum was processed. The ***thymus*** (Fig 7B) weighed approximately 1 g (n: 10 g) and on microscopic examination showed involution with Hassall's corpuscles, excess of macrophages, many of them pigmented and ill-formed histiocytic granulomas (Fig 7C). Adequate lymphoid tissue was present in the lymph nodes, spleen, small intestine and appendix. Stain for acid-fast bacilli (AFB), Periodic acid-Schiff (PAS) and Grocott done

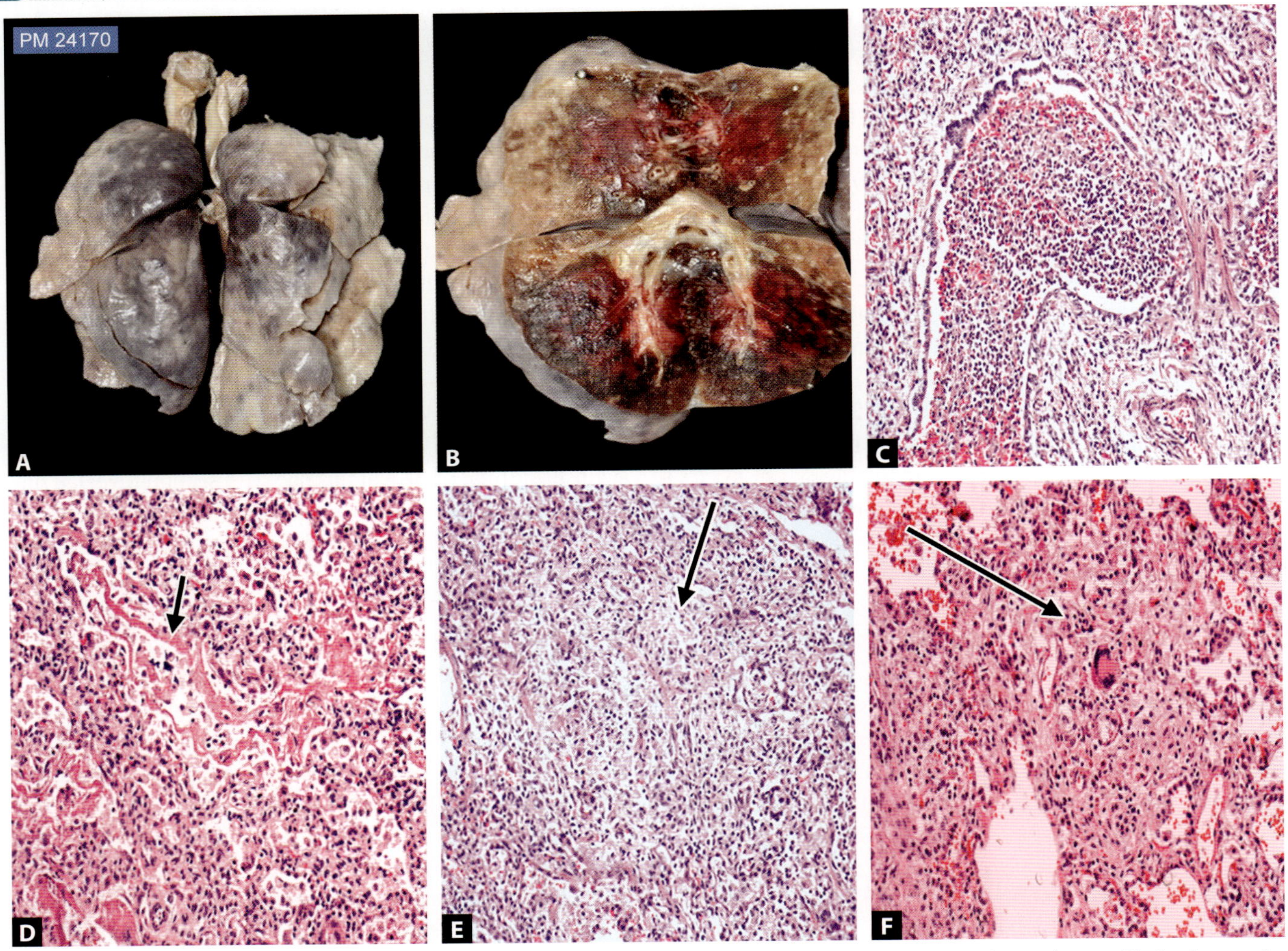

Figs 1A–F: (A) Lungs showing extensive pleural hemorrhages; (B) Cut section of the lung showing fresh hemorrhages. Photomicrographs of the lung showing; (C) Bronchopneumonia; (D) Diffuse alveolar damage with hyaline membrane formation (arrow); (E) Ill-formed histiocytic granuloma (arrow), and (F) Better defined granuloma with a giant cell.

on multiple sections of the lung, lymph nodes, spleen, liver and kidneys did not reveal any organism.

FINAL AUTOPSY DIAGNOSIS: PM 24170

7 Months Old Male with Previous Three Male Sibling Deaths

Consistent with Chronic granulomatous disease of childhood (CGD)–X-linked

- Florid active/chronic inflammation with histiocytic/suppurative granulomas in the lungs, lymph nodes, spleen, liver, kidneys, muscle and thymus.
- Confluent necrotizing pneumonia with diffuse alveolar damage.
- Acute pyelonephritis.

CHRONIC GRANULOMATOUS DISEASE OF CHILDHOOD

Chronic granulomatous disease of childhood[1] is a rare, inherited, primary disorder of the phagocyte/neutrophil function that was first described by Janeway et al in 1950s, when they described five children with recurrent infections and hyperglobulinemia. It was said to be a syndrome affecting the males who succumbed to their illness in the first decade of life with recurrent life-threatening infections (bacterial/fungal), hepatosplenomegaly, lymphadenopathy and hypergammaglobulinemia. In this condition the phagocytes are defective, are unable to kill organisms due to the paucity of oxidants.

CGD occurs due to a defect in the enzyme NADPH (reduced nicotinamide adenine dinucleotide phosphate) oxi-

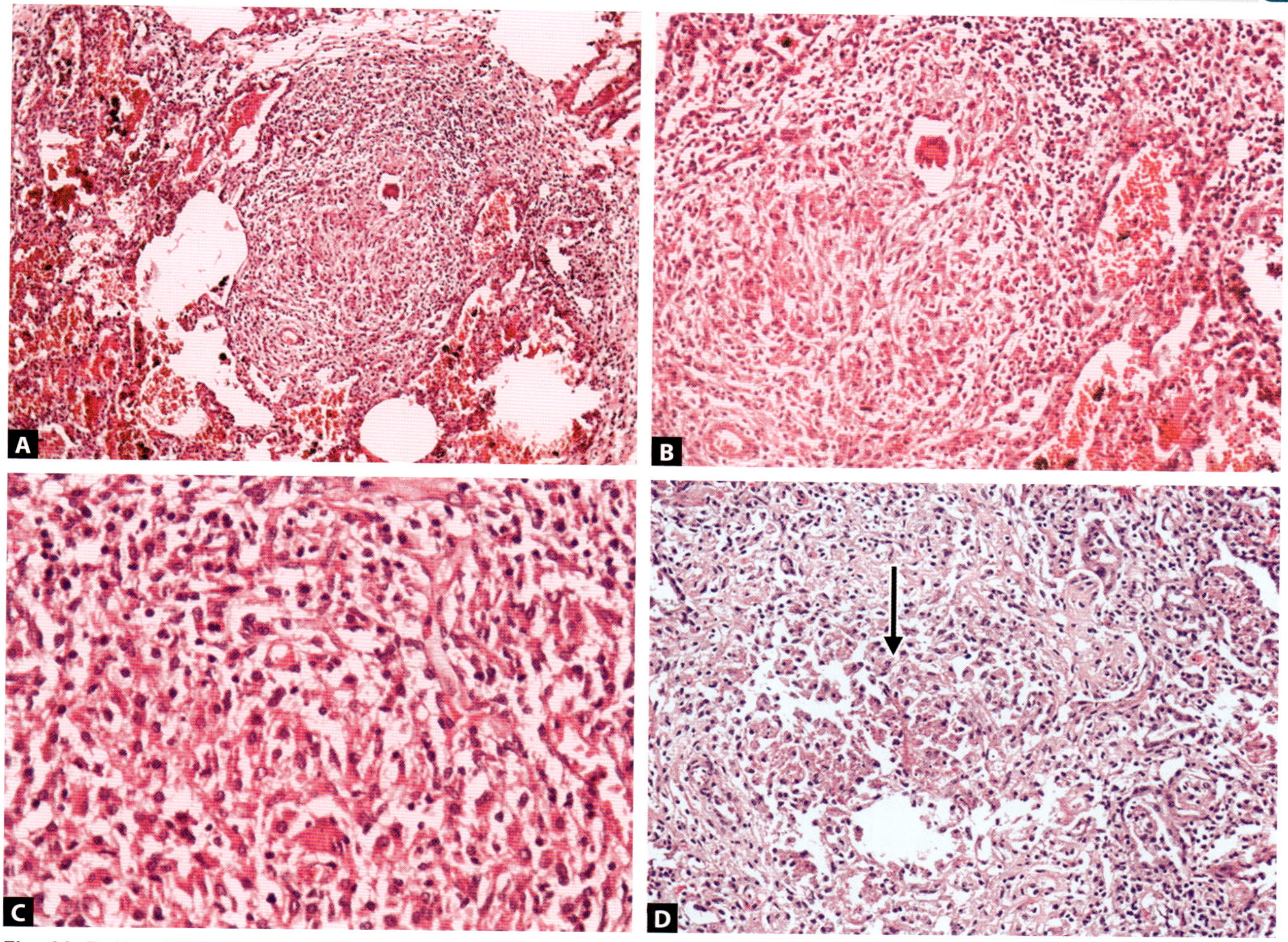

Figs 2A–D: (A and B) Lung showing well-formed histiocytic granulomas with giant cell; (C) High power of the granuloma composed of histiocytes and epithelioid-like cells; (D) Collection of pigmented macrophages surrounded by histiocytes.

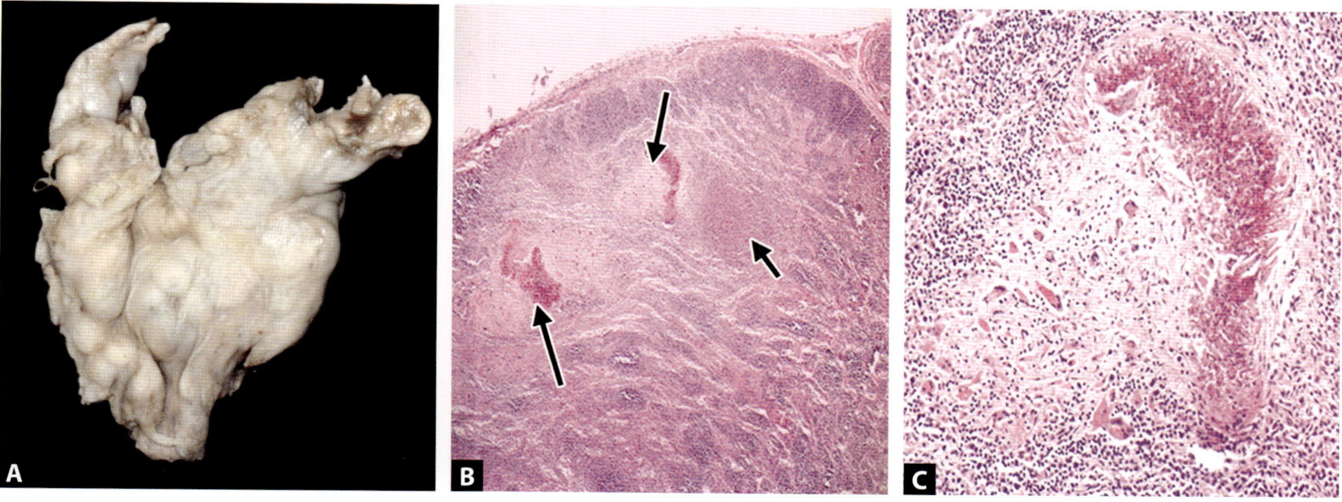

Figs 3A–C:

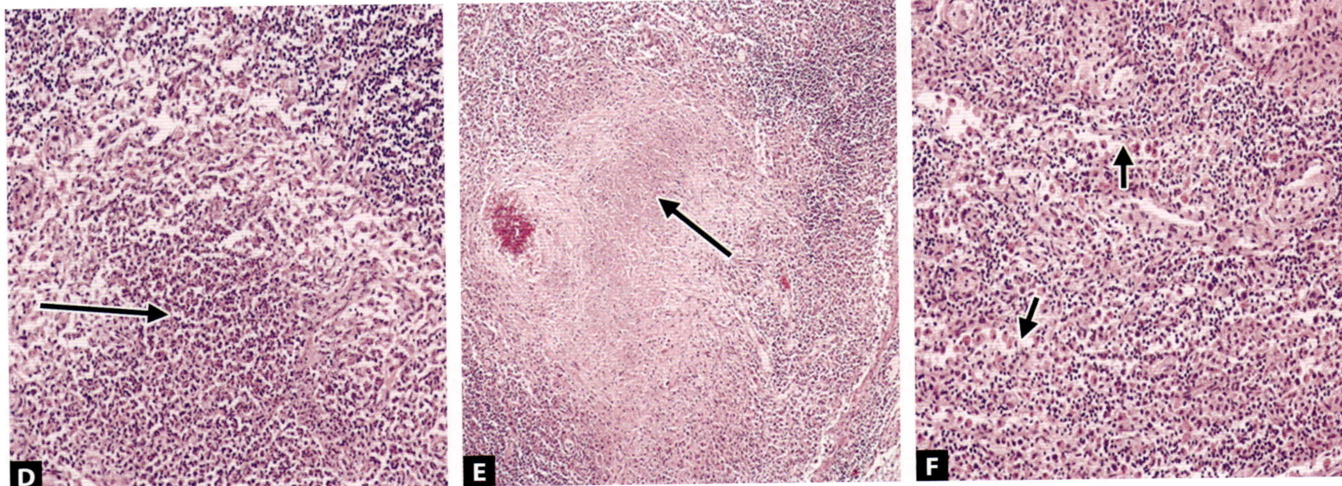

Figs 3A–F: (A) Enlarged mesenteric lymph nodes; (B) Low power view of the lymph node showing suppurative (small arrow) and histiocytic (long arrows) granulomas with pink amorphous material; (C) Histiocytic granuloma showing giant cells, histiocytes, and the pink undigested amorphous material; (D) Suppurative granuloma with polymorphs and nuclear debris in the center (arrow), surrounded by histiocytes; (E) Granuloma showing caseation like necrosis (arrow); (F) Pigmented macrophages in the sinuses of the lymph nodes (arrow).

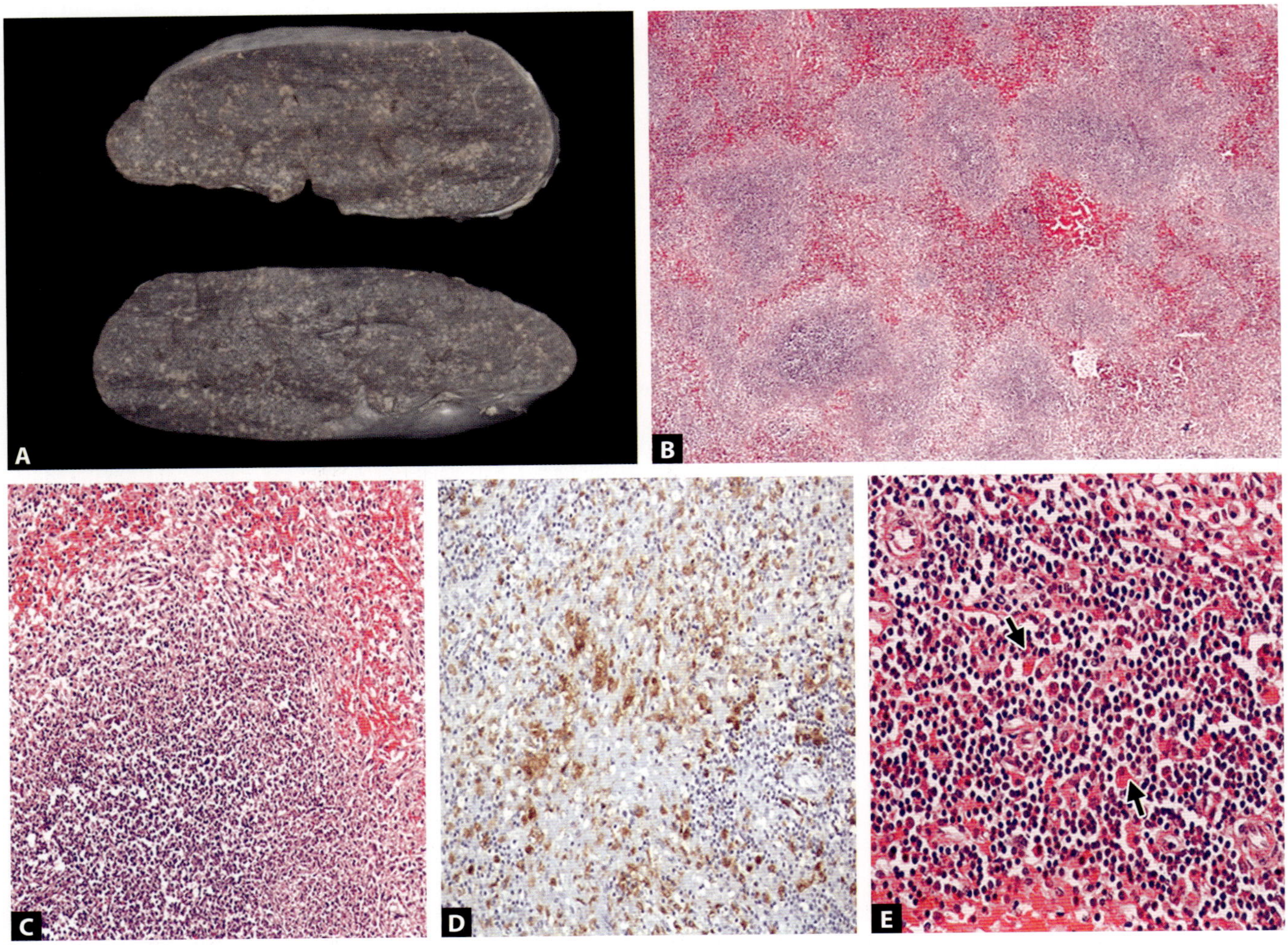

Figs 4A–E: (A) Coronal slices of the enlarged spleen showing millet-sized nodules present diffusely; (B) Photomicrograph of the spleen showing suppurative granulomas getting confluent; (C and D) Histiocytic granuloma replete with CD68 positive macrophages; (E) Spleen showing pigmented macrophages in between the lymphoid tissue.

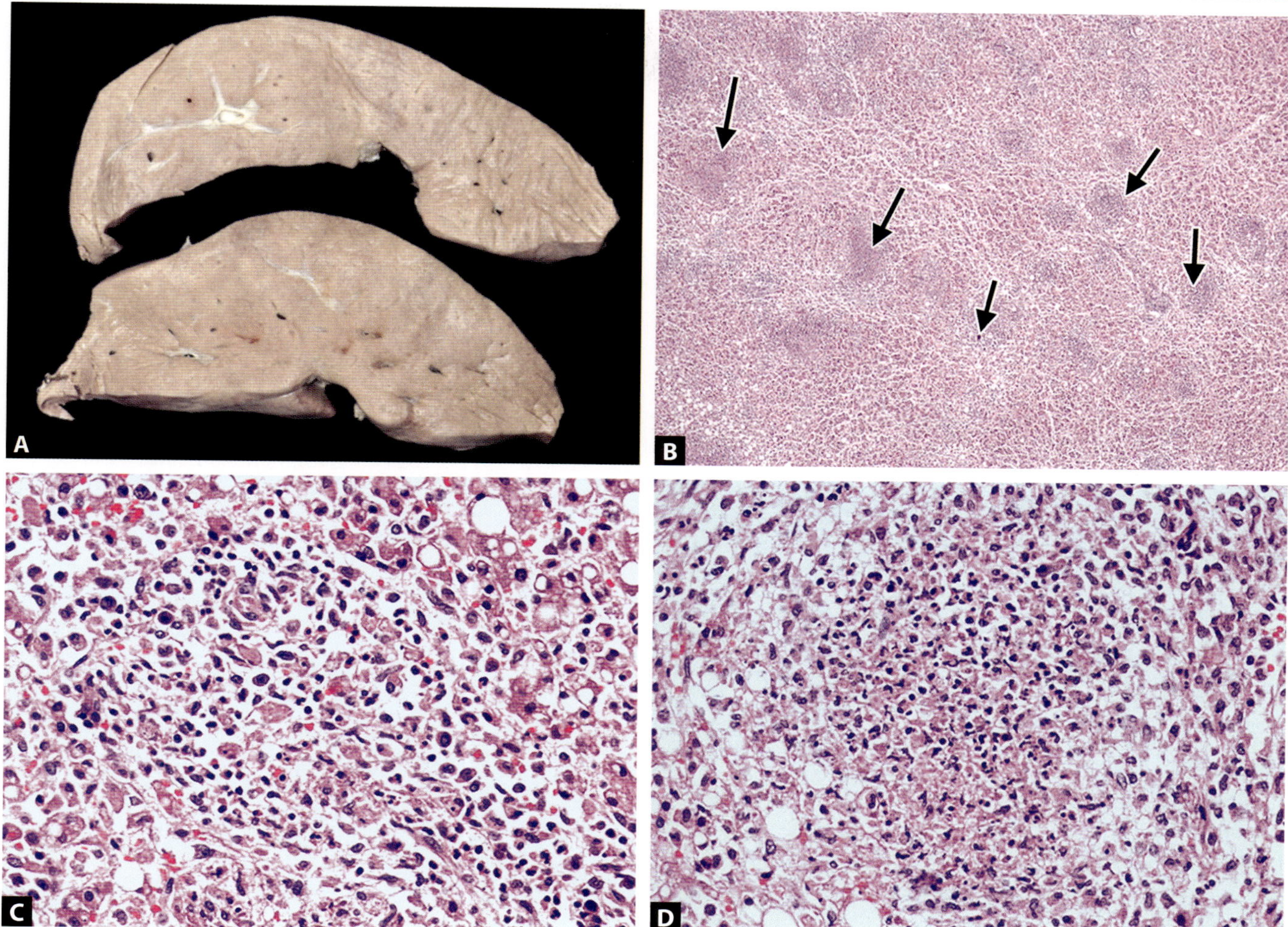

Figs 5A–D: (A) Coronal slices of the enlarged liver which are pale, but no focal lesion is seen; (B) Photomicrograph of the liver at low power, studded with granulomas (arrows); (C) Liver showing a granuloma composed of histiocytes and pigmented macrophages; (D) Liver showing a typical suppurative granuloma.

dase which is responsible for the respiratory burst and for the production of superoxide (O^{2-}) anion which is converted into reactive oxidants (hydroxyl radical (OH^-), hydrogen peroxide) which kill bacteria. The enzyme NADPH oxidase[2] is a complex of six proteins. It exists as two components in the basal state, a membrane bound structure present in the walls of the secondary granules ($gp91^{phox}$ and $p22^{phox}$) and as distinct cytoplasmic components ($p47^{phox}$, $p67^{phox}$, $p40^{phox}$ and rac). All except $p40^{phox}$ are needed for the production of superoxides. On activation of the cell, the cytoplasmic components relocate to the cytochrome in the membrane, thus forming an active NADPH oxidase. CGD occurs due to different mutations[3,4] in different genes coding for different components of the enzyme NADPH oxidase. This results in an inability to generate the superoxides and thereby the reactive oxygen species, i.e. hydroxyl radical and hydrogen peroxide. This in turn leads to a deranged microbial killing and repeated infections with catalase positive bacteria and fungi. The most common gene affected in CGD (in 70% cases) is the cytochrome B, β subunit (CYBB) gene present on the X chromosome which encodes for $gp91^{phox}$. So far, more than 350 mutations of the *CYBB* gene are known. The resultant syndrome is called the X-linked chronic granulomatous disease, i.e. X-CGD. Lyonization of the X-linked gene can occur in females. Heavy lyonization of the functional gene leads to the occurrence of X-linked CGD in females.[5] The second most common mutation occurs in the *NCF1* gene on chromosome 7 that encodes for the $p47^{phox}$. This accounts for 25% of all cases[6,7] of CGD and is the most common autosomal recessive form of the disease. In more than 90% cases, mutation in *NCF1* occurs as a single deletion. Other rare mutations occurring in 10% cases of CGD affect the genes

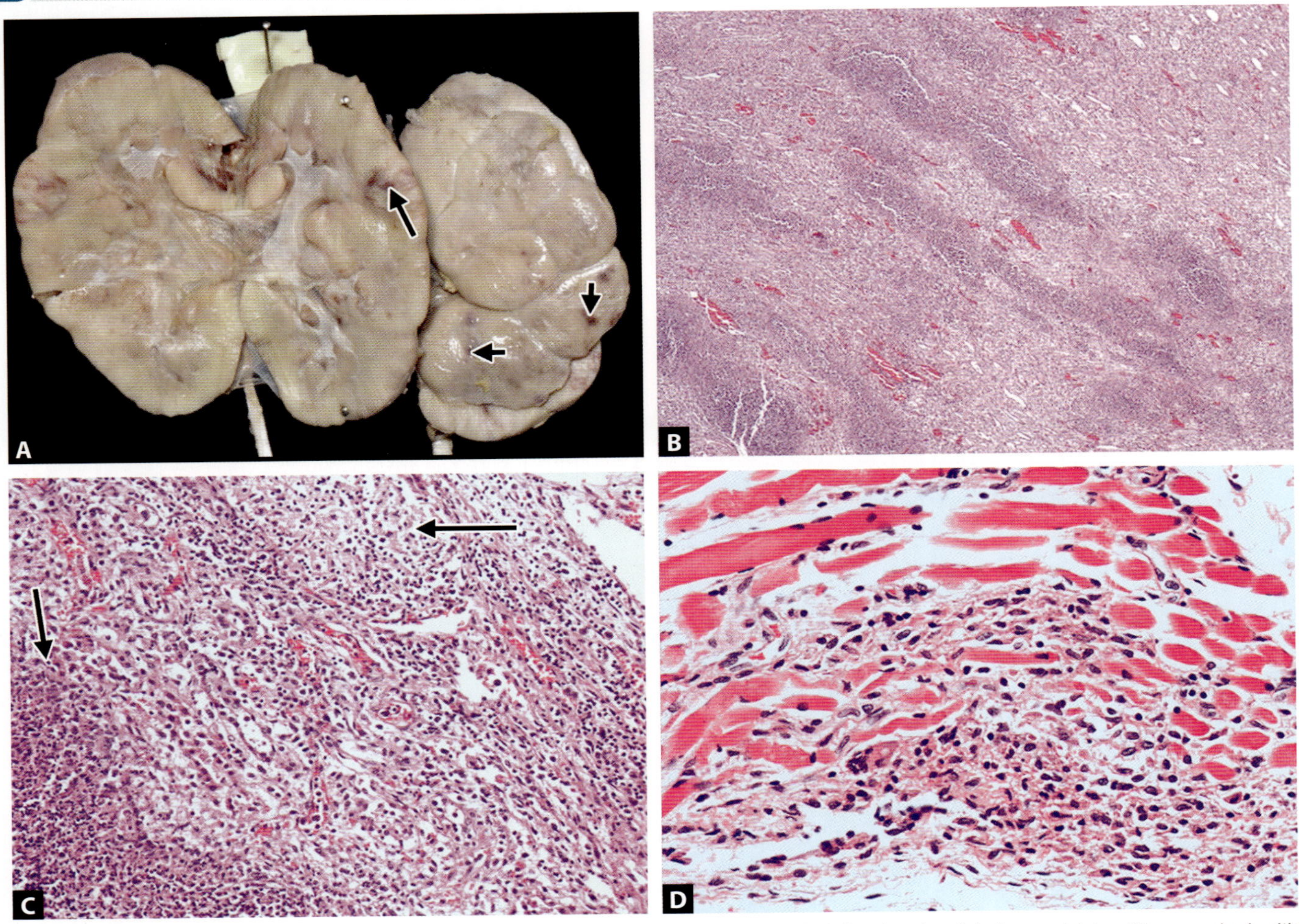

Figs 6A–D: (A) Both kidneys showing small areas of hemorrhages (arrows); (B) Medulla showing tubules and interstitium packed with polymorphs; (C) Ill-formed granulomas in the kidney (arrows); (D) Skeletal muscle showing histiocytic granuloma.

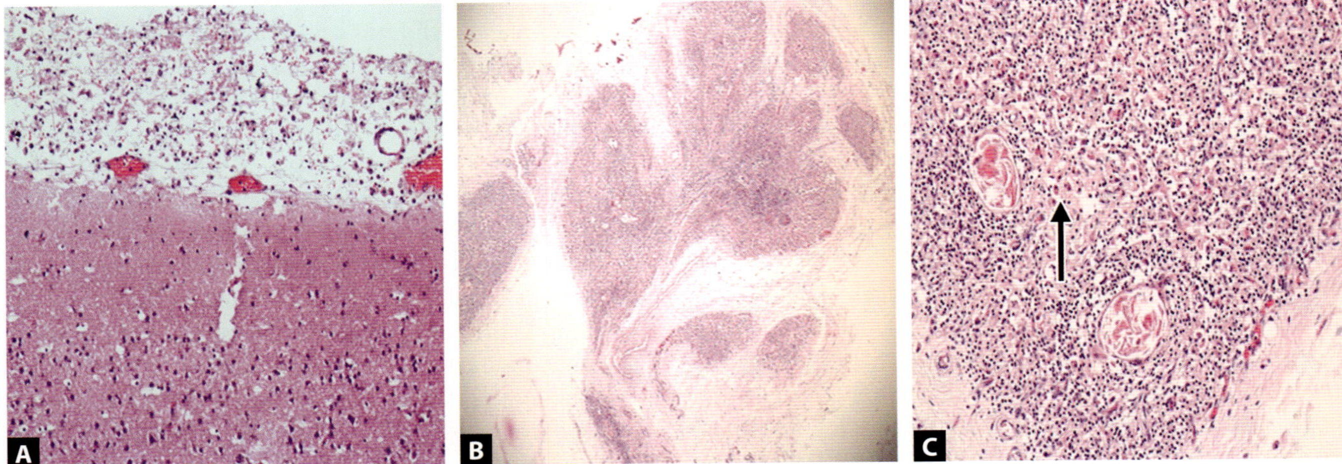

Figs 7A–C: (A) Brain showing histiocytes in the subarachnoid space; (B) Thymus showing marked involution; (C) Thymus showing Hassall's corpuscles and pigmented macrophages (arrow).

NCF2 (codes for P67) and *CYBA* (codes for p22) resulting in autosomal recessive disease. Approximately 95% of the mutations lead to a total absence or substantially decreased levels of the affected proteins. In rest of the cases, however a normal level of the defective protein is produced. Variant forms of X-linked or p47 CGD are seen in 10% cases and show residual phox activity leading to milder form of the disease. Here, the diagnosis of CGD may occur in adulthood. Carriers of CGD are asymptomatic. Mothers who are carriers of X-CGD and who have hyperlyonization have a less severe form of CGD. This occurs when the normal gene for gp91 is expressed in less than 10% phagocytes. They are at times misdiagnosed to have autosomal recessive disease which leads to a wrong guidance for family planning. Despite the defect, phagocytes from CGD patients can kill many microorganisms as the later produce endogenous hydrogen peroxide which is utilized by the defective phagocytes in killing them in the phagosomes.

Chronic granulomatous disease of childhood has no racial or ethnic predilection. Mortality or morbidity rates are highest in X-linked CGD, but have overall improved with early diagnosis and antibiotic prophylaxis. Two-thirds of the patients with CGD are males with X-linked form of the disease and the remaining have autosomal recessive disease. The hallmark of the disease is recurrent bacterial and fungal infections with granuloma formation. More than 75% cases are diagnosed less than 5 years of age. The organs involved are the lungs, skin, liver, spleen, lymph nodes, GI tract and bones. The microorganisms most frequently isolated are Staphylococcus aureus and *Aspergillus* species.[8] Other microorganisms encountered include E. coli, Nontyphoidal *Salmonella, Klebsiella, Burkholderia cepacia, Nocardia, Serratia, Actinomyces* and others. In CGD, catalase positive bacteria and fungi cause most of the infections and the catalase breaks down the endogenously produced hydrogen peroxide, thus needing the superoxide production by a normally functioning phox system to kill these infecting microorganisms. Catalase negative bacteria like *Streptococci* and *Pneumococci* are not usually pathogenic as the phagocytes are able to use H_2O_2 produced by the bacteria themselves. Patients with CGD, present with pneumonia (seen in 80% of patients), suppurative lymphadenitis and cutaneous disease or subcutaneous abscesses (seen in 50–60% patients), failure to thrive, lung abscesses, diarrhea, perianal/perirectal abscesses, hepatic/ splenic abscesses, osteomyelitis and septicemia. Manifestations of infections are peculiar, like frequent absence of fever and relatively milder inflammatory symptoms. So a very high index of suspicion is required for an early diagnosis. Obstruction is another manifestation of CGD that occurs as a result of granuloma formation in the gastrointestinal/genitourinary tract. Granulomas can present as nodular masses of inflammatory tissue as a result of the persistent antigenic stimuli due to the recurrent infections. Granulomas in the GI tract may lead to dysphagia, nausea, vomiting, abdominal pain and obstruction. GU tract obstruction causes dysuria, incontinence and urinary retention. Marciano et al[9] reviewed 140 patients with CGD and found GI involvement in 33%, which included granulomatous colitis, inflammatory bowel disease more like Crohn's disease, esophageal/gastric/duodenal obstruction and fistulas/abscesses around the anus. GI tract can be involved at any site right from the mouth to the anus. Cutaneous[10] disease includes granulomas with pigmented macrophages, aspergillus infection or nonspecific infection. Urological abnormalities[11] occur in 35–40% of cases and are seen as granulomatous inflammation in the urinary bladder, eosinophilic cystitis, ureteral strictures and infections of the urinary tract. Osteomyelitis[12] is a well-known complication of CGD.

The standard assay for enzyme NADPH oxidase is the NBT slide test which is a simple test and no specialized equipment is needed. The colorless compound NBT is reduced to blue formazan by the activity of the phox enzyme system. Slide test is carried out with phorbol ester or lipopolysaccharide coated slides. On placing a drop of blood, the phagocytes get activated, develop blue inclusions on incubation with NBT and their number is counted under a microscope. The NBT test can identify X-linked females who are carriers, when a two cell population, is seen i.e., one that reduces NBT to formazan and the other that does not. False negative test occurs when formazan accumulates in cells with low levels of active NADPH oxidase. These patients have the disease but their NBT test is negative. This test was initially used as a screening test, but is not used any more in the developed countries as it is a very subjective test. Dihydrorhodamine (DHR) test is a flow cytometric test and is now the preferred screening and diagnostic test for CGD. The phagocytic cells reduce DHR to form a strongly fluorescent compound rhodamine. Each fluorescent cell is counted and the amount of fluorescence per cell is quantified with flow cytometry. Genetic testing is not routinely done, as CGD is a rare disease and the number of mutations is too many. At present mutations can be identified in specialized laboratories, in nearly all patients and in about 90% of mothers of affected children. Gene therapy trials have started in CGD and the identification of the precise molecular defect is needed for it. Family history is very helpful and informative in X-linked CGD. Treatment involves the use of prophylactic or therapeutic antibiotics and newer therapies have been developed such as interferon gamma, bone marrow transplantation and gene therapy.

Histopathology of CGD[13-15] shows active chronic inflammation with suppurative granulomas comprising of polymorphs and nuclear debris in the center, bordered by histiocytes and epithelioid-like cells. More compact, noncaseating histiocytic granulomas are seen along with. Stain for AFB, PAS and Grocott done on multiple sections do not reveal any organisms. This type of granulomatous inflammation is very typical of CGD and is seen in the lungs, lymph nodes, liver and spleen. Characteristic pigmented macrophages are present, at times in clusters surrounded by histiocytes. These pigmented macrophages may also be seen in the mucosa of the GI tract. Granulomatous involvement of the gastrointestinal/genitourinary tract may be seen and at times obstructive pseudotumors occur, due to granulomas presenting as nodular masses of inflammatory tissue. At times one gets to see just inflammation, acute or chronic. On histopathology the main differential diagnosis is from other conditions which lead to granulomatous inflammation. In our setting, tuberculosis should be ruled out meticulously. In the study by Levine et al,[13] the histopathologic changes seen were a mixture of suppurative abscesses, acute necrotizing inflammation, granulomas with caseation and accumulation of pigmented macrophages. The pigmented material represents poorly digested intracellular debris due to the faulty microbial killing. However, in most biopsies there are no specific or diagnostic histopathologic features which can help us in making a diagnosis of CGD. An appropriate clinical setting and the above mentioned patterns can however suggest a diagnosis.

COMMENTARY—INDEX CASE: PM 24170

This 7-month-old male child had had multiple admissions due to recurrent infections (respiratory and urinary) since birth. An ischiorectal abscess had been drained. There was history of three male sibling deaths at the age of 3, 14 and 9 months. However, his five female siblings were alive and normal. Maternal aunt had also lost three male babies at 6 days, 12 months and 13 months of age. This points toward an X-linked disorder. There was a massive splenomegaly (spleen being six times enlarged) and moderate hepatomegaly. There was hyperglobulinemia and the NBT test was positive. Autopsy revealed a florid chronic active inflammation with both histiocytic/suppurative granulomas and pigmented macrophages in the lungs, lymph nodes, spleen, liver, kidneys and thymus. In the lungs, some of the histiocytic granulomas were ill-formed and difficult to discern, with collections of histiocytes and epithelioid-like cells merging with lung parenchyma. However, well-formed granulomas composed of histiocytes, epithelioid-like cells and giant cells were also seen. A few granulomas showed caseation like necrosis, strongly mimicking tuberculosis. Pigmented macrophages were seen in clusters surrounded by histiocytes. In the spleen and liver, the suppurative granulomas were more prominent and they showed a typical collection of polymorphs and nuclear debris in the center, surrounded by histiocytes and occasionally giant cells. Here the histiocytic granulomas were admixed with pigmented macrophages. In the lymph nodes pink amorphous material, which represented inadequate digestion of intracellular debris due to the faulty microbial killing, was seen in abundance within the granulomas. The baby was immunized for BCG at birth, but did not suffer from BCG infection, which was an odd point. So, taking into consideration the history and the histopathologic findings, the overall features are consistent with a diagnosis of X-linked CGD.

TAKE HOME MESSAGE

- Chronic granulomatous disease of childhood is a rare, inherited and primary disorder of the phagocyte/neutrophil function.
- It occurs due to a defect in the enzyme NADPH oxidase, which is responsible for the respiratory burst and for the production of bactericidal superoxide (O_2-) anions.
- There is an inability to generate the superoxides which leads to defective microbial killing and the hallmark of the disease, i.e. recurrent infections with catalase positive bacteria and fungi.
- Two-thirds of the patients with CGD are males, with X-linked form of the disease and the remaining have an autosomal recessive disease.
- The standard assay for enzyme NADPH oxidase, which is routinely used, is the nitroblue tetrazolium (NBT) test.
- Dihydrorhodamine test is a flow cytometric test and is now the preferred screening and diagnostic test for CGD.
- Histopathology of CGD shows active chronic inflammation with histiocytic/suppurative granulomas and pigmented macrophages in practically all the organs.

REFERENCES

1. Heyworth PG, Cross AR, Curnutte JT. Chronic granulomatous disease. Curr Opin Immunol. 2003;15:578-84.
2. Segal BH, Leto TL, Gallin JI, et al. Genetic, biochemical and clinical features of chronic granulomatous disease. Medicine (Baltimore). 2000;79:170-200.

3. Roos D. X-CGD base: a database of X-CGD causing mutations. Immunol Today. 1996;17:517-21.
4. Rae J, Newburger PE, Dinauer MC, et al. X linked chronic granulomatous disease: mutations in the CYBB gene encoding the gp91-phox component of the respiratory burst oxidase. Am J Hum Genet. 1998;62:1320-31.
5. Bolscher BG, ge Boer M, de Klein A, et al. Point mutations in the B-subunit of cytochrome b558 leading to X linked CGD. Blood. 1991;77:2482.
6. Clark RA, Malech HL, Gallin JL, et al. Genetic variant of chronic granulomatous disease: prevalence of deficiencies of 148- two cytosolic components of the NADPH oxidase system. N Engl J Med. 1989;321:647-52.
7. Winkelstein JA, Marino MC, Johnston RB Jr, et al. Chronic granulomatous disease. Report on a national registry of 368 patients. Medicine (Baltimore). 2000;79:155-69.
8. Gallin JI. Delineation of the phagocyte NADPH oxidase through studies of chronic granuloamtous disease of childhood. Int J Tissue Reac. 1993;15:99-103.
9. Marciano BE, Rosenzweig SD, Kleiner DE, et al. Gastointestinal involvement in chronic granulomatous disease. Pediatrics. 2004;114(2):462-8.
10. Dohil M, Prendiville JS, Crawford RI, et al. Cutaneous manifestations of CGD. A report of four cases and review of literature. J Am Acad Dermatol. 1997;36:899-907.
11. Walther MM, Malech H, Berman A, et al. The urological manifestations of CGD. J Urol. 1992;147:1314-8.
12. Dotis J, Roilides E. Osteomyelitis due to Aspergillus species in patients with CGD: comparison of Aspergillus nidulans and Aspergillus fumigates. Int J Infect Dis. 2004;8:103-10.
13. Levine S, Smith VV, Malone M, et al. Histopathological features of chronic granulomatous disease in childhood. Histopathology. 2005;47:508-16.
14. Nakhleh RE, Glock M, Snover DC. Hepatic pathology of chronic granulomatous disease of childhood. Arch of Pathol Lab Med. 1992;116(1):71-5.
15. Moskaluk CA, Pogrebniak HW, Pass HI, et al. Surgical pathology of the lung in chronic granulomatous disease. Am J Clin Pathol. 1994;102(5):684-91.

CONTRIBUTIONS BY:

1. Dr JL Mathew, Professor, Department of Pediatrics (Compilation of Clinical Details)
2. Prof. S Singhi, Ex-Professor and Head, Department of Pediatrics (Clinician In-Charge)

Post Graduate Institute of Medical Education and Research, Chandigarh, India.

CASE 57

Disseminated Nonreactive Tuberculosis, PCR-Proven Dual Positivity for *Mycobacterium Tuberculosis* and *Abscessus* ? Mendelian Susceptibility to Mycobacterial Disease: PM 25174

Nandita Bharadwaj Kakkar

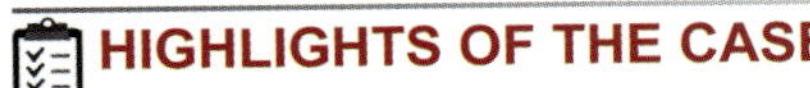

HIGHLIGHTS OF THE CASE

A 4-month-old male child had respiratory distress, fever, cough, skin rashes, tachycardia, tachypnea, anemia, polymorphonuclear leukocytosis, X-ray/contrast-enhanced CT (CECT) suggestive of pulmonary tuberculosis and acid-fast bacilli (AFB) were positive in the smears from the gastric aspirate, nasopharyngeal aspirate, endotracheal (ET) aspirate and pleural fluid. Work up for primary immunodeficiency was negative. Patient did not respond to anti-tubercular therapy (ATT). Four weeks after the start of the ATT, the pleural fluid smears were still positive for AFB. There was progressive respiratory failure, hypotensive shock leading to multiorgan failure and cardiac arrest. The clinical diagnosis was multidrug resistance (MDR) disseminated tuberculosis with healthcare-associated infection and severe sepsis ? underlying immunodeficiency. The final autopsy diagnosis was nonreactive pulmonary tuberculosis (AFB++++, PCR positive for ***Mycobacterium tuberculosis*** and Mycobacterium abscessus) with dissemination (to the lymph nodes, liver, spleen, small intestine and brain) and healthcare-associated confluent necrotizing pneumonia with diffuse alveolar damage ? Underlying Mendelian susceptibility to mycobacterial disease (MSMD).

Keywords: Mendelian susceptibility to mycobacterial disease, MSMD, non-tubercular mycobacteria, *M. abscessus*, *M. tuberculosis*, autopsy.

CLINICAL DETAILS

Date of Admission: 20.11.2012, Date of Death: 05.01.2013, Duration of Hospital Stay: 16 Days.

A 4-month-old male child came with presenting complaints of fever, cough and progressive rapid breathing, present since 15 days. Skin rashes were present since 10 days. The child was well till 3.5 months of age. The illness started with fever, which was of moderate grade (101–102°F) with no specific pattern. The cough was dry and rapid breathing was associated with lower chest indrawing and refusal to feed in the last 4 days. Skin rash was seen initially as reddish lesions over face and later as hypopigmented areas, involving upper chest and groin. There was no cyanosis or seizures. The child was born of a nonconsanguineous marriage with healthy parents. He was second in birth order with elder sibling being a girl, who was well. There was no history of any abortion or fetal loss. He was a term baby, who underwent an uneventful normal vaginal delivery. His development was normal and he was on breast feed, along with cows milk. He had received bacillus Calmette-Guérin (BCG) at birth and three doses of DPT and OPV. His grandmother had been treated for pulmonary tuberculosis 7 years ago but was presently fine. ***On physical examination*** the heart rate was 168/min, respiratory rate 84/min, BP: 94/60 mm Hg, SpO_2: 97%, weight: 5.5 kg, length 58 cm and head circumference 38.5 cm (all -2 Z score). There was no pallor or lymphadenopathy. There was grade II clubbing, oral thrush, desquamative papular rash over perianal and genital regions and hypopigmented macules over upper face. No BCG scar was present, despite BCG vaccination. On chest examination, there were subcostal and intercostal recessions, bilateral bronchial breathing and crepitations on the right side. The liver was palpable 3 cm below the costal margin with a span of 5.5 cm and the spleen was just palpable. Cardiovascular and central nervous systems were normal.

Investigations and Course of Management

Investigations revealed Hb of 6 g/dL, which went up to 11.2 g/dL (after transfusions) and nearing demise was

9.1 g/dL. The total leukocyte count was 4,300/μL, later rose to 31,200/μL and nearing demise was 21,500/μL. There was polymorphonuclear leukocytosis. The platelets were initially 2,66,000/uL and later rose to 4,19,000/uL. The coagulogram was within normal limits. Serum electrolytes, liver and renal function tests were within normal limits. CRP and ESR were raised. AFB were positive in the smears from the gastric aspirate, nasopharyngeal aspirate, endo-tracheal aspirate and from the pleural fluid. AFB cultures and the TB PCR done (gastric aspirate) turned out to be negative. Four weeks after the start of the ATT, the pleural fluid smears were still positive for AFB. Mantoux was negative. Blood culture, nearing demise grew *Acinetobacter* specis which was drug-resistant. Routine urine examination was normal. Pleural fluid—exudative picture, full of pus cells, proteins—2.9 g/dL, globulins—10 mg%, culture and sensitivity test (nearing demise)—*Acinetobacter* specis, CSF—40 cells, all lymphocytes; proteins—57 mg, globulins—65 mg, adenosine deaminase (ADA)—4.0 u/L, No AFB in smears, culture—sterile. ***Immunology workup:*** HIV—negative, IgG—631 (N: 240–880), IgA—112 (N: 10–50), IgM—145 (N: 20–100), NBT—normal. CD19 positive cells 643 (N: 600–3,000), CD3 positive cells—1,027 (N: 2,300–6,500). Echocardiography—normal. ***Radiology workup:*** X-ray chest revealed a diffuse lung disease with small nodules and diffuse consolidation. The CECT chest confirmed the findings of the X-ray i.e diffuse lung disease with nodules, consolidation, cavitary lesions and chest tube in situ. Mediastinal lymph nodes were enlarged, necrotic and revealed calcification. Soft tissue shadow was seen in the prevascular space which seemed to be the thymus. Overall features suggestive of pulmonary tuberculosis. USG abdomen—showed hepatosplenomegaly with the liver 6.8 cm and spleen 3.6 cm with normal echotexture, kidneys were normal and left minimal pleural effusion present.

The child was admitted with respiratory distress, started on nasal continuous positive airway pressure (CPAP), intercostal draining tube (ICDT) was placed for left sided pneumothorax, given intravenous (IV) antibiotics and amphotericin B. With AFB positivity in the various smears on day 3 and a very suggestive CECT, four-drug (HRZE) ATT with steroids was started on day 3 and antibiotics were stopped. He required mechanical ventilation for 3 days and was weaned to nasal O_2. Received packed red blood cells transfusion on day 3. He continued to have mild respiratory distress with persistent O_2 requirement and purulent drainage from ICDT. Fresh maculopapular rash was noted in second week. Attempts to remove ICDT failed with clinicoradiological evidence of left bronchopleural fistula. Work up for primary immunodeficiency was negative. Due to non-response after 4 weeks of ATT, ofloxacin and amikacin were added to treat MDR-TB. In the terminal week there was fresh onset fever with spikes and worsening respiratory distress. Blood culture grew Acinetobacter specis. There was progressive respiratory failure and hypotensive shock leading to multiorgan failure and cardiac arrest. ***Units final clinical diagnosis was***—MDR disseminated tuberculosis with healthcare-associated infection and severe sepsis, ? underlying immunodeficiency.

AUTOPSY FINDINGS: PM 25174

A complete autopsy was performed. The pleural cavities contained 100 mL of straw-colored fluid. There was adequate amount of lymphoid tissue (Figs 1A–C) in the lymph nodes, spleen, small intestine and appendix. The thymus was caught up in the mass of the matted lymph nodes, found behind the sternum and was involved by tuberculosis. Hence, it could not be assessed. Work up for primary immunodeficiency was negative. CD3 count was however low, i.e. 1,027 [N: 2,300–6,500, severe combined immunodeficiency (SCID) <600]. In view of the adequate lymphoid tissue and not so low CD3 counts, SCID was ruled out. NBT test was normal and the morphology of the case ruled out a chronic granulomatous disease of childhood. Cystic fibrosis was also ruled out as the pancreas was normal on microscopic examination. The ***lungs*** together weighed 183 g. They were adherent to the chest wall and were difficult to remove. Pleura showed hemorrhages and fibrinous tags (Fig 2A). On cut section (Fig 2B and C), the lungs were firm with large yellowish areas of consolidation showing breaking down. Cavities were noted containing necrotic debris. Microscopic examination of the lung (Figs 2D–F) revealed large geographic areas of caseation necrosis with calcification and replete with AFB (Ziehl–Neelsen stain). Periphery of the caseous areas revealed histiocytes and epithelioid-like cells. No well-formed granulomas or Langhans type of giant cell were seen. The cavities showed a fibrous wall and around them, were seen areas of fibrosis (Fig 3A). Adjoining lung showed a prominent adenomatoid change (Fig 3B). Some areas of the lung showed features of tubercular pneumonia with alveolar spaces packed with histiocytes forming nodules and were replete with AFB (Figs 3C and D). Other areas of the lung showed a confluent necrotizing bronchopneumonia with the bronchioles and alveolar spaces packed with polymorphs and nuclear debris (Figs 3E and F). Hyaline membranes (Fig 3F) were seen indicating a diffuse alveolar damage. Overall features were those of fibrocavitatory, nonreactive tuberculosis with tuberculous pneumonia and a heavy bacillary load.

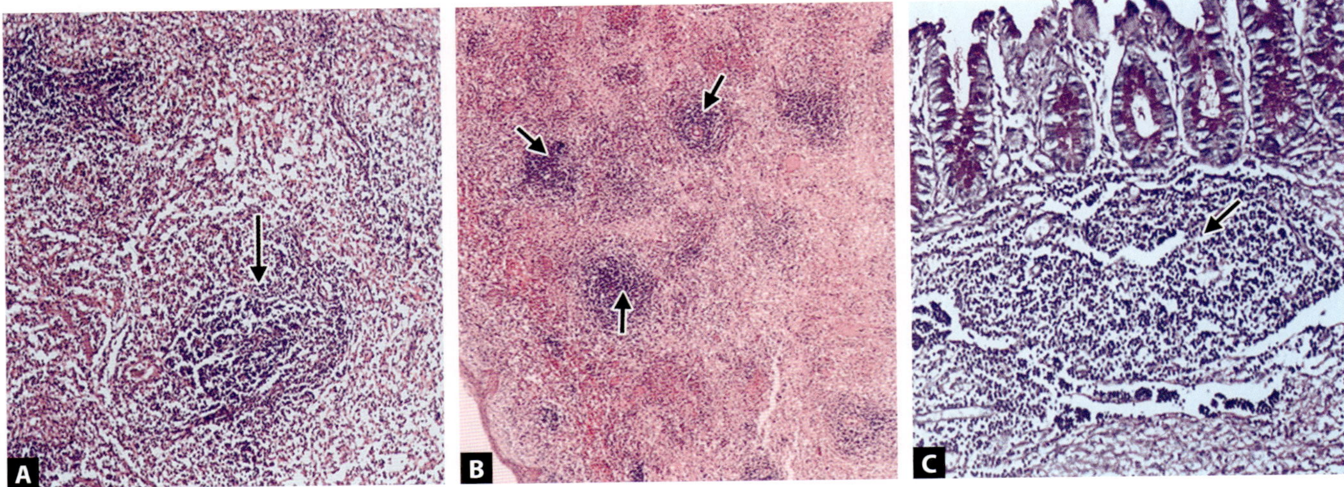

Figs 1A–C: Adequate lymphoid tissue (arrows) in the (A) Lymph nodes; (B) Spleen; and (C) Peyer's patches.

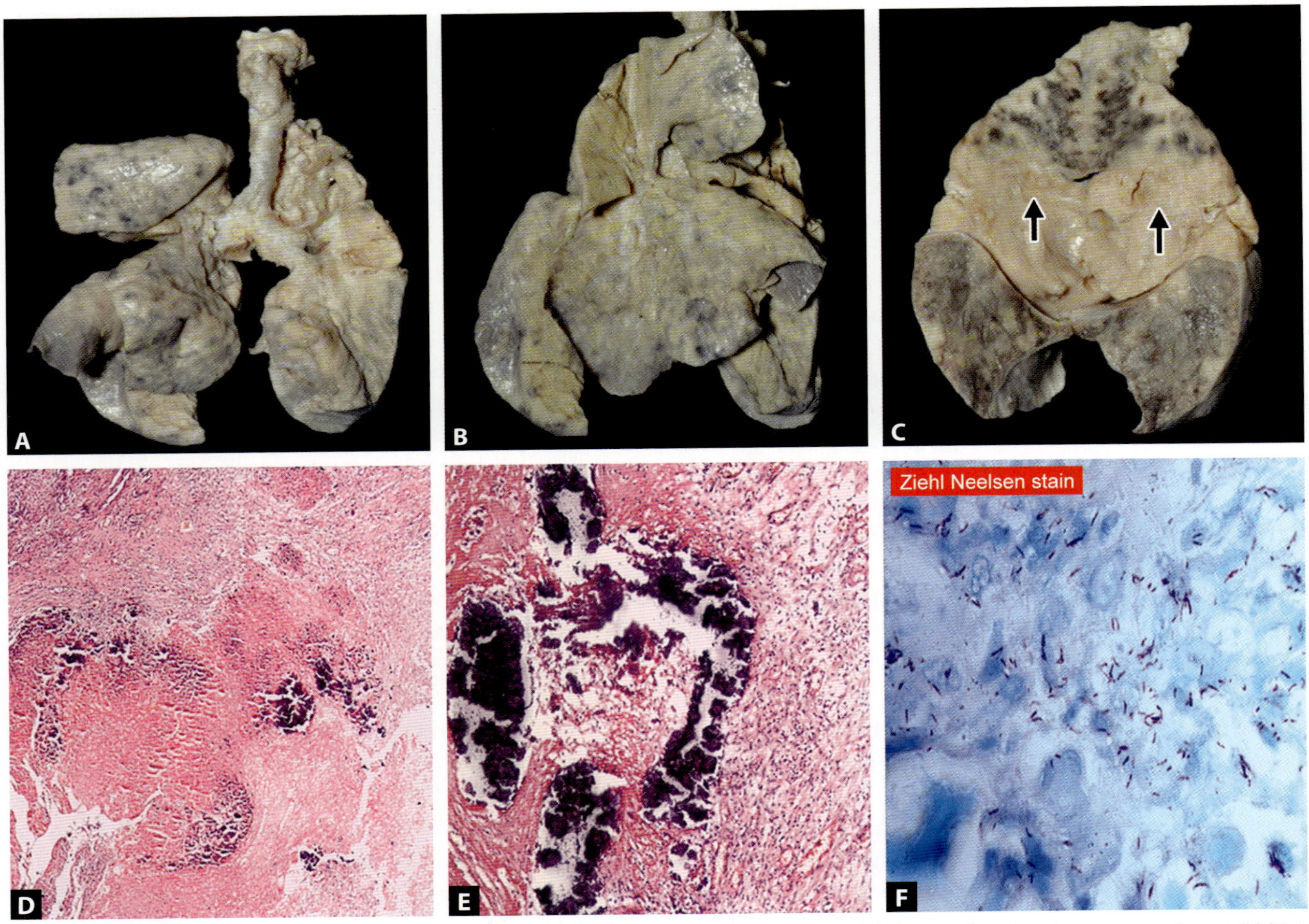

Ziehl Neelsen stain

Figs 2A–F: (A to C) Gross pictures of the lung. (A) Pleural aspect showing hemorrhages; (B) Cut section showing a pale yellow solid lung with small yellowish areas getting confluent; (C) Lower part of the left upper lobe showing diffuse yellowish consolidation with breaking down (arrows). Adjacent areas show hemorrhages. Photomicrographs of the lung; (D) Geographic areas of caseation necrosis. No granulomas seen; (E) Necrotic areas show extensive calcification; (F) Ziehl–Neelsen stain shows strong positivity for acid-fast bacilli.

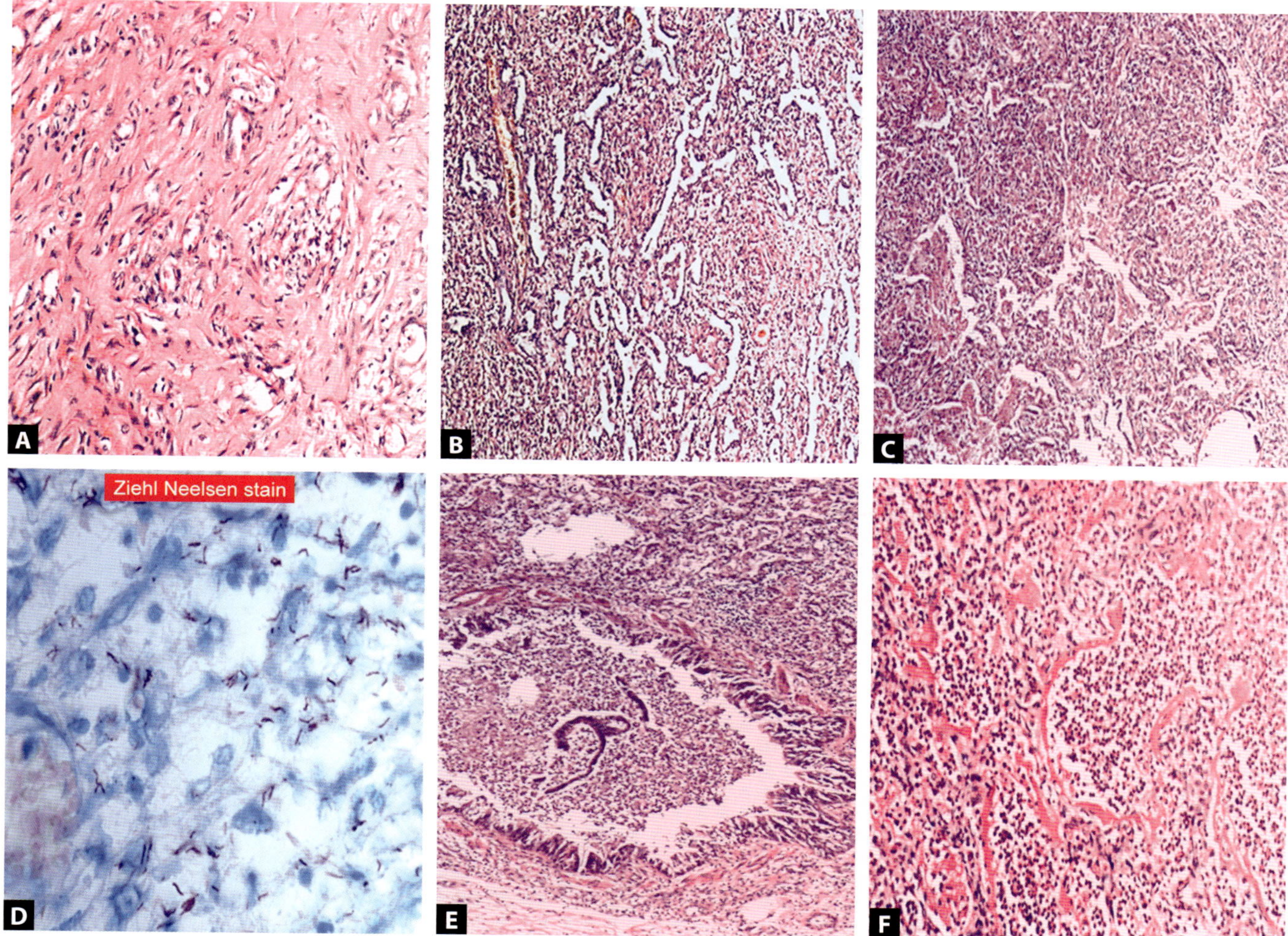

Figs 3A–F: Lung showing (A) Areas of fibrosis and (B) Adenomatoid change; (C and D) Alveolar spaces packed with histiocytes, replete with acid-fast bacilli; (E and F) Acute bronchopneumonia with hyaline membrane formation.

Superadded acute bronchopneumonia with diffuse alveolar damage was also noted. The hilar, carinal, paratracheal, mediastinal and peripancreatic ***lymph nodes*** were enlarged and revealed caseation necrosis. A matted lymph nodal mass was identified behind the sternum and the thymus was caught up in it. Microscopic examination (Figs 4A–D) of the lymph nodes revealed a picture very similar to that seen in the lungs, i.e. large areas of caseation necrosis, calcification, surrounding epithelioid-like cells and histiocytes. An occasional ill-formed granuloma was seen, but no Langhans type of giant cell were noted. Stain for AFB was strongly positive. The ***liver*** (Fig 5A) and ***spleen*** (Fig 5B) on microscopic examination revealed a few small epithelioid cell granulomas with no caseation or Langhans giant cells. Occasional AFB could be detected. The small intestine revealed prominent peyer's patches and few compact epithelioid cell granulomas with no caseation or giant cells in the submucosa (Fig 5C). Stain for AFB was strongly positive. The ***brain*** was grossly normal. However, microscopic examination of the standard sections showed a few compact epithelioid cell granulomas in the subependymal (Fig 5D) location and in the choroid plexus (Fig 5E). An occasional AFB was found in the choroid plexus. The ***kidneys*** on external and cut section showed blotchy congestion and microscopy revealed extensive tubular calcification (Fig 5F). The bone marrow, pancreas and heart were within normal limits. Polymerase chain reaction (PCR) from the lung tissue was positive for *Mycobacterium tuberculosis* and *Mycobacterium abscessus* (*Courtesy*: Dr Kusum Sharma, Department of Microbiology, PGIMER, Chandigarh).

IFNRG2 (4%) and NEMO (3%). Genetic etiology is identified in 50% of patients of MSMD.

Autosomal recessive, complete IFN-γR1 and IFN-γR2 deficiency is associated with severe, often fatal, infections with BCG and NTM in early childhood. The prognosis is poor and treatment with IFN-γ is ineffective due to the absence of functional receptors. Hematopoietic stem cell transplantation (HSCT) has been curative in a small number of patients, but rejection occurs with a high frequency. Less severe MSMD occurs after the age of 3, due to a different set of mutations, i.e. partial IFN-γR1/R2, complete IL-12R-beta1/IL12B, partial STAT1/IRF8 deficiencies and partial X-linked recessive (XR) mutations. The prognosis is generally good for patients who receive antimicrobial treatment and recombinant IFN-γ.

Patients with MSMD, typically present with infections with BCG, NTM and nontyphoid *Salmonella*. Disseminated NTM infection has nonspecific signs and symptom like fever, weight loss, sweating, diarrhea, generalized lymphadenopathy, cutaneous lesions, hepatosplenomegaly and diffuse abdominal tenderness. Disseminated BCG infection presents within weeks to months of the immunization. The draining lymph nodes may enlarge, form skin fistulas, soft tissue extension and may spread via the hematogenous route to distant sites. Meningitis, multifocal osteomyelitis, lung infection and extensive dissemination occurs. The type of mycobacterial strain and the mode of presentation is dependent upon the geographic location and whether BCG vaccine is routinely administered at birth. If the BCG vaccine is routinely given, infection with vaccine strain occurs. If not then the first encounter with mycobacteria is due to the environmental exposure with NTM. Patients with complete genetic defects typically present in early childhood with disseminated disease, whereas those with partial genetic defects or less severe defects such as *IRF8* or *IL12RB1* mutations may present in adolescence and/or with milder recurrent infections. In addition, patients with IL-12Rβ1 deficiency who live in highly *M. tuberculosis* endemic parts of the world may present with disseminated TB.

Diagnosis is made by measuring the levels of IFN-γ, IL-12p40 and IL-12p70 by ELISA. Further on, flow cytometric evaluation of cell surface receptor expression on monocytes and lymphocytes, as well as examining signaling either by intracellular staining or western blot can be done. The gene mutations can be pinpointed. The pathogenic strain causing the infection should be determined from the blood, bone marrow, liver, visceral lymph nodes or other normally sterile body site by culture or PCR. PCR can differentiate between NTM and *M. tuberculosis* and can usually distinguish which species of NTM is causing the infection. A positive culture is however required to perform drug-susceptibility testing. If the cultures or PCR is negative, a histopathologic demonstration of the AFB or granulomas supports the diagnosis. The value of the Mantoux test is debatable as the patients are overtly sick with disseminated *M. tuberculosis* or NTM disease and may be anergic, thus giving a false negative result. Differential diagnosis includes chronic granulomatous disease, SCID, cystic fibrosis, HIV infection and ectodermal dysplasia with immunodeficiency. Antenatal diagnosis and subsequent MTP can be done in families with documented cases of fatal complete IFNGR deficiencies. Genetic counseling is done in families where a specific mutation is identified. BCG vaccination should be avoided in cases of MSMD.

Nontubercular mycobacterial infection in MSMD patients, requires aggressive treatment with antimycobacterial antibiotics (same as those used for patients without MSMD). The treatment duration is however prolonged as the immune response and cure are slower. Once the infection is successfully cleared, patients are maintained on antibiotic prophylaxis. Cytokine replacement therapy with IFN-γ is an additional treatment option, but it has limited efficacy among patients with autosomal recessive complete defects of IFN-γ-R1/R2, (since lack of expressed receptors leads to a failure to respond to IFN-γ) and *STAT1* defects. Bone marrow transplantation has been used, with varying success, in several patients with the more severe forms of MSMD, i.e. autosomal recessive complete IFN-γ-R deficiencies, autosomal recessive complete STAT1 deficiency and GATA2 deficiency. Prognosis is variable and is related to the type of mutation present. Survival is poor in complete deficiencies of MSMD. Most NTM infections in patients with MSMD respond to prolonged courses of antimycobacterial therapy, with or without cytokine therapy.

MYCOBACTERIUM ABSCESSUS

Nonbacterial mycobacteria are acquired from the environment, but *M. abscessus* is a rapidly growing mycobacterium found in soil and water throughout the world. *M. abscessus* is very virulent, rapidly growing mycobacteria and an important human pathogen causing invasive lung disease. It generally leads to localized skin and soft tissue infections in the immunocompetent and disseminated infections in the immunocompromised. It is now considered an important pathogen leading to severe lung infections in cases of cystic fibrosis and chronic lung disease. This organism is a new antibiotic nightmare, as it is exceptionally resistant to antibiotics and a multidrug regimen is needed to combat it. It shares many traits with *M. tuberculosis*, i.e. it is acid-fast, is associated with caseous necrosis and can induce a persistent lung disease.

COMMENTARY—INDEX CASE: PM 25174

In the index case, florid pulmonary nonreactive tuberculosis with dissemination, resistance to ATT, a very heavy bacillary load, disseminated rashes and a terminal healthcare associated infection were seen. Highlights were:

- There was no response to anti-tubercular treatment despite 45 days of treatment with four drugs. Is it MDR tuberculosis or is there admixture with other non-tubercular mycobacteria? PCR from the lung tissue was positive for *M. tuberculosis* and *M. abscessus*. Hence admixture with NTM was present and this can explain the non-response to the given treatment.
- The nonreactive florid tuberculosis with a heavy bacillary load, seen at autopsy can be explained by:
    - Impaired granuloma formation and nonreaction is noted in NTM infections especially with *M. abscessus*.
    - The patient was not treated for *M. abscessus*, so the load became heavier.
- Mendelian susceptibility to mycobacterial disease is a strong possibility here, as it predisposes to NTM, leads to impaired IFN-γ-mediated immunity and also leads to poor granuloma formation. However, genetic studies at the molecular level for MSMD could not be carried out in the index case due to lack of facility.
- Index case was immunized with BCG, but there was no scar. So is it a *Mycobacterium bovis* infection? PCR done on the lung tissue, however ruled out this possibility. The absence of scar is probably due to MSMD, although he did not acquire BCG infection.
- In the index case, the entire immunodeficiency workup was negative and adequate lymphoid tissue was present in the various organs at autopsy. The possibility of chronic granulomatous disease and SCID were ruled out. In this child, the CD3 counts were low 1,027 (N: 2,300–6,500). However in patients of SCID, the CD3 counts are always less than 600. Cystic fibrosis was ruled out at autopsy, as the pancreas was within normal limits.
- Congenital tuberculosis is always a strong possibility in such a setting. It was however ruled out as the revised Cantwell criteria did not fit in here, i.e. presence of a proven tuberculous lesion and at least one of the following: (A) Lesions should be present in the first week of life. (B) Primary hepatic complex. (C) Tuberculous infection of placenta or maternal genital tract. (D) Exclusion of postnatal transmission by thorough contact investigation. The index child was doing well for the first 3.5 months of life. Primary hepatic complex was absent. The liver showed a few small epithelioid cell granulomas, which was a dissemination from the lungs. There was no documented tuberculous infection seen in the placenta and in the maternal genital tract. There was no history of any contact with a tuberculosis patient. The grandmother was treated for tuberculosis 7 years back, but was presently doing well.
- So, in the index patient, in a background of a ? MSMD there was a severe lung infection with both *Mycobacterium tuberculosis* and *abscessus*. The disseminated skin lesions also could be due to *M. abscessus*. The resistance to antitubercular treatment, presence of nonreactive tuberculosis on morphology and a heavy bacillary load was due to the admixture with nontubercular mycobacteria, i.e. *Mycobacterium abscessus*, for which he was not treated.

TAKE HOME MESSAGE

- Mendelian susceptibility to mycobacterial diseases is a rare congenital, immunodeficiency syndrome, where apparently healthy individuals are vulnerable to disease caused by poorly virulent mycobacteria like BCG and NTM.
- Genetic defects in the IFN-γ pathway result in MSMD.
- Host defense against *M. tuberculosis* and NTM, as well as *Salmonella*, depends heavily upon the functional integrity of IFN-γ/IL-12 pathway. IFN-γ is a principal factor in the elimination of both TB and NTM.
- Genetic mutations are identified in 50% patients of MSMD. It is a predominantly autosomal recessive condition, but can also be autosomal dominant or X-linked.
- Aggressive treatment with antimycobacterial antibiotics is the method for the management of patients with these disorders. Cytokine replacement therapy with IFN-γ can be done but has limited role in patients with autosomal recessive complete defects of IFN-γ-R1 and IFN-γ-R2.
- *M abscessus* is a rapidly growing mycobacterium found in soil and water throughout the world. It is very virulent, rapidly growing mycobacteria, an antibiotic nightmare and an important human pathogen causing invasive lung disease.

SUGGESTED READING

1. Al-Muhsen S, Casanova JL. The genetic heterogeneity of mendelian susceptibility to mycobacterial diseases. J Allergy Clin Immunol. 2008; 122(6):1043-51.
2. Altare F, Jouanguy E, Lamhamedi S, et al. Mendelian susceptibility to mycobacterial infection in man. Curr Opin Immunol. 1998; 10:413.
3. Casanova JL, Blanche S, Emile JF, Jouanguy E, Lamhamedi S, Altare F, et al. Idiopathic disseminated bacillus Calmette-Guerin infection: a French national retrospective study. Pediatrics. 1996;98:774--8.
4. Casanova JL, Jouanguy E, Lamhamedi S, Blanche S, Fischer Aet al. Immunological conditions of children with BCG disseminated infection. Lancet. 1995;346:581.
5. Cottle LE. Mendelian susceptibility to mycobacterial disease. Clin Genet. 2011; 79(1):17-22.
6. Dorman SE, Picard C, Lammas D, et al. Clinical features of dominant and recessive interferon gamma receptor 1 deficiencies. Lancet. 2004; 364:2113.
7. H Medjahed H, JL Gaillard JL, JM Reyrat JM. Mycobacterium abscessus: a new player in the mycobacterial field. Trends in Microbiology., 2010;18:117-23.
8. Han XY, De I, Jacobson KL. Rapidly growing mycobacteria: Clinical and microbiologic studies of 115 cases. Am J Clin Path. 2007;128:612-21.
9. Holland SM, Dorman SE, Kwon A, et al. Abnormal regulation of interferon-gamma, interleukin-12 and tumor necrosis factor-alpha in human interferon-gamma receptor 1 deficiency. J Infect Dis .1998; 178:1095.
10. Jean-Laurent Casanova JL. Mendelian susceptibility to mycobacterial infection in man. Swiss Med Wkly, 2001;131: 445-54.
11. Nessar R, Cambau E, Reyrat JM, et al . Mycobacterium abscessus : a new antibiotic nightmare. J Antimicrob Chemother., 2012; Jan 30 , doi:10.1093/jac/dkr57867(4):810-8.
12. Newport MJ, Huxley CM, Huston S, et al. A mutation in the interferon-gamma-receptor gene and susceptibility to mycobacterial infection. N Engl J Med. 1996; 335:1941.
13. Stenger S, Modlin RL. T cell mediated immunity to Mycobacterium tuberculosis. Curr Opin Microbiol. 1999; 2:89.
14. Wang LH, Yen CL, Chang TC, et al. Impact of molecular diagnosis on treating Mendelian susceptibility to mycobacterial diseases. J Microbiol Immunol Infect. 2012; 45:411.

CONTRIBUTIONS BY:

1. Dr Karthi N, Additional Professor, Department of Pediatrics (Compilation of Clinical Details)
2. Dr Kusum Sharma, Professor, Department of Microbiology (Performing PCR)
3. Dr Meenu Singh, Professor, Department of Pediatrics (Clinician In-Charge)

Post Graduate Institute of Medical Education and Research, Chandigarh, India.

SECTION 10

Infantile Nephrotic Syndrome

CASE 58

Congenital Nephrotic Syndrome of the Finnish Type: PM 23777

Nandita Bharadwaj Kakkar

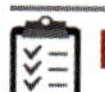

HIGHLIGHTS OF THE CASE

A 3½-month-old female child came with breath holding spells, rapid breathing and cough since 4 days. There was recent onset facial puffiness, which soon progressed to generalized edema. She was a preterm, small for date baby, born to a gravida 2 mother at 33 weeks gestation, the body weight at birth being 2 kg. The placenta was large weighing 900 g, i.e. 45% of the baby weight. There was one previous spontaneous abortion at 8 weeks gestation. Baby had dysmorphic facies, hypotension, tachycardia, edema, hypoproteinemia, hypoalbuminemia, nephrotic range proteinuria, deranged renal function tests and lipidogram, hypocalcemia, hyperphosphatemia, coagulopathy, bilateral lung infiltrates and peritonitis. A clinical diagnosis of congenital nephrotic syndrome—primary type with pneumonia, spontaneous bacterial peritonitis and refractory septic shock was made. Autopsy revealed congenital nephrotic syndrome of the Finnish type (CNF), organizing pneumonia, diffuse alveolar damage and shock.

Keywords: Congenital nephrotic syndrome, Finnish type, nephrin, podocyte, autopsy.

CLINICAL DETAILS

Date of Admission: 27.06.2010, Date of Death: 05.07.2010, Duration of Hospital Stay: 9 days.

A 3½-month-old female child came with history of breath holding spells, rapid breathing and cough since 4 days. There was recent onset facial puffiness which progressed to generalized edema during the hospital stay. The first episode of breath holding lasted for 5 minutes, it took place after an episode of prolonged crying, after which she became lethargic, stopped breathing, became dusky, but then responded to stimulation. There were three such episodes of breath holding in the 4 days, prior to admission. There was difficulty in breathing since the same duration, breathing was rapid, chest retraction was noted and breathing became more difficult during breast feeding. There was associated cough which was persistent, dry and paroxysmal. There was no history of fever, running nose, loose stools and cyanosis in the past. The mother was gravida 2, with one previous spontaneous abortion at 8 weeks gestation. The index case was a preterm, small for date baby, breach, born at 33 weeks gestation by a lower segment caesarean section, indication being fetal distress. The baby weighed 2 kg at birth. The placenta was large weighing 900 g, ratio being 900:2,000, i.e. 0.45. The baby was exclusively breastfed and was appropriately immunized for age. There was no history of renal disease or renal transplant in the family. The family was contacted in October 2015 and now they have a 3.5 years baby boy, who is doing well. ***Examination***: Baby was irritable, edematous, there was pallor, no icterus, respiratory rate—85-90/min, pulse—200-220/min with normal volume, normal blood pressure—62/35-68/47 mm Hg. CNS examination showed open anterior and posterior fontanelle, status E4M5V, no cranial nerve palsy was seen, deep tendon reflexes were present and meningeal signs were absent. Chest showed respiratory distress with tachypnea, nasal flaring and intercostal retractions. Liver was palpable 1 cm below the costal margin and splenomegaly was present. Dysmorphic facies was noted in the form of low set ears, depressed nasal bridge, small mouth, short neck and fingers.

Investigations

Hemogram—10.9 to 6.6 g/dl, TLC—18600/ul with polymorphonuclear leucocytosis, platelets—1,80,000/ul,

Coagulogarm—initially was within normal limits, towards the end—PT—33′ (N-13′), PTI—39%, INR—3.17 (N-2-3.5), APPT 80′ (N-25′-32′), D-dimers positive, Fibrinogen 2.08 gm/l (N-2-4g/l).

Blood Biochemistry: Serum bilirubin—0.7 mg%, AST—39 U/L, ALT—20 U/L, alkaline phosphatase-168–226 U/L, Total proteins/albumin/globulin—2.6/0.8/1.8 gm, serum creatinine—0.9–1.3 mg%, serum urea 11–40 mg%, uric acid—5.8 mg%, serum cholesterol—180 mg%, triglycerides 193 mg%, HDL 26 mg%, LDL—115.4 mg%, VLDL 38.6 mg%, electrolytes—Na^+—145 mEq/L, K^+ 2.9 mEq/L, Cl^- -119, Ca^{2+}—6.8 mg%, phosphatase—2.91 U/L. Routine urine—sp gravity 1.015, reaction 5, proteins 3+, 2-3 RBC/HPF, 2–3 WBC/HPF, 24 hour urinary protein—2.89 gm/day or 463 mg/m^2/hour.

Microbiology work up: TORCH workup negative, VDRL serology—negative, Blood culture negative, Ascitic tap—15–20 mL, white turbid, cells—4600, proteins—373 mg/dL, sugar—63 mg/dL, Culture grew acenitobacter species.

Other Investigations: X ray chest showed bilateral lung infiltrates. ECG—sinus tachycardia, Echocardiography—left systolic dysfunction with mild pulmonary artery hypertension, ABG—metabolic acidosis.

A ***clinical diagnosis*** of Congenital Nephrotic Syndrome- primary, pneumonia, spontaneous bacterial peritonitis, refractory septic shock, ARDS, acute kidney injury and multi organ dysfunction syndrome was made. She was put on antibiotics, inotropic and ventilatory support, transfused with packed RBC and given lasix. The baby however succumbed to her illness after a hospital stay of 9 days.

AUTOPSY FINDINGS: PM 23777

A partial autopsy was performed. The peritoneal cavity contained 500 mL of purulent fluid. The body was edematous. The ***kidneys*** (Figs 1A and B) together weighed 72 g, they were enlarged with prominent fetal lobulations and fine granularity. The cut section was pale and the cortex appeared thick. Microscopy at low power showed increased number of glomeruli (Fig 2A) of varying sizes (Fig 2B) and a striking tubular dilatation (Fig 2C). Some glomeruli were large whereas others were small. The small glomeruli (Figs 2D and E) were of the fetal type, covered by crowded cuboidal podocytes, lying in a dilated Bowman's space. The Bowman's space was strikingly prominent in many glomeruli, to the extent that in some, glomerular cysts (Fig 2F) were noted. Occasional glomeruli showed increased mesangial matrix and cellularity (Fig 3A). An occasional glomerulus was small and totally sclerosed (Fig 3B) and an occasional crescent (Fig 3C) was also noted. No podocyte hypertrophy or hyperplasia was noted. Striking tubular dilatation leading to the formation of tubular cysts containing hyaline casts (Fig 3D), interstitial inflammation (Fig 3E) and fibrosis better highlighted by

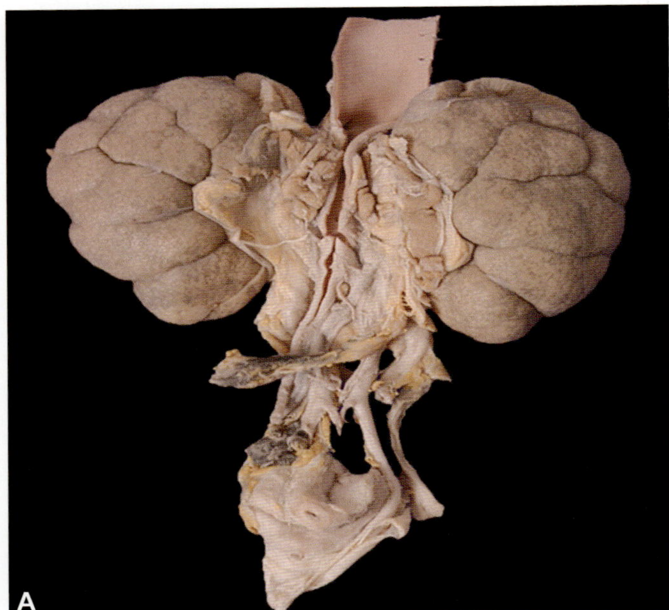

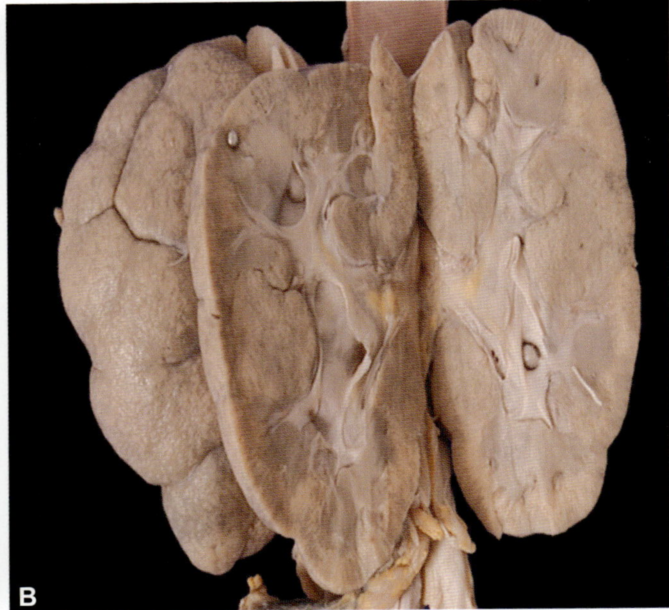

Figs 1A and B: (A) Gross picture of the kidneys, showing enlargement with prominent fetal lobulations and fine granularity; (B) Cut section is pale and the cortex is thick.

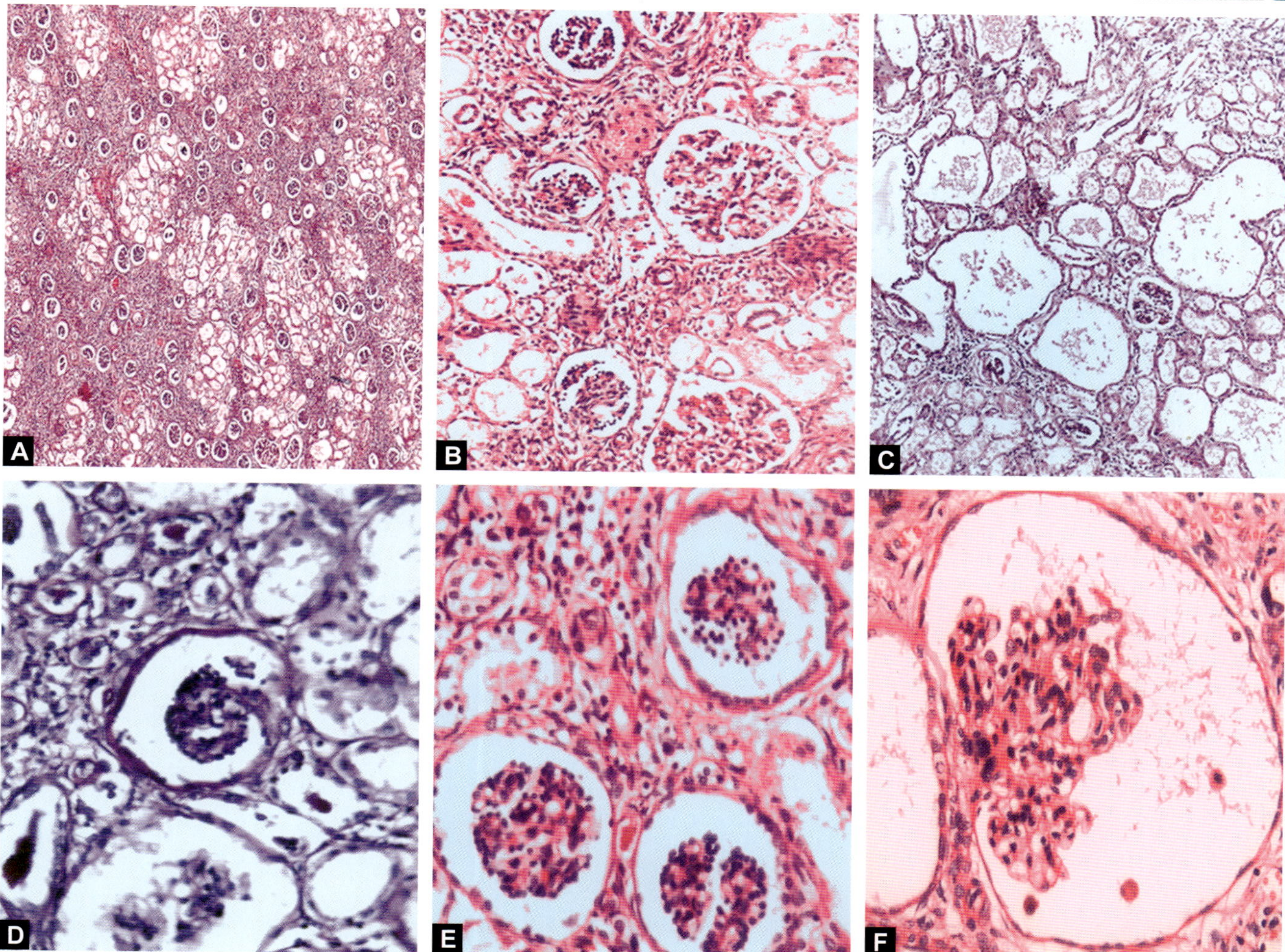

Figs 2A–F: (A) Low power photomicrograph shows increased number of glomeruli and a striking tubular dilatation; (B) Glomeruli of varying sizes; (C) Striking tubular dilatation; (D and E) Periodic acid–Schiff and H&E stain show fetal type of glomeruli, covered by cuboidal podocytes, lying in dilated Bowman's spaces; (F) Prominent Bowman's space forming a glomerular cyst.

Masson trichrome was seen (Fig 3F). Hypertensive changes were seen in the form of medial hypertrophy of the arterioles and intralobular arteries (Figs 4A and B). Tubular epithelial cells showed protein reabsorption (Fig 4C). Immunostain with WT1 showed strong positivity in the podocytes of the well-preserved large (Fig 4D) and small glomeruli and also in the few small sclerosed glomeruli (Fig 4E). Thus, there was no loss of WT1. Electron microscopy (Fig 4F) showed fusion of the foot processes with microvillous transformation. Immunofluorescence was negative for immunoglobulins and complement components. Overall features were consistent with the diagnosis of CNF. The ***lungs*** were firm to feel and showed features of organizing pneumonia with evidence of hyaline membrane formation, indicating diffuse alveolar damage (Fig 5A). Features of shock were seen in the form of centrizonal congestion in the liver and adrenal hemorrhage (Fig 5B). Thymus showed changes of marked stress involution (Fig 5C). Other organs were within normal limits.

FINAL AUTOPSY DIAGNOSIS: PM 23777

3½ Months Old Female

- Congenital Nephrotic Syndrome—Finnish type
- Organizing pneumonia with diffuse alveolar damage
- Shock—adrenal hemorrhage, centrizonal congestion in the liver
- Stress involution—thymus

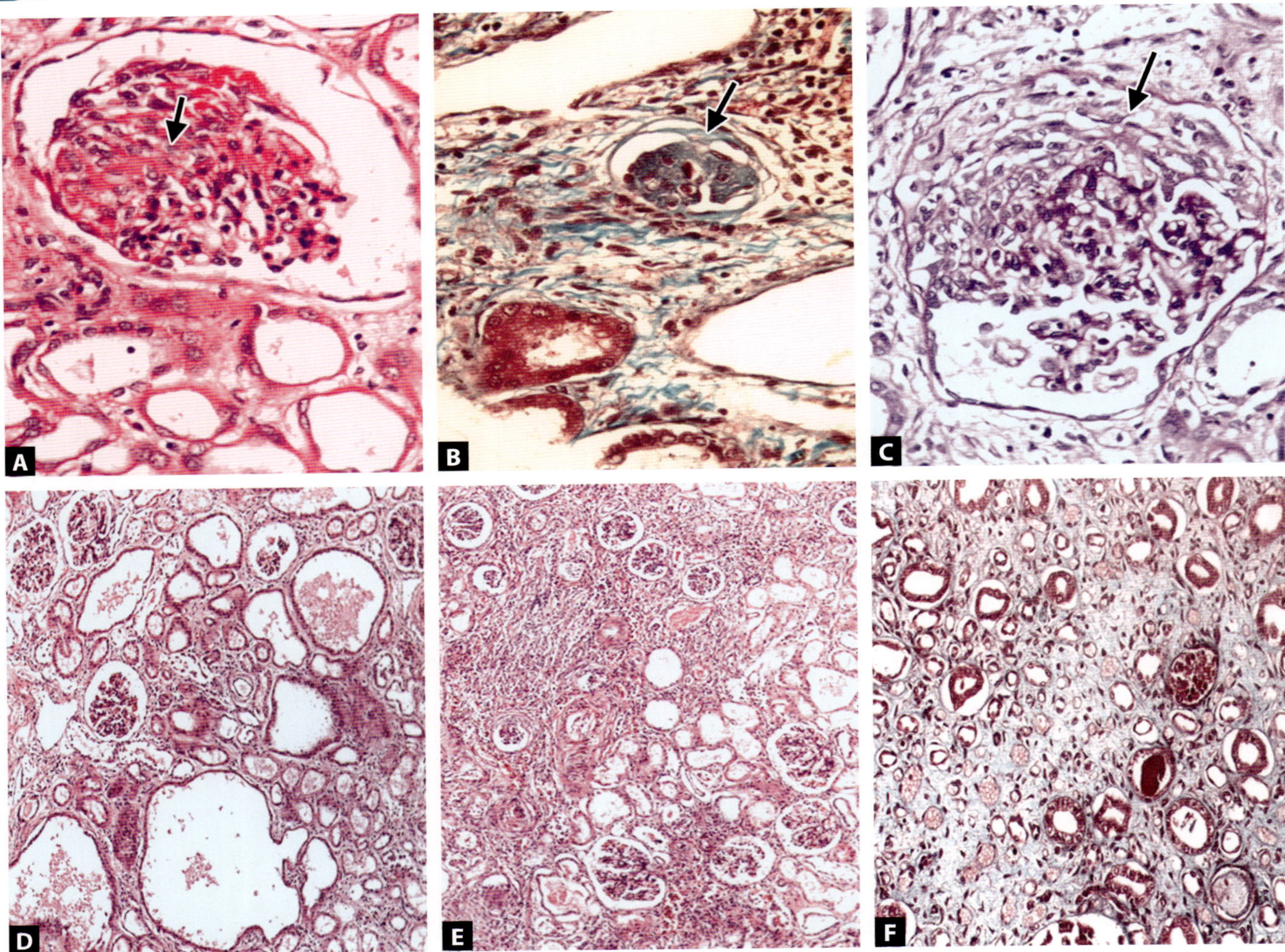

Figs 3A–F: (A) Glomerulus showing increased matrix and cellularity (arrow); (B) Masson trichrome stain showing a small sclerosed glomerulus (arrow); (C) Glomerulus showing a cellular crescent (arrow); (D) Tubular dilatation with hyaline casts; (E) Kidney showing interstitial inflammation; and (F) Fibrosis (Masson trichrome stain).

CONGENITAL NEPHROTIC SYNDROME—FINNISH TYPE

This entity is most commonly seen in Finland where it occurs in 1/8,000 births. It is however not restricted to the Finnish population and is also seen in other parts of the world.[1] It is autosomal recessive and thus has a recurrence rate of 25%. This entity was mapped to *NPHS1* gene at 19q13.1, which encodes the transmembrane protein in the slit diaphragm of the podocytes known as "nephrin". As a result of this mutation, the slit diaphragms are absent, leading to severe proteinuria, nephrotic syndrome and subsequent infections. Koziell[2] et al reviewed children with onset of proteinuria before 3 months of age, with histologic and electron microscopic findings consistent with CNF. They concluded that this phenotype could result from either *NPHS1* or *NPHS2* mutations. Mutations in *NPHS2* (which encodes "podocin") gene leads to autosomal recessive, steroid resistant nephrotic syndrome, which is histologically focal segmental glomerulosclerosis. They also concluded that triallelic mutations involving both the genes lead to congenital nephrotic syndrome with a focal segmental glomerulosclerosis phenotype.

In CNF, the nephrotic syndrome gets documented by 3 months of life, although proteinuria is present right from birth. Renal functions generally remain normal in the first 6 months of life and there are no extrarenal manifestations. Elevated α fetoprotein (AFP) levels in the amniotic fluid (15–18 weeks gestation) and in the maternal serum, form the basis of antenatal diagnosis in fetuses at risk. Elevated amniotic fluid AFP is a nonspecific finding, seen in many

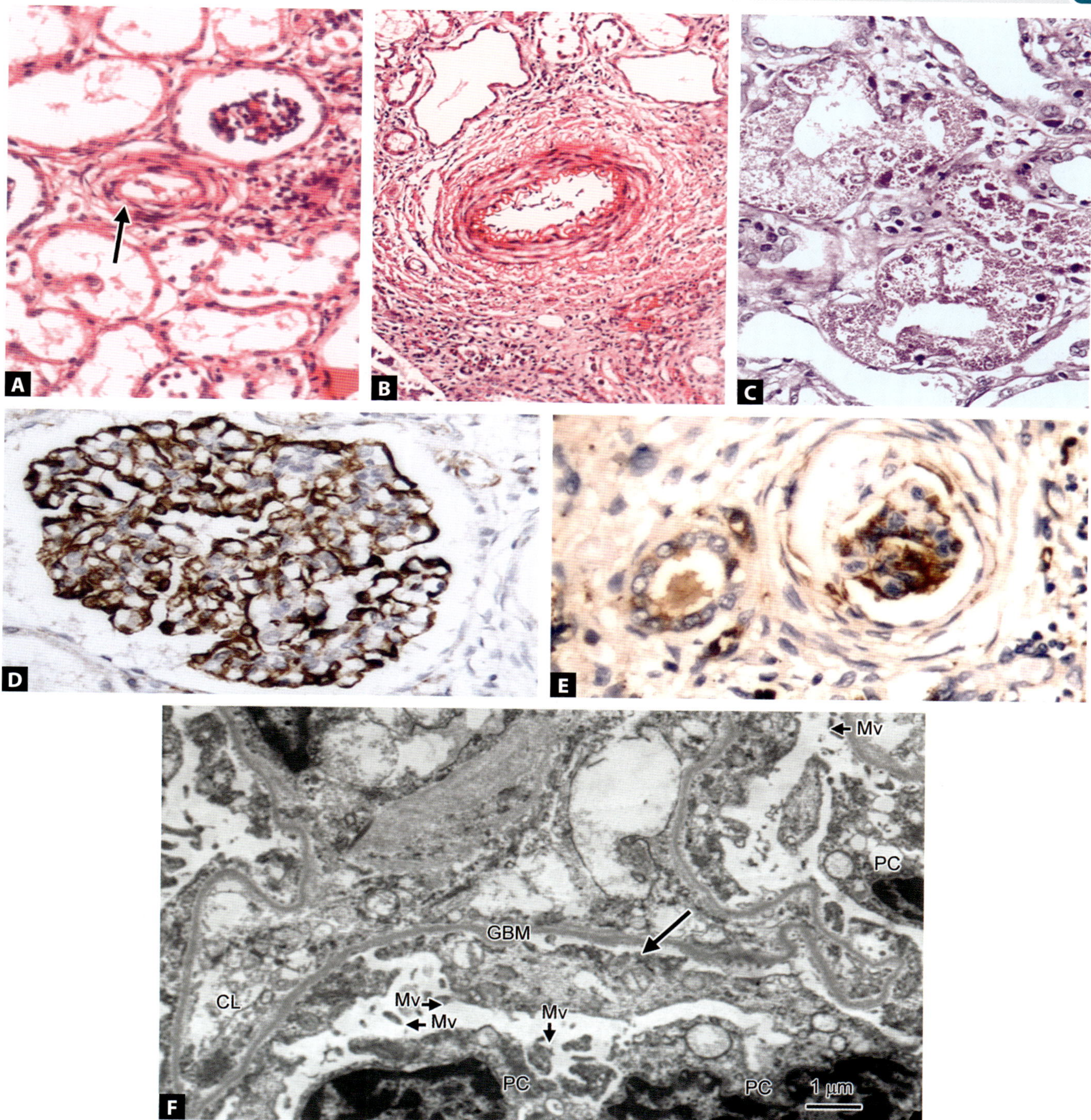

Figs 4A–F: (A and B) Photomicrograph of the kidney showing medial hypertrophy of the arterioles and intralobular arteries; (C) Tubular epithelial cells showing protein reabsorption—Periodic acid–Schiff stain; (D and E) WT1 immunostain showing strong positivity in the podocytes of the well-preserved and sclerosed glomeruli; (F) Electron micrograph through a segment of glomerulus showing microvilli (Mv) formation by podocytes (PC), loss of foot processes (arrow), glomerular basement membrane (GBM), and capillary lumen (CL). Stain: uranyl acetate and lead citrate, final magnification: 8,450x.

fetal disorders, but in CNF it occurs due to proteinuria. Thus, it can help only in fetuses at risk. CNF babies are born prematurely, are small for gestational age, edematous and have large placentas, weighing more than one-fourth of the

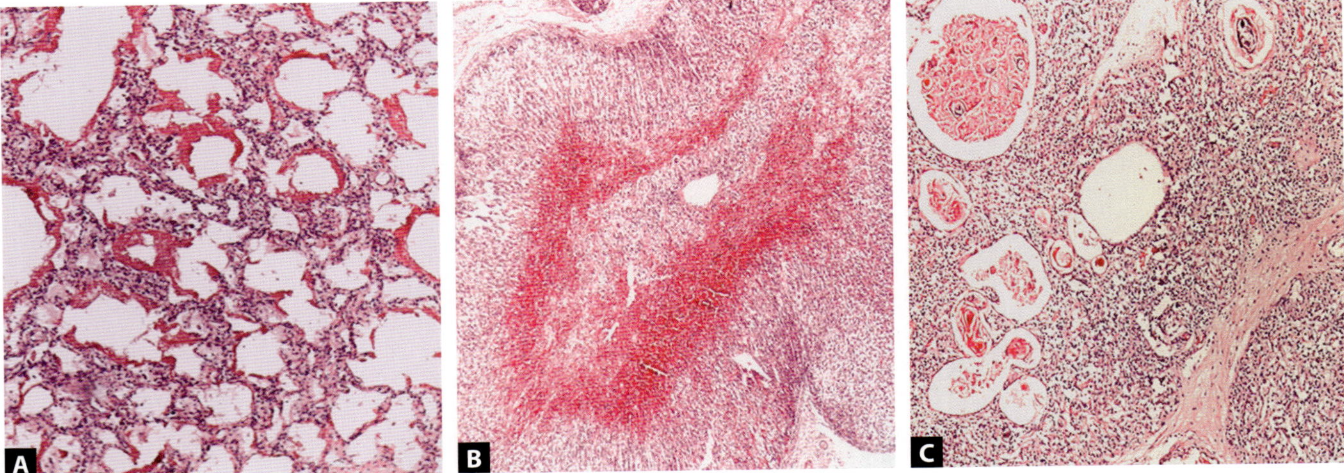

Figs 5A–C: (A) Photomicrograph of the lungs showing alveolar spaces lined by pink hyaline membranes; (B) Adrenal hemorrhage; (C) Stress involution of the thymus.

baby weight. The enlarged placenta leads to deformations of the skull, elbows, hips and knees. These babies have hypothyroidism due to urinary loss of thyroid binding globulin and this leads to abnormalities like delayed ossification, widely separated cranial sutures, large fontanelle and small nose with flat bridge.

On gross examination, kidneys in CNF are enlarged with thick cortices as they contain an increased number of nephrons. On microscopic examination, early in the course of the disease, the glomeruli are enlarged, may show increased mesangial matrix and cellularity and the Bowman's space is commonly dilated. At times glomerular cysts occur and the glomeruli in the cystic Bowman's space are small, covered by cuboidal podocytes, giving it a fetal appearance. With time the matrix increases, capillary walls become thick and the lumens become narrow. Advanced disease shows glomerular collapse, sclerosis, periglomerular fibrosis, solidification and crescents. Proximal convoluted tubules show a striking dilatation leading to the formation of tubular cysts containing hyaline casts. Electron microscopy shows fusion of the foot processes with microvillus transformation. The glomerular basement membrane may be thickened due to a wide rara interna but the lamina densa is thin. Immunofluorescence is negative for immunoglobulins and complement components. The CNF occurring outside Finland shows more clinical and morphologic heterogeneity and progresses to advanced disease more rapidly.[3] Morphology shows a combination of large and small fetal glomeruli with crowded podocytes, prominent Bowman's space, collapsed tufts, glomerular sclerosis, crescents, marked tubular dilatation, interstitial inflammation, medial hypertrophy of the arterioles and intralobular vessels.

Children with CNF die young, not due to renal failure but due to complications like malnutrition, infections and thromboembolism. Nephrin is a specific marker of podocytes in the kidney, but lately nephrin has been found in the lymphoid tissues (tonsils, adenoids), interdigitating cells of the germinal centers and T lymphocytes, brain and beta cells of the islets of Langerhans.[3] This explains why some patients develop infections and developmental delays. CNF is autosomal recessive, onset is congenital and babies are premature with large placentas, AFP is elevated in the amniotic fluid and mother's serum, there is late progression to renal insufficiency, normal blood pressure, massive proteinuria, steroid resistance and NPHS1 and 2 mutations are noted. On the other hand, diffuse mesangial sclerosis (DMS) is at times familial (AR), disease starts in the postnatal period, placenta is normal with exceptions in Drash syndrome, AFP is rarely elevated, blood pressure is elevated and there is early progression to renal failure.

COMMENTARY—INDEX CASE: PM 23777

This is a classical case of CNF in a 3½-month-old female child. She was a preterm, small for date baby, born to a gravida 2 mother at 33 weeks gestation, the body weight at birth being 2 kg. The placenta was large weighing 900 g, i.e. 45% of the baby weight. There was one previous spontaneous abortion at 8 weeks gestation. Baby had dysmorphic facies in the form of low set ears, depressed nasal bridge, small mouth and short neck and fingers. Dysmorphism occurs due to deformations because of a large placenta or due to hypothyroidism as a result of urinary loss of thyroid binding globulins. This baby was well till 3 months and 10 days of life. Thereafter, she presented with pneumonia, cough and breath holding spells. There was generalized edema, refractory hypotension, tachycardia, severe hypoproteinemia and hypoalbuminemia, nephrotic range proteinuria, deranged renal function tests and lipidogram, hypocalcemia, hyperphosphatemia, coagulopathy, bilateral lung infiltrates and peritonitis. A clinical diagnosis of congenital nephrotic syndrome—primary type with pneumonia, spontaneous bacterial peritonitis and refractory septic shock was made. She was treated with antibiotics, inotropic and ventilatory support, blood transfusions, intravenous proteins and lasix. The baby however succumbed to her illness after a hospital stay of 9 days. Autopsy revealed renal histology consistent with a diagnosis of CNF. There was morphologic heterogeneity as described as above.

TAKE HOME MESSAGE

- Congenital nephrotic syndrome of the Finnish type is seen predominantly in Finland, but it is also seen in other parts of the world.
- It is autosomal recessive, mapped to mutations in the *NPHS1* gene at 19q13.1, which encodes the transmembrane protein "nephrin" in the slit diaphragm of the podocytes.
- As a result of this mutation the slit diaphragms are absent leading to severe proteinuria, nephrotic syndrome and subsequent infections.

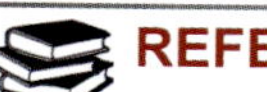

REFERENCES

1. Finn LS, Symons JM, Smith JM. Nephrotic syndrome in the newborn. Am J Kid Dis. 2003;42(6):1318-23.
2. Koziell A, Grech V, Hussain S, et al. Genotype or phenotype correlations of NPHS1 and NPHS2 mutations in nephrotic syndrome advocate a functional inter-relationship in glomerular filtration. Hum Mol Genet. 2002;11(4):379-88.
3. Shi Y, Ding J, Liu JC et al. NPHS1 mutations in a Chinese family with congenital nephrotic syndrome. Zhonghua Er Ke Za Zhi. 2005;43(11):805-9.

CONTRIBUTIONS BY:

1. Dr Charan Singh Rayat, Tutor, Department of Histopathology (Electron Microscopy)
2. Dr S Singhi, Ex-Professor and Head, Department of Pediatrics (Clinician In-Charge)

Post Graduate Institute of Medical Education and Research, Chandigarh, India.

CASE 59

Infantile Nephrotic Syndrome—Diffuse Mesangial Sclerosis in a 10-Month-Old Male Child: PM 26462

Nandita Bharadwaj Kakkar

 HIGHLIGHTS OF THE CASE

A 10-month-old male child, who was ill since 3 months, was referred from an outside facility in view of 4+ proteinuria and deranged renal function tests, having been started on oral prednisolone. He had loose stools, vomiting, generalized edema and rash. Four days prior to demise, there was difficulty in breathing and decreased urinary output. He was the first born child of an adequately supervised, primigravida mother, born at term with a birth weight of 2.6 kg. Investigations revealed a nephrotic range proteinuria, hyponatremia, hypokalemia, hypochloremia, deranged renal functions, hypoproteinemia, hypoalbuminemia, hyperlipidemia, deranged coagulogram and transition to pancytopenia within 5 days of hospital stay. ***Units clinical diagnosis*** was infantile nephrotic syndrome, chronic diarrhea, features of micronutrient deficiency, mucosal candidiasis and septic shock. Final autopsy diagnosis was infantile nephrotic syndrome consistent with diffuse mesangial sclerosis, along with early acute pancreatitis and bronchopneumonia with diffuse alveolar damage.

Keywords: Infantile, congenital, nephrotic syndrome, diffuse mesangial sclerosis, podocytopathy, autopsy.

 CLINICAL DETAILS

Date of Admission: 28.01.2015, Date of Death: 02.02.2015, Duration of Hospital Stay: 5 Days.

A 10-month-old male child was referred to our institute with complaints of loose stools and vomiting since 3 months. The stools were 10–20 per day, small volume, not containing blood or mucous and nonfoul smelling. There were 4–5 vomitings per day which were nonbilious and not blood stained. There was generalized swelling over the body and perianal rash since 1 month. The swelling started as periorbital puffiness which later became generalized. The rash initially started in the perianal area and gradually involved the thighs and genital area. Five days prior to demise, the stools were black-colored and there was hematemesis. Four days prior to demise there was difficulty in breathing and decreased urinary output. He was the first born child of an adequately supervised, primigravida mother. He was delivered at term, by emergency caesarean section in view of cephalopelvic disproportion, with a birth weight of 2.6 kg. There was no history of fever, poor feeding, feed intolerance, breathing difficulty, jaundice, seizures or altered sensorium. There was no similar illness in the family and no previous abortion. He was immunized for age and had received BCG, OPV and the BCG scar was present. He was on exclusive breast feed till 6 months of age and thereafter predominantly breastfed. He was admitted at an outside facility for 4 days and was referred to our institute in view of 4+ proteinuria and deranged renal function tests, having been started on oral prednisolone (2 mg/kg/day). On ***examination***—generalized body swelling, pitting edema, pallor, oral thrush, glossitis, cheilitis and rash with excoriation in the perianal and genital areas were present. The body weight was 10 kg (0 to +2 WHO), length: 72 cm (0 to −2 WHO) and occipito-frontal circumference: 45 cm (0 to −1 WHO). The abdomen was uniformly distended, umbilicus was horizontally slit and both kidneys were palpable and ballotable. Shifting dullness and bowel sounds were present. External genitalia were normal.

Investigations

Hemogram revealed transition to pancytopenia within five days of hospital stay. There was a progressive fall in hemoglobin (11.2–6.2 g/dL), TLC fell from 13,220/uL

(P 70, L 24, M 04, E 02) to 3200/uL (P 06, L73, M21) and platelets fell from 1,95000/uL to 16000/uL. Coagulogram was deranged (PT—20', PTI—70%, aPTT 56', INR—1.44).

Routine urine examination: proteins 4+, sugar 1+, pus cells—10–15 WBC's/HPF, RBC—nil, coarse granular casts and epithelial cell casts present. Urine osmolality—360 mosm/kg (normal—500 to 800); Serum osmolality—298 mosm/kg (normal—280 to 295); Urine electrolytes—Sodium-31, Potassium—27.2, Creatinine—20.5; Fractional excretion of sodium (FeNa) 22%, suggesting acute tubular necrosis; Transtubular potassium gradient 7.5 (high in the setting of hypokalemia).

Blood biochemistry: There was hyponatremia (122 mEq), hypokalaemia (2.2 mEq), hypochloremia (78 mEq), deranged renal functions (S urea 184 mg%—S creatinine 1.4 mg%), hypoproteinemia (3.1 gms), hypoalbuminemia (0.7 gms) and hyperlipidemia (S cholesterol—384 mg%, triglycerides—535 mg%).

Ultrasonography abdomen: Liver size 9 cms, normal echotexture, spleen: 3.7 cm, kidneys: Right: 7.9 cm, Left: 7.3 cm (normal 6 cm) with increased echogenicity of column of Bertini.

Microbiological investigations: Urine and blood cultures were sterile, HIV, HBV, HCV, VDRL-negative, TORCH serology-negative, Ascitic fluid—TLC-40 cells, DLC—predominantly polymorphs, culture-sterile.

The child was given antibiotics, fluconazole, micronutrients, Vitamin K, pantoprazole, lasix, fluid bolus, inotropes in view of shock, peritoneal dialysis and at the end was intubated. Preterminal events were seizures, altered sensorium, sepsis and shock. ***Units final clinical diagnosis*** was Infantile Nephrotic Syndrome, chronic diarrhoea, features of micronutrient deficiency, mucosal candidiasis and septic shock.

AUTOPSY FINDINGS: PM 26462

A partial autopsy was performed on this 10-month-old male child. The external appearance revealed a puffy face, distended abdomen with upturned umbilicus and sloughed off skin on both limbs. The peritoneal cavity contained 300 mL of straw-colored fluid. The ***kidneys*** together weighed 95 g as compared to a normal of 66 g at this age. They were enlarged with preserved fetal lobulations (Fig 1A). Cut section showed a distinct corticomedullary junction with medullary congestion (Fig 1B). Microscopic examination (Figs 1C–E and Figs 2A,C,D,E) showed a segmental/diffuse involvement of the glomeruli with characteristic sclerosis of the mesangial matrix by a fibrillary material, better highlighted by Masson trichrome stain. This was causing mesangial expansion leading to obliteration of the capillary lumina. Minimal mesangial cell proliferation was noted. The podocytes (visceral epithelial cells) were hypertrophied and showed a single layer of crown-like appearance over the sclerosed glomerular tufts (Figs 1C–E and Figs 2A,C,D,E). The podocytes in a few glomeruli showed hypertrophy and detachment giving a crowded appearance falsely mimicking hyperplasia. Immunohistochemistry with WTI showed positivity in the podocytes, i.e. there was no loss of WT1 (Figs 2F and G). The proliferation marker Ki67 was however negative in the prominent podocytes (Fig 3A). The Bowman's spaces were prominent. Some of the glomeruli were reduced to small sclerotic balls (Fig 2B), crowned by prominent podocytes, lying in a prominent Bowman's space (Figs 2E–G). The cortical glomeruli were more affected with diminishing severity toward the corticomedullary junction. Widespread tubular ectasia and dilation (Figs 3B and C) were noted with some tubules showing hyaline casts. Tubular epithelial cells also showed protein resorption droplets. Interstitium showed fibrosis, highlighted on Masson Trichrome stain and mild hypertensive changes were appreciated in the intralobular arteries. Some intralobular arteries show mild hypertensive changes. Immunofluorescence was negative for IgG, IgM, IgA, C3 and C1q. Electron microscopy (Figs 3D–F) showed collagen fibrils in the mesangium, irregular thickening of the glomerular basement membrane (GBM) with irregular contours and splitting in areas. The podocytes were prominent and showed effacement of foot processes, with detachment of the epithelial cell from the GBM. Overall features were consistent with a diagnosis of diffuse mesangial sclerosis (DMS). Morphologically the differential diagnosis of DMS is from collapsing glomerulopathy wherein the podocytes are de-differentiated leading to hyperplasia (> 2 cell layer). The hyperplastic podocytes in collapsing glomerulopathy show positivity with proliferation marker Ki67 and loss of WT1 nuclear expression, which was not seen in the index case. The ***pancreas*** (Figs 4A and B) was grossly normal with focal hemorrhage and chalky white deposits in peripancreatic region. Microscopic examination showed acute pancreatitis with acute inflammatory infiltrate in the acini and pancreatic ducts along with fat necrosis and hemorrhage in the peripancreatic region. The ***lungs*** (Fig 4C) showed acute bronchopneumonia with hyaline membrane formation indicating diffuse alveolar damage along with edema. The ***esophagus*** showed presence of blackish discoloration at gastro-esophageal junction, which on microscopy showed ulceration with presence of candidal spores and hyphae invading the wall. ***Adrenal*** hemorrhage was noted. All other organs were within normal limits.

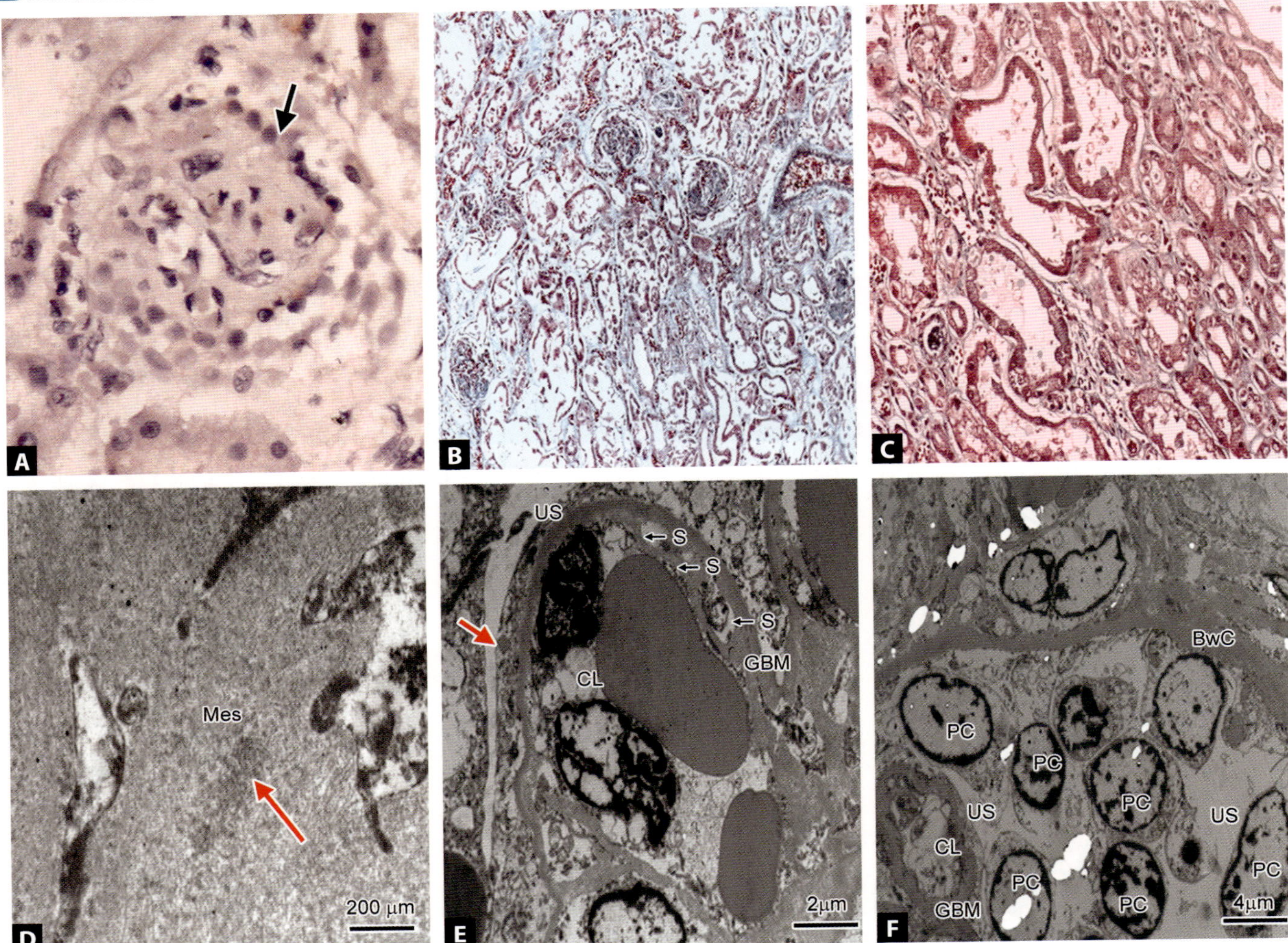

Figs 3A–F: (A) Ki67 immunohistochemistry negative in the hypertrophied podocytes (arrow); (B and C) Kidney showing prominent tubular dilatation; (D) Electron micrograph through mesangial (Mes) area of a glomerulus showing fibrillar material (arrow); stain: uranyl acetate and lead citrate, final magnification: 33,885x; (E) Electron micrograph through a segment of glomerulus showing splitting (S) of glomerular basement membrane (GBM), capillary lumen (CL), urinary space (US) and effacement of foot processes (red arrow); stain: uranyl acetate and lead citrate, final magnification: 5,650x; (F) Electron micrograph through a segment of glomerulus showing prominent podocytes (PC) in urinary space (US), Bowman's capsule (BwC), glomerular basement membrane (GBM) of a capillary loop and capillary lumen (CL); stain: uranyl acetate and lead citrate, final magnification: 2,800x.

umbrella of podocytopathies, which are caused by genetic or environmental factors. The clinical picture varies, depending on at what "time" during the glomerular development, the insult occurs and how rapidly it affects the glomerulus. The various clinical syndromes which occur due to the podocyte dysfunction of various types include congenital nephrotic syndrome of the Finnish type (CNF), diffuse mesangial sclerosis (DMS), Alport syndrome and variants, minimal change disease, FSGS, collapsing glomerulopathy (CG), immune/inflammatory glomerulopathy, hypertensive nephropathy, diabetic nephropathy and age-related glomerulopathy. These account for 90% of the end-stage renal diseases. WT1, a zinc finger protein transcription factor is critical to the development of podocyte architecture, regulates podocyte differentiation and maintains the integrity of the filtration barrier. It is initially expressed in all cell precursors, but in the mature nephron, its expression is limited to the podocytes only. It regulates key proteins including nephrin and podocalyxin. WT1 gene mutation leads to loss of podocyte WT1 protein content and an immature podocyte phenotype, which subsequently leads to various genetically determined or acquired podocytopathies like steroid resistant FSGS, DMS and CG. Other transcriptional regulators in podocyte injury include PAX2 and LIM homeobox transcription factor 1β.

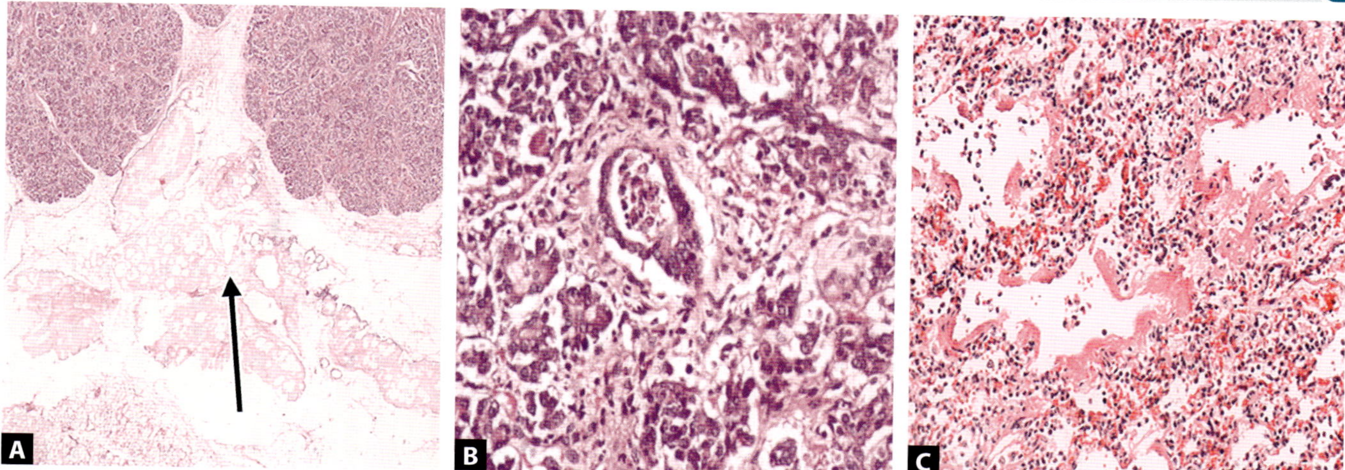

Figs 4A–C: (A) Photomicrograph showing fat necrosis around the pancreas; (B) Acute pancreatitis with polymorphs in the duct and interstitium; (C) Lungs showing pneumonia and hyaline membranes, indicating diffuse alveolar damage.

Injury to the podocytes alters their biology and leads to a spectrum of syndromes. Podocytopathies identify five patterns of glomerular injury:

1. ***Injury leading to developmental arrest of glomerulus*:**
   - Gene mutations leading to glomerular developmental arrest at an early stage lead to the clinical syndrome of *DMS* which includes proteinuria from birth and progression to end-stage renal disease within 6–12 months. Mutations in the WT1, PLCE1 and LAMB2 genes cause DMS.
   - Gene mutations leading to glomerular developmental arrest at a late stage lead to congenital nephrotic syndrome of the Finnish type (CNF), wherein life-threatening massive proteinuria occurs. The filtration machine prevents the loss of proteins into the glomerular filtrate and this job is done by the interdigitating foot processes of the podocytes and the slit diaphragms. Mutations in the genes which produce the various proteins and signaling system of the slit diaphragm is responsible for CNF. In CNF, mutations occur in the *NPHS1* gene coding for the slit diaphragm protein "nephrin" and *NPHS2* gene, coding for the foot process membrane protein "podocin".
2. ***Injury leading to podocyte depletion*:** FSGS has been associated with podocytopenia. In FSGS, the podocyte injury leads to podocyte death, denudation of the GBM, adhesions to Bowman's capsule, segmental sclerosis and global sclerosis. Mutations in genes *NPHS2* (podocin), *PLCE1, alpha-actinin 4* and *TRPC6,* leads to FSGS.
3. ***Injury leading to podocyte de-differentaition*** leads to collapsing glomerulopathy. This occurs in HIV-associated nephropathy and pamidronate toxicity. Here, mature podocyte markers like WT1, nephrin, GLEPP1, podocalyxin, p21, p27 and the foot processes are lost. With this de-differentiation and regression, markers of immaturity are acquired. Podocytes multiply and Ki67 immunohistochemistry shows positivity in the proliferating podocytes.
4. ***Injury leading to podocyte phenotype switch*:** The prototype of this type of injury leads to minimal change disease. This is triggered by allergic or immune events which produce circulating cytokines. Steroids can reverse the switch back to the normal podocyte phenotype. The podocyte number is normal.
5. ***Injury leading to defective GBM construction and maintenance*:** The GBM has to have specific characteristics, for performing its job. It has to be thin, strong and rugged. It is made of type 1V collagen—α3, α4, α5 chains, produced by the podocytes. Mutations in genes coding for the α3 and α4 chains lead to "thin GBM disease". Mutations in gene coding for α5 type IV collagen leads to Alport syndrome, which is sex-linked, causes defects in the GBM, eye lens and cochlear membrane leading to renal failure, deafness and visual defects.

Etiology of Congenital Nephrotic Syndrome

Infantile nephrotic syndrome has a genetic basis in approximately two-thirds of the cases.[4] Other causes are due to drugs (mercury), infections (TORCH, syphilis, HBV, HCV) and idiopathic. Hinkes et al[5] stated that two-thirds of cases of infantile nephrotic syndrome have mutations in four genes

(*NPHS1, NPHS2, WT1, LAMB2*) and they are resistant to steroid treatment. The four genes highlighted are:

1. *NPHS1*: This encodes a key component of the podocyte slit diaphragm, i.e. "nephrin" and leads to Finnish-type congenital nephrotic syndrome (CNS). The gene is present on the long arm of chromosome 19 (19q13.1).
2. *NPHS2*: This encodes a protein that interacts with nephrin at the slit diaphragm, i.e. "podocin" and leads to familial focal segmental glomerulosclerosis. The gene is present on the chromosome 1q25–1q31.
3. *WT1*, encodes a protein involved in the development of the kidney and gonads, i.e. the "transcription factor" and is responsible for the Denys-Drash syndrome.
4. *LAMB2*, encodes a component of the GBM, i.e. "laminin beta 2" and is responsible for the Pierson syndrome.

Mutations in *NPHS1* and *NPHS2* were the most common, accounting for approximately 95% of cases. Recently phospholipase C epsilon (PLCE1)[6] has been identified in cases of DMS. *PLCE1* mutation leads to abnormal glomerular development. Hinkes et al[7] highlighted that mutations in the *PLCE1* gene, which encodes phospholipase C epsilon, are responsible for the early onset of isolated DMS.

A common approach followed by practitioners is to separate cases into four categories:

- CNS of the Finnish type, i.e. CNF also known as primary CNS.
- Diffuse mesangial sclerosis including that occurring in Drash syndrome.
- Syndromic CNS other than Drash syndrome, which includes Frasier syndrome, Pierson syndrome, Galloway Mowat syndrome, Nail patella syndrome and Lowe syndrome.
- Secondary CNS, related to infections (CMV, hepatitis B and C, HIV, malaria, rubella, syphilis and toxoplasmosis), immune disorders (infantile systemic lupus erythematosus and alloimmunization to podocyte proteins) and drugs especially mercury (teething powder) toxicity.

Sibley et al[8] highlighted that patients who presented after 3 months of age had a better outcome than those in whom the same lesion presented before 3 months of age, regardless of the type of lesion. They further highlighted that DMS progressed to end-stage renal disease regardless of the patient's age at onset.

DIFFUSE MESANGIAL SCLEROSIS

Diffuse mesangial sclerosis[9] presents after birth, between 3 months and 11 months of life. It is the second hereditary cause of infantile nephrotic syndrome which is associated with glomerular injury leading to developmental arrest of glomerulus and progression to end-stage renal disease. It is divided into isolated DMS and Denys–Drash syndrome with DMS. There is severe proteinuria, often along with hematuria and this leads to hypoproteinemia and subsequent edema. There is elevated blood pressure and progressive renal failure begins at an early age. Amniotic fluid seldom shows elevated alpha-fetoprotein (AFP) levels and placentomegaly is not seen, exception being babies with DMS in Drash syndrome. In some cases, there is a familial occurrence and few of these indicate an autosomal recessive inheritance. None of these however demonstrate NPHS1 or NPHS2 mutations. Mutations in the WT1,[10] PLCE1,[6] and LAMB2 genes cause DMS. Mutations in WT1 lead to Denys–Drash syndrome, Frasier syndrome and Wilms tumor-aniridia (WAGR) syndrome. Drash syndrome consists of nephropathy, Wilms tumor and gonadal dysgenesis and is associated with point mutations in the Wilms tumor suppressor gene located at 11p13. Another gene implicated in DMS is PLCE1 gene located on chromosome 10q23 and it encodes for a protein PLCE1, which is a member of the phospholipase family of enzymes. Laminin beta 2 (LAMB2) mutations mapped to chromosome 3p14-p22 leads to Pierson syndrome, which shows DMS along with microconia. Galloway Mowat syndrome shows DMS, microcephaly, gyral abnormalities and hiatal hernia. The glomerular abnormality in DMS is the same, regardless of the syndromal association.

In DMS, grossly the kidneys may be enlarged. Microscopy reveals an increase in mesangial matrix without an increase in mesangial cellularity leading on to diminished patency of the capillary lumina, hypertrophy of podocytes and a crown like or crowded appearance of the hypertrophied vacuolated podocytes over the glomerular tuft (form the so called 'pseudocrescent'), prominent Bowmans space, variably thickened basement membrane and progressive sclerosis (segmental and global). In late stages (almost all glomeruli are involved), it progresses to transform the entire tuft into a shrunken, solidified ball with almost avascular glomerular tufts surrounded by crowded podocytes. The podocytes do not express Ki-67. The cortical glomeruli are more affected and the severity diminishes toward the corticomedullary junction. Tubular microcysts with hyaline casts are commonly present. There may be tubular atrophy along with interstitial fibrosis. The histopathologic differentiation of early DMS from CNF may be difficult. Immunofluorescence in DMS may be negative or may show nonspecific deposits of IgM and C3 and the abnormality is not immune-mediated. Electron microscopy shows mesangial collagen fibrils, irregular thickening of the GBM which has irregular contours and may show splitting and podocyte damage seen as effacement of foot processes with detachment of the epithelial cells from the GBM. The histopathologic appearance is however pathognomonic. Differential diagnosis of DMS includes collapsing variant of FSGS which is a focal process, causing de-differentiation of the podocytes in the form of hyperplasia (>2 cell layer) and tuft collapse. The podocytes show positivity with Ki-67 and there is loss of WT1 nuclear expression.

COMMENTARY—INDEX CASE: PM 26462

A 10-month-old male child, ill since 3 months, referred from an outside facility was diagnosed as a case of infantile nephrotic syndrome. He was the first born child of an adequately supervised, primigravida mother, born at term with a birth weight of 2.6 kg. There was no facial dysmorphism noted. Final autopsy diagnosis was infantile nephrotic syndrome consistent with diffuse mesangial sclerosis. Genetic work up could not be done in this case but the kidneys showed classical features of DMS. Both kidneys were enlarged. Microscopic examination showed characteristic sclerosis of the mesangial matrix, obliteration of the capillary lumina, minimal mesangial cell proliferation, hypertrophy of podocytes forming a single layer of crown-like architecture over the sclerosed glomerular tufts, podocytic detachment giving a crowded appearance falsely mimicking hyperplasia with the proliferation marker Ki67 being negative, prominent Bowman's space, few glomeruli reduced to small sclerotic balls crowned by prominent podocytes lying in a prominent Bowman's space and widespread tubular dilatation. Immunohistochemistry with WTI showed positivity in the podocytes thereby indicating that there was no loss of WT1. Electron microscopy also showed classical features of DMS. Morphologically the differential diagnosis of DMS is from collapsing glomerulopathy, which was ruled out in this case as discussed above

TAKE HOME MESSAGE

- Infantile nephrotic syndrome has a genetic basis in approximately two-thirds of the cases and show mutations in the following four genes—*NPHS1*, *NPHS2*, *WT1* and *LAMB2*.
- Mutations in the WT1, *PLCE1* and *LAMB2* genes cause diffuse mesangial sclerosis.
- Microscopy in DMS reveals mesangial sclerosis, hypertrophy of podocytes and a crown-like appearance of the hypertrophied vacuolated podocytes (negative for Ki67) over the glomerular tuft, prominent Bowman's space, diminished patency of the capillary lumina, prominent tubular dilatation and in late stages transforms the entire tuft into a shrunken, solidified ball with almost avascular glomerular tufts surrounded by crowded podocytes.

REFERENCES

1. Jameela A, Montini G, Bockenhauer D, et al. Clinic-pathological correlations of congenital and infantile nephrotic syndrome over twenty years. Pediatr Nephrol. 2014;29:2173-80.
2. Wiggens RC. The spectrum of podocytopathies: a unifying view of glomerular diseases. Kidney International. 2007;71: 1205-14.
3. Barisoni L, Schnaper HW, Kopp JB. Advances in the biology and genetics of the podocytopathies. Arch Path Lab Med. 2009;133:201-16.
4. Benoit G, Machuca E, Antignac C. Hereditary nephrotic syndrome: a systematic approach for genetic testing and review of associated podocyte gene mutations. Pediatr Nephrol. 2010;2:1621-32.
5. Hinkes BG, Mucha B, Vlangos CN, et al. Nephrotic syndrome in the first year of life: two thirds of cases are caused by mutations in 4 genes (NPHS1, NPHS2, WT1 and LAMB2). Pediatrics. 2007;119:e907–19.
6. Gbadegesin R, Hinkes BG, Hoskins BE, et al. Mutations in PLCE1 are a major cause of isolated diffuse mesangial sclerosis (IDMS). Nephrol Dial Transplant. 2008;23:1291-7.
7. Hinkes B, Wiggins RC, Gbadegesin R, et al. Positional cloning uncovers mutations in PLCE1 responsible for a nephrotic syndrome variant that may be reversible. Nat Genet. 2006;38:1397.
8. Sibley RK, Mahan J, Mauer SM, et al. A clinicopathologic study of 48 infants with nephrotic syndrome. Kidney International. 1985;27:544.
9. Vankalakunti M, Jha PK, Madraki RM, et al. Diffuse mesangial sclerosis- report of two cases. Indian J Nephrol. 2012;22(3):213-6.
10. Niaudet P, Gubler MC. WT1 and glomerular diseases. Pediatr Nephrol. 2006;21:1653-60.

CONTRIBUTIONS BY:

1. Dr Anand Bardia, Junior Resident, Department of Pathology (In taking Gross Pictures)
2. Dr Vani Bharani, Senior Resident, Department of Pathology (In taking Photomicrographs)
3. Dr Ashish Agarwal, Junior Resident, Department of Pediatrics (Compilation of Clinical Details)
4. Dr Charan Singh Rayat, Department of Histopathology (Electron Microscopy)
5. Dr Surjit Singh, Professor and Head, Department of Pediatrics (Clinician In-Charge)

Post Graduate Institute of Medical Education and Research, Chandigarh, India.

SECTION 11

Infections
Pediatric Cases

CASE 60

Disseminated Congenital Cytomegalovirus Infection with Islet Cell Hyperplasia as the Cause of Persistent Hypoglycemia in a Neonate: PM 23822

Nandita Bharadwaj Kakkar

HIGHLIGHTS OF THE CASE

A small for date, intrauterine growth retarded (IUGR) baby was born at 37 weeks gestation by an emergency lower segment caesarean section (LSCS) with a body weight of 1,000 g. The mother was 29-year-old, gravida 5, with no living issue. Baby was admitted to the NICU at 20 hours of life with chief complaints of hypoglycemia detected at 1 hour of life and jaundice detected at 8 hours of life. Ultrasonography at 25 weeks gestation had revealed gross oligohydramnios, thickened placenta, reversed umbilical artery flow and cytomegalovirus (CMV) infection was strongly suspected. The TORCH work up in the mother (antenatal) and in the baby during her stay in the NICU were negative. The clinical diagnosis was IUGR with persistent hypoglycemia and late onset neonatal sepsis. The autopsy revealed disseminated CMV with florid CMV pneumonia, hepatitis and tubulointerstitial nephritis. There was microcephaly, periventricular leukomalacia, patent ductus arteriosus (PDA) and pancreatic islet cell hyperplasia leading to persistent hypoglycemia.

Keywords: Congenital, cytomegalovirus infection, intrauterine growth retardation, neonatal, hypoglycemia, islet cell hyperplasia, CMV hepatitis, autopsy.

CLINICAL DETAILS

Date of Birth: 21.06.2010, 1.52 PM, Date of Admission: 22.06.2010, Date of Death: 29.07.2010, Duration of Hospital Stay: 38 Days.

A 39 days female baby was for the first time admitted to the NICU at 20 hours of life with chief complaints of hypoglycemia detected at 1 hour of life and jaundice detected at 8 hours of life. She was small for date with IUGR, was born at 37 weeks of gestation with a body weight of 1,000 g. The mother was 29-year-old with a bad obstetric history, with no living issue. She was gravida 5 with four abortions (G5P0040); G1—loss at 4 months Rubella positive, treated for 6 months; G2—loss at 3.5 months; G3—loss at 2.5 months; G4—loss at 2 months, antiphospholipid antibodies (APLA) positive, on ecosprin for 2 years and G5—index case. The mothers blood group was O +ve, was nondiabetic, she was APLA positive, was on heparin 40 U BD (APLA—Non reactive after treatment) and was hypothyroid [TSH—2.29] for which she was taking thyronorm 100 μg OD. Triple Screen/HIV/HbsAg/VDRL/TORCH IgM in the mother were all negative. This was a supervised pregnancy and she had received routine antenatal care. Ultrasonography at 25 weeks gestation revealed a hyperechoic bowel shadow, gross oligohydramnios, thickened placenta and umbilical artery showed a reversed flow. CMV infection was strongly suspected. Ultrasonography at 36 weeks gestation showed a breech presentation, absent end-diastolic flow (AEDF), oligohydramnios, IUGR approximately 27 weeks with an expected weight of 924 g. Baby was delivered by emergency LSCS, indication being severe IUGR, AEDF and the birth weight was 1.063 kg with an APGAR of 8, 9. On admission to NICU at 20 hours of life, serum bilirubin was 6.5 mg% with a packed cell volume (PCV) of 50% and phototherapy was started. The random blood sugar (RBS) at 1 hour after birth was low, for which intravenous infusion was started (5% dextrose at 4 mg/kg/min) and the RBS at 2 hour was 52 mg% and at 6 hour was 60 mg%. At 24 hours of life with RBS of 32 mg%, 10 % dextrose was added at 6 mg/kg/min. There was symmetrical IUGR with Ponderal index of 2.9, thus indicating a severe IUGR. On ***examination*** the cry, tone, activity was good and she was accepting minimal feeds well, dolichocephaly +, microcephaly +, non-blanchable purpuric spots +, hepatosplenomegaly + and ophthalmology evaluation showed persistent papillary membrane but no chorioretinitis or cataract. Rest of the systemic examination was clinically within normal limits. Echocardiography revealed a PDA of 1.5 mm, but she was clinically and hemodynamically stable.

Investigations and Course of Management

***Hemogram*:** Hb showed a progressive fall from 14.6 to 6.9 g/dL; TLC ranged from 7600 to 11,100 /uL, platelets fell from 82000 to 35000/uL, PBF- microcytic hypochromic anaemia, anisocytosis and NRBC's - 20/100 WBC's. Coagulogram: PT/PTI/aPTT/INR- 19s/68%/40s/1.58, Fibrinogen 4g/L, D-Dimer positive. G6PD deficiency present.

***Blood Biochemistry*:** Na^+ 155 to 123 mEq/L, K^+ 3.2 to 8 mEq/L, serum urea—13 to 42 mg%, S creatinine—2.7 mg%, total serum proteins/albumin—4.5/1.2 gm, total serum bilirubin/conjugated bilirubin—initially was 12.9/2.1 mg%, came down to 6.55/1.88 mg%, then again went up to 12.05/8.63 mg%, terminally SGOT/SGPT—262/91 U/L, alkaline phosphatase 161 U/L, CRP—135 mg/L, Random blood sugar ranged from 22–52 mg%, S ammonia—normal. Urine for reducing substances: Positive (Negative for glucose, fructose, galactose). GALT assay normal.

Microbiology*: *Blood culture was initially sterile and later at D25 grew Klebsiella Pneumoniae, ***CSF on D25***—20 cells, all polymorphs, proteins—183 mg%, sugar—10 mg % against RBS of 50 mg%, culture ***Klebsiella pneumoniae***, Ascitic fluid—20 cells, all lymphocytes, protein 5.94 gm%, sugar 41 mg% and culture was sterile.

Hormonal Assays*: *Serum Insulin—D11 < 2.00, D21—1.78 (Normal values—2.6-24.9 microunits per milliliter" mcU/mL), Serum cortisol—D11—944.4, D21—966 (N—AM range 171-536 nmol/L). Thyroid function tests—D22—T3: 2.13 ng/mL, T4:121.6 ng/mL, TSH: 3.77 IU/mL.

Radiology—D3-USG head: Bilateral periventricular leukomalacia, ventricles not dilated, USG Abdomen—Liver: 4 cm/Spleen: 4.2 cm/kidneys Rt: 3.1 cm Lt: 3 cm, moderate ascitis with few thin septations.

Course in Hospital

1. Baby had neonatal jaundice (NNJ) for which phototherapy was given till D7 of life. Double volume exchange transfusion ie DVET was done on D3.
2. Because of IUGR, hepatosplenomegaly, microcephaly, PDA and petechiae, intrauterine infection was suspected and TORCH work, including VDRL was sent, which was negative.
3. Persistent hypoglycaemia was present since birth and RBS was detected as low as 22 mg%. Glucose infusion rate (GIR) was hiked from 4 to 12 mg/kg/min till D7. Feeds were increased and glucose infusion rates were then decreased gradually till D13, when RBS was detected up till 91 mg%. Then at 4 mg /kg/min + feedsà, RBS again fell to 26 mg/kg/min. GIR were again hiked and titrated over next few days depending upon RBS values. As hypoglycaemia was nonresponsive, diazoxide was started on D23 and by D25, glucose infusion was stopped and child maintained on full feeds.
4. Sepsis came on D26, baby developed abdominal distention, tachypnea and tachycardia. Late onset neonatal sepsis was considered based on positive CRP, coagulopathy, thrombocytopenia, metabolic acidosis and hypoglycaemia. Antibiotics were started (Vancomycin + Piptaz) and blood products were transfused. On D25 blood and CSF culture grew Klebsiella. During this period, GIR had to be kept @ 16mg/kg/min to maintain RBS.
5. On D37, the baby developed shock, anasarca, DIC with hemoperitoneum. Baby was ventilated, ionotrops added and received transfusions. Antibiotics changed to Meropenam + flucanozole. Abdominal Xray showed distended bowel loops, no free gas in peritoneum. She developed cardiac arrest on D 38 from which she could not be revived.

***Unit's Final clinical diagnosis*:** Intra Uterine Growth Retardation with Persistent hypoglycaemia with hyperinsulinemia and late onset neonatal sepsis. Cause of Death: Septic shock with pulmonary hemorrhage.

AUTOPSY FINDINGS: PM 23822

A complete autopsy was performed on this 39 days female child who was admitted in NICU since D1 of life. The peritoneal cavity contained 70 mL of clear fluid. The weight at autopsy was 1,840 g, occipitofrontal circumference (OFC)—microcephaly 32 cm (<3rd percentile), chest circumference (CC)—25 cm, abdominal circumference (AC)—29 cm, crown rump length (CRL)—25 cm, crown heel length (CHL)—38 cm, foot length (FL)—5 cm. The ***lungs*** weighed 30 gm. The pleural aspect showed hemorrhages (Fig 1A). The cut section was firm with hemorrhages. No pulmonary thromboembolism was noted. Microscopic examination showed the classical basophilic intranuclear, owl eye inclusions of CMV in the cells lining the alveoli (Figs 1B–D). These inclusions were seen in plenty. Apart from this, there was bronchopneumonia, extensive alveolar hemorrhages (Fig 1E) and hyaline membrane formation (Fig 1F), indicative of diffuse alveolar damage. ***Liver*** was enlarged, weighed 72 gm and was bile stained (Fig 2A). There was porto-portal bridging fibrosis (Fig 2B), bile ductular proliferation

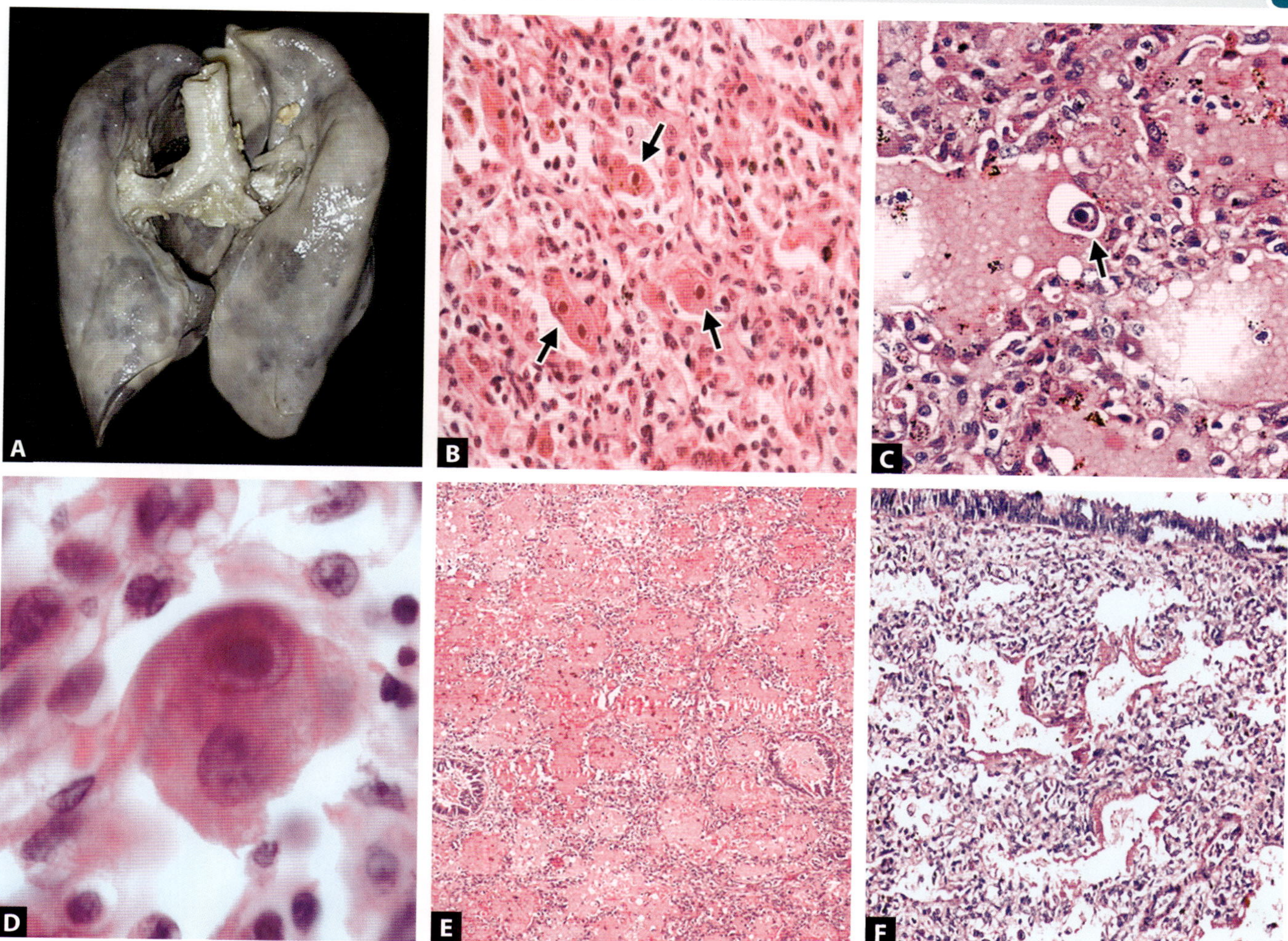

Figs 1A–E: (A) Gross photograph of the lungs showing hemorrhages. Photomicrographs of the lung; (B–D) Pneumocytes showing the characteristic intranuclear, owl-eyed cytomegalovirus inclusions with the halo around them (arrows); (E) Pulmonary hemorrhage; (F) Hyaline membrane formation.

(Fig 2C), cholestasis and CMV inclusions (Fig 2D) were seen in the hepatocytes and bile ductular epithelium. There was extensive centrizonal hemorrhagic necrosis indicative of shock (Fig 2E). Extramedullary hematopoiesis was prominent. Overall features were those of neonatal hepatitis due to CMV infection. The ***spleen*** was enlarged, weighed 14 gm and revealed CMV inclusions (Fig 2F) along with extramedullary hematopoiesis. The ***kidneys*** showed plenty of CMV inclusions in the tubular epithelial cells (Figs 3A and B), in the endothelial cells of the glomerular capillary loops (Fig 3C) along with interstitial inflammation and acute tubular necrosis (Fig 3D). Both ***adrenals*** were also replete with CMV inclusions (Fig 3E). The right adrenal in addition also showed cortical hyperplasia with a nodule formation (Fig 3F). The ***pancreas*** was normal in weight and texture and was blocked in toto. Microscopic examination from the body and tail showed prominent islet cell hyperplasia (Fig 4A) with strong immunohistochemical positivity with insulin (Figs 4B and C). Immunostain with glucagon showed normal alpha cells. ***Lymph nodes*** revealed infection associated erythrophagocytosis. The ***thymus*** showed stress-induced changes along with CMV inclusions. The ***brain*** weighed 310 g and coronal slicing did not reveal any significant hemorrhages apart from occasional pinpoint hemorrhages. One focus of softening was noted (Fig 4D) which on microscopy revealed periventricular leukomalacia, cystic type with no glial proliferation (Fig 4E). ***Heart*** revealed a PDA, measuring 0.5 cm in diameter (Fig 4F).

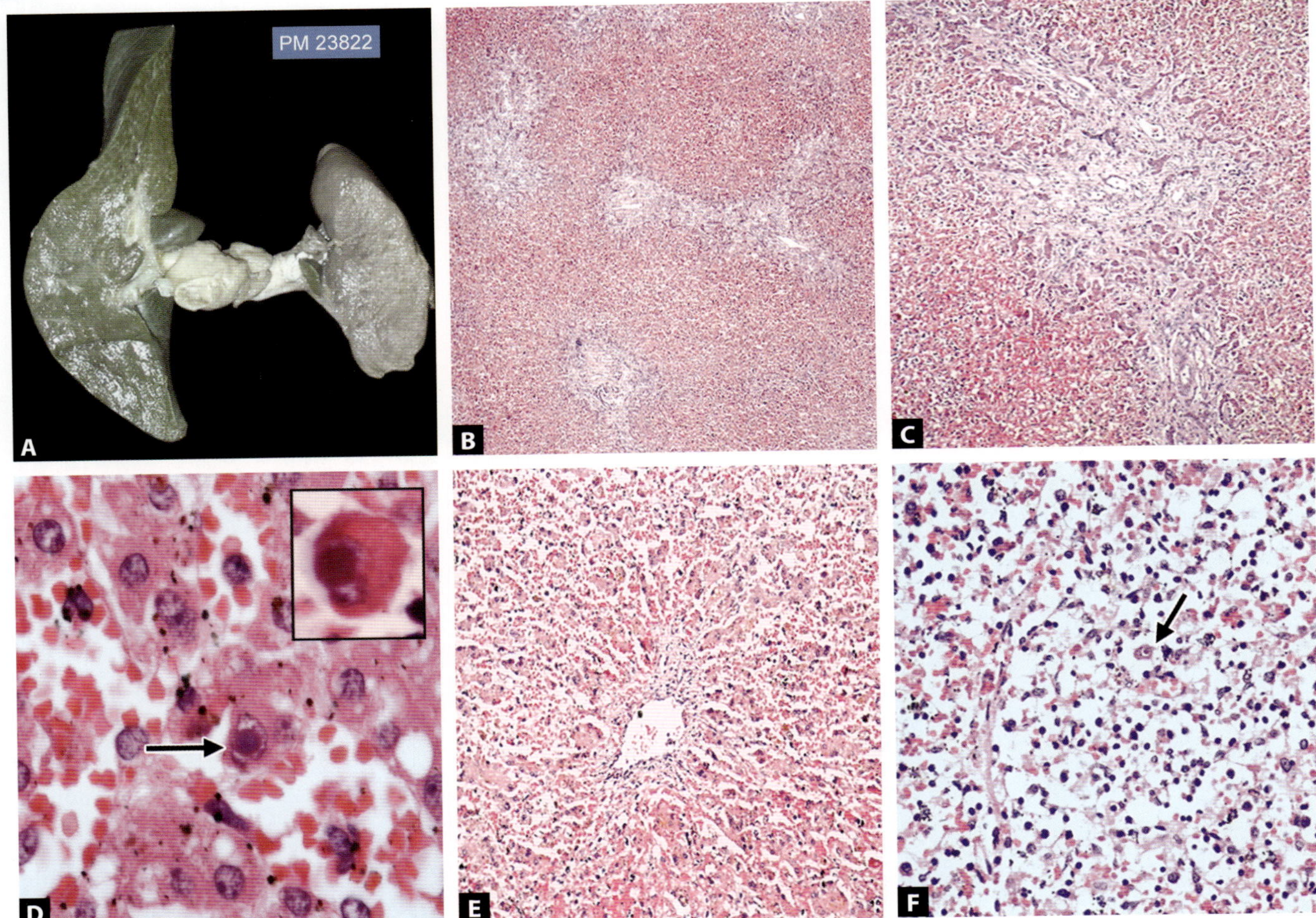

Figs 2A–F: (A) Organ complex of the enlarged, bile stained liver, enlarged spleen, and pancreas. Photomicrographs of the liver showing; (B) Porto-portal bridging fibrosis; and (C) Expanded portal tract with bridging showing bile ductular proliferation; (D) Characteristic cytomegalovirus inclusion in a hepatocyte (arrow); (E) Centrizonal hemorrhagic necrosis; (F) Spleen showing cytomegalovirus inclusion (arrow).

FINAL AUTOPSY DIAGNOSIS: PM 23822

A 39-day-female with severe IUGR, microcephaly, persistent hypoglycemia and recurrent fetal losses.

- Disseminated CMV infection involving the lungs, liver adrenals and spleen leading to:
    - CMV pneumonitis with diffuse alveolar damage and pulmonary hemorrhage
    - CMV hepatitis
    - CMV tubulointerstitial nephritis
- Islet cell hyperplasia—pancreas
- Dominant PDA
- Periventricular leukomalacia—brain
- Centrizonal hemorrhagic necrosis—liver
- Extramedullary hematopoiesis—liver, spleen
- Erythrophagocytosis—lymph nodes

CONGENITAL CYTOMEGALOVIRUS INFECTION[1]

Cytomegalovirus is a ubiquitous β-group herpesvirus and is the most common virus which infects the fetus and neonate. It has diverse manifestations which depend upon the age and immune status of the patient. It can be a potential killer or an innocent bystander. Latent infection resides in the monocytes and their progenitors in the bone marrow and can reactivate when the cellular immunity of the host becomes low. In healthy adults it causes an asymptomatic mononucleosis like illness, but in immunocompromised individuals and neonates it leads to a devastating infection, wherein, it infests many organs. This virus takes several routes for transmission—(1) Transplacental infection (congenital infection) from primary maternal infection who do not have protective antibodies or from recurrent infection. (2) Neonatal infection through the

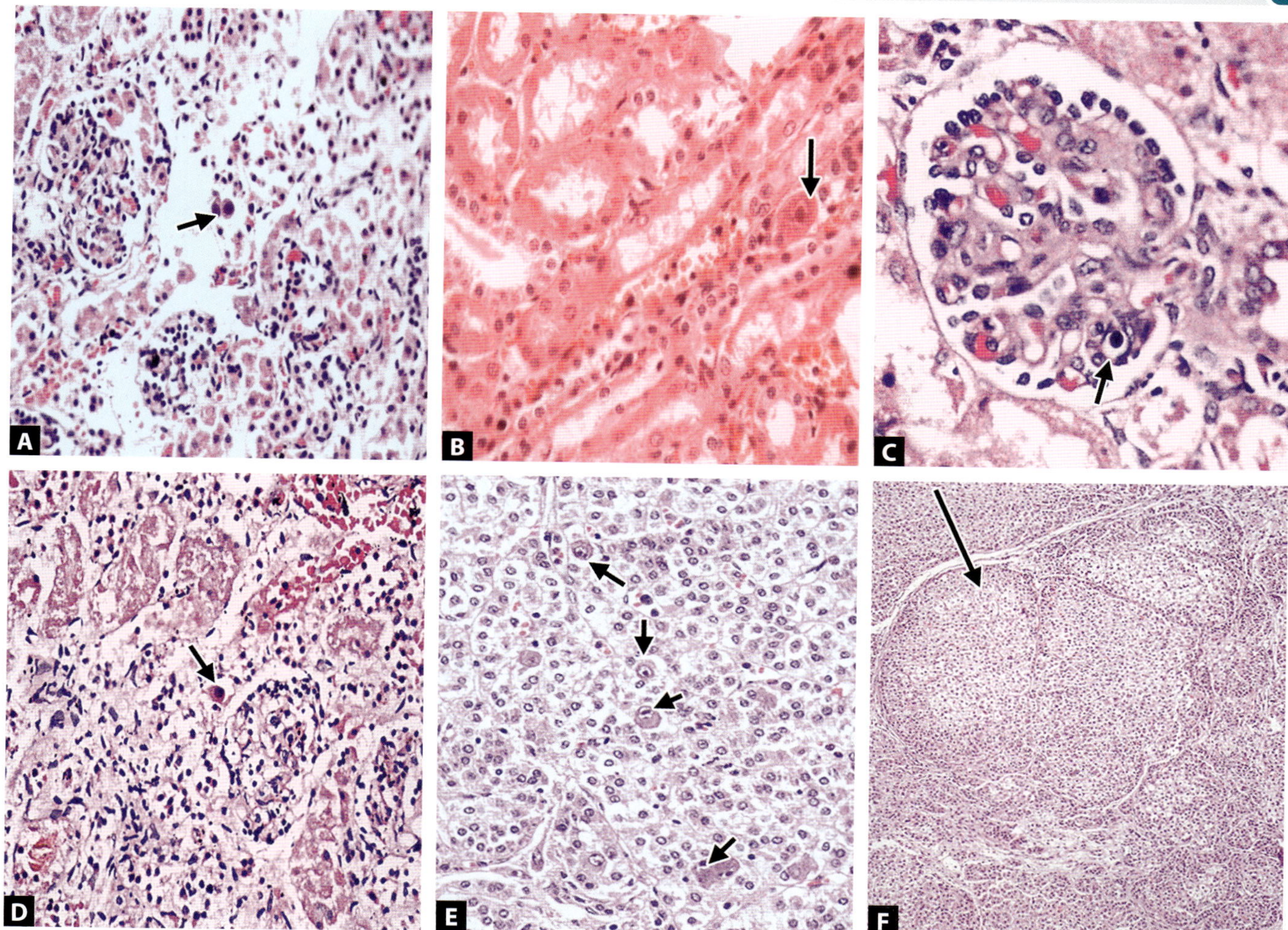

Figs 3A–F: Photomicrographs of the kidney showing (A and B) Cytomegalovirus inclusions in the renal tubular epithelial cells (arrows); (C) Cytomegalovirus inclusion in the endothelial cell of the glomerular capillaries (arrow); (D) Interstitial inflammation with tubular damage and cytomegalovirus inclusion (arrow); (E) Adrenal gland showing cytomegalovirus inclusions (arrows); (F) Adrenal showing cortical hyperplasia forming a nodule (arrow).

genital tract secretions at birth (intrapartum infection) or via the breast milk (postnatal infection). (3) Infection acquired through the saliva in the pre-school age group in day care centers, which can be further transmitted to the parents. (4) Transmission via the genital route, fecal–oral route and respiratory secretions. (5) Through blood transfusions and organ transplantation.

Cytomegalovirus infection is seen more in the developing countries. Neonates are infected via the placenta (in utero transmission, i.e. congenital infection), genital tract secretions (intrapartum transmission), breast milk and blood transfusions (postpartum transmission).

- ***Congenital CMV infection***: In women of childbearing age, CMV IgG antibodies are present in 80–90% cases.[2] Seroconversion during pregnancy occurs in 2.5% cases.

Fetus is worst affected when the infection occurs prior to 20 weeks gestation. In utero transmission can be due to primary or recurrent infection. Primary CMV infection is said to cause more fetal damage and is also said to be transmitted in a higher percentage, as compared to recurrent CMV infection. Some recent reports, have however emphasized that the outcome of recurrent maternal CMV infection can be as severe.[3] Approximately 90% of congenitally affected neonates are asymptomatic at birth and of these 20% develop neurologic deficits, hearing loss and chorioretinitis by 2 years of age. Amongst the 10% symptomatic neonates, 20% die and the rest manifest with severe sequelae[4] which includes intellectual disability, hearing loss and other neurological impairments. At times the congenital infection may manifest in a mild

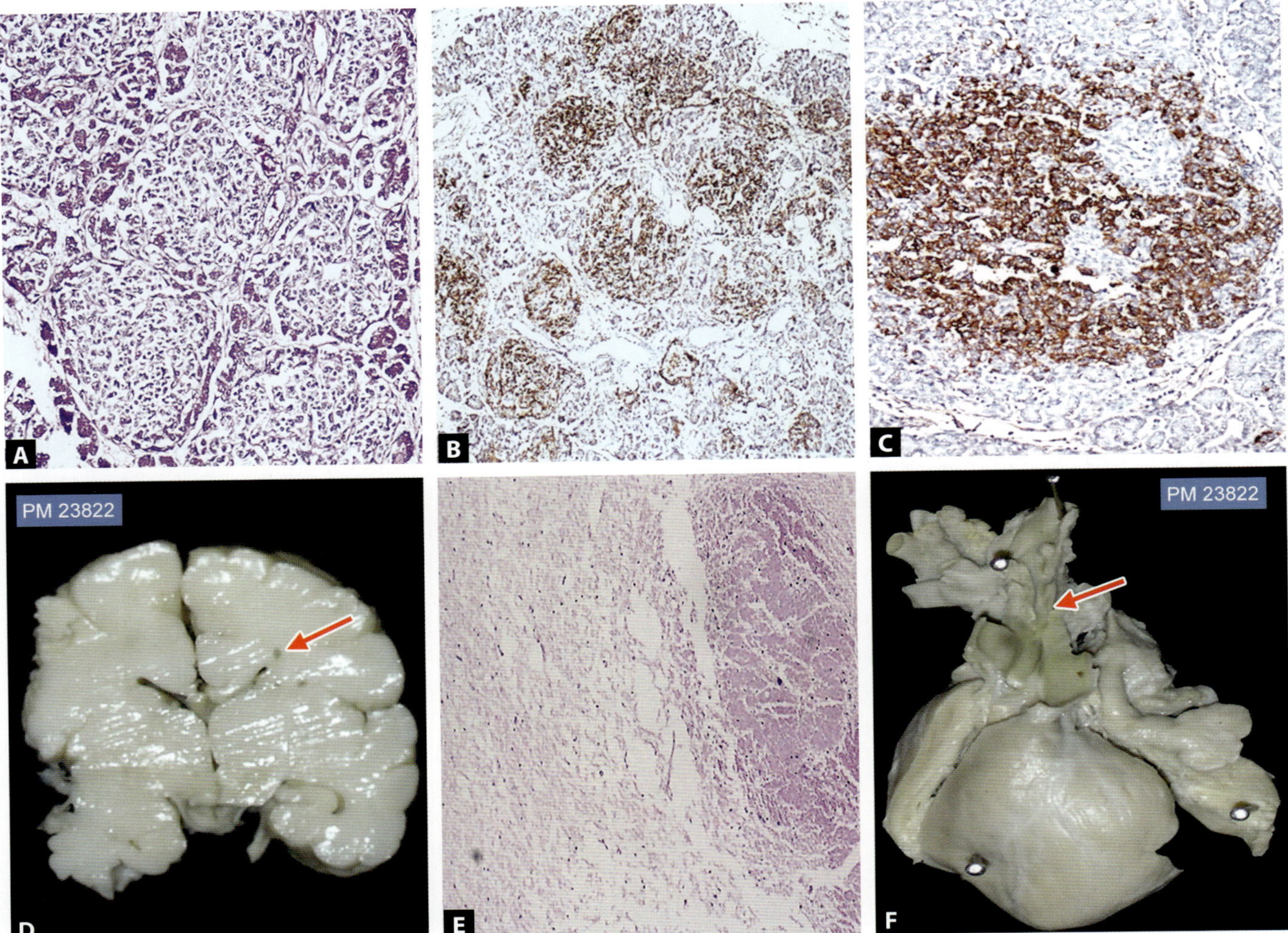

Figs 4A–F: (A) Section of the pancreas from the body showing islet cell hyperplasia (PAS stain); (B and C) Insulin immunostain showing strong positivity in the islets; (D) Coronal slice of the brain showing chalky white deposits in the periventricular area (arrow); (E) Photomicrographs of the brain showing periventricular leukomalacia; (F) Heart showing a patent ductus arteriosus (arrow).

form with interstitial pneumonitis, hepatitis or a hematological disorder. Most affected with this mild form of disease may recover but a few may develop intellectual disability later on. Rarely, an asymptomatic infection may manifest months or years later by neurologic sequelae which may include delayed onset intellectual disability and deafness.

- ***Perinatal CMV infections***: CMV infection acquired from the birth canal secretions (intrapartum) or from the breast milk (postpartum) is usually asymptomatic due to protective maternal anti-CMV antibodies, which are transmitted via the placenta to the fetus. It can however manifest (interstitial pneumonitis, rash, hepatitis or failure to thrive) in premature infants, although both clinical and pathologic features are much less severe as compared to congenitally acquired infection. Asymptomatic infants may continue to secrete CMV in the urine/saliva for months to years. They may develop subtle hearing or intellectual defects later on in life.

Cytomegalovirus disease resembles erythroblastosis fetalis and affected neonates can present with IUGR, effusions, microcephaly, hydrocephalous with calcification, chorioretinitis, hepatosplenomegaly, jaundice which could be cholestatic, hepatitis, pneumonitis, interstitial nephritis, anemia, purpura, thrombocytopenia and encephalitis. Cells which get infected are epithelial cells of glandular organs, neurons, cells of the biliary tree, alveolar macrophages/pneumocytes/endothelial cells of the lungs, tubular epithelial cells/glomerular endothelial cells of the kidney, exocrine cells and adrenal cortical cells. The morphologic hallmark of

CMV infection is a gigantic cell (30–40 μm) which shows a prominent basophilic, intranuclear inclusion with a halo separating it from the nuclear membrane, giving it a characteristic owl eye appearance. The cytoplasm of the infected cell show smaller basophilic inclusions. Affected organs show focal necrosis, minimal mononuclear cell infiltrate, vascular and parenchymal calcification particularly in the brain. Liver involvement is a common manifestation and can range from mild cholangitis to severe cholestatic hepatitis. Late sequelae, although rare include noncirrhotic portal fibrosis and portal hypertension which are fatal. Giant cell transformation is not commonly seen.

COMMENTARY—INDEX CASE: PM 23822

This baby was a small for date, with severe IUGR and microcephaly, born to a 29-year-old, gravida 5 mother (G5P0040), with no living issue, at 37 weeks gestation with a body weight of 1.06 kg. Mother had a bad obstetric history. G1 loss was at 4 months and the mother was detected to be positive for rubella infection and she was treated for 6 months. G2 and G3 losses were at 3.5 and 2.5 months, respectively and no cause could be identified at this point of time. G4 loss occurred at 2 months and at this point the mother was found to be APLA positive and has been on ecosprin for 2 years and was on heparin 40 U BD (APLA—Non reactive after treatment). The index baby was G5 and admitted to the NICU at 20 hours of life with chief complaints of hypoglycemia detected at one hour of life and jaundice (unconjugated hyperbilirubinemia attributed to IUGR and G6PD deficiency for which phototherapy was given) detected at 8 hours of life. There was a suspicion of CMV infection at 25 weeks gestation, when the ultrasonography revealed gross oligohydramnios, thickened placenta and reversed flow of the umbilical artery. The pitfall in this case was that the TORCH workup in the mother was found to be negative. The baby had persistent hypoglycemia since birth and RBS was detected as low as 22 mg%. The CMV workup, i.e. PP65 antigen in the baby was negative. The hemoglobin showed a progressive fall from 14.6g% to 6.9 g%, platelets were low and coagulopathy was present.

At autopsy, the baby had a disseminated congenital CMV infection involving the lungs, liver, kidneys, adrenals and spleen. There was CMV pneumonitis with diffuse alveolar damage, CMV hepatitis with porto-portal bridging fibrosis and CMV tubulointerstitial nephritis. There was microcephaly, periventricular leukomalacia in the brain with features of centrizonal hemorrhagic necrosis in the liver indicating shock. Apart from this there was a large PDA. Conditions associated with hyperplasia of the endocrine pancreas are—infants of diabetic mothers, erythroblastosis fetalis, Beckwith-Wiedemann syndrome, Zellweger syndrome, neonatal hepatitis, IUGR and persistent hyperinsulinemic hypoglycemia of infancy. In the index case, two of the above conditions were operating, i.e. severe IUGR and neonatal hepatitis. Both these could have contributed to the islet cell hyperplasia, which led to the persistent hypoglycemia.

TAKE HOME MESSAGE

- Cytomegalovirus is a ubiquitous β-group herpesvirus and is the most common virus which infects the fetus and neonates.
- It can be a potential killer or an innocent bystander.
- Neonates are infected via the placenta (in utero transmission, i.e. congenital infection), genital tract secretions (intrapartum transmission), breast milk and blood transfusions (postpartum transmission).
- The morphologic hallmark of CMV infection is a gigantic cell (30–40 μm) which shows a prominent basophilic, intranuclear inclusion with a halo separating it from the nuclear membrane, giving it a characteristic owl eye appearance.
- Neonates with congenital CMV infection can present with intrauterine growth retardation, effusions, microcephaly, hydrocephalous with calcification, chorioretinitis, hepatosplenomegaly, hepatitis, pneumonitis, interstitial nephritis, anemia, purpura, thrombocytopenia and encephalitis.

REFERENCES

1. Chakravarti A, Kashyap B, Matlani M. Cytomegalovirus infection: An Indian perspective. Indian J Med Microbiol. 2009;27(1):3-11.
2. Chakravarty A, Kashyap B, Rathi K. The seroepidemiological study on cytomegalovirus in women of childbearing age with special reference to pregnancy and maternal-fetal transmission. Indian J Pathol Microbiol. 2005;48:518-21.
3. Gaytant MA, Rours GI, Steegers EA, et al. Congenital cytomegalovirus infection after recurrent infection: case reports and review of literature. Eur J Pediatr. 2003;162:248-53.
4. Gandhoke I, Aggarwal R, Lal S, et al. Congenital CMV infection in symptomatic infants in Delhi and surrounding areas. Indian J Pediatr. 2006;73:1095-7

CONTRIBUTIONS BY:

1. Dr Praveen Kumar, Professor and Head, Department of Pediatrics—Neonatology Division (Clinician In-Charge) Post Graduate Institute of Medical Education and Research, Chandigarh, India.

CASE 61

Congenital Tuberculosis: An Underdiagnosed Entity: PM 24753

Nandita Bharadwaj Kakkar

HIGHLIGHTS OF THE CASE

A male baby was born to a primigravida, harboring undetected genital tuberculosis, at 28 weeks gestation with a weight (1,000 g) appropriate for gestational age. He developed respiratory distress soon after birth and in the 4 months that he lived, there was failure to thrive, increasing oxygen requirements, pulmonary nodules seen in both lungs on contrast-enhanced computed tomography (CECT) chest and raised transaminases. Autopsy of the baby revealed florid congenital/perinatal tuberculosis (AFB 5+) with primary complex in the lungs and hilar nodes, with miliary spread to the liver, kidneys, spleen and carinal lymph nodes. In the immediate postpartum period, the mother was detected to have a tubo-ovarian abscess which was drained. She took anti-tubercular treatment (ATT) for only 7 days. Immediately after the diagnosis of congenital tuberculosis was made on the baby, the family was contacted and it was learnt that the mother in the postpartum period had a downhill course, had been brought back to our institute and was diagnosed with tubercular meningitis but succumbed to her illness. The baby acquired tuberculosis by the aspiration of infected amniotic fluid during passage through the birth canal (due to presence of genital tuberculosis in the mother) and here the lungs were the primary focus of infection.

Keywords: Tuberculosis, congenital, underdiagnosed entity, Cantwell criteria, autopsy.

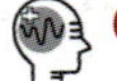

CLINICAL DETAILS

Date of Admission: 05.04.2012, Date of Death: 24.04.2012, Duration of Hospital Stay: 19 Days.

A 4-month-old male child presented with episodes of rapid breathing since birth. He was born to a primigravida mother by preterm vaginal delivery at 28 weeks of gestation with a birth weight of 1,000 g. The baby cried immediately but developed respiratory distress soon after birth and was kept in the incubator on oxygen in the NICU for 48 days. During this period he developed pneumonia and neonatal sepsis, had recurrent apneic spells, became oxygen dependent, gradually improved and was weaned off the oxygen. In the next 2 months, he had recurrent episodes of rapid breathing associated with chest indrawing requiring admission to the hospital thrice, labeled as pneumonia/septicemia each time and required oxygen supplementation and antibiotics. He was finally referred to PGIMER at the age of 4 months. There was no history of fever, lethargy, poor feeding, sweating on feeding, cough, loose stools, seizures, bleeding from any site or any delayed passage of meconium. In the antenatal period, the mother was having fever off and on since second trimester and in the third trimester she developed high grade, intermittent fever, was diagnosed as a case of typhoid and treated for the same. Postpartum, a tubo-ovarian abscess was detected which was drained. She was started on ATT which she took for only 7 days. The baby had not attained head holding by 4 months and there was no social smile. He was the first child from a nonconsanguineous marriage. There was no history of any family contact, overcrowding and was from a good socioeconomic status. The baby was not immunized. ***On examination***, the baby weighed 2.2 kg (< -3 z score), length was 47 cm (< -3 z score), OFC—31 cm (< -3 z score), pulse—118/min, BP—78 mm Hg (systolic), RR—50/min with normal efforts, SpO_2—80%, NpO_2—95%, anterior fontanelle 3 × 3 cm open, post fontanalle 1 × 1 cm open, no facial dysmorphism, no pallor, edema, jaundice, cyanosis and clubbing. Chest revealed bilateral equal and symmetrical movements with no chest retractions, normal vesicular breath sounds, with equal air entry and no added sounds. Abdomen was soft, there was no organomegaly and bowel sounds were present. CVS examination was within normal limits. CNS examination revealed a conscious state, he was alert, state to state variability was good, pupils were 3 mm ESRTL, tone/power/sensory examination were normal.

Investigations

Hemogram revealed Hb of 8 g/dL, TLC—30,000/uL with predominantly neutrophils, platelets—235000/uL; Serum Na^+, K^+, Cl^-, urea, creatinine, Ca^{2+}, total serum protein (TSP) and total bilirubin were within normal limits. AST—85 U/L, ALT—83 U/L, alkaline phosphatase—139 U/L, CRP—25.49 mg/L, ABG showed acidosis: pH—7.359, pO_2/pCO_2—62.9/53, HCO_3 - 26.1 and random blood sugar was 70 mg%. Blood culture grew *Staphylococcus aureus*, BACTEC was sterile; urine culture grew *E. coli*, VDRL/TORCH/Mantoux/HIV (mother and child) were negative. ***Chest X-ray*** (Fig 1A) showed normal volume lungs with evidence of multiple ill-defined diffusely scattered radio-opacities in both lung fields interspersed with lucent areas ? infection. There was no demonstrable pleural or pericardial effusion. ***CECT chest*** (Fig 1B) revealed areas of ground glass density, consolidations and variable-sized multiple nodules, scattered in both lungs. Thickened interlobular septae, patchy areas of air trapping and subsegmental atelectasis along with mild hilar lymphadenopathy were also seen in both lungs. ***Units final diagnosis***: Bronchopulmonary dysplasia, pneumonia, nosocomial sepsis with shock and cause of death being hypoxia. Other clinical possibilities were structural malformation of lung, cystic fibrosis and congenital heart disease.

AUTOPSY FINDINGS: PM 24753

A partial autopsy (brain and spinal cord not examined) was performed on this 4-month-old male child. The body weighed 2,300 g. Both pleural and peritoneal cavities contained 100 mL each of hemorrhagic and straw-colored fluid, respectively. The ***lungs*** weighed 125 g. The pleural surface was congested and studded with multiple nodules 0.3–1.5 cm. Cut section (Figs 2A and B) revealed multiple white nodules scattered all over, getting confluent with hardly any normal looking lung parenchyma. Enlarged lymph nodes were seen at the hilum and in the carinal region. On microscopic examination the nodules (Fig 2C) were composed of multiple confluent lymphohistiocytic granulomas (Figs 2D and 3A) with Langhans type of giant cells and epithelioid-like cells, some of them showing caseation necrosis. Alveolar spaces (Fig 3B) also contained similar collections of lymphohistiocytic cells. Apart from these, there were suppurative granulomas (Fig 3C) with collections of neutrophils in the center bordered by lymphohistiocytic cells, Langhans type of giant cells, epithelioid-like cells and calcification. Grade 1 pulmonary arterial hypertension was also noted. Ziehl–Neelsen stain (Fig 3D) for AFB (4+ positivity with AFB seen in clusters) and auramine rhodamine stain showed a very heavy bacillary load. Polymerase chain reaction was done from the lung tissue and was positive for *Mycobacterium tuberculosis* (Fig 4A). No atypical mycobacteria were identified. The ***lymph nodes*** (hilar/carinal) also revealed similar granulomas, lymphohistiocytic, with and without caseation necrosis (Figs 4B and C) and suppurative (Fig 4D), with a similar

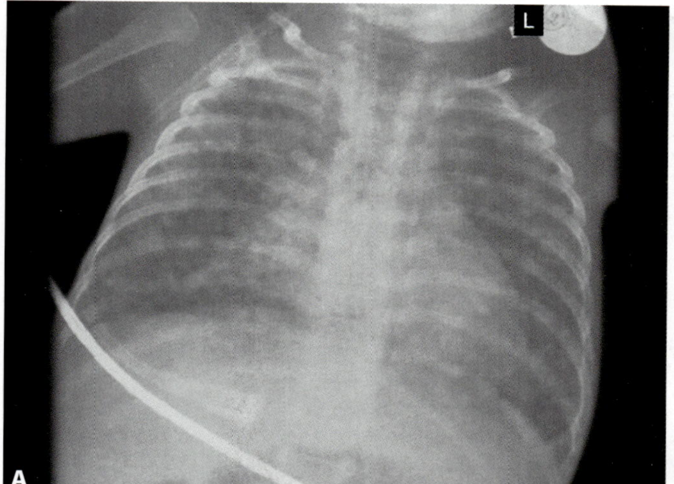

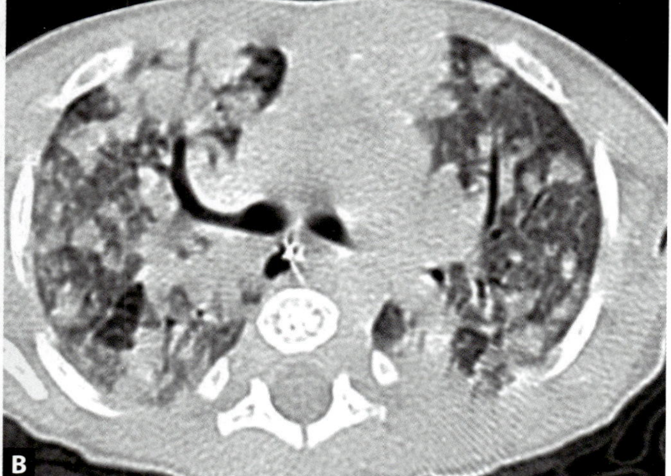

Figs 1A and B: (A) Chest X-ray reveals multiple ill-defined random nodules in both lungs; (B) CECT scan reveals bilateral pulmonary nodules with areas of ground glass density, consolidations and air trapping.

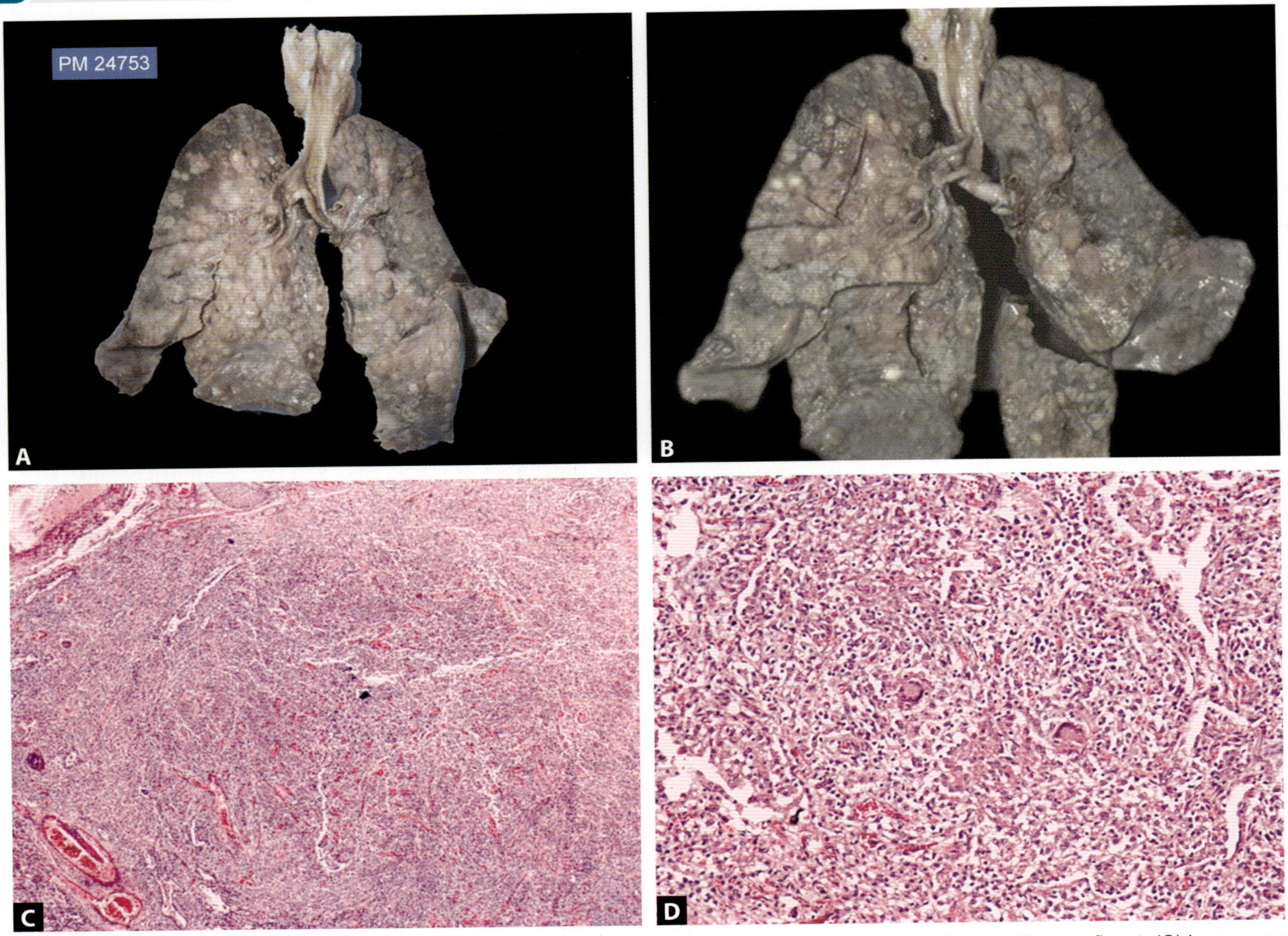

Figs 2A–D: (A and B) Gross pictures of the cut section of the lungs showing diffusely scattered white nodules getting confluent; (C) Low power view of a nodule composed of lymphohistiocytic infiltrate; (D) Granuloma at low power showing lymphohistiocytic cells, Langhans type of giant cells and epithelioid-like cells.

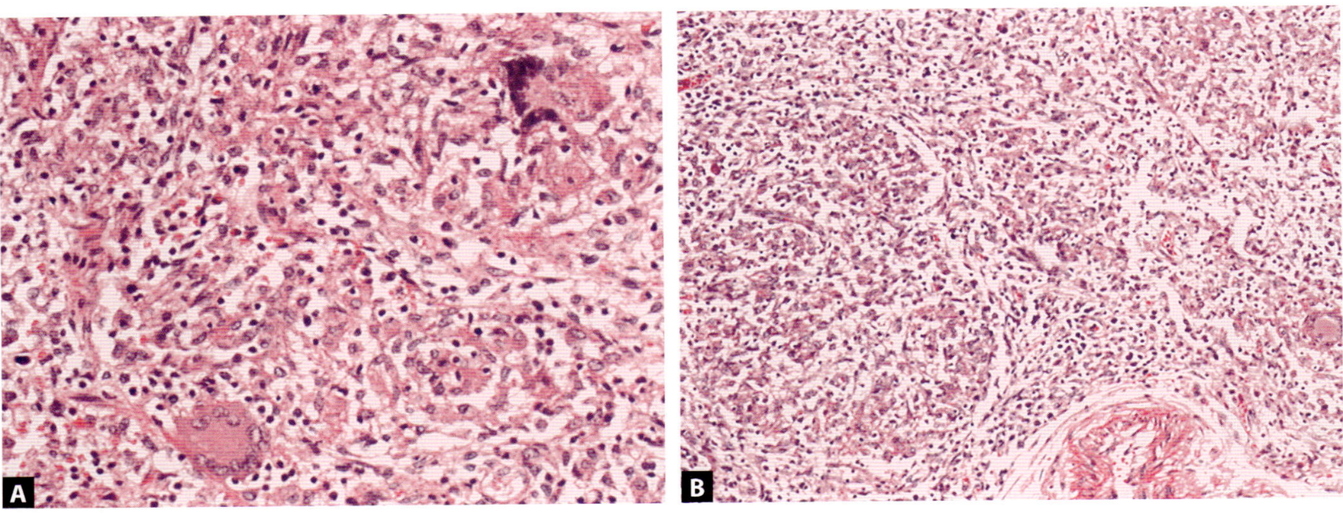

Figs 3A and B:

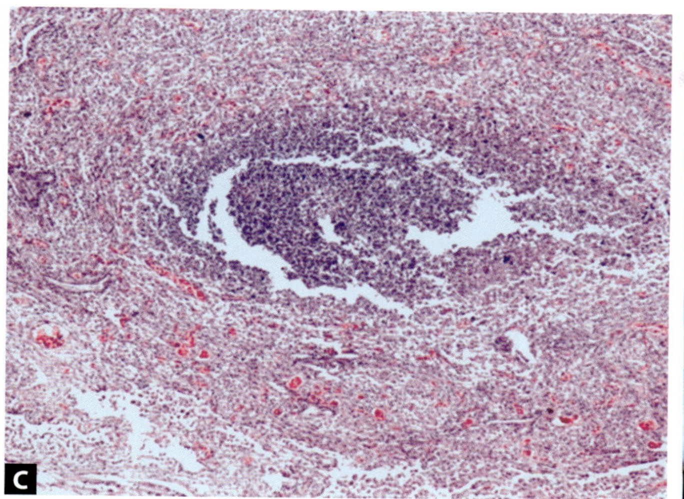

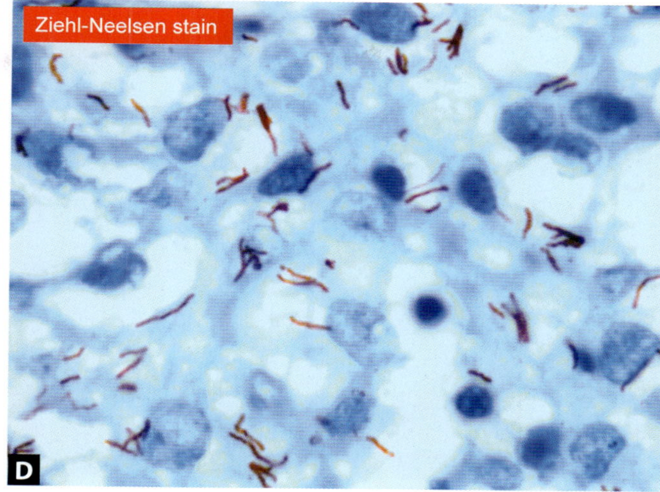

Figs 3A–D: Photomicrographs of the lung. (A) High power of the granuloma showing lymphohistiocytic cells, Langhans type of giant cells and epithelioid-like cells; (B) Lymphohistiocytic infiltrate in the alveolar spaces; (C) Low power view of a suppurative granuloma with collections of neutrophils in the center bordered by lymphohistiocytic cells, Langhans type of giant cells and epithelioid-like cells; (D) Ziehl-Neelsen stain replete with the typical beaded acid-fast tubercle bacilli.

heavy bacillary load. The ***liver*** weighed 110 g and coronal slicing (Fig 5A) did not show any gross lesion, but on microscopic examination sections were riddled with multiple small compact lymphohistiocytic granulomas with giant cells (Fig 5B). A large-sized portal vein showed infiltration by granulomas (Fig 5C). Stain for AFB showed 1 + positivity (Fig 5D). No portal adenopathy was noted and the lymph nodes did not reveal any granuloma on microscopic examination. The ***spleen*** weighed 15 g and no miliary tubercle was identified grossly (Fig 6A), but on microscopic examination it was riddled with small granulomas (Fig 6B). The kidneys were congested on gross examination (Fig 6C) and showed similar granulomas (Fig 6D). The ***thymus*** was normal grossly and microscopically (Figs 7A and B). There were no features of any immunodeficiency which was confirmed by CD3 (Fig 7C) and CD20 (Fig 7D) immunohistochemistry. Rest of organs were within normal limits.

 FINAL AUTOPSY DIAGNOSIS: PM 24753

4 Months Old Male

- *Congenital/perinatal tuberculosis*: AFB 5+, PCR positive for *Mycobacterium tuberculosis*
  - Primary complex in the lungs and hilar lymph nodes
  - Miliary spread to the liver, kidneys, spleen ,carinal lymph nodes.

Immediately after the autopsy diagnosis of congenital tuberculosis (1 month from the date of death of the baby) was made on the baby, the family was contacted. It was learnt that the mother in the postpartum period had a progressive downhill course and 20 days after the death of the baby, she was brought back to our institute and was diagnosed with tubercular meningitis but succumbed to her illness. The baby acquired tuberculosis by the aspiration of infected amniotic fluid during passage through the birth canal (due to presence of genital tuberculosis in the mother) and here the lungs were the primary focus of infection.

ABOUT CONGENITAL TUBERCULOSIS

Congenital tuberculosis is termed as infection with tubercle bacilli during intrauterine life or before the complete passage through the birth canal. Although, tuberculosis is rampant in the world today and is prevalent in pregnant women, yet there is a paucity of cases of congenital tuberculosis probably due to the fact that they are grossly under reported.[1-8] Placenta does form a protective barrier against the invasion of the fetus by tubercle bacilli. Literature says that perinatally acquired tuberculosis occurs rarely and is difficult to diagnose due to its overlap with the more common bacterial and viral infections. Till 1989, only 300 cases were reported in literature,[9] in 1994, 58 cases were reviewed by Abughali et al[10] and between 2001 till 2005, 18 more cases were added.[11]

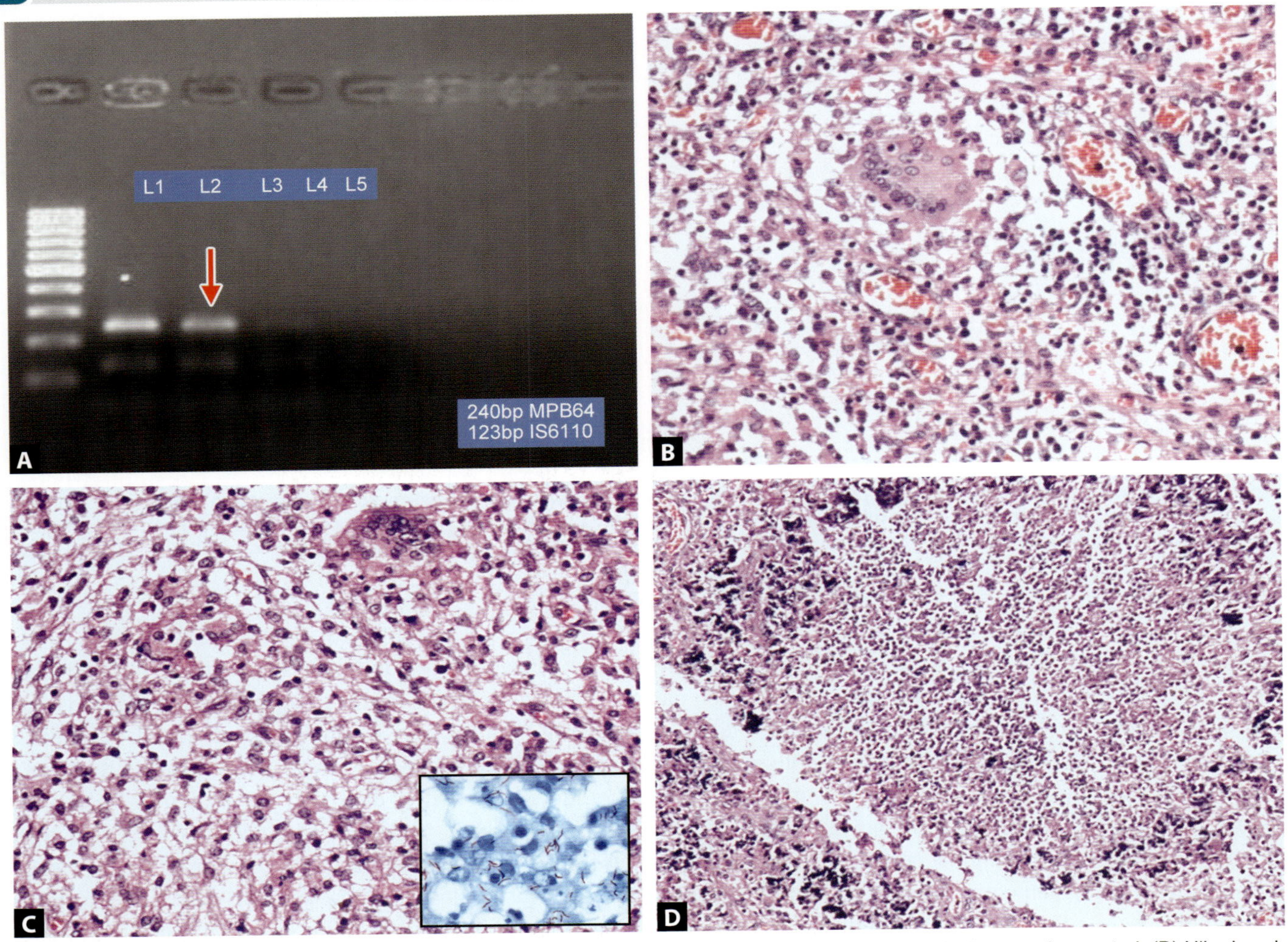

Figs 4A–D: (A) PCR showing L1—100 bp mm, L2—positive control, L3 and L4—DNA of lung tissue and L5—negative control; (B) Hilar lymph node showing a granuloma with lymphohistiocytic cells, epithelioid-like cells and a giant cell; (C) Lymph node-granuloma at a closer look. Inset shows Ziehl–Neelsen stain with abundant acid-fast bacilli; (D) Lymph node-suppurative granuloma with collections of neutrophils/nuclear debris in the center bordered by lymphohistiocytic cells and calcification.

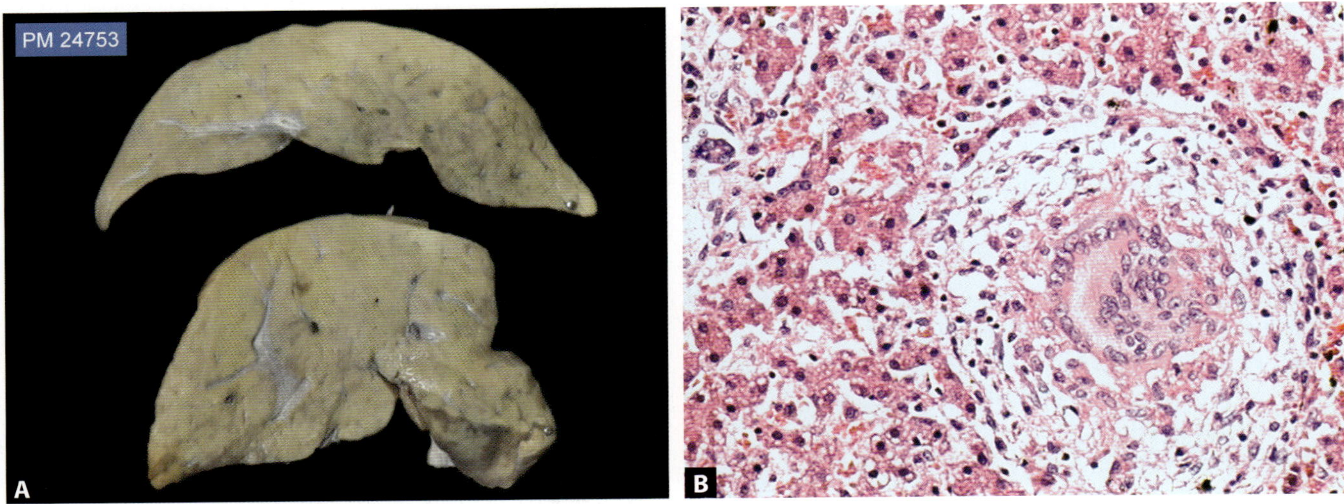

Figs 5A and B:

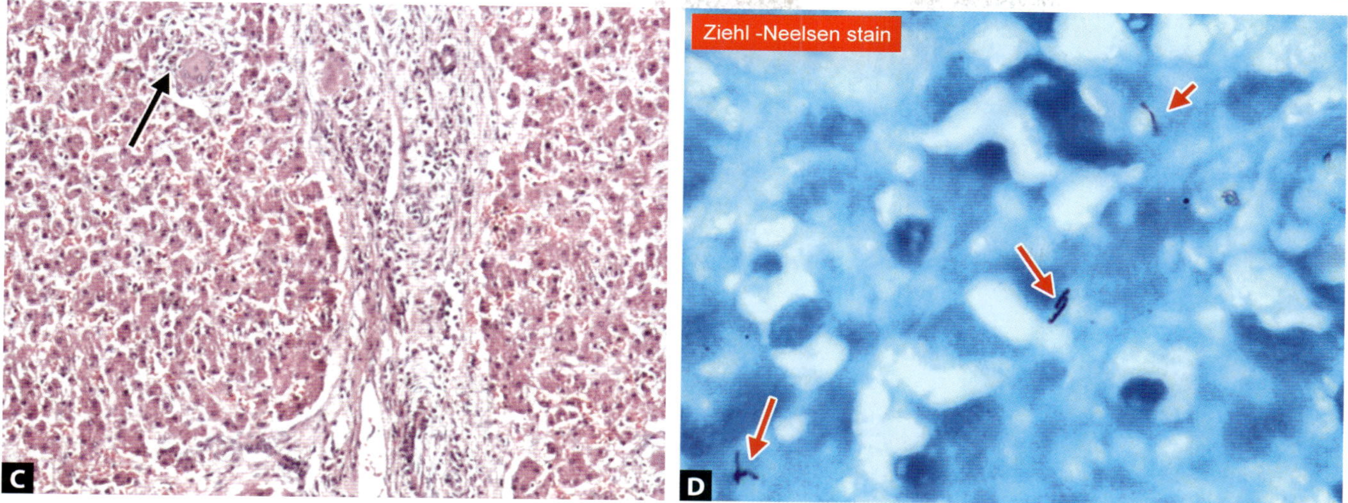

Figs 5A–D: Photographs of the liver. (A) Coronal slices of the liver showing congestion. No miliary tubercle was seen; (B) Photomicrograph showing a granuloma with lymphohistiocytic cells and a giant cell; (C) A large branch of the portal vein, infiltrated by granulomas; (D) Ziehl–Neelsen stain showing only a few tubercle bacilli.

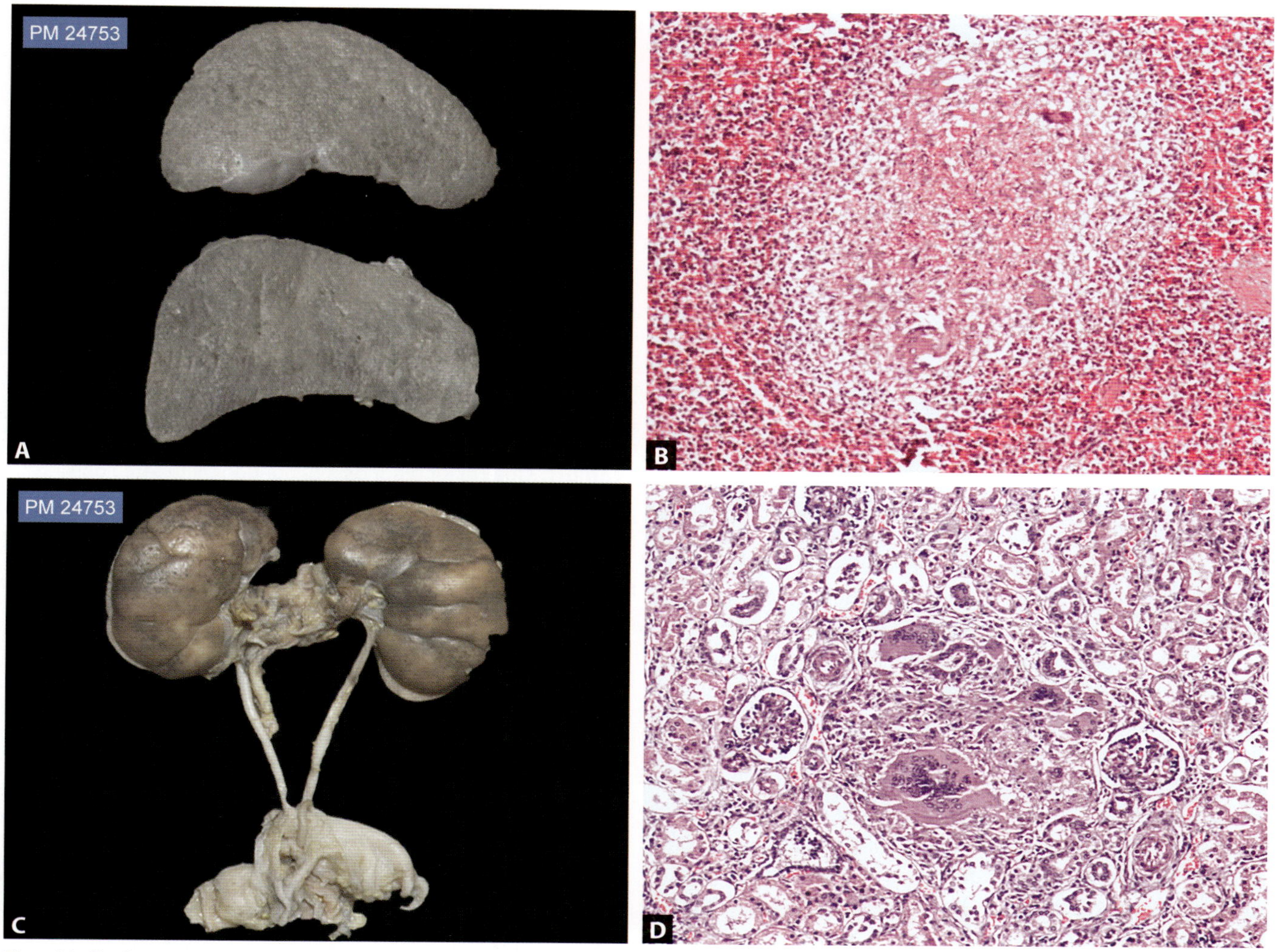

Figs 6A–D: Coronal slices of the spleen showing congestion. No tubercle was seen grossly; (B) Spleen showing a caseating granuloma; (C) Gross photograph of the kidneys showing congestion; (D) Photomicrograph of the kidney showing granuloma with giant cells and epithelioid cells.

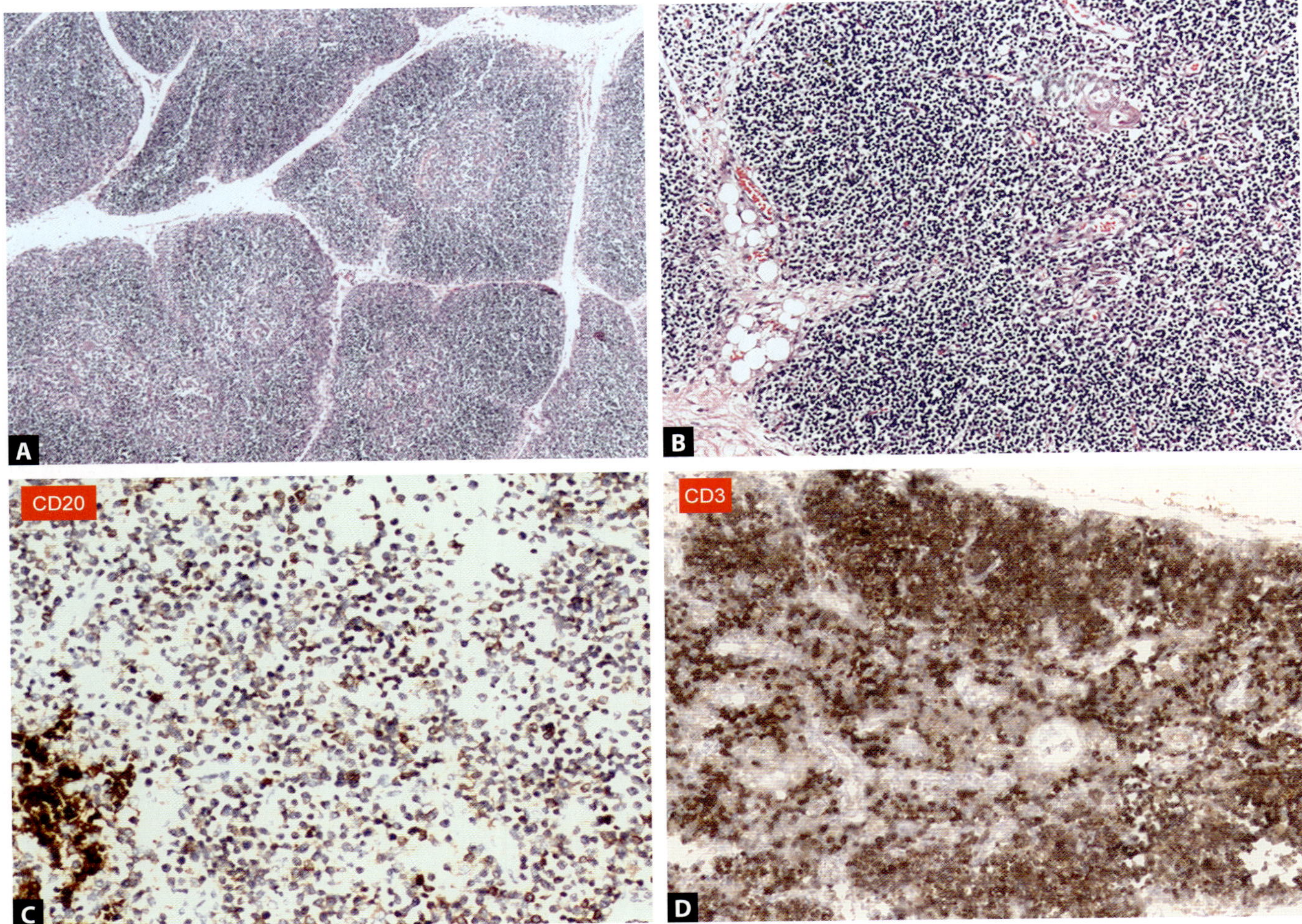

Figs 7A–D: (A and B) Photomicrographs of the thymus (low/high power view) showing normal thymic morphology with adequate amount of lymphoid tissue; (C) CD20 immunostain showing few B cells; (D) CD3 immunostain showing a predominance of T cells.

In 2011, Peng et al[12] analyzed 170 cases of congenital tuberculosis reported in literature between 1946 and 2009.

The criteria (Table 1) for the diagnosis of congenital tuberculosis were laid down by Beitzke, way back in 1935 and unfortunately these were very rigid. Beitzke's criteria[13,14] was modified by Cantwell et al.[15]

Congenital tuberculosis has three modes of transmission[1]—(1) Transplacental spread with primary complex in liver, (2) Aspiration of infected amniotic fluid during passage through birth canal, wherein the lungs are the primary focus of infection and (3) Ingestion of infected material, where the primary lesion lies in the gut. This is a highly underdiagnosed entity with a very high mortality. The consequences of delayed diagnosis and treatment are catastrophic, hence the importance of an early diagnosis. Awareness amongst doctors is very essential, who shoulder the responsibility

Table 1: Criteria for diagnosis of congenital tuberculosis.

Beitzki criteria, 1935[13,14]
▪ Tuberculosis diagnosed in the neonatal period (isolation of *M. tuberculosis*)
▪ Demonstration of primary hepatic complex
▪ In the absence of primary complex in the liver: • Evidence of tuberculosis within days after birth • Absence of contact with a case of tuberculosis after birth.
Revised criteria by Cantwell[15]
Proven tuberculous lesion and at least one of the following:
▪ Lesions should be present in the first week of life
▪ Primary hepatic complex
▪ Tuberculous infection of placenta or maternal genital tract
▪ Exclusion of postnatal transmission by thorough contact investigation.

of screening pregnant women at risk. Women with HIV infection in the childbearing age are at increased risk for tuberculosis, thereby increasing the risk for congenital tuberculosis. In a lot of cases cited in literature, the mothers have subclinical tuberculosis that comes to light only after tuberculosis in their babies is diagnosed. This further stresses the need for thoroughly evaluating all mothers of infants with tuberculosis. Congenital tuberculosis is underestimated because the criteria for its diagnosis laid down by Beitzke were very stringent. The demonstration of a primary hepatic complex is possible only with an open surgical procedure or an autopsy to confirm the liver involvement along with the regional nodes. Congenital tuberculosis presents with vague symptoms such as fever, distress, hepatosplenomegaly and are difficult to distinguish from the more common viral and bacterial infections, that occur at this age. Thus, it is easily misdiagnosed as pneumonia, sepsis or meningitis. Unusual signs and symptoms are reported, like skin rash, ear discharge, facial paralysis and bone deformities. Symptoms may be evident at birth, but usually present 2 weeks after birth. Cantwell's criteria[15] gave importance to the hepatic granulomas and the tuberculous infection of the placenta and the maternal genital tract. Peng et al[12] analyzed 170 cases of congenital tuberculosis reported in literature between 1946 and 2009. In their analysis, 70 were premature babies, average age of onset of disease was 20 days, mothers of 162 babies were diagnosed with active tuberculosis during pregnancy or after parturition, nonspecific signs and symptoms were found in all babies, abnormal chest radiographs were seen in 133 cases of whom in 83 cases, miliary tuberculosis and multiple pulmonary nodules were seen and 68 babies died amongst them. Mortality dropped to 21.7% after the ATT. Peng et al[12] highlighted that blood leucocyte count, anti-tubercular treatment, age of onset and presence of brain involvement affected the prognosis of congenital tuberculosis.

COMMENTARY—INDEX CASE: PM 24753

In the index case, the baby was born to a primigravida, harboring undetected genital tuberculosis, by vaginal delivery at 28 weeks gestation with a weight (1,000 g) appropriate for the gestational age. He was ill since birth with severe respiratory distress. There was marked failure to thrive and he weighed 2,300 g at 4 months of age. The baby had not attained head holding by 4 months and there was no social smile. Chest radiographs and CECT chest revealed diffusely scattered pulmonary nodules in both the lungs. During life, a diagnosis of congenital tuberculosis was not thought of and the various differentials thought of were bronchopulmonary dysplasia, pneumonia, nosocomial sepsis, shock, structural malformation of lung, cystic fibrosis, congenital heart disease, with the cause of death being hypoxia. There was evidence of infection in the mother which was undetected tuberculosis, evidenced from—(1) The postpartum detection of a tuberculous tubo-ovarian abscess from where the infection later spread to the lungs and brain, leading to her demise. (2) Documented fever in the mother, in the antenatal period since the 2nd trimester of pregnancy. After the postpartum drainage of the tubo-ovarian abscess, she was put on ATT, which she stopped after 7 days. The mother deteriorated postpartum and 5 months after the delivery, i.e. at the time the autopsy report was signed out, she developed tubercular meningitis and was hospitalized in our institute, was put on ATT, but succumbed to her illness. There was no history of contact in the family, no overcrowding, the child being from a good socio-economic status. At autopsy, tuberculosis was florid in the lungs and hilar lymph nodes with a very heavy (Ziehl–Neelsen stain for AFB 5+) bacillary load. In the liver, the quantum of infection was much less in degree with only a 1+ bacillary load and there was no portal adenopathy. There is no doubt in this case that the tuberculosis is "congenital". Applying the revised Cantwell criteria, the infant had florid proven tuberculous lesions and three of the remaining parameters, i.e. the infection was definitely present in the first week of life as he presented with severe respiratory distress, tuberculous infection was present in the maternal genital tract as there was a tubo-ovarian abscess that was drained and postnatal transmission was ruled out by thorough contact investigation. This infection was acquired by the aspiration of infected amniotic fluid during passage through the birth canal (due to presence of genital tuberculosis in the mother) and here the lungs were the primary focus of infection. The fact that the baby was born premature at 28 weeks gestation with a weight appropriate for gestational age, points toward the fact that the tuberculosis was acquired during parturition. As in other cases cited in literature, the infection in the mother was detected, after its detection in the child (at autopsy). The baby and the mother were HIV negative and there was no primary immunodeficiency as the thymus was normal both grossly and microscopically and on immunostaining with CD3 and CD20. So, this case highlights an undetected case of congenital tuberculosis, a highly underestimated entity with a very high mortality. Awareness amongst doctors is very essential, every pregnant woman should be screened and fever in the antenatal period should be taken very seriously.

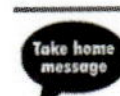

TAKE HOME MESSAGE

- Congenital tuberculosis is an under diagnosed entity.
- It is termed as infection with tubercle bacilli during intrauterine life or before the complete passage through the birth canal.
- Cantwell modification of Beitzke's criteria is less stringent and easier to apply.
- Symptoms of congenital tuberculosis are nonspecific and awareness leads to a correct diagnosis.
- Tuberculosis in the mothers is usually detected after its detection in the baby. Thus, the need for a thorough evaluation and ruling out tuberculosis in all pregnant mothers.
- Consequences of delayed diagnosis and treatment are catastrophic, hence the importance of an early diagnosis as it greatly brings down the mortality.

REFERENCES

1. Balasubramanian S, Shivram R, Padmasani LN, et al. Congenital tuberculosis. Indian J Pediatr. 1999;66:148-50.
2. Ray M, Dixit A, Vaipei K, et al. Congenital tuberculosis. Indian Pediatrics. 2002;39:1167-8.
3. Starke JR. Tuberculosis. An old disease but a new threat to the mother fetus and neonate. Clin Perinatol. 1997;24:107-27.
4. Hassan G, Waseem Q, Kadri SM. Congenital tuberculosis. JK Science. 2006;4:193-4.
5. Kang GH, Chi Je G. Congenital tuberculosis. J Korean Med Sci. 1990;5(1):59-64.
6. Chotpitayasunondh T, Sangtawesin V. Congenital tuberculosis. J Med Assoc Thai. 2003;86:689-95.
7. Bonnet C, Michel F, Nicaise C, et al. Congenital tuberculosis in preterm neonate: a cases report. Arch Pediatr. 2009; 16(5):439-43.
8. Machin GA, Honore LH, Fanning EA, et al. Perinatally acquired neonatal tuberculosis: report of two cases. Pediatr Pathol. 1992;12(5):707-16.
9. Seaton A, Seaton D, Leitch AG. Clinical features of tuberculosis. Crofton and Doughlas's Respiratory Diseases, 4th edition. London: Blackwell Scientific Publications; 1989. pp. 395-422.
10. Abughali N, Vander Kuyp F, Annable W, et al. Congenital tuberculosis. Pediatr Infect Dis J. 1994;13:731-41.
11. Grover SB, Pati NK, Mehta R, et al. Congenital tuberculosis: early diagnosis by imaging studies. Am J Perinatol. 2003; 20(3):147-52.
12. Peng W, Yang J, Liu E. Analysis of 170 cases of congenital tuberculosis reported in the literature between 1946 and 2009. Pediatr Pulmonol. 2011;46:1215-24.
13. Sri SS. Congenital tuberculosis. In: Textbook of Pulmonary and Extrapulmonary Tuberculosis, 2nd edition. New Delhi: Interprint; 1995. pp. 205.
14. Bahera D. Tuberculosis. In: Textbook of Pulmonary Medicine, 2nd edition. New Delhi: Jaypee Brothers Medical Publishers (P) Ltd.; 2010. pp. 495.
15. Cantwell M, Snider DE Jr, Cauthen GM, et al. Epidemiology of tuberculosis in the United States, 1985 through 1992. JAMA. 1994;272:535-9.

CONTRIBUTIONS BY:

1. Dr Pankaj C Vaidya, Professor, Department of Pediatrics (Compilation of Clinical Details)
2. Dr Kusum Sharma, Professor, Department of Microbiology (Providing Fig 4A)
3. Dr KS Sodhi, Professor, Department of Radiodiagnosis and Imaging (Providing Figs 4A and B)
4. Dr S Singhi, Ex-Professor and Head, Department of Pediatrics (Clinician In-Charge)

Post Graduate Institute of Medical Education and Research, Chandigarh, India.

CASE 62

Disseminated Cryptococcomas Mimicking Disseminated Malignancy, with Hepatic Dysfunction as the Initial Manifestation, in an Immunocompetent Child: PM 25744

Nandita Bharadwaj Kakkar

HIGHLIGHTS OF THE CASE

A 2-year-old, immunocompetent boy was ill since 3 months and presented with fever, obstructive jaundice, progressive abdominal distension with palpable masses, generalized lymphadenopathy, weight loss and decreased intake. Contrast enhanced computed tomography (CECT) scan showed generalized lymphadenopathy, multiple nodules and cavitation in both lungs with hypodense lesions in liver and spleen along with ascites. A diagnosis of disseminated tuberculosis or malignancy were thought of, till the time fine needle aspiration cytology (FNAC) from the cervical lymph node was done, which was suggestive of dual infection with cryptococcosis and histoplasmosis. Autopsy however revealed disseminated cryptococcomas (fibrotic granulomatous nodules) involving the lung, lymph nodes (generalized), liver, spleen, kidneys, adrenals and brain, ? *Cryptococcus gattii* infection in an apparently immunocompetent host. Disseminated cryptococcal infection is rare in immunocompetent hosts and hepatic dysfunction as the presenting manifestation is rarer.

Keywords: Cryptococcomas, disseminated, immunocompetent child, mimicker of malignancy, hepatic dysfunction, *Cryptococcus gattii*, fibrotic granulomatous nodules, autopsy.

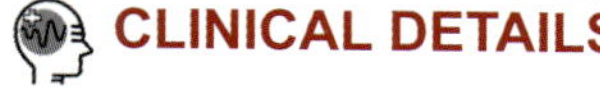

CLINICAL DETAILS

Date of Admission: 30.10.2013, Date of Death: 04.11.2013, Duration of Hospital Stay: 5 Days

A 2-year-old male child was admitted to PGIMER, Chandigarh with multiple complaints. He had fever since 3 months that was intermittent, with no rigors, chills or diurnal variation and was relieved by antipyretics. There was yellowish discoloration of eyes, with passage of high colored urine and clay colored stools, noticed for the same duration. Progressive abdominal distension was present, more in the upper abdomen, which was associated with palpable, multiple, discrete and hard masses since 2 months. Multiple lymph nodes were palpable in the axilla, neck and inguinal area since 1 month. There was history of weight loss (2 kg in last 3 months) with decreased intake and activity. However, there was no history of vomiting, loose stools, constipation, ear discharge, rashes, pyodermal lesions, seizure, altered sensorium, paucity of limb movements, vision impairment, bleeding manifestations, cough, rapid breathing, periorbital puffiness, dysuria, abnormalities in urinary stream and bone pain or any joint swelling. He was third in birth order with two elder female siblings, who were well. He belonged to low socioeconomic strata, but there was no contact with tuberculosis. He was a term, normal vaginal delivery, birth weight being 2.5 kg, baby cried immediately at birth and there was no perinatal asphyxia or jaundice. He was exclusively breast fed till one year. Baby had gained milestones appropriate for age and was immunized appropriately till 18 months of age. On ***examination*** he weighed 7 kg, height was 77 cm (< 3rd centile) and head circumference was 45 cm (-2 to-3Z score). Baby was emaciated with hollowing of temporal fossa, infected scalp lesions, thin, sparse and hypopigmented hair. There was pallor, knuckle hyperpigmentation, frontal bossing, anterior fontanelle 2 × 2 cm wide open, beading of ribs, icterus, excessive hair all over the body, bilateral pitting pedal edema, oral thrush and generalized lymphadenopathy with nodes 1–2 cm, hard, nontender, mobile and matted. Systemic examination revealed a distended abdomen with multiple, discrete hard nodules palpable all over, measuring 1 × 1 cm, nontender and mobile ? fecoliths. The liver was palpable 5 cm below right costal margin (span 8 cm) was hard, with sharp irregular margins and nodular surface. The spleen was not palpable and there was no free fluid. On chest examination, there was bronchial breathing in right upper zone with bilateral diffuse crepts. CNS revealed no meningeal signs or cranial nerve palsy.

This child had two admissions at an outside facility and then was referred to our institute. He was first admitted from 27th July till 14th August 2013, with the same complaints. Was found to have hepatomegaly and splenomegaly, chest X-ray was suggestive of progressive primary complex and so he was put on anti-tubercular treatment and discharged. He was readmitted at the same facility on 27th August 2013 with cold peripheries, decreased interaction and poor feeding. Investigations revealed—Hb 5.6 g/dL, PTI—60.4%, SGOT—149 U/L, SGPT—164 U/L, ALP—1442 U/L and HIV non-reactive. Aspiration cytology from the cervical lymph node revealed small mature lymphocytes, few follicular cells, occasional immunoblast and a single giant cell. Liver biopsy was suggestive of cholestasis with bridging fibrosis. He was managed with transfusions, broad spectrum antibiotics and referred to PGI on 29th Oct 2013.

Investigations (PGIMER)

Hemogram: Hb—10 g/dL, total leucocyte count—14400/μL, platelets 248000/μL. Serum bilirubin: conjugated/unconjugated—11.5/5.2 mg%, AST—277 U/L, ALT—179 U/L, ALP—1952 U/L, serum urea—75 mg%, serum creatinine -0.6 mg%, serum uric acid- 3.6 mg%, Ca^{2+}– 15.2 mg, iCa^{2+}– 2.4, HIV—nonreactive, blood culture and sensitivity test grew yeast and CSF examination was within normal limits. ***Ultrasonography*** of the abdomen showed multiple echogenic nodules in liver and spleen ? Calcified granulomas, enlarged lymph nodes with ? calcifications, mild ascites and bilateral raised renal cortical echogenicity. ***Chest X-ray*** revealed bilateral parenchymal infiltrates in the lung with two large cavities in right upper and lower zones. ***CECT chest*** showed necrotic mediastinal, hilar and abdominal lymphadenopathy, patchy consolidation with cavitations and nodules in both lungs, bilateral mild pleural effusion, hypodense lesions in liver/spleen and ascites. ***FNAC*** from the cervical lymph node was suggestive of dual infection with cryptococcosis and histoplasmosis. With the above clinical features and investigations, the child was initially started on two drug anti-tubercular therapy. After the FNA report, liposomal amphotericin B and flucytosine were started. Child had worsening respiratory distress and hemodynamic compromise requiring intubation and vasopressor support. In view of refractory shock, antibiotics were upgraded but the child continued to deteriorate and sustained cardiac arrest, from which he could not be revived. ***Units final diagnosis*** was severe protein energy malnutrition (PEM), disseminated histoplasmosis/cryptococcosis, sepsis and septic shock.

AUTOPSY FINDINGS: PM 25744

A complete autopsy was performed on this 2-year-old male child. On external examination, there was yellowish discoloration of the body and a distended abdomen. Peritoneal cavity revealed 700 mL of yellowish fluid and other serous cavities were within normal limits. The ***lungs*** were voluminous and weighed 210 g. On the pleural aspect, there were multiple nodules ranging in size from 0.5 cm to 2 cm in diameter (Fig 1A). Cut section of the lungs revealed multiple well-circumscribed nodules ranging in size from 3 mm to 2.5 cm in diameter, present diffusely (Figs 1B and C). The nodules were whitish in color, firm to feel and few of them were walled off from the lung parenchyma by thick fibrous walls. Some of them showed necrosis and cavitation. Microscopically the nodules at low power were well circumscribed and walled off from the lung parenchyma by fibrous tissue and revealed a foamy soap bubble appearance (Fig 2A). At a higher power the soap bubble appearance was better appreciated (Figs 2B–D) and along with it there was fibrosis (Fig 2B), plenty of giant cells (Figs 2B and C) and necrosis (Fig 2C). The empty spaces were replete with encapsulated, refractile, round to oval fungal profiles of cryptococci (Fig 2D). The Periodic acid-Schiff (PAS) stain (Figs 3A and B) showed deep pink staining of the entire organism. Mucicarmine (Fig 3C) and alcian blue stain (Fig 3D) stained the capsule magenta and deep blue, respectively. Grocott silver stain stained the body black. Morphology and staining characteristics of the fungal profiles conformed to the morphology of cryptococci. The normal looking adjacent lung parenchyma showed small granulomas composed of histiocytes, epithelioid-like cells, giant cells and plenty of cryptococci. There was generalized lymphadenopathy. All ***lymph nodes***, i.e. mesenteric (Figs 4A and B), cervical, hilar, carinal, mediastinal, paratracheal (Fig 1B), paraaortic along the ascending/abdominal aorta (Figs 4C and D), paraesophageal, peripancreatic, splenic, nodes at the porta hepatis, inguinal and those all along the gastrointestinal tract were enlarged, ranging in size from 0.5 cm to 3 cm in diameter. Cut section was yellowish. On microscopic examination, there was no lymphoid tissue identified and the lymph nodes (Figs 5A–E) were totally replaced by fibrosis, macrophages, giant cells, granulomas, areas of necrosis and replete with fungal profiles of cryptococci with similar morphology and staining characteristics as seen in the lung. Some of the lymph nodes however showed florid chronic granulomatous reaction (Fig. 5E). The ***liver*** (Figs 6A and B)

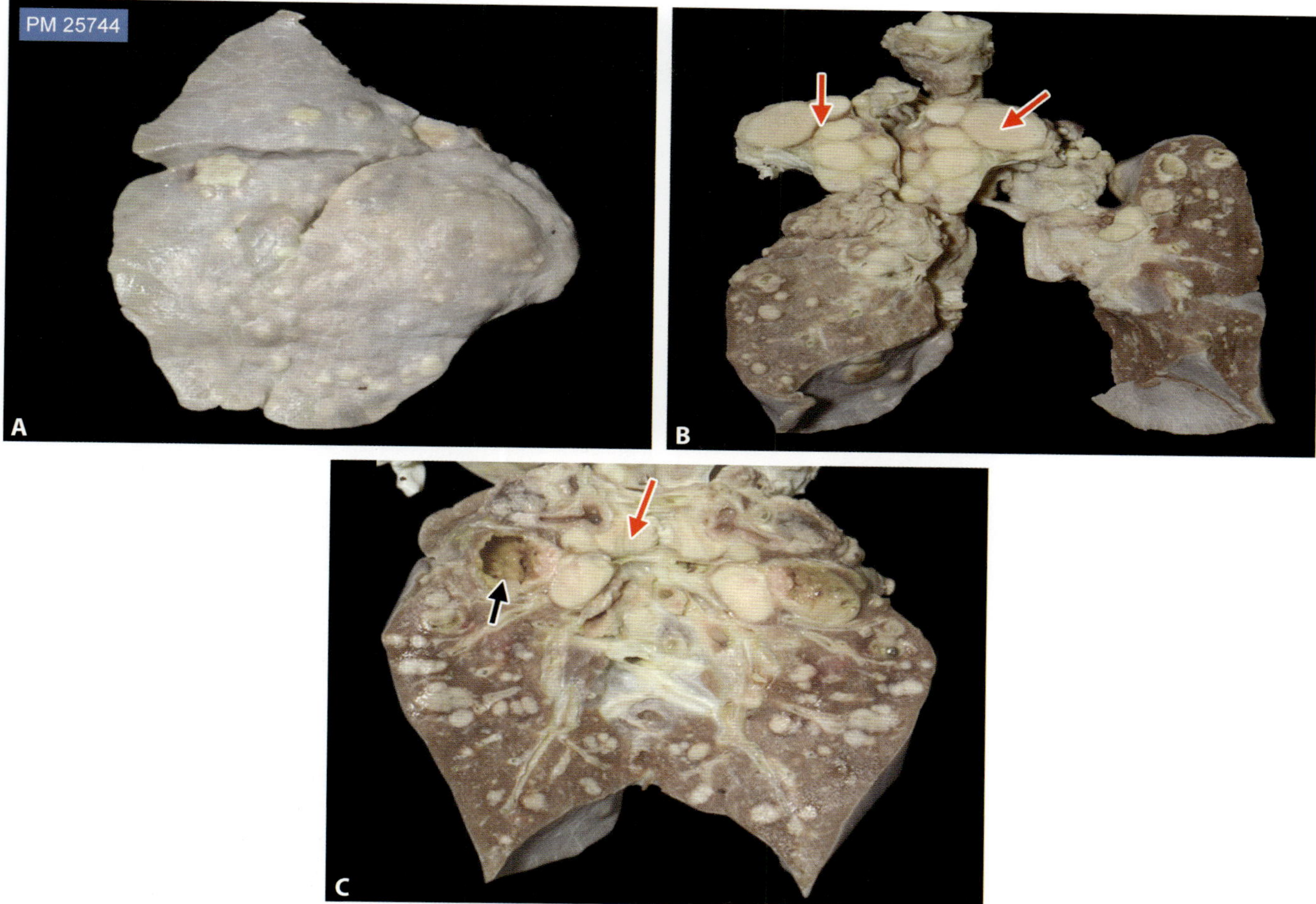

Figs 1A–C: (A) Pleural aspect of the lungs shows multiple nodules; (B and C) Cut section of the lungs show multiple well-circumscribed nodules, some with a thick fibrotic wall and some showing cavitation (arrow). The hilar, carinal and paratracheal nodes are enlarged (red arrows).

was enlarged, bile stained and weighed 540 g. Capsular aspect showed whitish firm areas. Cut section showed multiple white to yellowish nodules/masses some of which appeared longitudinal, as though growing along the major vessels, ranging in size from 0.5 cm to 6 cm in diameter. The lymph nodes at the porta, peripancreatic and splenic were enlarged (0.5–4 cm) forming a conglomerate mass. Microscopic sections from the nodular masses in the liver showed a sharp demarcation (Fig 6C) from the adjacent liver, dense fibrosis, areas of necrosis, calcification, macrophages, histiocytes, lymphocytes, giant cells and clear spaces were loaded with fungal profiles of cryptococci (Figs 6D and 7A) with similar morphology and staining characteristics as seen in the lungs. The adjacent liver (Figs 7B and C) showed features of extrahepatic biliary obstruction, i.e. expansion of portal tracts with bridging fibrosis, marked bile ductular proliferation with cholestasis, extensive hepatocytic (> in perivenular locations) and canalicular cholestasis. Some of the portal tracts (Fig 7D) revealed compact granulomas replete with cryptococci. The ***spleen*** was enlarged and weighed 105 g. Cut sections (Fig 8A) showed miliary nodules yellowish in color, scattered diffusely, some of them getting confluent to form bigger nodules. Microscopy (Figs 8B and C) was similar to that seen in the liver and lungs. The ***kidneys*** weighed 90 g and were grossly unremarkable. Microscopic examination shows multiple scattered granulomas with cryptococci (Fig 8D). The ***adrenals*** (Fig 8E) revealed granulomas with plenty of cryptococci. The ***brain*** was normal on gross examination. No slimy or mucoid exudate was visible, but there was slight opalescence (Fig 9A). Microscopy (Fig 9B), however showed small granulomas in the subarachnoid space. An occasional granuloma, deep in the depth of the sulcus was invading into the superficial cortex. Choroid plexus also showed small granulomas composed of epithelioid cells. PAS, alcian blue and mucicarmine stains revealed few cryptococci in the granulomas. Other organs, i.e. the bone

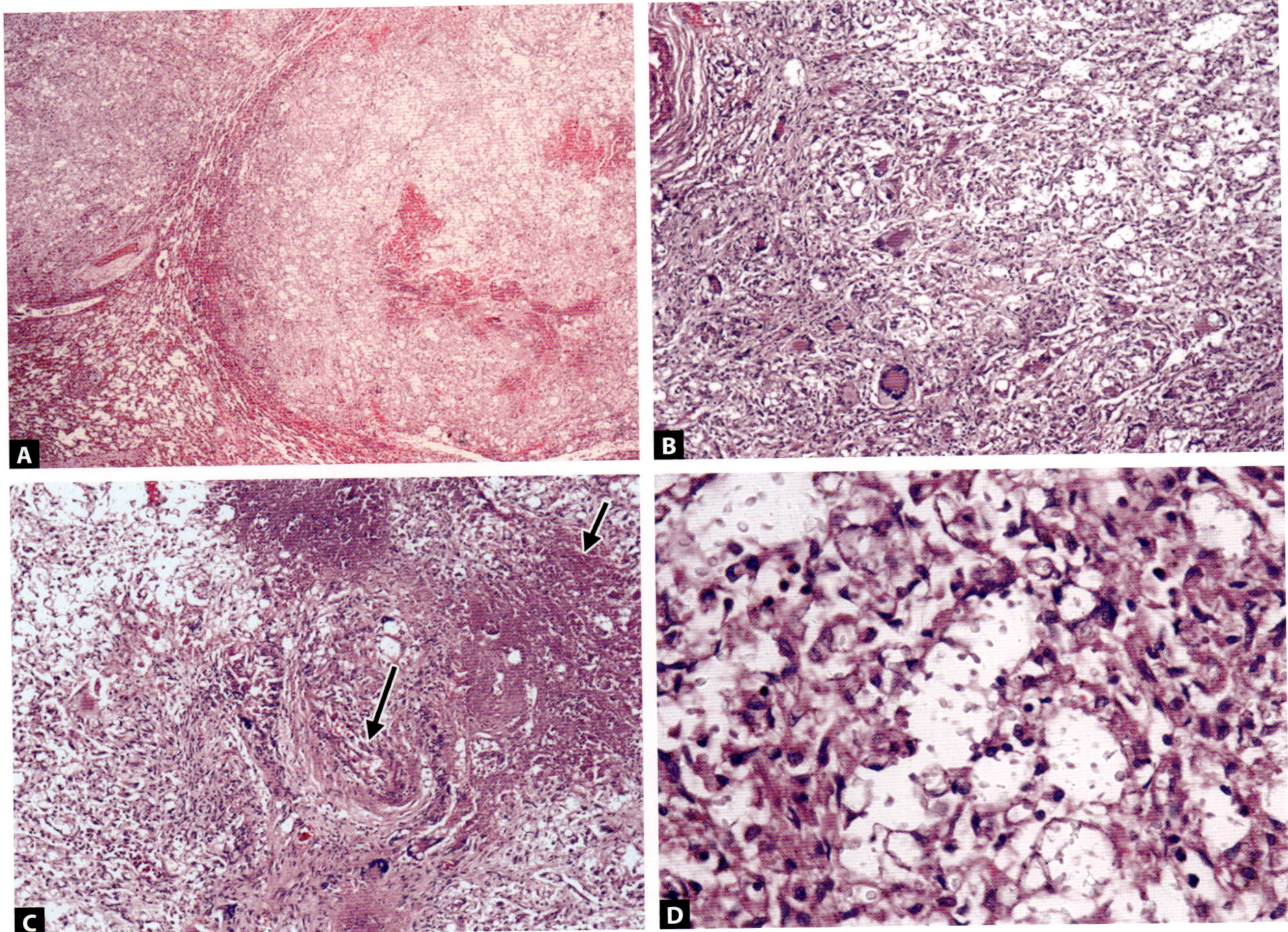

Figs 2A–D: (A) Photomicrograph of the lung at low power showing well-circumscribed nodules having a foamy soap bubble appearance with areas of necrosis; (B) The nodules are composed of giant cells, fibrosis and empty spaces containing cryptococci; (C) Nodule showing areas of necrosis (arrow) with a caught up vessel (arrow) and giant cells; (D) Empty spaces in the nodules containing refractile, empty looking fungal profiles of cryptococci.

marrow, heart, GIT and testis were within normal limits. Thymus was not discernable as it was caught up in the mediastinal mass and was involved by the disease process. Adequate lymphoid tissue was found in the spleen, peyer's patches and the appendix.

FINAL AUTOPSY DIAGNOSIS: PM 25744

2 Years Male Child

Disseminated cryptococcomas (fibrotic granulomatous nodules) involving the lung, lymph nodes (generalized), liver, spleen, kidneys and adrenals along with cryptococcal meningoencephalitis ? *Cryptococcus gattii* infection in an immunocompetent host.

Features of extrahepatic biliary obstruction—liver.

CRYPTOCOCCOSIS

Cryptococcosis[1] is a systemic infection caused by naturally encapsulated basidiomycetes of genus Cryptococcus. This yeast fungus infects humans, leading to asymptomatic or mild pulmonary colonization, to life-threatening meningoencephalitis or disseminated disease. Occurs predominantly as an opportunistic infection in immunocompromised individuals[2,3] with AIDS, lymphomas (Non-Hodgkins and Hodgkins), systemic lupus erythematosus, sarcoidosis and transplant recipients. These patients are on high dose corticosteroids, which is a major risk factor for cryptococcal infection. Cryptococcus can cause disease in immunocompetent hosts as well. Isolates of Cryptococcus[4] are of four distinct serotypes, A, B, C and D, on the basis of the immunologic properties

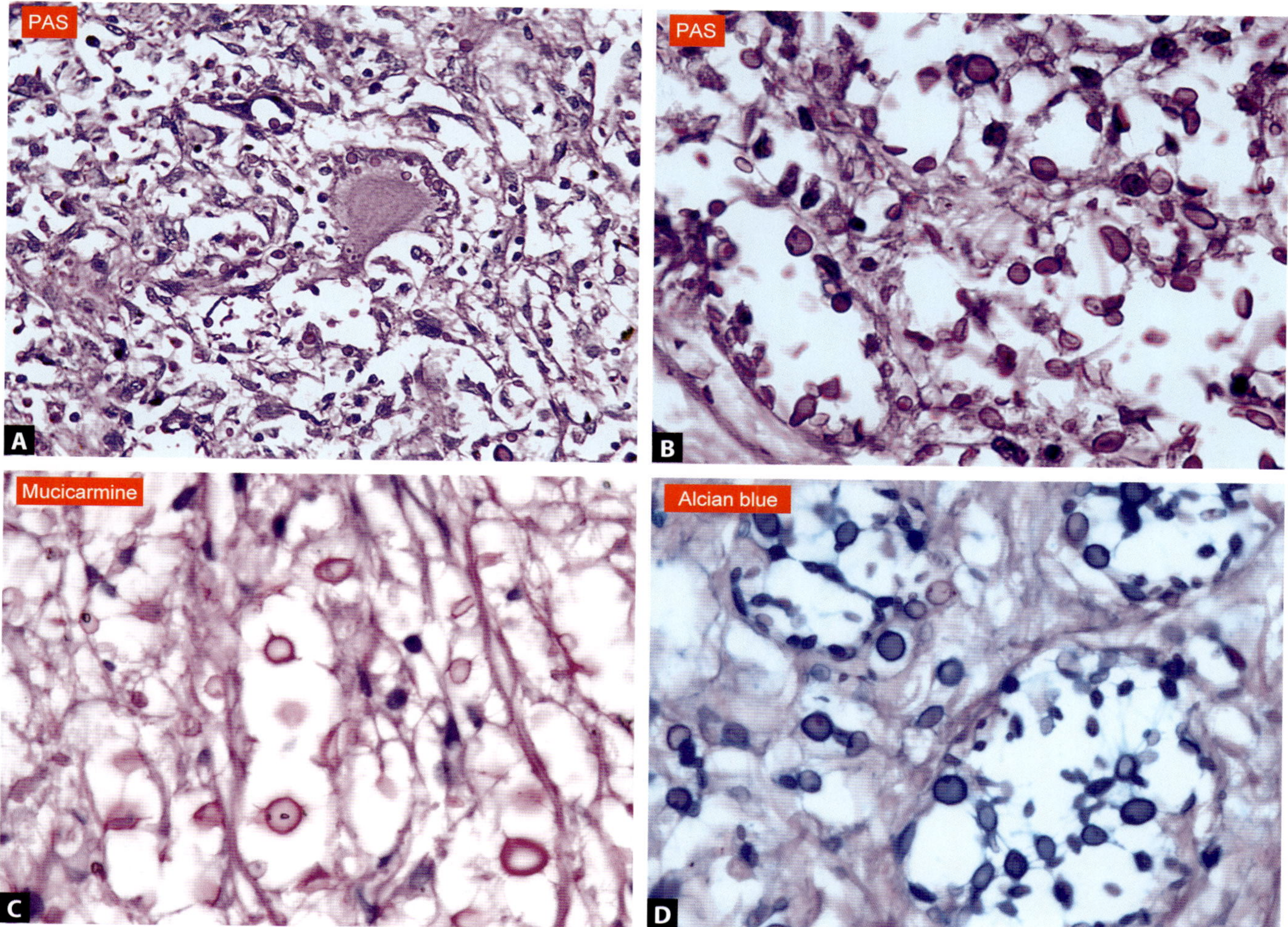

Figs 3A–D: Photomicrographs from the lung. (A and B) PAS stain shows deep pink staining of the entire cryptococcus with many within the giant cell; (C) Mucicarmine stain stains the capsule of the cryptococci magenta; (D) Alcian blue stain stains the capsule deep blue.

of their capsular polysaccharides. Pathogenic *Crypyococcus* species are presently divided into *C. grubii* (serotype A), *C. gattii* (serotypes B and C) and C. neoformans (serotype D). Both *C. neoformans* and *grubii* have a worldwide distribution, are commonly present in the soil, especially in places contaminated by pigeon droppings and infect patients when inhaled. *C. neoformans* is the most common among all the pathogenic species and is most widely studied as well. *C. grubii* has gained importance after HIV outbreaks, as infection with this fungus is considered as an AIDS defining illness. *C. gattii* infection has recently received widespread attention due to outbreaks in British Columbia,[5,6] Canada and the US Pacific Northwest.[7-9] It occurs in tropical and subtropical zones. It is common in Australia and California with occasional cases being reported from practically every country of the world. *C. gattii* is found in tree hollows especially of eucalyptus tree. The Vancouver Island outbreak of *C. gattii* infection from 1999–2004 was a result of import of eucalyptus trees from Australia. In addition, studies from South America have reported both species in the decaying heartwood of a number of trees. It generally causes disease in healthy hosts and is more likely to cause widespread cryptoccomas, which is mistaken for malignancy.

Cryptococci are spherical to oval, yeast, which is 5–20 µm in diameter, refractile structure, produces a single bud and has a thick gelatinous capsule. Unlike candida, there are no hyphal or pseudohyphal forms. It evades the host defenses due to its strong virulence factors, which include the polysaccharide capsule, enzymes and melanin production. The virulence factors are not very effective when the host defenses are good, but cause devastating disease in the immunocompromised individuals. The major virulence

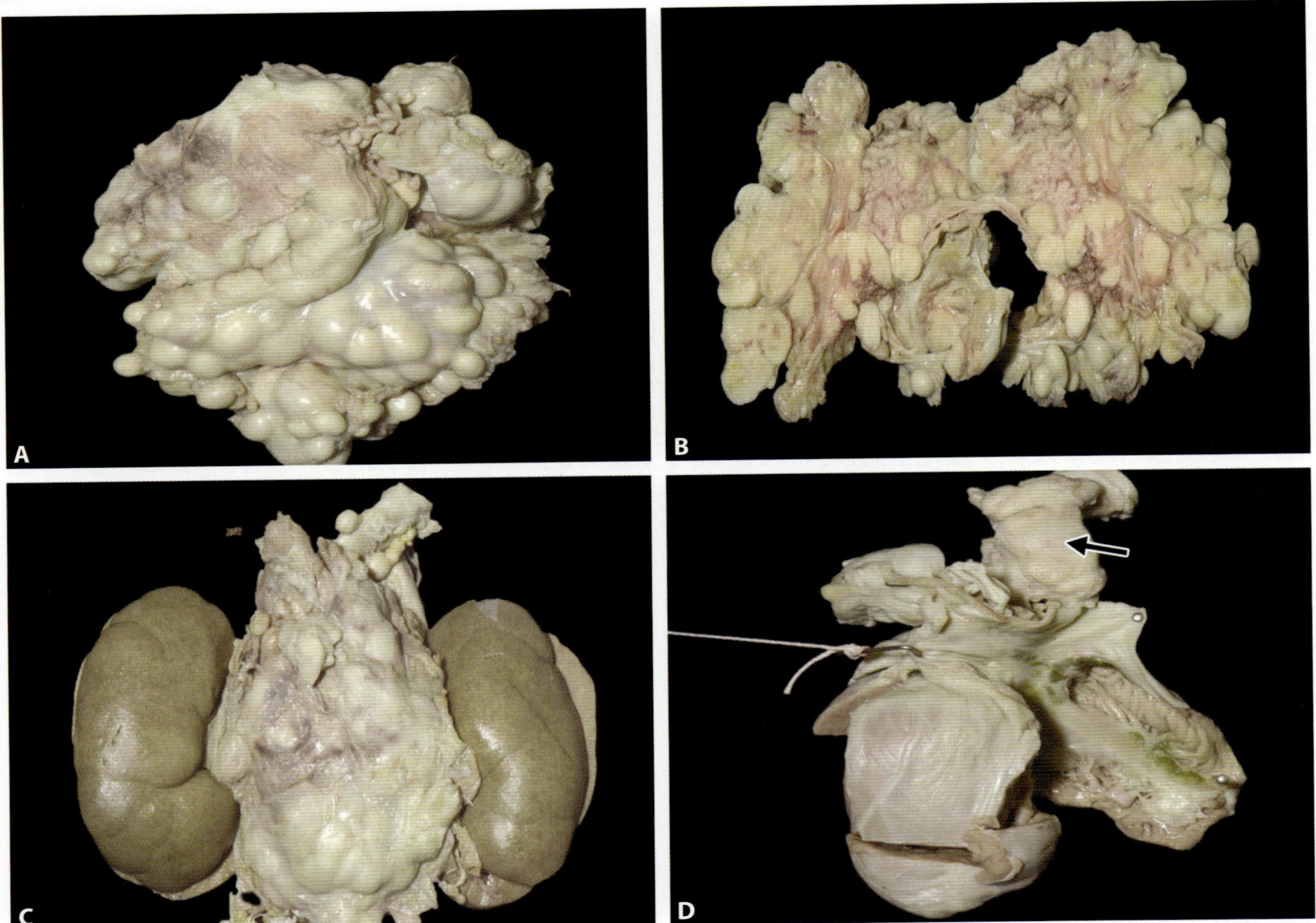

Figs 4A–D: Enlarged, well-circumscribed, firm and fibrotic lymph nodes in the (A and B) Mesentery; (C) Paraaortic, along abdominal aorta; and (D) Paraaortic, along the ascending aorta (arrow).

factor is the capsule, as the capsular polysaccharide inhibits phagocytosis, recruitment of inflammation and leucocyte migration. Acapsular strains are said to be less virulent. *C. neoformans* produces laccase, which catalyzes the formation of a melanin-like pigment, which protects the fungi from the epinephrine oxidative system in the host nervous system. These fungi also produce certain enzymes, which aid in tissue invasion. The thick gelatinous polysaccharide capsule has tremendous value, as it aids in the detection of this fungi. The capsule is stained by mucus stains such as Mayer's mucicarmine (deep pink) and alcian blue (deep blue colour). PAS stains the entire organism, i.e. the body and the capsule, magenta. Grocott silver stain stains the body black. With India ink, the unstained mucoid capsule of the fungi appears as a clear halo against a dark background. Mucicarmine staining of the capsule is diagnostic and this reaction is not given by any other pathogenic yeast like fungus. Cryptococcal antigen (CrAg) test detects the capsular antigen in the plasma or the CSF. Changes in the structure and size of the capsular polysaccharide can occur and lead to phenotypic switching, which leads to evasion of immune responses. So, demonstration of spherical to oval, refractile structures, 5–20 μm in diameter, producing a single bud with no hyphal or pseudohyphal forms, producing a clear halo against a dark background on India ink, capsule stained deep blue by alcian blue and deep pink colored with mucicarmine stain, entire body stained magenta with PAS and black with Grocott stain and demonstration of cryptococcal capsular polysaccharide antigen in titers more than 1:8 in serum or CSF, is confirmatory of the diagnosis.

In cryptococcosis, two types of tissue reactions are seen depending on the host immune status and the virulence of the

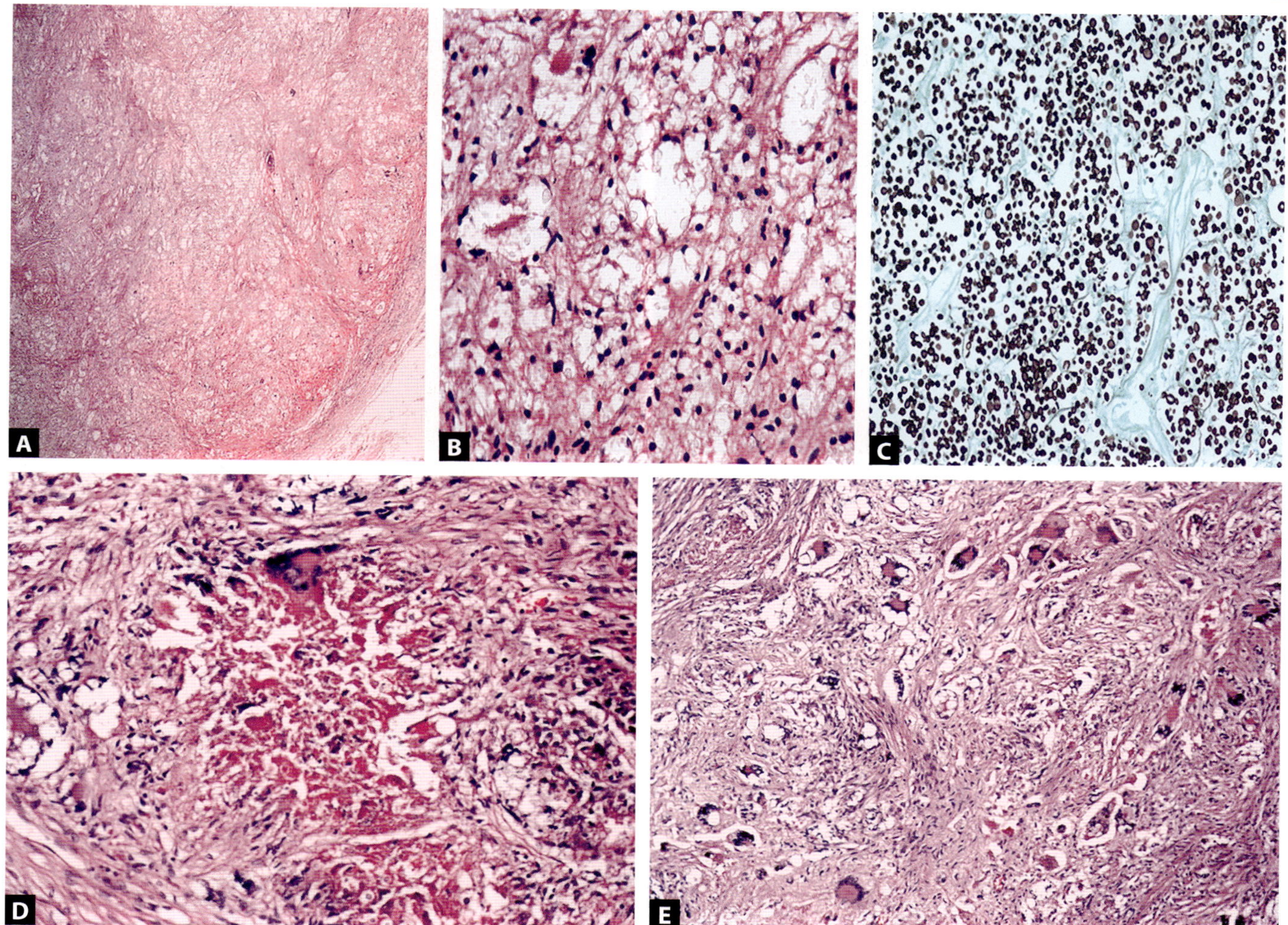

Figs 5A–E: Photomicrographs from the lymph nodes (A) At low power shows a foamy, bubbly and fibrotic appearance; (B) Clear spaces showing fungal profiles of cryptococci; (C) Grocott stain, stains the cryptococci black; (D) Areas showing necrosis, giant cells and fibrosis; (E) Chronic granulomatous reaction with giant cells, fibrosis and cryptococci.

organism. The reactions are either a chronic granulomatous reaction or a pauci-immune gelatinous type of reaction. The chronic granulomatous reaction occurs in immunocompetent individuals. To begin with, it shows necrotizing inflammation, suppuration and later the true granulomatous response comes up in the form of foreign body giant cells with phagocytosed organisms, macrophages, lymphocytes and fibrosis. The pauci-immune or gelatinous type of reaction occurs in immunosuppressed individuals, wherein there is a marked paucity of the inflammatory infiltrate and shows only sheets of cryptococci. The primary site of localization of ***C. neoformans*** is the lungs, where it causes a mild and usually an asymptomatic infection. The fungus then takes the hematogenous route to the brain leading to the causation of its most dreaded manifestation, i.e. cryptococcal meningitis. Concomitant lung infection is seen in 40–45% of cases and in many patients no evidence of the original lung infection is detectable. In cryptococcal meningitis, grossly the meninges may be distended by a slimy mucoid exudate, but more often they appear normal. Microscopically, in immunosuppressed individuals gelatinous masses of cryptococci with virtually no inflammatory reaction, are seen in the subarachnoid space (on the surface and deep in the sulci) and in the perivascular Virchow–Robin spaces within the gray matter, producing the characteristic soap bubble lesions. In immunocompetent individuals, cryptococci are accompanied by macrophages, lymphocytes and giant cells with ingested fungal profiles producing the granulomatous type of reaction. Acute necrotizing inflammation and at times fibrosis in the meninges, leading to obstruction in

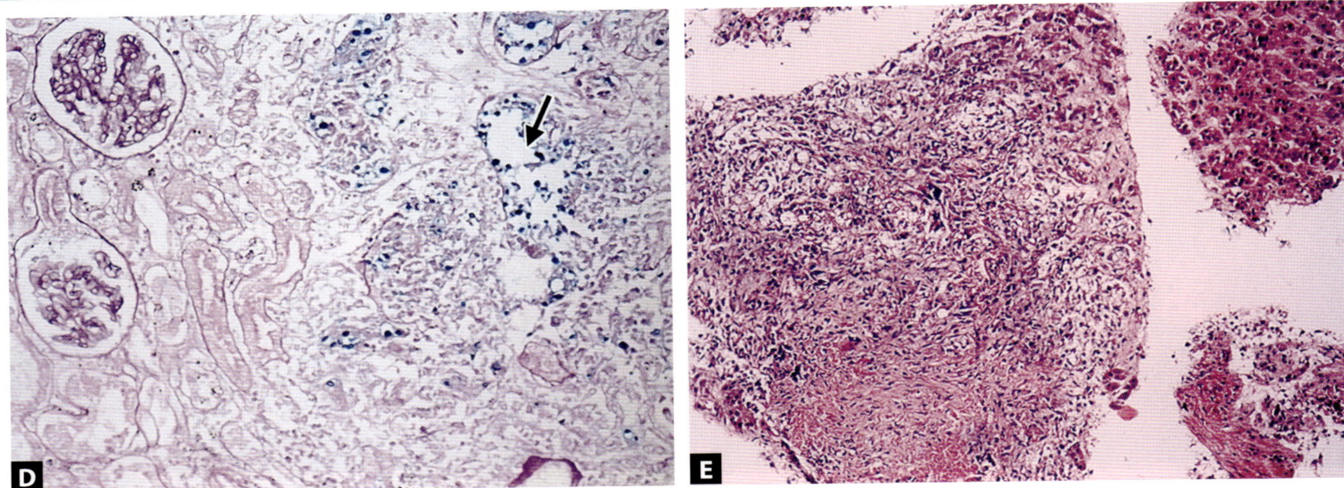

Figs 8A–E: (A) Coronal slices of the enlarged spleen showing whitish well-circumscribed nodules getting confluent; (B) Splenic cryptococcoma show plenty of giant cells containing cryptococci, inflammation and fibrosis; and (C) Spleen replete with cryptococci; (D) Alcian blue stain on the kidney shows plenty of cryptococci (arrow); (E) Adrenal gland shows cryptococcoma replete with 'cryptococci.

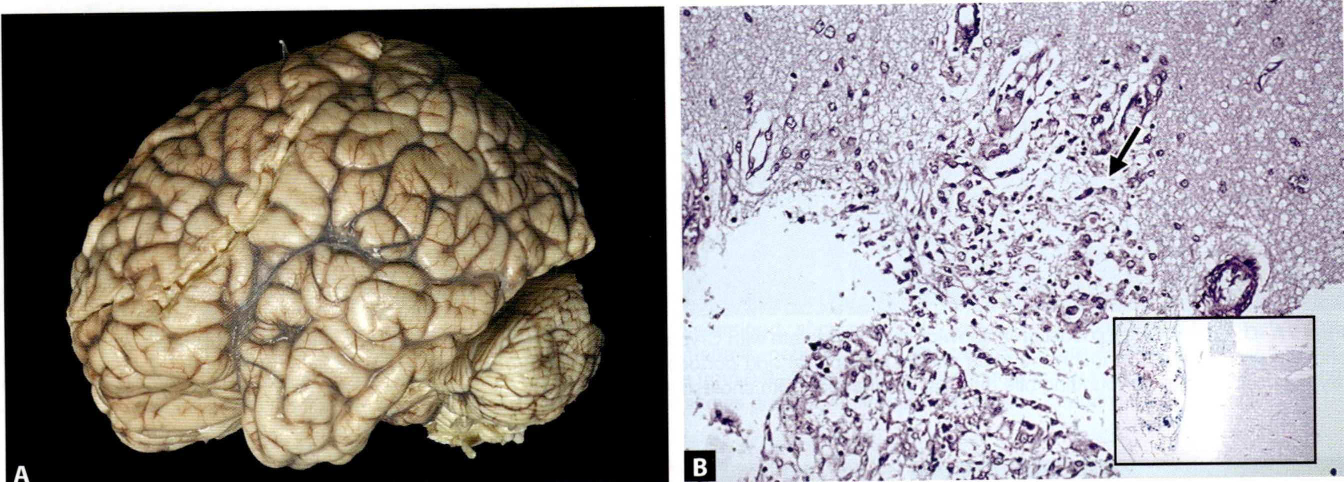

Figs 9A and B: (A) Gross picture of the brain showing slight meningeal opalescence; (B) Depth of a sulcus showing granulomas composed of macrophages, lymphocytes along with cryptococci in the subarachnoid space and invading the parenchyma (arrow). Alcian blue stain shows cryptococci (inset).

nodules', which can mimic a malignancy. ***Cryptococcus gattii*** is now considered as an emerging cause of pulmonary nodules.[11]

COMMENTARY—INDEX CASE: PM 25744

This 2-year-old male child was HIV negative. There was adequate lymphoid tissue in the spleen, appendix and ilium. Immunodeficiency workup was not done. He presented with hyperbilirubinemia, elevated transaminases AST > ALT, markedly elevated ALP, hypercalcemia, raised urea/creatinine, generalized lymphadenopathy, nodules in lungs, liver and spleen. Autopsy revealed disseminated cryptococcomas in the liver, lungs, lymph nodes and spleen which actually mimicked a malignancy. The type of reaction, seen in the index case i.e. the fibrotic granulomatous nodules replete with cryptococci, better known as cryptococcomas represent an infection in immunocompetent persons with an active cell-mediated immune response. Thus, it is highly unlikely that this child was immunocompromised. The histology was characterized by chronic granulomatous inflammation with giant cells, histiocytes, lymphocytes and a marked fibroblastic reaction. The immunocompetent state, presence of cryptococcomas, florid infection in the extracranial organs with minimal infection in the brain, strongly points toward *C. gattii* infection. This child presented with obstructive jaundice, because of the large lymph nodes pressing upon the extrahepatic biliary tract. Hepatitis, cholangitis and cholecystitis, as presenting manifestation of cryptococcal infection is seen in case reports.[12-14] Hence, hepatic dysfunction should be considered as one of the primary manifestations of disseminated cryptococcosis and should be given more importance in the era of effective antifungal therapy.

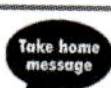

TAKE HOME MESSAGE

- Disseminated cryptococcomas (fibrotic granulomatous nodules) is a rare manifestation of cryptococcal infection and mimics a malignancy.
- ***C. gattii*** infection has recently received widespread attention due to outbreaks in British Columbia, Canada and the US Pacific Northwest.
- ***C. gattii*** occurs in tropical and subtropical zones. It is common in Australia and California with occasional cases being reported from practically every country of the world.
- ***C. gattii*** is found in tree hollows, especially of eucalyptus tree.
- ***C. gattii*** generally causes disease in healthy hosts and is more likely to cause widespread cryptococcomas, which is mistaken for malignancy.

REFERENCES

1. Shimodaira K, Okubo Y, Nakayama H, et al. Trends in the prevalence of invasive fungal infections from an analysis of annual records of autopsy cases of Toho University. Mycoses. 2012;55(5):435-43.
2. Shibuya K, Coulson WE, Wollman JS, et al. Histopathology of cryptococcosis and other fungal infections in patients with acquired immunodeficiency syndrome. Int J Infect Dis. 2001;5(2):78-85.
3. Shibuya k, Coulson WF, Naoe S. Histopathology of deep-seated fungal infections and detailed examination of granulomatous response against cryptococci in patients with acquired immunodeficiency syndrome. Japanese J Med Mycol. 2002;43(3):143-51.
4. Franzot SP, Salkin IF, Casadevall A. Cryptococcus neoformans var. grubii: separate varietal status for Cryptococcus neoformans serotype A isolates. J Clin Microbiol. 1999;37(3):838-40.
5. MacDougall L, Kidd SE, Galanis E, et al. Spread of Cryptococcus gattii in British Columbia, Canada and detection in the Pacific Northwest, USA. Emerg Infect Dis. 2007;13(1):42-50.
6. Kidd SE, Hagen F, Tscharke RL, et al. A rare genotype of Cryptococcus gattii caused the cryptococcosis outbreak on Vancouver Island (British Columbia, Canada). Proc Natl Acad Sci USA. 2004;101(49):17258-63.
7. Byrnes EJ, Li W, Lewit Y, et al. Emergence and pathogenicity of highly virulent Cryptococcus gattii genotypes in the northwest United States. PLoS Pathog. 2010;6(4):e1000850.
8. Dixit A, Carroll SF, Qureshi ST. Cryptococcus gattii: an emerging cause of fungal disease in North America. Interdiscip Perspect Infect Dis. 2009;2009:840452.
9. Walraven CJ, Gerstein W, Hardison SE, et al. Fatal disseminated Cryptocooccus gattii infection in New Mexico. PLoS One. 2011;6(12):e28625.
10. Popchai N, Chang Y, Sionov EL, et al. The primary target organ of C gattii is different from that of C. neoformans in a murine model. mBio. 2012;3(3):e00103-12.
11. Dewar GJ, Kelly JK. Cryptococcus gattii: an emerging cause of pulmonary nodules. Can Respir J. 2008;15(3):153-7.
12. Lin JI, Kabir MA, Tseng HC, et al. Hepatobiliary dysfunction as the initial manifestation of disseminated cryptococcosis. J Clin Gastroenterol. 1999; 28:273-5.
13. Kothari AA, Kothari KA. Hepatobiliary dysfunction as initial manifestation of disseminated cryptococcosis. Indian J Gastroenterol. 2004;23(4):145-6.
14. Rohtagi A, Aggarwal A, Chabra MK, et al. Disseminated cryptococcosis with hepatic dysfunction as the initial manifestation in an immunocompetent adult. Arch Iranian Med. 2013;16(5):303-5.

CONTRIBUTIONS BY:

1. Dr Jayashree M, Professor, Department of Pediatrics (Compilation of Clinical Details)
2. Dr KS Sodhi, Professor, Department of Radiodiagnosis and Imaging
3. Dr Sadhana Lal, Professor, Department of Gastroenterology (Clinician In-Charge)
4. Dr BR Thapa, Professor and Head, Department of Gastroenterology, Hepatology and Nutrition (Clinician In-Charge)

Post Graduate Institute of Medical Education and Research, Chandigarh, India.

Introduction to Tubercular Meningitis

Nandita Bharadwaj Kakkar

Tuberculosis (TB) is a highly prevalent disease, particularly in developing countries like India. Central nervous system (CNS) TB is a life-threatening, devastating disease with high mortality and morbidity, mainly affects young children and occurs in about 10% cases of TB. It may manifest as tubercular meningitis (TBM), tuberculomas, meningo-encephalitis, tubercular abscess, stroke due to vasculitis and tuberculous encephalopathy. Tuberculosis of the CNS causes a multitude of gross and microscopic changes, which although characteristic in a large majority of cases, may be a diagnostic challenge in some. The peculiar anatomy of the brain and spinal cord, duration of time elapsed since infection, the institution and adequacy of anti-tuberculous treatment, immune state of the individual, virulence of organism, age of patient etc. are all important determinants of the type of lesions seen in the CNS. The typical lesions seen in the brain are tuberculous meningitis (acute or chronic), vascular alterations, infarcts, borderzone encephalitis, ventriculitis, choroid plexitis, hydrocephalus, tuberculoma and tuberculous abscess. Edema and spinal arachnoiditis may be seen in a variable number of cases.

Mycobacterial tuberculosis is an aerobic, nonmotile, nonsporing and acid-fast bacilli which primarily infects the humans. TBM is mostly secondary to a primary involvement of the lungs. The alveoli of the lungs get infected by inhalation of droplet nuclei containing the bacilli. The bacilli are phagocytosed by the alveolar macrophages with the help of numerous receptors, block the formation of phagolysosomes and replicate unchecked in the vesicles. In a nonsensitized individual, in the early stages of primary tuberculosis, the bacteria proliferates in the macrophages and airspaces, with bacteremia leading to seeding at multiple sites like the draining lymph nodes and the highly oxygenated organs like the brain, i.e. the "Rich focus". This bacteremia causes a flu-like illness. Three weeks after the primary infection, cytokines/chemokines like IL12 lead to the activation of type 1 T helper cells (TH1) which mediate macrophage activation and killing of bacteria. These TH1 cells produce IFN-gamma, the key mediator in containing the M. tuberculosis infection. IFN-gamma stimulates maturation of phagolysosomes, thus making a lethal environment for the bacteria, stimulates the formation of nitric oxide, mobilizes antimicrobial peptides against the bacteria, stimulates autophagy and leads to granulomas and caseation necrosis, the morphologic hallmarks of tuberculosis. The activated macrophages are converted to "epithelioid histiocytes" which aggregate to form granulomas and some are converted into the characteristic Langhans type of giant cells. This halts the infection before significant tissue destruction or illness occurs.

TUBERCULAR MENINGITIS—GROSS EXAMINATION OF THE BRAIN

In TBM, gross examination of the brain shows a slight gray opacity of the meninges over the cerebral convexities and a thick, gelatinous exudate on the basal aspect, where the structures in the interpeduncular fossa and on the anterior surface of the brain stem are obscured. The infundibular and optic recesses of the third ventricle can be seen bulging through the exudates, suggesting the presence of hydrocephalus. The exudate engulfs the optic chiasm, mammillary bodies, infundibulum and anterior surface of the brain stem particularly the pons extends along the Sylvian fissures and may be seen over the superolateral surfaces of the cerebral hemispheres. The spinal cord may be engulfed by the exudate. Small tubercles can be seen particularly along the Sylvian fissures, orbital surfaces of the frontal lobes and tip of temporal lobe. It may be noted that the receding exudates may leave behind tiny specks, which may resemble tubercles. This thick gelatinous exudate entraps the various arteries and nerves at the base of the brain like the basilar or middle cerebral artery and their branches. It also compromises the flow of cerebrospinal fluid (CSF) at the tentorial opening leading to hydrocephalus. The gyri are flattened and the sulci may be obliterated as a result of edema. On slicing the brain, hydrocephalous, infarcts and tuberculomas may be seen.

TUBERCULAR MENINGITIS—MICROSCOPIC EXAMINATION OF THE BRAIN

Microscopy in TBM shows acute serofibrinous exudates in the subarachnoid space, separating the two layers of the leptomeninges. Enclosed within this exudate are dilated congested blood vessels and irregular geographical areas of caseous necrosis. Granulomas composed of epithelioid cells and giant cells may be present. The cellular reaction consists largely of lymphocytes, plasma cells and histiocytes, though neutrophils may form a significant population, early in the course of the disease. Direct contact of the exudates with the brain surface leads to borderzone encephalitis, where the underlying brain parenchyma shows a reaction comprising of edema, perivascular infiltration and a microglial reaction. Ependymal surface of the ventricles, unlike in pyogenic meningitis, is rarely lined by the exudate. More frequent finding is the granular ependymitis which microscopically is seen either as true involvement by the tubercles or as a nonspecific subependymal proliferation of glial cells with erosion of the overlying ependyma. Choroid plexitis with inflammation and foci of necrosis is seen very frequently. Different regions of the brain are likely to show different stages of the inflammatory process. Treated cases of tuberculous meningitis show more fibrous exudates with gross hydrocephalus, fibroblastic proliferation and large meningeal tuberculomas.

TUBERCULAR MENINGITIS—COMPLICATIONS

Vasculitis: The most serious consequence of TBM is vasculitis occurring in the vessels of the circle of Willis, vertebrobasilar system and the perforating branches of the middle cerebral artery with resultant infarctions and strokes, leading to a high morbidity and mortality. Ischemic stroke is an important clinical outcome of tubercular arteritis. It is estimated that around 20% patients of TBM develop stroke during the course of their illness. Pasticci et al evaluated 26 patients of TBM and found stroke in six cases. In five cases, the anterior circulation was involved and in one case, the posterior circulation. Middle cerebral artery and internal carotid artery were involved as major large vessels. TBM shows a unique spectrum of vascular lesions like vascular spasm, arteritis, arterial thrombosis and compression by the thick exudate, seen more in the middle cerebral artery territory followed by the basilar artery territory. Arteritis mainly affects the perforating branches of the major arteries at the base of the brain leading to basal ganglia infarction, which is seen most frequently. The larger arteries are also affected but to a lesser degree. The vascular lesions are of three types, i.e. infiltrative, necrotizing and proliferative. The pattern of involvement depends on the caliber of the vessel and the duration of the disease. The necrotizing lesions are seen more in the smaller vessels and the proliferative lesions more in the larger-sized vessels. Grossly, these may look congested, dilated, narrowed, visibly thrombosed, cord-like or even aneurysmal. This is particularly true for the main branches of the middle cerebral artery. On microscopic examination, the large arteries may show subintimal edema, intimal fibrous hyperplasia or eccentric pillows representing subintimal fibrosis following inflammation. Advanced vascular changes may be seen as convoluted elastic lamina with prominent infolding, medial fibrosis or fibrous obliteration of the vessel. Smaller arteries show the most marked histological changes which may consist of adventitial proliferation, medial necrosis, inflammation, subintimal edema, thrombosis, endothelial proliferation and endarteritis obliterans. Veins and venules may also be involved. Only rarely a true tuberculous granuloma is seen in the vessel wall. Streptomycin treatment is known to result in replacement of necrotizing vasculitis by a fibrous endarteritis with compromise of the lumen.

Infarcts: Infarcts are seen in up to 37–72.5% cases in various autopsy studies. These are generally multiple and may be superficial or deep in location, in the territory supplied largely by the middle cerebral artery (57.1%). Several studies have reported that basal ganglia and internal capsule are the most common sites of infarction in TBM. The anterior circulation involving middle cerebral artery territory is more frequently found to be affected in TBM, than the posterior circulation. This could be attributed to the basal exudates which affect the branches of middle cerebral artery in the sylvian fissure. The infarcts are generally pale, but hemorrhagic infarcts have been described. Dastur et al, in their review of 100 brains with TBM, found infarcts in 41% cases and Thomas et al found them in 55% cases. Chatterjee et al in their autopsy study found infarcts in 72.5% cases, grossly in 52.9% cases. In their study, macroscopic infarcts were seen predominantly in the middle cerebral artery territory, whereas microscopic infarcts in basilar artery territory. Thus, they highlighted that in TBM, there is a consistent involvement of smaller arteries and arterioles in both the anterior and posterior circulation.

Hydrocephalous: Hydrocephalus is seen frequently at autopsy (55–78%) and is more frequent in children. Even a small amount of fibrous exudate may be associated with huge hydrocephalus. In acute stages, it results from mechanical blockage of basal cisterns, especially the cisterna pontis. In more chronic cases, the fibrous obliteration of the leptomeningeal space is responsible for gross communicating type of hydrocephalus. Occasionally, obstructive hydrocephalus develops following narrowing or occlusion of the cerebral aqueduct by compression caused by either the thick exudates around the brain stem or presence of a subependymal tuberculoma.

TUBERCULAR MENINGITIS—PATHOGENESIS

The pathogenesis of TBM comes from the meticulous work done by Rich and McCordock in 1933 at the John Hopkins hospital. They demonstrated that the key pathway in the origin of tubercular meningitis lies in direct spread of tubercle bacilli into the subarachnoid space either from a subpial focus called "Rich focus" or a subependymal small focus. The tubercle bacilli cannot escape freely into the meninges from the blood stream. It was however seen that not all cases of tubercular meningitis show evidence of preexisting Rich focus. This suggested alternate sources of spread like choroid plexus tuberculoma or a tuberculous focus in the middle ear or vertebral column. Rich and McCordock stressed the difficulties in finding the "Rich focus". They put forward that—(1) The small size of the lesion (3–5 mm) can be found if the entire brain is cut into translucent slivers not more than 3 mm thick. (2) These caseous nodules are difficult to see macroscopically as the brains are formalin fixed and the color of these nodules is virtually identical with that of the brain substance. (3) The caseous meningeal plaque is often masked macroscopically by the surrounding meningitis and which in many cases, can be recognized as being clearly older than the meningitis only by microscopic examination. Thus, it is very important to study microscopically all strikingly dense meningeal foci. All studies have clearly indicated that tubercular meningitis is not caused by a sudden diffuse infection of the meninges by bacilli escaping from the blood stream, but rather by a direct extension of the infection from a local lesion. The resultant picture is an acute inflammatory caseous meningitis, proliferative meningitis, disseminated miliary tubercles or focal caseous plaques, which depends on the number of bacilli and the host resistance. The cytokine tumor necrosis factor alpha (TNFα) is very critical in the pathogenesis of CNS tuberculosis. TNFα plays an important role in the granuloma formation and containment of mycobacterial infection. But in the CNS, local production of TNFα in experimental animals leads to alteration in the permeability of the blood–brain barrier leading to leukocytosis in the CSF, which causes progression of TBM. In the CNS, the macrophages are the microglia and these are infected by *M. tuberculosis* and seem to be the principal targets. Microglia infected by *M. tuberculosis* produce several cytokines and chemokines in vitro like TNFα, IL6, IL-1β, CCL2, CCL5 and CXCL10.

TUBERCULAR MENINGITIS—VARIOUS TYPES

Disseminated miliary tuberculosis: This occurs as a result of generalized dissemination of bacilli in miliary tuberculosis. The miliary tubercles may be of the compact epithelioid cell types or of the acute caseating type, corresponding with the type of tubercles elsewhere in the body.

The degree to which a given tissue is involved in miliary tuberculosis depends upon the ability of the tissue to arrest circulating foreign particulate matter. Due to the inherent property of the meninges and the fact that the tubercle bacilli do not escape freely into the meninges from the blood stream, miliary tuberculosis does not lead to diffuse meningitis. Thus, cases in which the lung, liver, spleen etc. are virtually riddled with tubercles, one finds with a meticulous search just an occasional small tubercle in the meninges with no diffuse meningitis. No experimental study has been able to produce diffuse inflammatory meningitis as a result of intravascular injection of tubercle bacilli, even when the injection has been made directly into the carotid artery. It is seen that miliary tuberculosis and TBM often occur together, but the age and character of the visceral miliary tubercles do not correspond with the age and character of the meningitis.

Focal caseous plaques: This is a meningeal lesion, which frequently is a source of origin of diffuse meningitis. These lesions vary in size from 1 or 2 mm to a cm in diameter. They are commonly globular in shape or irregularly outlined, flattened, plaque-like masses. They occur deep in the sulcus but can occur on the surface as well. They may lie in an arrested state as a caseous mass encapsulated by connective tissue, which may be hyalinized. These lesions represent small and solitary tuberculomata of the meninges, just as that seen in the brain and other tissues. These lesions may develop due to the transient bacillemia that occurs at the time of primary infection or develop during post primary progressive infection. This caseous plaque is said to be a source of diffuse meningitis.

Acute inflammatory caseous meningitis: This occurs if the tubercle bacilli are directly introduced into the subarachnoid space. It can be localized or diffuse. The localized meningitis occurs when a caseous tubercle in the cortex extends to the overlying meninges and infects it or when a meningeal plaque extends. If the number of bacilli is small or if the resistance is good enough, the inflammatory reaction remains localized. This localized exudate gets organized in due course of time and one may encounter this as an encapsulated, caseous cortical nodule in contact with the densely scarred meninges. Diffuse inflammatory caseous meningitis appears as a thick, gelatinous exudate in the pia-arachnoid, more abundant at the base of the brain. Minute cheesy nodules can be seen along the blood vessels. Microscopically, the characteristic features are abundant serofibrinous exudates, predominance of mononuclear phagocytes, necrosis, arteritis, granulomas and caseation. In a few cases, polymorphonuclear leukocytes predominate in the exudates. The infection invariably extends into the superficial layers of the cortex producing borderzone encephalitis. In addition, the endarteritic occlusion of the vessels leads to small superficial infarction of the cortex.

Proliferative meningitis: Meningitis in which tubercles, fibroblasts and connective tissue are present in striking amounts. This usually occurs as a focal process localized at the meningeal margin of a tuberculous lesion in the cortex, or at the periphery of a local lesion in the meninges. Diffuse proliferative meningitis is uncommon.

SUGGESTED READING

1. Anuradha HK, Garg RK, Agarwal A. Predictors of stroke in patients of tuberculous meningitis and its effect on the outcome. Q J Med. 2010;103:671-8.
2. Chatterjee D, Radotra BD, Vasishta RK, et al. Vascular complications of tuberculous meningitis: An autopsy study. Neurol India. 2015;63:926-32.
3. Dustur DK, Lalitha VS, Udani PM, et al. The brain and meninges in tuberculous meningitis. Gross pathology in 100 cases and pathogenesis. Neurology India. 1970;18:86-100.
4. Finsterer J, Kladosek A, Nagelmeier IE, et al. Chronic granulomatous meningitis with multiple cranial nerve lesions hydrocephalus, stroke ,sinus thrombosis and epilepsy. South Med J. 2000;93:1108-11.
5. Garg RK. Tuberculosis of the central nervous system. Postgrad Med J. 1999;75:133-40.
6. Jacobs RF, Starke JR. Mycobacterium tuberculosis. In: Long SS, Pickering LK, Prober CG (Eds). Principles and Practice of Pediatric Infectious Diseases. New York, NY: Churchill Livingstone; 2003.
7. Kalita J, Misra UK, Nair PP. Predictors of stroke and its significance in the outcome of tuberculous meningitis. J Stroke Cerebrovasc Dis. 2009;18:251-8.
8. Lalitha VS, Dastur DK. Histopathology of blood vessels in neurotuberculosis: a tuberculous meningitis. In: Kapila CC, Dastur DK, Singh B, Tandon PN (Eds). Tuberculosis of Nervous System. India: Indian Academic Medical Sciences; 1974. pp. 74-115.
9. Nair PP, Kalita J, Kumar S, et al. MRI pattern of infarcts in basal ganglia region in patients with tuberculous meningitis. Neuroradiology. 2009;51:221-5.
10. Nicholas A Be, Kwang Sik Kim, William R Bishai, et al. Pathogenesis of CNS tuberculosis. Curr Mol Med. 2009;9: 94-9.
11. Rich AR, McCordock HA. The pathogenesis of tuberculous meningitis. Bull Johns Hopkins Hosp. 1933;52:5-37.
12. Rich AR. Pathogenesis of Tuberculosis. Springfield: Charles C Thomas; 1951.
13. Rock RB, Olin M, Baker CA, et al. CNS tuberculosis: pathogenesis and clinical aspects. Clin Microbiol Rev. 2008; 21(2):243-61.
14. Siva A. Vasculitis of the nervous system. J Neurol. 2001; 248:451-68.
15. Thomas MD, Chopra JS, Banerjee AK, et al. Tuberculous meningitis: A clinicopathological study. Neurology India. 1997;25:26-34.

CASE 63

Catastrophic Posterior Circulation Tubercular Arteritis with Infarcts and Cortical Venous Thrombosis—A Rare Co-existence: PM 26344

Nandita Bharadwaj Kakkar

HIGHLIGHTS OF THE CASE

A 14-year-old boy was admitted with sudden onset fever, headache, vomiting and altered sensorium. He was diagnosed as a case of tubercular meningitis with bilateral basal ganglia and thalamic infarcts. Child was started on anti-tubercular treatment (ATT) with hydrocortisone, a ventriculoperitoneal shunt was performed but he continued to deteriorate with CT showing expanding infarcts. Autopsy revealed tubercular meningitis (AFB ++), extensive arteritis with dominant involvement of the right main posterior cerebral artery, i.e. the posterior circulation, extensive infarction along with cortical venous thrombosis involving the superior longitudinal sinus/superficial cortical veins.

Keywords: Tubercular meningitis, arteritis, infarcts, post circulation, cortical venous thrombosis, autopsy.

CLINICAL DETAILS

Date of Admission: 6.11.14, Date of Death: 12.11.14, Duration of Hospital Stay: 6 days

A 14-year-old school going boy was admitted with chief presenting complaints of fever, headache, vomiting for 10 days and altered sensorium for 4 days. Fever was high grade (103–104°F), intermittent in nature and not associated with rigors and chills. Headache was throbbing, severe in intensity, holocranial, with no history of diurnal or postural variation. The vomiting was episodic, nonprojectile, nonbilious and nonbloody. The child developed reduced responsiveness and was not recognizing family or friends. There was no history of seizures, motor weakness, dysphagia, dysarthria and bowel/bladder abnormalities. There was neither a preceding history of viral exanthema or vaccination nor any significant past or family history. On ***examination***, pulse rate—94/min, regular, BP—110/60 mm Hg, respiratory rate—18/min and SpO_2—98%, there was no pallor, icterus, cyanosis, clubbing, lymphadenopathy and edema. ***CNS examination*** revealed—patient was $E_1V_2M_5$, pupils were sluggishly reactive to light, neck rigidity and right hemiparesis (power 4/5) was noted. Rest of the systemic examination was within normal limits.

Investigations

Hemogram: Hb—10.6 g/dL, TLC—12,700/µL, DLC—N75, L20, M03, E02. Blood biochemical profile revealed significant hypernatremia, normal liver/renal function tests and normal coagulogram. ***CSF examination*** revealed elevated total WBC count—140 cells, with 90 lymphocytes, raised protein concentration and low sugar. CSF adenosine deaminase (ADA) levels were also elevated (23.0), however, culture was sterile. ***Chest X-ray*** revealed bilateral reticulo-nodular opacities in upper and mid-zones. ***CT scan*** head revealed bilateral basal ganglia and thalamic infarcts with diffuse meningeal enhancement and hydrocephalus. In view of above clinical, laboratory and radiological findings, a clinical diagnosis of tubercular meningitis was made and child was started on ATT and hydrocortisone. Subsequently a ventriculoperitoneal shunt was performed to relieve hydrocephalus. However, the patient's Glasgow coma scale (GCS) continued to deteriorate with CT showing expanding infarcts. Finally after a hospital stay of 7 days, the child succumbed to his illness.

AUTOPSY FINDINGS: PM 26344

A brain only autopsy was performed after a written informed consent from the parent of the deceased child. After giving a bitemporal incision, the prosector noted an area of extradural hemorrhage (4 × 3 cm).

Gross examination: The brain weighed 1,407 g, was swollen with bilateral tonsillar and uncal herniation. Thick grayish leptomeningeal exudates were seen over cerebral convexities along the cortical veins (Fig 1A) and cerebellum (Fig 1B). The base of the brain also showed thick leptomeningeal exudates over ventral surface of pons, midbrain, interpeduncular fossa, mammillary bodies encasing oculomotor nerve, optic nerve and olfactory tracts extending up to inferior frontal cortex and laterally into sylvian fissures encasing the branches of middle cerebral artery (Fig 1C). The lateral surface of the brain showed multiple tiny meningeal tubercles of 0.1–0.3 cm (Fig 1D). The right temporal lobe was soft and damaged during removal. The coronal slice of the brain at the level of thalamus and basal ganglia showed focal areas of brownish discoloration (Fig 2A). The brain stem including midbrain, pons and medulla were soft with areas of infarction. Coronal slice at the level of the mammillary bodies showed thick exudates (Fig 2B). The right main posterior cerebral artery (Fig 2C) was encased in the thick exudate and its territory showed infarction. In addition, the superior sagittal sinus was distended with a thrombus in its middle part, however, the superficial cortical veins appeared congested.

Microscopic findings: Multiple sections were examined from cerebral cortex, cerebellum, midbrain, medulla and pons. The subarachnoid space was expanded by a thick fibrinous exudate comprising of polymorphs, lymphocytes, areas of necrosis and the arteries were seen encased within it (Figs 3A and B). Amidst the meningeal inflammation, multiple caseating and non-caseating granulomas composed of epithelioid histiocytes, Langhans giant cells and lymphocytes were seen (Figs 3C and D). This granulomatous inflammation

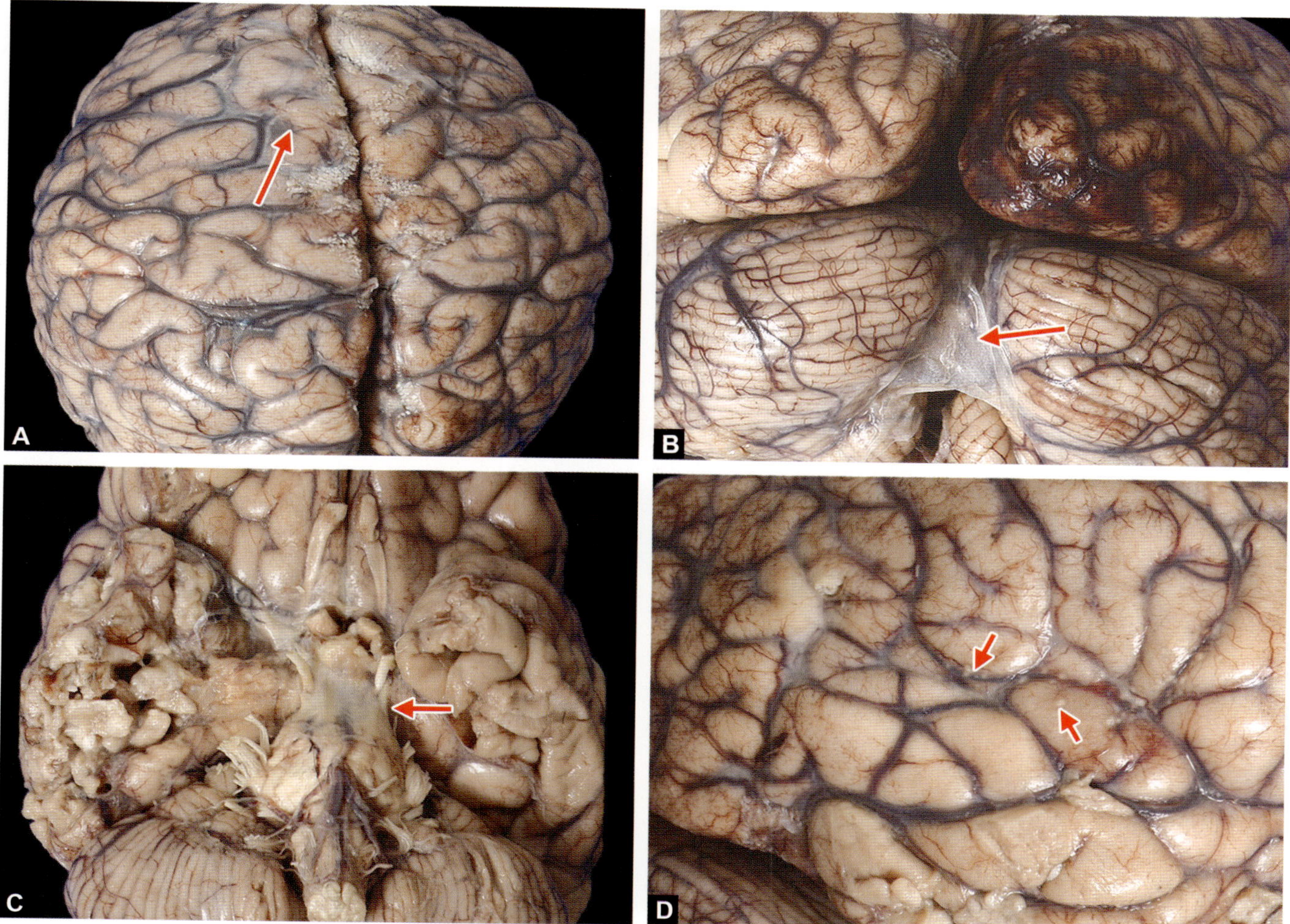

Figs 1A–D: Gross photographs of brain showing thick leptomeningeal exudates over the (A) Cerebral convexities; (B) Cerebellum; (C) Base of brain; (D) Tiny meningeal tubercles on the superolateral surface (arrows).

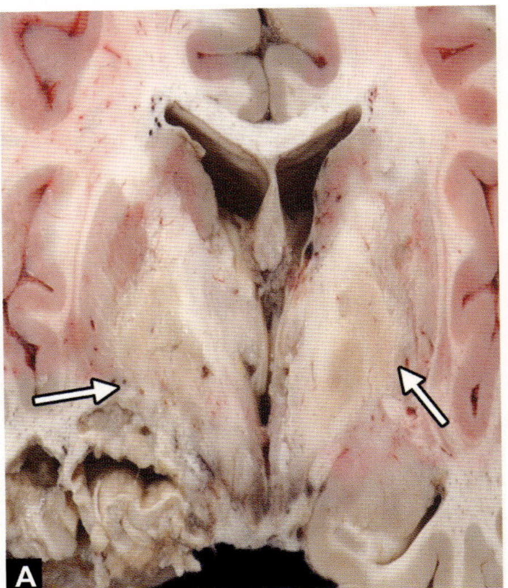

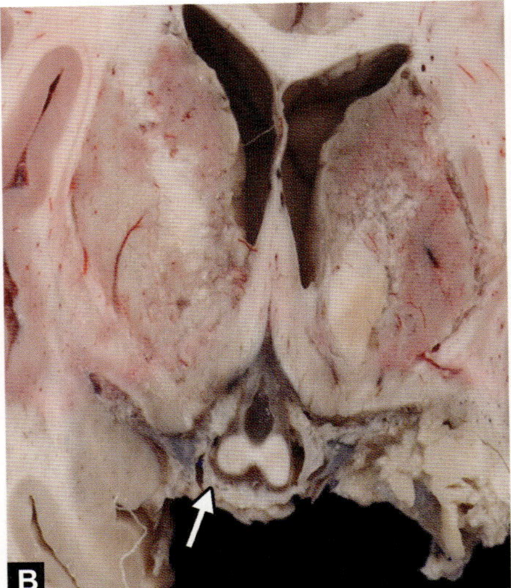

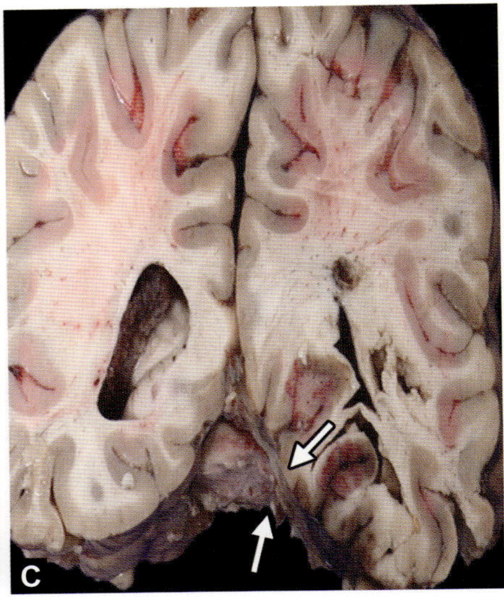

Figs 2A–C: (A) Gross photographs of coronal slice of brain showing bilateral basal ganglia infarcts (arrows); (B) Thick leptomeningeal exudate at the level of mammillary bodies and optic chiasma (arrow); (C) Exudate encasing the right posterior cerebral artery (arrows).

was also extending into the adjacent brain parenchyma causing borderzone encephalitis (Fig 3E). Ziehl-Neelsen stain for acid-fast bacilli (AFB) was positive (Fig 3F). The exudate was encasing the basilar artery and the main right posterior cerebral artery (Fig 4A) leading to transmural acute inflammation with nuclear debris in the wall (Fig 4B). AFB stain in the adventitial inflammatory infiltrate of both of these arteries was strongly positive (Fig 4C). The entrapped small arteries also showed varying degree of vasculitis in the form of necrotizing, inflammatory and proliferative lesions causing endarteritis obliterans (Figs 4D–F). The extensive arteritis involving the larger arteries like the basilar artery, the main right posterior cerebral artery, branches of the middle cerebral arteries and other smaller arteries led to widespread infarction in the territories of the brain supplied by them. Multiple infarcts were present in the midbrain, pons, medulla (brain-stem), cerebral cortex, cerebellum, thalamus and internal capsule (Figs 5A–D). Both old infarcts comprising of macrophages and proliferating capillaries and acute infarcts comprising of ischemic neurons, neutrophils and axon retraction bulbs were noted. Myelin stain performed accentuated the infarcts. The thrombus occluding the superior sagittal sinus (Fig 5E) and in the superficial cortical veins (Fig 5F) were confirmed on the microscopy.

FINAL AUTOPSY DIAGNOSIS: PM 26344

14 Years Male

- Tubercular meningitis (AFB ++) with complications:
  - Borderzone encephalitis
  - Tubercular arteritis leading to acute and old infarcts involving the cerebral cortex, basal ganglia, thalamus, midbrain, pons, medulla and cerebellum.
  - Cortical venous thrombosis involving the superior longitudinal sinus or superficial cortical veins.

Tubercular meningitis—See preceeding chapter on "Tubercular meningitis"

CORTICAL VENOUS THROMBOSIS

Cerebral venous thrombosis (CVT) is less frequently encountered than arterial thrombosis. It occurs due to occlusion of central veins and sinuses by thrombus, thrombophlebitis or tumor. CVT occurs due to varied predisposing causes like hypercoagulable state, severe dehydration, oral contraceptives, pregnancy and puerperium, infections, congenital heart diseases, malignancies, red blood cell disorders and liver disorders. Among infectious causes bacterial, fungal and parasitic infections predominate. Association of CVT with extracranial tuberculosis is a rare occurrence and is limited to only a few case reports. The pathogenesis of CVT in TB may be explained by endothelial injury to the intracranial veins, stasis of blood flow due to intracranial low pressure system and increased blood coagulability as a result of platelet hyperaggregability. There is enough evidence in literature to suggest that tuberculosis is a hypercoagulable state. MRI and magnetic resonance venography combined together form the current gold standard for diagnosis of CVT. It is important to diagnose this entity early in TBM, since the patient

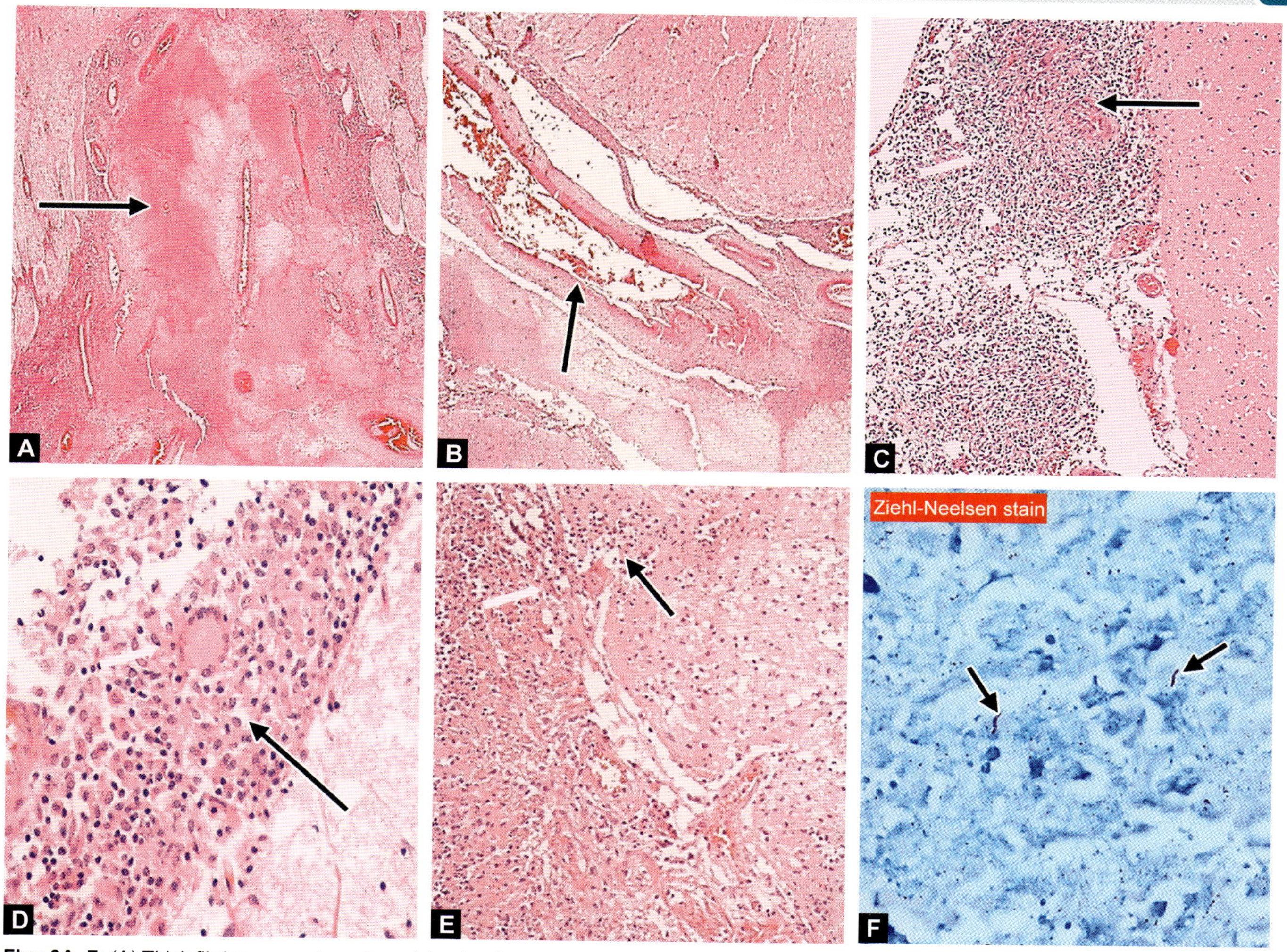

Figs 3A–F: (A) Thick fibrinous meningeal exudate showing caseous necrosis, causing expansion of subarachnoid space; (B) Exudate encasing the posterior cerebral artery causing periarteritis (arrow); (C and D) Meningeal granulomas; (E) Meningeal inflammation extending into the underlying brain parenchyma causing borderzone encephalitis (arrow); (F) Ziehl-Neelsen stain showing acid-fast bacilli (arrows).

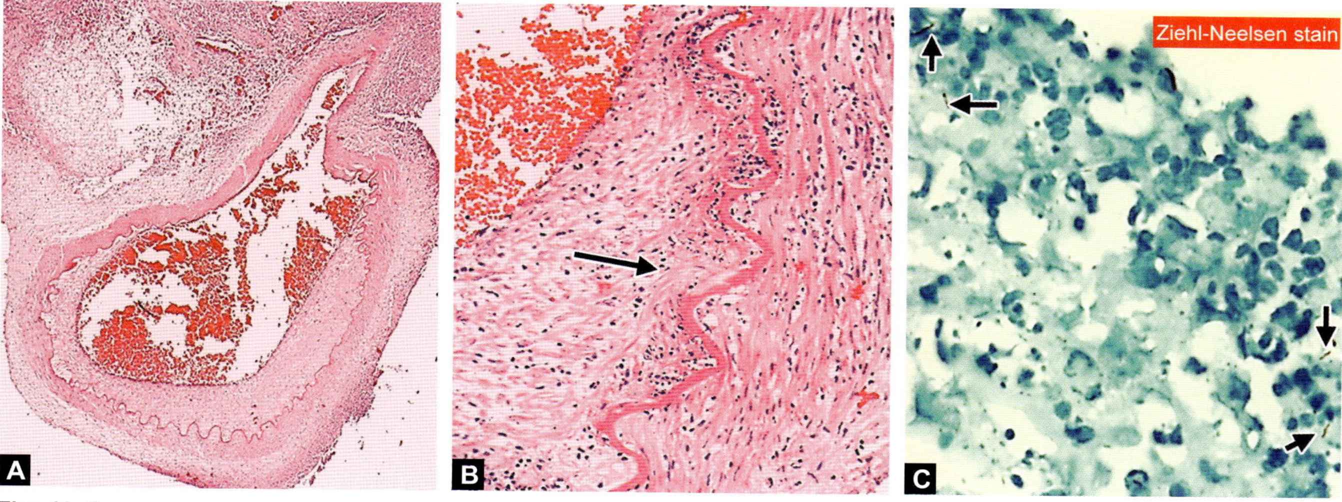

Figs 4A–C:

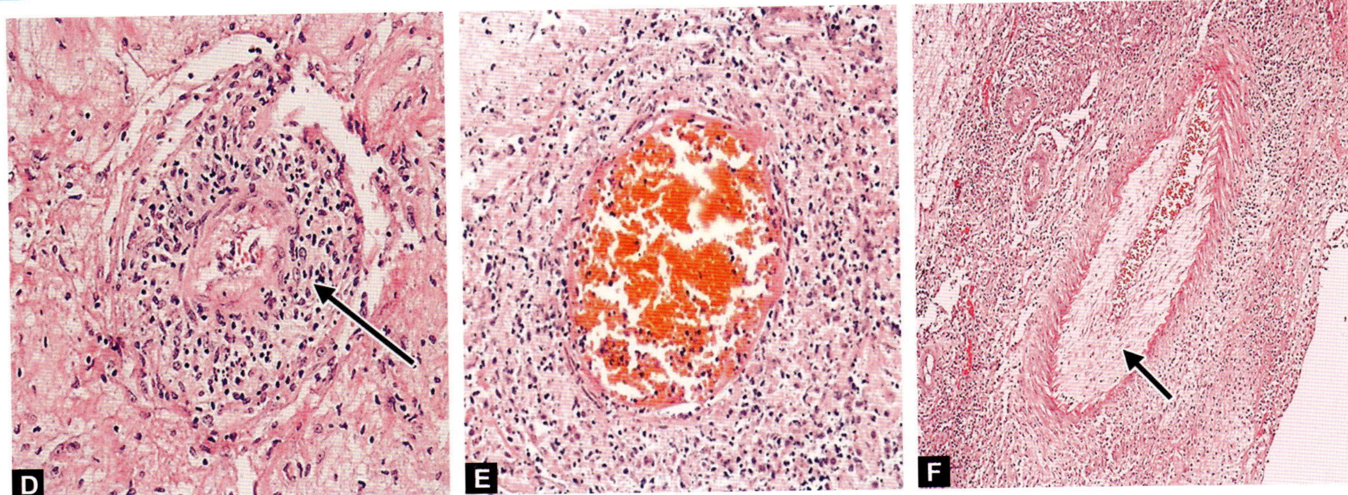

Figs 4A–F: (A) Photomicrograph of the right main posterior cerebral artery caught in the exudate; (B) High power view of the posterior cerebral artery showing transmural acute inflammation with nuclear debris (arrow); (C) Ziehl-Neelsen stain showing acid-fast bacilli in the adventitial infiltrate of the posterior cerebral artery (arrows); (D and E) Small arteries in the meningeal exudate showing arteritis (arrow); (F) Artery amidst the dense inflammation showing showing endarteritis obliterans (arrow).

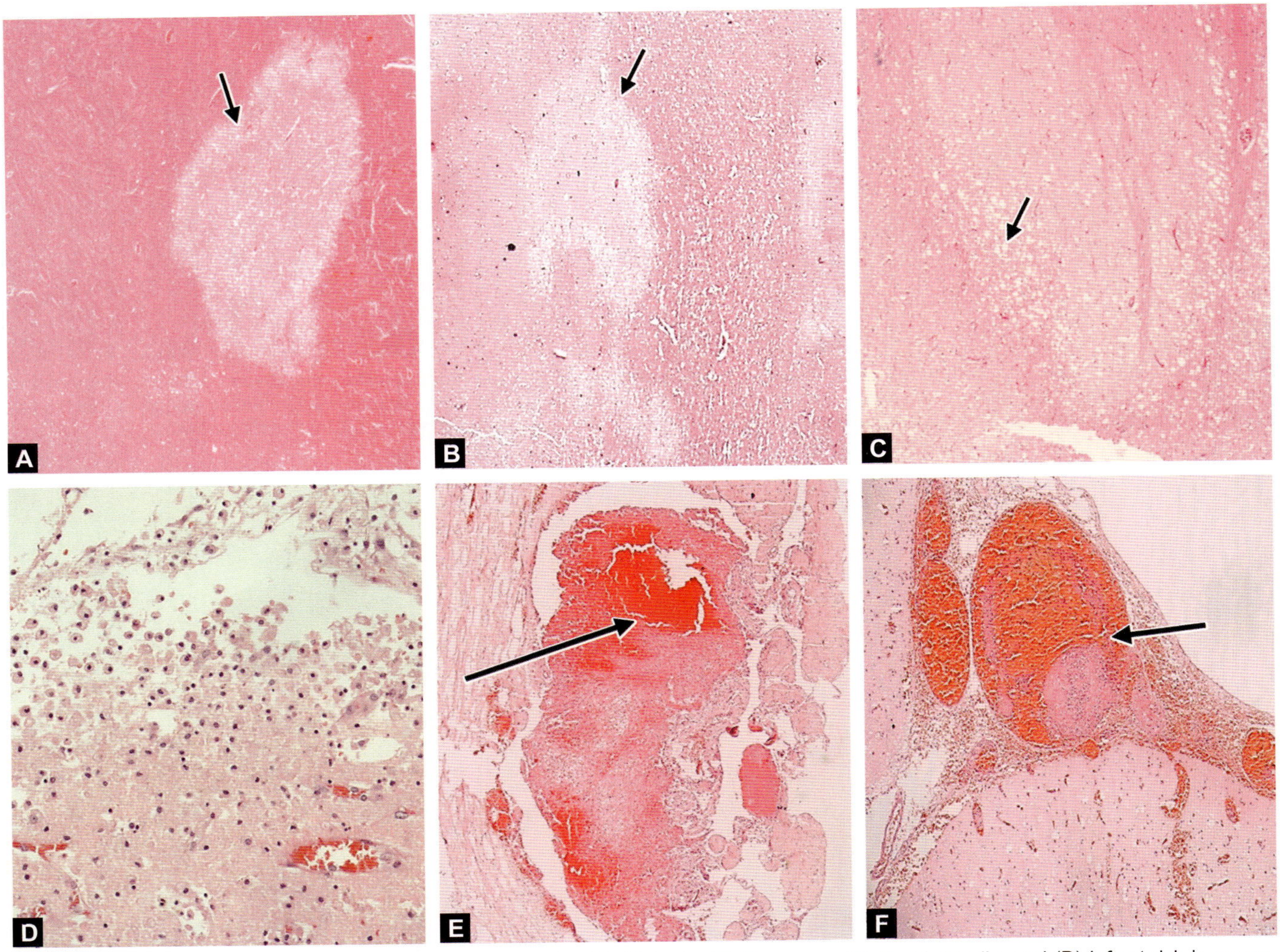

Figs 5A–F: Photomicrographs showing infarcts (arrows) in the (A) Midbrain; (B) Thalamus; (C) Basal ganglia; and (D) Infarct rich in macrophages; (E and F) Photomicrographs showing thrombus (arrows) in the superior longitudinal sinus and superficial cortical veins.

may develop stroke like manifestations and therefore, an aggressive treatment needs to be started. Most cases cited in literature are associated with extracranial tuberculosis, but an occasional case of meningitis with CVT has been reported.

COMMENTARY—INDEX CASE: PM 26344

The present case is rare since there is a coexistence of both posterior circulation tubercular vasculitis leading to infarcts in the brain stem and CVT involving superior longitudinal sinus/superficial cortical veins leading to early cortical infarcts. Though, the anterior circulation was also involved, as there were infarcts in the basal ganglia, cortex and thalamus, the right main posterior cerebral artery was dominantly affected and was encased by the thick exudate and showed transmural arteritis. Both the arterial and venous involvement proved catastrophic in this young child despite the early institution of ATT along with steroids. This was a partial autopsy and the extracranial organs were not examined and hence the presence of tuberculosis in the lungs cannot be ruled out. But X-ray chest did show bilateral reticulonodular opacities in upper and mid-zones.

TAKE HOME MESSAGE

- Tubercular meningitis leads to extensive arteritis and infarction involving most frequently the basal ganglia and internal capsule. Widespread infarction can involve the cortex, thalamus, hippocampus and midbrain. Infarcts are seen in up to 37%–72.5% cases in various autopsy studies. Anterior circulation is involved more than the posterior circulation.
- Tubercular meningitis leading to cortical venous thrombosis is rare and limited to few cases reports only.

SUGGESTED READING

1. Fiorot JA, Felicio AC, Fukujima MM, et al. Tuberculosis – an uncommon cause of cerebral venous thrombosis. Arq Neuropsiquiatr. 2005;63(3-B):852-4.
2. Kakkar N, Banerjee AK, Vasishta RK, et al. Aseptic cerebral venous thrombosis associated with abdominal tuberculosis. Neurol India. 2003;51:128-9.
3. Sarode R, Bhasin D, Marwaha N, et al. Hyperaggregation of platelets in intestinal tuberculosis: role of platelets in chronic inflammation. Am J Hematol. 1995;48:52-4.
4. Verma R, Lalla R, Patil TB, et al. A rare presentation of cerebral venous sinus thrombosis associated with tubercular meningitis. BMJ Case Rep. 2013;2013. pii:bcr2013009892.

CONTRIBUTIONS BY:

1. Dr Saniya Sharma, Senior Resident, Department of Pathology (Helping with the Manuscript)
2. Dr Mukin Kumar S, Junior Resident, Department of Pathology (Helping within Gross Photographs)
3. Dr Dhananjay Zutshi, Professor, Department of Internal Medicine (Compilation of Clinical Details)
4. Dr BD Radotra, Professor, Department of Histopathology (Consultation)
5. Dr SN Mathuriya, Ex-Professor and Head, Department of Neurosurgery (Clinician In-Charge)

Post Graduate Institute of Medical Education and Research, Chandigarh, India.

CASE 64

Child with Disseminated Miliary Tuberculosis, Tubercular Meningitis with Extensive Arteritis, Infarction and Ischemic Hepatitis: PM 25901

Nandita Bharadwaj Kakkar

HIGHLIGHTS OF THE CASE

A 5-year-old female child was diagnosed as a case of tubercular meningitis on the basis of clinical history, examination, CT and cerebrospinal fluid (CSF) findings. She was put on anti-tubercular treatment (ATT) with steroids and a ventriculoperitoneal (VP) shunt was inserted to reduce the raised intracranial pressure. Autopsy revealed disseminated miliary tuberculosis (TB), tuberculous meningitis with extensive arteritis, infarction and ischemic hepatitis.

Keywords: Miliary tuberculosis, tuberculous meningitis, arteritis, infarction, ischemic hepatitis, shock liver, autopsy.

CLINICAL DETAILS

Date of Admission: 24.01.2014, Date of Death: 05.02.14, Duration of Hospital Stay: 13 Days.

A 5-year-old female child presented with complaints of fever and headache for 20 days with altered sensorium for 10 days and multiple seizure episodes for 1 day. She also had history of contact with pulmonary TB in the family. The child was immunized as per age and was developmentally normal. She was put on intermittent positive pressure respiration (IPPR). On examination, she was E2M3VT with nonreactive pupils, bilateral optic atrophy, hypertonia, dystonia, brisk deep tendon reflexes, bilateral extensor plantars, positive meningeal signs and power of 1/5 on right side and 2/5 on left side.

Investigations (Table 1)

Coagulogram on day 1: PT—16′, aPTT—32′, PT1—81%, INR—1.2

Coagulogram on day 11: PT—100′, aPPT—74′, PTI—13%

CSF examination revealed 130 cells with 98% lymphocyte count, increased protein (632 mg/dL) and reduced glucose level (40 mg/mL). CSF was negative for acid-fast bacilli (AFB) on Ziehl–Neelsen (ZN) stain, TB-PCR (polymerase chain reaction), TB culture, Gram stain and for cryptococcal antigen. Mantoux test was negative, gastric lavage for AFB—negative, blood/urine cultures were negative and the child was human immunodeficiency virus (HIV) negative.

MRI showed thick exudates along the basal cisterns, dilatation of both temporal horns, multiple infarcts in the right frontal, bilateral basal ganglia and internal capsules along with mild ventriculomegaly.

A clinical diagnosis of tuberculous meningitis with nosocomial sepsis with multiorgan dysfunction was kept. The child was given ATT with steroids to treat tuberculous meningitis and a VP shunt was inserted to reduce the raised intracranial pressure. After a hospital stay of 13 days, the child succumbed to her illness.

AUTOPSY FINDINGS: PM 25901

A complete autopsy was performed. The serous cavities wee within normal limits. ***Brain: Gross examination***—the dura mater appeared normal. No sagittal sinus thrombosis was seen. The superolateral surface (Fig 1A) of the brain did not show any exudate, was shiny with congested vessels. The base of the brain (Fig 1B) however showed a dense, greyish white, firm exudate covering the optic nerves, optic chiasm, inferior frontal surface, interpeduncular fossa and ventral surface of the pons. No meningeal tubercles were identified. Mild bilateral tonsillar herniation was seen. The pineal gland was enlarged, 10 × 12 × 8 mm and was surrounded by exudates. The gland was partly cystic and yielded gelatinous translucent material on cut section. Coronal slicing of the brain revealed areas of brownish discoloration with softening and breakdown indicating infarction in both basal

Table 1: Investigations

	Day 1	*Day 3*	*Day 5*	*Day 9*	*Day 12*
Hb (mg/dL)	12.1	11.4	11.0	10.3	8.7
TLC/uL	13,900	14,700	16,600	24,300	28,300
DLC-P/L/M/E	60/37/2/1	–	82/12/4/2	90/7/2/1	93/5/1/1
Platelets/μL	3,62,000	–	3,78,000	3,68000	2,47000
Creatinine mg%	0.7	–	0.9	1.6	1.9
Urea mg%	16	24	–	40	41
Bilirubin total/conjugated—mg%	1.1	–	–	2.2/1.4	3.9/2.9
Serum glutamic oxaloacetic transaminase—U/L	68	–	196	6804	9818
Serum glutamic pyruvic transaminase —U/L	64	–	68	3432	5210
Alkaline phosphatase—U/L	–	–	173	252	272
Lactate dehydrogenase—U/L	–	–	–	10534	–
Total proteins/albumin (gm)	–	6.4/3.4	–	4.2/2.5	3.8/2.5
C-reactive protein (mg/L)	–	–	–	3.01	–

(DLC: Differential leukocyte counts; Hb: Hemoglobin; TLC: Total lymphocyte counts)

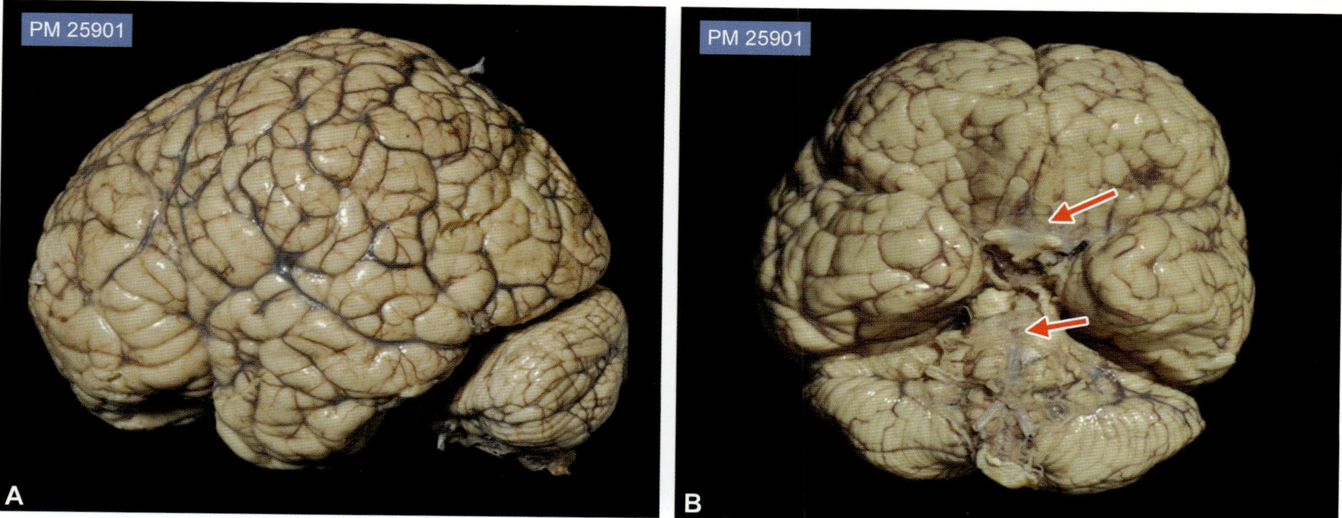

Figs 1A and B: (A) Gross picture of the left superolateral aspect of the brain which is shiny with no exudate; (B) Base of the brain showing a thick exudate over the optic nerves, optic chiasm (arrow), inferior frontal surface, interpeduncular fossa, pons and cerebellum (arrow).

ganglia which were appreciated better on the left side (Fig 2A). Similar areas of softening were seen in the thalamus, midbrain, left inferior frontal cortex, occipital cortex and the hippocampus. Many sulci in the depths showed brownish discoloration indicating recent infarction. The splenium of the corpus callosum also showed an area of ischemic infarct. The sylvian fissure contained exudates, entrapping the arteries (Fig 2B). No significant hydrocephalus was noted and no tuberculomas were seen. ***Microscopic examination***: Sections examined from the basal meninges (Figs 2C and D; Figs 3A–D) showed a dense thick fibrinous, lymphohistiocytic infiltrate with polymorphs, entrapping the vessels, with large areas of fibrinoid necrosis and multiple epithelioid cell granulomas with Langhans type of giant cells. The infiltrate was making its way into the underlying brain parenchyma leading to borderzone encephalitis (Figs 3E and F). Small

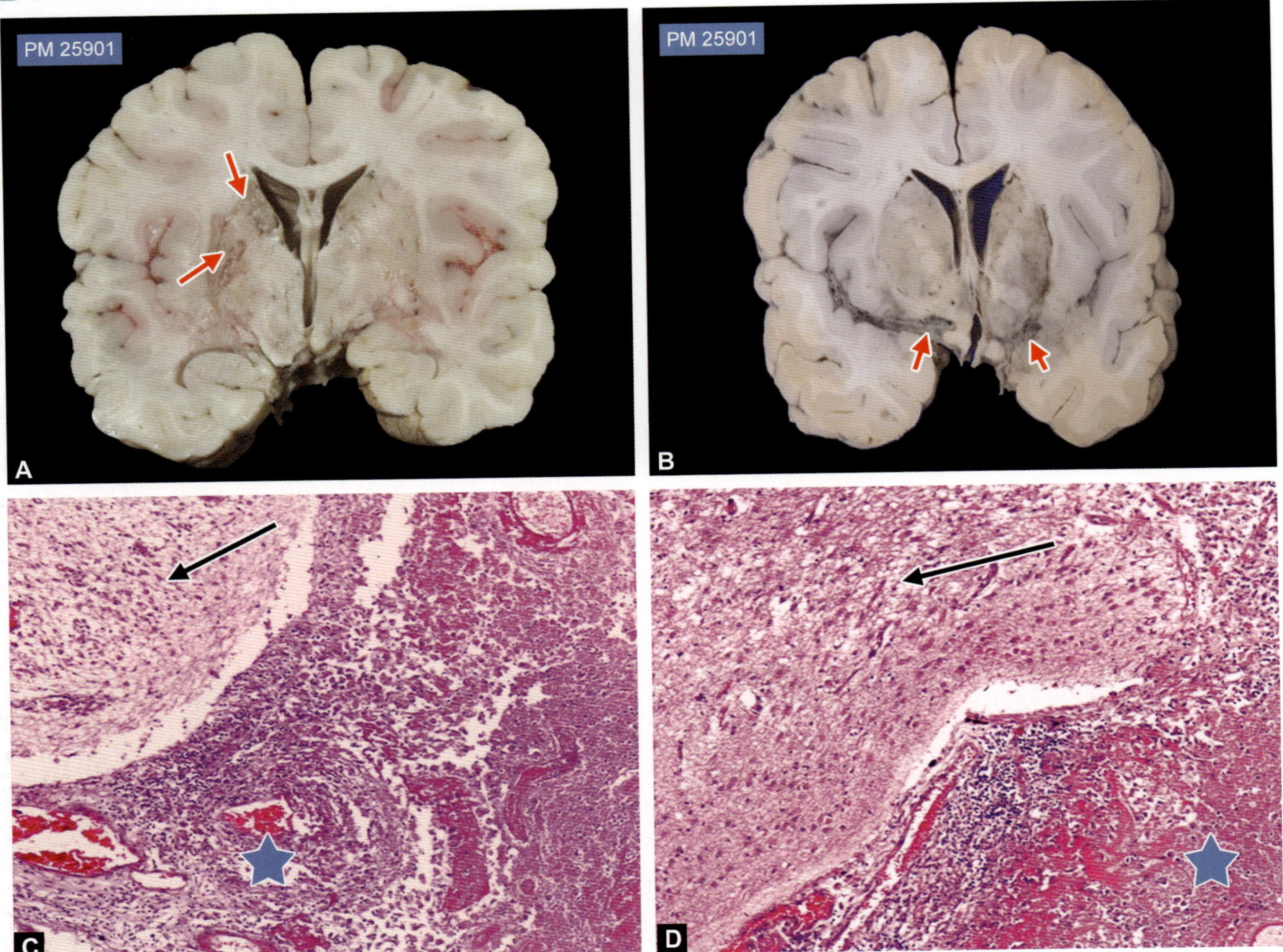

Figs 2A–D: (A) Coronal slice of the brain at the level of the mammillary bodies showing two infarcts involving the left caudate nucleus and left putamen (arrows) encroaching upon the internal capsule; (B) Coronal slice of the brain at the level of the optic chiasm showing thick exudate in the sylvian fissures (arrows); (C and D) Photomicrographs from the base of the brain showing a dense, fibrinous, lymphohistiocytic meningeal infiltrate (stars) with plenty of neutrophils and caught up vessels. Adjacent brain parenchyma (arrows) shows edema.

subpial granulomas (Figs 4A and B) were noted in the superficial brain parenchyma and in the depths of the sulci. These are the pathogenetic lesions of tubercular meningitis known as the "Rich foci". The exudates (Figs 4C–F) were also seen in the meninges of the cerebellum, anterior aspect of the pons, choroid plexus leading to choroid plexitis and around the cranial nerves especially the oculomotor and optic nerves. Blood vessels (Figs 5A–C) embedded within meningeal exudates showed spectrum of changes ranging from transmural fibrinoid necrosis leading to total destruction/thrombosis and periartertis in some. Multiple infarcts (Figs 5D–F) were noted in the cortex (laminar infarction), basal ganglia, thalamus, hippocampus and midbrain. Areas of infarction revealed neuronal/myelin loss, capillary proliferation and marked macrophage infiltration (Figs 6A and B). Neurofilament protein (NFP) stain showed loss of neurons and CD68 highlighted macrophage infiltration. Ziehl Neelsen stain (Fig 6C) for AFB was strongly positive in the meningeal exudate. Section examined from cyst in pineal region showed eosinophilic material, reactive glial tissue in the wall, peripherally compressed pineal gland, consistent with a diagnosis of glial cyst. ***Lungs*** (Figs 7A and B) weighed 340 gm, were heavy and firm. The mucosa of the tracheobronchial tree showed mild discoloration. Pleural surface was dull and showed millet-sized tubercles. Cut section of the lung revealed areas of consolidation along with

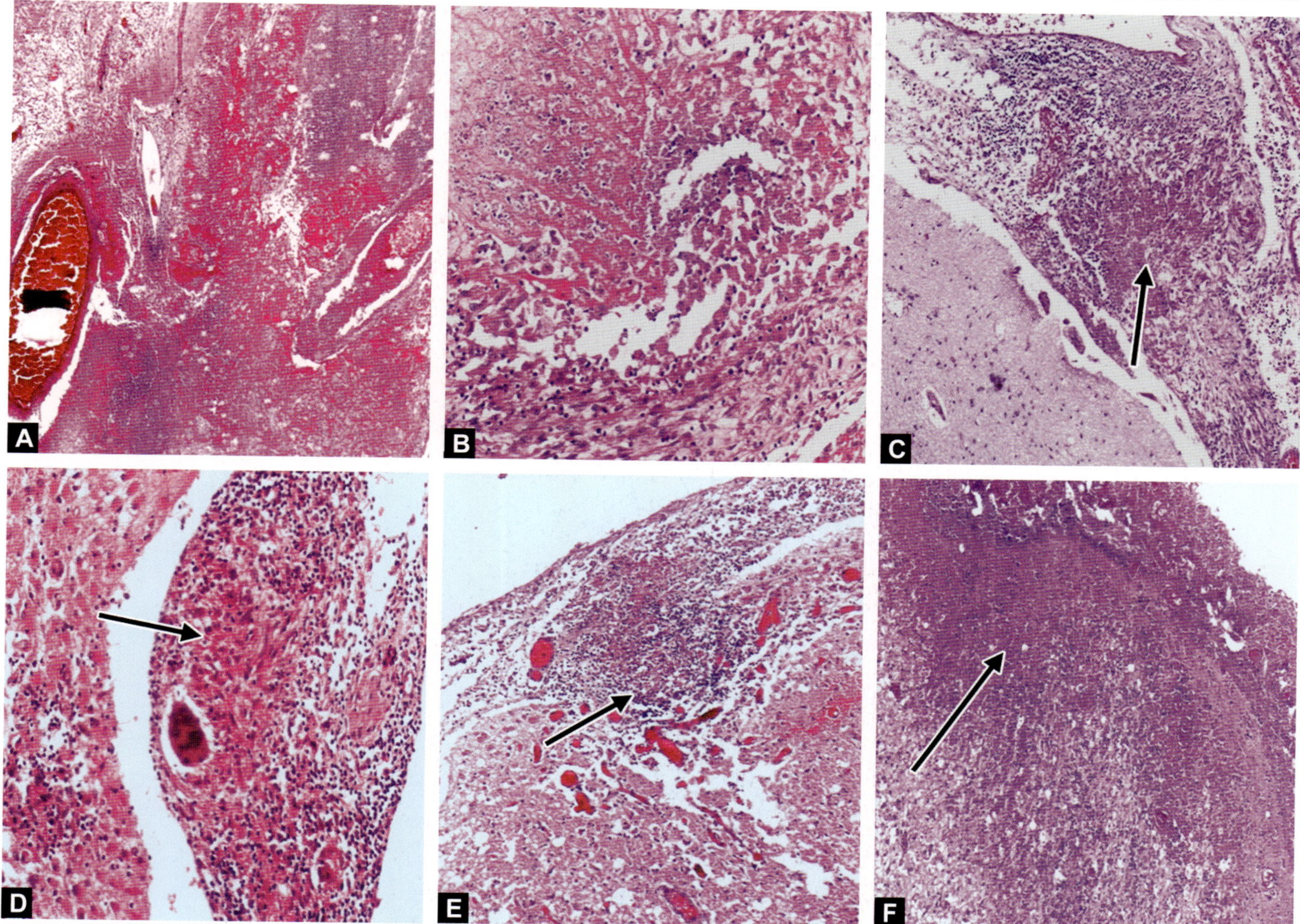

Figs 3A–F: The thick meningeal exudate shows (A) Caught up vessels; (B) Areas of acute necrosis with nuclear debris; (C and D) Epithelioid cell granulomas with giant cells; (E and F) Infiltrate going into the adjacent brain parenchyma leading to borderzone encephalitis (arrows).

miliary tubercles ranging in size from 0.1 cm to 0.5 cm. Hilar lymph nodes were enlarged and showed caseous necrosis. Microscopy (Figs 7C and D) revealed diffusely scattered, single as well as confluent, epithelioid cell granulomas with caseation necrosis, giant cells and surrounding lymphocytes. ZN stain for AFB showed positivity. Sections (Figs 7E and F) studied from the areas of consolidation revealed a confluent necrotizing bronchopneumonia with alveolar spaces packed with acute inflammatory infiltrate. In addition, intra-alveolar edema and hemorrhage were also noted. The hilar lymph nodes were enlarged and showed caseous necrosis. On microscopy they revealed multiple caseating epithelioid cell granulomas. The ***liver*** (Figs 8A–E) was shrunken and weighed 430 g, as against a normal of 600 g, at this age. Coronal slicing revealed a nutmeg appearance in which dark congested and hemorrhagic discolored areas alternated with relatively preserved paler areas. Microscopic examination showed few portal tract granulomas. There was extensive centrizonal hemorrhagic necrosis, sparing only the periportal hepatocytes and in areas destroying even them. These areas of necrosis showed reticulin collapse. Thus, liver showed features consistent with ischemic hepatitis or what is known as shock liver. The ***spleen*** weighed 30 g, capsule was thickened, capsular aspect and coronal slices showed small millet-sized nodules. Microscopy revealed multiple caseating epithelioid cell granulomas. The mesenteric, peri-pancreatic, gastric, celiac and paraaortic ***lymph nodes*** were enlarged and showed caseous necrosis, which on microscopy showed caseating epithelioid cell granulomas. Small and large ***intestines*** showed mucosal roughening and sections confirmed few caseating epithelioid cell granulomas. An occasional granuloma was seen in the section from the

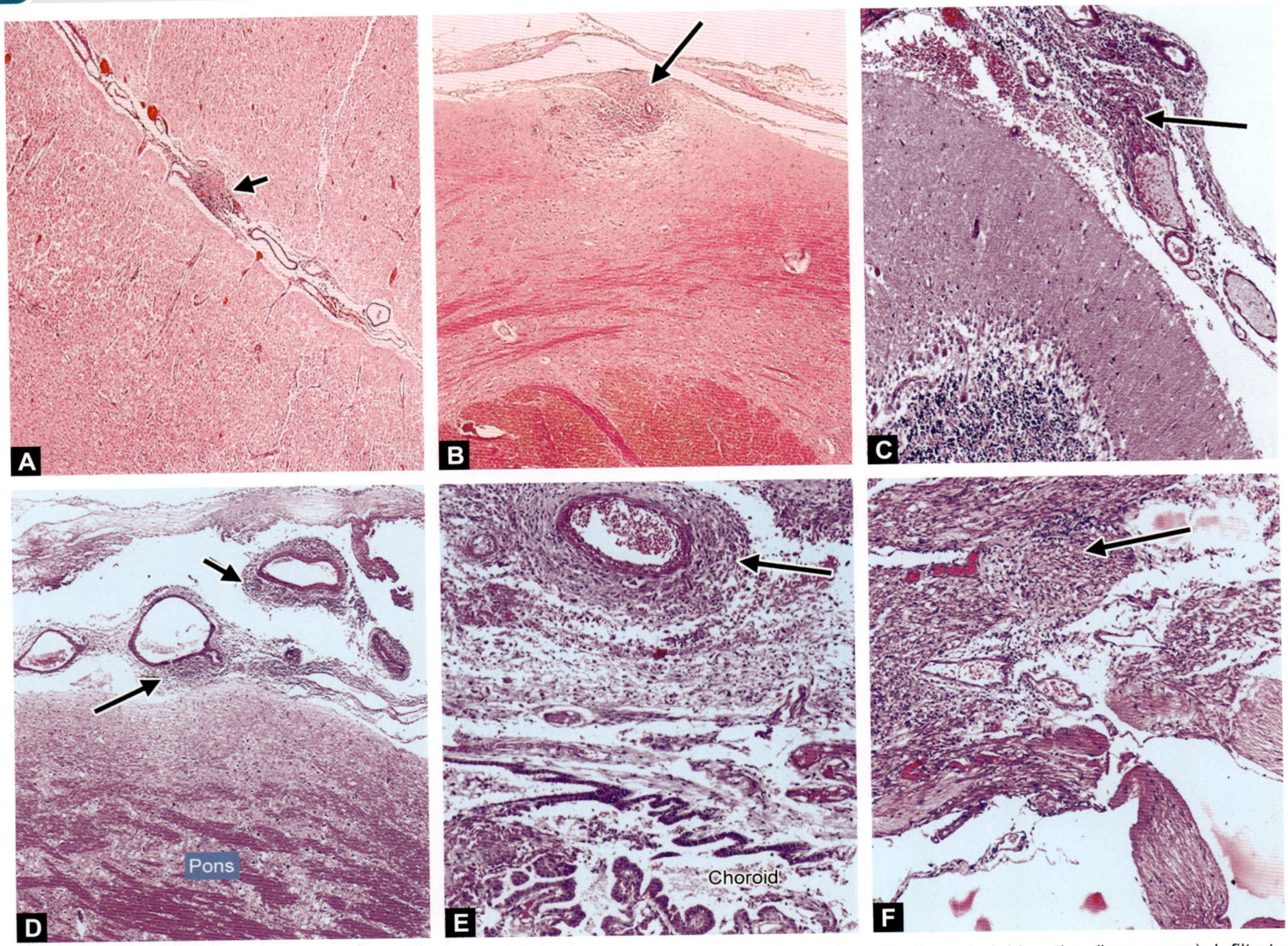

Figs 4A–F: (A and B) Rich focus, i.e. small granulomas seen deep in the sulci (small arrow) and in the subpial location (long arrow). Infiltrate seen in the (C) Cerebellar meninges; (D) Anterior aspect of pons; (E) Choroid plexus; (F) Around the oculomotor nerve (arrow).

pancreas. ***Thymus*** showed features of stress involution. Adequate lymphoid tissue was present in the spleen, lymph nodes, appendix and the GIT. This negates the possibility of an underlying immunodeficiency.

FINAL AUTOPSY DIAGNOSIS: PM 25901

5 Years Old Female

- Tubercular meningitis (AFB +++) with borderzone encephalitis, choroid plexitis, extensive arteritis, infarction involving bilateral basal ganglia, thalamus, hippocampus, midbrain and cerebral cortex.
- Incidental glial cyst of pineal gland.
- Disseminated miliary TB involving lungs, liver, spleen, lymph nodes, small intestine and pancreas.
- Necrotizing bronchopneumonia with alveolar hemorrhage and edema.
- Ischemic hepatitis/shock liver—extensive centrizonal hemorrhagic necrosis.

Tubercular Meningitis—See chapter on "Tubercular meningitis".

MILIARY TUBERCULOSIS

Miliary TB is a complication of either primary or secondary TB, when the body defenses fail or if the treatment is inadequate. Here, there is entry of the tubercle bacilli into the blood stream leading to small granulomas in many organs like the liver, spleen, lymph nodes, bone marrow, meninges and kidneys. The granulomata are 1–4 mm in size, i.e. the size of a millet seed. Microscopically

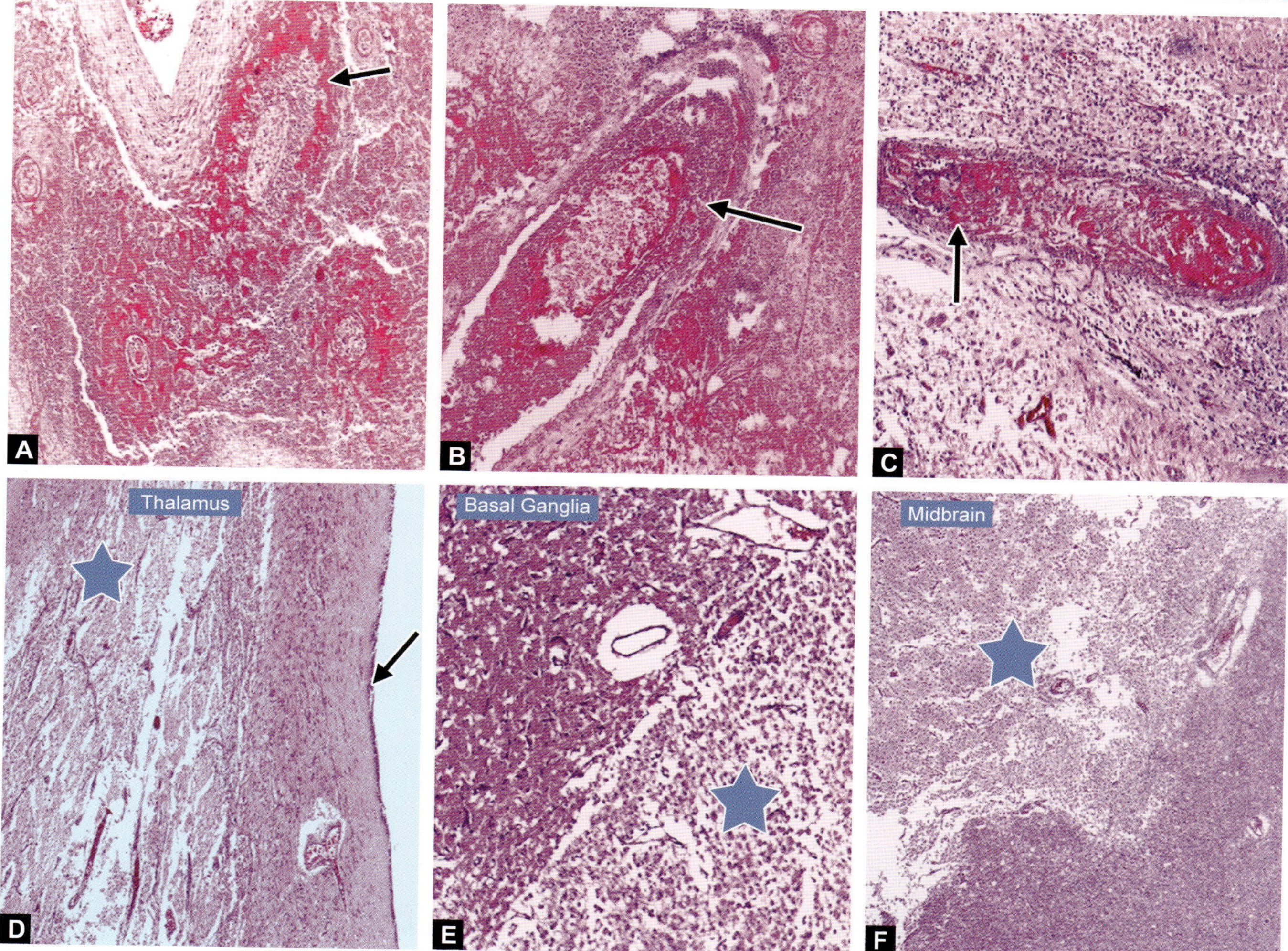

Figs 5A–F: (A to C) Arteries (arrows) caught up in the thick fibrinous necrotic meningeal exudate showing total destruction with fibrinoid necrosis and thrombosis. Infarcts (stars) seen in the (D) Thalamus; (E) Basal ganglia; (F) Midbrain.

the miliary tubercles may be of the compact epithelioid cell type or of the acute caseating type. In children, the miliary tubercles are seen more in the lungs where high oxygen tension favors the growth of the *M. tuberculosis*.

ISCHEMIC HEPATITIS OR SHOCK LIVER

Shock is a state wherein a decreased cardiac output or a decreased effective circulating blood volume impairs tissue perfusion and leads to cellular hypoxia, which if uncorrected leads to death. Shock can be labeled as cardiogenic shock (myocardial infarction, ventricular arrhythmia, cardiac tamponade and pulmonary embolism), hypovolemic shock (massive hemorrhage, fluid loss from severe burns), shock associated with systemic inflammation (burns, trauma, pancreatitis and microbial sepsis), anesthetic shock, neurogenic shock and anaphylactic shock. Shock associated with systemic inflammation can be triggered by both microbial (septic shock) and non-microbial factors and leads to a similar set of clinical findings referred to as systemic inflammatory response syndrome. The pathogenesis lies in the activation of cytokine cascades, peripheral vasodilatation, vascular leakage, pooling of blood, leukocyte-induced damage, endothelial activation/injury, induction of a procoagulant stage and disseminated intravascular coagulation. This leads to hypotension, tissue hypoperfusion, cellular hypoxia, metabolic derangements, organ dysfunction, organ failure and death.

Septic shock due to overwhelming microbial infections (bacterial or fungal), ranks first among the causes of death in hospitals, worldwide. A group of secreted bacterial proteins,

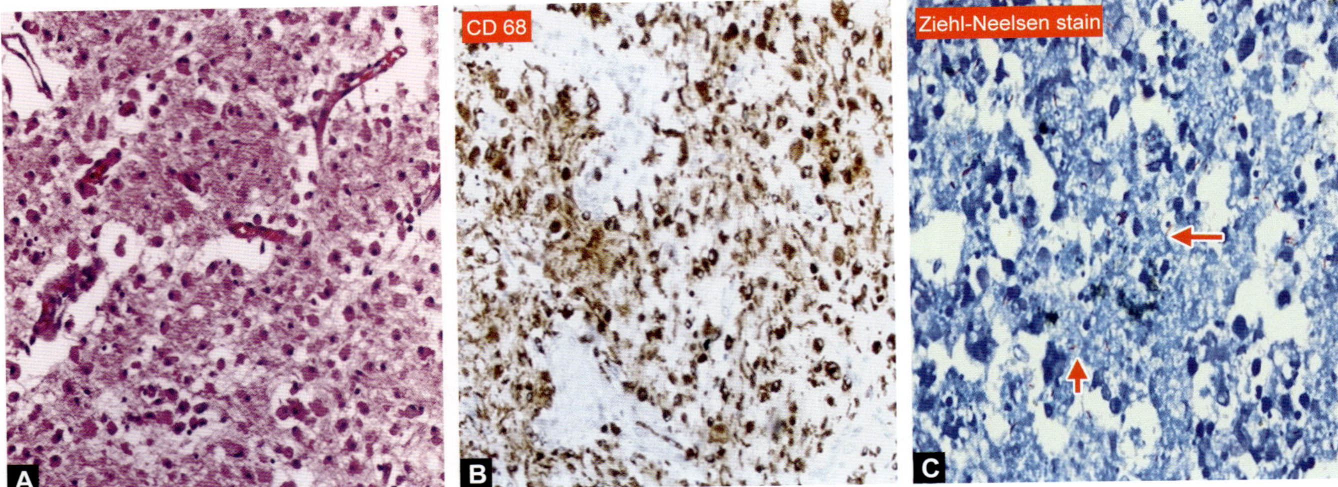

Figs 6A–C: (A and B) Areas of infarcts showing sheets of macrophages positive for CD68 immunostain; (C) Ziehl–Neelsen stain showing plenty of acid-fast bacilli in the meningeal exudate.

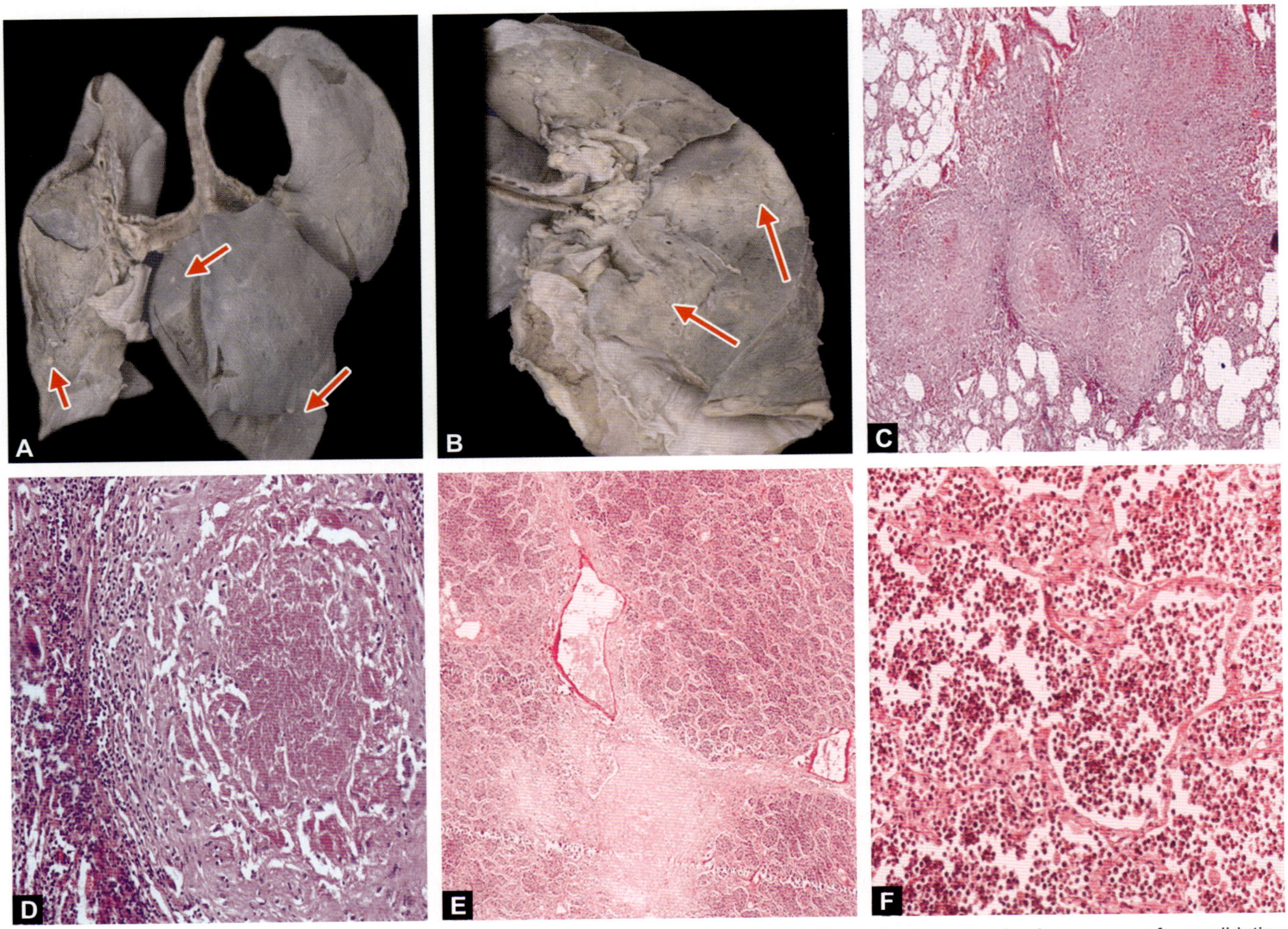

Figs 7A–F: (A) Pleural aspect of the lungs showing miliary tubercles (arrows); (B) Cut section of the lung showing large areas of consolidation (arrows) and miliary tubercles; (C and D) Photomicrograph of the lung showing small epithelioid cell granulomas with central caseation necrosis and giant cells; (E and F) Lung showing alveolar spaces packed with polymorphs.

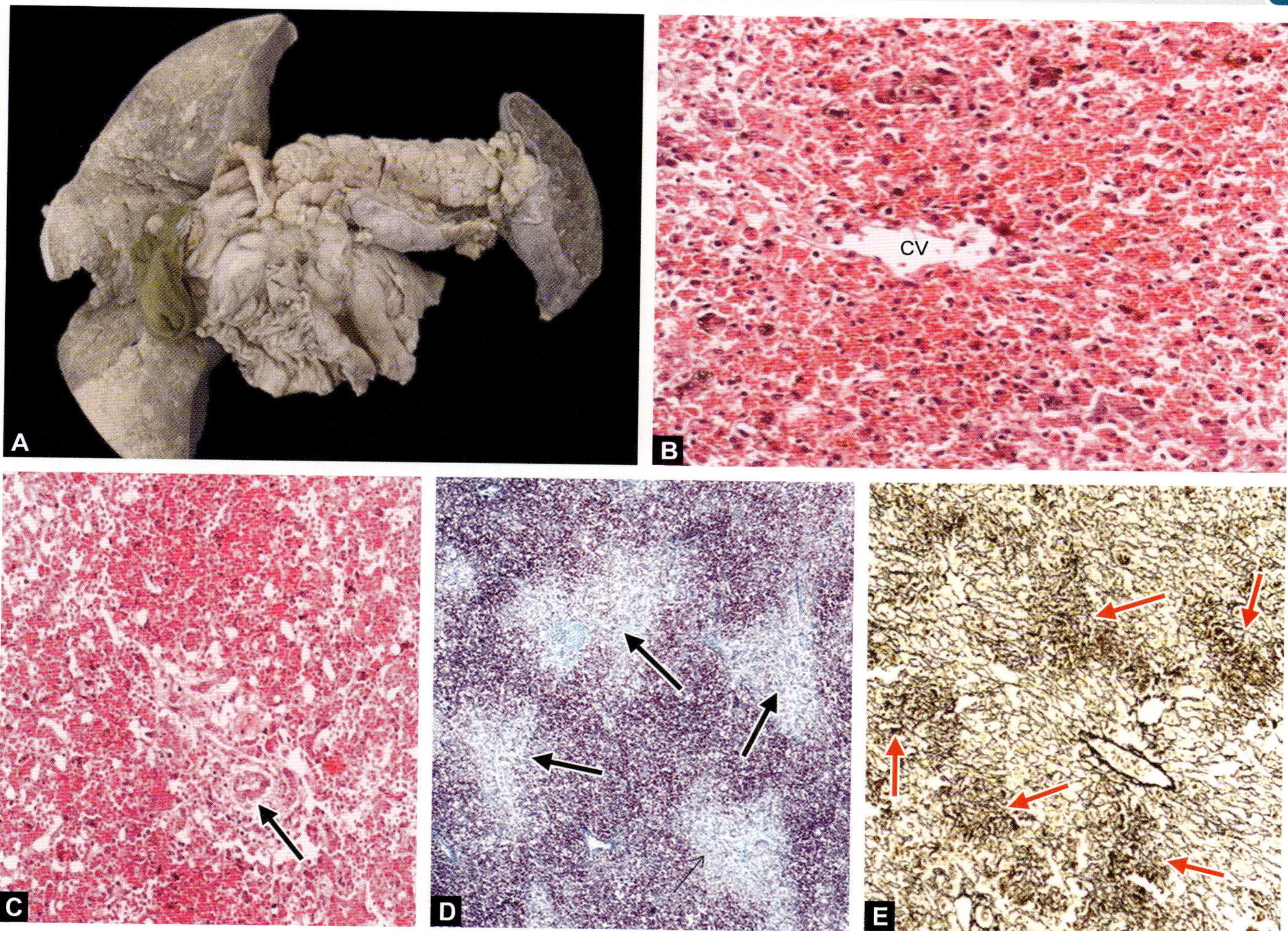

Figs 8A–E: (A) Organ complex of a slice of the shrunken liver, pancreas, C-loop of duodenum, gallbladder and slice of spleen. Photomicrographs of the liver showing; (B) Extensive hemorrhagic necrosis around the central vein (CV); (C) Extensive hemorrhagic necrosis reaching right up till the portal tract (arrow); (D) Masson trichrome stain showing lighter areas (arrows) which are the preserved periportal hepatocytes. Rest of the area shows hemorrhagic necrosis; (E) Reticulin stain showing areas of reticulin collapse (arrows).

known as "superantigens" which are polyclonal T lymphocyte activators, which release high levels of cytokines, leads to numerous manifestations like diffuse rash, vasodilatation, hypotension, shock and death. The incidence of septic shock is on the rise due to the better life support systems for critically ill patients, increasing numbers of immunocompromised individuals as a result of chemotherapy, longevity, HIV infection, etc and due to the multidrug resistant strains in hospital settings. Gram positive bacterial infection is the biggest trigger of septic shock, followed by gram negative bacterial infection and fungal infections. The outcome of septic shock depends on a number of factors like associated co-morbidities, immune status of the host, virulence of the organism and the level of cytokine storm.

Morphological changes of shock are seen in many organs like brain, heart, lungs, liver, kidneys, adrenals and depends on the type and the degree of shock. Cardiogenic or hypovolemic shock leads to lipid depletion of the cortical cells of the adrenals, acute tubular necrosis in the kidneys, neuronal loss in the brain and myocyte loss in the heart. Lungs are generally not affected in pure hypovolemic shock as they are resistant to the ischemic injury. But in septic shock or trauma, they manifest with diffuse alveolar damage where microscopically the alveolar spaces are lined by hyaline membranes.

Hepatic injury in acute heart failure and peripheral circulatory shock occurs due to hypoperfusion. On coronal slicing of the liver, there is a nutmeg appearance wherein dark congested and hemorrhagic discolored areas alternate with relatively preserved paler areas. Microscopic examination shows widespread hemorrhagic/coagulative necrosis of the hepatocytes in the perivenular/centrizonal location, also known as the microcirculatory periphery of the acinus. This loss of liver cells is apparent on reticulin stain, as reticulin collapse and condensation of the perivenular reticulin framework. Cholestasis may be apparent at the periphery of the necrotic hepatocytes. In severe shock, zone 2 hepatocytes may be involved and show hemorrhagic or coagulative necrosis, sparing only a single rim of periportal hepatocytes. In very severe shock, the periportal or zone 1 hepatocytes may also get affected. In ischemic hepatitis there may be mild rise of serum bilirubin and a dramatic and rapid rise in serum aminotransferases.

COMMENTARY—INDEX CASE: PM 25901

A 5-year-old female child came with recent onset of fever and headache along with altered sensorium and multiple seizures. She was diagnosed as a case of tubercular meningitis on the basis of clinical history, examination, CT and CSF findings. She was put on ATT with steroids and a VP shunt was inserted to reduce the raised intracranial pressure. Clinicopathological correlation brings out the following in the index case:

- There was tubercular meningitis with extensive arteritis and infarction involving bilateral basal ganglia, thalamus, hippocampus, midbrain and cerebral cortex. The pathogenetic lesion of tubercular meningitis, i.e. the subpial "Rich focus" was identified.
- There was miliary TB predominantly involving lungs and lymph nodes (hilar, carinal, mesenteric, peripancreatic, gastric, celiac and para-aortic). There were granulomas seen in the liver, spleen and GIT. Disseminated TBin this child also contributed to the septic shock. This was a 5-year-old child with a tuberculous contact in the family. This could well be a case of primary or secondary TB with miliary spread.
- There was nosocomial or hospital acquired infection which also contributed to septic shock and reflected clinically as a rapid rise in total leukocyte count with predominant polymorphs and as confluent necrotizing bronchopneumonia at autopsy.
- There was an irreversible stage of septic shock due to disseminated tuberculosis and nosocomial sepsis which reflected as classical ischemic hepatitis/shock liver in this case. At admission the liver function tests showed a minimal rise in serum transaminases (SGOT: 68, SGPT: 64) and serum bilirubin was normal. But soon there was a dramatic rise in the serum aminotransferases and terminally, they were in thousands. The coagulogram was normal at admission, but got totally deranged during the course of the hospital stay. This irreversible shock, led to a shrunken nutmeg liver which on microscopy showed a florid centrizonal (zone1) hemorrhagic necrosis, along with involvement of zone 2 (most areas) and with involvement of the periportal hepatocytes, i.e. zone 1 in many areas.

TAKE HOME MESSAGE

- Tubercular meningitis can lead to extensive arteritis and infarction involving bilateral basal ganglia and internal capsule most frequently. Widespread infarction can occur to involve the cortex, thalamus, hippocampus and midbrain.
- Infarcts are seen in up to 37%–72.5% cases in various autopsy studies. Anterior circulation is involved more than the posterior circulation.
- Rich and McCordock in 1933 at the John Hopkins hospital demonstrated that the key pathway in the origin of tubercular meningitis lies in direct spread of tubercle bacilli into the subarachnoid space from a subpial focus called "Rich focus". The tubercle bacilli however cannot escape freely into the meninges from the blood stream.
- Ischemic hepatitis or shock liver leads to widespread hemorrhagic/coagulative necrosis of the hepatocytes in the perivenular/centrizonal location, also known as the microcirculatory periphery of the acinus.

CONTRIBUTIONS BY:

1. Dr Saniya Sharma, Senior Resident, Department of Pathology (In preparing the manuscript)
2. Dr Kumar Sangam, Junior Resident, Department of Pathology (In taking Gross Photographs)
3. Dr Aparna Mishra, Junior Resident, Department of Pediatrics (Compilation of Clinical Details)
4. Dr BD Radotra, Professor, Department of Histopathology (Consultation)
5. Dr S Singhi, Ex-Professor and Head, Department of Pediatrics (Clinician In-Charge)

Post Graduate Institute of Medical Education and Research, Chandigarh, India.

CASE 65

Disseminated Cryptococcal Infection in an HIV-positive Child: PM 23563

Nandita Bharadwaj Kakkar

 HIGHLIGHTS OF THE CASE

A 14-year-old, human immunodeficiency virus (HIV) positive child (CD4 absolute count 29), was admitted with fever, cough, shortness of breath, loose stools, loss of weight and appetite. He was symptomatic since 4 years and was treated for tuberculosis, after which he improved, till his present illness. He had received a directed blood transfusion from his father, at the age of one year, as he was severely anemic. His mother was HIV negative, but the father was detected to be HIV positive later on. There was generalized lymphadenopathy and splenohepatomegaly. X-ray chest showed bilateral interstitial infiltrates. Autopsy revealed disseminated cryptococcal infection (gelatinous type) with a heavy fungal load, involving lungs, lymph nodes, spleen, liver, lungs, kidneys and gastrointestinal tract (GIT). The unique features in this case were presentation with generalized lymphadenopathy, very heavy cryptococcal load and total absence of inflammation, cryptococcal lymphangiectasia and sinusoidal localization of cryptococci in the liver.

Keywords: Cryptococcosis, disseminated, generalized lymphadenopathy, HIV-positive, intestinal lymphangiectasia, autopsy.

 CLINICAL DETAILS

Date of Admission: 26.02.2010, Date of Death: 28.02.2010, Duration of Hospital Stay: 2 Days

A 14-year-old boy was admitted in February 2010, with complaints of fever, productive cough and breathing difficulty since 1 month. The fever was moderate grade, intermittent, associated with rigors and chills, with evening rise and responded to antipyretics. There was cough with mucopurulent expectoration of small volume (1 teaspoon), nonfoul smelling, with no hemoptysis and with no postural and diurnal variation. Shortness of breath, New York Heart Association (NYHA) II–III was present since 1 month. There was no history of orthopnea or paroxysmal nocturnal dyspnea (PND). There were episodes of loose stools, loss of weight/appetite, nausea and occasional vomiting. There was however, no headache or any visual symptoms. Oral ulcers and difficulty in swallowing were present. This child had been symptomatic for 4 years with fever and cough with expectoration. He was treated for tuberculosis in 2008 (? duration) and in 2009 (for 9 months). Symptoms improved with treatment, till his present illness. He had received a directed blood transfusion from his father, at the age of one-year, as he was severely anemic. Both grandparents were treated for tuberculosis, his parents were both healthy and he was their only child. In February 2010, the child was admitted in a private hospital and he was detected to be HIV positive and referred to our institute. On examination he was conscious, oriented and cooperative. On examination his pulse was 90 beats/min, respiratory rate 26 breaths/min, BP 116/78 mm Hg and weight was 34 kg (expected 48 kg). There was pallor, cervical, axillary and inguinal lymphadenopathy. There was however no cyanosis, edema, icterus, clubbing or raised jugular venous pressure (JVP). On auscultation, there were normal vesicular breath sounds, occasional wheeze and crepitations in bilateral mammary regions. The abdomen was soft, nontender, liver and spleen were palpable 4 cm below their respective costal margins and there was no free fluid. Central nervous system (CNS) examination was within normal limits.

Investigations and Course of Management

Investigations revealed Hemoglobin of 8 g/dL, TLC of 5,000/ul platelets 84,000/ul and ESR of 96 in 1st hour. Coagulation profile was within normal limits. Blood biochemistry revealed raised aspartate aminotransferase (AST) 97.9 U/L, alanine aminotransferase (ALT) 47.4 U/L and alkaline phosphatase 625 U/L, but serum bilirubin was normal. There was hypoalbuminemia (2.4 g). HIV serology was positive, CD4 absolute count was 29 (N-410-1590) and % of CD3 lymphocytes were 3 (N-31-60%). The mother was HIV negative, but the father was HIV positive. HbsAg was negative and VDRL was nonreactive. Routine urine examination—albumin 1+, sugar nil, RBC 2–4/hpf and pus cells 10–15/hpf. X-ray chest showed bilateral interstitial infiltrates with hilar prominence and ground-glass opacity. Ultrasonography revealed hepatosplenomegaly with mesenteric, peripancreatic and perisplenic lymphadenopathy. The kidneys were of normal echotexture. The patient succumbed to his illness within 3 days of hospitalization. The units clinical diagnosis was HIV disease (AIDS) with *Pneumocystis carinii* pneumonia.

AUTOPSY FINDINGS: PM 23563

A partial autopsy was performed on this 14-year-old, HIV-positive male child. All serous cavities were within normal limits. There was ***lymphadenopathy*** (Figs 1A–C) involving the cervical, axillary, hilar, carinal, tracheal, mesenteric, peripancreatic, perisplenic, porta hepatic, para-aortic and inguinal lymph nodes. Cut section of the lymph nodes was fleshy and mucoidy. On microscopic examination (Figs 1D–F) there was a severe depletion of lymphoid tissue with total replacement by refractile, empty looking fungal profiles, ranging in size from 5 μm to 12 μm, showing

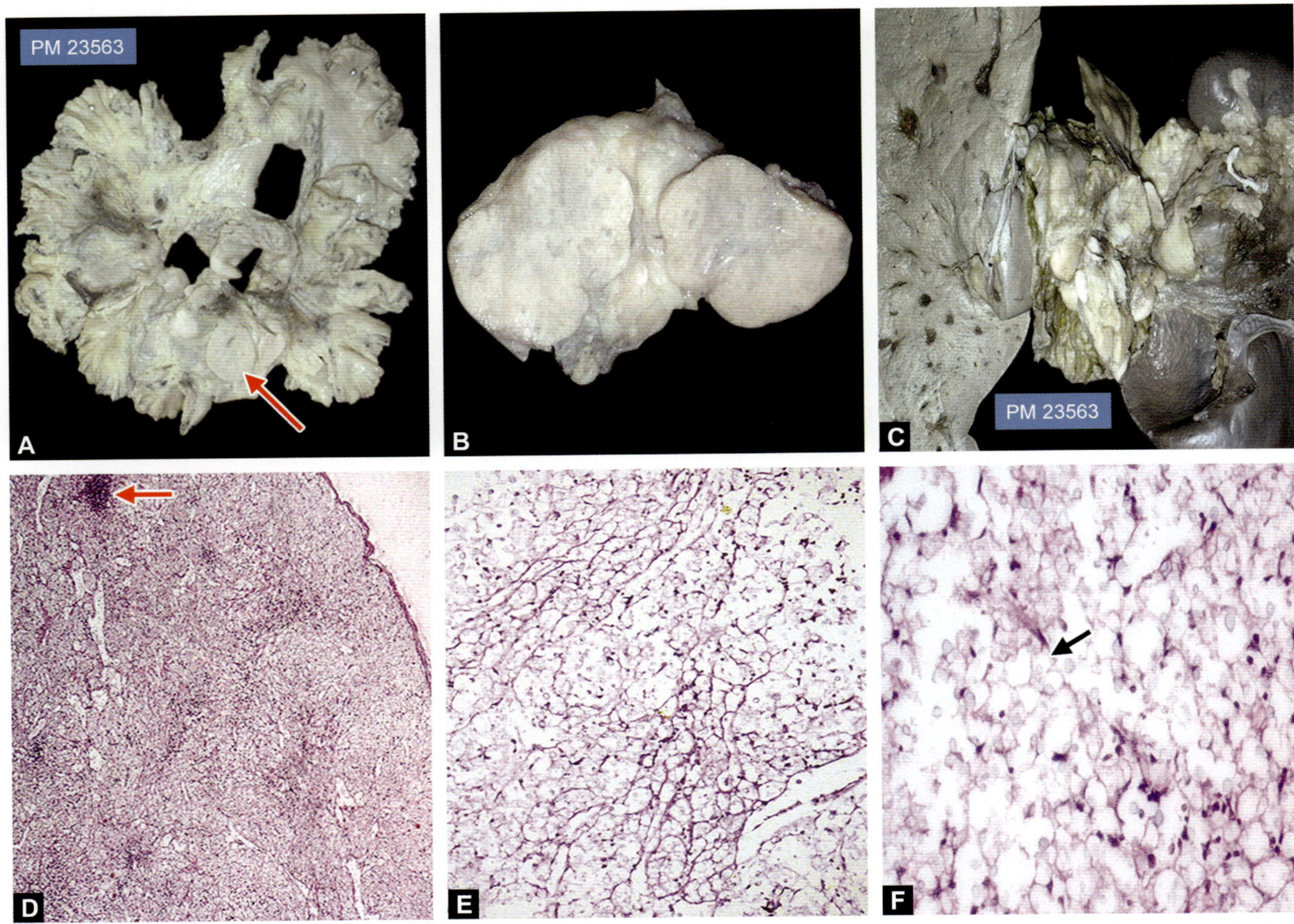

Figs 1A–F: (A–C) Enlarged mesenteric, para-aortic, peripancreatic, splenic lymph nodes; (D) Low-power view of a lymph node showing total loss of lymphoid tissue with a tiny left over remnant at one edge (arrow); (E and F) Same node at a higher power shows bland foaminess and is replete with round to oval refractile fungal profiles of cryptococci (arrow). No inflammation is noted.

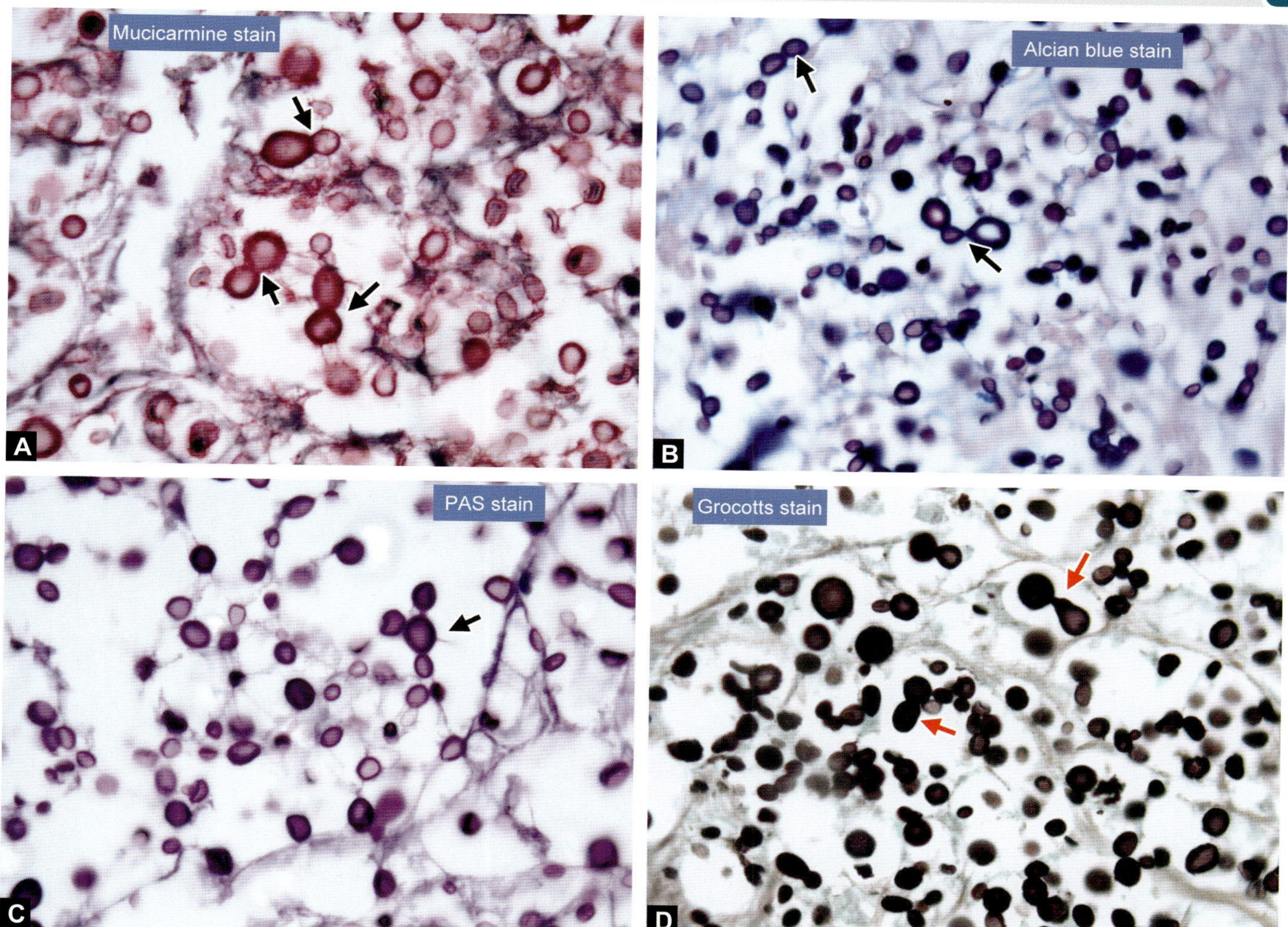

Figs 2A–D: Cryptococci showing prominent budding (arrows). (A) Mucicarmine stain—stains the capsule deep pink; (B) Alcian blue stain—stains the capsule deep blue; (C) PAS stain—stains the entire organism magenta; (D) Grocotts stain—stains the entire organism black.

prominent budding, morphology consistent with that of *Cryptococcus*. No accompanying inflammatory cells, giant cells or fibrosis was noted and the reaction was consistent with the gelatinous type of reaction, which is the hallmark reaction seen in immunocompromised hosts. The capsule (Figs 2A and B) stained with mucicarmine (deep pink) and alcian blue (deep blue). The entire organism stained magenta with PAS (Fig 2C) and black with Grocott's stain (Fig 2D). The ***liver*** (Fig 3A) was enlarged and weighed 1,300 g. Cut section did not show any focal lesion and was slimy to feel. Microscopy, revealed areas of hepatocytic loss replaced by sheets of cryptococci (Figs 3B and C), along with sinusoids (Figs 3D–F) packed with cryptococci. No inflammation was noted. The ***spleen*** weighed 520 g. On cut section there was a diffuse enlargement and the surface was slimy (Fig 3A). Microscopic examination (Figs 4A and B) revealed total depletion of white pulp and replacement of the entire spleen by sheets of cryptococci with an absent inflammatory reaction. The ***lungs*** (Fig 4C) together weighed 800 g, pleurae were dull and the cut section did not reveal any focal lesion but was slimy to feel. Microscopy (Figs 4D–F) revealed abundant cryptococci lying in the alveolar spaces along with plenty of macrophages and hemorrhage. The ***kidneys*** (Fig 5A) were enlarged and showed petechial hemorrhages on capsular and cut surface. Abundant cryptococci were seen in the glomerular capillaries (Figs 5B–D) and in the dilated vasa recta forming cysts (Fig. 5E). The ***stomach*** showed prominent rugae and on microscopy the lamina propria contained spaces full of cryptococci. The ***small intestine*** (Fig 6A) also showed marked prominence of villi and on microscopy (Figs 6B–D) the villi were bulbous and markedly expanded by sheets of cryptococci with no inflammation. The cryptococci

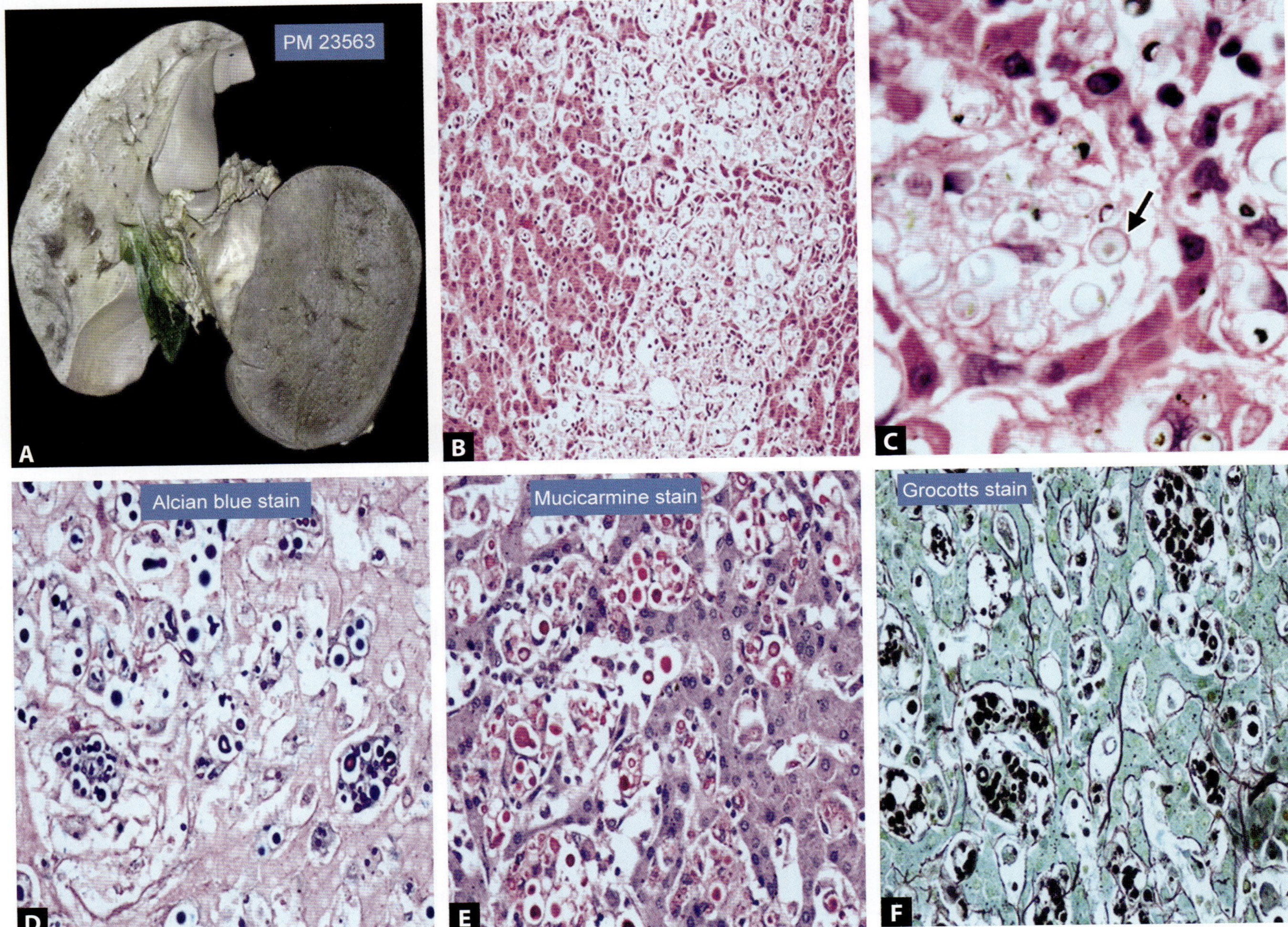

Figs 3A–F: (A) Organ complex comprising of a slice of the enlarged liver, spleen along with gallbladder, C loop of duodenum and pancreas. The liver and spleen show diffuse enlargement; (B and C) Liver shows areas of bland hepatocytic loss replete with cryptococci (arrow); (D–F) Alcian blue, mucicarmine and Grocotts stain, stain the cryptococci swimming in the sinusoids of the liver.

seem to be within dilated lymphatics. The morphology looks akin to lymphangiectasia and the term cryptococcal lymphangiectasia would be appropriate. No Peyer's patches were however seen. The ***large intestine*** revealed only a few cryptococci in the lamina propria. Lymphoid tissue was absent in the intestine and in the appendix. The ***thymus*** also showed marked lymphoid depletion but no cryptococci were identified. The heart was within normal limits.

FINAL AUTOPSY DIAGNOSIS: PM 23563

A 14 Years Old Male, HIV-Positive

Disseminated Cryptococcal infection (gelatinous type) with heavy fungal load, involving the lymph nodes, spleen, liver, lungs, kidneys and GIT. Marked lymphoid depletion.

CRYPTOCOCCAL INFECTION IN HIV-POSITIVE INDIVIDUALS

Human immunodeficiency virus is the causative agent of acquired immunodeficiency syndrome (AIDS), but 80% patients die of opportunistic infections rather than from HIV. Cryptococcosis is the most common fungal disease in HIV-infected individuals, it being the AIDS-defining illness in 60–70% cases. In a study by Currie et al,[1] the annual prevalence of cryptococcosis among HIV-infected in New York City is estimated to be 6.1–8.5%. A study[2] on AIDS-related opportunistic mycoses in a tertiary care hospital in North India, revealed candidiasis (41.7%) as the most common fungal infection, followed by cryptococcosis (10%), pneumocystinosis and apergillosis (8.3% each). In a study by French et al,[3] cryptococcal infection is an important

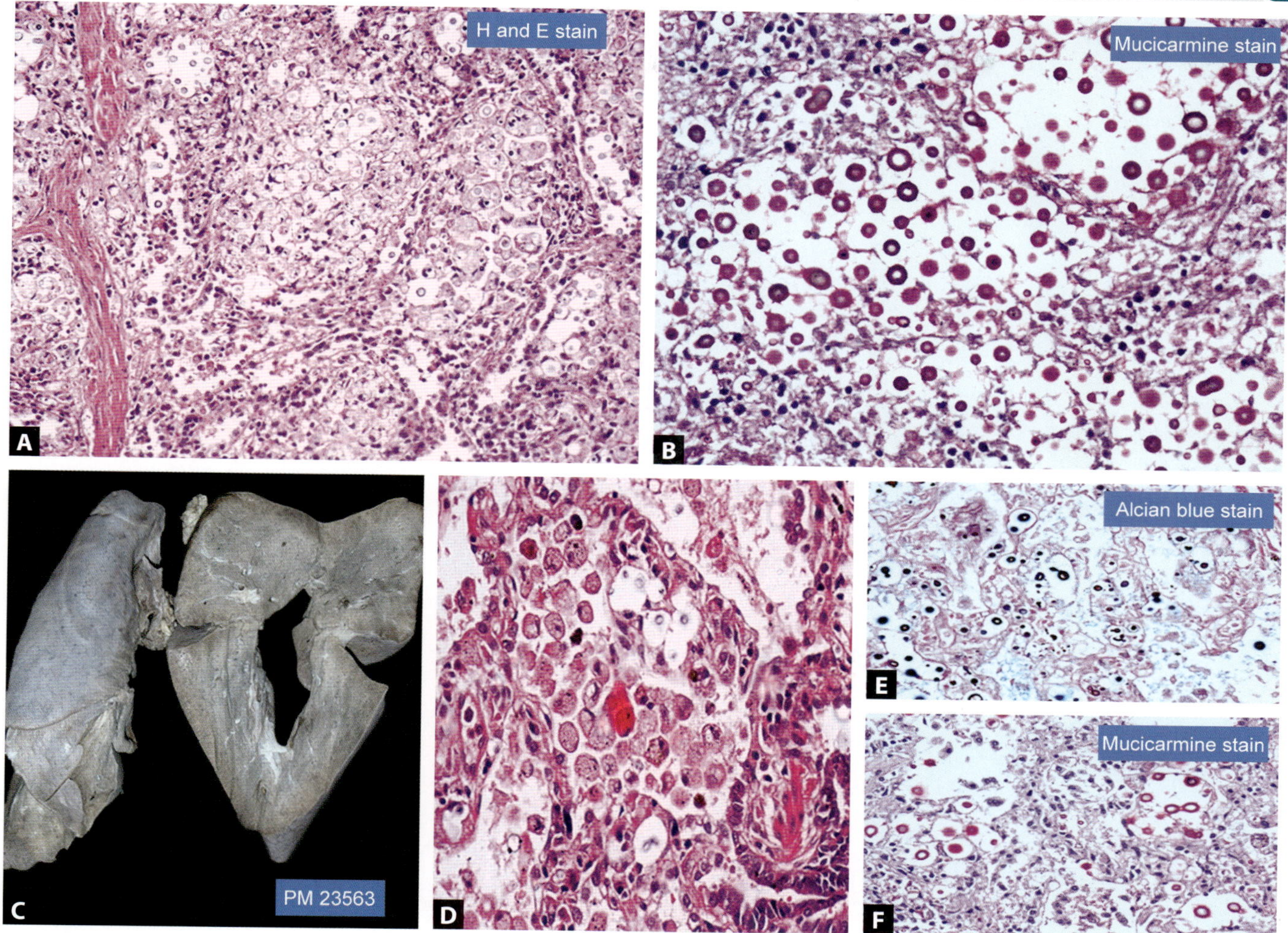

Figs 4A–F: (A and B) Spleen showing total replacement by cryptococci. The capsule stains deep pink with mucicarmine; (C) Pleural and cut surface of the lungs was firm and slimy. No hemorrhage or any lesion was noted; (D–F) Alveolar spaces packed with macrophages (D) along with plenty of cryptococci stained with alcian blue (E) and mucicarmine stain (F).

contributor to mortality and suffering in HIV-infected Ugandans. Antiretroviral therapy given to HIV patients has brought down the number of cases of cryptococcal infection, but still, the yearly occurrence of cryptococcosis is one million and the maximum cases are seen in Africa.[4]

Cryptococcus neoformans[5] an encapsulated basidiomycetous yeast, is the frequently seen organism in HIV-positive patients. Before the HIV era, it was a rare disease but is now a leading cause of pulmonary, CNS (meningitis, meningoencephalitis, space occupying lesions) or disseminated disease.[2] ***C. neoformans*** is classified into four serotypes on the basis of the type of polysaccharide present in the capsule i.e. glucuronoxylomannan.[1] They are capsular types A (variety ***grubii***), B and C (variety ***gattii***) and D (variety ***neoformans***). ***C. neoformans*** is genetically distinct from ***C. gattii*** and so the latter is labeled as a distinct species. ***Cryptococcus*** has a worldwide distribution and is seen in the droppings of pigeons and chickens. Human infection however can occur without a history of direct contact with birds. ***C. gattii*** is seen in the tropics and subtropics and is found in decaying vegetation and in eucalyptus tree.[6] The Vancouver Island outbreak of ***C. gattii*** infection from 1999-2004 was a result of import of eucalyptus trees from Australia.[7] ***C. neoformans*** and ***grubi*** predominantly affect the immunocompromised individuals and ***C gattii*** predominantly affect the immunocompetent hosts.

Cryptococcus survives in the sexual form in the environment. It produces hyphae with chains of unbudded yeast at the terminal ends also, called basidiospores. The basidiospores separate off into 3 micron sized yeast and get aerosolized and get deposited in the alveolar spaces. This

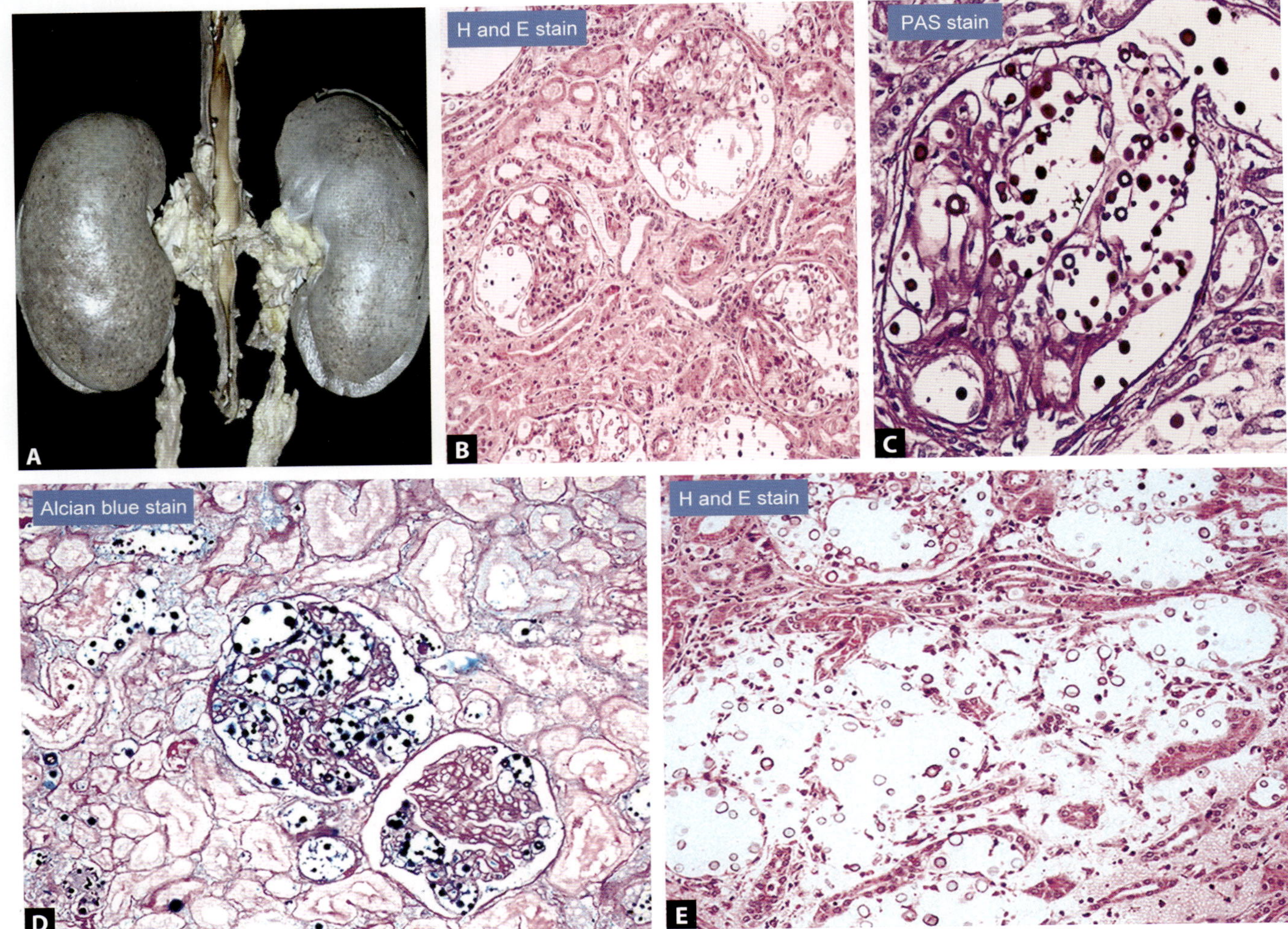

Figs 5A–E: (A) Enlarged kidneys showing blotchy congestion; (B–D) Dilated glomerular capillaries packed with cryptococci, which stain strongly with PAS and alcian blue stains; (E) Interstitium of the kidney showing dilated spaces packed with cryptocoocci.

infestation is asymptomatic, but in cases with cell-mediated immunodeficiency, the organisms enter the circulation leading to dissemination. Virulence factors[8] permitting its survival in the host include:

- Cryptococcal phagocytosis is prevented by the polysaccharide capsule.
- Enzyme phenol oxidase which uses catecholamines as substrate to produce melanin that accumulates in the cell wall.

Cryptococcus[9] generally involves the lungs and the brain, although it can be disseminated, involving practically every organ of the body. Pulmonary disease occurs as granulomas which are noncalcified and not detected on X-rays or as acute pneumonia. Antiretroviral therapy has reduced mortality in HIV-positive patients, but cryptococcal meningitis[10] still remains an important cause of mortality. It presents with a slowly creeping headache of several-weeks duration. Fever occurs late in the course of the disease and neck rigidity is often absent. Extracranial manifestations are seen in approximately 50% cases which involve the lungs, skin (molluscum-like lesions), bone marrow, bone and genitourinary tract. Lymphadenopathy can occur at any stage of HIV infection, with multiple etiologies including reactive, infectious and malignant. The GIT is a major site of disease in HIV patients and a large number of infections like bacterial, viral and fungal can be seen. Cryptococcal infection can be seen, where in, the mucosa of the GIT is thick and the lamina propria contains the fungal profiles in abundance.

The diagnosis of cryptococcosis is made by the latex agglutination test for capsular polysaccharide antigen, either from the

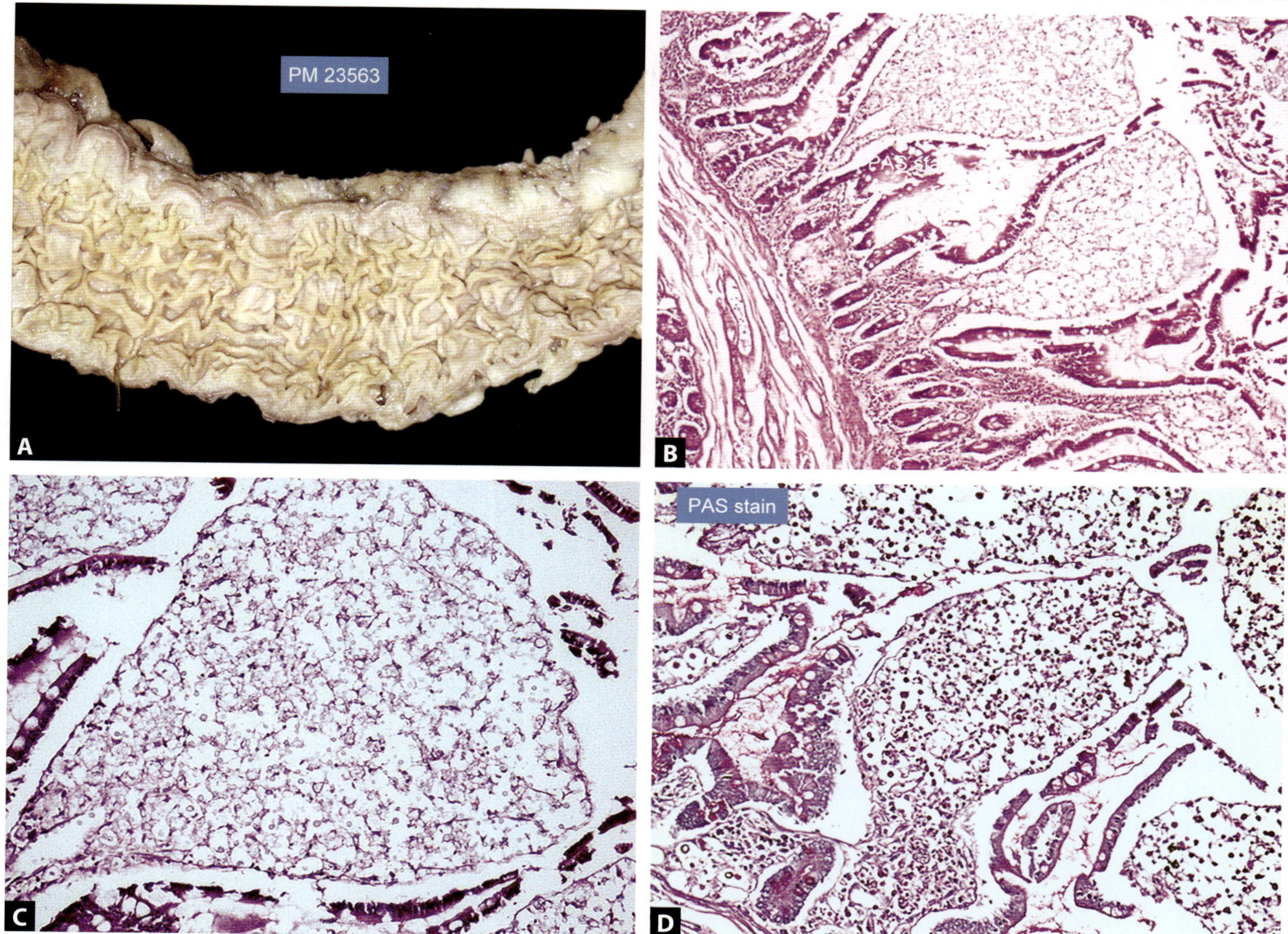

Figs 6A–D: (A) Small intestine showing prominent rugae; (B and C) Photomicrographs from the small intestine show bulbous villi, wherein the lymphatics are dilated and replete with cryptococci; (D) Bulbous villi show plenty of PAS-positive cryptococci.

cerebrospinal fluid (CSF) or serum. In the CSF, it is over 90% sensitive and specific for the diagnosis of cryptococcal meningitis. Two types of histologic pattern occur with cryptococcal infection:

- Gelatinous
- Granulomatous.

Both types may coexist in the same lesion. The gelatinous lesions are seen in immunocompromised hosts and are characterized by sea/masses of organisms with mucoid degeneration and no inflammation.

COMMENTARY—INDEX CASE: PM 23563

This young boy acquired HIV at the age of one, after receiving a directed blood transfusion from his father, who was HIV positive. He was symptomatic since 4 years and was treated for tuberculosis, after which he improved, till his present illness. He was detected to be HIV positive and was referred to our institute. He came with fever, shortness of breath and loose stools. HIV positivity was confirmed. There was generalized lymphadenopathy and splenohepatomegaly. X-ray chest showed bilateral interstitial infiltrates. Liver enzymes were raised, but serum bilirubin was normal. There was hypoalbuminemia (2.4 g). The CD4 (29) and CD3 (3) counts were markedly decreased. A clinical diagnosis of HIV disease (AIDS) with Pneumocystis carinii pneumonia was made. But autopsy revealed disseminated cryptococcal infection (gelatinous type) with a very heavy fungal load, involving lymph nodes, spleen, liver, lungs, kidneys and GIT. Marked lymphoid depletion was noted. The morphology was consistent with the gelatinous type of cryptococcal reaction, which occurs in immunocompromised hosts, wherein, there is no inflammatory reaction to the cryptococci, which are present in sheets, mimicking an ocean and totally distorting the architecture of the parent organ. Every organ that was involved in this case was like a culture plate of cryptococci. There was a marked sinusoidal localization of the cryptococci in the liver, along with small cysts. The small intestinal villi were expanded, markedly bulbous and packed with cryptococci, which seemed to be within the dilated lymphatics. Thus, the term cryptococcal lymphangiectasia is appropriate. This explains the presence of loose stools and the hypoalbuminemia. The brain was not examined in this case as the permission for brain removal was not given by the relatives. There could be cryptococcal CNS disease as well, because the absence of signs and symptoms do not negate the presence of pathological disease. The unique features in this case were presentation with generalized lymphadenopathy, very heavy cryptococcal load, total absence of inflammation, cryptococcal lymphangiectasia and sinusoidal localization of cryptococci in the liver.

TAKE HOME MESSAGE

- The practice of directed blood transfusions should be strictly prohibited.
- Human immunodeficiency virus is the causative agent of AIDS, but 80% patients die of opportunistic infections, rather than from HIV.
- Cryptococcosis is the AIDS-defining illness in 60–70% cases.
- A study on AIDS-related opportunistic mycoses from North India, revealed candidiasis (41.7%) as the most common fungal infection, followed by cryptococcosis (10%).
- The unique features in the index case were presentation with generalized lymphadenopathy, very heavy cryptococcal load, total absence of inflammation, cryptococcal lymphangiectasia and sinusoidal localization of cryptococci in the liver.

REFERENCES

1. Currie BP, Casadevall A. Estimation of the prevalence of cryptococcal infection among patients infected with the human immunodeficiency virus in New York City. Clin Infect Dis. 1994;19(6):1029-33.
2. Wadhwa A, Kaur R, Agarwal SK, et al. AIDS-related opportunistic mycoses seen in a tertiary care hospital in North India. J Med Microbiol. 2007;56(Pt.8):1101-6.
3. French N, Gray K, Watera C, et al. Cryptococcal infection in a cohort of HIV-1-infected Ugandan adults. AIDS. 2002; 16(7):1031-8.
4. Park BJ, Wannemuehler KA, Marston BJ, et al. Estimation of the current global burden of cryptococcal meningitis among persons living with HIV/AIDS. AIDS. 2009;23(4):525-30.
5. Tyler Warkentien, Nancy F, Crum-Cianflone. An Update on cryptococcosis among HIV-infected persons. Int J STD AIDS. 2010;21(10):679-84.
6. Ellis DH, Pfeiffer TJ. Natural habitat of *Cryptococcus neoformans* var. *gattii*. J Clin Microbiol. 1990;28(7):1642-4.
7. Fyfe M, MacDougall L, Romney M, et al. *Cryptococcus gattii* infections on Vancouver Island, British Columbia, Canada: Emergence of a tropical fungus in a temperate environment. Can Commun Dis Rep. 2008;34(6):1-12.
8. Perfect JR, Wong B, Chang YC, et al. *Cryptococcus neoformans*: Virulence and host defences. Med Mycol. 1998; 36(Suppl 1):79-86.
9. Jarvis JN, Harrison TS. HIV-associated cryptococcal meningitis. AIDS. 2007;21(16):2119-29.
10. Bekondi C, Bernede C, Passone N, et al. Primary and opportunistic pathogens associated with meningitis in adults in Bangui, Central African Republic, in relation to human immunodeficiency virus serostatus. Int J Infect Dis. 2006; 10(5):387-95.

CONTRIBUTIONS BY:

1. Dr Devi Dayal, Professor, Department of Pediatrics (Compilation of Clinical Details)
2. Dr Surjit Singh, Ex-Professor, Department of Internal Medicine (Clinician In-Charge)

Post Graduate Institute of Medical Education and Research, Chandigarh, India.

SECTION 12

Cardiovascular System Pediatric Case

CASE 66

Transposition of Great Arteries: PM 24027

Nandita Bharadwaj Kakkar

HIGHLIGHTS OF THE CASE

A 41-day-old male child, born to a primigravida, at term, with a birth weight of 2.5 kg, came with complaints of respiratory distress from early neonatal period with worsening by day 31 of life in the form of fever, cyanosis and increasing respiratory distress. There was a bluish discoloration of the body, on excessive cry, first noticed on day 37 of life in hospital. Chest X-ray showed cardiomegaly with increased pulmonary flow. Echocardiogram revealed transposition of great arteries (TGA) with normal atrioventricular connections, a large patent ductus arteriosus (PDA) and patent foramen ovale (PFO). Autopsy fingings were concordant with the echocardiographic findings.

Keywords: TGA, Transposition of great arteries, patent ductus arteriosus, patent foramen ovale, autopsy.

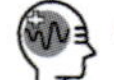

CLINICAL DETAILS

Date of Admission: 15.11.2010, Date of Death: 25.11.2010, Duration of Hospital Stay: 10 days

A 41-day-old male child was referred from an outside facility with complaints of rapid breathing on and off since birth, in the form of increased respiratory rate. Fever along with cough was present since 10 days. There was a bluish discoloration of the body, developed on excessive cry, first noted on day 37 of life in hospital, associated with worsening of respiratory distress in the form of increased rates and retractions. Echocardiography done in the outside facility revealed a bicuspid aortic valve, small PDA more than 2:1 with left-to-right shunt and patent foramen ovale. She was an unbooked, supervised, primigravida with two antenatal ultrasonography reported as normal. No antenatal echocardiography was done. She was not a known hypertensive or diabetic. It was a normal vaginal delivery, baby cried immediately after birth and the birth weight was 2.4 kg. He was appropriately vaccinated. On ***examination***, the respiratory rate was 66/min, subcostal/intercostal retractions were noted, bilateral crepitations were heard, S1 S2 were audible, pansystolic murmur was heard all over the precordium with maximal intensity over the left parasternal area. No organomegaly was present.

Investigations

Hb—19.4g%, TLC—12,900/μL, DLC—P80, L16, M02, E02, platelets—63,000/μL, PT—17′, PTI—76%, aPTT—26′, INR—1.44, D-dimer +; blood culture grew *Acinetobacter* sensitive to piptaz; Na+—149 mEq/L; K+—6.7 mEq/L; Cl^-—108 mEq/L; serum urea—71 mg%; creatinine—1.0 mg%; ***Chest X-ray*** showed cardiomegaly with increased pulmonary flow. ***Echocardiogram*** revealed dextro-transposition of great arteries (d-TGA), PFO 3 mm (L-R), PDA 5 mm (L-R), no coarctation, no significant pulmonary stenosis, normal LV systolic function, LV free wall thickness 4.2 mm, coronaries arising from opposing sinuses and no ventricular septal defect (VSD). There was excessive oxygen lability even on minimal stimulation. Preductal saturation was 65% and postductal saturation was 95%. There was decreased air entry into the left lower zones. The PaO_2 was less than 50 even on 100% FiO_2. The child was adequately treated and there was improvement of SpO_2 on starting prostaglandin E1 (PGE1) infusion. But on the 9th day, he suffered a cardiorespiratory arrest and could not be revived. ***Units clinical diagnosis*** was Congenital cyanotic heart disease—d-TGA with PDA, PFO, sinus rhythm, congestive cardiac failure, pulmonary arterial hypertension (secondary), pneumonia and shock (septic + cardiogenic).

AUTOPSY FINDINGS: PM 24027

A complete autopsy was performed on this 50-day-old male child, with a clinical diagnosis of cyanotic congenital heart disease. No dysmorphic facies was seen and the body weight was 2,180 g. All serous cavities were within normal limits. The ***heart*** (Figs 1A and B; Figs 2A and B) was egg-shaped, with apex formed by both right and left ventricles. The right atrial appendage was on the right side and left atrial appendage on the left side. The right atrium was placed (as should be) on the right side and was connected to the morphological right ventricle through the tricuspid valve, which was normal. The left atrium was placed (as should be) on the left side and was connected to the morphological left ventricle, through the mitral valve, which was normal. Thus, there was no atrioventricular discordance. However, the aorta was arising from the morphological right ventricle and was placed to the right and anteriorly. The main pulmonary artery was arising from the morphological left ventricle and was placed to the left of the aorta and posteriorly. Thus, there was ventriculoarterial discordance. The right pulmonary artery was connected to the aorta by a large PDA measuring 0.6 cm. The right atrium and left atrium were dilated and connected via a PFO. There was right ventricular hypertrophy noted. All the valves were within normal limits. No VSD was noted. Features were those of TGA with a large PDA and PFO. Lungs were normal grossly and revealed features of pulmonary arterial hypertension (Figs 3A and B) in the form of medial hypertrophy of the intra-acinar arterioles. There was ulceration of the lining epithelium of the bronchioles with lumen filled with inflammatory infiltrate, predominantly composed of neutrophils and macrophages, which were extending into adjacent alveolar spaces, indicating acute bronchopneumonia. Features of passive venous congestion, as a result of congestive cardiac failure, were seen in the lungs, liver and spleen.

FINAL AUTOPSY DIAGNOSIS: PM 24027

50 Day Old Male with Cyanotic Congenital Heart Disease

- Transposition of great arteries, with normal atrioventricular connections, with a patent foramen ovale (PFO), large patent ductus arteriosus (PDA) and without ventricular septal defect (VSD).
- Bronchopneumonia with pulmonary edema.
- Pulmonary arterial hypertension.
- Passive venous congestion—liver, lungs and spleen.

TRANSPOSITION OF GREAT ARTERIES

Transposition of the great arteries is a common cause of cyanotic congenital heart diseases, constitutes 5% of all

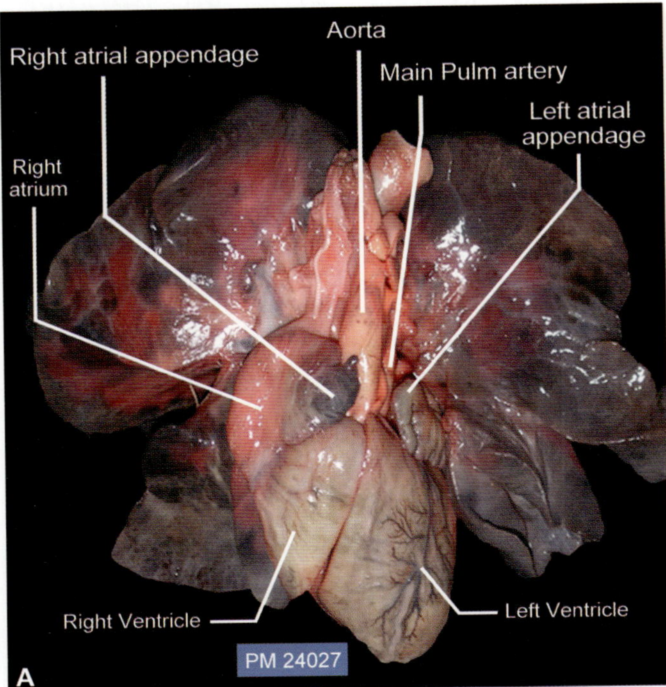

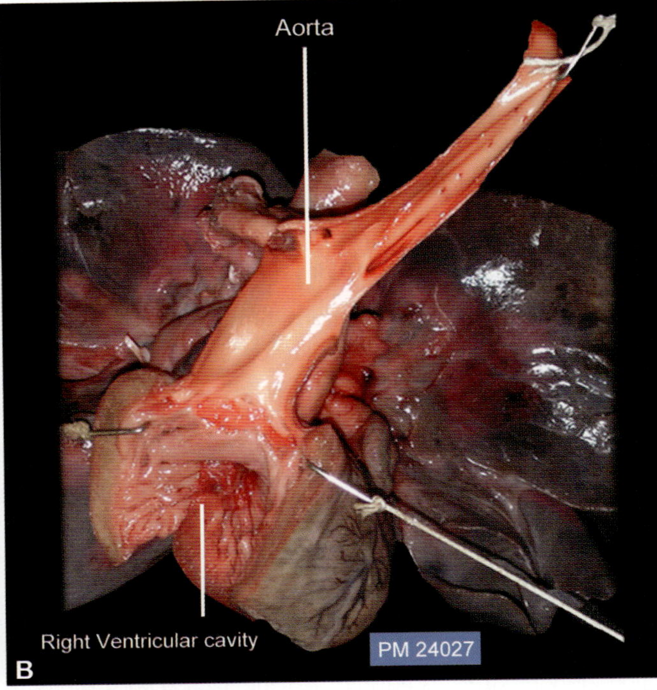

Figs 1A and B: (A) Organ complex of the heart and both lungs. The aorta is arising from the right ventricle and the main pulmonary artery (hidden behind the aorta) from the left ventricle; (B) Opened up right ventricle giving rise to the aorta.

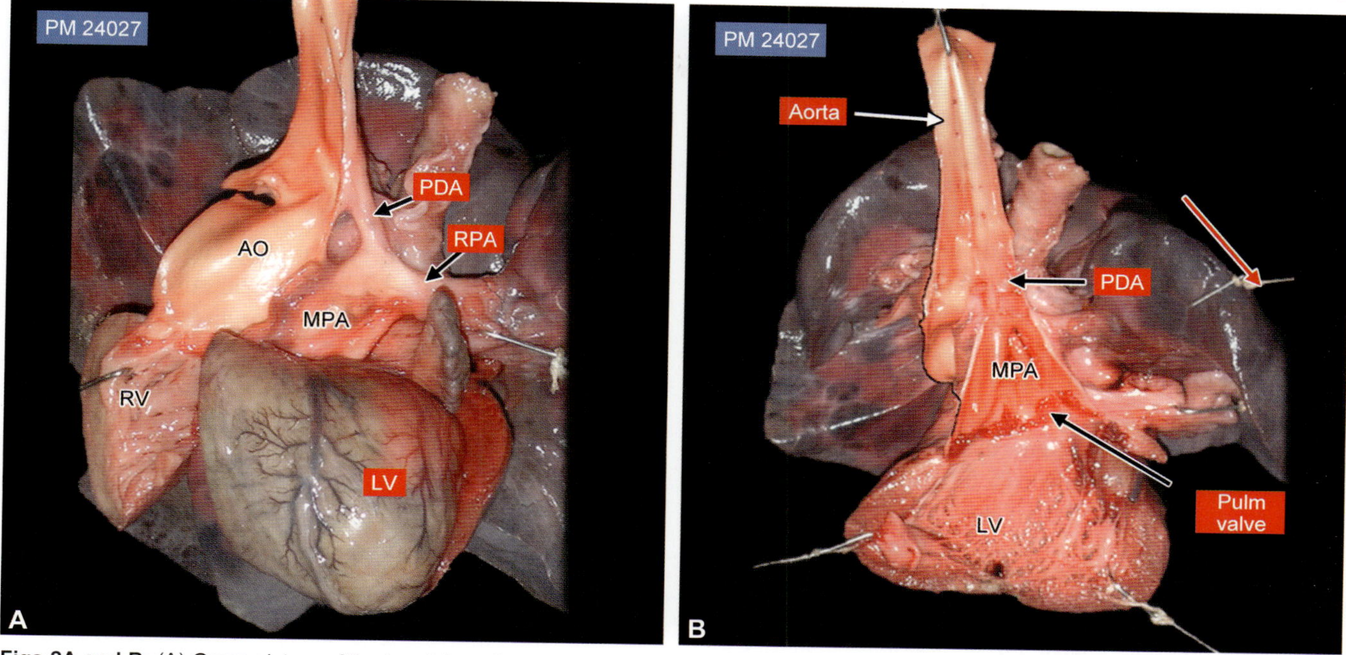

Figs 2A and B: (A) Gross picture of the heart from the posterior side showing the opened up right ventricle (RV) giving rise to the aorta (AO). The main pulmonary artery (MPA) is arising from the left ventricle (LV). A large PDA connects the right pulmonary artery (RPA) to the aorta; (B) Opened up left ventricle giving rise to the main pulmonary artery (MPA). The pulmonary valve is tricuspid.

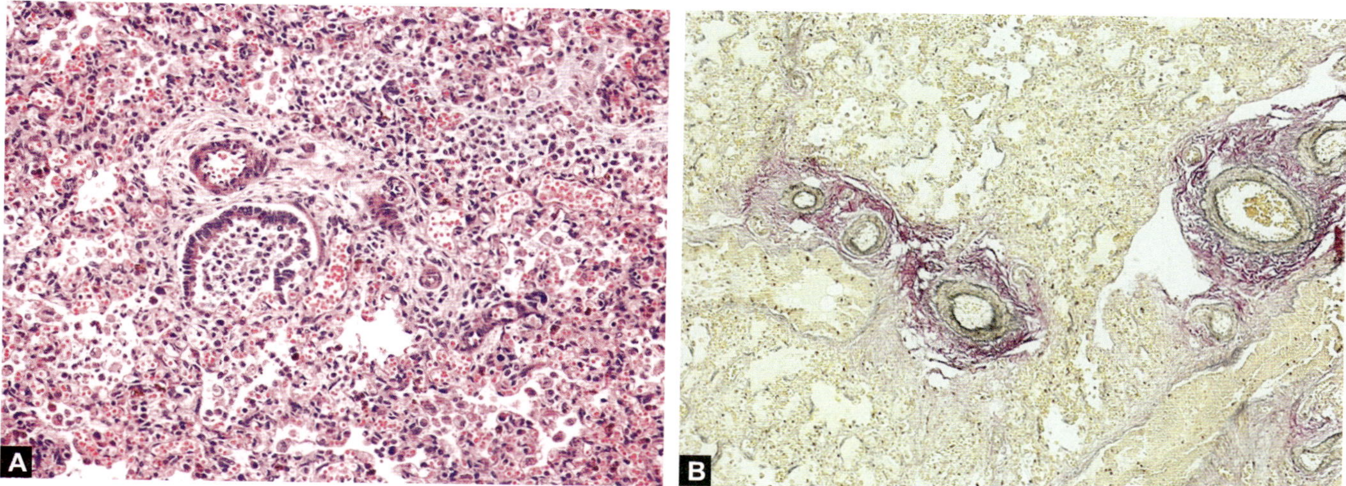

Figs 3A and B: (A) Photomicrograph of the lung showing bronchopneumonia; (B) Elastic van Gieson stain showing medial hypertrophy of the small arteries of the lung.

congenital heart disease, predominantly occurs as an isolated anomaly and shows a multifactorial inheritance. There is no racial predilection, but shows a male predominance. It is however, seen more in mothers having diabetes, age older than 40 years, poor nutrition, excessive consumption of alcohol during pregnancy, inflicted with viral infections during pregnancy and in babies with Down syndrome. The hallmark of TGA is ventriculoarterial discordance. The aorta arises from the morphologic right ventricle and is placed to the right and anteriorly and the pulmonary artery arises from the morphologic left ventricle and is placed to the left of the aorta and posteriorly known as d-TGA. The atrium to ventricular connections are concordant, i.e. the right atrium is connected to the morphologic right ventricle and the left atrium is connected to the morphologic left ventricle. The embryologic defect is due to the abnormal formation of the truncal and aortopulmonary septa leading to a total separation of both the circulations. The deoxygenated systemic venous blood returning to the right atrium goes to the right ventricle from where it is pumped to the systemic circulation, thus by passing the lungs. The oxygenated pulmonary venous blood, returns to the left atrium, goes into the left ventricle, but is then recirculated back to the lungs. Here, the right ventricle is functioning as the left ventricle and hence gets hypertrophied. The left ventricle on the other hand becomes thin-walled, as it sends blood to the low resistance pulmonary circulation. The saving grace is the mixing of blood via a shunt like atrial/ventricular septal defects or patent ductus arteriosus.

Babies with TGA are born at term, show no intrauterine growth retardation or any dysmorphic facies. Clinical manifestations however depend on the degree of mixing of the oxygenated blood from the left to the right side of the heart. (1) TGA with no shunts present with progressive cyanosis on day 1 of life and this situation is incompatible with life. (2) TGA with a substantial VSD or PDA may not show any symptoms except for mild cyanosis, particularly while crying. But within about 4 weeks, signs and symptoms of congestive heart failure sets in. (3) TGA with VSD and left ventricular outflow tract obstruction present with extreme cyanosis at birth which is proportional to the degree of the obstruction. (4) TGA with VSD and pulmonary vascular obstructive disease, present with progressive cyanosis, despite an early successful palliative procedure, but no congestive heart failure, despite a large ASD.

The survival is dependent on the type of TGA and the surgery resorted to. Arterial switch surgery has the best long-term prognosis and more than 95% patients are alive and do well at 25 years of age. Atrial switch operation has significant long-term morbidity due to complications like right ventricular failure, tricuspid regurgitation and atrial brady or tachy arrhythmias. TGA without a shunt is incompatible with life. A combination of TGA with a VSD is seen in 35% cases and they often have a stable shunt. A combination of TGA with PDA and PFO occur in 65% cases and in them the scenario is not that good. In untreated patients of TGA with shunts, survival depends on the type and the degree of shunting. Majority however die by one month of age. Congestive heart failure occur more in patients with large VSD or PDA or both as the pulmonary vascular resistance falls with increasing age.

Differential diagnosis includes double outlet right ventricle with malposed great arteries, Tetralogy of Fallot, pediatric tricuspid atresia, pulmonary atresia with intact ventricular septum, total anomalous pulmonary venous connection and truncus arteriosus. Diagnosis is established by echocardiography.

COMMENTARY—INDEX CASE: PM 24027

A 41-day-old male child, born to a primigravida, at term, with a birth weight of 2.5 kg, came with history of respiratory distress from early neonatal period with worsening by day 31 of life in the form of fever, cyanosis and increasing respiratory distress. There was a bluish discoloration of the body, on excessive cry, first noticed on day 37 of life. No dysmorphic facies was noted. Chest X-ray showed cardiomegaly with increased pulmonary blood flow. Echocardiogram revealed d-TGA, a large PDA and PFO. Autopsy findings were concordant with the echocardiographic findings. There was polycythemia and platelets were low (seen commonly in patients with coronary heart disease), although no bleeding manifestations were present. There was a d-TGA with a large PDA and PFO and hence a good degree of intermixing of the blood was going on. Thus, as happens in such cases, there were complaints of on and off rapid breathing from early neonatal period and cyanosis was first detected during an episode of excessive cry, on day 37 of life, while he was admitted at an outside facility. As the pulmonary blood flow increased, signs of congestive heart failure like tachypnea, tachycardia and failure to gain weight set in.

TAKE HOME MESSAGE

- Transposition of the great arteries is a cyanotic CHD, presents at birth and its hallmark is ventriculoarterial discordance.
- This situation is incompatible with survival, unless there is a shunt present like an atrial or ventricular septal defect or a PDA.

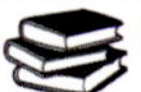

SUGGESTED READING

1. Clark EB. Cardiovascular system. In: Gilbert-Barness E (Ed). Potter's Pathology of the Fetus, Infant and Child, 2nd edition. US: Mosby Elsevier; 2007. p. 994.
2. Martins P, Castela E. Transposition of the great arteries. Orphanet J Rare Dis. 2008;3:27.

CONTRIBUTIONS BY:

1. Dr Ashim Das, Professor, Department of Histopathology (Consultation)
2. Dr Praveen Kumar, Professor and Head, Department of Pediatrics—Neonatology Division (Clinician In-Charge)

Post Graduate Institute of Medical Education and Research, Chandigarh, India.

SECTION 13

Hematological Disorders Pediatric Cases

CASE 67

Child with Acute Lymphoblastic Leukemia on Induction Therapy with Febrile Neutropenia and Disseminated *Aspergillus* Infection: PM 25927

Nandita Bharadwaj Kakkar

HIGHLIGHTS OF THE CASE

This 4-year-old female child presented with history of fever and progressive pallor, since 3 months and developed petechiae, generalized lymphadenopathy and hepatosplenomegaly. A diagnosis of pre-B cell acute lymphoblastic leukemia was made and she was put on induction chemotherapy. She developed febrile neutropenia on day 6 and this persisted till her demise. All measures were taken to avoid infection, but despite everything, she developed a disseminated *Aspergillus* infection and succumbed to her illness.

Keywords: Acute lymphoblastic leukemia, disseminated aspergillosis, febrile neutropenia, opportunistic infection, autopsy.

CLINICAL DETAILS

Date of Admission: 21.01.2014, Date of Death: 18.02.2014, Duration of Stay: 27 days

A 4-year-old female child presented with history of fever and progressive pallor since 3 months, abdominal distension since 4 days and petechial spots over the lips, oral mucosa and tongue, since one day. She had received three units of blood transfusion during last 3 months, prior to referral to our institute. She was the only child of a nonconsanguineous marriage, was exclusively breast fed and adequately immunized. On ***examination***: Heart rate—136/min, respiratory rate—30/min, temperature—38°C, BP—100/60 mm Hg. There was ecchymosis, oral petechiae, generalized lymphadenopathy and hepatosplenomegaly (6 cm and 3 cm, respectively).

Investigations and Course of Management

Sequential hemograms (Table 1): The hemogram (10 days before admission) done at an outside facility, revealed a very low hemoglobin, thrombocytopenia and 86% lymphocytes. The blasts were counted as lymphocytes. In PGI, at admission the total leukocyte count was high and there were 33% blasts in the peripheral blood (Fig 1A).

Bone marrow examination (P-41/14 done on 21/01/14): Bone marrow aspiration revealed 95% blasts which were myeloperoxidase (MPO) negative (Figs 1B and C).

Flow cytometry: Positive markers—HLA-DR, TdT, CD19, CD10, cCD22, cCD79a, CD34 and CD38. *Negative markers*: MPO, CD13, CD33, CD117, CD20, CD3, CD4, CD8, CD5, CD7 and cCd3.

Final report: Pre-B cell acute lymphoblastic leukemia.

Blood biochemistry: Serum urea went up from 49 mg% to 160 mg%, serum creatinine went up from 0.7 mg% to 1.3 mg%, Na^+/K^+—135/5.1 mEq/L, Ca—8.7 mg% and uric acid—11.1 mg%.

She was started on induction chemotherapy (Regimen B UK ALL protocol) on day third of admission, following which she developed febrile neutropenia on day sixth. Her blood cultures were sterile and galactomannan level was within normal range. Her antibiotics were upgraded to cefoperazone-sulbactam/amikacin. She also developed tumor lysis syndrome on day eight, which was managed with fluids/allopurinol/rasburicase. Febrile neutropenia persisted in the 2nd week, so the antibiotics were further upgraded on day 10 to vancomycin, imipenem and amphotericin B. Induction chemotherapy was stopped on day 14, following which bone marrow examination was repeated on day 15 to look for remission status. The repeat marrow was diluted with blood and no definite opinion was given. Neutropenia persisted in the 3rd week of hospital stay and she developed amphotericin B-induced renal dysfunction. Voriconazole was added, but soon it had to be withdrawn because she developed skin

Table 1: Sequential Hemograms.

Date	*11/01/14 Outside facility*	*21/01/14 PGI*	*Day 13 of induction PGI*	*Day 16 PGI*	*Day 20 PGI*	*Day 24 PGI*
Hb g/dL	3.7	6.4	8.1	8.2	9.8	9.4
TLC/uL	20,600	69,500	700	700	400	400
DLC	P10, L86, M02 E01	BL-33, P09, L50, M07 E01	L10	L8		
Platelets/uL	45,000	35,000	31,000	30,000	41,000	30,000

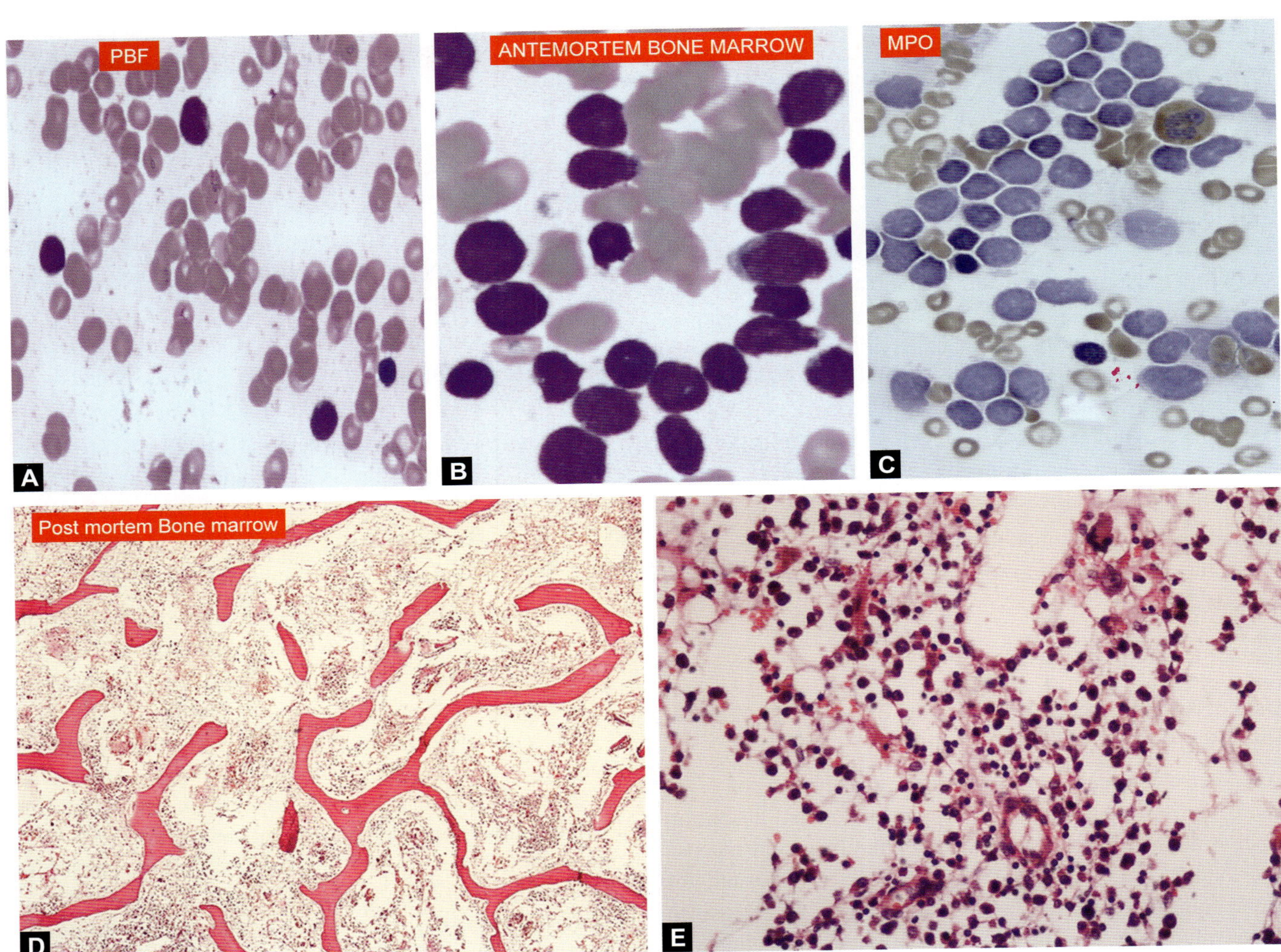

Figs 1A–E: (A) Peripheral blood smear stained with Giemsa shows presence of blasts; (B) Antemortem bone marrow aspirate smear showing sheets of blasts with high N:C ratio, opened up chromatin, conspicuous nucleoli, and scanty agranular cytoplasm. No Auer rods seen; (C) Myeloperoxidase cytochemistry on the aspirate, showing these blasts to be MPO negative; (D) Post mortem bone marrow biopsy showing hypocellular marrow spaces; (E) Higher magnification shows no excess of blasts or immature cells. (Figs 1A–C. *Courtesy* Dr Shano Naseem)

rashes. Skin biopsy was done on day 2 of onset of rash, but did not reveal any granuloma/fungus/leukemic infiltration. On day 20, she developed seizures which were recurrent. Noncontrast computerized tomography of the head was done which was not contributory. Her condition continued to worsen in the 4th week of hospital stay and preterminally was confounded by sepsis/multiple organ dysfunction syndrome (MODS). Galactomannan level was repeated and was found

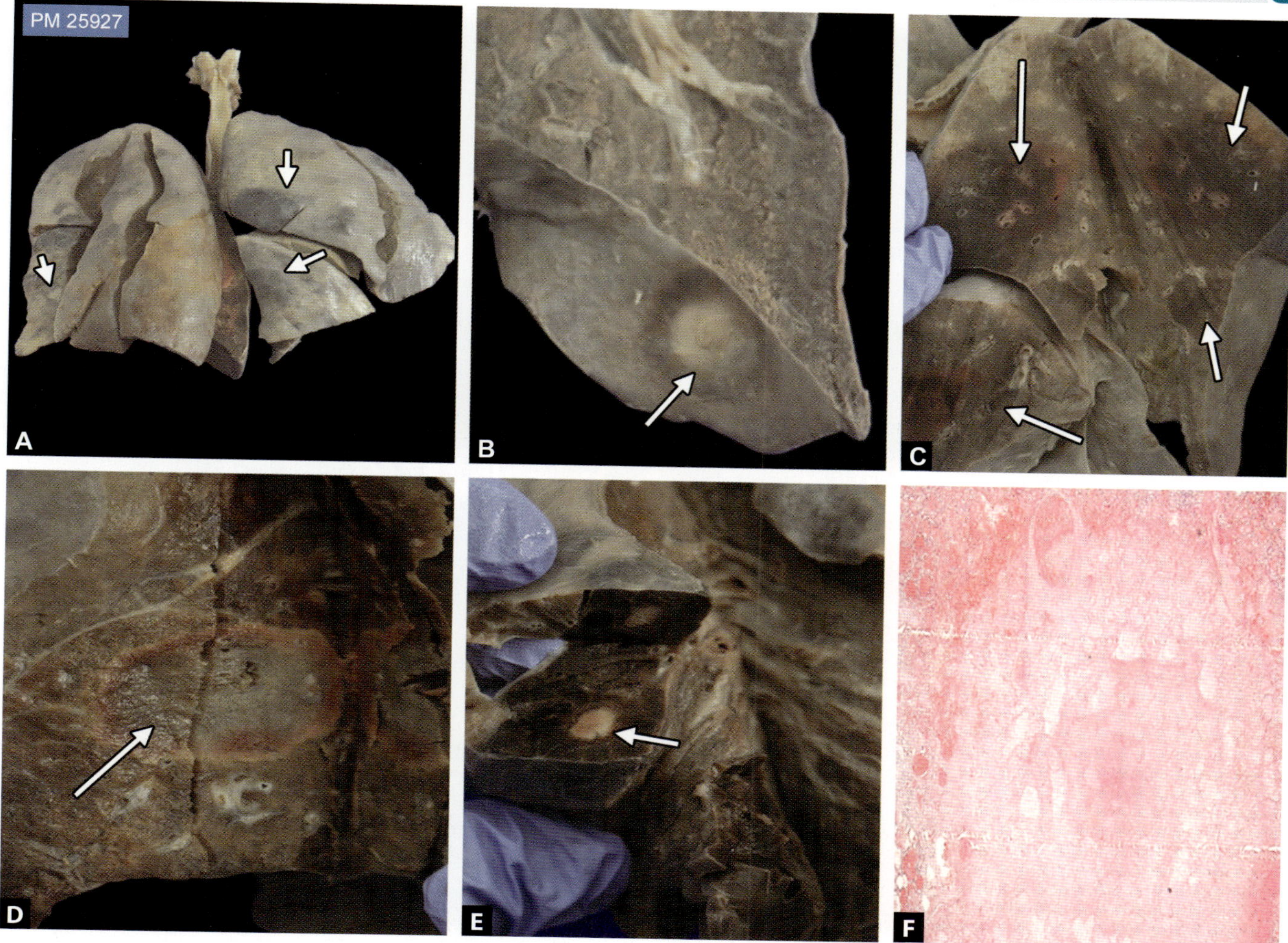

Figs 2A–F: (A) External surface of both the lungs showing nodular grayish-white areas (arrows); (B) Diaphragmatic surface of right lung showing a well-circumscribed grayish white nodular lesion (arrow) measuring 3 × 2.5 cm with surrounding hemorrhagic border; (C) Cut surface of left lung showing diffuse hemorrhagic consolidation (arrow); (D) Cut surface of left lower lobe showing a circumscribed necrotic area (arrow) with hemorrhagic border measuring 2.5 × 2 cm; (E) A subpleural grayish white nodular lesion (arrow) measuring 0.8 cm in diameter; (F) Photomicrograph of the lung showing area of infarction.

to be high, but this report was available after her demise. Final clinical diagnosis was acute lymphoblastic leukemia on treatment, with febrile neutropenia, fungal pneumonia, focal seizure ? CNS Aspergillosis, typhlitis, drug rash, acute respiratory distress syndrome (ARDS) and septic shock. .

AUTOPSY FINDINGS: PM 25927

A complete autopsy was performed on this 4-year-old female child. A diffuse maculopapular skin rash was noted. There was 200 mL of straw-colored fluid in each pleural cavity and 1,000 mL of hemorrhagic fluid in the peritoneal cavity. The pericardial cavity was within normal limits. The post mortem ***bone marrow*** (Figs 1D and E) was hypocellular with no excess of blasts. The ***lungs*** (Figs 2A–E) weighed 424 g and were subcrepitant to feel. The pleural aspect was dull and showed areas of thickening and nodular firm lesions. Cut section showed well-circumscribed necrotic lesion, with surrounding hemorrhagic border measuring 3 × 2.5 cm. In addition scattered, whitish nodules measuring 0.8–1.2 cm in diameter were seen in both the lungs. On microscopy, large areas of bland necrosis (Fig. 2F) bordered by hemorrhagic areas were seen. These necrotic areas (Figs. 3A to C) were replete with long, thin, slender, fungal hyphae showing septations and acute angle branching, conforming to the morphology of *Aspergillus*. The fungal profiles were better highlighted by periodic acid–Schiff

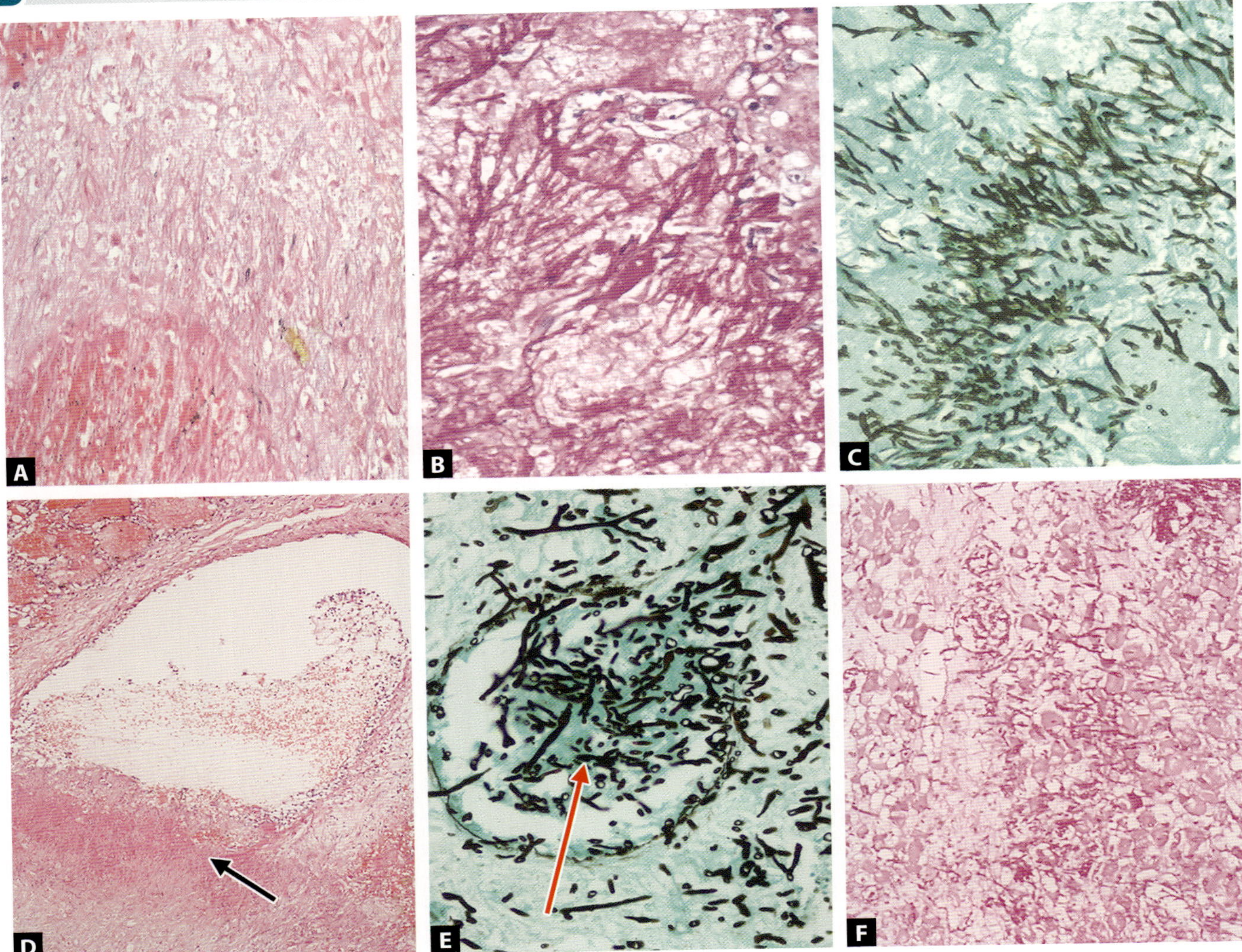

Figs 3A–F: Photomicrographs of the lung show (A) Areas of infarction replete with fungal profiles; (B) Periodic acid–Schiff (PAS) stain highlights the fungal hyphae, which are long, thin with septations and acute angle branching, conforming to morphology of *Aspergillus*; (C) Grocott stain showing acute angle branching fungal hyphae; (D) Fungal profiles seen invading and destroying the wall of vein (arrow); (E) Grocott stain showing fungal hyphae invading the blood vessel (red arrow); (F) PAS stain showing similar fungal profiles in the wall of the diaphragm.

and Grocotts stains. These fungal hyphae were seen to invade the pulmonary vessels (Figs. 3D and E). Giant cell reaction, pulmonary hemorrhage and pulmonary edema were also seen. The ***diaphragm*** (Fig. 3F) showed similar well-circumscribed necrotic lesions and microscopically showed muscle necrosis and invasion by *Aspergillus*. The ***esophagus*** (Fig. 4A) showed multiple superficial ulcers which on microscopy revealed fungal hyphae of *Aspergillus*. The mucosa of ***stomach*** (Figs. 4B to D) was congested and the serosal aspect showed a well-circumscribed necrotic lesion measuring 2.5 cm in diameter, which on microscopy showed serosal vessels clogged with fungal hyphae (arrows), which were making their way into the muscularis propria and the submucosa. The ***small and large intestine*** (Figs. 4E and F; Figs. 5A to C) showed multiple ulcers ranging in size from 2 cm to 4 cm in diameter. The ulcer base was necrotic, at times rimmed by hemorrhagic area. Microscopy revealed transmural hemorrhagic necrosis replete with fungal hyphae of *aspergillus*, showing extensive angioinvasion. The ***liver*** weighed 880 g and was normal grossly. There was mild portal inflammation, macrovesicular steatosis, centrizonal hemorrhagic necrosis indicating shock, hemosiderin laden macrophages (Perl's positive) in the sinuses and no

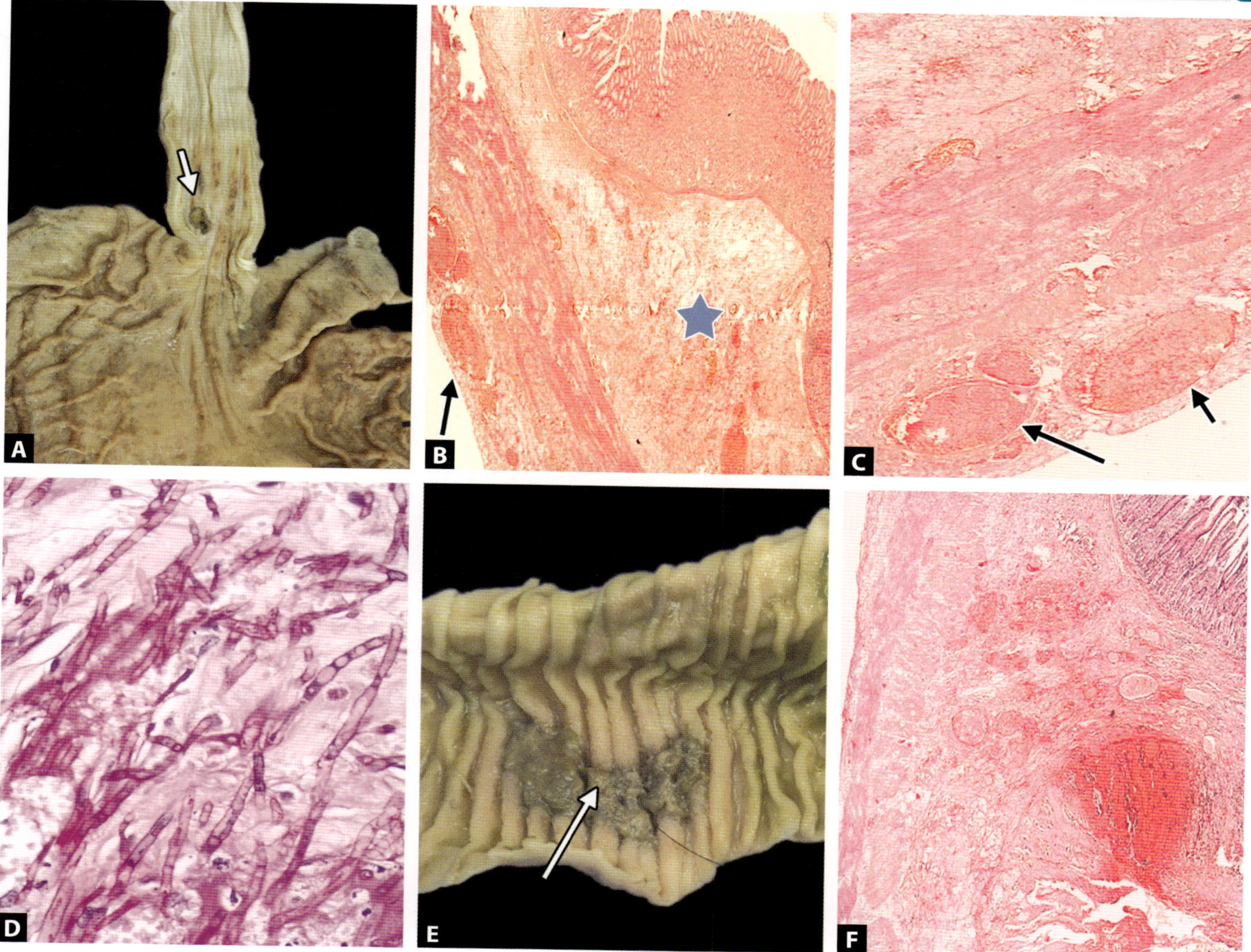

Figs 4A–F: (A) Hemorrhagic ulcer (arrow) seen at gastroesophageal junction measuring 5 mm. Mucosa of stomach is congested and shows pin point hemorrhages; (B) Photomicrograph of stomach shows infarcted muscularis propria and serosa (arrow). Submucosa is edematous (star); (C) Higher magnification of 4B showing serosal vessels (arrow) clogged with thrombi containing fungal profiles; (D) Periodic acid–Schiff stain showing *Aspergillus hyphae* in the wall of the stomach; (E) Jejunum showing a deep mucosal ulcer (arrow) covered with necrotic slough; (F) Photomicrograph of the jejunum showing transmural infarction of the wall. The submucosal vessels are completely occluded with thrombi replete with fungal profiles.

infiltration by any atypical cell. The ***spleen*** was enlarged and weighed 106 g. Microscopy revealed marked congested red pulp with relative depletion of white pulp. The ***kidneys*** showed blotchy congestion. On microscopy the glomeruli were normal and tubules showed shedding of tubular epithelial cells indicating acute tubular necrosis. Peritubular capillaries were congested and showed nucleated red cells. Interstitium showed hemosiderin laden macrophages. The brain was normal grossly and on microscopic examination. The lymph nodes were not enlarged and did not reveal any atypical cell.

FINAL AUTOPSY DIAGNOSIS: PM 25927

4 Years Female, c/o Pre B All on Induction Therapy

- Hypocellular bone marrow with no excess of blasts.
- Disseminated angioinvasive aspergillosis: Lungs, gastrointestinal (esophagus, stomach, small and large intestine) and diaphragm
- Alveolar hemorrhages and pulmonary edema
- Centrizonal hemorrhagic necrosis and steatosis—liver
- Secondary hemosiderosis—liver and kidneys
- Early acute tubular necrosis—kidneys.

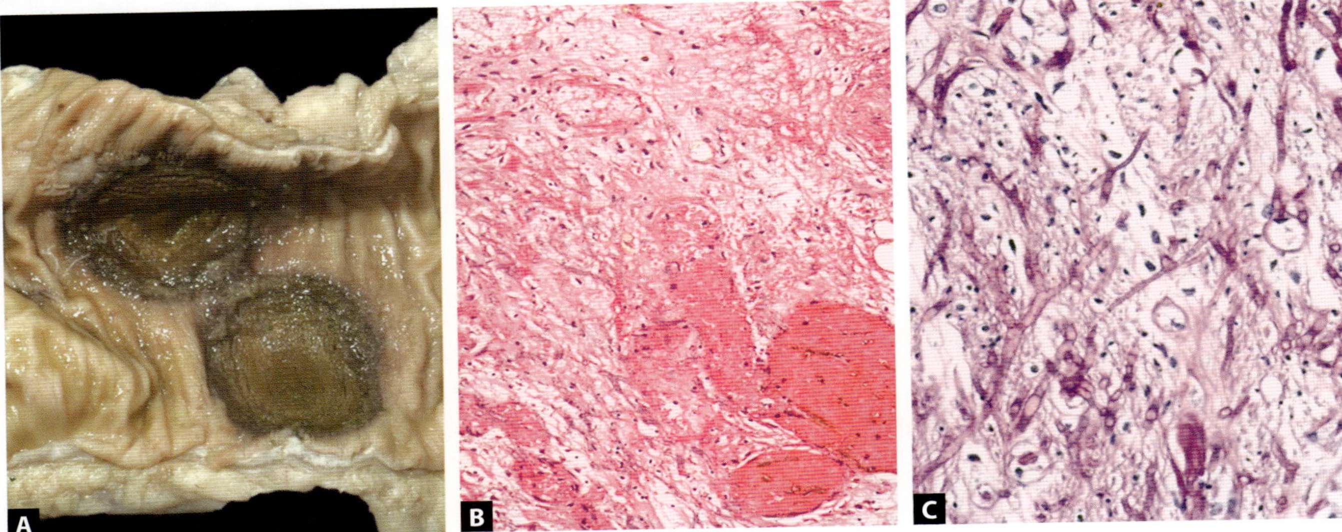

Figs 5A–C: (A) Large intestine showing multiple well-circumscribed deep mucosal ulcers with necrotic centre and hemorrhagic border measuring 3-4 cm in diameter; (B and C) Microphotographs of the ulcers show bland necrosis, vascular thrombi, and Aspergillus hyphae.

FEBRILE NEUTROPENIA

Neutropenia is an abnormally low level of neutrophils, in adults less than 1,500 neutrophils/μL and in children it varies with age. However, counts less than 500 are always considered to be neutropenia (Mayo clinic). Profound neutropenia is said to be present when absolute neutrophil count (ANC) is less than 100/μL of blood. Febrile neutropenia is one of the most devastating complications of cancer chemotherapy. It increases the incidence of bacterial and fungal infection. The risk of infection is directly related to degree and the duration of neutropenia. Studies have shown that infection is the major cause of treatment-related mortality in pediatric acute lymphoblastic leukemia and is greatest during the induction phase. Absolute neutrophil counts less than 500, predisposes to infection. Recovery of counts within a week has lesser complications. The spectrum of causative organisms among bacterial infection ranges from Gram-positive cocci, including methicillin-resistant *Staphylococcus aureus* and coagulase negative *Staphylococcus species* to Gram-negative bacilli including *Escherichia coli*, Klebsiella species and *Pseudomonas aeruginosa*. Prolonged neutropenia leads to fulminant fungal infections with Candida, *Aspergillus*, Cryptococcus neoformans and the Phycomycetes. An estimated cause specific mortality due to invasive fungal infection is found to be around 35%.

COMMENTARY—INDEX CASE: PM 25927

This 4-year-old female child presented with history of fever and progressive pallor since 3 months and petechiae since one day. She had generalized lymphadenopathy and hepatosplenomegaly. At admission the peripheral blood revealed 33% blasts and the bone marrow showed 95%, MPO negative blasts. Flow cytometry was performed and a diagnosis of Pre-B cell acute lymphoblastic leukemia was made and she was put on induction chemotherapy (Regimen B UK ALL protocol). She was detected to have febrile neutropenia on day 6 and this persisted till her demise. All measures were taken to avoid infection, but despite everything she developed a disseminated *Aspergillus* infection and succumbed to her illness. The galactomannan level was initially negative, but the sample tested just before her demise was positive. She also had renal dysfunction and seizures. Autopsy revealed a disseminated angioinvasive aspergillosis involving the lungs and the gastrointestinal tract along with acute tubular necrosis and features of shock.

TAKE HOME MESSAGE

- Febrile neutropenia is one of the most devastating complications of cancer chemotherapy.

- High-risk patients are those who have persistent neutropenia for more than 7 days and are most vulnerable to bacterial and fungal infections. .

SUGGESTED READING

1. Auberger J, Lass-Florl C, Ulmer H, et al. Significant alterations in the epidemiology and treatment outcome of invasive fungal infections in patients with hematological malignancies. Int J Hematol. 2008;88:508-15.
2. Bhatt VR, Viola GM, Ferrajoli A. Invasive fungal infections in acute leukemia. Ther Adv Hematol. 2011;2:231-47.
3. Kern WV. Risk assessment and treatment of low-risk patients with febrile neutropenia. Clin Infect Dis. 2006;42:533-40.
4. O'Connor D, Bate J, Wade R, et al. Infection-related mortality in children with acute lymphoblastic leukemia: an analysis of infectious deaths on UKALL2003. Blood. 2014;124:1056-61.
5. Sharma A, Lokeshwar N. Febrile neutropenia in haematological malignancies. J Postgrad Med. 2005;51:S42-8.

CONTRIBUTIONS BY:

1. Dr Khushboo, Junior Resident, Department of Pathology (In taking Photographs)
2. Dr Aseem Bassha M, Junior Resident, Department of Pediatrics (Compilation of Clinical Details)
3. Dr Sudha Sharma, Senior Resident, Department of Pathology (In working up the Case)
4. Dr Shano Naseem, Associate Professor, Department of Hematology (Figs 1A–C)

Post Graduate Institute of Medical Education and Research, Chandigarh, India.

CASE 68

Myeloid Sarcoma of Lacrimal Sac as the First Manifestation of AML-M1 with Acute Diffuse Colorectal Neutropenic Colitis in a Child: PM 23395

Nandita Bharadwaj Kakkar

HIGHLIGHTS OF THE CASE

This is a story of a 10-year-old female child who presented to the ophthalmology department of PGIMER in May 2009, with watering and inner canthal swelling of the right eye, since 3 months. Biopsy of the swelling revealed a low-grade mucosa-associated lymphoid tissue (MALT) lymphoma and the patient was referred to the radiotherapy department. Three months later, the peripheral blood film revealed atypical cells, a bone marrow was done which confirmed a diagnosis of acute myeloid leukemia-without maturation (AML-M1) and she was put on treatment. The lacrimal mass was reviewed and the diagnosis was revised to a myeloid sarcoma (MPO++). She was started on chemotherapy and went into febrile neutropenia by the end of the induction therapy. Repeat bone marrow at this point showed her to be in remission. She recovered from neutropenia and became afebrile. She was then given the second course of chemotherapy. She again developed fever, 10 days after start of second course and within 11 hours succumbed to her illness. At the time of death, she was severely neutropenic, but was not on antibiotics. Autopsy in this child, a case of AML-M1 on treatment with first presentation as a blastic type of myeloid sarcoma of the lacrimal gland, showed florid acute diffuse colorectal neutropenic colitis.

Keywords: Acute myeloid leukemia, myeloid sarcoma, chloroma, granulocytic sarcoma, extramedullary myeloid tumor, neutropenic colitis, diffuse, colorectal, autopsy.

CLINICAL DETAILS

Date of Admission: 22.08.09, Date of Death: 30.10.09, Duration of Hospital Stay: 68 Days.

A 10-year-old female child presented to the ophthalmology department of PGIMER in May 2009 with watering and inner canthal swelling of the right eye since 3 months. The watering was persistent and unilateral with no visual disturbances. The swelling was insidious in onset, slowly progressive and lemon-sized. There was no history of fever, nasal symptoms or any headache. There was no report of a hemogram at this time. Computerized tomography of the nose/paranasal sinuses/orbit was done on the 12th May 2009 which revealed a soft tissue lesion in region of right lacrimal sac with contiguous bony thinning and extension into the nasolacrimal duct and right orbit, ? chronic dacryocystitis, ?? neoplastic. An endoscopic biopsy of the swelling was done on the 7th July 2009 which was diagnosed as a low grade MALT lymphoma and the patient was referred to the radiotherapy department in August 2009. A CT chest/abdomen (12.8.09, for staging) was normal except for the presence of small pretracheal and right hilar lymph nodes, largest measuring 1.3 cm. At this point of time, a hemogram was done which revealed atypical cells and she was then referred to the pediatric oncology department. ***On examination***: heart rate—90/min, RR—22/min, afebrile, BP—88/62 mm Hg, weight—22 kg (67% of expected), height—134 cm (97% of expected), mild pallor and no icterus/cyanosis. There was a 3 × 3 cm hard, lobulated swelling in right nasolacrimal region with no signs of inflammation. Right pre-auricular/submandibular lymph nodes were mildly enlarged (0.5–1 cm) and firm/hard to feel. The chest, CVS, CNS and abdomen were within normal limits. There was no organomegaly.

Investigations

Hemogram—Table 1. On 6th August, the peripheral blood film revealed atypical cells and low platelets. On the 24th August 2009, there were 77% blasts in the peripheral blood, a bone marrow (P 303/2009) was done and a diagnosis of AML–M1 was given (Figs 1D).

Table 1: Serial hemograms.

Date	*Time course*	*Hb g/dL*	*TLC/μL*	*DLC*	*Platelets × 10³*
6.8.09	Radiotherapy OPD	10.3	5,400	$N_4L_{64}M_2$ Atypical$_{30}$	135
24.8.09	Pediatric oncology	9.4	4,800	$N_6L_{15}M_1E_1$ Blasts$_{77}$	82
13.9.09	Start of induction	10.6	5,900	$N_{67}L_{23}M_3E_2$ Blasts$_3$	39
23.9.09	Induction completed	7.3	1,200	N_4L_{21}	13
1.10.09	Febrile neutropenia	11.2	800	N_5L_{45}	2
5.10.09	Febrile neutropenia	9.1	1,100	$N_{15}L_5M_5$	37
19.10.09	Start: 2nd course chemotherapy	11.4	13,800	$N_{72}L_{21}M_4E_2My_1$	606
26.10.09	End of chemo-2	10.1	4,300	$N_{66}L_{30}M_2E_2$	181
29.10.09	1 day prior to death	10.4	500	Too low	60

(DLC: Differential leukocyte count; Hb: Hemoglobin; OPD: Oligoprogressive disease; TLC: Total lymphocyte counts).

She was started on chemotherapy and went into febrile neutropenia (Table 1).

Antemortem Right Lacrimal Sac Biopsy (S-9286/09)

Lacrimal mass showed a small blue round cell tumor and a whole lot of immunostains were done initially—CD99, desmin, pan-cytokeratin (pan-CK), myogenin, CD68, CD34, CD20 and CD3 were all negative. CD79a was focally positive and these cells were seen to infiltrate the lining epithelium and a suggestion of low grade MALT lymphoma was given. Myeloid sarcoma was not thought of initially. After a diagnosis of AML-M1 was made, on the bone marrow immunostain for myeloperoxidase was done 'on the lacrimal mass' which was strongly positive and the diagnosis was revised to myeloid sarcoma (Figs 1A–C).

Check bone marrow P-371/2009 (19.10.2009, 5 weeks from first chemotherapy): In remission. ***CSF for malignant cytology***: 13.9.2009; No malignant cells. 19.10.2009: Traumatic tap. ***Blood biochemistry***: serum Na+ ranged from 143–137 U/L, K+ 4.3–3.4 U/L, serum urea—18–108 mg%, serum creatinine—0.6–1.1 mg% and liver function tests were within normal limits.

Course in Hospital

After the induction therapy, there was febrile neutropenia which took 26 days to recover. The second course of chemotherapy was given and a day prior to her death, the TLC was 500/μL with undetectable neutrophils. She was given UK MRC AML XII protocol: daunorubicin—3 doses, cytarabine—10 days, etoposide—5 days and triple intrathecal chemotherapy (methotrexate, cytarabine and hydrocortisone). There was fever on day 4 of chemotherapy along with swelling/pain in the left arm. Cefoperazone, sulbactam, amikacin and cloxacin were started. There was mild cough, but the chest X-ray was normal. Antimicrobials were switched to vancomycin/meropenem/amphotericin after 7 days, as fever was persisting, with worsening neutropenia. Cellulitis (induration and tenderness) of arm continued to be a problem. Amphotericin was stopped after 6 days for deranged renal functions and then restarted after a gap of 8 days. Chloroquine was given empirically. Chest X-ray (7.10.09): left upper zone opacity, CT lungs (14.10.09): 1 × 1 cm cavitary lesion in the anterior segment of left upper lobe with evidence of soft tissue contents within it ? fungal ball. The child became afebrile after 3 weeks, counts recovered, vancomycin and meropenem were stopped and the eye swelling subsided completely. Blood culture done six times were sterile. Urine culture (8.10.09) grew Candida albicans. She was given septran and itraconazole prophylaxis, nasogastric feeds and physiotherapy for contracture in arm, blood transfusions and platelets. Second course of chemotherapy was given (19.10.2009 onward) which was uneventfully over 8 days. She was afebrile throughout. Amphotericin was switched to oral voriconazole (for ? fungal ball) after a duration of 20 days. She developed fever 10 days after start of second course and within 11 hours there was sudden worsening of sensorium, vacant look and gasping respiration. She was intubated, went into shock, inotropes were administered but she succumbed to her illness. At the time of death, she was severely neutropenic and was not on antibiotics. ***Units final clinical diagnosis*** was AML-M1, Bone marrow in remission following first course of chemotherapy, cavitary lesion—left upper lobe lung ? fungal ball. Cause of death— ? intracranial bleed ? invasive CNS fungal infection.

AUTOPSY FINDINGS: PM 23395

A complete autopsy was performed. The serous cavities did not reveal any excess of fluid. The postmortem bone marrow

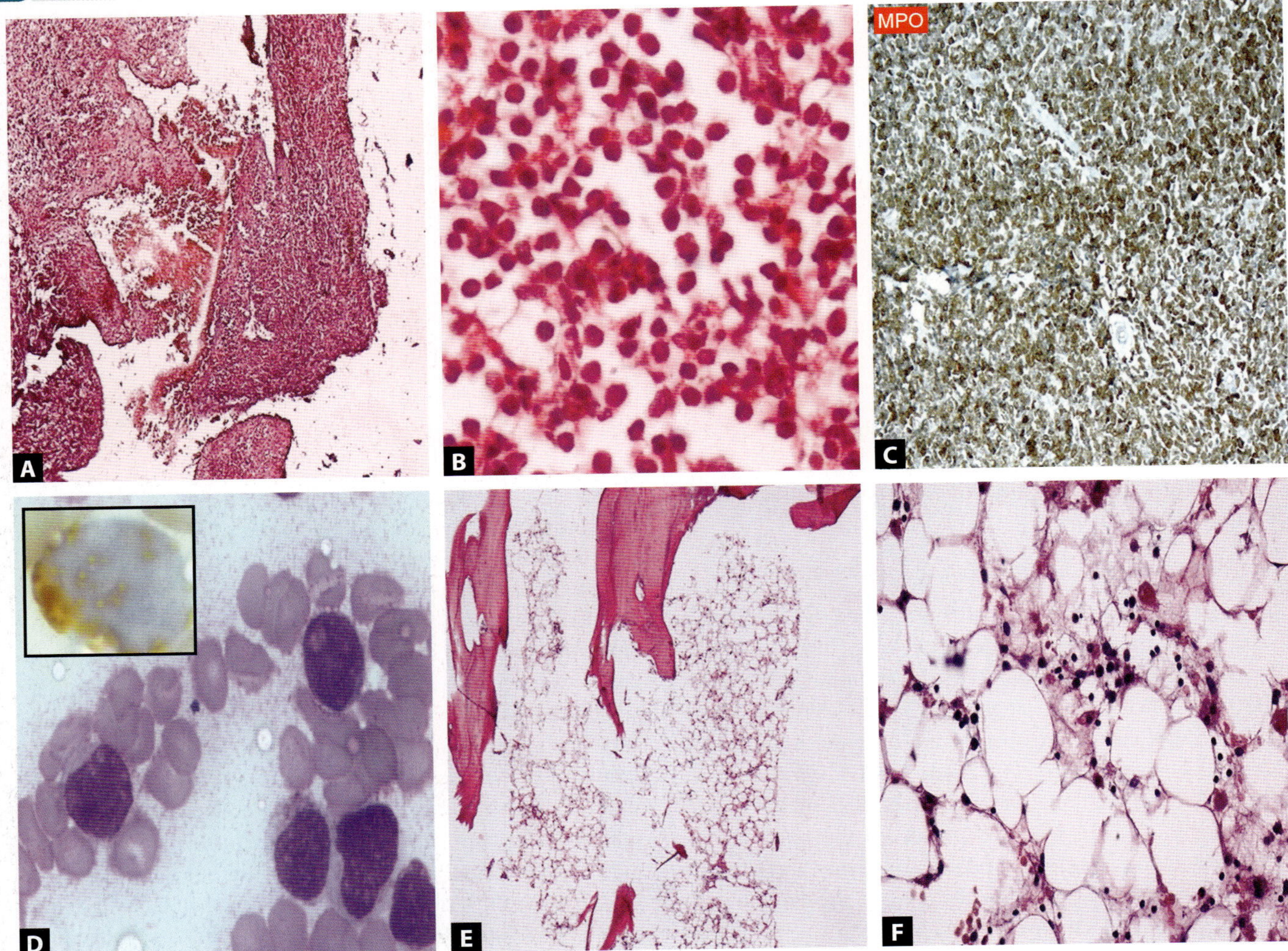

Figs 1A–F: (A and B) Photomicrograph from the lacrimal mass show sheets of small blue round cells with high N/C ratio; (C) Myeloperoxidase stain showing positivity in the small blue round cells; (D) Bone marrow (antemortem) shows presence of myeloid blasts positive for myeloperoxidase (inset); (E and F) Postmortem bone marrow section shows a markedly hypocellular marrow showing few lymphocytes and erythroid series of cells. No atypical cell seen.

(Figs 1E and F) was markedly hypocellular. Few lymphocytes, macrophages and erythroid series of cells were seen. No megakaryocyte was appreciated, Prussian blue stain for iron was 1+ and reticulin was 1+. The ***liver*** weighed 640 g (Figs 2A and B) and ***spleen*** weighed 40 g (Figs 2A, C and D), were grossly and microscopically normal. No atypical cells were seen. The spleen showed focal extramedullary hematopoiesis and increased iron on Perl's stain. ***Lymph nodes*** showed sinus histiocytosis. No atypical cells were seen. Lungs on the pleural surface showed hemorrhages. Cut section (Fig 2E) showed extensive hemorrhages and a 1 cm diameter cavity containing whitish material in the left upper lobe (white arrow). There was no thromboembolism. Microscopic examination (Figs 2F and G) revealed extensive edema and pulmonary hemorrhages (left > right), evidence of aspiration and aspergilloma in the left upper lobe (Fig 2H). ***Gastrointestinal tract***—the stomach and esophagus showed areas of congestion and areas of submucosal hemorrhages. The entire colon (Fig 3A) was involved starting from the ileocecal valve right till the rectum, in a diffuse manner. The wall of the colon was thickened, but the serosa was normal. The small intestine (Fig 3B) was unremarkable. Grossly the mucosa of the colon (Figs 3C and D, Figs 4A and B) showed diffuse areas of hemorrhagic necrosis, raised umbilicated well-circumscribed hemorrhagic lesions 0.2–0.6 cm in diameter with intervening normal mucosa. There were diffuse areas of fibrinopurulent exudates adherent over the necrotic and edematous mucosa, forming yellowish membranes. Microscopic examination (Figs 5A–D) revealed a bland (no inflammation) hemorrhagic/nonhemorrhagic necrosis

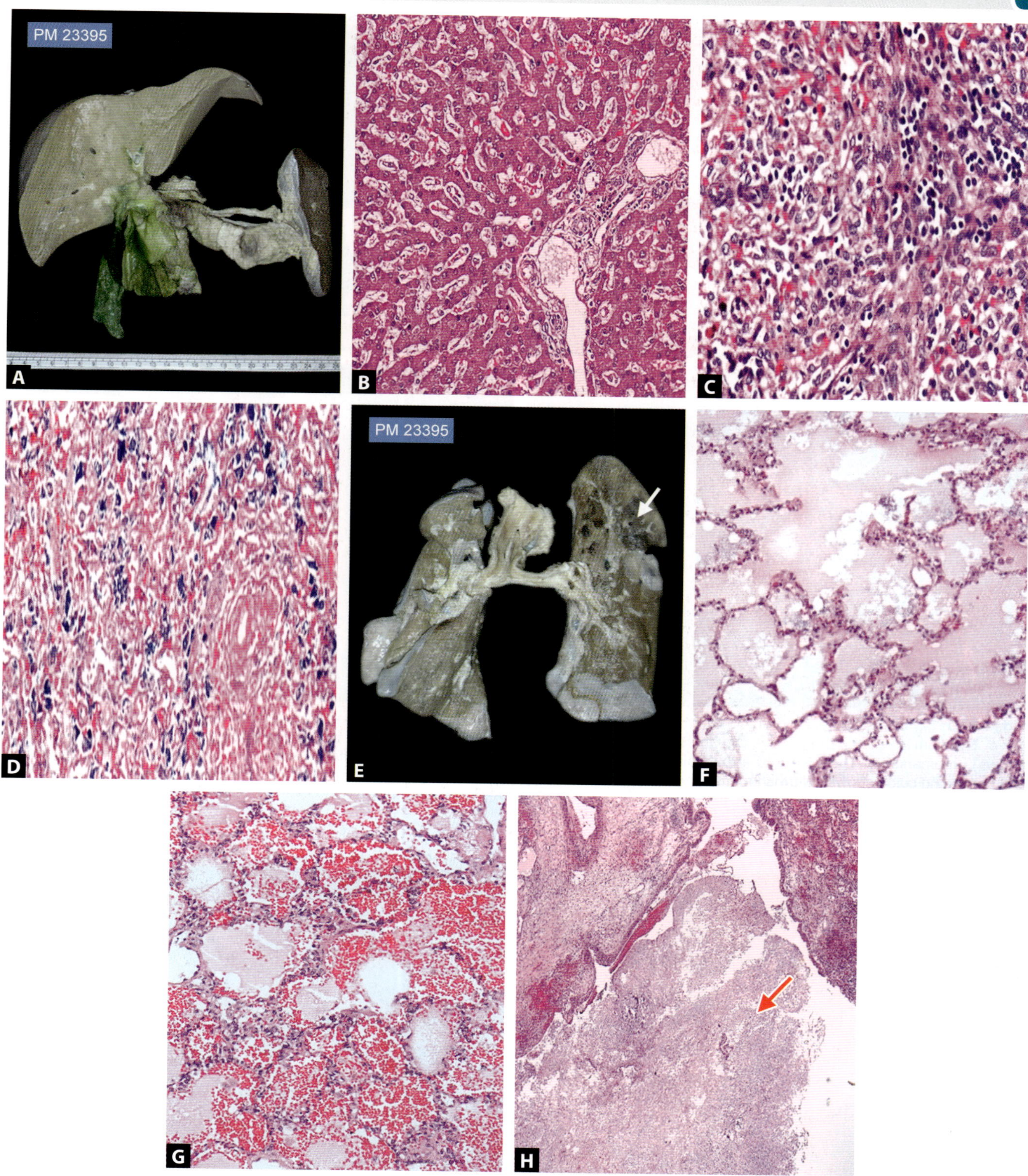

Figs 2A–H: (A) Organ complex comprising of slice of liver, spleen, gall bladder, and pancreas. No focal lesion seen; (B) Photomicrograph of the liver shows no atypical cell in the portal tract/sinusoids; (C) Section of spleen shows foci of extramedullary hematopoiesis. No atypical cell seen; (D) Spleen shows 2–3 + Fe (Prussian blue stain); (E) Cut section of lungs shows areas of hemorrhage in the left upper lobe and a cavity (arrow). Photomicrographs of the lung showing; (F) Pulmonary edema; (G) Alveolar hemorrhage; and (H) Cavity with fungal ball (aspergilloma) (red arrow).

CASE 69

Niemann–Pick Disease Type B Presenting with Massive Splenohepatomegaly and Hypertensive Crisis in a 12-year-old Child: PM 27096

Nandita Bharadwaj Kakkar

HIGHLIGHTS OF THE CASE

This is the story of a 12-year-old female child, a clinically diagnosed case of Niemann–Pick type B (NPB). She had a 9-year-old male sibling with similar disease who died one week after her demise. The index child was neurodevelopmentally normal, had stunted growth, coarse facial features, massive splenomegaly, hepatomegaly, mitral valve prolapse and hypertensive blood pressure record. Investigations revealed pancytopenia, transaminitis and deranged lipidogram. Autopsy showed characteristic Niemann–Pick (NP) cells widely distributed in almost all organs, sparing however the brain. The degree of lung involvement was out of proportion to the mild exertional dyspnea that this patient had. The mitral valve prolapse was present and microscopy of the valve revealed a unique finding of myxomatous degeneration with clusters of NP cells. Liver revealed stage 4 fibrosis, with occasional nodule formation. The mesangium of the glomeruli showed the presence of clusters of NP cells. Could this be the cause of hypertension, is a speculation. The terminal event in the index case was a hypertensive crisis followed by abdominal bleed. Large blood clots were found in the abdomen at autopsy, but the source of the bleed could not be ascertained. The male sibling also presented with hypertensive crisis, but an autopsy was not done.

Keywords: Niemann–Pick type B, hypertensive crisis, mitral valve prolapse showing Niemann–Pick cells, mesangial Niemann–Pick cells, abdominal bleed, autopsy.

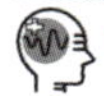

CLINICAL DETAILS

Date of Admission: 16.12.2015, Date of Death: 19.12.2015, Duration of Hospital Stay: 3 Days

A 12-year-old female child, who was developmentally normal, presented with progressive abdominal distension which started at one year of age. The distension was gradually progressive, localized to the upper part of abdomen and was not associated with abdominal pain, vomiting, urinary retention or respiratory difficulty. Since past one year mild periorbital puffiness was noted. There was a history of poor linear growth, but there was no history of jaundice, bleeding manifestations, previous blood transfusions, decreased visual acuity, seizures, loss of consciousness, hypoglycemia, paraesthesia, pedal edema, anasarca, pains or any previous hospitalization. She was born to a nonconsanguineously married couple and her birth and development history was normal. She had a similarly affected younger brother who was also noticed to have progressive abdominal distension form infancy. Both the siblings were developmentally normal and attended regular school. On examination she weighed 26 kg (<3rd centile), height was 129 cm (< 3rd centile) and head circumference was 51 cm (between mean and -2SD). The blood pressure was 130/90 mm Hg. There was mild periorbital puffiness, thickened skin, absence of subcutaneous fat and subtle facial dysmorphism in the form of receding hairline, prominent forehead, long philtrum and thin upper lip. Massive firm hepatomegaly (span 16 cm) and splenomegaly (span 21 cm) was present. Cardiovascular examination showed short systolic murmur at cardiac apex. Other systemic examination was normal.

Investigations and Course of Management

Hemogram: Hemoglobin—11.8 g/dL, TLC—3,500/µL, DLC—N32, L65, M3, platelet counts—67,000/µL, ESR—35. ***Biochemistry:*** Na^+—137 mEq/L, K^+—4.7 mEq/L, Cl—107 mEq/L, urea—16 mg%, creatinine—0.2 mg%, Total serum protein - 7.1 gms, albumin - 4.2 gms. Aspartate aminotransferase (AST)—56 U/L, alanine aminotransferase (ALT)—67 U/L, alkaline phosphatase (ALP)—151 U/L, uric acid—2.8 mg% and serum amylase—445 U/L. Coagulogram: PT—18 seconds, aPTT—43 seconds, PTI—72%, INR—1.35, Rendom blood sugar - 192 mg%. Lipid profile: cholesterol—187 mg%, LDL—121 mg%, HDL—very low, triglycerides—243 mg%, Routine urine examination: normal. ***Radiology:*** Chest X-ray—mildly increased interstitial infiltrates and X-ray spine was normal. ***USG abdomen*** showed hepatomegaly (size 21 cm, normal echotexture), gall bladder was distended and splenomegaly (size 22 cm and normal echotexture). Right kidney measured 9.8 cm and left kidney 9.9 cm, both were normal in size and shape. Portal vein was normal in size. ***Electrocardiogram*** was normal, ***Echocardiogram*** showed mitral valve prolapse with moderate mitral regurgitation and normal left ventricular ejection fraction. ***Upper GI endoscopy:*** showed normal esophagus, nodularity of antral mucosa. Duodenum showed thickened mucosal folds with nodularity. Duodenal biopsy showed collection of large foamy cells with finely vacuolated cytoplasm in the lamina propria.

The child underwent upper gastrointestinal endoscopy. Subsequently after few hours, she started having intractable vomiting. Blood pressure at that time was 160/140 mm Hg and she soon became encephalopathic. She was started on intravenous labetalol infusion for hypertensive crisis. Blood pressure was controlled and her encephalopathy and irritability improved for few hours. Within 6 hours of infusion she had precipitous fall in blood pressure, infusion was stopped, fluid boluses were given and dopamine infusion was started. She became pale, unresponsive and her blood pressure was not recordable. She required intubation however, had bradycardia and cardiac arrest. ***Units final diagnosis:*** Lysosomal storage disorder ? Niemann–Pick disease type B ?? glycogen storage disorder ??? and mucopolysaccharidoses. ***Cause of death:*** accelerated hypertension with possible cardiac event/ intracranial/major internal hemorrhage.

Investigations in Sibling of Index Patient

Younger brother (9 years old) of the index child also had a similar problem with abdominal distention noticed from infancy. He was admitted in pediatric emergency at the same time with acute severe headache and seizures Anthropometry was suggestive of short stature and normal head size. He also had massive hepatosplenomegaly and hypertensive blood pressure records (BP 218/135 mm Hg). He was managed in pediatric intensive care unit for hypertensive emergency and subsequently had worsening respiratory distress and required intubation and mechanical ventilation. Investigations revealed anemia (Hb: 9.7 g/dL), leucopenia (TLC: 3,900/µL) and thrombocytopenia (29,000/µL). Biochemistry revealed elevated urea—130 mg% and creatinine—0.76 mg%. Total serum protein was 7.2 gm%, serum albumin was 2.2 gm%, total serum bilirubin was 2.2 mg% and conjugated fraction was 1.1 mg%. AST was 113 U/L, ALT was 59 U/L and ALP was 71 U/L. Lipid profile total cholesterol—171 mg%, triglycerides—281 mg%, LDL—60 mg% cholesterol and HDL—5 mg%.

Bone marrow biopsy showed normocellular marrow with abundant large periodic acid–Schiff (PAS) negative foamy histiocytes suggestive of Niemann–Pick disease (NPD). Further investigation showed negative urinary glycosaminoglycans (GAGs), normal levels of enzyme acid sphingomyelinase (ASM) assay and enzyme beta-glucosidase. He had worsening respiratory distress and required high frequency ventilation. He showed features of restrictive interstitial lung disease and died with respiratory failure, one week after the demise of his sister. Autopsy was not on him.

AUTOPSY FINDINGS: PM 27096

A complete autopsy was performed on this 12-year-old female child. She was a short-statured child. The pericardial and pleural cavities were within normal limits. The abdomen yielded 50 mL of blood and large blood clots were present adherent to the intestine, kidney, ureter and urinary bladder. The ***bone marrow*** (Figs 1A–C) showed plenty of characteristic NP cells, which are large lipid laden, foamy histiocytes, 40–75 µm in size, having an eccentric nucleus. These cells contained innumerable small vacuoles of uniform size, which are the distended lysosomes containing sphingomyelin, cholesterol, glycolipid and acylglyceropyrophosphate. The ***liver*** (Figs 1D and E) weighed 2,600 gm. It was pale and no focal lesion was identified. The portal vein and the biliary system were within normal limits. Microscopic examination revealed expansion of the portal tracts and porto-portal and porto-central bridging fibrosis (Stage 4) with occasional nodule formation (Figs 2A and B). The fibrosis was highlighted on reticulin and Masson trichrome stains (Figs 2C and D). The sinusoids were dilated and packed with the characteristic NP cells (Figs 3A and B), forming nodules in

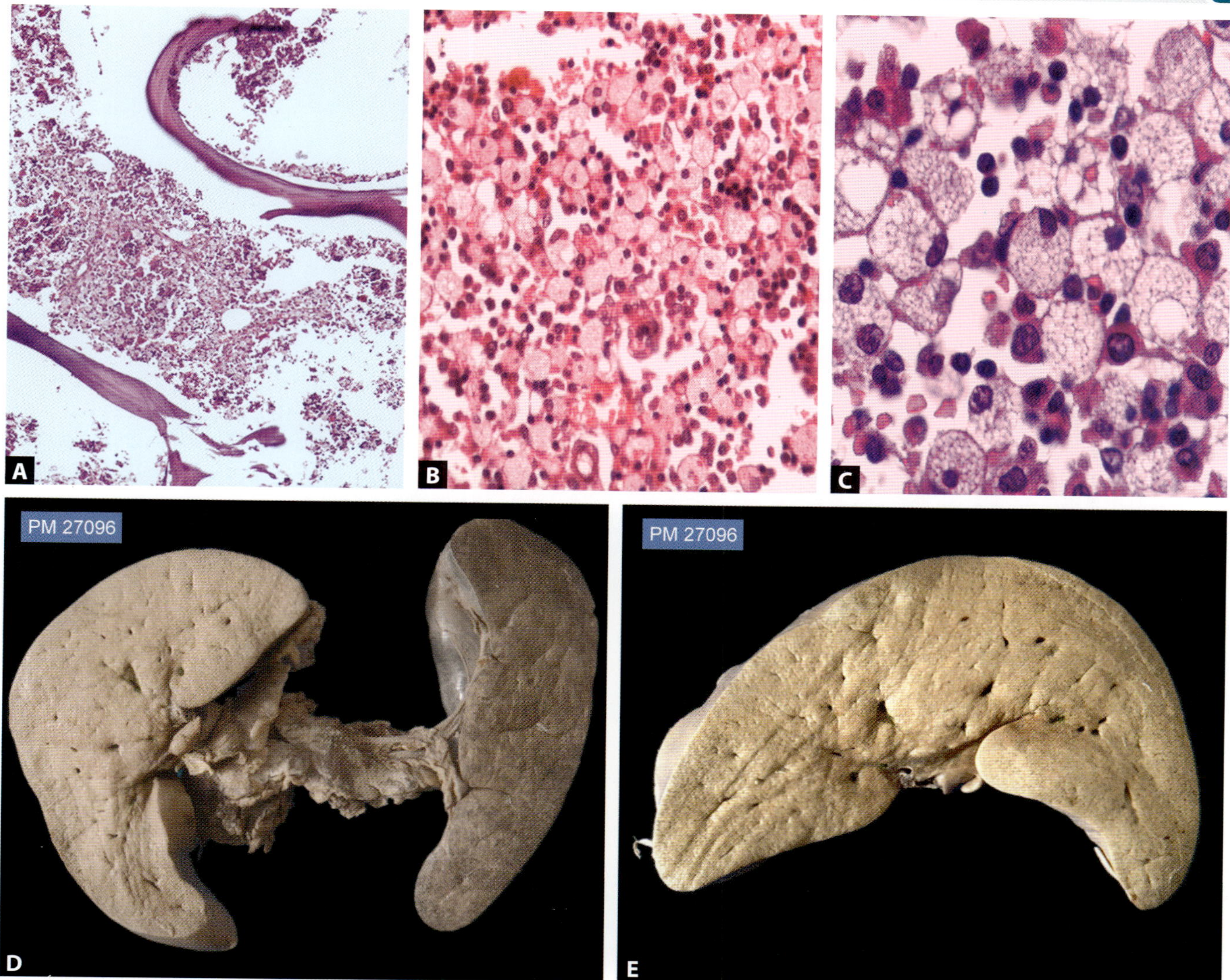

Figs 1A–E: (A to C) Bone marrow at various powers showing characteristic Niemann–Pick cells admixed with hematopoietic elements; (D) Organ complex comprising of slice of the diffusely enlarged liver and spleen along with the pancreas and gall bladder. The spleen is as big as the liver; (E) Coronal slice of the diffusely enlarged pale liver. No focal lesion is seen.

areas. These are the Kupffer cells, wherein the lysosomal accumulation of sphingomyelin, cholesterol, glycolipid and acylglyceropyrophosphate has imparted the characteristic foaminess. The NP cells were PAS negative (Fig 3C) and stood out very prominently with Masson trichrome stain (Fig 3D). No cholestasis was noted. The hepatocytes also exhibited a foamy cytoplasm indicating lipid accumulation. But the NP cells could be demarcated from the foamy hepatocytes. The ***spleen*** weighed 1,500 g (Fig 4A). The cut section showed diffuse enlargement with no focal lesion. Microscopic examination showed sheets of PAS negative, characteristic NP cells in the red pulp (Figs 4B–D). The white pulp was compressed and also showed presence of these cells. The ***lymph nodes*** (mesenteric, peripancreatic, aortic, carinal, hilar) were minimally enlarged and showed total replacement by NP cells (Figs 5A and B). A few follicles could be seen pushed towards the capsule. The ***lungs*** (Figs 5C and D) were heavy and on cut section showed hemorrhages. Microscopic examination confirmed the hemorrhages, amidst which NP cells glared out prominently (Fig 5E). The alveoli were distended and packed with the characteristic NP cells (Fig 6A). Overall features were those of lipoid pneumonia. No infection was however seen. The ***heart*** weighed 112 g. The right ventricular wall measured 0.5 cm indicating

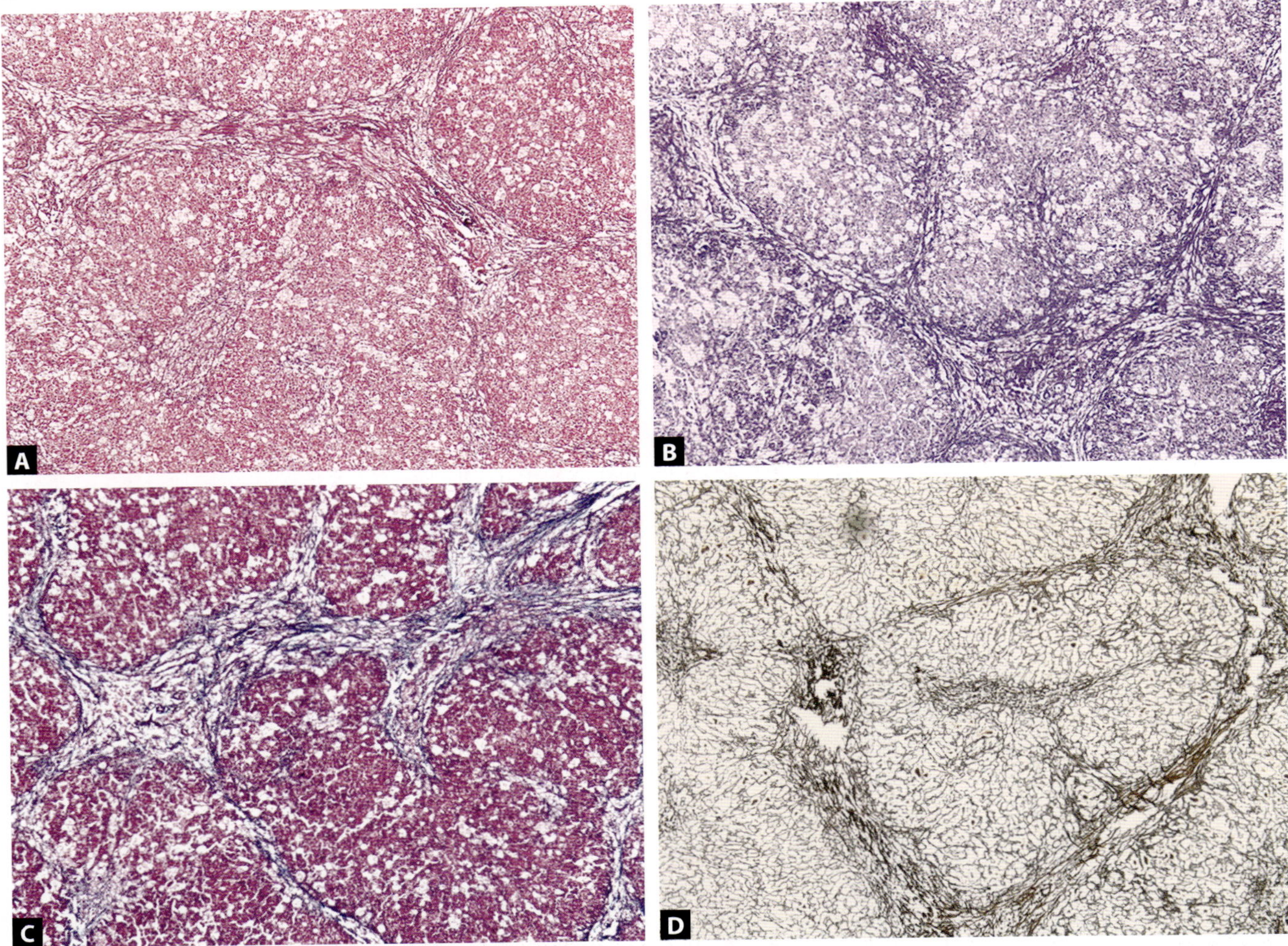

Figs 2A–D: Photomicrographs (H&E, periodic acid–Schiff, Masson trichrome, reticulin stain, respectively) of the liver showing porto-porto and porto-central bridging fibrosis forming nodule. Pale staining cells can be seen amidst the hepatocytes.

hypertrophy. The posterior leaflet of the mitral valve showed hooding and this leaflet was enlarged, redundant, thick and rubbery (Fig 6B arrow). Microscopy revealed thickening of the spongiosa layer with deposition of myxomatous material (Fig 6C). Amidst the myxomatous degeneration were seen clusters of large foamy macrophages with morphology consistent with NP cells (Figs 6D and E). Hence, mitral valve does show features of prolapse with presence of NP cells amidst the myxomatous degeneration. Right coronary artery and left circumflex artery were within normal limits but the left anterior descending (LAD) artery (Fig 6F) showed atherosclerotic narrowing (40%). The aorta also showed atherosclerosis (Fig 6G). ***Gastrointestinal tract—Stomach*** on gross examination showed nodularity (Fig 7A) and on microscopy revealed NP cells in the lamina propria (Fig 7B). The ***small intestine*** also showed nodularity and NP cells in the lamina (Figs 7C and D) and in the villi, clogging and distending them (Figs 7E and F). The ***colon*** however did not show any NP cells. The ganglion cells also revealed foaminess, indicating deposition of lipid. The ***kidneys*** were normal grossly and the renal arteries did not show any atherosclerotic narrowing. Microscopy showed presence of NP cells in the mesangium (Figs 8A and B). ***Pancreas*** showed congestion on cut section and microscopic examination revealed presence of NP cells amidst the acini (Fig 8C). ***Electron microscopy*** (Fig 8D) from the liver and spleen showed large cells packed with distended lysosomes, the cytoplasm of which contained the Zebra bodies, which are myelin figures showing lamillations. The serosal aspect (Figs 9A and B) of some portions of the small intestine, rectum,

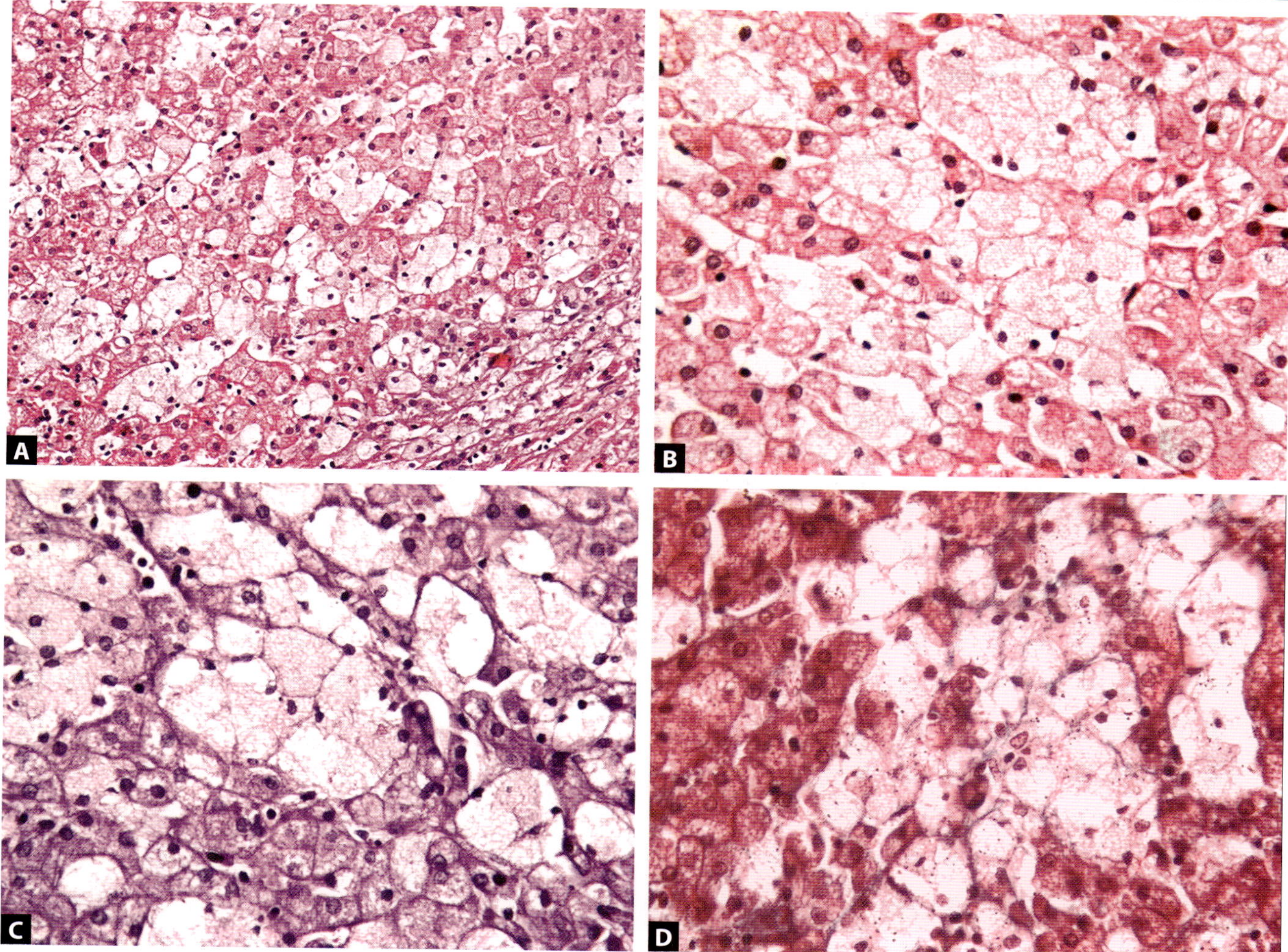

Figs 3A–D: (A and B) Liver showing the characteristic multivacuolated Niemann–Pick cells in the sinusoids; (C) The foamy Niemann–Pick cells are periodic acid–Schiff negative; (D) Niemann–Pick cells better appreciated in the Masson trichrome stain.

periureteric soft tissue and posterior aspect of the urinary bladder revealed hemorrhage and blood clots. However the site of the bleed could not be identified. The ***brain*** (Figs 9C and D) weighed 1,270 g and was normal grossly and on microscopic examination. There was death of another sibling, 9-year-old male, one week after the demise of the index case. This child had presented with similar clinical features and antemortem bone marrow done was consistent with a diagnosis of NPD.

FINAL AUTOPSY DIAGNOSIS: PM 27096

12 Years Old Female

- Niemann–Pick disease (non-neuronopathic) type B—bone marrow, liver, spleen, lymph nodes, lungs, stomach, small intestine, mitral valve, kidney and pancreas.
- Lipoid pneumonia and pulmonary hemorrhage.
- Liver fibrosis—stage 4.
- Mitral valve prolapse.
- Intra-abdominal bleed ? site.
- Atherosclerosis—Aorta: grade 1; LAD: 40% occlusion.

NIEMANN–PICK DISEASE

Niemann–Pick disease type A and B (NPA and NPB),[1-3] are both due to the inherited deficiency of a specific enzyme, acid sphingomyelinase (ASM), found within the lysosomes due to which the sphingomyelins cannot be metabolized properly and this leads to their accumulation within the cell, causing cell death and malfunction of major organ systems. NPA and NPB represent two ends of the same spectrum, wherein NPA has little or no ASM production (less than 1% of normal)

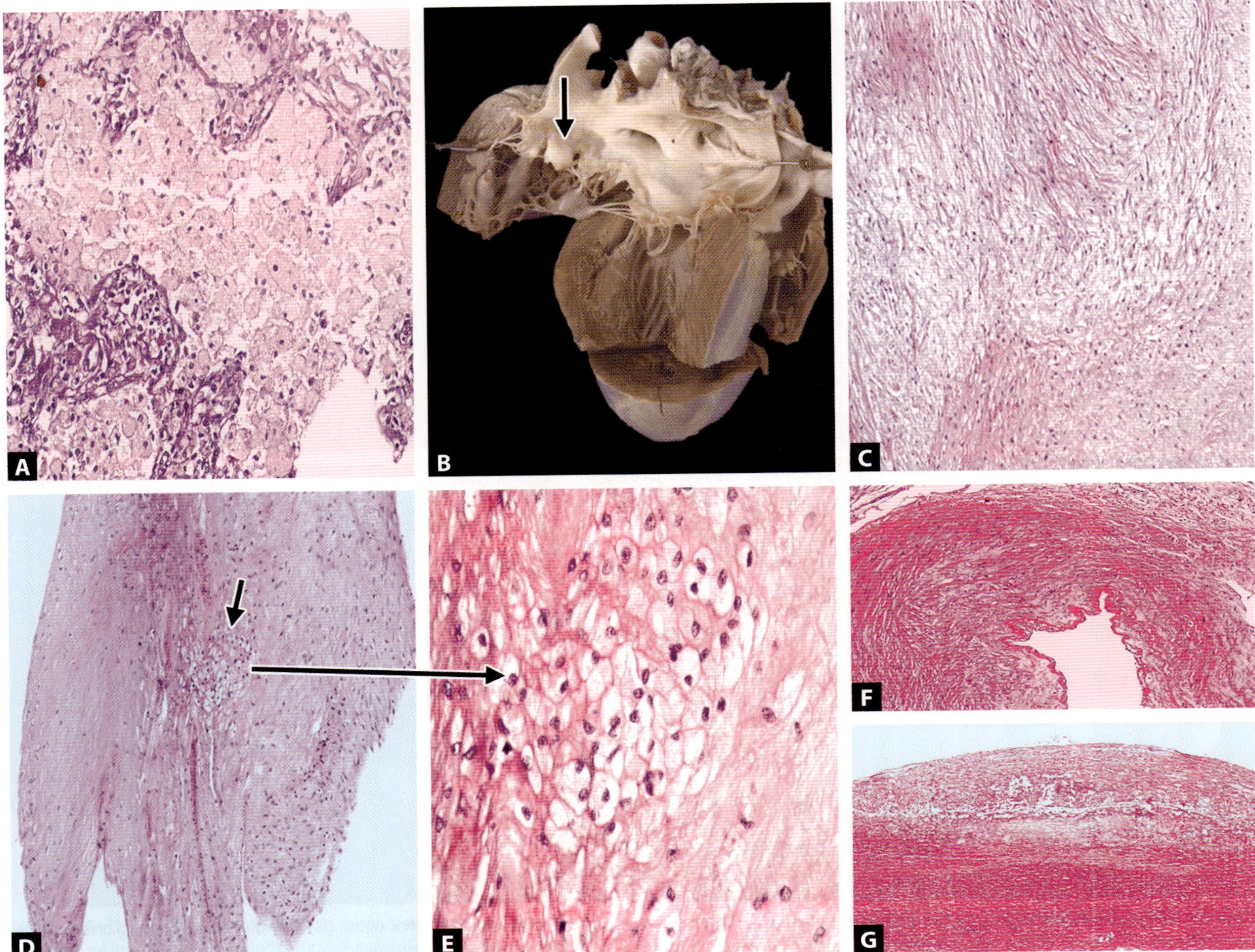

Figs 6A–G: (A) Photomicrograph of the lung showing Niemann–Pick cells in the alveolar spaces; (B) Gross picture of the left inflow tract showing enlarged, redundant, thick and rubbery posterior leaflet of mitral valve (arrow); (C–E) Photomicrograph of the mitral valve showing myxomatous degeneration amidst which can be seen Niemann–Pick cells (arrow); (F) Left anterior descending artery showing atherosclerosis; (G) Aorta showing atherosclerosis..

together. In NPC, mutations are seen in two genes, *NPC1* and *NPC2* with *NPC1* mutation contributing 95% of the patients. *NPC* is due to a defect in the lipid transport, wherein there is a defect in the transport of free cholesterol to the cytoplasm from the lysosomes. It shows clinical heterogeneity and presents with hydrops fetalis, neonatal hepatitis or most commonly with progressive neurologic damage. Niemann–Pick type D is the subacute juvenile or adult neuronopathic type of disease.

COMMENTARY—INDEX CASE

This 12-year-old girl presented with progressive abdominal distension from infancy. On examination, she was short-statured, had facial dysmorphism, massive splenohepatomegaly, mitral valve prolapse and hypertensive blood pressure record. Investigations revealed pancytopenia, transaminitis and very low HDL. Clinically, a diagnosis of lysosomal storage disorder, i.e. Niemann Pick disease Type B was considered. Autopsy showed characteristic NP cells widely distributed in almost all organs, sparing however the brain. Pulmonary involvement[4-6] is well-documented in NPD wherein a picture like lipoid pneumonia is seen with distended alveolar spaces packed with NP cells. In the index case, the degree of lung involvement was out of proportion to the mild exertional dyspnea that this patient had. This discrepancy however can be seen in NPD Type B. The mitral valve prolapse was present and microscopy of the valve

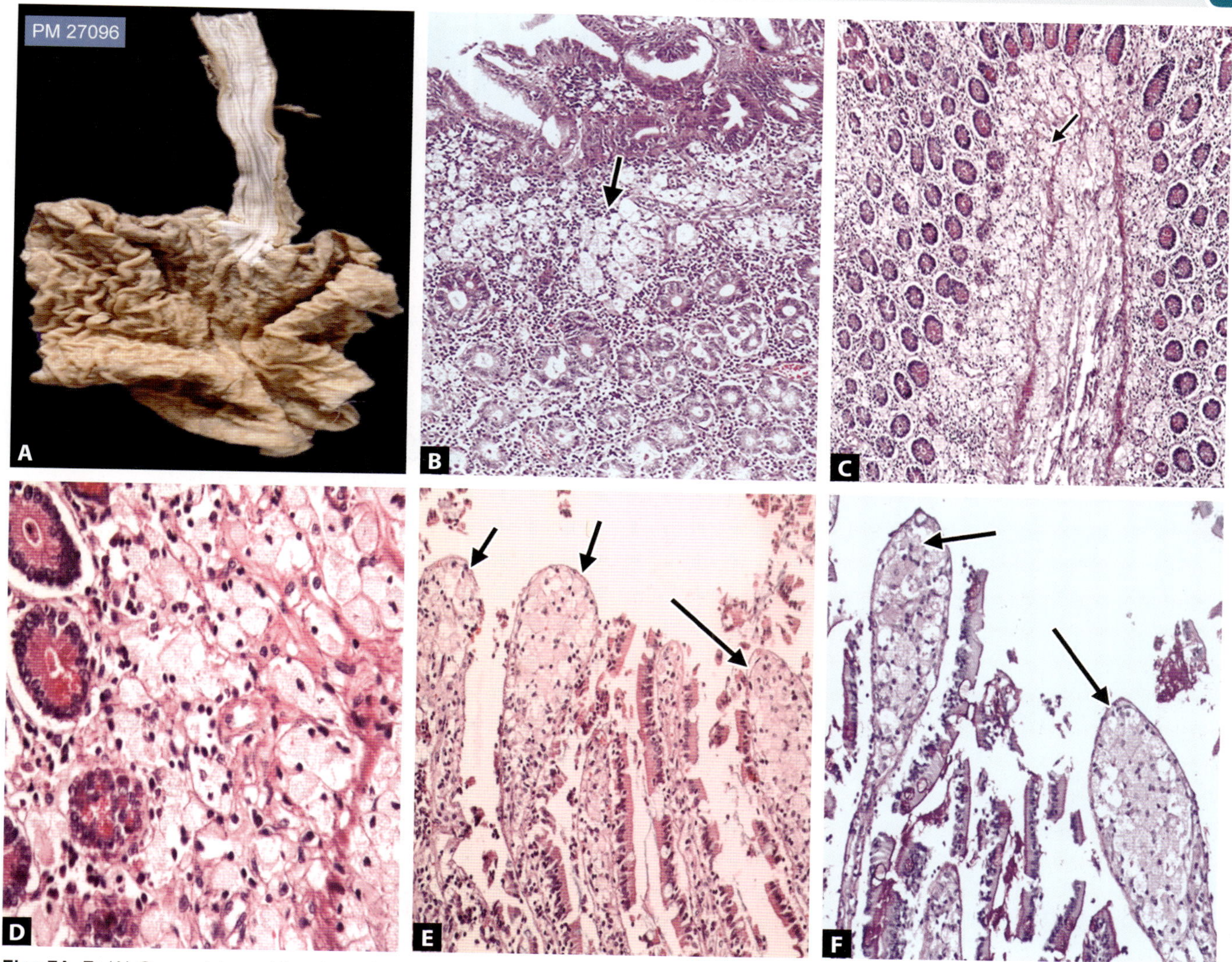

Figs 7A–F: (A) Gross picture of the stomach showing tiny pinhead sized nodules; (B) Niemann–Pick cells in the lamina propria of the stomach (arrow); (C and D) Niemann–Pick cells in the lamina propria of the small intestine; (E and F) Niemann–Pick cells clogging the villi of the small intestine (arrow).

revealed a unique finding of myxomatous degeneration with clusters of NP cells. McGovern et al[1] documented valvular involvement in five of their patients of NPD, but the cause was not documented. This is the first case in literature, where valvular involvement was due to mitral valve prolapse with histopathologic documentation of NP cells amidst the myxoid degeneration. Liver[7-9] in NPD can show varying degrees of fibrosis. The liver in the index case revealed stage 4 fibrosis with occasional nodule formation, along with abundant NP cells in the sinusoids. This has been reported in literature wherein liver biopsies from a cohort of 17 adult patients with NPD type B revealed some degree of fibrosis ranging from minimal to frank cirrhosis.[9] Studies in the mouse model of NPD have shown that inactivation of acid sphingomyelinase leads to overexpression of cathepsin B, that promotes liver fibrosis.[9] McGovern et al[1] reported cirrhosis in three of their patients. These observations have postulated that intralysosomal storage of sphingomyelin may provoke a fibrotic reaction in the surrounding tissue. The other unique feature in the index case, not reported in literature, was the presence of clusters of NP cells in the mesangium of the glomeruli. Could this be the cause of hypertension, is a speculation. The terminal event in the index case was a hypertensive crisis followed by abdominal bleed. Large blood clots were found in the abdomen, but the source of the bleed could not be ascertained. Clinically significant bleed has been reported in seven patients by McGovern et al.[1] The sibling of the index case also had a hypertensive crisis and died 1 week after the death of his sister.

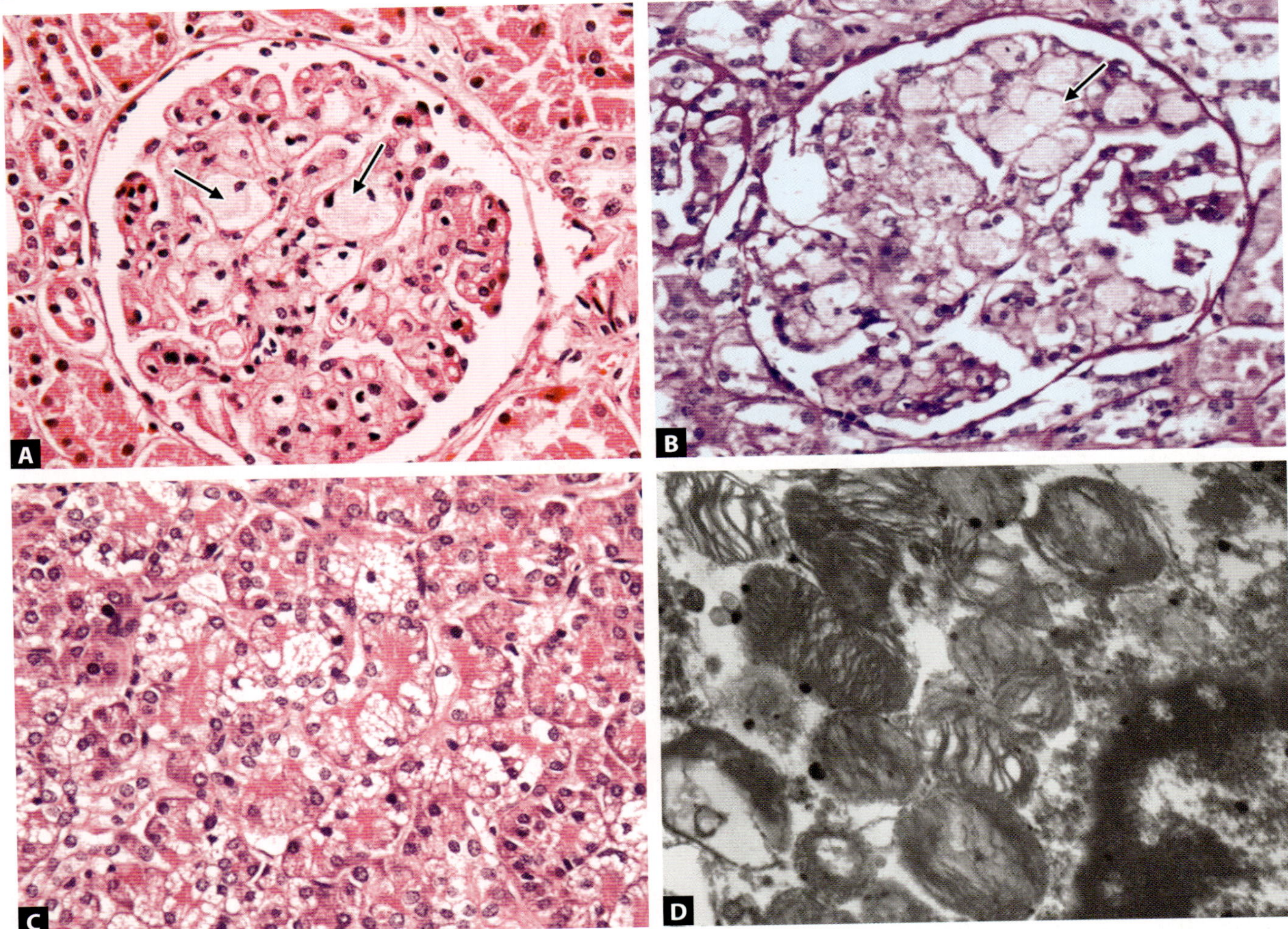

Figs 8A–D: (A and B) NP cells in the mesangium of the glomeruli (arrows) (H&E/PAS stains); (C) Photomicrograph from the pancreas showing presence of NP cells; (D) Electron microscopy of the liver showing lysosomes with lamellated structures i.e the Zebra bodies.

TAKE HOME MESSAGE

- Niemann–Pick types A and B are both due to the inherited deficiency (autosomal recessive) of a specific enzyme, acid sphingomyelinase.
- Niemann–Pick type A is a severe neuronopathic infantile form with extensive visceral and neuronal accumulation of sphingomyelin, leading on to severe neurologic involvement, progressive wasting, failure to thrive and death within 3 years of life.
- Niemann–Pick type B is non-neuronopathic, has visceral involvement and patients can survive to adulthood.
- The index case of NPB was very unique both clinically and on microscopic examination. It presented with hypertensive crisis and microscopically showed mitral valve prolapse due to infiltration by NP cells, extensive lung involvement with alveolar spaces packed with NP cells, stage 4 liver fibrosis and glomerular mesangium showing presence of large NP cells.

Acknowledgement

This case has been published as a 'Clinicopathologic conference' in the Journal of Postgraduate Medicine Education and Research, Chandigarh, India - Official Journal of PGIMER Chandigarh.

REFERENCES

1. McGovern MM, Lippa N, Bagiella E, et al. Morbidity and mortality in type B Niemann–Pick disease. Genet Med. 2013; 15:618-23.
2. Wasserstein MP, Aron A, Brodie SE, et al. Acid sphingomyelinase deficiency: prevalence and characterization of an intermediate phenotype of Niemann–Pick disease. J Pediatr. 2006;149:554-9.

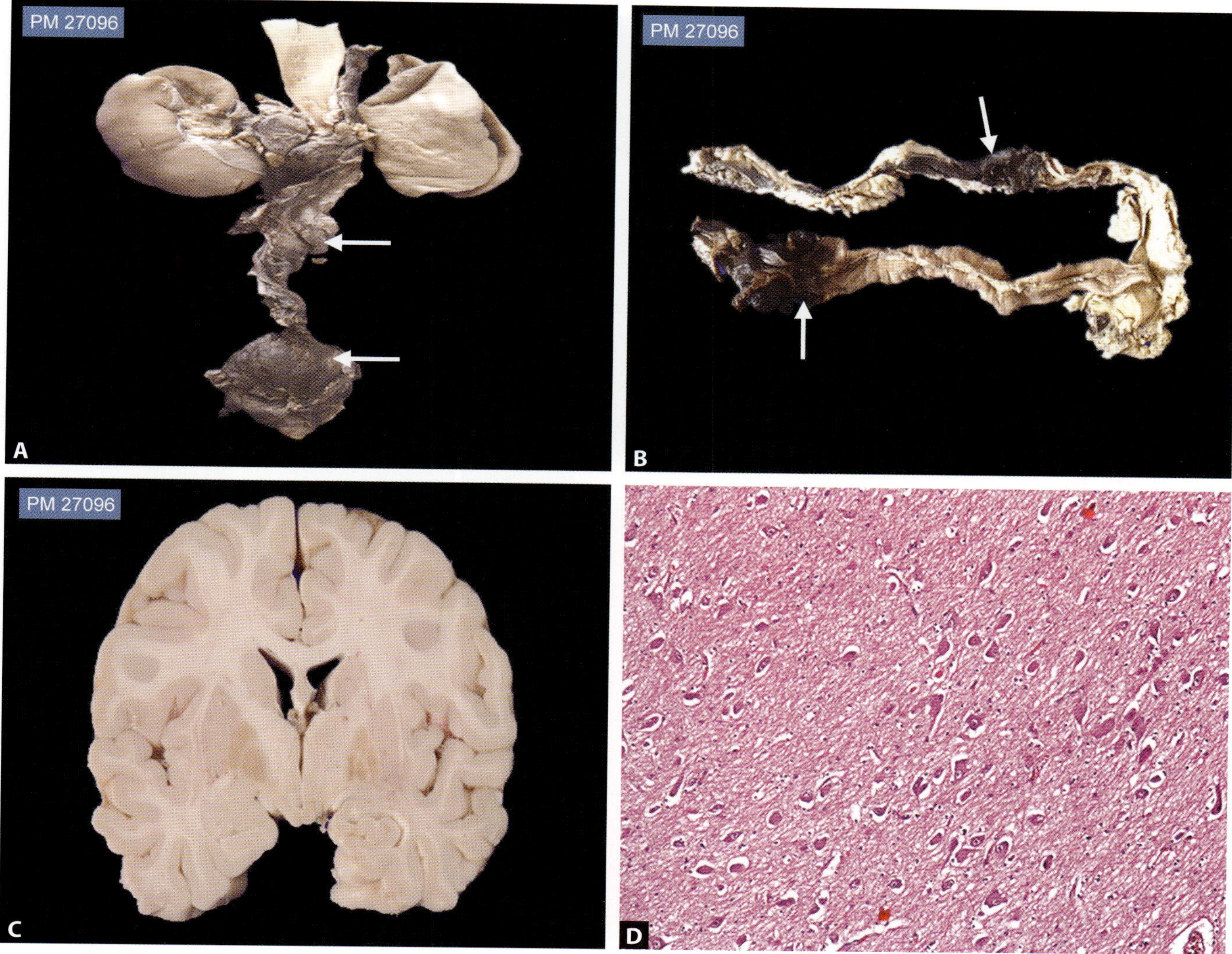

Figs 9A–D: (A) The outer aspect of the urinary bladder (lower arrow) and periureteric connective tissue, with caught up ureters (upper arrows) show hemorrhage. Both kidneys are pale; (B) The serosal aspect of the large intestine showing attached blood clots (arrows); (C) Coronal slice of the brain which is normal; (D) Brain showing normal neurones and glia. No storage material seen in the brain.

3. Wasserstein MP, Desnick RJ, Schuchman EH, et al. The natural history of type B Niemann–Pick disease: results from a 10-year longitudinal study. Pediatrics. 2004;114:e672-7.
4. Niggemann B, Rebien W, Rahn W, et al. Asymptomatic pulmonary involvement in 2 children with Niemann–Pick disease type B. Respiration. 1994;61:55-7.
5. Guillemot N, Troadec C, de Villemeur TB, et al. Lung disease in Niemann–Pick disease. Pediatr Pulmonol. 2007;42:1207-14.
6. Nicholson AG, Florio R, Hansell DM, et al. Pulmonary involvement by Niemann–Pick disease. A report of six cases. Histopathology. 2006;48:596-603.
7. Tassoni JP Jr, Fawaz KA, Johnston DE. Cirrhosis and portal hypertension in a patient with adult Niemann-Pick disease. Gastroenterology. 1991;100:567-9.
8. Thurberg BL, Wasserstein MP, Schiano T, et al. Liver and skin histopathology in adults with acid sphingomyelinase deficiency (Niemann-Pick disease type B). Am J Surg Path. 2012;36:1234-46.
9. Moles A, Tarrats N, Fernandez-Checa JC, et al. Cathepsin B overexpression due to acid sphingomyelinase ablation promotes liver fibrosis in Niemann-Pick disease. J Biol Chem. 2012;287:1178-88.

CONTRIBUTIONS BY:

1. Dr Renu Suthar, Assistant Professor, Department of Pediatrics (Compilation of Clinical Details)
2. Dr Sadhana Lal, Professor, Department of Gastroenterology-Pediatric (Clinician In-Charge)

Post Graduate Institute of Medical Education and Research, Chandigarh, India.

SECTION 15

Pediatric Renal Cystic Disease (Developmental/ Genetic/Syndromes)

Pediatric Cystic Disease (Developmental/ Genetic) of Kidney—Introduction

Nandita Bharadwaj Kakkar

PEDIATRIC RENAL DEVELOPMENTAL DISORDERS

Pediatric renal cystic lesions of the kidney are classified into two main groups, i.e. developmental and genetic. The acquired lesions are not considered here. Till date, classification is based on several classifications, notably those of Bernstein/Gardner, Risdon et al, Gary S Hilland Bisceglia et al. Over the years, other entities have come up and need a slot in the classification system. We at PGIMER, Chandigarh, India, perform nearly 350 stillbirths/neonatal autopsies per year and encounter a large number of renal developmental/hereditary lesions and malformation syndromes. We follow the following listing as it is reproducible and clinician-friendly. This listing is a conglomerate of the above listed classification systems and we feel is very straight forward and clinician-friendly. Embryology, developmental disordersand hereditary renal adysplasia (HRA) will be addressed in this chapter. Others would be addressed with the respective cases.

DEVELOPMENTAL DISORDERS

Renal Hypoplasia

- Simple hypoplasia (PM 27245, PM 25677)
- Oligomeganephronic hypoplasia
- Segmental hypoplasia: secondary to vesicoureteric reflux (s-14525/2008).

Renal Dysplasia

- Hypodysplasia (PM 19521, PM 25711)
- *Multicystic dysplasia*: Unilateral (PM 22428, PM 22393, PM 26428) or bilateral (PM 20505, PM 24340, PM 26207)
- *Renal agenesis*: Unilateral (PM 26824), bilateral (PM 24019, PM 27025)
- *Segmental dysplasia*: Upper pole of duplex kidney (PM 19965)
- Congenital hydronephrosis with or without dysplasia:
  - *Unilateral*: Ureteropelvic junction obstruction (PM 26291)
  - *Bilateral with hydroureteronephrosis and hypertrophied urinary bladder*: Posterior/anterior urethral valves (PM 18485, PM 26118), urethral stricture and Prune belly syndrome (PM 23424, PM 25509).

GLOMERULOCYSTIC DISEASE

- This can be genetic, sporadic or associated with other cystic diseases or syndromes (PM 28154, PM 28255).

MISCELLANEOUS DISORDERS—QUANTITY/POSITION/FORM

- Multiple or supernumerary kidneys, renal or ureteric duplications, renal ectopia, renal fusion—horse shoe kidney and renomegaly.

HEREDITARY LESIONS

Polycystic Disease

- Autosomal recessive polycystic kidney disease (ARPKD): PM 22879
- Autosomal dominant polycystic kidney disease (ADPKD): PM 22828.

Medullary Cysts

- Medullary cystic disease
- Familial juvenile nephronophthisis
- Medullary sponge kidney.

Renal Cysts in Chromosomal Abnormalities and Hereditary Syndromes

- Trisomy 21/13/18/4p, Turner syndrome
- *Syndromes with cerebral malformations*: Autosomal recessive conditions—Meckel syndrome and variants [Meckel Gruber (PM 20070, PM 26190), Goldston's, Miranda's, Simopoulos], tuberous sclerosis, von Hippel-Lindau disease, Lissencephaly syndrome, Smith-Lemli-Opitz syndrome and Zellweger syndrome

- *Syndromes with skeletal abnormalities*:
    - *Autosomal recessive*: Jeune syndrome, chondrodysplasia punctata (rhizomelic type), Winter syndrome, Elejalde syndrome, short rib-polydactyly type I/II syndromeand Ellis-van Creveld syndrome.
- *Autosomal dominant*: Orofacial—digital syndrome, Syndromes with primary urologic abnormalities—renal retinal dysplasias, Prune belly syndrome (PM 23424, PM 25509), hereditary renal adysplasia (PM 20505, PM 25677) and familial hydronephrosis.
- *Miscellaneous syndromes*: Ivemark, Glutaric acidemia (type 2), Laurence-Moon-Bardet-Biedl, Beckwith-Wiedemann, Perlman, Brachiootorenal, Ehlers-Danlos, Fryns, Kallmann, Dieker, Townes, nail-patella, Apert and Rokitansky-Küster-Hauser.

Renal Abnormalities with Various Associations:

- *Vacterl/Vater*: Vertebral defects, anal atresia, cardiac, tracheoesophageal fistula, renal (renal agenesis, cystic dysplasia, ectopia, fusion, hydronephrosis—occasional), limb defects.
- *Charge*: Coloboma, congenital heart defects, atresia choanae, retarded development and growth, genitourinary abnormalities (renal agenesis, ectopia, dysplasia—occasional), ear abnormalities, i.e. deafness. Two-thirds of cases are due to a CHD7 mutation. Important cause of congenital deafness and blindness.
- *DiGeorge syndrome*: thymic hypoplasia, hypoplasia or absence of parathyroids, Fallot's tetralogy or other heart defects, aortic arch or great vessel abnormalities, renal (microcysts or dysplasia—occasional)
- *MURCS*: Müllerian duct aplasia (absence of vagina or uterus), renal (agenesis, ectopia—occasional) and cervicothoracic vertebral defects.
- *Sirenomelia*: Lower limb fusion (mermaid), genitourinary defects (renal agenesis—frequent), imperforate anus and lower vertebral defects (PM 27027).
- *Schisis*: Neural tube defects (anencephaly, encephalocele, meningomyelocele). Diaphragmatic hernia, cleft palate, omphalocele, heart defects and renal agenesis (frequent).

EMBRYOLOGY

Both the urinary and the genital systems are anatomically and embryologically interconnected. They are derived from the intermediate mesoderm and initially their excretory ducts open in a common cavity i.e the cloaca. After the folding of the embryonic disc and the formation of the peritoneal cavity, the intermediate mesoderm forms a bulge called the "nephrogenic cord" on the posterior abdominal wall. This cord extends from the cervical to the sacral region of the embryo. A number of important structures are formed in relation to the nephrogenic cord, which are—excretory tubules (mesonephros) associated with the development of the kidney, the mesonephric duct formed in relation to the excretory tubules, paramesonephric duct and the gonads. The cloaca divides into the rectum and the primitive urogenital sinus. The primitive urogenital sinus further divides into the cranial vesicourethral canal (which forms the urinary bladder and the primitive urethra) and the caudal definitive urogenital sinus (which divide into pelvic and phallic parts). The mesonephric duct opens into that part of the cloaca which forms the urogenital sinus. The definitive human kidney arises from two distinct sources—(1) The nephrons are derived from the metanephros (lowest part of the nephrogenic cord), the cells of which form the metanephric blastema. (2) The collecting part of the kidney is derived from a diverticulum called the ureteric bud, which arises from the lower part of the mesonephric duct. The ureteric bud grows cranially toward the metanephric blastema and its growing end dilates to form an ampulla. This ampulla divides repeatedly to form the pelvis (by fusion of first, three to five divisions), major calyces (next divisions), minor calyces and the collecting tubules (further divisions). The growing tip of each branch of the ureteric bud is dilated to form an ampulla. The cells of the metanephric blastema in contact with an ampulla, undergoes differentiation to form a nephron. This differentiation is induced by the ampulla. Loosely arranged cells of the metanephric blastema form solid clumps in relation to the ampulla. Each solid clump is converted into a vesicle. The vesicle soon becomes pear-shaped and opens into the ampulla, after this it becomes an S-shaped tube with its distal end invaginated by a tuft of capillaries, which form the glomerulus. From 7 weeks to 14 weeks of gestation, the ureteric bud divides dichotomously. From 14 weeks to 22 weeks, three to four ranks of glomeruli form, the first one being the inner most, i.e. juxtamedullary. From 22 weeks to 36 weeks, there is no branching of the ureteric bud, but the nephrons are formed taking the number to 13–14 ranks. After 36 weeks no new nephrons are formed.

It is known that the mesonephric duct opens into that part of the cloaca which forms the urogenital sinus. The ureteric buds arise from the mesonephric duct a little above the cloaca. The part of the mesonephric duct caudal to the origin of the ureteric bud gets absorbed into the vesicourethral canal (forms the trigone of the bladder) and thus both the mesonephric duct and the ureteric bud have independent openings into the cloaca. Soon the opening of the ureteric buds move cranially and laterally. The ureter is derived from that part of the ureteric bud that lies between the pelvis of the kidney and the vesicourethral canal.

Detailed descriptions of all entities listed above are beyond the scope of this book. However, the postmortem cases listed above would be discussed in brief.

RENAL HYPOPLASIA

By definition, renal hypoplasia is defined as small kidney, weighing less than 50% of the expected weight or less than two standard deviation of the normal and histologically shows reduction in the total number of nephrons. It is of three types:

1. ***Simple hypoplasia*:** This is also known as miniature kidney and is rare. Grossly the kidney has a normal shape, is small in size and weighs less than 50% of the expected weight. There is a reduction in the number of renal calyces and renal lobes to less than or equal to 5 (normal kidney has more than or equal to 10 lobes). Ectopia of ureteric orifices may be seen and microscopically there are just 2–3 ranks of glomeruli, disarray with reduction of tubules seen more in the medulla. This is probably due to the inadequate branching of the ureteric bud. No parenchymal maldifferentiation, i.e. dysplasia is noted. Unilateral hypoplasia occurs sporadically, is rarely associated with lower urinary tract anomalies and may present with recurrent infections, reflux nephropathy and hypertension. Severe bilateral hypoplasia leads to renal failure and early death. Less severe cases however show growth or mental retardation and chronic renal insufficiency. Congenital CNS lesions may show some degree of renal hypoplasia.
2. ***Segmental hypoplasia (Ask Upmark kidney)*:** This condition is generally unilateral, but can be bilateral and can occur in utero or after birth or both. It occurs more in the females. The kidney is small in size, with a transverse groove on the capsular surface at the upper pole, overlying an area of marked parenchymal thinning. Microscopy shows scarred zones called areas of segmental hypoplasia with absent glomeruli, atrophic thyroid-like tubules, thick-walled blood vessels, occasional minute focus of cartilage but no dysplasia. It occurs due to vesicoureteric reflux, as the pattern of distribution of lesions are consistent with reflux damage. The compound papillae most susceptible to damage, are concentrated at the upper pole and hence it occurs at the upper pole. It may lead to hypertension or recurrent urinary tract infections and in this scenario, nephrectomy is done. Renal insufficiency occurs in 50% cases.
3. ***Oligomeganephronic hypoplasia*:** Bilateral renal hypoplasia or oligomeganephronia was first described by Habib et al in 1962 in French literature. It typically presents in infancy with polyuria, proteinuria, vomiting, dehydration and has a protracted course. It slowly progresses to renal failure, with failure to thrive and renal osteodystrophy. Patients usually reach end-stage renal failure by 12–14 years of age. Grossly, the kidneys are very small, both together weigh less than 20 g and measure 4–5 cm each. On histological examination, it shows a reduction in the count of glomeruli along with an increase in the size of the existing glomeruli and tubules, as compared to age matched controls. The glomeruli show changes like increase in mesangial cellularity or matrix and focal/segmental glomerulosclerosis. Interstitial inflammation can be seen and changes can resemble those seen in advanced pyelonephritis. No primitive duct (hallmark of dysplasia) is however seen. With time, glomerulosclerosis, tubular atrophy and fibrosis sets in. The cause is generally said to be an arrest of metanephric induction by the ureteric bud, between 14 weeks and 20 weeks of fetal life. Chromosome 4 abnormalities and mutations in PAX2 and hepatocyte nuclear factor-1 beta (HNF-1 beta) have been reported.

RENAL DYSPLASIA

Renal dysplasia can be unilateral (more common) or bilateral, can be cystic (more common) or noncystic. Enlarged multicystic variety is the most common bilateral cystic disease in the newborn and the most common cause of palpable abdominal masses in this age group. Bilateral disease is incompatible with life. They present with "Potter's sequence", i.e. (1) Peculiar facies—face contorted into a permanent grimace, prominent fold extending from the inner canthus of the eye to the cheek, bags under eye, parrot-beaked nose and low set ears. (2) Oligohydramnios leading to flexion at knees and hips along with clubbed feet. (3) Hypoplastic lungs. When these findings are associated with bilateral renal agenesis, the term "Potter's syndrome" is used, as highlighted by Potter way back in 1946. Unilateral dysplasia may go undetected or is incidentally detected by the mother or the physician as an abdominal mass. There may be no symptoms and if present, are due to the involvement of the opposite kidney with pyelonephritis or hydronephrosis. Dysplasias with upper urinary tract abnormalities are seen equally in males and females, but dysplasias with lower urinary tract abnormalities, like posterior urethral valve, are seen more in the males. Patients with renal dysplasias have increased incidence of malformations in other systems like gastrointestinal tract (anorectal malformations, esophageal atresia, tracheaesophageal fistula), central nervous system (spina bifida occulta, meningomyelocele, hydrocephalous, Dandy-Walker deformity), respiratory system (lung hypoplasia) and cardiovascular system (ventricular septal defect, tetralogy of Fallot). Other abnormalities include cleft lip, cleft palate, congenital talipes equinovarus, etc. Kakkar et al, in an autopsy study of 4,099 cases, found 158 cases of developmental and genetic renal lesions, wherein associated malformations were seen in 100% cases. These associated malformations were seen in the genitourinary tract (95%), respiratory tract (42%), musculoskeletal system (36%), gastrointestinal tract (20%), CNS (19%) and CVS (11.4%).

PATHOGENESIS OF RENAL DYSPLASIA

Potter was the pioneer in this field and formulated the theory that dysplasia occurred due to the failure of the ureteric bud to induce formation of nephrons in the apposed metanephric mesenchyme, i.e. the ureteric bud does not meet the metanephric mesenchyme at the right time and place. ***Bernstein*** formulated the theory of obstruction and said that obstruction is the primary event in producing dysplasia. Obstruction after nephrogenesis is complete, leads to simple hydronephrosis (without dysplasia) as seen in postnatal life. Obstruction prior to the end of nephrogenesis leads to hydronephrosis with dysplasia. In early obstruction, there is more prominent parenchymal disarray and dysplasia is seen with mesenchymal stromal proliferation and cuffing of ducts. This is because the glomeruli are most susceptible at the primitive "S" stage of development. ***Schwarz et al*** formulated that complete obstruction leads to severe degree of hypodysplasia. Partial ureteral obstruction in utero leads to marked hydronephrosis with or without dysplastic changes. Partial urethral obstruction leads to hydronephrosis and dysplasia depends on the location of the ureteral orifices. If the orifice is normally placed, dysplasia is minimal or absent. Malplaced orifices lead to increased hypodysplastic changes. So there are two important things—obstruction (time, speed and severity) and aberrant location of the ureters, which govern the degree of hypodysplasia. ***Bud theory*** states that ectopic ureteric orifice reflects the misplaced origin of the ureteric bud and so the union of the bud and the metanephric mesenchyme does not occur at the right time and place. A ureteric bud arising from the correct position, i.e. the "normal" zone of the mesonephric duct, will ultimately hit the metanephric blastema at the right place leading to a perfect development of the kidney. But if the ureteric bud originates either too cranially or too caudally, it will not meet the metanephric blastema properly, leading to the formation of a dysplastic kidney. Failure of nephron formation can also occur due to unresponsiveness of the mesenchyme or due to deficient inductive action. ***Extracellular matrix*** (ECM) plays an important role in nephrogenesis. Inductive tissue interactions, that is one cell population significantly altering the behavior of an adjacent cell population, are common in organ development. Major event in nephrogenesis is the conversion of metanephric mesenchyme into epithelial structures. In the 5th week of intrauterine life, rapid changes occur in ECM proteins and these are critical and the first detectable response of the nephrogenic mesenchyme to the inducing signal. ECM is composed of fibrous structural proteins (collagen, elastin), adhesive glycoproteins (laminin and fibronectin) and proteoglycans (syndecan). Cells grow and differentiate in intimate contact with the ECM, which critically influences the cell functions. At about 5th week of intrauterine life, normal induction occurs and there is a shift in the intercellular matrix from an interstitial type (fibronectin and collagen type 1 and III) to basement membrane type (laminin, collagen type IV, proteoglycans, syndecan). This means that collagen I and III, fibronectin, NCAM are lost and laminin, collagen type IV, uromodulin and syndecan are acquired. Regulatory genes for conversion of mesenchyme into epithelial structures involve *PAX2* and *WNT4*. Menon and Kakkar et al studied the expression of laminin and fibronectin in renal dysplasia and found that there was a persistence of fibronectin and absence of laminin in dysplastic kidneys. They concluded that in dysplastic kidneys, there is no shift in the intercellular matrix from an interstitial type to basement membrane type. ***Genes*** have a role to play in nephrogenesis. *WT1* is a tumor suppressor gene, encodes a transcription factor and is expressed in mesenchyme of the metanephric blastema and in the podocytes (epithelial) of the glomeruli. Thus, the metanephric blastema becomes responsive to the ureteric bud in normal nephrogenesis. The ureteric bud branches normally in the presence of glial derived neurotrophic factor (GDNF) and hepatocyte growth factor, whose production is regulated by *WT1*. The epithelium of the ureteric bud produces the tyrosine kinase receptors RET and MET for GDNF and hepatocyte growth factor respectively and this establishes a signaling pathway between the two tissues leading to normal nephrogenesis. Homozygous null mutations of *WT1* produced in mice, lead to renal agenesis. Other genes which play a role are *PAX2, PAX8, BCL2, WNT4, GATA3, SIX homeobox 1(SIX1) and growth differentiation factor 11 (GDF11)*. Early induction of renal mesenchyme and growth factors for inducing growth of ureteric buds is done by *WT1*. Late induction, i.e. conversion of metanephric mesenchyme into epithelial structures, is done by *PAX2*. In normal nephrogenesis, *WT1*, *PAX2/8* and *BCL2* gene expressions are most important. When the kidney becomes mature, both *WT1* and *PAX2* get down regulated. Thus, the pathogenesis of renal dysplasia is multifactorial and includes the bud theory, ectopia of the ureteric orifices, intrauterine obstruction, inductive effect of the ECM proteins and genetic aberrations.

PATHOLOGY OF RENAL DYSPLASIA

Renal dysplasia shows abnormal differentiation of metanephric parenchyma. It can be cystic or noncystic. There is complete lobar disorganization with jumbling of nephron elements, distortion of normal corticomedullary relations, rudimentary medullary development, inability to produce a countercurrent gradient and hence such kidneys are incapable of function. Morphologically the hallmark of dysplasia is the "***primitive duct***" which is pathognomic of dysplasia and without which the term "dysplasia" cannot be used. "Primitive duct" is a small duct-like structure, usually lined by tall columnar epithelium, at times by low cuboidal epithelium or pseudostratified epithelium. At times, the epithelium is non-descript or may be ciliated. Characteristically, they are surrounded by a circumferential fibromuscular cuffing of immature mesenchyme. Typically they are found in the medulla of the dysplastic kidney, but in the severely dysplastic kidneys, they are seen right from the cortex till the medulla. They may be found singly or in groups, amidst the immature mesenchyme, giving it a nodular configuration. Other morphological elements seen in dysplastic kidneys are varying sized cysts, abortive glomeruli, rudimentary tubules, foci of cartilage, bone, foci of extramedullary hematopoiesis (EMH), basement membrane thickening of the primitive ducts, proliferating nerves/vessels and occasionally foci of nodular renal blastema. The cysts are derived from the primitive ducts and may be large/small or numerous/few. The cysts thus decide the gross appearance i.e. multicystic dysplasia (bunch of grapes appearance), hypoplastic dysplasia or aplastic dysplasia. Cartilage is usually seen in the would be cortex or at the corticomedullary junction. Rarely cartilage has been seen in patients with trisomies or even in normal kidneys. The abortive glomeruli and the rudimentary tubules are scattered throughout the dysplastic kidney in the loose connective tissue. An important part of renal dysplasia is the loss of cohesion or lack of interrelation between the parenchymal elements, which becomes more evident with increasing dysplasia. Foci of EMH are seen in the would be medulla and in kidneys with segmental dysplasia, it is seen only in the dysplastic portions. The dysplastic elements are derived both from ureteric bud and metanephric blastema. Ureteric bud gives rise to the primitive ducts and their surrounding mesenchyme. Metanephric blastema gives rise to the primitive glomeruli, tubular structures and metaplastic cartilage.

TYPES OF RENAL DYSPLASIA

- ***Multicystic dysplasia—bilateral or unilateral*****:** This is the most common dysplasia variant and the most common bilateral cystic disease in the newborn. Unilateral multicystic dysplasia is more common, but autopsy data claims that the bilateral multicystic dysplasia is more common. This is because the unilateral dysplasia can be compatible with life and is the most common form of cystic disease throughout childhood. Grossly, the kidneys appear as large irregular cystic masses with varying sized cysts ranging in size from 0.5 cm to 5 cm in diameter, resembling a bunch of grapes. Amidst the cysts, classic features of dysplasia (listed above) are seen. Pelvis is fused with the mass and the ureters are atretic, malformed, absent or may even be dilated and tortuous. Urinary bladder is malformed, can be large, small, hypertrophied and distorted. Bilateral disease is fatal and the child presents with Potters facies, deformed lower limbs and history of oligohydramnios. Unilateral multicystic dysplastic kidney with a normal contralateral kidney has a good prognosis, but this situation is seen in only half of the cases. In unilateral dysplasia, the status of the opposite kidney is very important. Here, assessment of the pelvis and ureters of the dysplastic kidney is done. Isolated renal pelvic atresia without ureteral abnormality occurs in 48% and in them the contralateral kidney is abnormal in 7% and this has a better prognosis. Ureteral atresia with or without renal pelvic atresia occurs in 52% and in these the contralateral kidney is abnormal in 40% cases, which thus has a worse prognosis. The abnormalities, which can be seen in the contralateral kidney, are ureteropelvic junction obstruction with hydronephrosis, ureteral abnormalities, segmental dysplasia, horseshoe kidney, etc.
- ***Hypodysplasia*****:** Hypoplastic kidneys are small in size and show hypoplastic areas, mixed with areas of frank dysplasia. Cysts are infrequent or scattered peripheral cysts may be present. Ureters are nearly always patent but are malformed (megaureters, stenosis and ectopia). Some residual renal function is present. Unilateral hypodysplasia is asymptomatic and prognosis depends upon the status of the opposite kidney. Hypodysplastic kidney is frequently associated with an abnormal opposite

kidney which may show the following—ureteropelvic junction obstruction with hydronephrosis, horseshoe kidney, segmental dysplasia or ureteral abnormalities.

- ***Segmental dysplasia***: In segmental dysplasia, a portion of the kidney at upper pole is dysplastic. There is an association with duplication of renal pelvis and ureter (exhibiting obstruction, ectopia or terminating in an ectopic ureterocele). Ten percent have duplex kidney on the opposite side. There is a female preponderance and the patients present with recurrent urinary tract infection. On microscopy, dysplastic segments are clearly demarcated from the adjacent normal parenchyma.
- ***Renal agenesis***: Renal agenesis is either bilateral (incompatible with life) or unilateral. Unilateral agenesis could be totally asymptomatic or may show a wide range of abnormalities of the urinary tract like ureteral abnormalities, fusion of the pelvis, vesicoureteric reflux along with anomalies of the reproductive, cardiovascular, skeletal and gastrointestinal systems. Renal agenesis is a sporadic developmental abnormality, but some cases of unilateral or bilateral agenesis are genetic with an autosomal dominant inheritance, known as hereditary renal adysplasia (HRA). Pathogenesis of renal agenesis is considered to be failure of the ureteric bud to sprout from the lower part of the mesonephric duct, or it atrophies after budding, or it does not meet the metanephric blastema or it does meet, but due to some reason, there is a failure of induction of the blastema. When associated anomalies are present, it signifies more extensive developmental field defects, wherein a region or a part of an embryo responds as a coordinated unit to embryonic interaction, leading to maldevelopment. Potter divided cases of renal agenesis into three zones of regional disturbance, which leads to maldevelopment and Buchta et al further modified these concepts. Field A: Here the abnormality is limited to the lower part of the mesonephric or paramesonephric duct which leads to agenesis of the kidneys and ureters with variable maldevelopment of the genital tract. Field B: Here the abnormality involves the hindgut and the cloacal membrane which along with the field A abnormalities, also show imperforate anus, atresia of terminal hind gut with or without rectovesical or rectovaginal fistula and abnormalities of the external genitalia. Field C: This includes the entire caudal end of the embryo. Here spinal and limb abnormalities are seen along with sirenomelic monsters.
- ***Unilateral renal agenesis***: Unilateral agenesis has an incidence of 1:450 to 1:1,800 (three times more common than bilateral renal agenesis) and may be compatible with life. It is seen more frequently in males with a male to female ratio is 2:1. But the incidence of genital abnormalities is more common in females than males. Ipsilateral ureter and hemitrigone of the bladder is absent. Females have ipsilateral absence of fallopian tube and uni or bicornuate uterus in 50% cases. Males have ipsilateral absence of vas and testes in 10% cases. In unilateral agenesis, abnormality may not be limited to the ureteral bud, but may show more extensive field defect, wherein abnormalities are seen in other structures derived from the mesonephric duct and also from neighboring structures like the paramesonephric duct. In males, seminal vesicle cyst due to a blind ending ejaculatory duct, absence of vas deferens/epididymis /seminal vesicle and rarely duplication of the vas deferens/epididymis can be seen. In females, Gartner's duct cyst can be seen due to abnormality of the distal mesonephric duct. The paramesonephric duct (also known as Müllerian duct) which lies lateral to the mesonephric duct in the nephrogenic cord gives rise to the uterine tubes, uterus and possibly part of the vagina. Thus, due to the close proximity of the paramesonephric and mesonephric ducts, malformations of the female genital system are common. Common abnormalities are uterine duplication, vaginal duplication, cervical atresia, absent tube on the affected side and imperforate vagina. The opposite solitary kidney may show ureteropelvic junction obstruction, vesicoureteric reflux etc. and hence start the lifelong problems of recurrent urinary tract infections and hydronephrosis. Thus, Müllerian abnormalities and unilateral renal agenesis have a close association and if one is present, then abnormalities in the other should be looked for. Duncan et al described MURCS- Müllerian duct (MU) aplasia, i.e. uterine hypoplasia or aplasia, renal aplasia (R), cervicothoracic somite dysplasia (CS) manifesting as 2–4 anomalous vertebrae between C5–T1. Another severe anomaly described is VATER, which includes vertebral defects, anal atresia, tracheoesophageal fistula with esophageal atresia, radial dysplasia and renal defects. Others seen are VSD and single umbilical artery. This is explained by disruption of structures lying in close proximity before 5 weeks of gestation.
- ***Bilateral renal agenesis***: Bilateral agenesis shows total absence of any renal structures, ureters, renal artery, hypoplastic or absent urinary bladder and a defective urethra. Potter estimated the incidence to be approximately 1 per 4,800 births. The M:F ratio is 3:1, but the females have a higher incidence of associated genitourinary abnormalities. It appears to be sporadic but genetically determined in some cases. Half of the cases are stillborns

and the liveborns are small for gestational age, generally have Potter's syndrome and die within 1–2 days, due to pulmonary hypoplasia. Autopsy reveals absence of both kidneys and the space is occupied by the adrenals, which look like flattened oval discs. In more than 50% cases, there is no remnant of renal tissue and absent ureters and urinary bladder. Very occasionally, there may be a small nubbin of renal tissue attached to the adrenal glands without any ureters which microscopically show glomeruli and tubules, without any collecting ducts and pelvis (Fig. 1). This proves that metanephric blastema is not wholly dependent on the inducing capacity of the ureteric bud. At times few nubbins of renal tissue composed of abortive glomeruli and tubules may show some degree of ureteral development which ends at the pelvis. The bladder may be absent or so hypoplastic, that it may not be recognizable. At times, it may be a tube-like structure with scanty or absent smooth muscle, due to the absence of stretch by the urine. In males, testis are absent in 10% cases and in 33%, are cryptorchid. Penis may show hypospadias in some cases, but mostly is normal. However, the vas deferens is absent in most cases. Genital abnormalities are common in the females and may show absent or bicornuate uterus and absent or blind vaginas in most cases. The ovaries and fallopian tubes are generally normal. Ovarian hypoplasia or aplasia may occur. Abnormalities of the gastrointestinal tract are seen in most patients and include absence of sigmoid colon and rectum with imperforate anus, malrotation of the bowel, Meckel diverticulum, duodenal atresia and tracheoesophageal fistula. Other abnormalities include atrial septal defect, VSD, meningomyelocele, hydrocephalous, microgyria, microphthalmia and cataract.

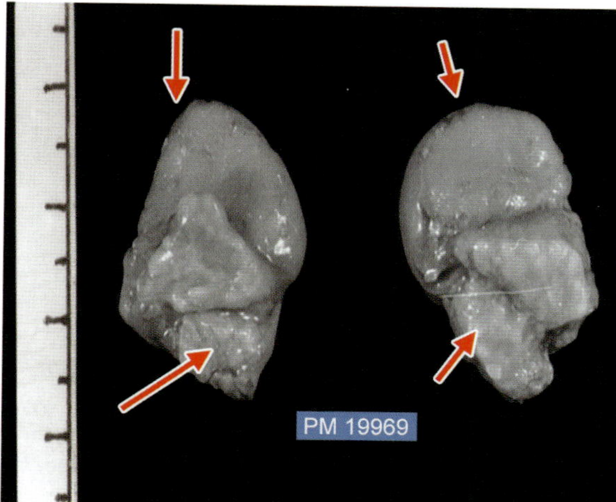

Fig. 1: Gross photograph showing adrenals (upper arrows) along with attached nubbins composed of renal tissue which have been cut open (lower arrows).

Potter's syndrome: Potter described a collection of characteristic abnormalities, which she labeled as Potter's syndrome, in babies with bilateral renal agenesis. It is also seen in cases of severe bilateral cystic dysplasia, urethral obstruction and in chronic leakage of amniotic fluid. Potter's syndrome has a distinctive facies, bent and deformed extremities and a bell-shaped chest due to hypoplastic lungs. The face has a haggard look and shows a contorted grimace, bags under the eye, broad and flat nose with a hooked parrot beaked appearance and prominent cleft between the lower lip and chin along with low set ears. There is flexion at the hips and knees and legs are bowed with clubbed feet. The skin is dry and loose folds are seen under the chin, around the abdomen, extremities and on the hands. There is a bell-shaped chest due pulmonary hypoplasia and if the child is born live, they die within 24 hours due to pulmonary insufficiency. Oligohydramnios causes Potter's syndrome.

- ***Congenital hydronephrosis with or without dysplasia*:** Congenital hydronephrosis occurs due to intrauterine obstruction at any level of the urinary tract. In obstructive uropathy, four factors which play an important role in ascertaining the degree of maldevelopment are—time, rapidity, degree (complete or partial) and site of obstruction. Complete and early obstruction, i.e. before the nephrogenesis is complete, leads to marked hydronephrosis with cyst formation in the thinned out rim of the cortex, along with features of dysplasia. Presence of dysplastic changes is also proportional to the degree of ectopia of the ureteral orifice. Obstruction late in gestation, i.e. after nephrogenesis is complete, leads to simple hydronephrosis of varying degrees without dysplastic changes. In partial obstruction, renal development continues and has a better prognosis. The site of obstruction decides the unilaterality or bilaterality of the hydroureteronephrosis and the involvement of the bladder. In severe urethral obstruction, there is bilateral hydroureteronephrosis with bladder involvement. There is generally a variation in the severity of involvement of the two sides. The kidneys retain their basic reniform shape and the capsular aspect is studded with innumerable tiny cysts. On cut section, the kidneys show dilatation of the renal pelvis, obliteration of the calyces, loss of corticomedullary distinction, with the cysts confined to the peripheral cortex. Ureters are dilated and the urinary bladder is hypertrophied. On microscopy, the cortex shows hydronephrotic atrophy with widespread disarray and dysplastic changes. Cysts are lined by low to columnar epithelium and may show remnant of an atretic glomerular tuft indicating that cysts are the dilated "S-shaped" portion of the nephron and thus the insult took place at the most vulnerable "S stage" of nephrogenesis. Cysts are small and may show a fibromuscular collar around it and should be differentiated from primitive ducts. Intervening glomerular and tubular remnants are sparse with varying degrees of atrophy. The most common cause of bilateral congenital hydroureteronephrosis is posterior urethral valve followed by Prune belly syndrome. Less common are urethral atresia and urethral fibroelastosis.

HEREDITARY RENAL ADYSPLASIA (HRA)

- Renal developmental disorders, i.e. hypoplasia or dysplasia as such are considered to be sporadic, noninherited malformations. But this is not always true, as there are a large number of reports in literature stating the familial nature of these disorders. So, the familial occurrence of renal abnormalities like agenesis, dysplasia or hypoplasia either unilateral or bilateral is a group referred to as HRA, the term first described by Buchta et al. The kidney is generally small and rudimentary, but can be multicystic. Mode of inheritance in most cases is autosomal dominant with incomplete penetrance and variable expression, can also be autosomal recessive and occasionally X-linked. Multifactorial inheritance remains a possibility. McPherson et al described seven families and reviewed literature wherein they found 65 families with renal developmental disorders like agenesis or dysplasia showing a repetition, but not fitting into any syndrome. They, thus stressed on the fact that all cases of renal agenesis or dysplasia should have a comprehensive assessment with ultrasonographic study of the kidneys (and uterus) along with family details of their parents and siblings. McPherson et al came to the conclusion that the most likely pattern of transmission of HRA is autosomal dominant with incomplete penetrance (50% and 90%). In pedigrees with HRA, the risk for acquiring grave disease in the offspring of affected or obligate heterozygotes is 15–20%. McPherson et al also stated that in the presence of a negative family history along with normal renal findings in both parents, the risk for recurrence of bilateral renal agenesis /dysplasia/hypoplasia in siblings of the affected infant is 3.5%. In unilateral renal agenesis/dysplasia/hypoplasia, if the family history suggests HRA, the risk of acquiring disease in both the kidneys of offspring or other family members is low.

SUGGESTED READING

1. Battin J, Lacombe D, Leng JJ. Familial occurrence of hereditary renal adysplasia with mullerian anomalies. Clin Genet. 1993;43(1):23-4.
2. Bernstein J. A classification of renal cysts. In: Gardner KD (Ed). Cystic Diseases of the Kidney. New York: John Wiley & Sons Publishers; 1976. pp. 7-30.
3. Bernstein J. Developmental abnormalities of the renal parenchyma-hypoplasia and dysplasia. Pathol Annu. 1968; 3:213-47.
4. Bernstein J. Hepatic and renal involvement in malformation syndromes. Mt Sinai J Med. 1986;53:421-8.
5. Bernstein J. The classification of renal cysts. Nephron. 1973;11:91.
6. Bernstein J. The morphogenesis of renal parenchymal maldevelopment (renal dysplasia). Pediatr Clin North Am. 1971;18:395-407.
7. Bernstein J. The multicystic kidney and hereditary renal adysplasia. Am J Kidney Dis. 1991;18(4):495-6.
8. Buchta RM, Viseskul C, Gilbert EF, et al. Familial bilateral renal agenesis and hereditary renal adysplasia. Z Kinderheilkd. 1973;115(2):111-29.
9. Cain DR, Griggs D, Lackey DA, et al. Familial renal agenesis and total dysplasia. Am J Dis Child. 1974;128:377-80.
10. Duncan PA, Shapiro LR, Stangel JJ, et al. The MURCS association: Müllerian duct aplasia, renal aplasia and cervico-thoracic somite dysplasia. J Pediatr. 1979;95(3):399-402.
11. Fletcher J, Hu M, Berman Y, et al. Multicystic dysplastic kidney and variable phenotype in a family with a novel deletion mutation of PAX2. J Am Soc Nephrol. 2005;16:2754-61.
12. Glassberg KI, Stephens FD, Lebowitz RE, et al. Renal dysgenesis and cystic disease of the kidney: A report of the committee on terminology, nomenclature and classification, section on urology. Am Acad Pediatr J Urol. 1987;138:1085.
13. Hill GS. Cystic and Dysplastic diseases of the kidney: Developmental lesions. In: Hill GS (Ed). Uropathology, Volume 1. Edinburgh, New York: Churchill Livingstone; 1989. pp. 81-133.
14. Kakkar N, Menon S, Radotra BD. Histomorphology of renal dysplasia – An autopsy study. Fetal Pediatr Pathol. 2006;25(2):73-86.
15. Kakkar N, Menon S, Radotra BD. Spectrum of pediatric development and genetic renal lesions and associated congenital malformations- an autopsy study from North India. Fetal Pediatr Pathol. 2006;25(1):35-49.
16. McPherson E, Carey J, Kramer A, et al. Dominantly inherited renal adysplasia. Am J Med Genet. 1987;26(4):863-72.
17. Menon S, Kakkar N, Radotra BD. Expression of laminin and fibronectin in renal dysplasia. Pediatr Dev Pathol. 2004; 7(6):568-76.
18. Moerman P, Fryns JP, Sastrowijoto SH, et al. Hereditary renal adysplasia: new observations and hypotheses. Pediatr Pathol. 1994;14(3):405-10.
19. Murugasu B, Cole BR, Hawkins EP, et al. Familial renal adysplasia. Am J Kidney Dis. 1991;18(4):490-4.
20. Risdon RA, Young LW, Crispin AR. Renal hypoplasia and dysplasia: A radiological and pathological correlation. Pediatr Radiol. 1975;3:312.
21. Schwarz RD, Stephens FD, Cussen LJ. The pathogenesis of renal dysplasia. III Complete and in-complete urinary obstruction. Invest Urol, 1981;19:101.

CASE 70

Recurrent Bilateral Multicystic Dysplastic Kidneys, Consistent with Hereditary Renal Adysplasia: PM 20505

Nandita Bharadwaj Kakkar

HIGHLIGHTS OF THE CASE

A 25-year-old female, gravida 3, with two previous pregnancy losses at 12 weeks and 28 weeks, came with ultrasonographic detection of oligohydramnios with enlarged multicystic kidneys. G2 at ultrasonography (USG) revealed bilateral multicystic kidneys. Index baby, i.e. G3 was a spontaneous abortion at 22 weeks gestation. Autopsy revealed bilateral multicystic dysplastic kidneys with megaureters. In view of the recurrence of renal disease, diagnosis was consistent with familial or hereditary renal adysplasia.

Keywords: Recurrence, bilateral, multicystic dysplasia, bunch of grapes, familial or hereditary renal adysplasia, megaureters, autopsy.

CLINICAL DETAILS

Date of Still Birth: 03.03.2005.

A 25-year-old female, G_3P_{0110}, with two previous pregnancy losses at 12 weeks and 28 weeks, was admitted with ultrasonographic detection of oligohydramnios along with fetal cystic kidneys. She conceived 4 years after her marriage. ***G1***: A missed abortion at 12 weeks of gestation. ***G2***: There was history of taking some medication, the nature of which is not known. USG at 3 months was apparently normal. At 28 weeks, there were decreased fetal movements. USG revealed intrauterine fetal death and bilateral multicystic kidneys. She delivered a macerated female baby with no external abnormality. Autopsy was not done. ***G3*** (index baby): one year later she conceived again while being on some unknown medication, the first trimester was uncomplicated and no early USG was done. Blood pressure at 21 weeks was 140/90 mm Hg and blood sugar was within normal limits. ***USG at 21 + 2 weeks***—Single live fetus, placenta anterior marginal, oligohydramnios present, fetal kidney show multiple cysts and no urinary bladder seen. Other congenital malformation cannot be ruled out. ***USG—level 3 at 22 weeks***: Right kidney: 5.9 × 4.8 cm, left kidney: 4.0 × 2.0 cm, both kidneys multicystic and no liquor present. The patient aborted spontaneously 4 hours after admission. It was a male baby, 700 g, with a distended abdomen. Baby was sent for autopsy.

AUTOPSY FINDINGS: PM 20505

A complete autopsy was performed on this 700 g male baby. The abdomen was distended. There was flexion deformity at the hips and knees along with congenital talipes equino varus (CTEV). No other external abnormality was noted. There was an asymmetrical enlargement of both kidneys with multiple cysts, giving the classical bunch of grapes appearance (Fig 1A). The right kidney measured 8 × 5 × 4 cm and the left measured 5 × 4 × 3 cm. The ureters were dilated, tortuous and showed aberrant insertion into the distorted urinary bladder (Fig 1A). Cut section of the kidney revealed cysts of varying sizes (Fig 1B) ranging between 0.5 cm and 2 cm in diameter, containing clear fluid. Solid areas could be identified in between the cysts. No pelvicalyceal system was identified, as it was fused with the mass. Microscopic examination (Figs 1C and D) revealed total lobar disorganization with cysts lined by flattened epithelium. The solid areas in between contained the diagnostic hallmark of dysplasia known as "primitive ducts" (Fig 1E), which are small tubular structures, lined by columnar epithelium and surrounded by a collar of concentrically placed immature mesenchyme. They were present singly and in clusters. Apart from this, the solid areas showed hypocellular loose

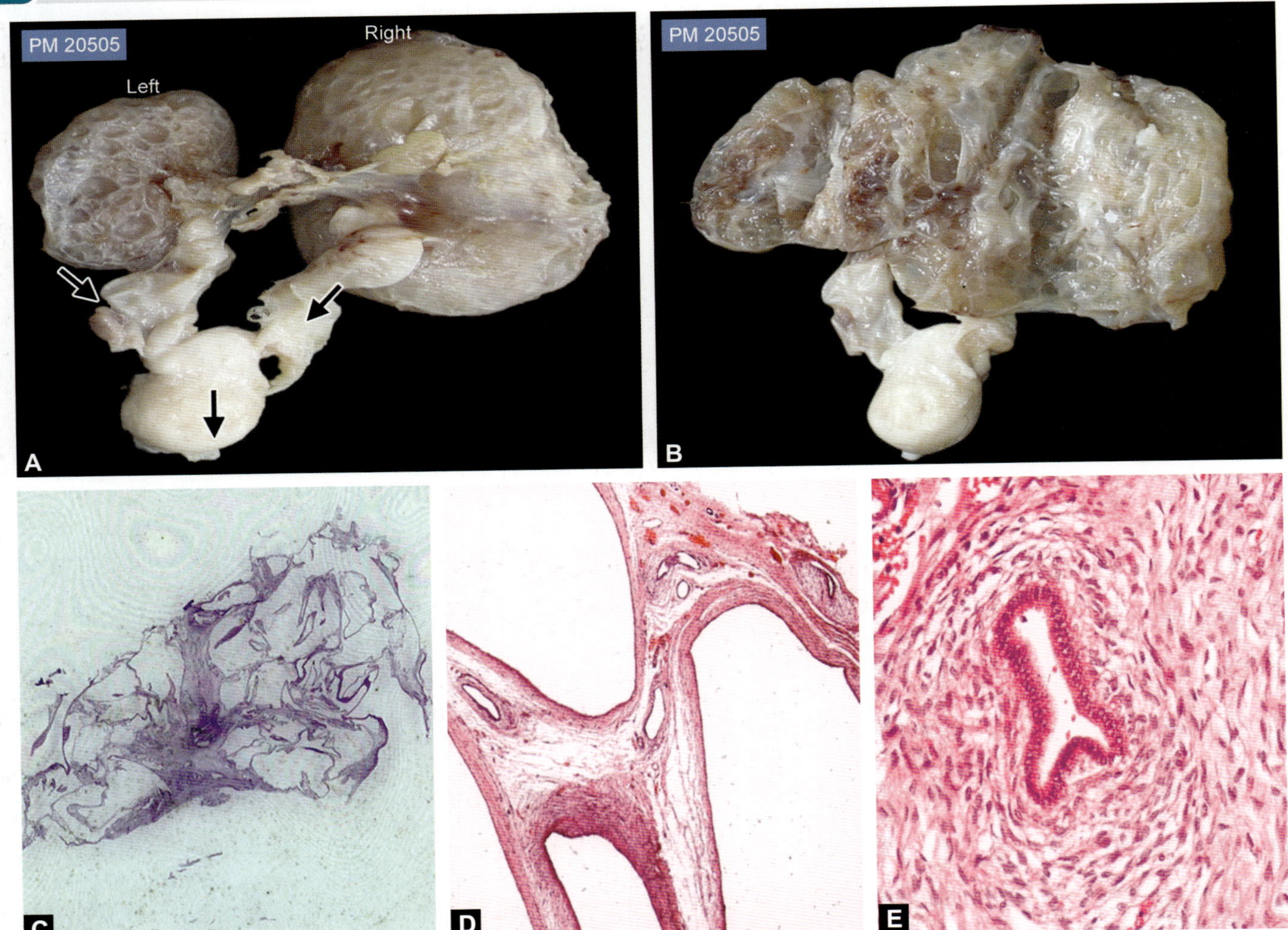

Figs 1A–E: (A) Gross photograph of the enlarged multicystic kidneys resembling "bunch of grapes", along with distorted mega ureters (upper arrows) and urinary bladder (lower arrow); (B) Cut section of both kidneys showing multiple cysts of varying sizes, ranging between 0.5 cm and 3 cm in diameter. Solid areas can be appreciated in between. No pelvis is appreciated; (C) Photomicrographs at low power showing multiple cysts; (D) Photomicrograph showing cysts with flattened lining epithelium and intervening septae show loose connective tissue; (E) Primitive duct lined by columnar epithelium and surrounded by a collar of immature mesenchyme.

mesenchyme, abortive glomeruli, rudimentary tubules, proliferating vessels/nerves, immature cartilage and foci of extramedullary hematopoiesis. Overall features were those of bilateral multicystic dysplastic kidneys. The lungs weighed 28 g and did not show any hypoplasia. The liver was normal and did not show any features of ductal plate malformation.

FINAL AUTOPSY DIAGNOSIS: PM 20505

22 Weeks Gestation, Spontaneous Expulsion. Case of Recurrent Fetal Death

Bilateral multicystic dysplastic kidneys with megaureters consistent with hereditary renal adysplasia.

***For renal multicystic dysplasia and herditary renal adysplasia*:** Refer to "Pediatric cystic disease (developmental/genetic) of kidney- Introduction".

COMMENTARY—INDEX CASE: PM 20505

This was a gravida 3 mother, with no living issue. There was a recurrence of multicystic, dysplastic renal disease and this is known as hereditary renal adysplasia. Although multicystic dysplasia is a developmental, sporadic disorder, it is seen to occur in families and recur in the same family, known as hereditary or familial renal adysplasia, which in most cases has an autosomal dominant mode of inheritance. Once a diagnosis of renal agenesis or dysplasia is made in a case, a thorough evaluation is undertaken. Detailed family history and ultrasonographic study of the kidneys and uterus of all parents and siblings of affected individuals is mandatory. In pedigrees with HRA, the risk for acquiring grave disease in the offspring of affected or obligate heterozygotes is 15–20%. So, serial USG during pregnancy is strongly recommended. In the presence of a negative family history along with normal renal findings in both parents, the risk for recurrence of bilateral renal agenesis/dysplasia/hypoplasia in siblings of the affected infant is 3.5%.

TAKE HOME MESSAGE

- Renal developmental disorders, i.e. renal dysplasias are considered to be sporadic, non-inherited malformations. However, there are a large number of reports in literature stating the familial nature of these disorders.
- The familial occurrence and increased risk of recurrence in a subsequent pregnancy, of renal developmental abnormalities like renal agenesis or dysplasia is a group referred to as familial or hereditary renal adysplasia.
- The kidney in hereditary renal adysplasia is usually tiny and rudimentary (renal aplasia) but can be multicystic (index case).
- Mode of inheritance in HRA is predominantly autosomal dominant with incomplete penetrance and variable expression, but can also be autosomal recessive and occasionally X-linked.
- "Primitive duct" is the morphological pathognomonic hallmark of dysplasia. Without this, the term "dysplasia" cannot be used.

CONTRIBUTIONS BY:

1. Dr Sarla Gopalan, Ex-Professor and Head, Department of Obstetrics and Gynaecology (Clinician In-Charge) Post Graduate Institute of Medical Education and Research, (PGIMER) Chandigarh, India.

CASE 71

Symmetrically Enlarged, Solid Dysplastic Kidneys with Intrauterine Growth Retardation: PM 24340

Nandita Bharadwaj Kakkar

HIGHLIGHTS OF THE CASE

This was a female baby, born at term to a primigravida, weighed 1,472 g, had severe birth asphyxia requiring extensive resuscitation. Ultrasonography done at 25+4 weeks revealed severe intrauterine growth retardation, oligohydramnios and enlarged kidneys with few cysts. Autopsy revealed bilateral predominantly solid, dysplastic kidneys with pulmonary hypoplasia.

Keywords: Solid, symmetrical enlargement, dysplastic kidneys, lung hypoplasia, Potter's facies, autopsy, intrauterine growth retardation.

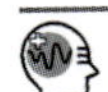

CLINICAL DETAILS

Date of Birth and Death: 29.6.2011, Lived for 1.5 Hours

A female baby was born at 37 weeks gestation (birth weight—1,472 g), to a 22-year-old primigravida mother, by an assisted breech vaginal delivery. There was severe birth asphyxia with a very low APGAR score of 1,1,1,1. The baby required extensive resuscitation with positive pressure ventilation and chest compression. She expired at 90 minutes of life. The pregnancy was supervised in PGI since 24 weeks gestation. The first trimester was however uncomplicated and no early ultrasonography was done. Ultrasonography done at 25+4 weeks revealed severe intrauterine growth retardation, oligohydramnios, enlarged kidneys with few cysts and a small urinary bladder. Cord revealed two vessels only. There was no history of radiation, drug exposure or any fever. Gestational diabetes mellitus was detected at 29 weeks, for which she was put on a diabetic diet. The blood pressure records were normal. After birth, the baby was put on intermittent positive pressure respiration (IPPR). Baby had a dysmorphic, i.e. Potter's facies with low set ears, depressed nasal bridge, flat facies, retrognathia, abnormal palmar creases, congenital talipes equino varus (CTEV) of right foot and a single umbilical artery. There was no renal mass palpable and the genitalia were normal. The clinical diagnosis was severe birth asphyxia, intrauterine growth retardation, Potter's facies, enlarged kidneys with small cysts, lung hypoplasia ? autosomal recessive polycystic kidney disease (ARPKD).

AUTOPSY FINDINGS: PM 24340

External appearance*:** Baby had a Potter's facies, retrognathia, abnormal palmar creases and CTEV of right foot. The abdomen was distended. ***Anthropometric measurements: body weight at autopsy—1,450 g, crown heel/crown-rump length—41/25 cm, femur/foot length—8/6 cm, head/chest/abdominal circumference—30/25/27 cm. The abdomen was distended. The kidneys (Fig 1A) were symmetrically enlarged with discernable fetal lobulations, measuring 4.5 × 1.5 × 0.8 cm. Capsular surface showed few small cysts. The right ureter was mildly dilated all along its length and the left ureter showed skip areas of atresia. The urinary bladder was distorted with ectopia of the ureteric orifices. Cut- section of the kidneys (Fig 1B) was predominantly solid with small scattered cysts, no corticomedullary differentiation and a fused pelvis. Microscopic sections (Figs 1C–E) from the kidney revealed complete lobar disorganization, small cysts, abortive glomeruli, rudimentary tubules and clusters of classical primitive ducts, lined by columnar epithelium and surrounded by the characteristic collar of immature mesenchyme. The lungs weighed 12 g and were hypoplastic. No ductal plate malformation was present.

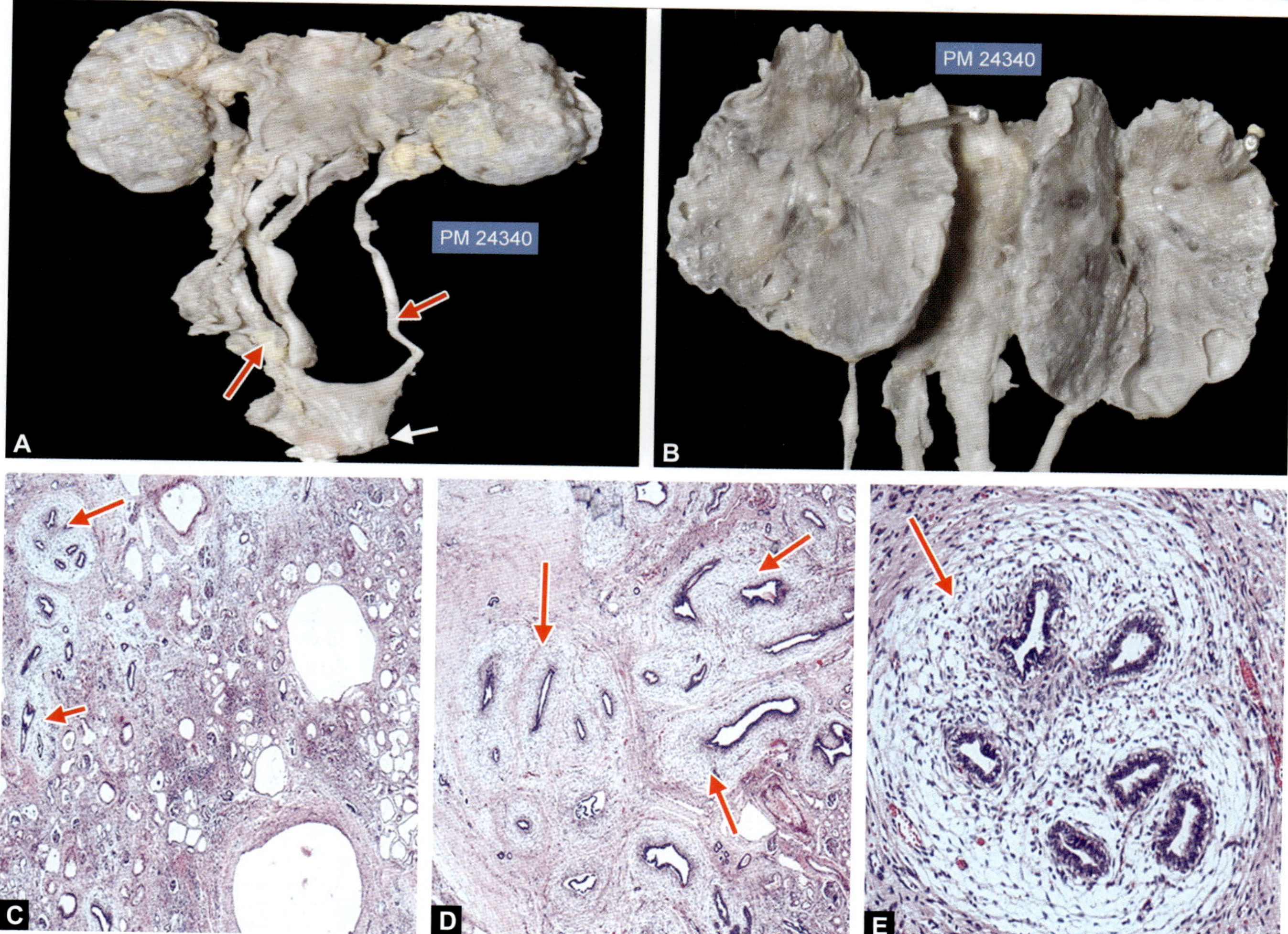

Figs 1A–E: (A) Gross photograph of both kidneys showing cysts on the surface, abnormal ureters, i.e. right is (arrow) dilated and left shows skip areas of narrowing (arrow) and the small and distorted urinary bladder (white arrow) with abnormally placed ureteric orifices; (B) Cut section of both kidneys showing few scattered cysts and no corticomedullary differentiation. Pelvis is fused with the kidney; (C–E) Photomicrograph of the kidney showing complete lobar disorganization, few small-sized cysts, rudimentary glomeruli/tubules, and primitive ducts in clusters (red arrows), surrounded by collars of immature mesenchyme.

FINAL AUTOPSY DIAGNOSIS: PM 24340

Neonate Born at 37 Weeks Gestation and Lived for 1.5 Hours

- Bilateral symmetrically enlarged, solid dysplastic kidneys with bilateral ureteric and bladder abnormality.
- Bilateral pulmonary hypoplasia.

For renal dysplasia—Refer to "Pediatric cystic disease (developmental/genetic) of kidney- Introduction".

COMMENTARY—INDEX CASE: PM 24340

Bilateral symmetrical enlargement of the kidneys with maintained reniform shape is the diagnostic hallmark of ARPKD and Meckel-Gruber syndrome (MGS). In ARPKD, on a closer look of the kidneys, there is a myriad of pinhead sized cysts on the capsular surface and the cut section reveals linear cysts, running from the medulla to the cortex, giving the classical sunray appearance. No dysplasia is seen on microscopy. In MGS, cut section of the kidneys show rounded cysts present diffusely and on microscopy, dysplasia is noted. The liver in both conditions show ductal plate malformation. MGS is an autosomal recessive condition and in addition shows polydactyly and CNS malformation (mostly encephalocele). Dysplastic kidneys are generally distorted, show an asymmetrical enlargement, bunch of grapes appearance and the reniform shape is not maintained. Very occasionally one can encounter a bilateral symmetrical enlargement with maintained reniform shape, as seen in the index case. Absence of ductal plate malformation, polydactyly and CNS malformation differentiates it from MGS. Absence of the typical sunray appearance, ductal plate malformation and presence of dysplasia differentiates it from ARPKD.

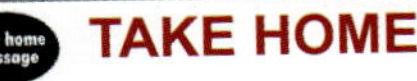

TAKE HOME MESSAGE

- Bilateral symmetrical enlargement of the kidneys with maintained reniform shape is the diagnostic hallmark of autosomal recessive polycystic kidney disease and Meckel Gruber syndrome. However, it can be occasionally seen in predominantly solid dysplastic kidneys.

CONTRIBUTIONS BY:

1. Dr Vikrant, Junior Resident, Department of Pathology
2. Dr Rohit Bhowmick, Junior Resident, Department of Pediatrics (Compilation of Clinical Details)
3. Dr Praveen Kumar, Professor and Head, Department of Pediatrics—Neonatology Division (Clinician In-Charge)

Post Graduate Institute of Medical Education and Research, Chandigarh, India.

CASE 72

Multicystic Dysplastic Kidneys with Dilated Ureters and Hypertrophied Urinary Bladder Leading to Obstructed Labor and Uterine Rupture: PM 26207

Nandita Bharadwaj Kakkar

 HIGHLIGHTS OF THE CASE

This was a 22-year-old, gravida 2, lady, who underwent an unsupervised pregnancy. At term, she was diagnosed with oligohydramnios and bilateral multicystic kidneys were detected in her baby. She had obstructed labor followed by uterine rupture. The baby weighed 5 kg, had Potter's facies and a markedly distended abdomen. Autopsy revealed bilateral multicystic dysplastic kidneys with bilateral hydroureters and an enlarged hypertrophied urinary bladder along with hypoplastic lungs.

Keywords: Kidneys, bilateral, multicystic dysplasia, still birth, term, uterine rupture, obstructed labor.

 CLINICAL DETAILS

Date of Still-birth: 14.08.2014

A 22-year-old female, G2P1001, at 40 weeks period of gestation was admitted at an outside facility in Kurukshetra, on 13th August 2014 at 10 PM with labor pains. At 11:30 PM, she was fully dilated and there was spontaneous delivery of the head after which there was shoulder dystocia. Ultrasonography done at term revealed bilateral multicystic kidneys with severe oligohydramnios. She was immediately referred to our institute, where she reached at 4 AM on 14th August 2014. Past history revealed that G1 was a normal vaginal delivery and the baby is doing well. On ***examination*** at admission, the mother was afebrile and dehydrated. The pulse was—116/min, respiratory rate—24/min and BP—150/100 mm Hg. There was no pallor. The baby was dead and its head and shoulders were lying outside the vagina. Urethral hematoma was present. Mother was catheterized and the urine was hemorrhagic. The contractions were moderate and regular and half of the baby up till the diaphragm was delivered. There was impending uterine rupture. She was being prepared for the surgery when she expelled the baby at 6:50 AM. It was a male baby, weighing 5 kg with a markedly distended abdomen. On per vaginal examination, a large vent was felt in the posterior uterine wall. Ultrasonography revealed free fluid in the abdomen and the placenta was in the peritoneal cavity. She was immediately taken up for surgery. There was hemoperitoneum, with 800 mL of hemorrhagic fluid. The uterus, cervix and the vaginal tears were repaired meticulously. The mother survived the catastrophe.

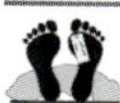 AUTOPSY FINDINGS: PM 26207

A complete autopsy was performed. Baby (Fig 1A) had Potter's facies (low set ears, contorted grimace, mongoloid slant, short neck, bags under the eye, talipes equinovarus) and a markedly distended abdomen. Anthropometric measurements: crown-heel/crown-rump length—53/38 cm, head/chest/abdominal circumference—35/34/52 cm and foot length—8 cm. Weight at birth was 5 kg. All serous cavities were within normal limits. There was no cryptorchidism. The scrotum was enlarged and the penis was small with an identifiable urethral meatus. Imperforate anus was noted. Both the kidneys (Fig 1B) were asymmetrically enlarged and markedly distorted with multiple cysts, giving the classical bunch of grapes appearance. The left kidney measured 15 × 10 × 7 cm and the right kidney 8 × 7 × 4 cm. The ureters were markedly dilated, tortuous and measured 2 cm in diameter and the urinary bladder was markedly hypertrophied. No posterior urethral valve was identified. The gut was ending blindly on the surface of the urinary bladder, but was not communicating with it. Cut section of

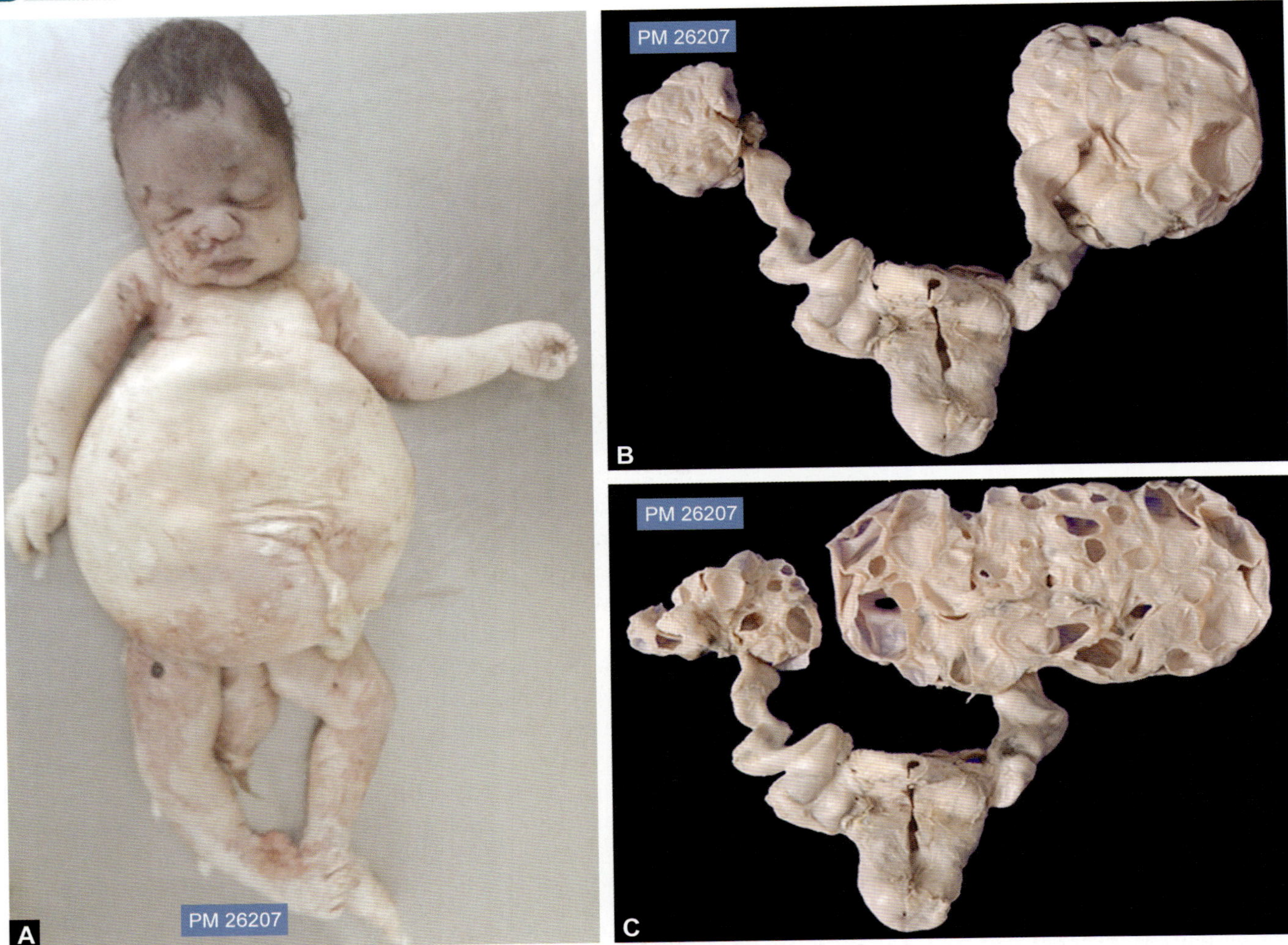

Figs 1A–C: (A) Still born male, showing Potter's facies and a markedly distended abdomen; (B) Gross photograph of both the kidneys—bunch of grapes appearance, asymmetrical enlargement, multiple cysts, dilated tortuous ureters and hypertrophied urinary bladder; (C) Cut section of the kidneys showing multiple cysts present diffusely.

the kidneys (Fig 1C) revealed cysts of varying sizes ranging between 0.5 and 3 cm in diameter, containing clear fluid present diffusely both in the cortex and medulla. Solid areas could be identified in between the cysts. Microscopic examination revealed total lobar disorganization with cysts lined by flattened epithelium (Figs 2A and B). The solid areas in between the cysts contained "primitive ducts", the diagnostic hallmark of dysplasia which are small structures, lined by columnar epithelium and surrounded by a collar of concentrically placed immature mesenchyme (Figs 2B and C-arrows). They were present singly or in clusters. Apart from this, the solid areas showed hypocellular loose mesenchyme, rudimentary tubules, immature cartilage (Fig 2D), proliferating nerves (Fig 2E) and foci of extramedullary hematopoiesis. The urinary bladder and the ureters showed hypertrophied muscle (Figs 2F and G). Overall features were those of bilateral multicystic dysplastic kidneys with dilated tortuous ureters and hypertrophied urinary bladder. The liver showed extramedullary hematopoiesis, but did not show any feature of ductal plate malformation. The lungs were hypoplastic, together weighed 27 g and the right lung was hemorrhagic. The adrenals showed hemorrhage. The brain was within normal limits.

FINAL AUTOPSY DIAGNOSIS: PM 26207

Fresh Still-birth at 40 Weeks Gestation with Uterine Rupture

- Bilateral multicystic dysplastic kidneys with bilateral hydroureters and an enlarged hypertrophied urinary bladder.
- Bilateral hypoplastic lungs.
- Anorectal malformation.

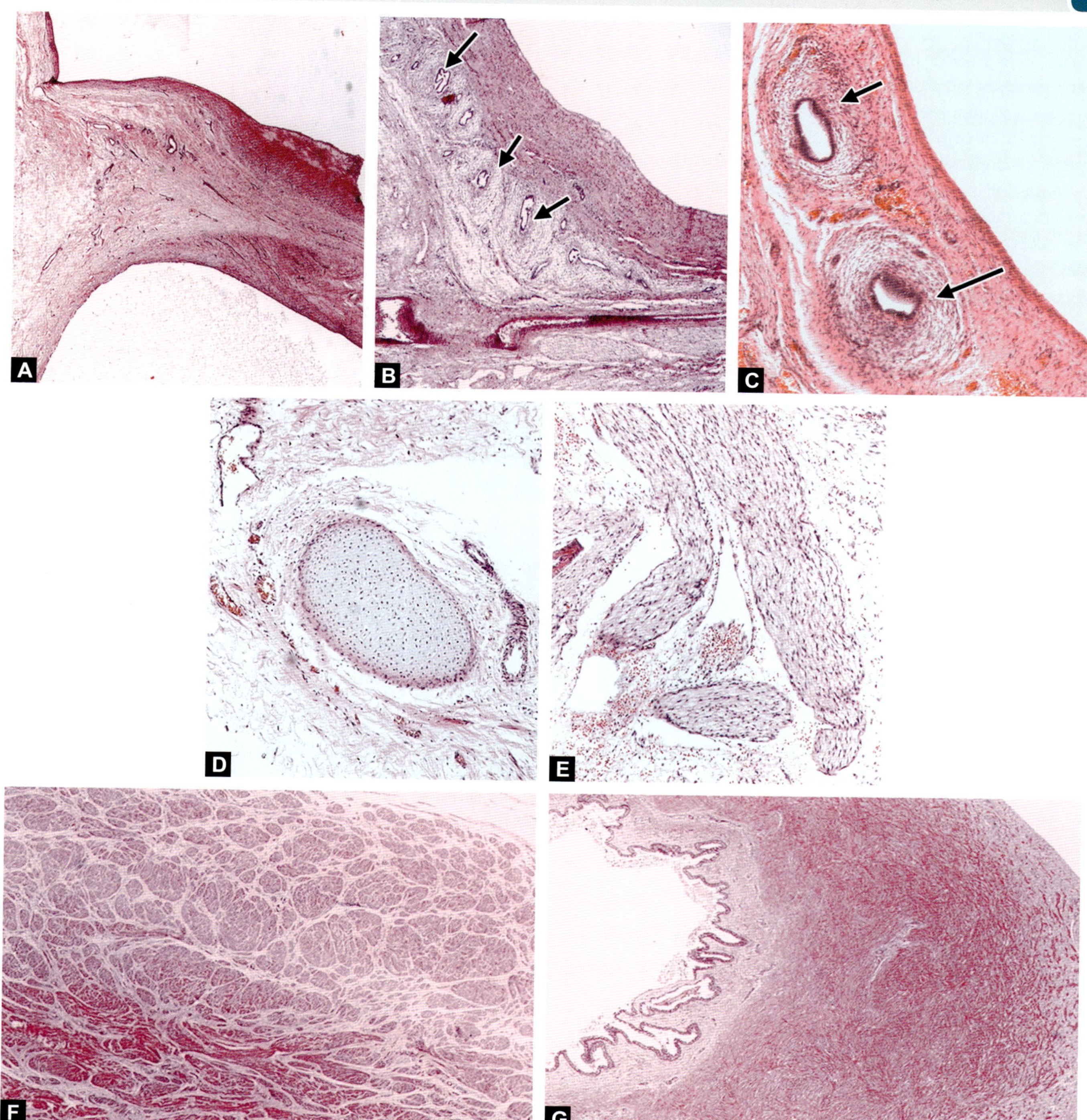

Figs 2A–G: Photomicrographs of the kidney showing (A) Cysts lined by non-descript epithelium with intervening septae; (B and C) Septae show primitive ducts (arrows) surrounded by a collar of immature mesenchyme; (D) Immature cartilage; (E) Proliferating nerves; (F) Photomicrograph of the bladder showing hypertrophied muscle bundles; (G) Ureter showing transitional lining and hypertrophied muscle.

COMMENTARY—INDEX CASE: PM 26207

This was a 22-year-old, second gravida mother, who did not avail antenatal care. She was diagnosed to have bilateral multicystic kidneys and oligohydramnios at term. She had obstructed labor followed by uterine rupture, which was repaired. Autopsy revealed bilateral multicystic dysplastic kidneys, hydroureters and hypertrophied urinary bladder along with hypoplastic lungs and anorectal malformation. Dilated tortuous ureters and a hypertrophied urinary bladder are always seen in cases of posterior urethral valve/urethral obstruction and not so often seen with multicystic dysplasia. In the index case, both kidneys revealed the classic bunch of grapes appearance as is classically seen in multicystic dysplastic kidneys. In posterior urethral valve/urethral obstruction, the kidneys maintain their reniform shape, show cysts on the surface and cut section shows hydronephrosis with thinned out cortical rim. So, the gross appearance of the kidneys in the index case negates a diagnosis of posterior urethral valve/urethral obstruction.

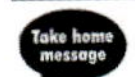

TAKE HOME MESSAGE

- Markedly dilated and tortuous ureters with hypertrophied urinary bladder at times can be seen in cases of multicystic dysplasia but always seen in cases of posterior urethral valve/urethral obstruction. The gross appearance of the kidneys, however clinches the diagnosis.
- Classical bunch of grapes with fused pelvis is diagnostic of multicystic dysplasia and maintained reniform shape with hydronephrosis is seen in posterior urethral valve/urethral obstruction.

CONTRIBUTIONS BY:

1. Dr L Dhaliwal, Ex-Professor and Head, Department of Obstetrics and Gynecology (Clinician In-Charge)
2. Dr Suravi Mohanty, Fellow, Post-doctoral Course, Pediatric Pathology

Post Graduate Institute of Medical Education and Research, Chandigarh, India.

CASE 73-74

Renal Hypodysplasia: PM 19521, PM 25711

Nandita Bharadwaj Kakkar

HIGHLIGHTS OF THE CASES

Both cases show bilateral hypodysplastic kidneys, with patent malformed ureters and imperforate anus with blind ending large gut. The lungs were not hypoplastic. Both babies died of lung complications, although their prognosis was as such poor due to the bilateral renal hypodysplasia.

Keywords: Bilateral, renal hypodysplasia, patent or malformed ureters, hyaline membrane disease, congenital pneumonia.

CASE 73: PM 19521

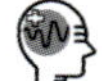

CLINICAL DETAILS

Date of Birth and Death: 09.10.2003, Lived for 5 hours

A 24-year-old lady, primigravida came with preterm rupture of membranes at 33 weeks gestation. There was leakage per vaginum for the last 36 hours. She delivered a male baby by an assisted breech delivery. The facies was normal. Baby weighed 1.4 kg, had severe respiratory distress and was put on ventilatory support. The APGAR at birth was 2,2,1,1. Baby expired at 5 hours of life and was sent for autopsy after permission from the parents. ***Units clinical diagnosis was:*** Severe hyaline membrane disease with tension pneumothorax ?? pulmonary hypoplasia.

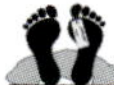

AUTOPSY FINDINGS CASE 73: PM 19521

The baby weighed 1,462 g (33 weeks gestation) and on external examination there was an imperforate anus. Bilateral pneumothorax was confirmed. Both the kidneys (Figs 1A and B) were small, left measured 0.8 × 0.5 × 0.2 cm and right measured 1.5 × 1 × 0.3 cm. The ureters were patent, but malformed. The urinary bladder was enlarged and hypertrophied and the large intestine was ending blindly on its surface (Figs 1A and B-red arrows). Cut section of the kidneys revealed discernable pelvis and few tiny cysts (more in the right kidney). Microscopy of the tiny left kidney (Fig 1C) revealed 2–3 ranks of glomeruli, loose connective tissue, foci of extramedullary hematopoiesis and primitive ducts embedded in immature mesenchyme (seen toward the medulla-black arrows in Fig 1C). The right kidney (Figs 1D and E) showed a larger number of peripheral cysts, 2–3 ranks of glomeruli and primitive ducts embedded in loose immature mesenchyme seen toward the medullary region (black arrows in Figs 1D and E). Overall features were consistent with hypodysplastic kidneys. Lungs were normal in weight and no hypoplasia was noted. Cut section was firm, liver like, with areas of hemorrhage. Microscopy (Fig 1F) revealed hyaline membrane disease, alveolar hemorrhage, congenital pneumonia and bilateral pneumothorax. The ductus was patent. Other organs were within normal limits.

FINAL AUTOPSY DIAGNOSIS: PM 19521

5 Hour Male Baby

- Bilateral hypodysplastic kidneys, patent malformed ureters and hypertrophied urinary bladder.
- Congenital pneumonia, hyaline membrane disease, pulmonary hemorrhage, congenital pneumonia and bilateral pneumothorax.
- Imperforate anus with blind ending large gut.

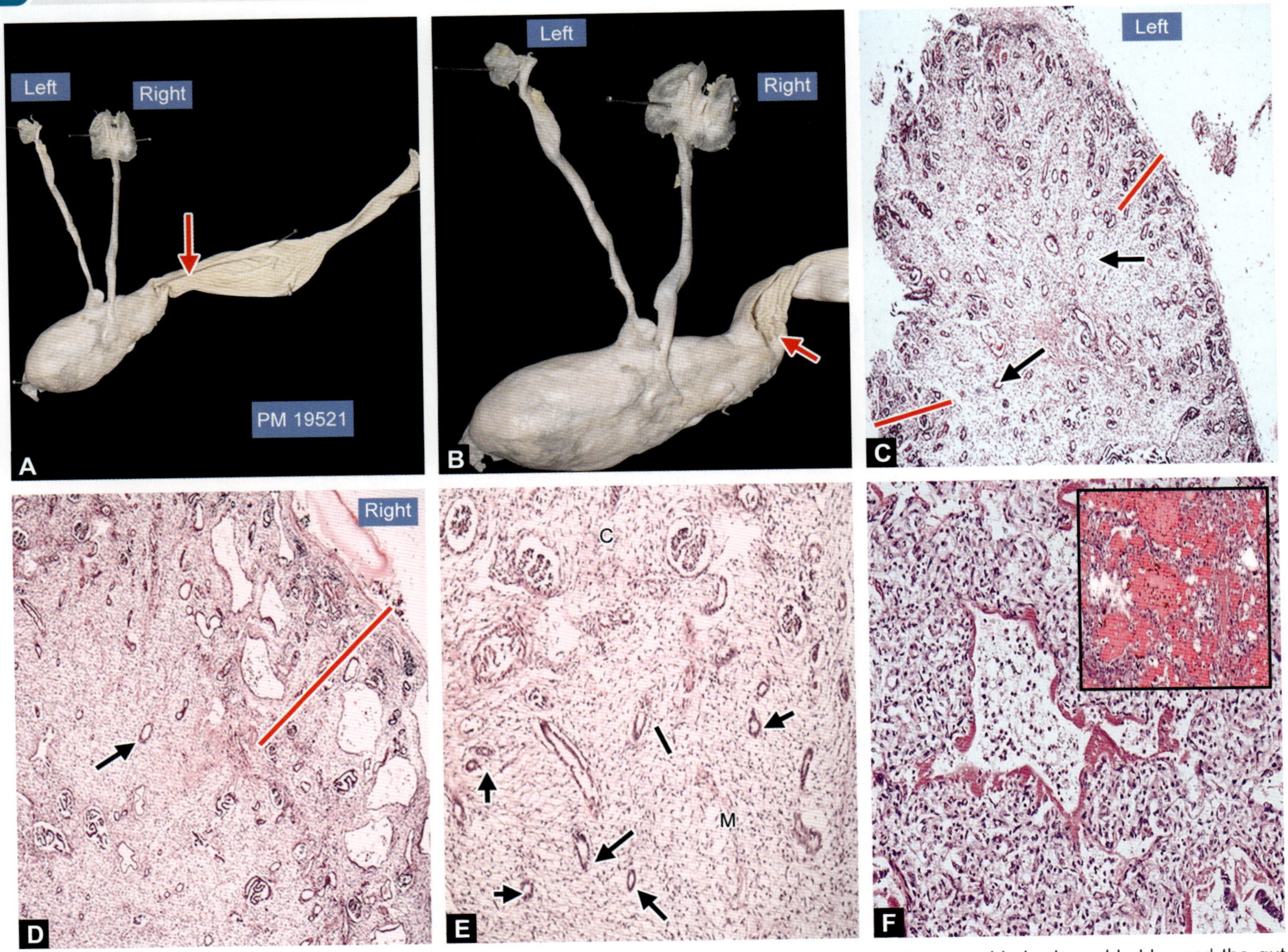

Figs 1A–F: (A and B) Gross photographs shows small-sized kidneys, patent/malformed ureters, hypertrophied urinary bladder and the gut ending blindly on its surface (arrows); (C and D) Photomicrographs of the left and right kidney—cortex shows 2–3 ranks of glomeruli (red lines) with few cysts and medulla shows small primitive ducts (black arrows) embedded in loose immature mesenchyme; (E) Photomicrograph of the right kidney shows cortex "C" and medulla "M" shows primitive ducts (black arrows) embedded in loose immature mesenchyme; (F) Photomicrographs of the lung showing hyaline membranes lining the dilated alveolar space along with neutrophils indicating congenital pneumonia. Inset shows areas with alveolar hemorrhage.

CASE 74: PM 25711

CLINICAL DETAILS

Day 2 Male Child, Baby Lived for 28 Hours

A 23-year-old lady, G2P1001, with one live child doing well, came with spontaneous onset of labor at 35 weeks gestation. She delivered a male baby (vaginal delivery), weighing 1,820 g. APGAR was 8,9. But the baby soon developed respiratory distress and had to be ventilated. Ultrasonography at 28 + 6 weeks had revealed oligohydramnios, small kidneys, left—1.8 cm and right 2.4 cm, with no corticomedullary differentiation and with increased echogenicity. Urinary bladder was visualized. Baby died at 28 hours of life. Clinical diagnosis was bilateral renal hypoplasia and pulmonary hemorrhage.

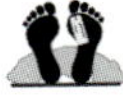

AUTOPSY FINDINGS: PM 25711

The baby had low set ears and weighed 1,800 g (35 weeks gestation). Both kidneys (Figs 2A and B) were small measuring 2.5 × 2 × 1 cm and showed small cysts on the capsular aspect as well as on cut section. The ureters were patent, but malformed and the urinary bladder appeared normal. Microscopy (Figs 2C–E) revealed well-preserved cortical renal parenchyma "C" showing 2–3 ranks of

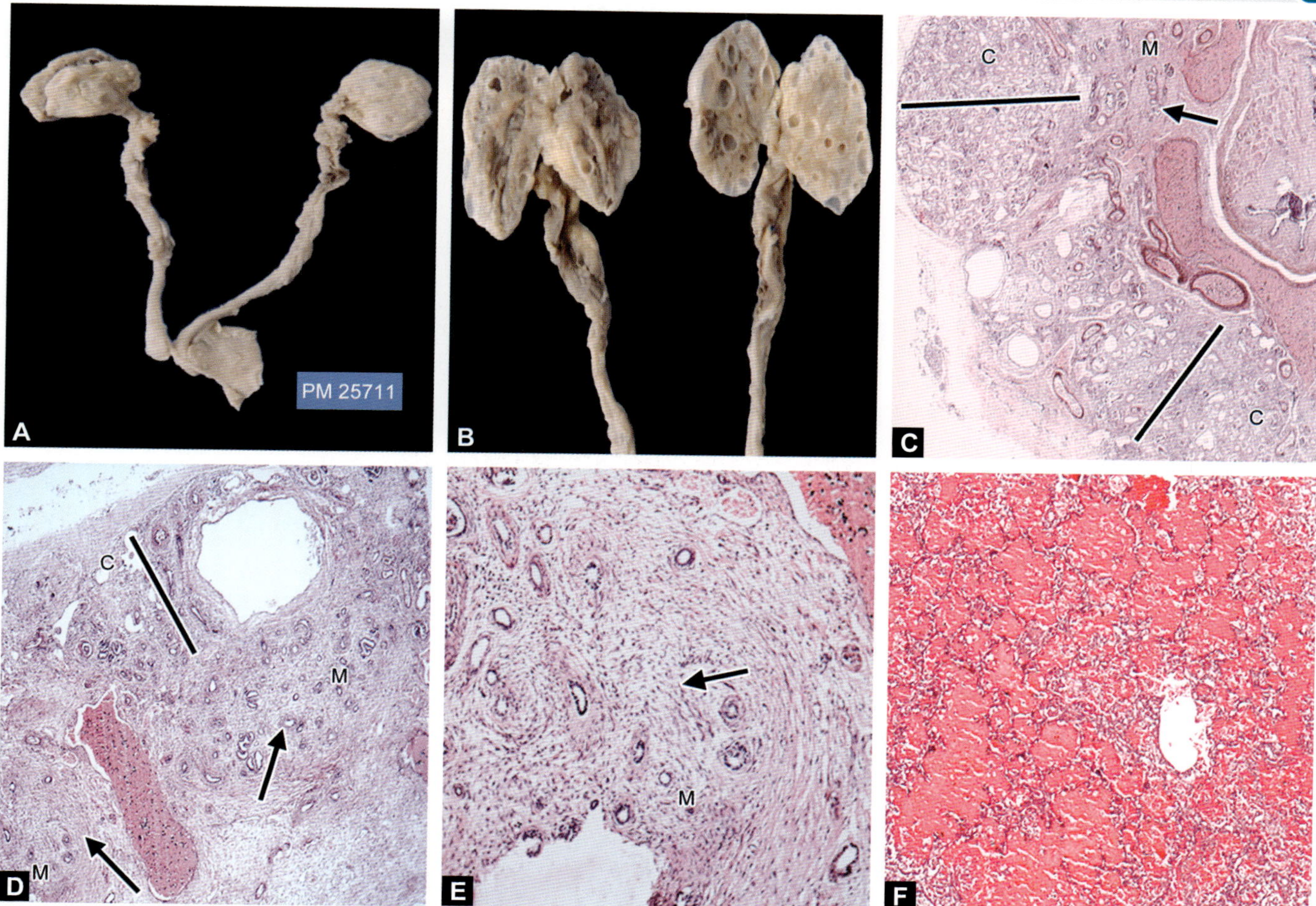

Figs 2A–F: (A and B) Both kidneys are small in size, show cysts on the surface and on cut section (mostly cortical), ureters are patent but malformed and the urinary bladder is normal sized; (C and D) Photomicrographs of the kidney show well-preserved cortical renal parenchyma showing 2–3 ranks of glomeruli (Lab 'C' -black lines), cysts and the medullary areas (Lab 'M'- arrows) show many primitive ducts embedded in immature mesenchyme; (E) Photomicrograph of the medulla "M" showing primitive ducts embedded in immature mesenchyme; (F) Lung showing florid alveolar hemorrhage.

glomeruli (lab "C"-black lines), cysts and the medulla "M" showed primitive ducts embedded in immature mesenchyme (black arrows), features consistent with hypodysplastic kidneys. The lungs were not hypoplastic, weighed 37 g and on microscopy exhibited diffuse alveolar hemorrhage (Fig 2F). There was anal atresia and imperforate anus.

FINAL AUTOPSY DIAGNOSIS: PM 25711

Day 2 Male Baby

- Bilateral hypodysplastic kidneys, patent malformed ureters with normal urinary bladder.
- Pulmonary hemorrhage.
- Imperforate anus with blind ending large gut.

Renal hypodysplasia—Refer to "Pediatric cystic disease (developmental/genetic) of kidney—Introduction".

COMMENTARY—INDEX CASES: PM 19521, PM 25711

Both babies were born premature (33/35 weeks gestation) and were growth retarded. They developed respiratory distress, were ventilated but died at 5 hours and 28 hours of life respectively. Hypodysplastic kidneys have some renal function, although feeble. Gastrointestinal malformations are known to occur with renal dysplasias. Both babies died of lung complications, although their prognosis as such was poor due to the bilateral renal hypodysplasia. Parents were sent for genetic counseling

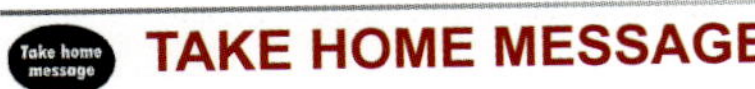

TAKE HOME MESSAGE

- Hypodysplastic kidneys have some renal function, although feeble.

CONTRIBUTIONS BY:

Case 73

1. Dr Praveen Kumar, Professor and Head, Department of Pediatrics, Neonatology Division, (Clinician In-Charge)

Case 74

1. Dr Venkataseshan S, Professor, Department of Pediatrics, Neonatology Division (Clinician In-Charge)

Post Graduate Institute of Medical Education and Research, Chandigarh, India.

CASE 75

Bilateral Renal Agenesis: PM 24019

Nandita Bharadwaj Kakkar

 HIGHLIGHTS OF THE CASE

A gravida 2 mother, with one previous abortion, delivered a male baby at 38 weeks gestation, by a breech assisted vaginal delivery. The baby weighed 2,400 g and the APGAR score was low. Antenatal ultrasonography (USG) revealed non-visualization of both kidneys and severe oligohydramnios. Baby had Potter's syndrome, respiratory distress, hypoxic-ischemic encephalopathy (HIE) and died at 15 hours of life. Autopsy revealed bilateral renal agenesis with absent ureters and urinary bladder, bilateral lung hypoplasia and bilateral absence of vas deferens.

Keywords: Bilateral renal agenesis, Potter's facies, absent vas deferens, autopsy.

 CLINICAL DETAILS

Date and Time of Birth: 17.11.2010 at 07:52 Hours; Date and Time of Death: 17.11.2010 at 11,00 Hours; Lived for: 15 Hours

A 26-year-old, G2P0010, at 38 weeks gestation was referred to PGIMER. Antenatal ultrasonography revealed nonvisualization of both kidneys and severe oligohydramnios. She underwent a breech assisted vaginal delivery. It was a male baby, 2,400 g with low APGAR of 2,1,1 at 1 minute, 5 minutes and 10 minutes and there were high pressure requirements during resuscitation. G1 was a spontaneous abortion due to bleeding per vaginam at 15 weeks gestation. Ultrasonography details were not known and autopsy was not done. In the index case, USG at 24 weeks revealed oligohydramnios, at 28 weeks the kidneys were not visualized and kyphoscoliosis was noted and at 30 weeks gestation, bilateral kidneys and urinary bladder was not seen. ***On examination*** of the baby, there was Potter's facies, low set ears, kyphoscoliosis, congenital talipes equinovarus (CTEV), tachypnea, intercostal retractions, decreased air entry and HIE stage 3. Parents were told of the situation and were not willing for medical care. Thus, compassionate care was given and the baby expired at 15 hours of life. Body was sent for autopsy.

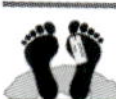 AUTOPSY FINDINGS: PM 24019

A complete autopsy was performed on this 15-hour-old male baby. The baby weighed 2,380 g (38 weeks gestation). Anthropometric measurement: crown-heel length—37 cm, crown rump—25 cm, OFC—34 cm, chest circumference—28 cm, abdominal circumference—19 cm and foot length—7 cm. External examination (Figs 1A–C) revealed a Potter's facies with the characteristic contorted grimace, bags under eye, broad, flat, parrot-beaked nose, low set ears, flexion at knees and hips, kyphoscoliosis and CTEV. On opening, there was bilateral renal agenesis (Figs 2A and B) with absent ureters and urinary bladder. The adrenal glands (Figs 2A and B-arrows) were present and appeared slightly enlarged. Both lungs were hypoplastic and together weighed 21 g (Fig 2C). The vas deferens was absent. All other organs were within normal limits.

 FINAL AUTOPSY DIAGNOSIS: PM 24019

15 Hour Old Male Baby

- *External appearance*: Potter's facies, flexion at knees and hips, kyphoscoliosis and CTEV.
- Bilateral renal agenesis with absent ureters and urinary bladder.

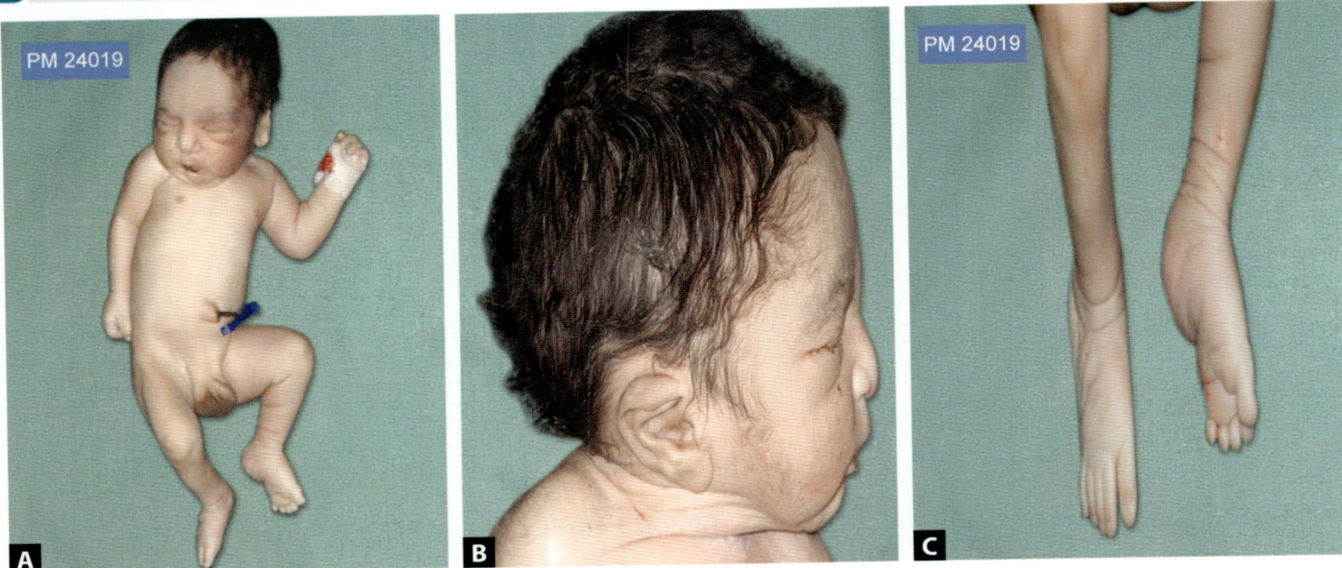

Figs 1A–C: Photographs of the baby showing: (A) Potter's facies with characteristic grimace, bags under eye, broad, flat parrot-beaked nose, flexion at knees and hips; (B) Low set ears and a broad, flat-beaked nose; (C) Congenital talipes equinovarus.

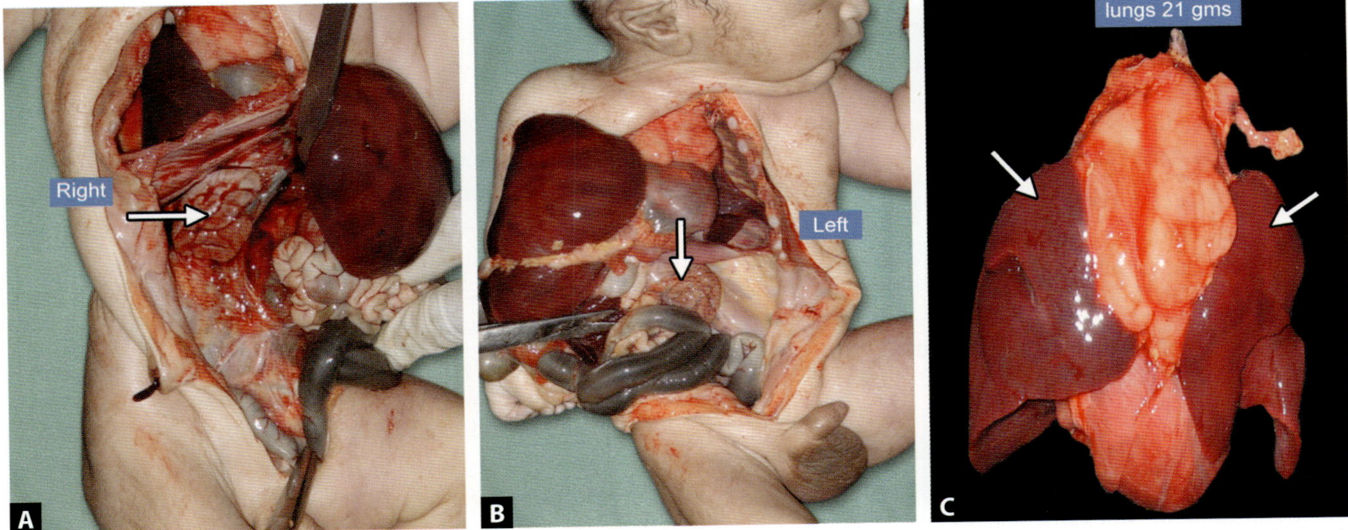

Figs 2A–C: (A and B) Photographs shows absence of both kidneys, ureters and the urinary bladder. Both adrenal glands are present (arrows). The liver and gastrointestinal tract are retracted to the opposite side to confirm the finding; (C) Heart and lung complex showing bilateral hypoplastic lungs (arrows), weighing 21 g. Thymus is seen on the anterior aspect.

- Bilateral lung hypoplasia.
- Absent vas deferens.

COMMENTARY—INDEX CASE: PM 24019

This is a classical case of Potter's syndrome with the characteristic Potter's facies, CTEV, flexion at knees and hip, kyphoscoliosis and hypoplastic lungs. Both kidneys, ureters and urinary bladder were absent. The genitalia were normal except for the absence of vas deferens. Baby died of pulmonary insufficiency before renal failure set in. There was one previous abortion in this case and hence genetic counseling is mandatory.

Renal agenesis—See "Pediatric cystic disease (developmental/genetic) of kidney-Introduction".

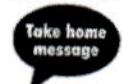

TAKE HOME MESSAGE

- Edith Potter estimated the incidence of bilateral renal agenesis to be approximately 1 per 4,800 births.
- The M:F ratio is 2.5 to 3:1, but the females have a higher incidence of associated genitourinary abnormalities.
- In most cases it occurs sporadically, but is genetically determined in some cases.
- Babies show Potter's syndrome—distinctive facies, bent and deformed extremities, a bell-shaped chest due to hypoplastic lungs along with bilateral renal agenesis.

CONTRIBUTIONS BY:

1. Dr Kanya Mukhopadhyay, Professor, Department of Pediatrics (Neonatology Division) (Clinician In-Charge) Post Graduate Institute of Medical Education and Research, (PGIMER) Chandigarh, India.

CASE 76-80

Unilateral Renal Developmental Malformations: PM 22428, PM 22393, PM 26428, PM 26291, PM 26824

Nandita Bharadwaj Kakkar

HIGHLIGHTS OF THE CASES

Unilateral renal developmental malformations are more common than bilateral. But at autopsy, bilateral malformations are more common, as unilateral defect may be compatible with life. The prognosis of unilateral renal malformation depends on the status of the contralateral kidney. The first three cases show unilateral multicystic dysplasia with ureteral abnormality, the fourth case shows unilateral congenital hydronephrosis with ureteric stenosis and the fifth case shows unilateral renal agenesis.

Keywords: Unilateral, malformation, renal, dysplasia, hydronephrosis, ureteral, abnormality, agenesis.

CASE 76: PM 22428

CLINICAL DETAILS

Date of Still-birth: 30.01.2008

A 24-year-old female, G2P1001, at 28 weeks gestation, came with preterm rupture of membranes with antepartum hemorrhage going on since 2 days. Ultrasonography revealed right multicystic kidney. Heart beat could not be localized. A day later she delivered a baby girl per vaginally. Baby was sent for autopsy after proper consent from the parents.

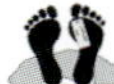

AUTOPSY FINDINGS: PM 22428

A complete autopsy was performed. The baby weight was 960 g (normal for the period of gestation). No external abnormality was noted. The right kidney (Fig 1A) was enlarged, multicystic, pelvis was fused with the mass, right upper part of the ureter was atretic and the lower part was dilated (Fig 1A-arrows). The left kidney (Fig 1A) showed normal fetal lobulations and its pelvis/ureter were normal. The urinary bladder was normal with orthotopically placed ureters. On microscopic examination (Fig 1A-inset), the right kidney showed multicystic dysplasia with lobar disorganization, cysts, primitive ducts, immature mesenchyme and rudimentary tubules/glomeruli. The left kidney was normal on microscopic examination. The lungs were normal in weight and no other abnormality was detected.

FINAL AUTOPSY DIAGNOSIS: PM 22428

- Right multicystic dysplastic kidney with ureteral abnormality.
- Normal left kidney with normal ureter.
- Normal urinary bladder.

COMMENTARY—INDEX CASE: PM 22428

This is a case of right multicystic dysplastic kidney with ureteral abnormality. The contralateral kidney and ureter were normal. The urinary bladder was normal with normally placed ureters. This situation has a good prognosis. In the index case, the right kidney had a fused pelvis along with ureteral abnormalities, which occurs in over 50% cases of unilateral dysplasia and is an indicator of the contralateral kidney or ureter being abnormal in 40% cases. But the contralateral kidney and ureter were normal. Thus, the index case was compatible with life as far as the renal malformation was concerned and there was no lung hypoplasia. The still birth occurred due to antepartum hemorrhage.

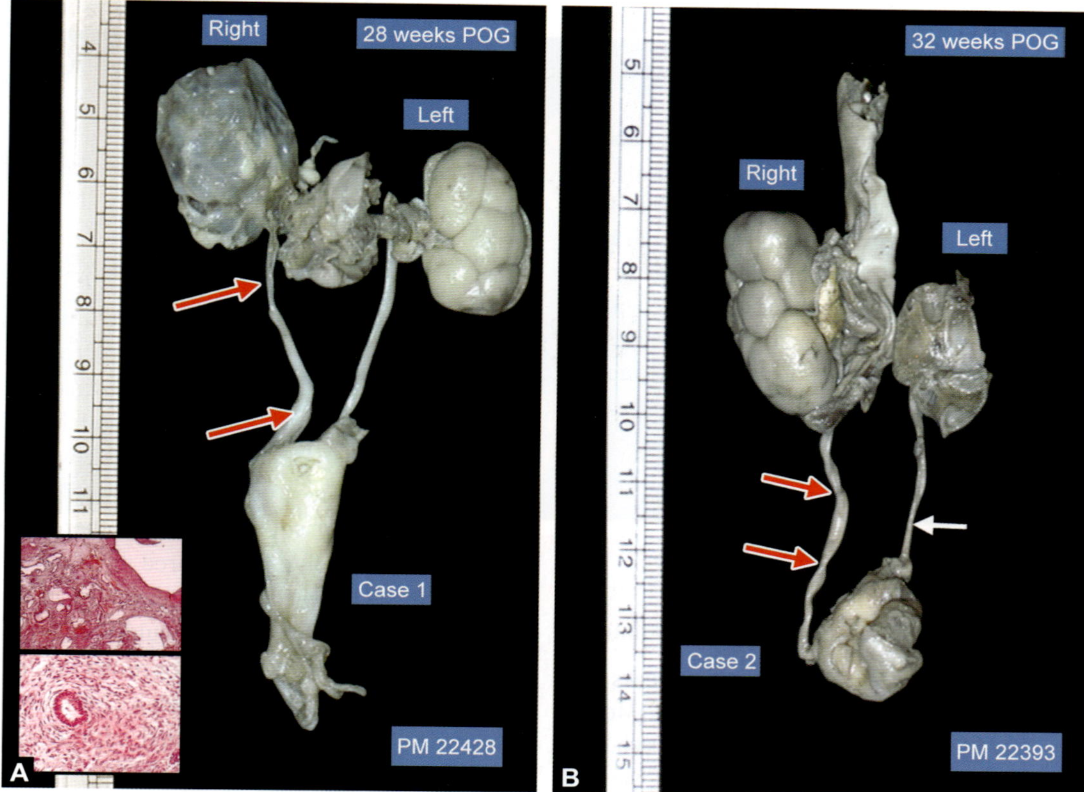

Figs 1A and B: Right kidney is enlarged, multicystic, right upper part of the ureter is atretic (upper arrow) and the lower part is dilated (lower arrow). The left kidney and ureter are normal. Both the ureters open orthotopically into the urinary bladder which is normal. Inset shows right kidney showing cysts and primitive duct; (B) Left kidney is small and multicystic with the ureter showing narrowing in the lower one-third (white arrow). The right kidney shows normal fetal lobulations and the ureter shows multiple areas of narrowing with dilatation (red arrows).

CASE 77: PM 22393

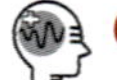

CLINICAL DETAILS

Date of Birth: 06.01.2008, Date of Death: 07.01.2008, Lived for 14 Hours

This was an unbooked but supervised twin pregnancy (diamniotic/dichorionic). The mother was a primigravida, delivered a male baby (Twin 2) weighing 1,300 g at 32 weeks gestation, with an APGAR of 2,5,6,7. The baby was appropriate for gestational age. There was meconium stained liquor, baby was not vigorous at birth, suction was done and no meconium was found below the vocal cords. Baby was intubated and put on ventilation. At 14 hours of life he suffered cardiac arrest and could not be revived. The clinical diagnosis was—Prematurity, Birth asphyxia (unclassified HIE) ? meconium aspiration syndrome ? congenital heart disease ? esophageal atresia. Baby was sent for autopsy after proper consent from the parents.

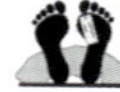

AUTOPSY FINDINGS CASE 77: PM 22393

A complete autopsy was performed. No external abnormality was noted. The left kidney (Fig 1B) was small in size, cut section revealed multiple cysts, pelvis was fused and the ureter showed narrowing in the lower one-third (Fig 1B-white arrow). The right kidney (Fig 1B) showed normal fetal lobulations, pelvis was normal but the ureter revealed multiple areas of narrowing with dilatation (Fig 1B-red arrows). The urinary bladder was normal with normally placed ureters. Microscopy of the right kidney was consistent with a diagnosis of multicystic dysplasia. The lungs were normal in weight. The heart revealed a single common atrium.

FINAL AUTOPSY DIAGNOSIS: PM 22393

- Left multicystic dysplastic kidney with ureteral abnormality.
- Normal right kidney with ureteral abnormality
- Congenital heart disease—common atria.

Section 15C: Renal Hypoplasia

CASE 84

Neonate with Bilateral Simple Renal Hypoplasia, Lung Hypoplasia and Hydrocephalus: PM 27245

Nandita Bharadwaj Kakkar

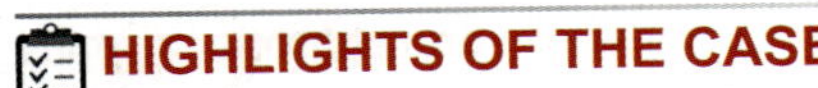

HIGHLIGHTS OF THE CASE

This was a neonate who lived for one hour and was born to a primigravida at 37 weeks gestation. Ultrasonography at 28 weeks gestation revealed Dandy–Walker syndrome, single umbilical artery and absent stomach bubble. The renal malformation was not picked up on ultrasonography. Autopsy revealed a classic picture of bilateral renal hypoplasia with associated lung hypoplasia, hydrocephalus and a single umbilical artery. Mother did reveal history of her sister having lost her baby with renal malformation. Mother was sent for genetic counseling.

Keywords: Renal hypoplasia, simple, bilateral, miniature kidney, lung hypoplasia, hydrocephalus.

CLINICAL DETAILS

Date of Birth and Death: 25.02.2016, lived for 1 hour

A primigravida delivered a baby with ambiguous genitalia, vaginally, at 37 weeks gestation. The baby weight was 1,815 g (SGA—2). The APGAR was 1,6 and baby had severe birth asphyxia, hypoxic ischemic encephalopathy stage 3 with gasping efforts and died within an hour of birth. Ultrasonography at 28 weeks gestation revealed Dandy–Walker syndrome, single umbilical artery and absent stomach bubble. No comment on liquor was given. Examination of the baby revealed a flat forehead, broad nasal bridge, abnormal genitalia, sacral sinus, cleft palate and bilateral congenital talipes equinovarus. Clinical diagnosis was—Major congenital malformation, Dandy–Walker syndrome. Baby was sent for autopsy after taking permission from the parents.

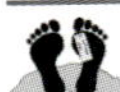

AUTOPSY FINDINGS: PM 27245

A complete autopsy was performed. The baby weighed 1,800 g. On external examination, there was a Potter's facies with low set ears, flat forehead, Mongolian slant, broad nasal bridge, abnormal genitalia, cleft palate and bilateral congenital talipes equinovarus. The brain revealed hydrocephalus with a patent aqueduct. No features of Dandy–Walker syndrome were noted, i.e. the posterior fossa was normal, cerebellar vermis was present and the fourth ventricle did not show any dilatation. The kidneys (Figs 1A–D) were hypoplastic measuring $1 \times 1 \times 0.5$ cm, weighed 4 g ($<50\%$ of expected weight), ureters were patent and showed mild ectopic insertion into the urinary bladder. No fetal lobulations were seen and the capsular aspect was smooth. The left ureter was slightly dilated in its mid portion (Fig 1D-arrow). The bladder appeared normal. Cut section of the kidneys revealed a reduction in the number of renal calyces and renal lobes. Tiny peripheral cysts could be appreciated under a magnifying glass. The adrenals appeared enlarged and disc-shaped (Fig 1A-white arrows). Microscopic examination of the kidneys (Figs 2A–F) revealed peripheral small cysts, cortex showed 2–3 ranks of glomeruli (term baby should show 12–14 ranks) of normal morphology, few peripheral glomeruli showed glomerulocystic change and foci of extramedullary hematopoiesis was seen. The interstitium showed hemorrhage and loose connective tissue. The interlobular vessels were prominent and showed medial hypertrophy (Fig 2F-arrow). No primitive duct was present, i.e. there was no element of dysplasia. The lungs (Fig 3A-arrows) together weighed 10 g and were hypoplastic. Microscopy (Fig 3B) confirmed the hypoplasia in the form of

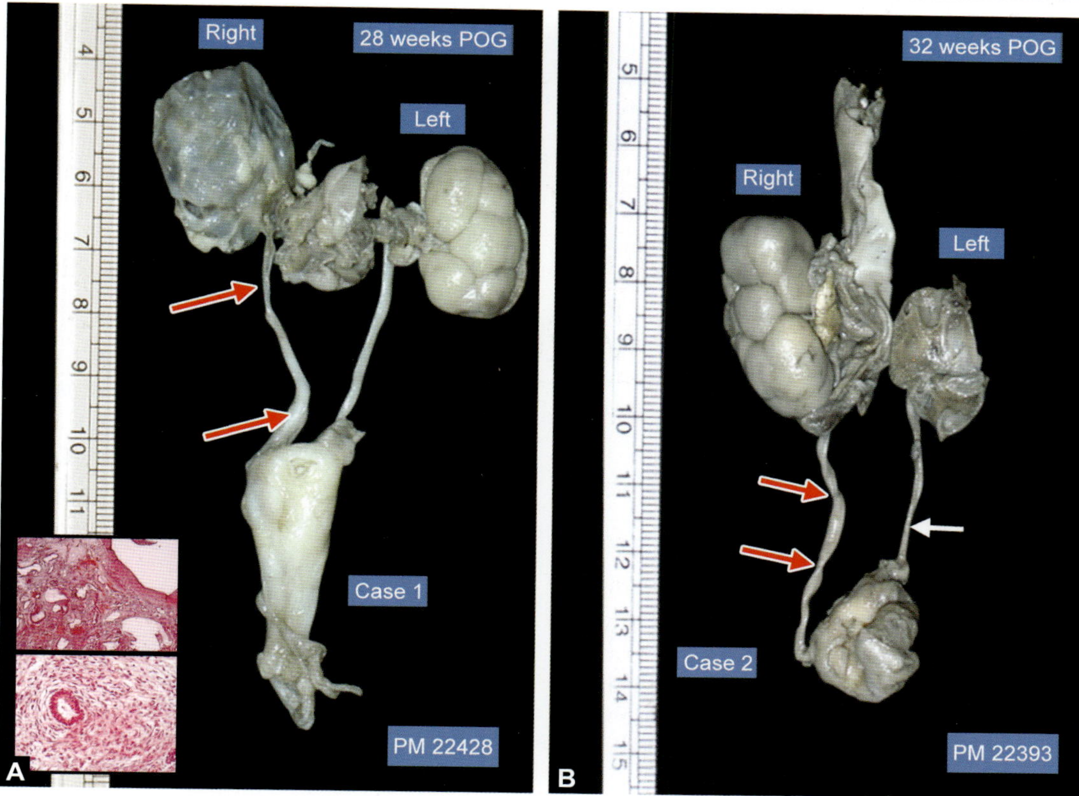

Figs 1A and B: Right kidney is enlarged, multicystic, right upper part of the ureter is atretic (upper arrow) and the lower part is dilated (lower arrow). The left kidney and ureter are normal. Both the ureters open orthotopically into the urinary bladder which is normal. Inset shows right kidney showing cysts and primitive duct; (B) Left kidney is small and multicystic with the ureter showing narrowing in the lower one-third (white arrow). The right kidney shows normal fetal lobulations and the ureter shows multiple areas of narrowing with dilatation (red arrows).

CASE 77: PM 22393

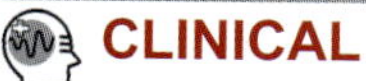

CLINICAL DETAILS

Date of Birth: 06.01.2008, Date of Death: 07.01.2008, Lived for 14 Hours

This was an unbooked but supervised twin pregnancy (diamniotic/dichorionic). The mother was a primigravida, delivered a male baby (Twin 2) weighing 1,300 g at 32 weeks gestation, with an APGAR of 2,5,6,7. The baby was appropriate for gestational age. There was meconium stained liquor, baby was not vigorous at birth, suction was done and no meconium was found below the vocal cords. Baby was intubated and put on ventilation. At 14 hours of life he suffered cardiac arrest and could not be revived. The clinical diagnosis was—Prematurity, Birth asphyxia (unclassified HIE) ? meconium aspiration syndrome ? congenital heart disease ? esophageal atresia. Baby was sent for autopsy after proper consent from the parents.

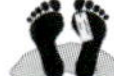

AUTOPSY FINDINGS CASE 77: PM 22393

A complete autopsy was performed. No external abnormality was noted. The left kidney (Fig 1B) was small in size, cut section revealed multiple cysts, pelvis was fused and the ureter showed narrowing in the lower one-third (Fig 1B-white arrow). The right kidney (Fig 1B) showed normal fetal lobulations, pelvis was normal but the ureter revealed multiple areas of narrowing with dilatation (Fig 1B-red arrows). The urinary bladder was normal with normally placed ureters. Microscopy of the right kidney was consistent with a diagnosis of multicystic dysplasia. The lungs were normal in weight. The heart revealed a single common atrium.

FINAL AUTOPSY DIAGNOSIS: PM 22393

- Left multicystic dysplastic kidney with ureteral abnormality.
- Normal right kidney with ureteral abnormality
- Congenital heart disease—common atria.

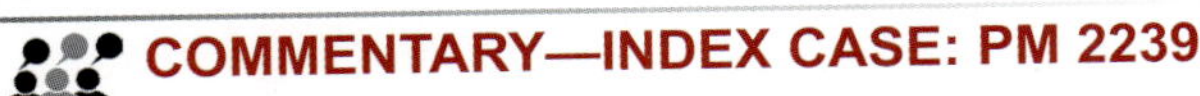

COMMENTARY—INDEX CASE: PM 22393

This is a case of left multicystic dysplastic kidney with normal contralateral kidney, bilateral ureteral abnormality and normal bladder. This situation has a bad prognosis and in unilateral dysplastic kidneys, is seen in 50% cases and is an indicator of the contralateral kidney being abnormal in 40% cases. In the index case, the renal malformation would have been compatible with life, but problems would have arisen in childhood due to the right ureteric abnormality. The index baby died due to the cyanotic congenital heart disease, i.e. common atria. Extra renal malformations are very common in renal developmental disorders. Twin 1 died of sepsis at day 4 of life. No autopsy was done on him.

CASE 78: PM 26428

CLINICAL DETAILS

Date of Birth and Death: 15.01.2015, Lived for 30 minutes.

This was an extremely premature female, born at 28 weeks gestation to a multigravida (G4P0030) with no live issue. Mother did not avail any antenatal care. It was an assisted breech delivery as a result of preterm-onset of labor and the baby weighed 1,063 g. The APGAR was 1,0,0,0. There was failure of resuscitation and baby expired within 30 minutes of life. Baby was sent for autopsy after proper consent from the parents.

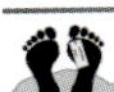

AUTOPSY FINDINGS: PM 26428

A complete autopsy was performed. The baby weight was 1,050 g (normal for the period of gestation). No external abnormality was noted. The right kidney (Fig 2A) was normal sized with a near maintained reniform shape, but small cysts were appreciable diffusely on the capsular surface. The ureter was patent but abnormal, showing mild dilatation all along its length. It was orthotopically placed in the urinary bladder. Cut section of the right kidney (Fig 2B) was solid with tiny cysts and a fused pelvis. The left kidney (Figs 2A and B) showed normal fetal lobulations, cut section revealed normal corticomedullary distinction and no cysts were appreciated. The ureter was patent but appeared abnormal with portions showing dilatation (Fig 2B-white arrow). The urinary bladder was normal with normally placed ureters. On microscopic examination, the right kidney (Figs 2C–F) showed features of multicystic dysplasia and the left kidney (Fig 3A) was normal. Both lungs were hypoplastic (Figs 3B and C). The ductus was patent. Patches of subarachnoid hemorrhage were seen.

FINAL AUTOPSY DIAGNOSIS: PM 26428

- Right multicystic dysplastic kidney with patent, malformed ureter.
- Normal left kidney with patent but malformed ureter.
- Bilateral hypoplastic lungs, subarachnoid hemorrhage and patent ductus.

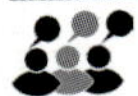

COMMENTARY—INDEX CASE: PM 26428

This is a case of unilateral (right) renal dysplasia with tiny cysts, a normal contralateral kidney, patent but malformed ureters, orthotopically placed in the urinary bladder. The baby had low APGAR due to bilateral lung hypoplasia, which was incompatible with life and was the cause of death. Bilateral lung hypoplasia with unilateral dysplastic kidney is generally not seen. The mother was a multigravida (G4) with no live issue, three previous abortions and a still birth at 28 weeks gestation (index case). For some reason, the file of this patient could not be traced and the cause for the previous three abortions could not be discerned. But this mother has a high chance of being labeled as a case of "hereditary renal adysplasia" and needs proper counseling.

CASE 79: PM 26291

CLINICAL DETAILS

Date of Medical Termination of Pregnancy: 10.10.2014

This was a multigravida (G4P2102) with two living children doing well. In the index pregnancy, unilateral hydronephrosis was detected at 18 weeks on ultrasonography. The family opted for medical termination of pregnancy.

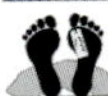

AUTOPSY FINDINGS: PM 26291

A complete autopsy was performed. The baby weighed 380 g. No external abnormality was noted. The left kidney (Fig 4A) was enlarged (4 × 3 × 2 cm) and showed tiny pinhead-sized cysts on the surface. Cut section of the kidney (Fig 4B) revealed marked hydronephrosis with dilated pelvicalyceal system and a thin rim of cortex. The left ureter (Fig 4C) showed stenosis in its mid portion with dilatation above that point. The right kidney and ureter were within normal limits (Figs 4A–D). The urinary bladder was normal with orthotopic insertion of both ureters. Microscopy of the left kidney (Figs 4E and F, Figs 5A and B) revealed a thin

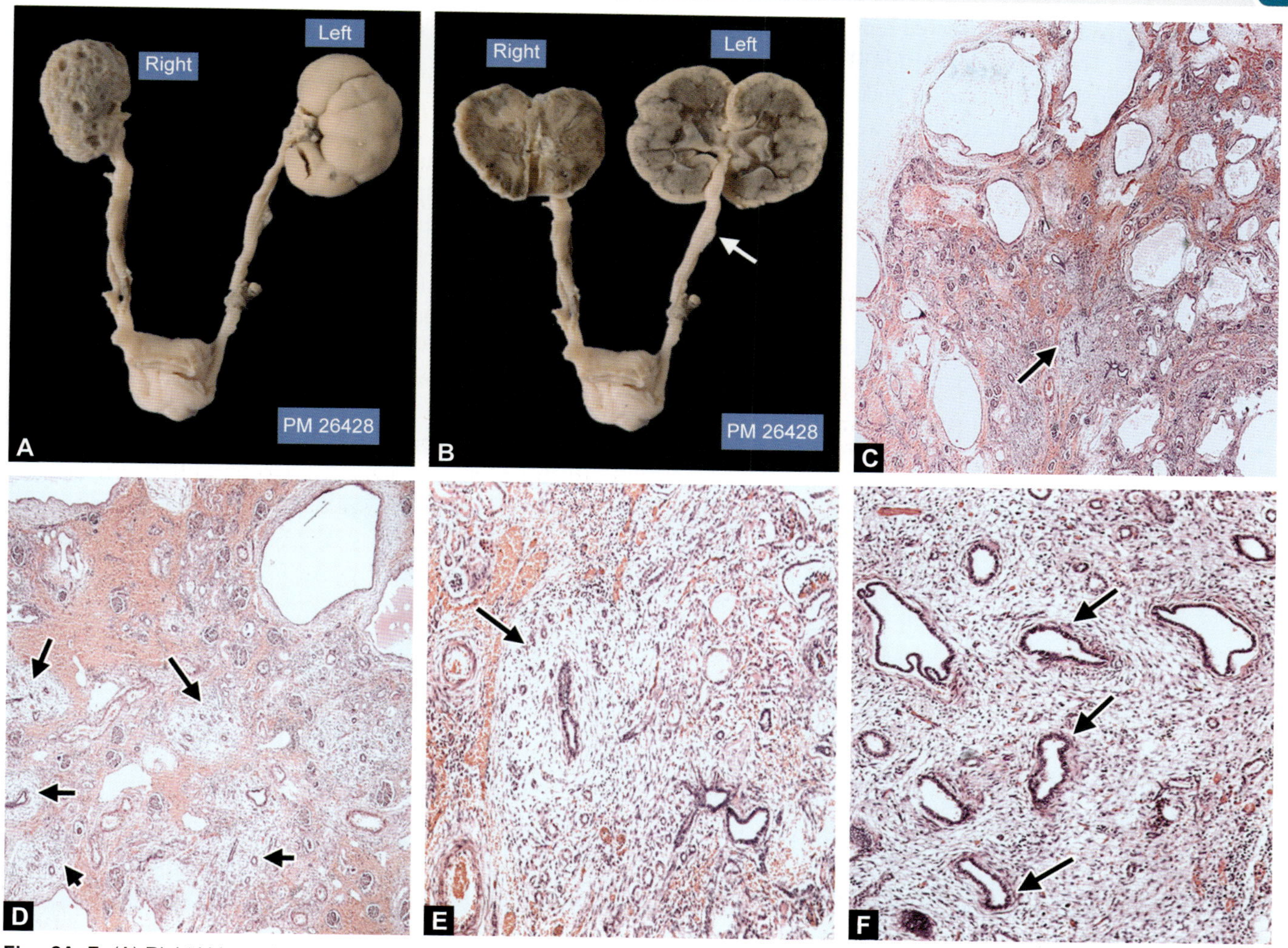

Figs 2A–F: (A) Right kidney showing small cysts on the capsular surface, fused pelvis and the right ureter shows mild dilation. The left kidney shows normal fetal lobulations but the ureter shows areas of dilatation. The urinary bladder is normal; (B) Cut section of right kidney shows tiny cysts and fused pelvis. Cut section of left kidney is normal. Photomicrographs of the right kidney (C–F) Show multiple cysts, lobar disorganization and clusters of primitive ducts (arrows) surrounded by immature mesenchyme.

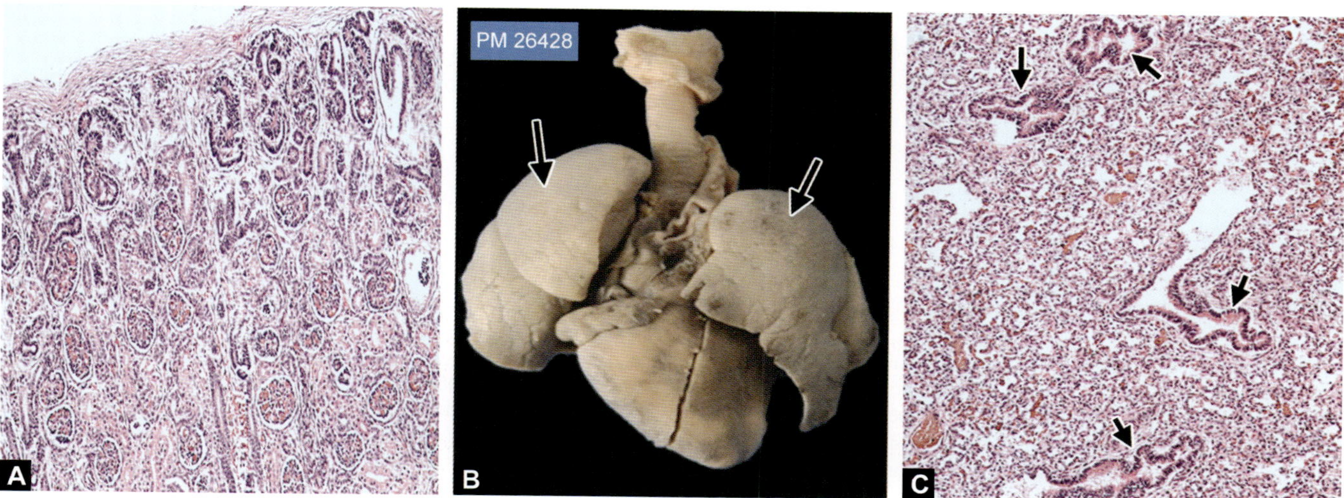

Figs 3A–C: (A) Left kidney shows normal morphology with ongoing subcapsular neoglomerulogenesis; (B) Heart lung complex showing hypoplastic lungs (arrows); (C) Photomicrograph of the lung showing hypoplasia with closely placed bronchioles (arrows).

rim of cortex showing well-preserved renal parenchyma with peripheral cysts. The medullary portion (Figs 4E and F and 5A-black arrows) showed primitive ducts with surrounding immature mesenchyme, indicating the presence of dysplasia. Glomerulocystic change was noted in the peripheral glomeruli (Fig 5B). Other organs were within normal limits. There was no lung hypoplasia.

FINAL AUTOPSY DIAGNOSIS: PM 26291

- Left congenital hydronephrosis with dysplasia with mid ureteric stenosis and proximal hydroureter.
- Right kidney, right ureter and urinary bladder—within normal limits

COMMENTARY—INDEX CASE: PM 26291

This is a case of unilateral (left) renal congenital hydronephrosis with dysplasia with mid ureteral stenosis and proximal hydroureter. There was dysplasia indicating that the obstruction must have occurred very early in nephrogenesis. The contralateral kidney was normal with normal ureter. This case would have been compatible with life as the contralateral kidney/ureter was within normal limits, lungs were normal and there was no oligohydramnios.

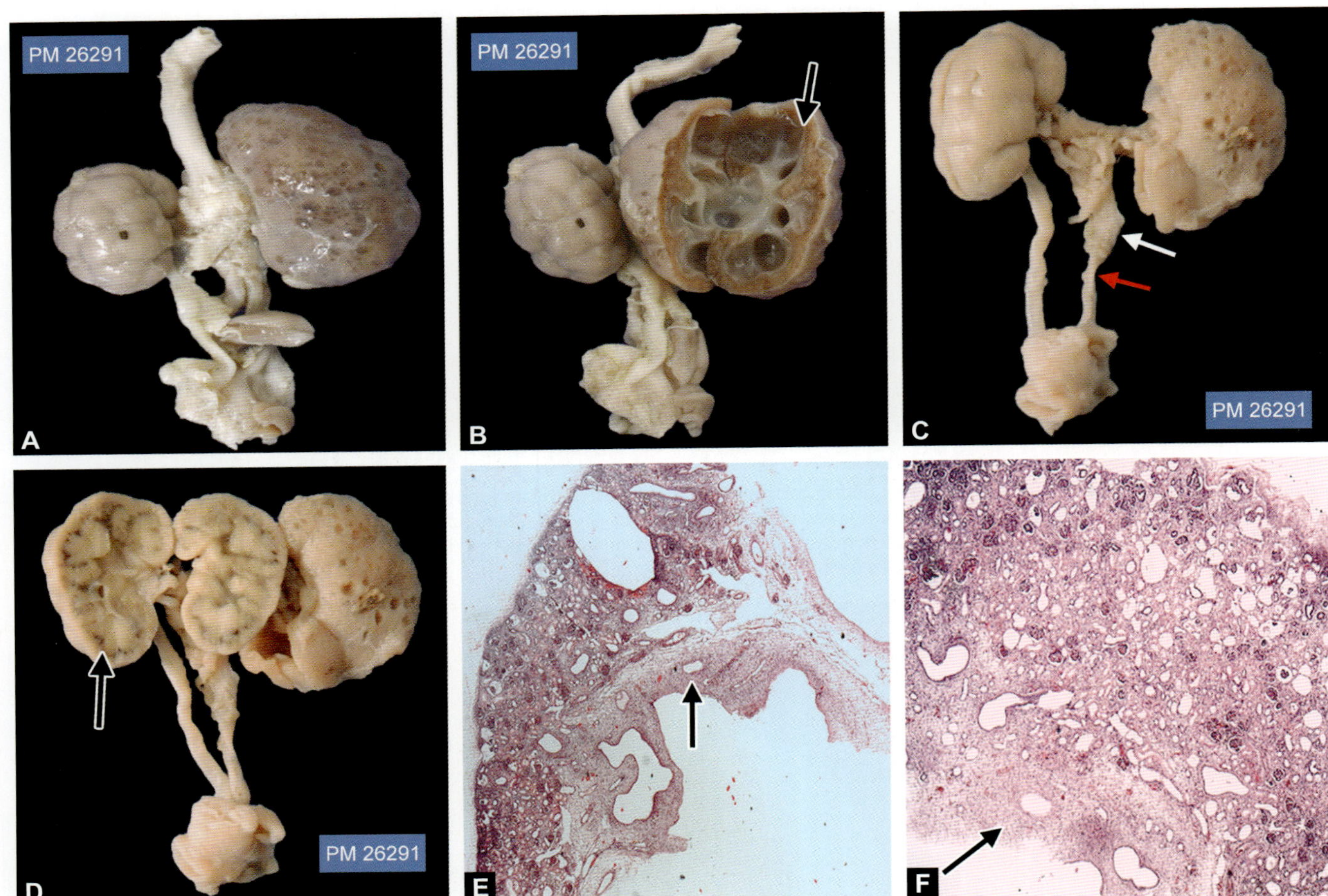

Figs 4A–F: Gross photographs of both kidneys, ureters and urinary bladder. (A) The left kidney is enlarged and shows small cysts all over the capsular aspect. The right kidney is normal; (B) Cut section of the left kidney shows marked hydronephrosis with dilated pelvicalyceal system and a thin rim of cortex (arrow); (C) The left ureter shows stenosis (red arrow) in its mid portion with dilatation above that point (white arrow); (D) Cut section of the right kidney is normal (arrow); (E and F) Photomicrographs of the left kidney showing thinned out cortex, normal renal parenchyma, scattered small cysts and primitive ducts in the medullary areas (arrows).

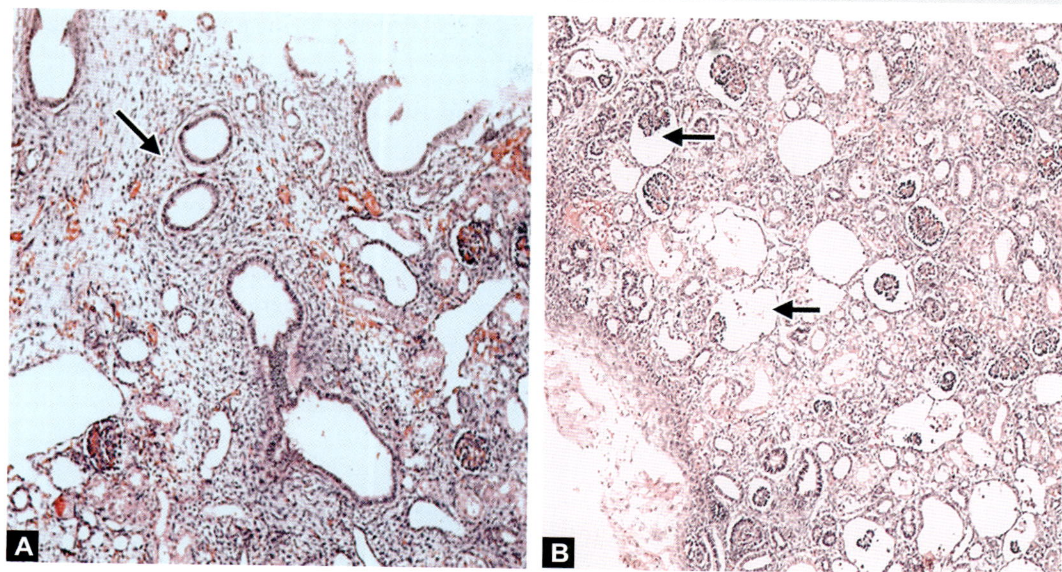

Figs 5A and B: (A) Photomicrographs of the left kidney showing primitive ducts surrounded by immature mesenchyme in the medullary areas (arrow); (B) Some of the glomeruli showed glomerulocystic change (arrows).

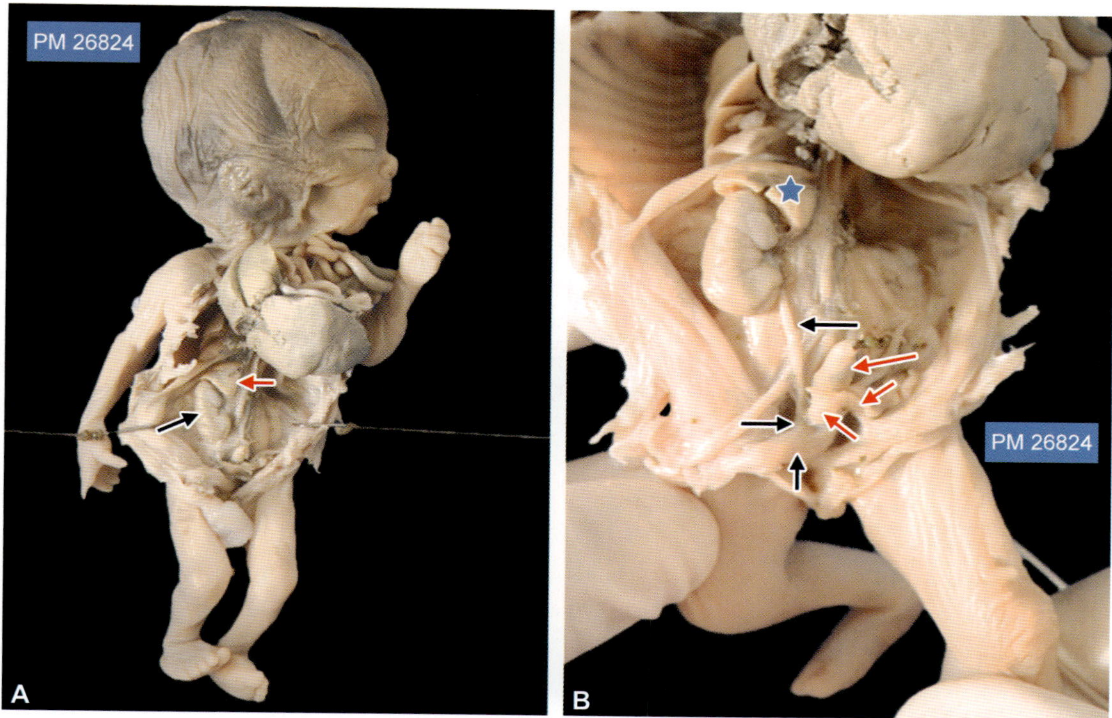

Figs 6A and B: (A) Abortus with the abdominal organs reflected upward, showing absent left kidney/ureter and left adrenal gland. The right kidney/adrenal gland are seen (arrows); (B) In situ dissection shows adrenal gland (star), right kidney, right ureter (upper black arrow) opening (middle black arrow) into the urinary bladder (lower black arrow). The posteriorly placed gut (upper red arrow) with meconium oozing out, fallopian tube (mid red arrow) and the uterus (lower red arrow) can also be seen.

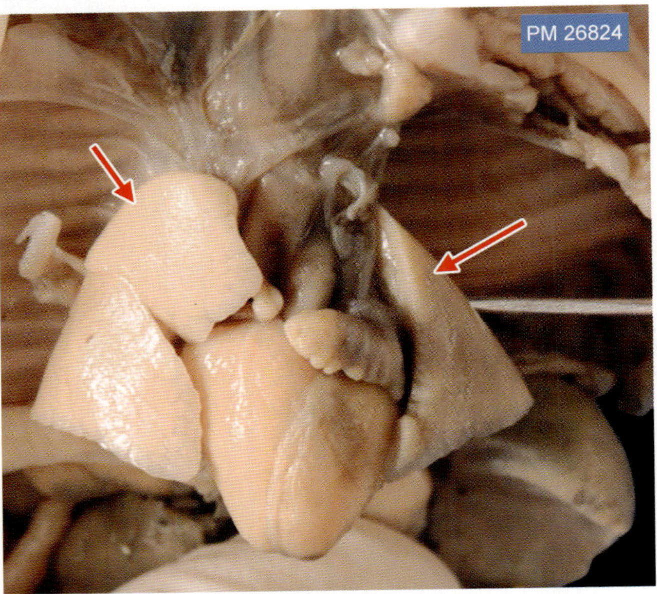

Fig 7: Heart lung complex showing hypoplastic lungs (red arrows).

CASE 80: PM 26824—UNILATERAL RENAL AGENESIS

CLINICAL DETAILS

Date of Medical Termination of Pregnancy: 03.08.2015

This was a medical termination of pregnancy done at 19 weeks gestation, in view of severe oligohydramnios and nonvisualization of left kidney and urinary bladder on ultrasonography. The right kidney was however visualized, was small and anechoic. The mother was 24-year-old, G2P0010, with one previous abortion and no live issue. Details of the previous abortion were not available.

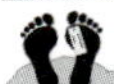

AUTOPSY FINDINGS: PM 26824

This was a female abortus and weighed 250 g. No external abnormality was noted. The left kidney (Figs 6A and B) along with the ureter and left adrenal gland were absent. The right kidney and the right ureter opening into the urinary bladder could be appreciated on meticulous in situ dissection and were within normal limits (Figs 6A and B). The uterus along with the fallopian tube could be seen behind the urinary bladder and posterior to that, the gut could be appreciated from which meconium was seen to be oozing out (Fig 6B). The right adrenal gland was present (Fig 6A-star). The lungs were hypoplastic (Fig 7).

COMMENTARY—INDEX CASE: PM 26824

This was a gravida 2 mother with one previous abortion, details of which were not available. Ultrasonography at 19 weeks revealed severe oligohydramnios and nonvisualization of left kidney and urinary bladder. At autopsy, the right kidney, ureter and urinary bladder were seen and were within normal limits. Left renal agenesis was present. Medical termination of pregnancy was justifiable as there was severe oligohydramnios and hypoplasia of the lungs.

TAKE HOME MESSAGE

- Unilateral renal malformations are more common than bilateral.
- At autopsy, however, bilateral malformations are more common as unilateral defect is compatible with life.
- The prognosis of unilateral renal malformation depends on the status of the contralateral kidney/ureter.
- Meticulous in situ dissection of small fetuses can clinch the correct diagnosis.
- Genetic counseling is mandatory.

CONTRIBUTIONS BY:

Case 76

1. Dr Vanita Suri, Professor and Head, Department of Obstetrics and Gynecology (Clinician In-Charge)

Case 77

2. Dr Saurabh Datta, Professor, Department of Pediatrics (Neonatology Division) (Clinician In-Charge)

Case 78

3. Dr Shiv Sajan Saini, Assistant Professor, Department of Pediatrics (Neonatology Division) (Clinician In-Charge)

Case 79

4. Dr L Dhaliwal, Ex-Professor and Head, Department of Obstetrics and Gynecology (Clinician In-Charge)

Case 80

5. Dr Vanita Jain, Professor, Department of Obstetrics and Gynecology (Clinician In-Charge)

Post Graduate Institute of Medical Education and Research, (PGIMER) Chandigarh, India.

CASE 81

Segmental Renal Dysplasia with Duplex Kidney and Ureterocele: PM 19965

Nandita Bharadwaj Kakkar

HIGHLIGHTS OF THE CASE

This was a fresh still birth at 34 weeks gestation. Autopsy revealed a right duplex kidney with the upper moiety showing segmental dysplasia along with a ureterocele.

Keywords: Duplex kidney, ureterocele, segmental renal dysplasia.

CLINICAL DETAILS

Date of Still-birth: 22.05.2004

A 26-year-old female went into preterm labor at 34 weeks gestation. There was hand prolapse with intrauterine fetal death. A fresh still born, growth retarded male baby, weighing 870 g was delivered. No external malformation or abnormal facies was noted. The mother was gravida 3 (G3P1101), with one live child (G1) born at term, doing well and one preterm still birth (G2) at 28 weeks gestation. G2 was not autopsied. G3 was the index case which was an unsupervised pregnancy. Baby was sent for autopsy after taking parental permission.

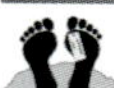

AUTOPSY FINDINGS: PM 19965

A complete autopsy was performed. The baby weighed 860 g (34 weeks gestation). There was no external abnormality or any abnormal facies. Both kidneys were enlarged, left more than the right. The ***right kidney*** appeared more bulky in its upper half (Fig 1A-middle red arrow) but the lower half appeared normal. The difference in texture could be visibly appreciated. There were two ureters (Fig 1A-upper and lower red arrows) draining the right kidney at the upper and lower pole. The right upper pole ureter (Fig 1A) was dilated and distorted all along its length and was ectopically placed in the bladder. On further dissection, the upper pole ureter revealed a cystic dilatation at its lower end, at the point of insertion into the urinary bladder, what is known as ureterocele. The lower pole ureter appeared normal. The cut section of the right kidney showed two pelvicalyceal systems. The upper pole pelvicalyceal system was dilated and revealed rudimentary calyces and the draining renal parenchyma showed small cysts and appeared dysplastic. The lower pole pelvicalyceal system was within normal limits and the draining renal parenchyma looked grossly normal. Microscopy from the upper part of the right kidney (Fig 1B upper part, Fig 2A) revealed features of dysplasia with classical primitive ducts, immature mesenchyme, rudimentary glomeruli/tubules and scattered small cysts. Microscopy from the lower pole of the right kidney revealed normal renal parenchyma along with on going neoglomerulogenesis (Fig 1B-lower part). The sharp transition between the dysplastic upper pole and normal lower pole renal parenchyma could be well appreciated (Fig 1B). The ***left kidney*** (Fig 1A) was enlarged and showed cysts on the capsular aspect and a markedly distorted ureteral system consistent with morphology of a bifid ureter. Cut section revealed multiple cysts and a fused pelvicalyceal system. Microscopy (Figs 2B and C) revealed multicystic dysplasia, i.e. complete lobar disorganization, multiple large cysts, primitive glomeruli/tubules and plenty of classical primitive ducts surrounded by collar of immature mesenchyme. No lung hypoplasia was seen.

FINAL AUTOPSY DIAGNOSIS: PM 19965

Still-birth at 34 Weeks Gestation

- Right duplex kidney with upper pole segmental dysplasia and ureterocele.
- Left multicystic dysplastic kidney with ureteric abnormalities (Bifid ureter).

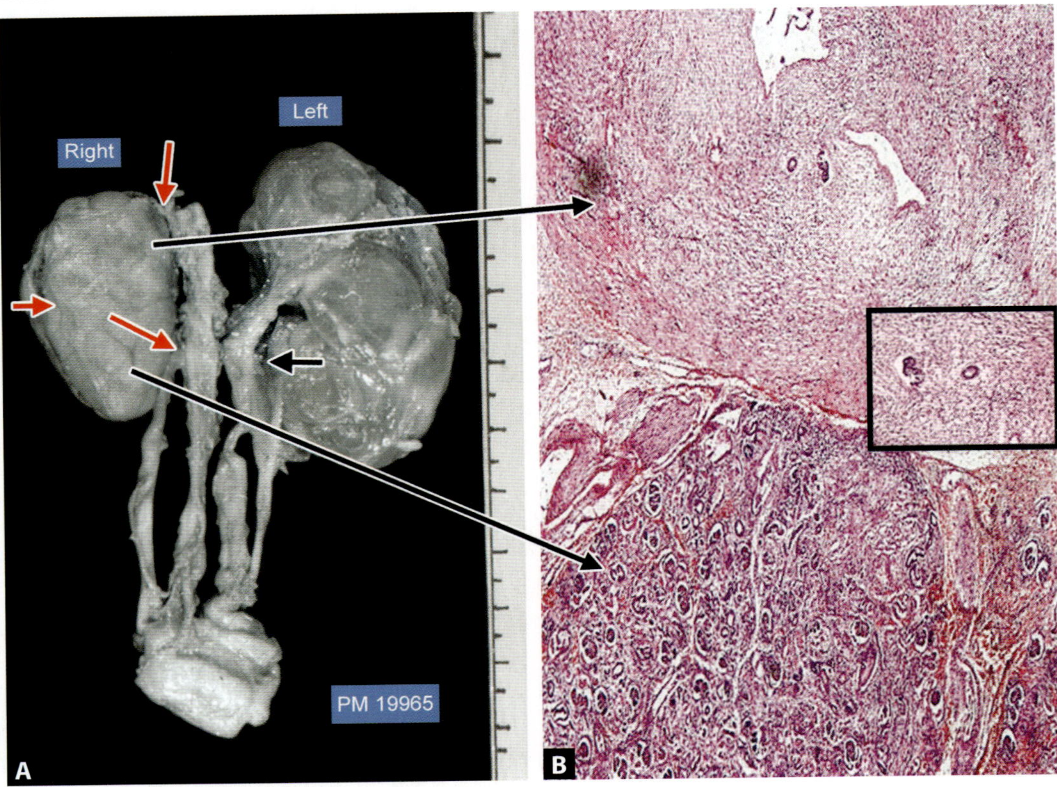

Figs 1A and B: (A) Right kidney shows two ureters (upper and lower red arrows). The upper half is bulky and there is a distinct difference in texture between the upper and lower part with a sharp transition (middle red arrow). Left kidney is enlarged, shows cysts on the surface and a distorted ureteral system (small black arrow); (B) Photomicrograph of the right kidney from the transition shows dysplasia of the upper moiety showing primitive ducts embedded in immature mesenchyme. The lower moiety shows normal renal parenchyma.

SEGMENTAL RENAL DYSPLASIA AND DUPLEX KIDNEY

In segmental renal dysplasia, a portion, i.e. generally the upper part of the kidney shows dysplasia and this segment is associated with duplicated renal pelvis, i.e. a duplex kidney. The ureter draining the upper portion of the kidney shows partial or complete duplication and is obstructed due to an ectopic insertion into the bladder. It may end into the bladder with a ureterocele or at times may have a normal insertion. Duplex kidneys have two pelvicalyceal systems with complete or partial duplication of the ureters, with more than the normal reniculi and may be associated with ureterocele. When associated with a ureterocele (as seen in the index case), the pelvicalyceal systems are completely duplicated, the upper moiety is dysplastic and its draining ureter is dilated or distorted and ectopically inserted into the urinary bladder. The ureter may even end in the urethra or in the Gartner's ducts, vagina or vas deferens. This causes obstruction of the upper ureter, reflected as dilatation of the pelvicalyceal system of the kidney with a thinned out cortex and dysplasia. The lower moiety however has a normal ureter, inserted into the trigone with a normal pelvicalyceal system most of the time, but may have vesicoureteric reflux due to the upward displacement of the ureteral orifice as a result of the ectopic ureterocele of the upper ureter. Microscopically the upper moiety shows complete dysplasia in the form of lobar disorganization, primitive ducts, immature mesenchyme, metaplastic cartilage, rudimentary glomeruli/tubules and few scattered cysts. Pyelonephritic changes at times are prominent. There is a sharp transition between the upper pole dysplastic renal parenchyma and lower pole normal renal parenchyma. The lower moiety is generally normal, but when a vesicoureteric reflux is present, may show hydronephrosis, pyelonephritic changes or even segmental hypoplasia. In most cases, however, removal of the upper dysplastic kidney and the ureterocele gives excellent results. Ectopic ureterocele is approximately six times more common in the females, is bilateral in 10% cases and causes recurrent urinary tract infections in infancy. It may lead to hematuria, acute retention or incontinence. Diagnosis is made by excretion urography.

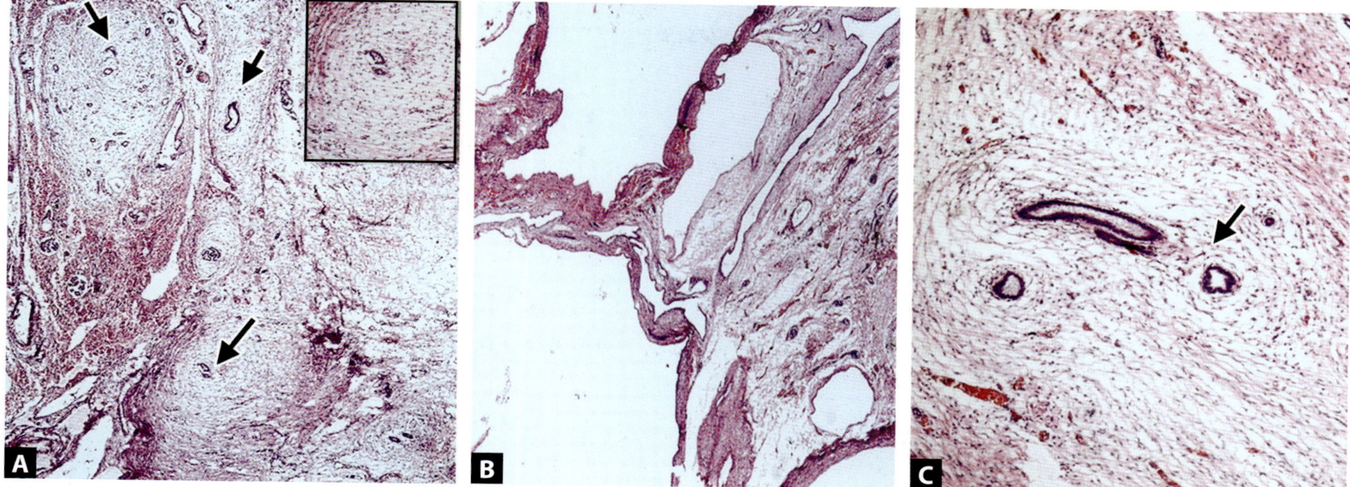

Figs 2A–C: (A) Photomicrographs from the right kidney—upper moiety shows clusters of primitive ducts (arrows) embedded in immature mesenchyme (Inset shows primitive duct with surrounding immature mesenchyme); (B and C) Left kidney shows cysts and primitive ducts (arrow) with collar of immature mesenchyme.

As we know that the kidney is formed when the ureteric bud (which arises from the lower part of the mesonephric duct) meets the metanephric blastema and induces reciprocal induction. Premature branching of the ureteric buds leads to incomplete duplex kidney and duplicate budding leads to a complete duplex kidney with two separate ureters. Abnormal origin of the ureteric bud leads to ectopia of the ureteric orifice and this leads to dysplasia of the renal parenchyma, which it drains. The Weigert–Meyer law is applicable here which states that due to the rotation and caudal migration of the upper pole ureteric bud, the upper pole ureter takes a more medial and caudal location in the urinary bladder. Thus this leads to insertion of the ureter either in the—(1) Urogenital canal, i.e. in the urinary bladder or prostatic urethra, or (2) Mesonephric duct structures like ejaculatory duct/seminal vesicle/vas deferens/epididymis in males, wherein they do not lead to incontinence as these structures are above the external urethral sphincter. In females, the ureter may have its opening in the urogenital canal, i.e. in the urinary bladder, urethra or distal vagina and when regression of the mesonephric duct takes place (only in females), it leads to insertion into paramesonephric duct structures like the upper vagina, uterus and fallopian tubes. Thus an ectopic ureter in the females may lead to urinary incontinence.

COMMENTARY—INDEX CASE: PM 19965

This was a classical case of right duplex kidney with two separate ureters and two pelvicalyceal systems. The right upper ureter was dilated and distorted all along its length with ectopic insertion into the bladder, ending in a ureterocele. The upper moiety showed segmental dysplasia and the lower moiety revealed normal renal parenchyma with a sharp transition. The left kidney showed multicystic dysplasia along with bifid ureters.

TAKE HOME MESSAGE

- In segmental renal dysplasia, a portion, i.e. generally the upper part of the kidney shows dysplasia and this segment is associated with duplicated renal pelvis, i.e. a duplex kidney with duplicated ureters. The ureter draining this part shows ectopic insertion into the urinary bladder and may show a ureterocele.

SUGGESTED READING

1. Abel C, Lendon M, Gough DCS. Histology of upper pole in complete urinary duplication—does it affect surgical management. Br J Urology. 1997;80:663-5.
2. Jeon A, Cramer BC, Walsh E, et al. A spectrum of segmental multicystic renal dysplasia. Pediatr Radiol. 1999;29:309-15.

CONTRIBUTIONS BY:

1. Dr Sarla Malhotra, Ex-Professor and Head, Department of Obstetrics and Gynecology (Clinician In-Charge) Post Graduate Institute of Medical Education and Research, (PGIMER) Chandigarh, India.

CASE 82-83

Posterior Urethral Valve Leading to Congenital Hydroureteronephrosis and Hypertrophied Urinary Bladder: PM 18485, PM 26118

Nandita Bharadwaj Kakkar

HIGHLIGHTS OF THE CASE 82 AND 83

Both these cases show posterior urethral valve (PUV) leading to bilateral hydronephrosis with dysplasia, bilateral hydroureters and hypertrophied urinary bladder with dilated posterior urethra. The first case was a young primigravida with an unsupervised pregnancy, came at 36 weeks gestation with leaking per vaginam and ultrasonography revealed the malformation. The second case is of a fourth gravida with three previous abortions and no live issue, was antenatally diagnosed to have oligohydramnios, bilateral hydronephrosis and lumbar meningomyelocele.

Keywords: Congenital hydroureteronephrosis, dysplasia, hypertrophied urinary bladder, posterior urethral valve, hypoplastic lungs, autopsy.

CASE 82: PM 18485

CLINICAL DETAILS: PM 18485

Date of Birth and Death: 29.05.2002, Baby Lived for 5 Hours

A 24-year-old primigravida, with an unsupervised pregnancy came at 36 weeks gestation with leaking per vaginum. Ultrasonography at admission revealed oligohydramnios, breech presentation, hydroureteronephrosis and a hypertrophied large urinary bladder ? PUV. A male baby, weighing 2.6 Kg was born by an assisted breech delivery. The APGAR was 2, 2, 5 at 1, 5, 10 minutes. On ***external examination*** the baby had a Potter facies and other components of oligohydramnios complex, i.e. flat facies, short neck, beaked nose, low set ear, epicanthic folds, ill-formed small chest, abdominal distention and congenital talipes equinovarus (CTEV). The skin over the abdomen was not wrinkled or prune-like and the testes were undescended. X-ray chest revealed pulmonary hypoplasia and bilateral pneumothorax. The baby was started on bag mask ventilation to which he did not respond, there was persistent cyanosis with saturation of 35–40%. Parents were told about the expected outcome and were not willing for further care. Compassionate care with intravenous fluid and O_2 was given and the baby expired at 5 hours of life.

AUTOPSY FINDINGS: PM 18485

A complete autopsy was performed on this D1 (5 hours) male baby. Baby weighed 2,690 g (36 weeks gestation). Anthropometric measurements: crown-heel/crown-rump length—50/35 cms, head/chest/abdomen circumference—32/28/40 cms (abdominal circumference normal for this age is 28 cm), foot length—8 cm. The head, chest and abdominal circumference normally decrease caudally, but in the index case the abdominal circumference was more than the others. There was Potters facies with a flat face, beaked nose, bags under the eyes, low set ears and short neck. The chest was ill-formed and small. The abdomen was distended, but skin over it did not show any wrinkled appearance. Bilateral CTEV was present. There was no cryptorchidism, penis was normal and the urethral meatus could be identified. The kidneys (Fig 1A) were symmetrically enlarged, together weighed 90 g against a normal of 21 g at this age, reniform shape was maintained and external surface was studded with innumerable cysts of varying sizes. Cut section of the kidneys (Fig 1B) revealed marked dilatation of the pelvicalyceal system, with a rim of preserved cortex showing small cysts, ranging in size from 0.4 cm to 0.6 cm. The ureters (Fig 1A) were markedly dilated and tortuous. The urinary bladder (Fig 1A) was enlarged and hypertrophied. The posterior urethra was dilated and distal to it a membrane-like structure

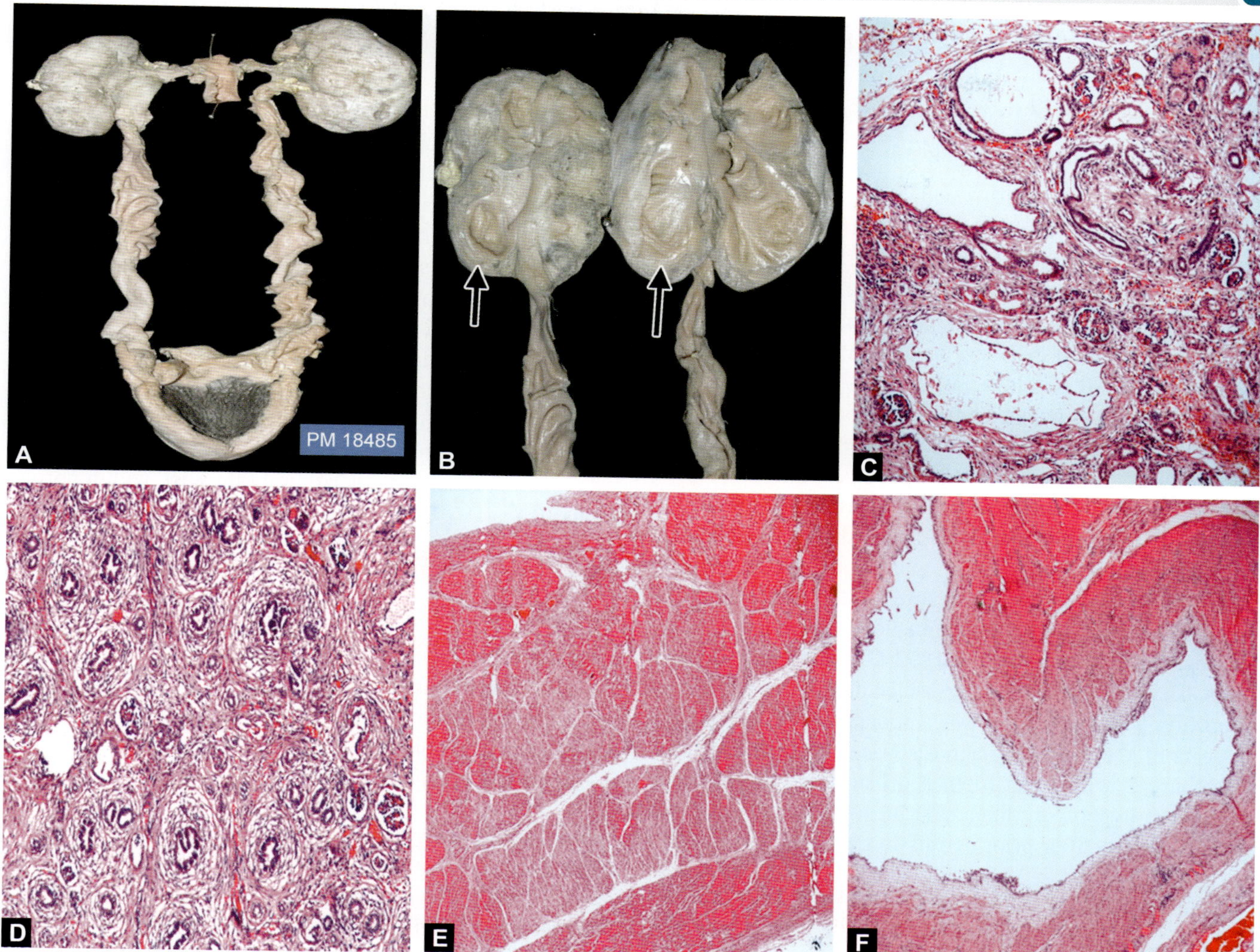

Figs 1A–F: (A) Gross photograph of the symmetrically enlarged kidneys with maintained reniform shape, showing cysts on the surface. Also seen are dilated, tortuous ureters and hypertrophied urinary bladder; (B) Cut section of the kidneys showing marked dilatation of the pelvicalyceal system with a thin rim (arrows) of cortical tissue; (C) Photomicrograph of the kidney showing peripheral cysts with interspersed glomeruli and tubules; (D) Photomicrograph of the kidney showing clusters of primitive ducts lined by cuboidal epithelium with a collar of immature mesenchyme; (E) Urinary bladder showing marked hypertrophy of the detrusor muscle; (F) Ureter showing dilatation, tortuosity and hypertrophy of the muscle.

was identified which got severed during the dissection. On microscopy (Figs 1C–F), the cortex shows hydronephrotic atrophy with widespread disarray and dysplastic changes. Cysts (predominantly peripheral) were lined by a flattened to low columnar epithelium and occasional one showed remnant of an atretic glomerular tuft. Interspersed between the cysts were seen glomeruli, rudimentary tubules, foci of extramedullary hematopoiesis, proliferating nerves and classical primitive ducts with a collar of mesenchyme around them. Clusters of primitive ducts were seen more toward the medullary area (Fig 1D). Sections from the urinary bladder (Fig 1E) showed marked hypertrophy of the detrusor muscle. Sections from the ureters (Fig 1F) showed dilatation, tortuosity and hypertrophy of the muscle. The prostate was normal on microscopic examination. Both lungs together weighed 22 g and were hypoplastic. Other organs were within normal limits.

FINAL AUTOPSY DIAGNOSIS: PM 18485

5 Hours Male 36 Weeks Gestation, 2,690 gms

- Congenital bilateral hydroureteronephrosis with dysplasia, hypertrophied urinary bladder with dilated posterior urethra, consistent with Posterior Urethral Valve.
- Bilateral hypoplastic lungs.

CASE 83: PM 26118

CLINICAL DETAILS: PM 26118

Date of Birth and Death: 16.06.2014

A fourth gravida (G4P0030) with three previous abortions (cause unknown) and no live issue was antenatally diagnosed (at 29 weeks gestation) to have bilateral hydronephrosis, lumbar meningomyelocele and oligohydramnios. She delivered a male baby at 33 weeks gestation, weighing 2,100 g by a breech assisted delivery, indication being breech footling. The APGAR was low, i.e. 2, 2, 2, 1, baby had cyanosis, gasping efforts with a heart rate of less than 60/min. Bag and mask ventilation was started and then he was intubated and kept on manual intermittent positive pressure respiration (IPPR). Baby suffered cardiac arrest at 40 minutes of life. On examination, the baby had a distended abdomen, flat facies and a 3 cm lumbar meningomyelocele. Mother had increased blood pressure records in the third month and was put on medication. Random blood sugar and glucose tolerance tests were normal. G1/G2/G3 were born 12/11/10 years back, respectively after which there was secondary infertility. The index baby was a spontaneous conception at 36 years of age. Clinical diagnosis was congenital hydroureteronephrosis with hypertrophied urinary bladder consistent with PUV, hypoplastic lungs and birth asphyxia. Baby was sent for autopsy after prior permission.

AUTOPSY FINDINGS CASE 83: PM 26118

A complete autopsy was performed on this D1 (40 min) male baby. Baby weighed 2,100 g (33 weeks gestation). Anthropometric measurements: crown heel-crown-rump length—48/32 cm, head/chest/abdominal circumference—31/28/35 cm, foot length—8 cm. There was Potters facies. The abdomen was distended, but skin over it did not show any wrinkled appearance. Bilateral CTEV was present. There was no cryptorchidism, penis was normal and the urethral meatus could be identified. Meningomyelocele (3 cm) was seen in the lumbar region. The kidneys (Fig 2A) were asymmetrically enlarged, right measuring 5 × 4 × 3 cm and the left measuring 12 × 8 × 5 cm, reniform shape was maintained and external surface were studded with innumerable cysts of varying sizes. The ureters were markedly dilated and tortuous. The urinary bladder was enlarged and markedly hypertrophied and the posterior urethra was dilated. Cut section of the kidneys (Figs 2B and C) revealed marked dilatation of pelvicalyceal system (arrows), with a rim of preserved cortex, showing small cysts, ranging in size from 0.2 cm to 0.4 cm. On microscopy (Figs 3A–E), sections from the thinned out rim of the cortex showed small peripherally placed cysts with few well-developed glomeruli/tubules. The inner cortex or medullary areas showed widespread disarray and dysplastic changes. The cysts were lined by a flattened epithelium. Medullary areas revealed immature mesenchyme, classical primitive ducts (single and in clusters) with a collar of mesenchyme around them, primitive glomeruli, rudimentary tubules and foci of extramedullary hematopoiesis. The tubules showed dilatation and few glomeruli showed glomerulocystic changes (Fig 3D). Sections from the urinary bladder (Fig 3E) and ureters showed marked hypertrophy of the muscle. Both lungs (Fig 3F) together weighed 18 g and were visibly hypoplastic. The liver showed extensive extramedullary hematopoiesis. No ductal plate malformation was seen. Other organs including brain were within normal limits.

FINAL AUTOPSY DIAGNOSIS: PM 26118

40 Minute Male, 33 Weeks Gestation 2,100 gms

- Congenital bilateral hydroureteronephrosis with dysplasia, hypertrophied urinary bladder with dilated posterior urethra consistent with posterior urethral valve (PUV).
- Bilateral hypoplastic lungs.
- Lumbar meningomyelocele (3 cm).

COMMENTARY—INDEX CASE: PM 26118

Both are classical cases of PUV with bilateral severe hydronephrosis, widespread disarray/dysplastic changes seen in the renal parenchyma, markedly dilated and tortuous ureters showing hypertrophy of the muscle, enlarged and hypertrophied urinary bladder with marked hypertrophy of the detrusor muscle and a dilated posterior urethra. In this condition, there is generally a variation in the severity of involvement of the two kidneys, which is not seen in case 82 (kidneys were symmetrically enlarged) but seen in case 83. In addition a neural tube defect was detected in case 83. The degree of renal parenchymal dysgenesis was proportionate to the degree of hydroureters and hypertrophy of the urinary bladder.

Case 83 was a gravida 4 mother (G4P0030) with no live child. She had had three previous abortions but the cause was unknown. The index case was supervised at an outside facility. Her level III ultrasonography revealed normal kidneys and urinary bladder with normal liquor. At 22 weeks gestation, ultrasonography revealed a suspicion of a distended bladder, prominence of left renal pelvis and decreased liquor. At 26 weeks, there was severe oligohydramnios with hydronephrosis and distended urinary bladder and at 28

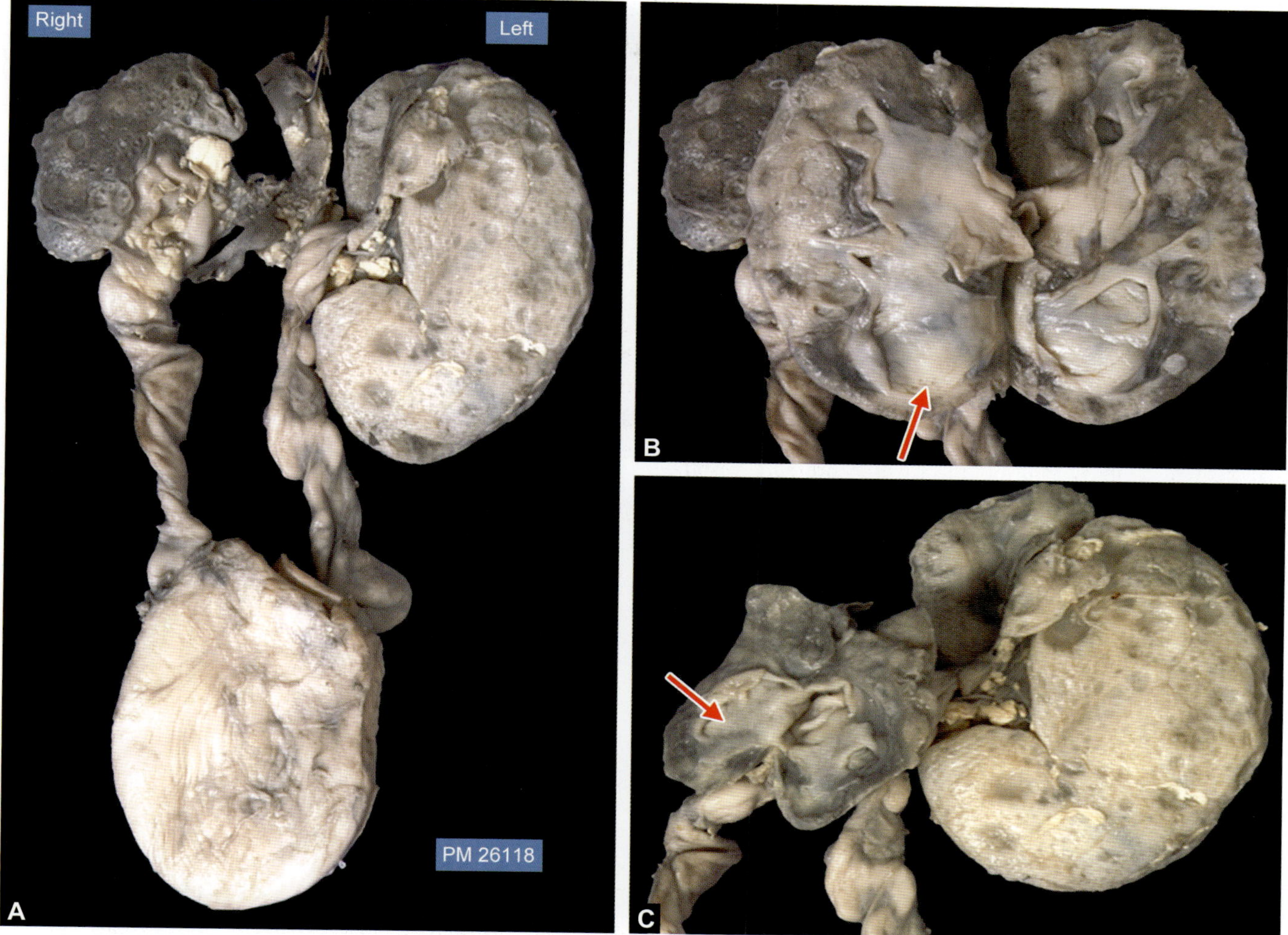

Figs 2A–C: (A) Gross photograph of the asymmetrically enlarged kidneys with maintained reniform shape and cysts of varying sizes on the capsular aspect. The ureters are dilated, tortuous and the urinary bladder is markedly hypertrophied; (B and C) Cut section of the kidneys shows markedly dilated pelvicalyceal systems with a thin rim of cortical tissue showing small cysts.

weeks similar findings were detected with a dilated urinary bladder (key sign positive) and enlarged hydronephrotic kidneys. PUV is a developmental problem and hence most cases are sporadic, but PUVs occurring in families have been reported. Case 83 did not give any history of similar kidney disease in the family. There was an accompanying neural tube defect, but this case cannot be fitted into any syndrome. Thereafter, six months later this mother conceived again and had a supervised pregnancy at our institute. She had hypertension and gestational diabetes mellitus for which she was on insulin. She delivered a normal male baby, 2.4 kg by a normal vaginal delivery on the 3rd August 2015. Baby is doing well.

POSTERIOR URETHRAL VALVE

The most common cause of bladder outlet obstruction in male babies is a PUV, which is an obstructing membrane, occurring due to an abnormal embryologic development, located in the posterior male urethra. Posterior urethral valve is also known as congenital obstructing posterior urethral membranes (COPUM). Its incidence is 1:10,000 to 25,000 live births. Young et al in 1919 categorized PUVs into type 1, type 2 and type 3. Dewan et al believed that the three types of valves probably represent a single diaphragm-like structure that can give a different look, due to antenatal rupture or postnatal instrumentation. The valve causes mechanical obstruction to bladder emptying, increases the voiding pressures and further distorts the fetal bladder and kidney

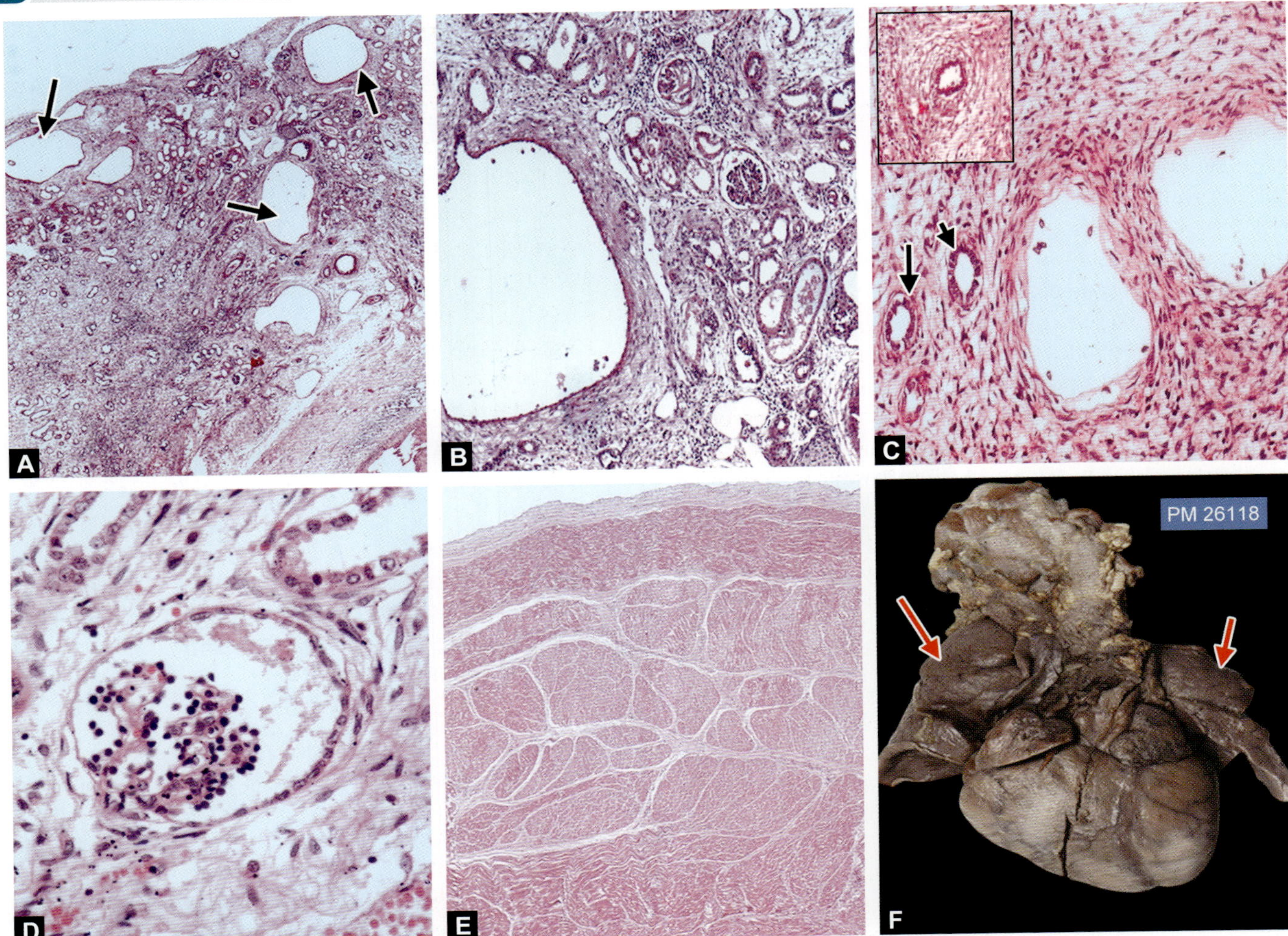

Figs 3A–F: Photomicrographs of the kidneys. (A and B) Showing peripheral cysts (arrows) with interspersed well-developed glomeruli and tubules; (C) Classical primitive ducts surrounded by a collar of immature mesenchyme, seen interspersed between the cysts. Inset shows a primitive duct; (D) Glomeruli showing glomerulocystic change; (E) Urinary bladder showing marked hypertrophy of the detrusor muscle; (F) Heart lung complex showing markedly hypoplastic lungs (arrows).

development. Thus, at one end of the spectrum, are cases with severe obstruction occurring early in development. In them, the outcome is poor with renal failure, lung hypoplasia oligohydramnios and these babies are either still born or die soon after birth. However, mild-to-moderate obstruction is compatible with life and these babies suffer from symptoms of voiding dysfunction like vesicoureteric reflux. Varying degrees of hydronephrosis occurs, depending on the severity of obstruction. Hydronephrosis occurs due to—(1) Bladder dysfunction with high back pressures on the ureter; (2) Ureter may develop an abnormal musculature due to chronic distention from high pressure or high urine flow and this further lead to hydronephrosis; (3) Dilatation of the kidneys and ureters can further occur due to high urinary flow, which occurs due to the lack of urinary concentrating ability of the nephron; (4) Vesicoureteric reflux and rarely ureterovesical obstruction also cause hydronephrosis. In approximately 50% cases of PUV, vesicoureteral reflux is present and is thought to be physiologic, with high bladder pressure combating the competence of the ureterovesical junction. Reflux may also be anatomic, secondary to abnormal position of the ureteric orifices, as a result of abnormal ureteral bud development during embryogenesis. Urinary bladder dysfunction is thought to be caused by alterations in the development of detrusor smooth muscle cells, which lead to myogenic failure. Few protective mechanisms like bladder diverticula, urinary ascites and massive unilateral vesicoureteral reflux help to lower the intraluminal pressures and allow at least one kidney to develop more normally.

Posterior urethral valve is a valve-like membrane arising from the tissue of the Wolffian duct, as a result of the failure of regression of the mesonephric duct. This membrane courses from the verumontanum to the most distal portion of the prostatic urethra. This insult occurs around 5–7 weeks of gestation. This is a developmental problem and hence most cases are sporadic, but PUVs occurring in families have been reported. Association with other congenital malformations includes craniospinal defects, bowel atresia, abdominal wall defects and chromosomal abnormalities like Down syndrome. Antenatal diagnosis of PUV is becoming increasingly common with routine obstetric ultrasonography. In severe cases it shows oligohydramnios, distension/hypertrophy of the urinary bladder, hydroureteronephrosis and a dilated posterior urethra. Assessing the degree of renal dysplasia is difficult antenatally, but increased echogenicity of the kidneys with loss of corticomedullary differentiation is an indicator of renal dysplasia. Key hole sign on ultrasound can be seen, which is the result of distension of the urinary bladder and the posterior urethra, proximal to the valve. In less severe cases, the hydroureteronephrosis may or may not be present. In postnatal life ultrasonography confirms the hydroureteronephrosis and examination of the posterior urethra can be performed longitudinally through the perineum. This is best done during micturition, where the proximal urethra is seen to dilate and a diameter of more than 6 mm is highly specific and sensitive to the diagnosis of a PUV. Postnatal voiding cystourethrography (VCUG) is the best technique for the diagnosis of PUV, wherein the diagnosis is best made during the micturition phase in a lateral or oblique view, so that the dilated and elongated posterior urethra can be imaged properly. VCUG also assesses the bladder for associated findings of trabeculation, diverticula and vesicoureteral reflux.

TAKE HOME MESSAGE

- The most common cause of bilateral congenital hydroureteronephrosis is Posterior urethral valve (PUV) followed by Prune belly syndrome.
- In obstructive uropathy, four factors which play an important role in ascertaining the degree of maldevelopment are—time, rapidity, degree (complete or partial) and site of obstruction.
- Posterior urethral valve is a developmental disorder, most cases are sporadic, but PUVs occurring in families have been reported.
- The kidneys (with PUV) are enlarged, retain their reniform shape and show cysts on the surface. There is generally a variation in the severity of involvement of the two sides.
- Microscopy (in PUV) shows hydronephrotic atrophy of the cortex with widespread disarray and dysplastic changes. Marked hypertrophy of the detrusor muscle of the urinary bladder and ureters is seen.

SUGGESTED READING

1. Chatterjee SK, Banerjee S, Basak D, et al. Posterior urethral valve: the scenario in a developing country. Pediatr Surg Int. 2001;17:2-7.
2. Dewan PA, Zappata SM, Ransley PG, et al. Endoscopic reappraisal of the morphology of congenital obstruction of the posterior urethra. British J Urol. 1992;70:439-44.
3. Duffy PG, Chowdhary SK. Posterior urethral valve: current perspective. J Indian Association Pediatr Surg. 2003;8:169-74.
4. Haekar F, Wehrmann M, Hacker H, et al. Renal dysplasia in children with posterior urethral valves: a primary or secondary malformation. Pediatr Surg Int. 2002;18:119-22.
5. Hill GS. Cystic and dysplastic diseases of the kidney: developmental lesions. In: Hill GS, (Ed). Uropathology, Volume 1. Edinburgh, New York: Churchill Livingstone; 1989. pp. 107-10.

CONTRIBUTIONS BY:

Case 82

1. Dr Anil Narang, Ex-Professor and Head, Department of Pediatrics (Clinician In-Charge)

Case 83

1. Dr Kanya Mukhopadhyay, Professor (Clinician In-Charge)
2. Dr Shiv Sajan Saini, Assistant Professor (Clinician In-Charge)

Post Graduate Institute of Medical Education and Research, Chandigarh, India.

Section 15C: Renal Hypoplasia

CASE 84

Neonate with Bilateral Simple Renal Hypoplasia, Lung Hypoplasia and Hydrocephalus: PM 27245

Nandita Bharadwaj Kakkar

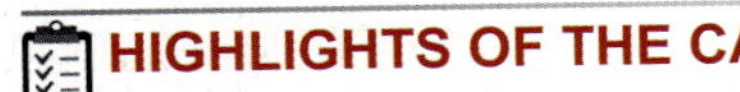

HIGHLIGHTS OF THE CASE

This was a neonate who lived for one hour and was born to a primigravida at 37 weeks gestation. Ultrasonography at 28 weeks gestation revealed Dandy–Walker syndrome, single umbilical artery and absent stomach bubble. The renal malformation was not picked up on ultrasonography. Autopsy revealed a classic picture of bilateral renal hypoplasia with associated lung hypoplasia, hydrocephalus and a single umbilical artery. Mother did reveal history of her sister having lost her baby with renal malformation. Mother was sent for genetic counseling.

Keywords: Renal hypoplasia, simple, bilateral, miniature kidney, lung hypoplasia, hydrocephalus.

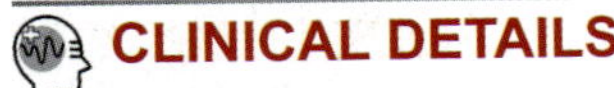

CLINICAL DETAILS

Date of Birth and Death: 25.02.2016, lived for 1 hour

A primigravida delivered a baby with ambiguous genitalia, vaginally, at 37 weeks gestation. The baby weight was 1,815 g (SGA—2). The APGAR was 1,6 and baby had severe birth asphyxia, hypoxic ischemic encephalopathy stage 3 with gasping efforts and died within an hour of birth. Ultrasonography at 28 weeks gestation revealed Dandy–Walker syndrome, single umbilical artery and absent stomach bubble. No comment on liquor was given. Examination of the baby revealed a flat forehead, broad nasal bridge, abnormal genitalia, sacral sinus, cleft palate and bilateral congenital talipes equinovarus. Clinical diagnosis was—Major congenital malformation, Dandy–Walker syndrome. Baby was sent for autopsy after taking permission from the parents.

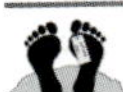

AUTOPSY FINDINGS: PM 27245

A complete autopsy was performed. The baby weighed 1,800 g. On external examination, there was a Potter's facies with low set ears, flat forehead, Mongolian slant, broad nasal bridge, abnormal genitalia, cleft palate and bilateral congenital talipes equinovarus. The brain revealed hydrocephalus with a patent aqueduct. No features of Dandy–Walker syndrome were noted, i.e. the posterior fossa was normal, cerebellar vermis was present and the fourth ventricle did not show any dilatation. The kidneys (Figs 1A–D) were hypoplastic measuring $1 \times 1 \times 0.5$ cm, weighed 4 g (<50% of expected weight), ureters were patent and showed mild ectopic insertion into the urinary bladder. No fetal lobulations were seen and the capsular aspect was smooth. The left ureter was slightly dilated in its mid portion (Fig 1D-arrow). The bladder appeared normal. Cut section of the kidneys revealed a reduction in the number of renal calyces and renal lobes. Tiny peripheral cysts could be appreciated under a magnifying glass. The adrenals appeared enlarged and disc-shaped (Fig 1A-white arrows). Microscopic examination of the kidneys (Figs 2A–F) revealed peripheral small cysts, cortex showed 2–3 ranks of glomeruli (term baby should show 12–14 ranks) of normal morphology, few peripheral glomeruli showed glomerulocystic change and foci of extramedullary hematopoiesis was seen. The interstitium showed hemorrhage and loose connective tissue. The interlobular vessels were prominent and showed medial hypertrophy (Fig 2F-arrow). No primitive duct was present, i.e. there was no element of dysplasia. The lungs (Fig 3A-arrows) together weighed 10 g and were hypoplastic. Microscopy (Fig 3B) confirmed the hypoplasia in the form of

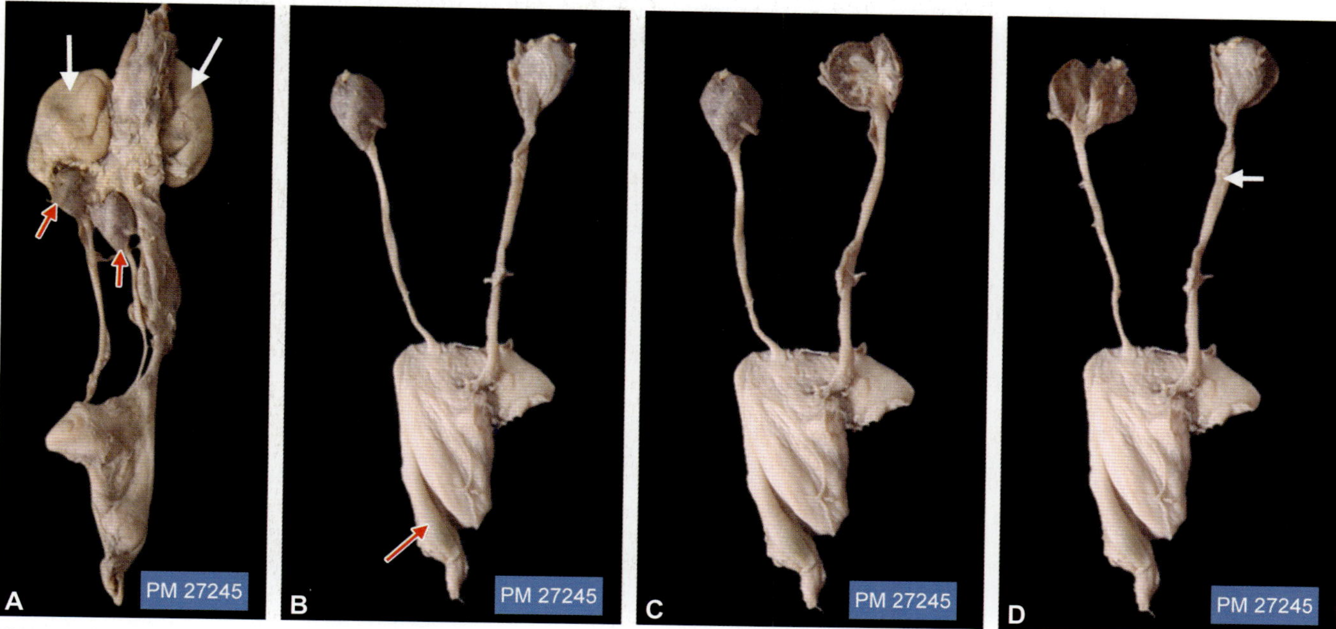

Figs 1A–D: Gross photographs showing (A) Organ complex comprising of both the hypoplastic kidneys (red arrows), ureters, urinary bladder, and adrenals (white arrows); (B) Both kidneys are small 1 × 1 × 0.5 cm, do not show fetal lobulations and show patent ureters with mild ectopic insertion into the urinary bladder. A part of the uterus is seen attached to the urinary bladder (red arrow); (C and D) Cut section of the left and right kidneys shows cortex with tiny cysts, reduced renal lobes/calyces. The left ureter shows dilatation (arrow).

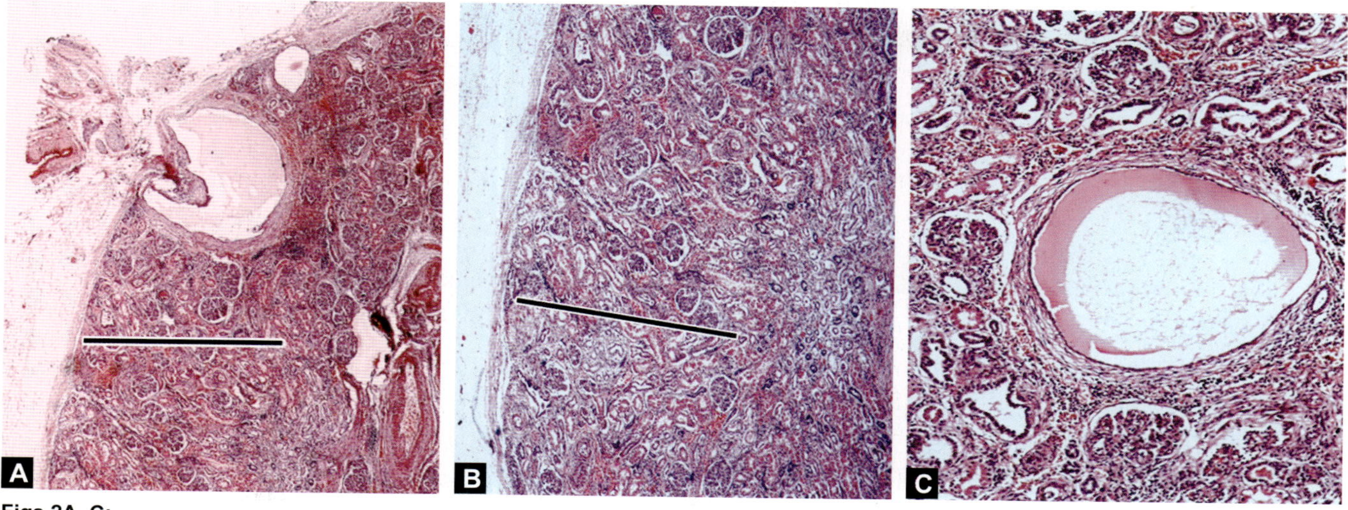

Figs 2A–C:

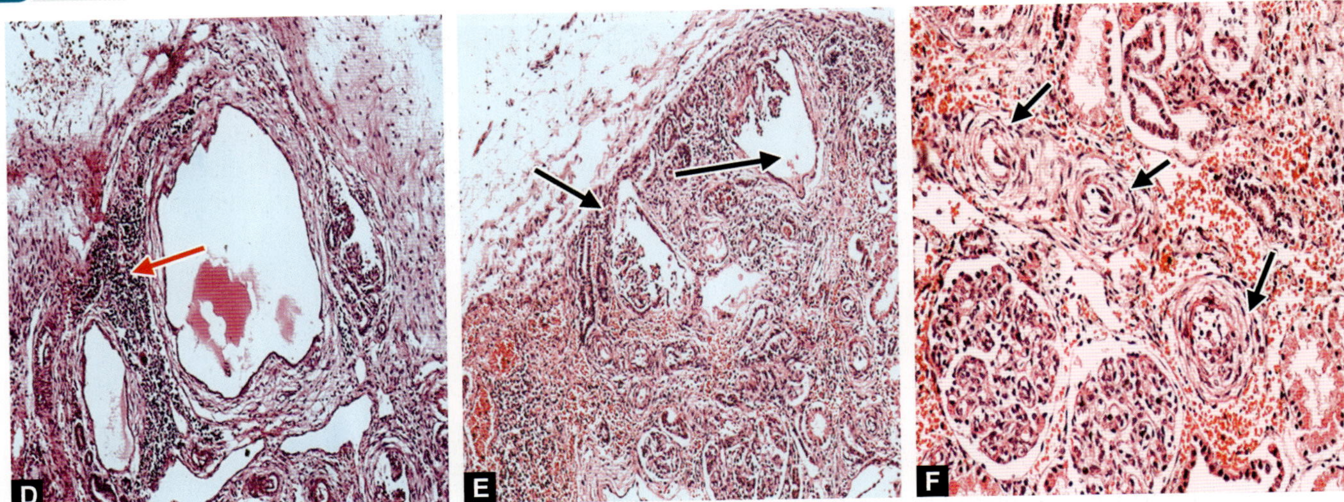

Figs 2A–F: Photomicrographs of the kidneys (A and B) Show peripheral cyst, cortex (black line) with 2–3 ranks of glomeruli which show normal morphology; (C and D) Cysts with surrounding normal looking glomeruli and foci of extramedullary hematopoiesis (red arrow). Interstitium shows loose connective tissue; (E) Few peripheral glomeruli show glomerulocystic change (arrows); (F) Interlobular vessels appear prominent and show medial hypertrophy (arrows). Interstitium shows hemorrhage.

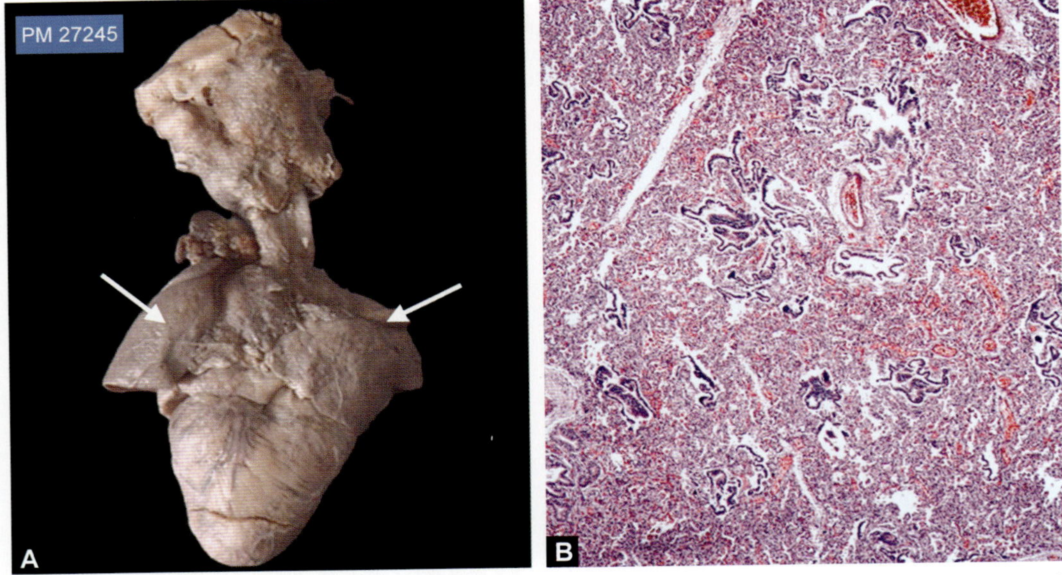

Figs 3A and B: (A) Heart–lung complex showing hypoplastic lungs (arrows) weighing 10 g. Normally the lungs cover the entire heart; (B) Photomicrograph of the lung shows hypoplasia manifesting as approximation of the bronchioles.

marked approximation of the bronchioles. Single umbilical artery was noted. Gastrointestinal tract was within normal limits. Uterus, tubes and ovary were found and were normal.

FINAL AUTOPSY DIAGNOSIS: PM 27245

Term baby with Potter's Facies and Abnormal Genitalia

- Bilateral simple Hypoplasia - Miniature kidney
- Bilateral hypoplastic lungs.
- Hydrocephalus with patent aqueduct
- Single umbilical artery.

For renal hypoplasia—refer to "Pediatric cystic disease (developmental/genetic) of kidney: Introduction".

COMMENTARY—INDEX CASE: PM 27245

This was a neonate, born to a primigravida at 37 weeks gestation, weighed 1,815 g, had low APGAR score, Potter's facies, ambiguous genitalia and died one hour after birth. Ultrasonography at 28 weeks gestation revealed Dandy–Walker syndrome, single umbilical artery and absent stomach bubble. The renal malformation was not picked up on ultrasonography. Autopsy revealed a classic picture of bilateral renal hypoplasia with associated lung hypoplasia, hydrocephalus and a single umbilical artery. Uterus, tubes and ovaries were found. Baby died due to lung hypoplasia. Mother did reveal history of her sister having lost her baby with renal malformation. Mother was sent for genetic counseling.

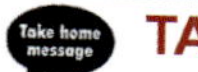

TAKE HOME MESSAGE

- Simple renal hypoplasia (Miniature kidney) shows small-sized kidneys without fetal lobulations, patent ureters which may show abnormalities, reduced calyces/lobes, 2–3 ranks of glomeruli and few peripheral cysts.

CONTRIBUTIONS BY:

1. Dr Venkataseshan S, Professor, Department of Pediatrics (Neonatology Division) (Clinician In-Charge)
Post Graduate Institute of Medical Education and Research, Chandigarh, India.

CASE 85

Bilateral Simple Renal Hypoplasia, Cystic Periventricular Leukomalacia with Hydrocephalus ex vacuo in Surviving Twin, after Death of Monochorionic Co-twin: PM 25677

Nandita Bharadwaj Kakkar

 HIGHLIGHTS OF THE CASE

A 49-day-old male baby, 2nd of the twin, with loss of a monochorionic co-twin in the 2nd trimester, was autopsied as was advised by the pediatricians, at the time of discharge from NICU, when he was 1-week-old. He was born to a 27 years, third gravida mother, G3 P1210, who had two previous fetal losses with no living issue. Ultrasonography (USG) revealed repeated renal malformations in all three pregnancies, bilaterally enlarged hydronephrotic kidneys in G1, bilateral enlarged multicystic kidneys in G2 and bilateral hypoplastic kidneys with noncommunicating hydrocephalus in G3 (Twin 2). G3 (index case) was a monochorionic twin pregnancy with death of its co-twin (twin 1) in the second trimester (30–32 weeks). The index case at autopsy revealed two major problems—recurrent renal developmental malformation and periventricular leukomalacia (PVL) subsequent to the death of the monochorionic co-twin.

Keywords: Cystic leukomalacia, surviving twin, monochorionic twins, renal hypoplasia, renal developmental disorders, recurrent, hereditary renal adysplasia, autopsy.

 CLINICAL DETAILS

Date of Birth: 14.08.2013

A 49-day-old male baby, 2nd of the twin, was brought dead to pediatric emergency for autopsy as was advised by the pediatricians, at the time of discharge from NICU, when he was one week old. This baby was 2nd of the twin, born to a 3rd gravida mother on 14.08.2013, the mother having been referred to PGIMER Chandigarh at 31 + 5 weeks of gestation with a provisional diagnosis of congenital malformation with two previous pregnancy losses.

G1—2010: USG at 18 weeks showed bilateral pelvi ureteric junction obstruction with gross hydronephrosis ? polycystic kidneys. Medical termination of pregnancy was done (at an outside facility) at 18 weeks gestation, a male abortus was expelled but autopsy was not done.

G2—February 2012: In this pregnancy, she was booked and supervised in PGIMER Chandigarh. USG at 9 weeks—single live fetus with adequate liquor. USG at 21 + 2 weeks (12.10.11) revealed bilateral enlarged cystic (small fluid filled noncommunicating cysts) kidneys with a nonvisualized bladder and reduced liquor. Lateral ventricles 8 mm (normal). She delivered at term, a live baby boy who expired soon after birth. Autopsy was refused by the parents.

G3—August 2013: Twin gestation, USG at ***16 weeks*** was normal with two gestational sacs, a single large placenta and oligohydramnios. USG at ***18 weeks*** did not reveal any abnormality. Lateral ventricles were 10 mm. USG at ***28 weeks*** showed both live fetuses, two gestational sacs, T2—mildly dilated lateral ventricles, 12 mm, third ventricle 4.7 mm and ? aqueductal stenosis. USG at ***32 weeks*** showed T1—IUD, T2—dilated lateral ventricles 20 mm - hydrocephalus. No other congenital malformation seen.

Birth history: T2 delivered in PGIMER at 33 weeks gestation on 14th August 2013, assisted breech delivery and APGAR scores were 8 and 9 at 1 and 5 minutes, respectively. T1 was a macerated still birth. On examination the birth weight of T2 was 1.5 kg (<10th centile), head circumference—29 cm (<10th centile) and no external abnormality was detected. There was no facial dysmorphism, polydactyly, any skeletal deformity or cleft lip/palate. Family history did not reveal similar problem in any other family member. ***Investigations*** for TORCH group of infections were negative. ***Postnatal***

USG of the cranium (14.8.13 and 20.8.13) revealed normal posterior fossa structures, dilatation of the supratentorial ventricular system (50% VHR) with small cystic lesions in bilateral frontal regions in periventricular location, suggestive of multicystic encephalomalacia with noncommunicating hydrocephalus. ***Postnatal USG of the abdomen*** showed bilateral small kidneys (right 1.3 cm, left 1.8 cm) with raised cortical echogenicity, no cysts, pelvicalyceal system not dilated, lost corticomedullary differentiation, renal parenchymal disease and bladder not distended. ***Echocardiography*** was normal; ***ABG*** (day 8); pH: 7.4, PaO_2: 34, $PaCO_2$: 35, HCO_3: 21, Lactate: 1.1, ***Blood Biochemistry***: Random blood sugar—64 mg%, Na^+ 134 mEq/L, K^+ 5.3 mEq/L, serum creatinine—6.9 mg%, serum urea—44 mg%. Routine urine examination normal. Parents' karyotyping was normal and USG did not reveal any renal malformation in them. ***Course in hospital:*** Baby was started on full tube feeds which he tolerated well. Neurological examination was normal and he was passing urine. He developed neonatal jaundice for which phototherapy was given for 2 days. His blood pressure was high, systolic 101–120, diastolic 55–71 (>95th centile) and was started on hydrochlorothiazide. Prognosis was explained to the parents in view of kidney disease/brain abnormality and he was discharged on D10. His stay at home had poor weight gain, but activity was said to be good and he was passing urine. He became very irritable on the day of demise. He was taken to a local doctor and he expired within 2 hours of hospitalization. The body was brought for autopsy to PGIMER, Chandigarh. ***Units Clinical Diagnosis*** was recurrent (third pregnancy) renal malformation—bilateral small kidneys with renal parenchymal disease, multicystic encephalomalacia with noncommunicating hydrocephalus ? Meckel-Gruber syndrome ? Zellweger syndrome. Cause of death—Chronic kidney disease with hyperkalemia and anemia.

AUTOPSY FINDINGS: PM 25677

A complete autopsy was performed on this 49-day-old male baby who was born at 33 weeks gestation (corrected age 40 weeks gestation). Externally the prosector did not find any facial dysmorphism, or any other abnormality. The head was not enlarged. The baby weighed 1,890 g. ***Anthropometric measurements*** revealed crown heel - 45 cm, crown rump 28 cm, head/chest/abdominal circumference - 31/28/26 cm and foot length 7.5 cm. On opening, all serous cavities were within normal limits. Both the ***kidneys*** were small measuring 1.3 × 1 × 0.5 cm each and together weighed 10 g which is <50% of expected weight (normal for age 28 g). Fetal lobulations were present, but no cysts were seen on the surface (Fig 1A). Ureters were moderately dilated with normal ureteric orifice position and the urinary bladder was normal. Cut section of the kidneys (Fig 1B) did not show any cysts or dilatation of pelvicalyceal system. Microscopy showed a thinned out cortex with extensive ineffective neoglomerulogenesis in the superficial cortex, decrease in the number of renal lobes and in few of the lobes, not a single glomerulus was identified (Figs 1C and D). In other lobes, sparse glomeruli (Fig 1E) could be seen (2–3 ranks against a normal of 12–14 ranks) and the peripheral cortical tubules showed mild degree of dilatation. The sparse glomeruli which were present showed a variety of features—increased mesangial cellularity and matrix (Fig 2A), focal segmental glomerulosclerosis (Fig 2B) and occasional large glomeruli (Fig 2C). Apart from this interstitial inflammation (Fig 2D), fibrosis, calcification, tubular dilatation and periglomerular fibrosis (Fig 2E) was noted. No features of dysplasia, i.e. primitive ducts (hallmark of dysplasia), cartilage, proliferating nerves, extramedullary hematopoiesis, primitive glomeruli/tubules or any cysts could be seen. Overall features were those of bilateral renal hypoplasia along with features of tubulointerstitial nephritis. The ***brain*** weighed 320 g (normal for this age—356 g). On external examination, there was no exudate, no subarachnoid hemorrhage, base of the brain/sulci/gyri were within normal limits, no pachygyria or microgyria noted, brain was soft and cystic on the superolateral/temporal surfaces and the occipital lobes were thinned out and cystic (left>right). On coronal slicing, the lateral ventricles were markedly dilated (Figs 3A–E) in its entirety, i.e. central, anterior and posterior horns were maximally affected. The third ventricle (Fig 3A), aqueduct of Sylvius (Fig 4A) and fourth ventricle (Fig 4B) were not dilated. Bilateral cortical cysts were seen more so in the frontal lobes and involving the periventricular, central and subcortical white matter (Figs 3A and B). The right insular cortex showed laminar necrosis and was separating from the underlying white matter. No intraventricular/germinal matrix/ parenchymal/subarachnoid hemorrhage was seen. Microscopy of the affected brain revealed extensive white matter atrophy with cystic change (Figs 5A and B). The sulci were dilated with marked approximation to the dilated ventricles, due to white matter atrophy and gliosis was appreciated (Figs 5C and D). Neuronal migration disarray with clusters of neurons caught up in the cysts, in the central breaking down white matter (Figs 6A and B) and in the wall of the dilated ventricles were noted (Fig 5D). Apart from this, there was extensive myelin loss (Fig 6C), proliferating astrocytes, microgemistocytes, oligodendroglia and macrophages (Fig 6D). The extensive white matter damage had resulted in hydrocephalus ex vacuo with mark-

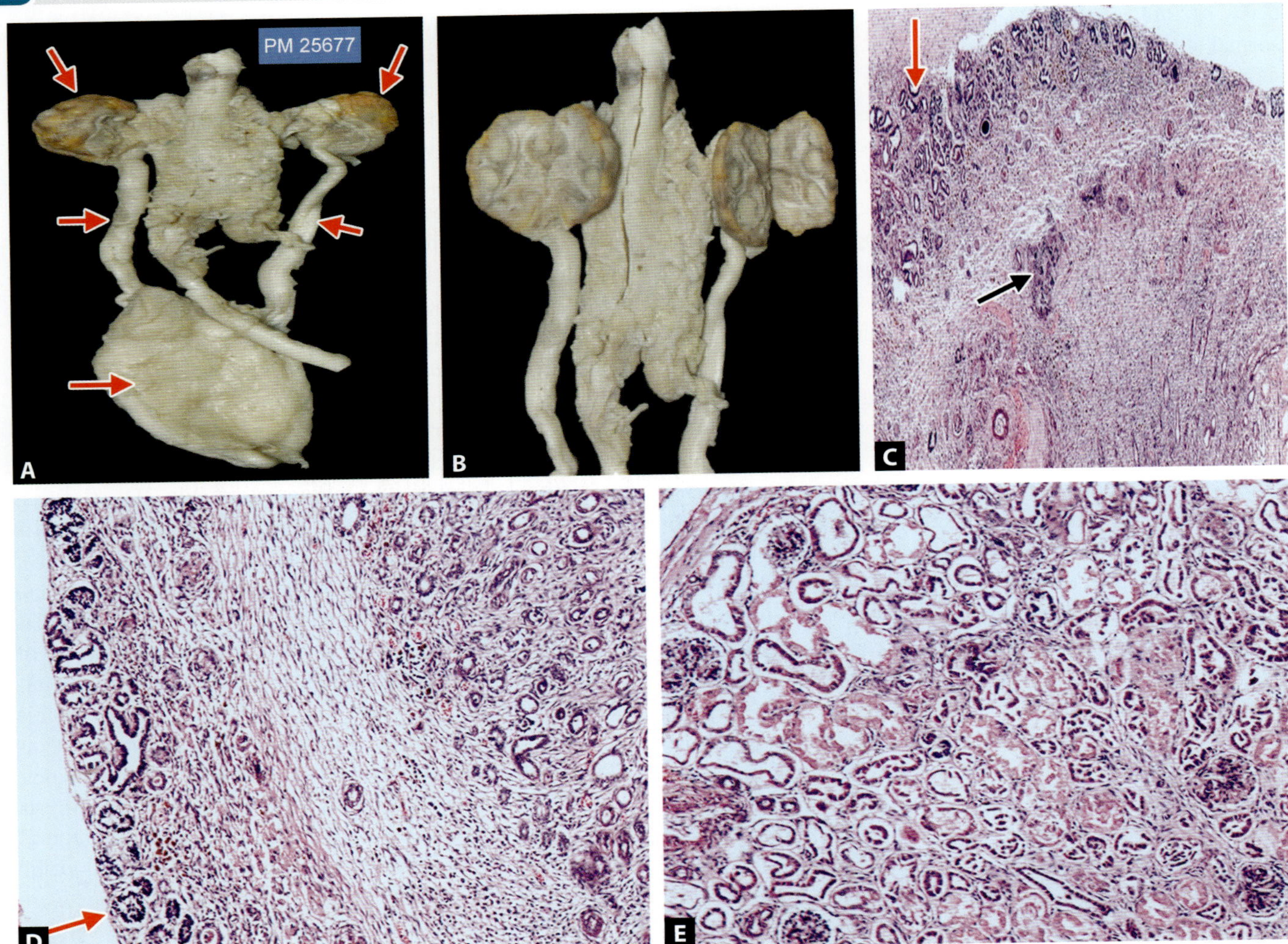

Figs 1A–E: (A) Gross photographs of both the kidneys (upper arrows) which are small and show fetal lobulations, without any cyst. Both ureters are dilated (middle arrows). Urinary bladder is normal (lower arrow); (B) Cut section of both kidneys showing absence of cysts and no dilatation of the pelvicalyceal system; (C and D) Photomicrographs of the kidney showing a thin cortex with ongoing ineffective neoglomerulogenesis (red arrows). No glomeruli can be seen. Foci of calcification (black arrow) and prominent vessels are noted; (E) Photomicrographs of the kidney showing sparse glomeruli (2–3 ranks). Tubules show dilatation.

edly dilated lateral ventricles. Features in the brain were consistent with multicystic PVL with hydrocephalus ex vacuo. No features suggestive of Zellweger syndrome were seen, i.e. there was no cerebellar, dentate or olivary nucleus dysplasia, microgyria/pachygyria, lissencephaly and agenesis or hypoplasia of corpus callosum or any optic nerve atrophy. The ***liver*** weighed 70 g and was normal both grossly and microscopically. No ductal plate malformation or any fibrosis was seen. The ***heart*** was slightly overweight (28 g). Coarctation of aorta was present along with dilated ascending/arch of aorta (Fig 7A), left ventricular hypertrophy with dilatation and a patent ductus arteriosus (Fig 7B). The ***lungs*** weighed 48 g and were not hypoplastic. Microscopically there was no pneumonia or hemorrhage, however persistent pulmonary hypertension was noted. Bone marrow showed erythroid hyperplasia. The pancreas, adrenals, thymus, gastrointestinal tract and testis were within normal limits.

FINAL AUTOPSY DIAGNOSIS: PM 25677

Fourty-nine Days Male, c/o Gravida 3 with Recurrent Fetal/infant Deaths due to Recurrent Renal Malformations.

- ***Kidneys:*** Bilateral simple renal hypoplasia with tubulointerstitial nephritis. Recurrent (third) renal developmental malformation consistent with hereditary renal adysplasia.
- ***Brain:*** Multicystic encephalomalacia with hydrocephalus ex vacuo in surviving twin (monochorionic, diamniotic placenta).

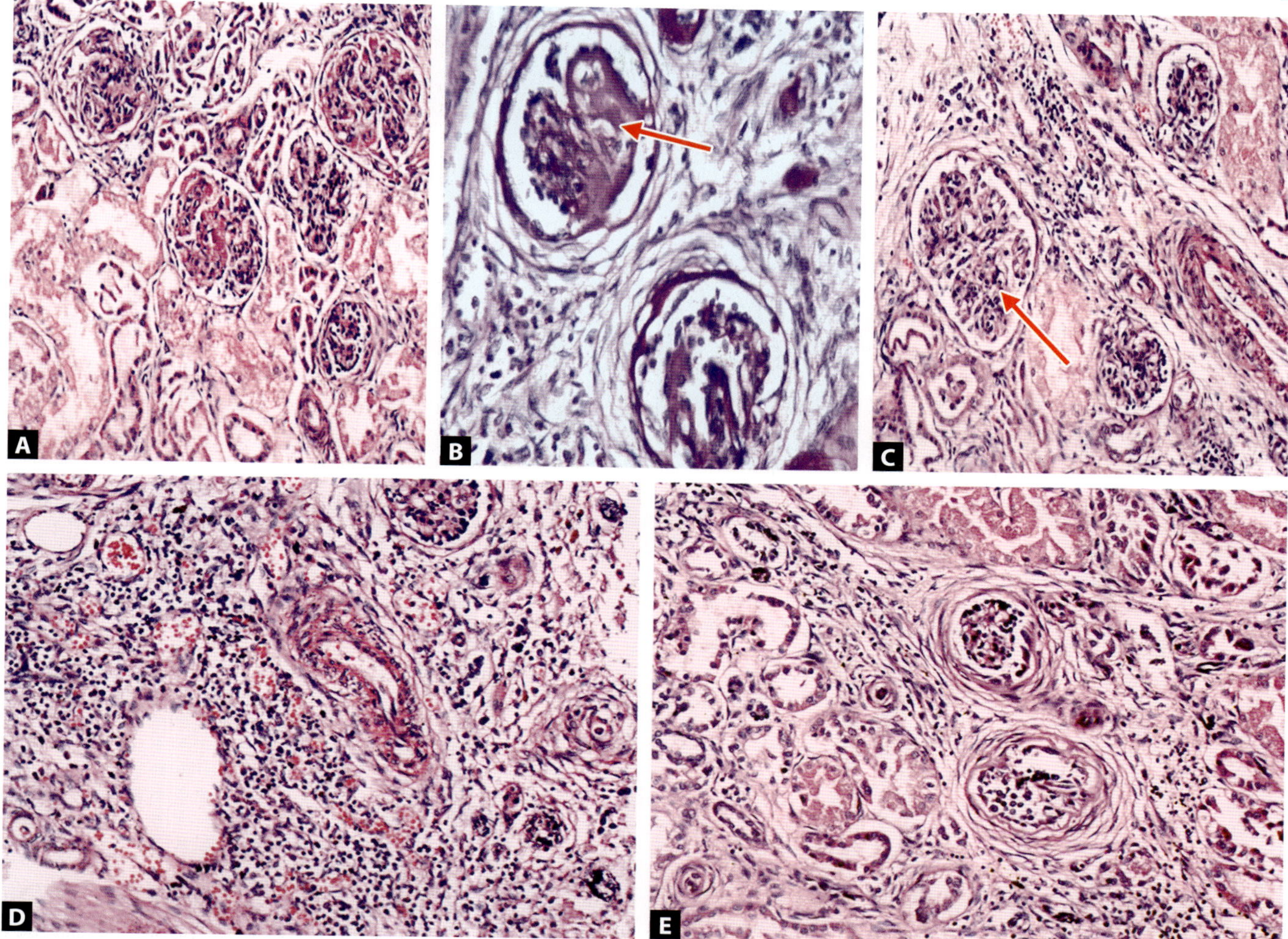

Figs 2A–E: Photomicrographs of the kidney showing glomerular changes. (A) Glomeruli show increased mesangial cellularity and matrix; (B) Glomeruli showing sclerosis—periodic acid-Schiff stain; (C) Occasional large glomerulus was noted; (D) Photomicrograph showing dense interstitial inflammation and tubular destruction; (E) Photomicrograph showing periglomerular fibrosis.

- ***Heart:*** Coarctation of aorta, dilated ascending/arch of aorta, left ventricular hypertrophy with dilatation, patent ductus arteriosus.
- Persistent pulmonary artery hypertension (PPHN).

Pathology Findings of Twin 1: PM 25586, Dead Fetus

Baby weighed 560 g, was badly autolysed, but there was no malformation.

PERIVENTRICULAR LEUKOMALACIA

Periventricular leukomalacia is defined as an ischemic lesion present in the periventricular white matter of a preterm infant and is characterized by infarction of the deep white matter. It occurs due to hypoxia incurred between 24 weeks and 32 weeks gestation before the myelination starts. Preterm infants are at a very high risk for developing PVL or white matter damage in the neonatal period, a contributor of cerebral palsy later in infancy. This was observed way back in 1867 by Virchow,[1] who described whitish yellow spots in the periventricular white matter. Banker and Larroche[2] in 1962 framed the term PVL as white (leukos) spots and softening (malacia) in the periventricular white matter. In the last decade, due to the medical advancements, preterms of as low as 24 weeks are surviving and autopsy studies on them have shown a diffuse pattern of white matter damage.[3] Histological findings depend on the time period between death and the occurrence of the insult. Microscopy shows pallor, myelin loss, proliferating astrocytes, microgemistocytes, macrophages and breakdown of the central necrotic area (occurs after 10–20 days) leading to the formation of small

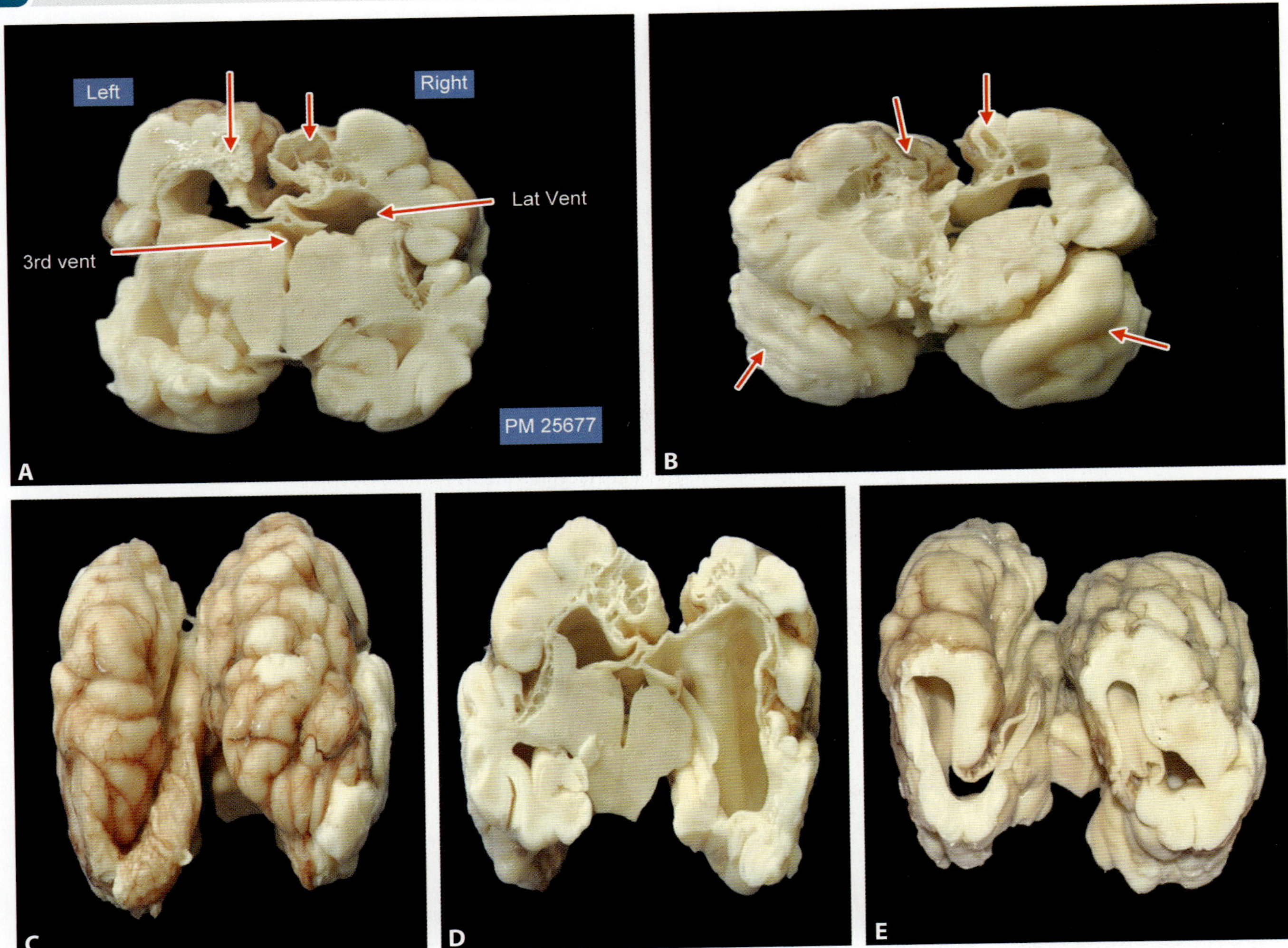

Figs 3A–E: (A) Coronal slice of the brain showing dilated lateral ventricles (middle red arrow) with a normal third ventricle (long red arrow). Bilateral cortical cysts are seen in the frontal lobes, involving the periventricular, central, and subcortical white matter (upper red small arrows); (B) Brain showing dilated lateral ventricles, multiple white matter cysts (upper red arrows), and large cystic occipital lobes (lower arrows); (C) Occipital lobes which are large and cystic; (D and E) Marked dilatation of the posterior horns of the lateral ventricles. In "E", the occipital lobes are sliced from the posterior aspect.

cavities in the periventricular white matter, gliosis, calcification and eventually hydrocephalus ex vacuo. Although ischemia plays a major role in its pathogenesis, there are other contributing factors as well. The immature oligodendrocyte are highly vulnerable to glutamate.[4] Cytokines[5] released during ischemia play a major role in the damage of the white matter and this may also play a role in intrauterine life. Raised interleukins[6] (IL-1b, IL-6 and TNF-α) found in the amniotic fluid or cord blood, in cases of white matter disease is now a well-established cause. High frequency ventilation leading to hypocarbia, which further leads on to vasoconstriction, is a common risk factor for PVL.

In monochorionic pregnancies,[7-10] 20% of surviving co-twins, after second or third-trimester intrauterine fetal death of one twin, develop cystic PVL or multicystic encephalomalacia. Bernischke[11] was the first to describe neurologic damage in a surviving twin and attributed it to the passage of thromboplastin from the dead fetus to the surviving twin, through the existing placental anastomosis, causing multiple infarctions. Or it occurs as a result of acute hypotension due to the blood loss from the surviving twin and its flow into the placenta and then into the dead twin, which is said to occur at the time of the death of the co-twin. The latter proposition is however, more acceptable. This has been substantiated by Nicolini et al[12] wherein they assessed the hematocrit levels

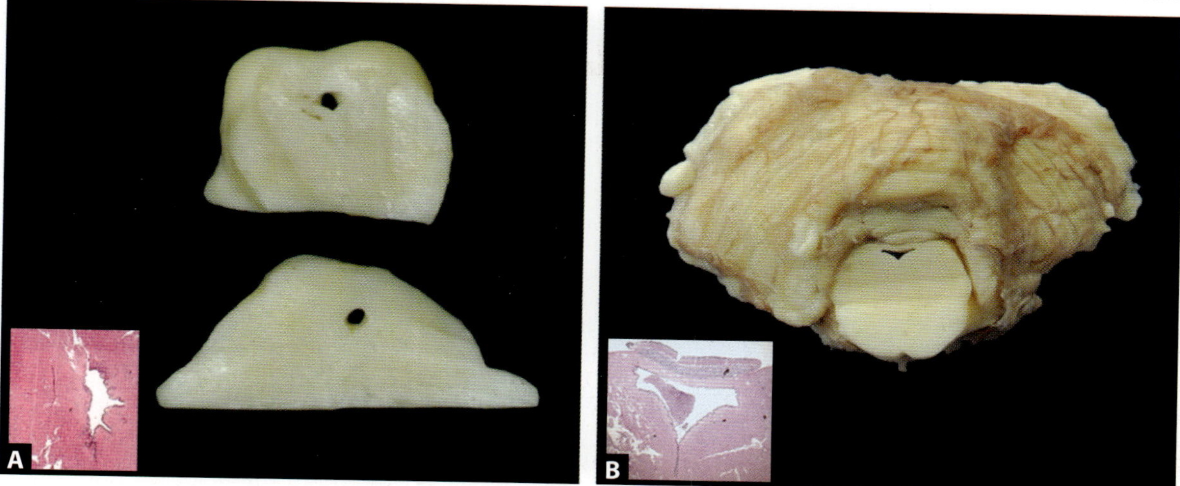

Figs 4A and B: (A) Slice of the midbrain with a normal patent aqueduct of Sylvius. Inset shows the microscopy of the normal aqueduct; (B) Slice of cerebellum with upper pons along with the fourth ventricle, which is not dilated. Inset shows the microscopy of the normal fourth ventricle.

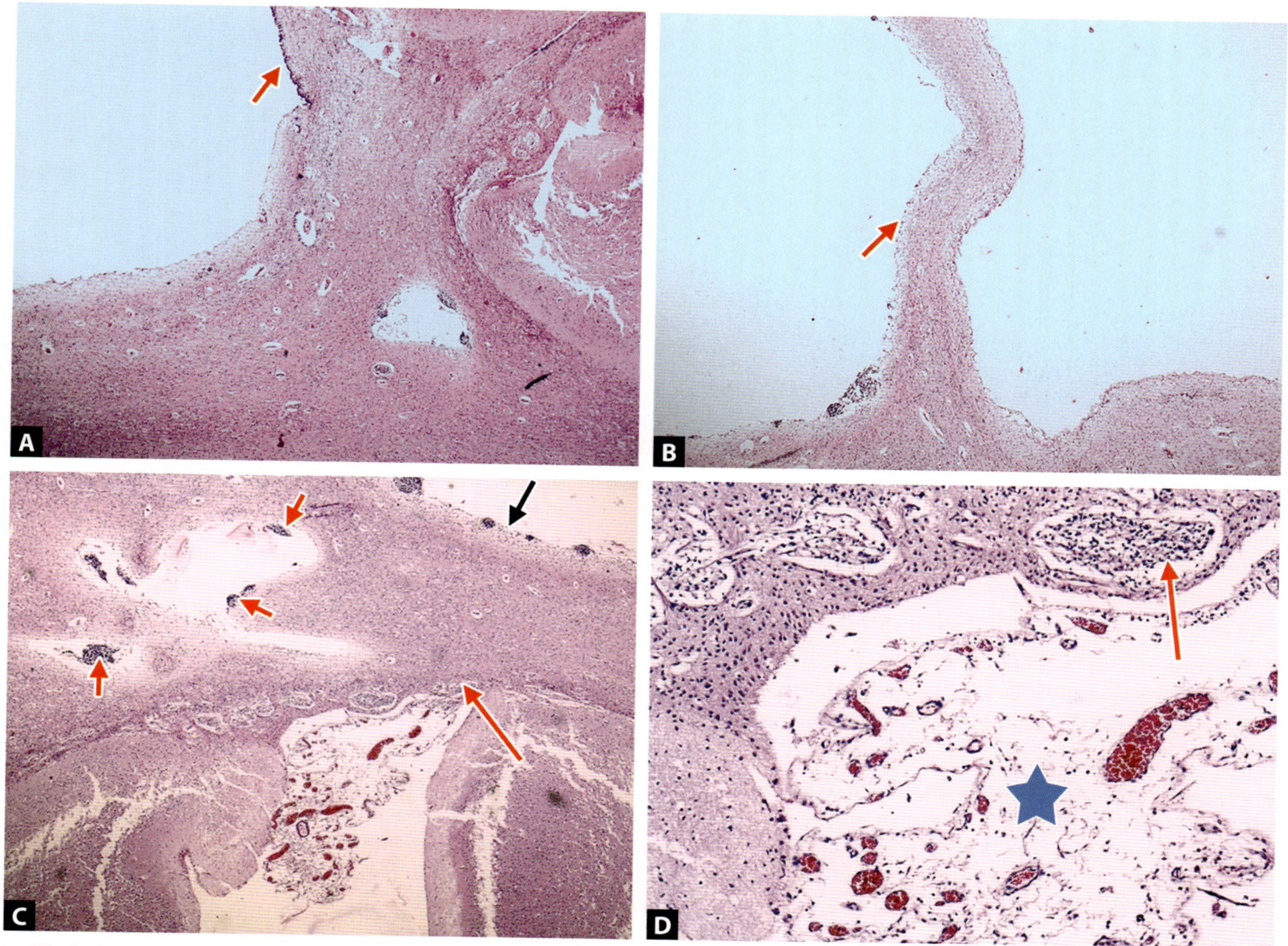

Figs 5A–D: (A and B) Photomicrograph from the cortex of the brain showing multiples cysts. The ventricular lining is partially evident (arrow) in the dilated ventricle; (C) Photomicrograph of the brain showing the depth of the sulcus (long red arrow) with marked approximation to the dilated ventricle (black arrow) due to white matter atrophy and gliosis. Small cysts present in the white matter show caught up neurons (small red arrows); (D) Dilated sulcus (star) showing caught up neurons in the white matter (red arrow).

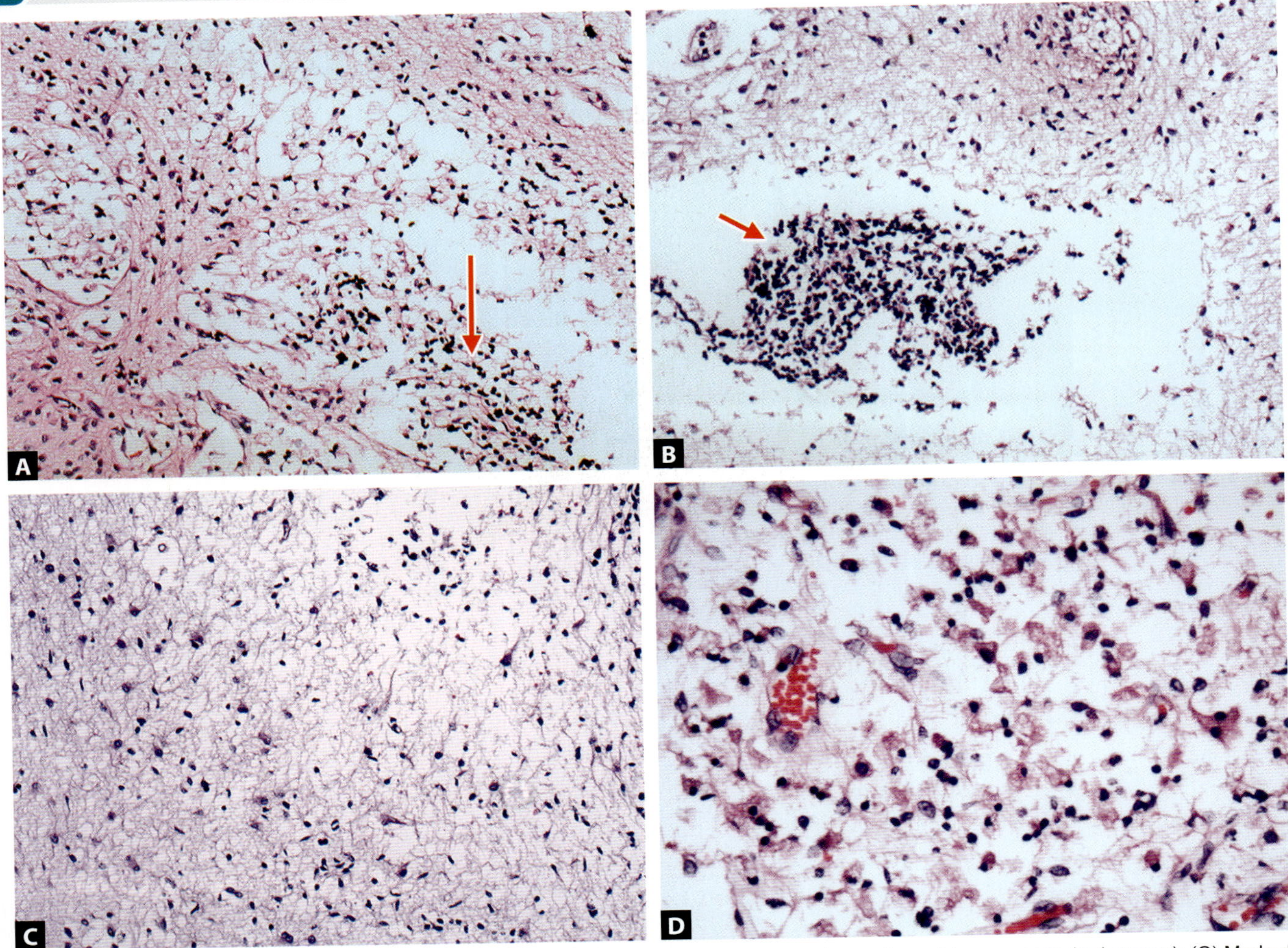

Figs 6A–D: Photomicrographs of white matter of the brain. (A and B) Showing cysts, atrophy, and caught up neurons (red arrows); (C) Marked pallor with loss of myelin, proliferating astrocytes, and macrophages; (D) Marked loss of myelin with proliferating microgemistocytes and oligodendroglia.

of a twin before and after death of its co-twin and found a reduction in hematocrit from 54% to 31%. Postnatal CT scan of the head revealed diffuse areas of low attenuation. Thus, hypotension, anemia and emboli may all contribute to the abnormalities seen in the surviving twin of a monochorionic pregnancy. In children surviving preterm birth, cystic PVL[13-16] is the most common cause of cerebral palsy. It is said to occur due to the necrosis of the periventricular white matter, as a result of hypoxia or ischemia, due to impaired perfusion in the watershed areas. Another hypothesis of PVL is intrauterine infection leading to cytokine (interleukin-1β, 6 and TNF-α) production which in turn damages the fetal oligodendrocytes and astrocytes. Cystic PVL occurs in the setting of prematurity, asphyxia, respiratory distress, septicemia, chorioamnionitis/premature rupture of the membranes, maternal hemorrhage, arterial hypotension, persistent ductus arteriosus, hypocarbia and multiple gestations. Medically assisted reproductive techniques have increased the occurrence of multiple gestations in the present era, which has been identified as an important risk factor for the development of cystic PVL and subsequent cerebral palsy. Monochorionic pregnancies have even greater problems, as a result of the vascular connections in the shared placenta, leading to imbalanced placental blood supply, twin to twin transfusion syndrome (TTS) and complications due to the intrauterine death of the co-twin. In TTS, there is volume overload or hydrops of the recipient twin and growth retardation of the donor twin along with oligohydramnios. If the monochorionic co-twin dies in second or third trimester, the surviving twin has a very high rate of morbidity or

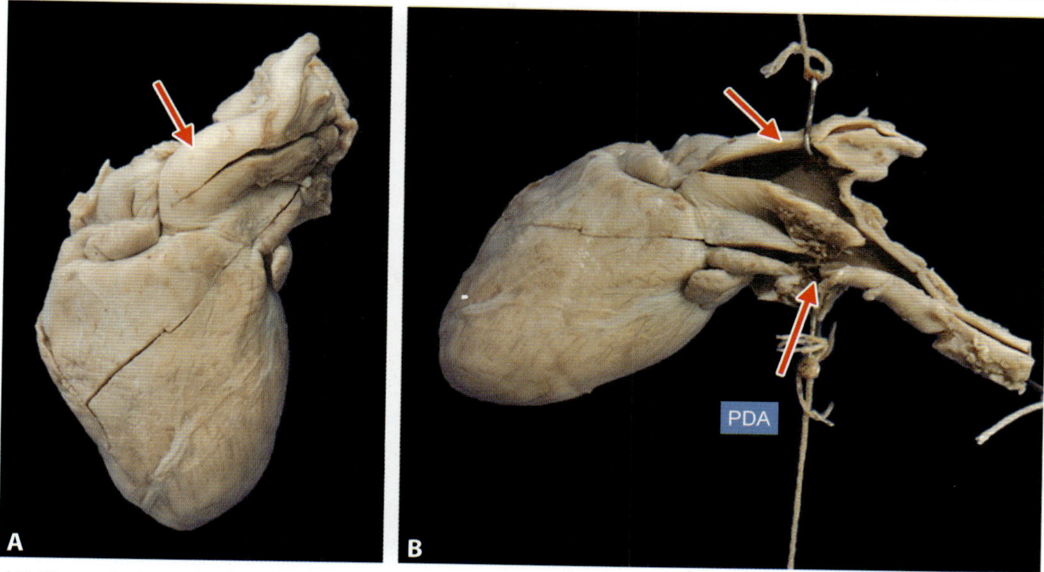

Figs 7A and B: (A) Gross photograph of the heart showing dilated ascending/arch of aorta (arrow); (B) Opened up aorta and pulmonary artery showing dilated aorta (small arrow) proximal to the coarctation and patent ductus arteriosus (lower long arrow).

mortality, as they can suffer from multicystic encephalomalacia, porencephaly, renal cortical necrosis and small bowel atresia as a result of the shared placenta. It is known that PVL and associated cerebral palsy are more common in preterms and amongst them seen more in twins (monochorionic > dichorionic 33% vs. 3.3%) than in singletons.

Hereditary renal adysplasia and simple hypoplasia—See "Pediatric cystic disease of kidney (developmental/genetic): Introduction."

COMMENTARY—INDEX CASE: PM 25677

The index baby was the second twin of a 27-year-old, third gravida mother, with no living issue. The earlier two pregnancy losses were due to developmental renal malformations proven on ultrasound. Third pregnancy, i.e. G3 was twins with a monochorionic and diamniotic placenta. USG at 16 weeks was normal with two gestational sacs, a single large placenta and oligohydramnios. USG at 18 weeks did not reveal any abnormality, lateral ventricles being 10 mm. USG at 28 weeks showed both live fetuses, two gestational sacs, T2 revealed borderline lateral ventricles (12 mm) with no CMF. USG at 32 weeks showed T1—IUD, T2—hydrocephalus with markedly dilated lateral ventricles (20 mm each) and no other CMF was seen. The mother delivered per vaginally at 33 weeks gestation, T1 being a macerated still birth and T2 a live born male with a birth weight of 1.5 kg with no external abnormality. The postnatal USG of the cranium revealed normal posterior fossa structures, marked hydrocephalus with multicystic periventricular encephalomalacia. Postnatal USG of the abdomen showed bilateral small kidneys (right-1.3 cm, left-1.8 cm) with raised cortical echogenicity, no cysts, pelvicalyceal system not dilated, lost corticomedullary differentiation, renal parenchymal disease and nondistended urinary bladder. So, the clinical details clearly highlight the fact that the co-twin died after 28 weeks gestation and the entire damage to the brain of the live born, i.e. T2 took place after the death of T1. The renal abnormality was not detected in the antemortem USG (the last done at 28 weeks gestation) but was diagnosed at birth. The baby was in renal failure in the first week of life. The grim prognosis was explained to the parents and the baby was sent back home at D10 of life. They were counseled to get an autopsy done in case the baby expires. At autopsy, there was bilateral renal hypoplasia with tubulointerstitial nephritis, multicystic encephalomalacia with hydrocephalus ex vacuo, coarctation of aorta, patent ductus arteriosus and persistent pulmonary artery hypertension.

The index case has three aspects:

1. Bilateral simple renal hypoplasia ie miniature kidneys, a rare renal developmental disorder. This shows a reduction in the number of calyces and shows 2–3 ranks of glomeruli, against a normal of 13–14 ranks. In the index case, infection led to tubulointerstitial nephritis and the variety of glomerular changes ie compensatory enlargement of few glomeruli and occasional focal segmental glomerulosclerosis like lesions.

2. The case fits into hereditary renal adysplasia (recurrent renal developmental abnormality), an autosomal dominant condition with incomplete penetrance and variable expression.
3. The multicystic encephalomalacia with hydrocephalus ex vacuo occurred after the death of the monochorionic co-twin, a well documented complication, which occurs in 20% of surviving co-twins, after 2nd or 3rd trimester death of one twin, in monochorionic twin pregnancies.

This mother was counselled that she has a nearly 50% risk of recurrence of the renal abnormality in her subsequent pregnancy. But she insisted on taking another chance. Two months back, I got a mail from this couple that they have been blessed with a baby boy, who is doing well and has no congenital malformation.

TAKE HOME MESSAGE

- Renal developmental disorders, i.e. hypoplasia or dysplasia were initially considered to be sporadic, noninherited malformations. But this is not the case now.
- The familial occurrence or recurrences of renal developmental disorders is referred to as hereditary renal adysplasia. Mode of inheritance is predominantly autosomal dominant with incomplete penetrance and variable expression.
- Periventricular leukomalacia is defined as an ischemic lesion present in the periventricular white matter of a preterm infant and is characterized by infarction. It occurs due to hypoxia incurred between 24 weeks and 32 weeks gestation.
- In monochorionic pregnancies, 20% of surviving co-twins, after second or third-trimester intrauterine fetal death of one twin, develop cystic PVL or multicystic encephalomalacia.

REFERENCES

1. Virchow R. Zur pathologischen Anatomie des Gehirns I: congenitale encephalitis und myelitis. Arch Pathol Anat. 1867;38:129-42.
2. Banker BQ, Larroche J-L. Periventricular leukomalacia in infancy: a form of neonatal anoxic encephalopathy. Arch Neurol. 1962;7:386-410.
3. Paneth N, Rudelli R, Monte W, et al. White matter necrosis in very low birth weight infants: neuropathologic and ultrasonographic findings in infants surviving six days or longer. J Pediatr. 1990;116:975-84.
4. Back SA, Gan X, Li Y, et al. Maturation-dependent vulnerability of oligodendrocytes to oxidative stress-induced death caused by glutathione depletion. J Neurosc. 1998;18: 6241-53.
5. Savman K, Blennow M, Gustafson K, et al. Cytokine response in cerebrospinal fluid after birth asphyxia. Pediatr Res. 1998; 43:746-51.
6. Yoon BH, Jun JK, Romero R, et al. Amniotic fluid inflammatory cytokines (interleukin-6, interleukin-1beta and tumor necrosis factor-alpha), neonatal brain white matter lesions and cerebral palsy. Am J Obstetr Gyn. 1997;177:19-26.
7. Weiss JL, Cleary-Goldman J, Tanji K, et al. Multicystic encephalomalacia after first-trimester intrauterine fetal death in monochorionic twins. Am J Obstet Gynecol. 2004; 190(2):563-5.
8. Karageyim Karsidag AY, Kars B, Dansuk R, et al. Brain damage to the survivor within 30 min of co-twin demise in monochorionic twins. Fetal Diagn Ther. 2005;20(2):91-5.
9. Levine D. Encephalomalacia in surviving twin after death of monochorionic co-twin. Radiology. 2002;223(2):392-5.
10. Fusi L, McParland P, Fisk N, et al. Acute twin-twin transfusion: a possible mechanism for brain-damaged survivors after intrauterine death of a monochorionic twin. Obstet Gynecol. 1991;78:517-20.
11. Bernischke K. Twin placenta in prenatal mortality. N Y State J Med. 1961;61:1499-1508.
12. Nicolini U, Pisoni MP, Cela E, et al. Fetal blood sampling immediately before and within 24 hours of death in monochorionic twin pregnancies complicated by single intrauterine death. Am J Obstet Gynecol. 1998;179:800-3.
13. Resch B, Vollaard E, Maurer U, et al. Risk factors and determinants of neurodevelopmental outcome in cystic periventricular leucomalacia. Eur J Pediatr. 2000;159:663-70.
14. Bejar R, Wozniak P, Allard M, et al. Antenatal origin of neurologic damage in newborn infants. I. Preterm infants. Am J Obstet Gynecol. 1988;159:357-63.
15. Zupan V, Gonzalez P, Lacaze-Masmontail T, et al. Periventricular leukomalacia: risk factors revisited. Dev Med Child Neurol. 1998;38:1061-7.
16. De Vries LS, Reger R, Dubowitz LM, et al. Perinatal risk factors for the development of extensive cystic leukomalacia. Am J Dis Child. 1988;142:732-5.

CONTRIBUTIONS BY:

1. Dr RK Vasishta, Professor and Head, Department of Histopathology (Consultation)
2. Dr Kanya Mukhopadhyay, Professor, Department of Pediatrics-Neonatology Division (Clinician In-Charge)
3. Dr Shalini Gainder, Additional Professor, Department of Obstetrics and Gynecology (Obstetrician In-Charge)
4. Professor S Singhi, Ex-Professor and Head, Department of Pediatrics (Clinician In-Charge)

Post Graduate Institute of Medical Education and Research, Chandigarh, India.

CASE 86

Segmental Hypoplasia (Ask-Upmark Kidney): S-14525/2008

Nandita Bharadwaj Kakkar

HIGHLIGHTS OF THE CASE

This was an 11-year-old male who was diagnosed to have a duplex kidney with the lower moiety showing vesicoureteric reflux. Partial nephrectomy of the lower moiety revealed segmental hypoplasia.

Keywords: Segmental hypoplasia, vesicoureteric reflux.

CLINICAL DETAILS

A 11-year-old male child came with history of repeated urinary tract infections. He also had hypertension. On investigations, the right kidney was found to be duplex with two ureters. Vesicoureteric reflux was present in the lower moiety. The upper moiety appeared normal. The left kidney was also normal. Partial nephrectomy of the right lower moiety was done.

HISTOPATHOLOGY DETAILS

The partial nephrectomy specimen (Fig 1A) measured 5 × 3 × 2 cm and the ureter measured 5 cm in length. Fetal lobulations were present and a deep groove was appreciated at the upper pole of the specimen (Fig 1A–left arrow). The pelvis was extrarenal and dilated (Fig 1A–right arrow). The ureter was also dilated more so in the lower part. Cut section of the kidney (Fig 1B) showed a dilated pelvicalyceal system (PCS) with thinning of the cortex, more so at the groove, seen near the upper pole. Microscopy from the grooved area revealed a dilated PCS with a thinned out cortex (Fig 1C). Section from the deep groove showed hypoplasia blending abruptly with the adjacent normal renal parenchyma (Fig 1D). The area of hypoplasia showed loss of glomeruli, occasional thyroid-like tubules, thick-walled arteries and fibrosis along with mononuclear cell infiltrate (Figs 1E and F). No primitive duct or cartilage was noted. Other part of the cortex showed normal morphology.

DIAGNOSIS

Overall features in this partial nephrectomy specimen (lower moiety of a complete duplex kidney) are consistent with segmental hypoplasia (Ask-Upmark kidney) with hydronephrosis, deep groove, at the upper pole and extrarenal pelvis with ureteric dilatation all features seen subsequent to a vesicoureteric reflux disease of some duration.

SEGMENTAL HYPOPLASIA (ASK UPMARK KIDNEY)

This condition is generally unilateral, but can be bilateral and can occur in utero or after birth or both. It occurs more in the females. It occurs due to vesicoureteric reflux as the pattern of distribution of lesions, are consistent with reflux damage. The compound papillae most susceptible to damage are concentrated at the upper pole and hence it occurs at the upper pole. It may lead to hypertension and recurrent urinary tract infections, wherein a nephrectomy is done. Renal insufficiency occurs in 50% cases. Grossly the kidney is small in size, with a transverse groove on the capsular surface at the upper pole, overlying an area of marked parenchymal thinning. Microscopy shows scarred zones called areas of segmental hypoplasia with absent glomeruli, atrophic thyroid-like tubules, thick-walled blood vessels, occasional minute focus of cartilage but no dysplasia.

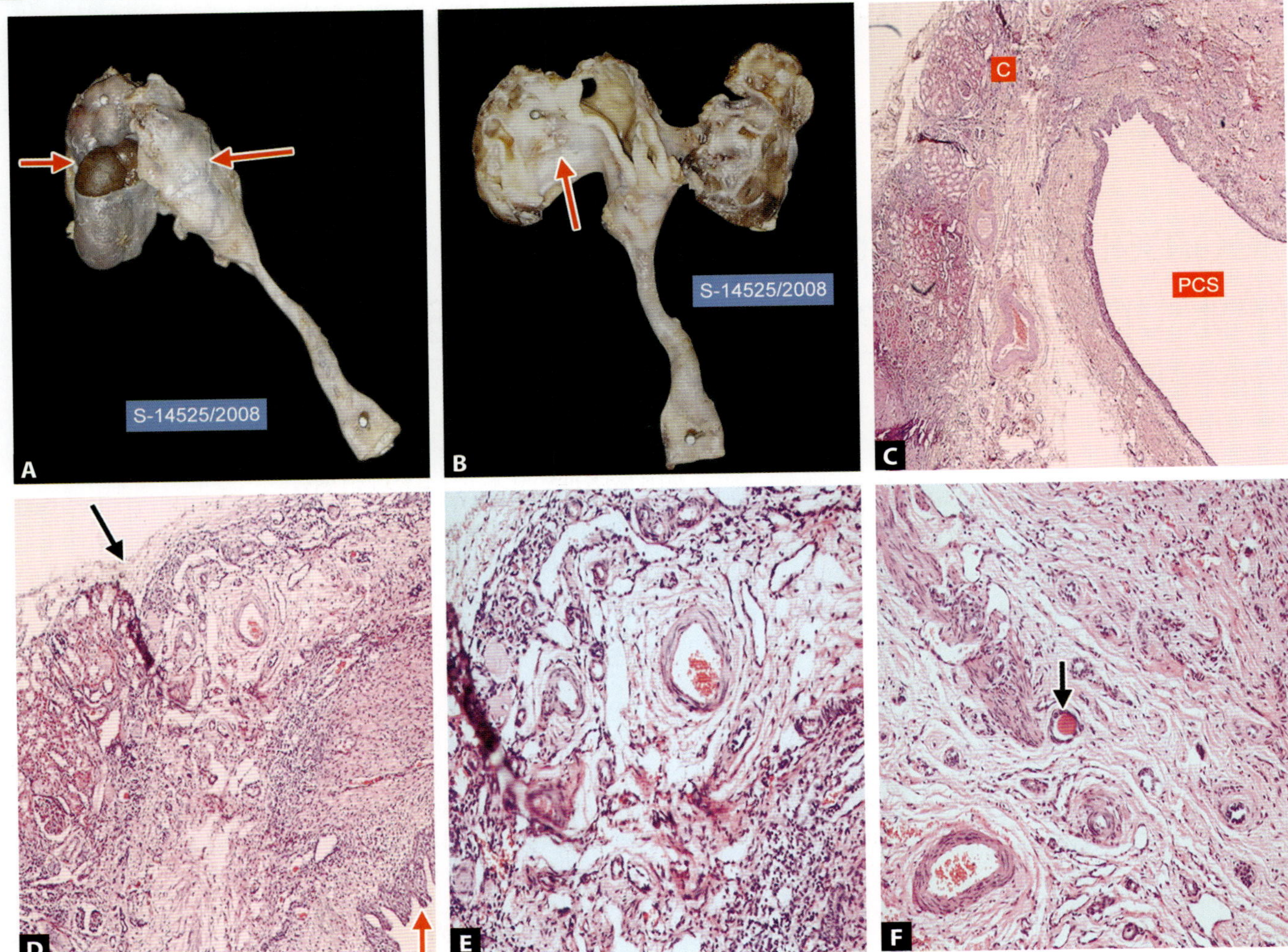

Figs 1A–F: (A) Partial nephrectomy specimen shows fetal lobulations, deep groove at the upper pole (left arrow), extrarenal dilated pelvis (right arrow), and dilated ureter, more in the lower part; (B) Cut section of the kidney shows dilated pelvicalyceal system. Microphotographs of the kidney show; (C) Dilated pelvicalyceal system (PCS) and thinned out cortex; (D) Cortex shows hypoplastic area in the right upper part and normal renal parenchyma on the left side separated by the arrow. Lining of the PCS can be seen in the lower right segment (red arrow); (E and F) Hypoplastic area showing absent glomeruli, prominent vessels, occasional thyroid-like tubule (arrow), inflammation and fibrosis.

TAKE HOME MESSAGE

- Segmental hypoplasia occurs due to vesicoureteric reflux, can be uni/bilateral, can occur in utero or after birth, leads to hypertension and recurrent urinary tract infections.
- Kidney shows a transverse groove at the upper pole, which overlies an area of marked parenchymal thinning, which shows absent glomeruli, atrophic thyroid-like tubules and thick-walled blood vessels.

CONTRIBUTIONS BY:

1. Dr JK Mahajan, Professor, Department of Pediatric Surgery (Clinician In-Charge)
Post Graduate Institute of Medical Education and Research, Chandigarh, India.

Section 15D: Genetic Disorders

CASE 87

A Classical Case of Autosomal Recessive Polycystic Kidney Disease: PM 22879

Nandita Bharadwaj Kakkar

HIGHLIGHTS OF THE CASE

A 35-year-old female, G8, P2142 with four abortions, one preterm loss and two live females doing well, came at 40 weeks gestation with sluggish/loss of fetal movements since 2 days. Ultrasonography revealed hyperechoic enlarged kidneys, empty fetal urinary bladder, oligohydramnios and intrauterine fetal death. Autopsy revealed a classical case of autosomal recessive polycystic kidney disease (ARPKD) with nonimmune hydrops fetalis.

Keywords: Autosomal recessive polycystic kidney disease, oligohydramnios, ductal plate malformation, congenital hepatic fibrosis, pulmonary hypoplasia, autopsy.

CLINICAL DETAILS

A 35-year-old female, G8 P2142 was admitted to PGIMER, Chandigarh, at term (40 weeks gestation) with history of sluggish/loss of fetal movements since 2 days. The mother in the current pregnancy had gestational diabetes mellitus, chronic hypertension and oligohydramnios. Ultrasonography done after admission, revealed hyperechoic enlarged kidneys, empty fetal urinary bladder, oligohydramnios and intrauterine death. She delivered a fresh still born male baby, weighing 4 kg. No facial dysmorphism was noted. The baby was edematous, abdomen was distended and congenital talipes equinovarus (CTEV) was noted. The mother was from a rural background and had not been supervised in any of the eight pregnancies. G1 was a preterm loss, G2 and G3 were normal vaginal deliveries, conducted at home by a midwife, both were female babies, are alive and doing well, G4 was a spontaneous abortion at 20 weeks gestation, G5,6,7 were all first trimester abortions between 8 and 12 weeks gestation and G8 was the index case. A diagnosis of recurrent fetal death with bilateral enlarged kidneys ? ARPKD was made. The baby was sent for autopsy.

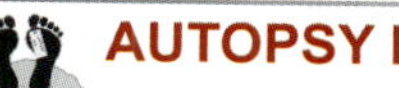

AUTOPSY FINDINGS: PM 22879

Date of Autopsy: 27.10.2008

A complete autopsy was performed. The body was edematous, abdomen was distended and the body weight was 4 kg. The pleural and peritoneal cavities yielded 200 and 300 mL of straw-colored fluid. Both ***kidneys*** were markedly, symmetrically enlarged, but maintained their reniform shape and fetal lobulations (Fig 1A). They together weighed 203 g against a normal of 24 g at this age. There were myriads of pin head-sized cysts (1 mm) recognizable just below the capsular surface (Fig 1B). The ureters and urinary bladder were normal. Cut section revealed radially oriented cysts, extending from the medulla to the cortex giving the classical "sunray" appearance (Fig 1C). Microscopy (Figs 1D and 2A) revealed radially oriented cysts, perpendicular to the cortex, extending from medulla to the cortex. Cysts were lined by nondescript cuboidal epithelium and occupied more than 90% of the renal parenchyma. Interspersed between the cysts, normal glomeruli and tubules could be seen. The number of glomeruli were normal, but appeared sparse due to interspersed cysts. No primitive ducts were seen, despite studying multiple sections. Overall features were consistent with a diagnosis of ARPKD. The ***liver*** (Fig 2B) was enlarged and weighed 172 g against a normal of 120 g at this age. It was firm to feel and cut section revealed prominent streaks of fibrosis. Microscopy (Figs 2C and D) revealed expanded portal tracts and porto-portal bridging fibrosis. Increased number of abnormally angulated biliary channels were present, conspicuously at the periphery of the expanded

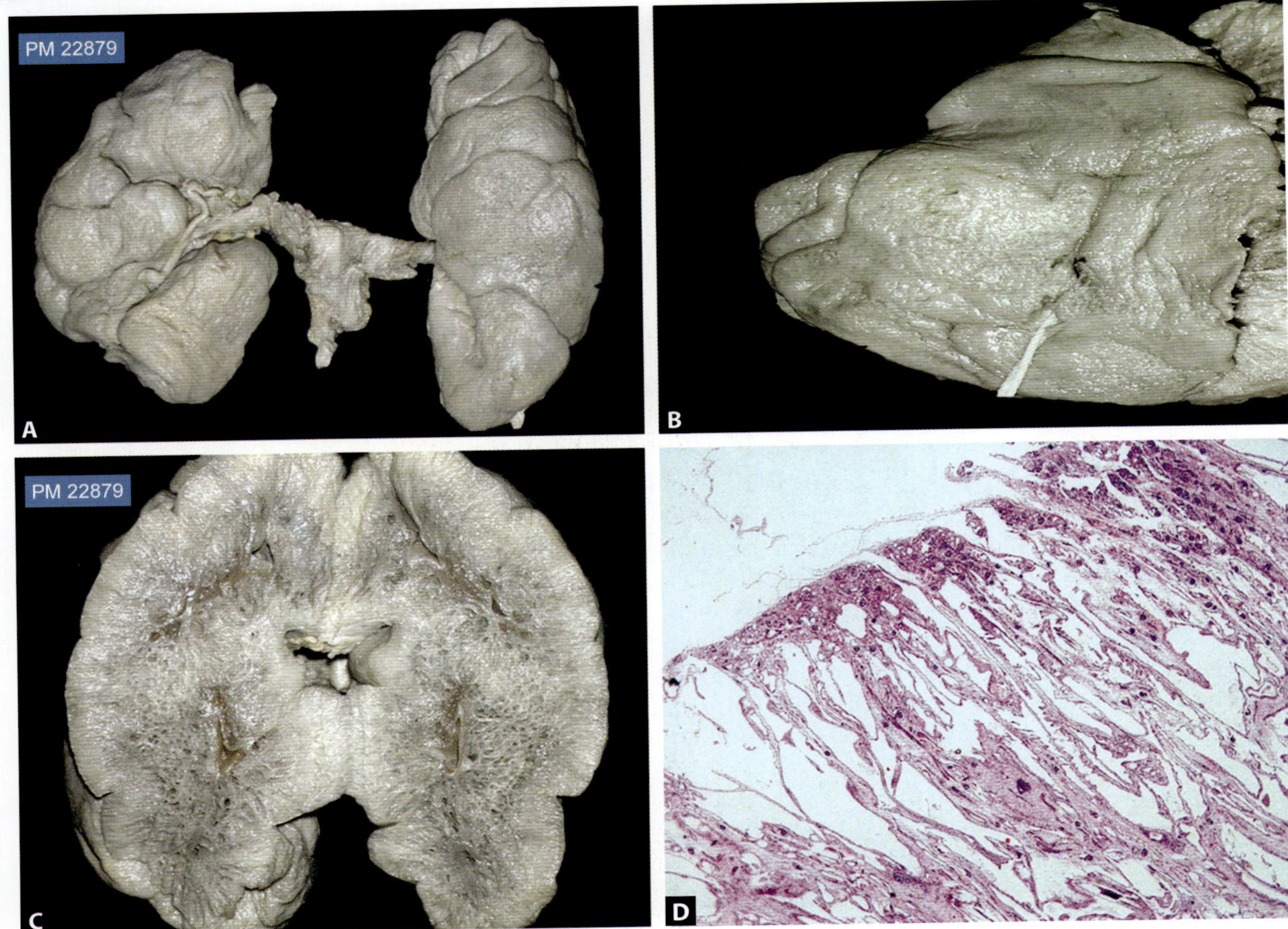

Figs 1A–D: (A) Both kidneys are symmetrically enlarged and show preserved fetal lobulations; (B) Capsular aspect shows pinhead-sized cysts beneath the capsule; (C) Cut section shows radially oriented cysts, elongated in the cortex, i.e. sunray appearance and rounded in the medulla; (D) Photomicrograph of the kidney shows radially oriented cysts.

portal tracts. Features were consistent with a diagnosis of ductal plate malformation (DPM). The lungs weighed 22 g and revealed bilateral hypoplasia. Other organs, including the brain, were within normal limits.

FINAL AUTOPSY DIAGNOSIS: PM 22879

Gravida 8, with 4 Abortions, One Preterm Loss and Two Live Females Doing Well. G8- Still-born, Male at 40 Weeks Gestation

- Autosomal recessive polycystic kidney disease—Perinatal variety
- Ductal plate malformation
- Nonimmune hydrops fetalis with ascites and bilateral pleural effusion
- Bilateral lung hypoplasia.

AUTOSOMAL RECESSIVE POLYCYSTIC KIDNEY DISEASE AND CONGENITAL HEPATIC FIBROSIS

Autosomal recessive polycystic kidney disease and congenital hepatic fibrosis (CHF) are two ends of the same spectrum, are inseparably intertwined entities and constitute a single disease process with a wide spectrum of expression. Incidence varies from 1:6,000 to 1:55,000 in various studies. This entity is divided into four groups—perinatal, neonatal, infantile and juvenile (Table 1). This division is based on

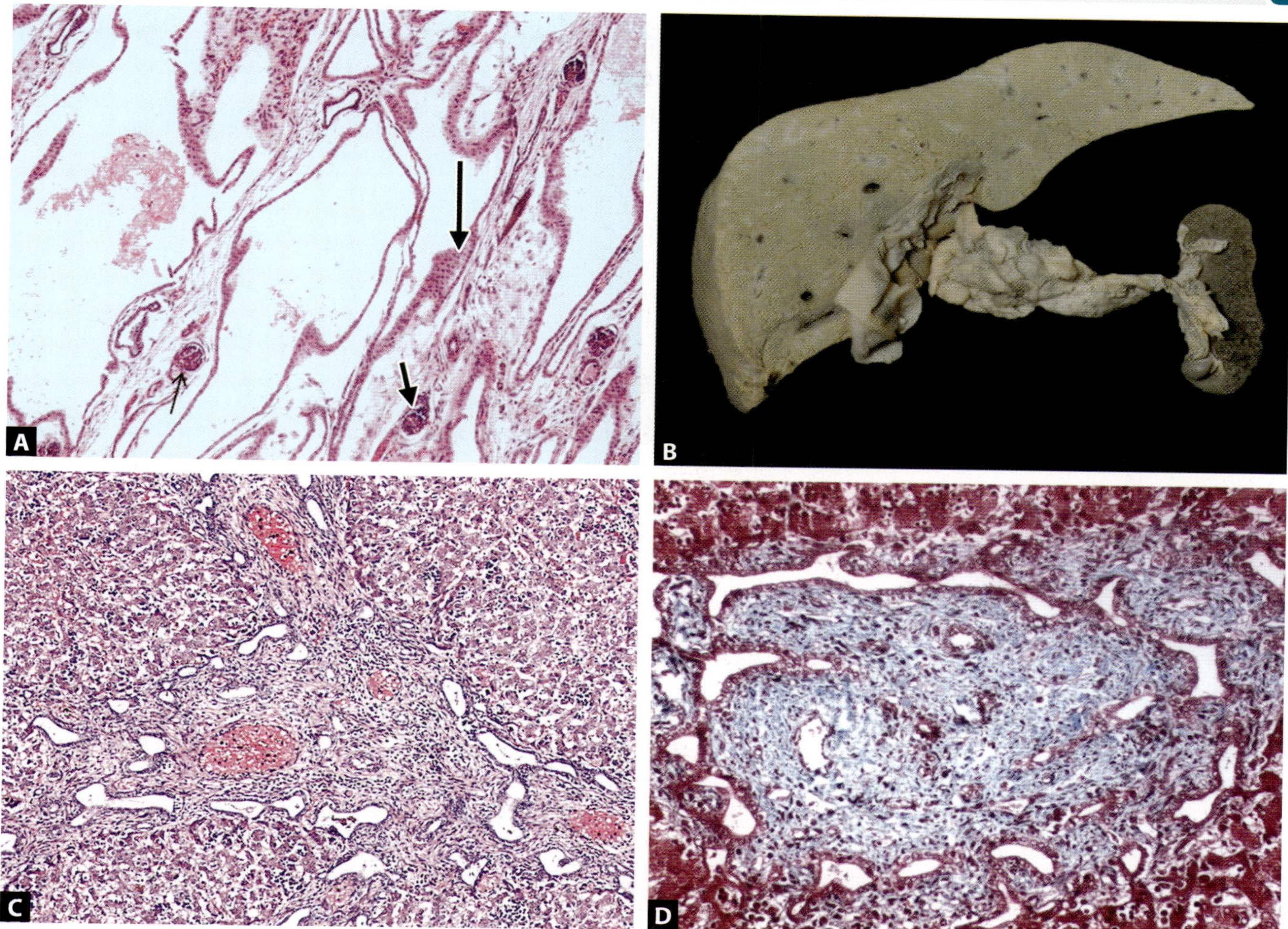

Figs 2A–D: (A) Photomicrograph of the kidney shows longitudinal cysts lined by nondescript cuboidal epithelium with interspersed glomeruli (small arrows). At places, the epithelium shows stratification (long arrow); (B) Organ complex of the slice of liver, spleen, and pancreas. The liver shows prominent streaks of fibrosis; (C) Photomicrograph of the liver showing expanded and fibrotic portal tracts with porto-portal bridging fibrosis and abundant angulated bile ductules seen at their periphery; (D) Massons trichrome stain brings out the portal fibrosis better. Also seen are the angulated bile ductules.

the age at presentation, mode of presentation or progress, proportion of renal tubules involved, proportion of abnormal bile ducts and extent of periportal fibrosis in the liver. One end of the spectrum, i.e. perinatal and neonatal varieties, shows extensive renal lesions with minimal hepatic lesions. The other end of the spectrum, i.e. the juvenile variety, shows extensive fibrosis of the portal tracts along with portal hypertension, but show only trivial renal lesions in the form of few cysts. In the middle of these extremes are children who have a moderate involvement of both the kidney and liver, i.e. the infantile variety. In the juvenile variety of ARPKD, the hepatic lesion is termed as congenital hepatic fibrosis (CHF) and in the other three variants it is referred to as ductal plate malformation (DPM).

The most severe form, i.e. the perinatal and neonatal forms of ARPKD, present with Potter's facies, oligohydramnios, lung hypoplasia and bilateral, massive, symmetrical, enlargement of the kidneys. These babies are either still born or die in early neonatal period due to respiratory insufficiency, either due to hypoplastic lungs or due to compression by the large abdominal masses. They show bilateral, symmetrical, renal enlargement with a smooth surface and tiny cysts recognizable just below the capsular surface. The kidneys maintain their reniform shape and show fetal lobulations. On cut surface, the kidneys show diffusely dilated tubules, radially arranged in a regimented parallel manner from the calyx to the capsule, imparting a characteristic "sunray" appearance. These radially oriented

Table 1: Varieties of autosomal recessive polycystic kidney disease.

	Perinatal	*Neonatal*	*Infantile*	*Juvenile*
Age of presentation	At birth	< 1 month	3–12 months	1–5 years
Mode of presentation	Huge bilateral renal masses	Huge bilateral renal masses	Renal masses bilateral + hepatosplenomegaly	Hepatomegaly
Progress	Progressive renal failure	Progressive renal failure	Chronic renal failure + portal hypertension	Portal hypertension
Survival time	Still-born to 6 weeks	< 6 weeks to 1 year	< 10 years	> 12 years
Kidneys Percentage of parenchyma affected	All effected 90%	All affected 60%	All affected 25%	All affected 10%
Liver	All affected Fibrosis: minimal	All affected Fibrosis: mild	All affected Fibrosis: moderate	All affected Fibrosis: gross

cysts are elongated in the cortex and somewhat rounded in the medulla. On microscopic examination, the cysts occupy more than 90%, 60%, 25% and 10% of the renal parenchyma in the perinatal, neonatal, infantile and juvenile varieties, respectively. The cystic structures are lined by a nondescript low cuboidal epithelium and in areas may show stratification. Interspersed between the cysts are seen normal glomeruli, which appear sparse due to the presence of cysts, but actually are present in normal numbers. Absence of dysplasia, i.e. absence of primitive ducts is an important diagnostic feature. The cysts are of collecting duct origin.

Liver shows congenital hepatic fibrosis, a developmental disorder of the portobiliary system, wherein there is an abnormal remodeling of the ductal plate, known as ductal plate malformation (DPM) along with defective branching of the intrahepatic portal veins. This results from faulty development, i.e. disturbance in epithelio-mesenchymal inductive interactions The liver shows expansion of the portal tracts with fibrosis and abundant angulated bile ducts along with porto-portal bridging fibrosis. These biliary channels are lined by a bland cuboidal epithelium. During development, the liver cells surrounding the portal tracts undergo a phenotypic change, as and when they come in contact with the mesenchyme of the portal tracts and form the intrahepatic bile ducts. To begin with, an uninterrupted double layered ductal plate is formed around each portal tract. This plate remodels in the presence of appropriate epithelio-mesenchymal inductive interactions. Defective remodeling leads to the formation of a large number of abnormally angulated bile ducts, which are weak, immature structures and undergo a progressive destructive cholangiopathy leading to fibrosis. In ARPKD, 100% cases show DPM or CHF, but only 60% cases of CHF have ARPKD. Congenital hepatic fibrosis can also be seen in cases of autosomal dominant polycystic kidney disease (ADPKD), nephronophthisis, medullary cystic disease, occasionally renal dysplasia, Ivemark syndrome (100% cases) and Meckel–Gruber syndrome (MGS) (100% cases). Since ARPKD is an autosomal recessive disorder, siblings of either sex have a 25% chance of being affected and neither parents show evidence of the disease. The genetic locus for ARPKD is present in chromosome 6.

Diagnosis of ARPKD can be made as early as 16–18 weeks of gestation. Characteristic ultrasonographic findings are bilateral, enlarged hyperechoic kidneys with poor differentiation between cortex and medulla. However, these findings can also be seen prenatally in infants with autosomal dominant polycystic kidney disease (ADPKD). It is now a well-known fact that ADPKD can occur in neonates. On intravenous urography, ARPKD shows a sunburst appearance (due to dilatation of collecting tubules). A picture of puddle formation with quick excretion of the contrast on excretory urogram suggests ADPKD. Finding of a normal ultrasonogram in both parents, particularly if they are over 30 years of age, supports the diagnosis of ARPKD. History of oligohydramnios or a genetic history of ARPKD is strong indicator of ARPKD. Once the diagnosis of ARPKD is suspected, referral for genetic counseling is mandatory. A detailed history should be taken of at least three generations.

The most important differential diagnosis of ARPKD is from MGS. MGS is also an autosomal recessive disorder, which is a tetrad of CNS malformation, mostly occipital encephalocele, bilateral multicystic dysplastic kidneys, ductal plate malformation and polydactyly. The kidneys in MGS also show bilateral symmetrical enlargement with maintained reniform shape and fetal lobulations, as seen in ARPKD.

Cut section however, does not show radially oriented cysts (seen in ARPKD), but rounded small cysts, uniformly distributed in the cortex and the medulla. Microscopy shows dysplastic kidneys with presence of classical primitive ducts (not seen in ARPKD). Congenital hepatic fibrosis is seen in both conditions. CNS malformation and polydactyly are seen in MGS and not in ARPKD.

COMMENTARY—INDEX CASE: PM 22879

This was a 35-year-old female, G8 P2142 with four abortions, one preterm loss and two live females, doing well. She came at 40 weeks gestation with sluggish/loss of fetal movements since 2 days. Fetal ultrasonography revealed hyperechoic enlarged kidneys, empty fetal urinary bladder, oligohydramnios and intrauterine fetal death ? ARPKD. At autopsy it was a classical case of ARPKD—Perinatal variety with ductal plate malformation, nonimmune hydrops and pulmonary hypoplasia.

TAKE HOME MESSAGE

- Autosomal recessive polycystic kidney disease is an autosomal recessive disorder affecting the kidneys along with the liver and leading to a spectrum of clinical presentations.
- Autosomal recessive polycystic kidney disease and CHF/DPM are two ends of the same spectrum. All cases of ARPKD have CHF/DPM, but not vice versa.
- Autosomal recessive polycystic kidney disease is of four types—perinatal, neonatal, infantile and juvenile.
- Perinatal and neonatal presentations have a predominance of renal symptoms and the infantile and juvenile varieties present later in life with liver disease.

SUGGESTED READING

1. Desmet VJ. What is congenital hepatic fibrosis? Invited review. Histopathology. 1992;20:465-77.
2. Gang DL, Herrin JT. Infantile polycystic disease of the liver and kidney. Clin Nephrol. 1986;25(1):28-36.
3. Guay-Woodford LM, Muecher G, Hopkins SD, et al. The severe perinatal form of ARPKD maps to chromosome 6p21. 1-p12: Implications for genetic counselling. Am J Hum Genet. 1995;56:1101-7.
4. Hill GS. Cystic and dysplastic disease of the kidney: genetic lesions. In: Hill GS (Ed). Uropathology. New York: Churchill Livingstone; 1989. pp. 141-51.
5. Kakkar N, Vasishta RK, Lamba A, et al. Recessive polycystic kidney disease with congenital hepatic fibrosis. Pediatr Pathol Mol Med. 2001;20(3):227-34.
6. Lipschitz B, Berdon WE, Defelice AR, et al. Association of congenital hepatic fibrosis with autosomal dominant polycystic kidney disease. Report of a family with review of literature. Pediatr Radiol. 1993;23(2):131-3.
7. Matsuda O, Ideura T, Shinoda T, et al. Polycystic kidney of autosomal dominant inheritance, polycystic liver and congenital hepatic fibrosis in a single kindred. Am J Nephrol. 1990;10:237-41.
8. Proesmans W, Moerman P, De Praetere M, et al. Association of bilateral renal dysplasia and CHF. Int J Pediatr Nephrol. 1986;7:113-6.
9. Vankalakunti M, Gupta K, Kakkar N, et al. Renal – hepatic – pancreatic dysplasia syndrome (Ivemarks Syndrome). Diagn Pathol. 2007;2(2):24.
10. Zerres K, Muecher G, Bachner L, et al. Mapping of the gene for autosomal recessive polycystic kidney disease (ARPKD) to chromosome 6p21-cen. Nat Genet. 1994;7:429-32.

CONTRIBUTIONS BY:

1. Dr L Dhaliwal, Professor, Department of Obstetrics and Gynaecology (Clinician In-Charge)
Post Graduate Institute of Medical Education and Research, Chandigarh, India.

CASE 88

Autosomal Dominant Polycystic Kidney Disease with Cyst Infection: PM 22828

Nandita Bharadwaj Kakkar

 HIGHLIGHTS OF THE CASE

This is a case of autosomal dominant polycystic kidney disease with tubulointerstitial nephritis, hypertension and cyst infection. Septic shock led to the demise of the patient.

Keywords: Autosomal dominant, polycystic kidney, sepsis, cyst infection, hypertension.

 CLINICAL DETAILS

Date of Admission: 16.09.2008, Date of Death: 24.09.2008, Duration of Hospital Stay: 8 days

A 47-year-old male, presented with complaints of hiccoughs, low grade fever and abdominal pain since 7 days. He had burning micturition along with generalized weakness of body since 4 days. There was no history of hematuria or decreased urine output. Past history revealed acquisition of a bulbar urethral stricture after a road traffic accident in 1991, was diagnosed with hypertension in 1993, was operated for urethral stricture at PGIMER in early 2008 and at that time detected to have autosomal dominant polycystic kidney disease (ADPKD) with a positive family history. Three months before his demise, he was admitted under our nephrology services with a diagnosis of ADPKD with cyst infection and was discharged with advice to complete a 4 weeks course of Inj meropenem. ***Examination***: He was conscious, oriented, febrile, pulse rate—108/min, BP—106/80 mm Hg, respiratory rate—22/min and pallor was present. Abdomen revealed enlarged ballotable kidneys, palpable in both flanks along with tenderness. Other organ systems were within normal limits.

Investigations and Course of Management

Hemogram: Hb—8.2 g/dL; TLC—23,400/μL with polymorphonuclear leukocytosis and platelets—2,80,000/μL. Peripheral blood revealed mild anisocytosis with hypochromia. ***Blood biochemistry:*** Serum urea/creatinine—−29/1.85 mg%, total proteins fell from 7.22 to 4.38 g, albumin fell from 3.1 to 1.8 g, liver function tests—normal, Ca^{2+}/PO_4—6.5/3 mg%, corrected Ca^{2+}—8.26 mg%, Na^+ 104–115 mEq/L, K^+—2.66–3.44 mEq/L. ***Urine examination:*** proteins+, sugar negative, pus cells—35–45/HPF, RBCs—8–10/HPF, spot Na—67. ***Blood culture*** was initially sterile and 2 days before his demise, it grew *E. coli*. ***Urine culture*** initially grew *E. coli* and 5 days before his demise grew *Klebsiella pneumoniae*. ***USG abdomen (20.09.2008):*** Liver—17.5 cm in size, no cysts seen, right kidney—20.3 cm, left kidney—21.2 cm, both kidneys replaced by cysts of varying sizes, few of the cysts show internal echoes and septal thickening, spleen—12.4 cm. ***Contrast-enhanced CT abdomen (22.09.2008):*** right kidney—22 cm, left kidney—23 cm, multiple cysts of varying sizes seen in both kidneys, largest cyst on right side—7.5 × 7 × 5 cm at inferior pole and largest cyst on the left side—5 × 4.5 × 3 cm at upper pole, some of the cyst walls show evidence of calcification, small calculi are present in both kidneys and few cysts show hyperdense contents. Retroperitoneal, paraaortic, aortocaval and paracaval lymph nodes are enlarged. Liver 15 cm in size and cysts are seen in both lobes. ***Compression USG:*** No evidence of deep vein thrombosis. A **2D echocardiography**—ejection fraction 55–60%, no clot or vegetations seen, left ventricular hypertrophy noted.

It was a case of ADPKD with hypertension and stricture urethra. He was being treated for cyst infection and started on inj. ciprofloxacin. There was no symptomatic relief and his sensorium worsened and he succumbed to his illness.

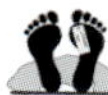 AUTOPSY FINDINGS: PM 22828

Both the ***kidneys*** (Figs 1A and B) were massively enlarged and distorted with a vague appreciable reniform shape, each measuring 21 × 12 × 6 cm and together weighing 1,480 g. The capsular aspect showed multiple cysts of varying sizes ranging from 0.5 to 2.5 cm in diameter. Few cysts showed hemorrhage (Fig 1B–black arrows). The ureters and urinary bladder appeared normal. A part of the pelvis was extrarenal on both sides (Fig 1B–red arrow). Cut section of the kidneys (Fig 2A) showed multiple rounded cysts, present both in the cortex and medulla, ranging in size from 1 cm to an occasional one being 6 cm in diameter, containing straw-colored as well as hemorrhagic fluid. Some of the cysts were stained with hemosiderin and few of them contained small calculi. The renal arteries were normal and the abdominal aorta showed atherosclerosis. Microscopy revealed the cysts to be lined by simple cuboidal to flattened epithelium (Figs 2B and C). The renal parenchyma (Figs 3A–F) showed florid tubulointerstitial nephritis in the form of dense inflammation, tubular atrophy, periglomerular fibrosis with few sclerosed glomeruli, interstitial fibrosis, few abscesses and cysts filled with polymorphs and macrophages. The vessels showed changes of hypertension. The ***liver*** (Fig 4A) was normal grossly and on coronal slicing, did not show any cysts. On microscopic examination, there was perivenular congestion and hemorrhagic necrosis indicating shock. The sinusoids contained polymorphs indicating septicemia. Many von Meyenburg complexes (bile duct hamartoma) were seen composed of clusters of proliferating, angulated bile ducts in a fibrous stroma (Figs 4B and C). ***Lungs*** were edematous and on microscopy showed extensive edema (Fig 4D). The pancreas was within normal limits and no cysts were noted. The ***heart*** was enlarged, weighed 350 g. All valves and chambers were normal. No mitral valve prolapse was

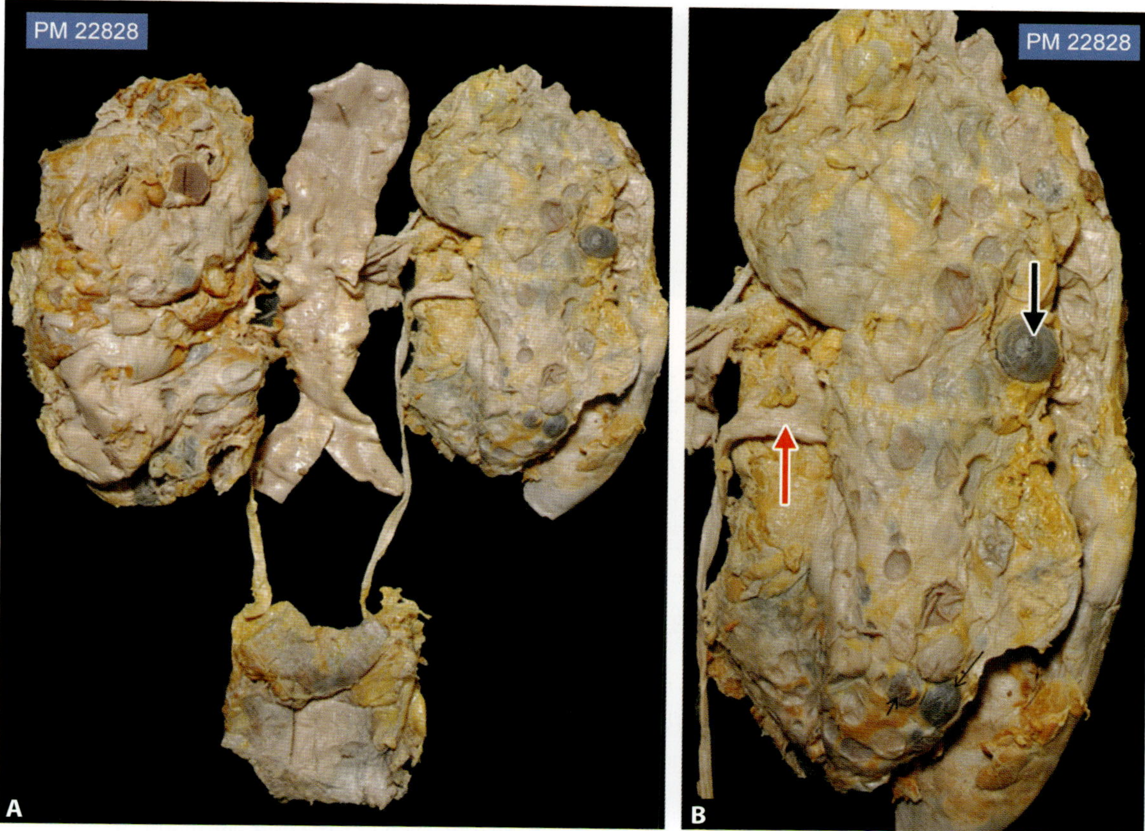

Figs 1A and B: (A) Gross photograph of both kidneys which are massively enlarged and studded with multiple cysts. Ureters and urinary bladder are normal. The opened up abdominal aorta shows atherosclerosis; (B) Close-up of the left kidney showing multiple cysts, few containing hemorrhagic fluid (black arrows). The pelvis is partly extrarenal (red arrow).

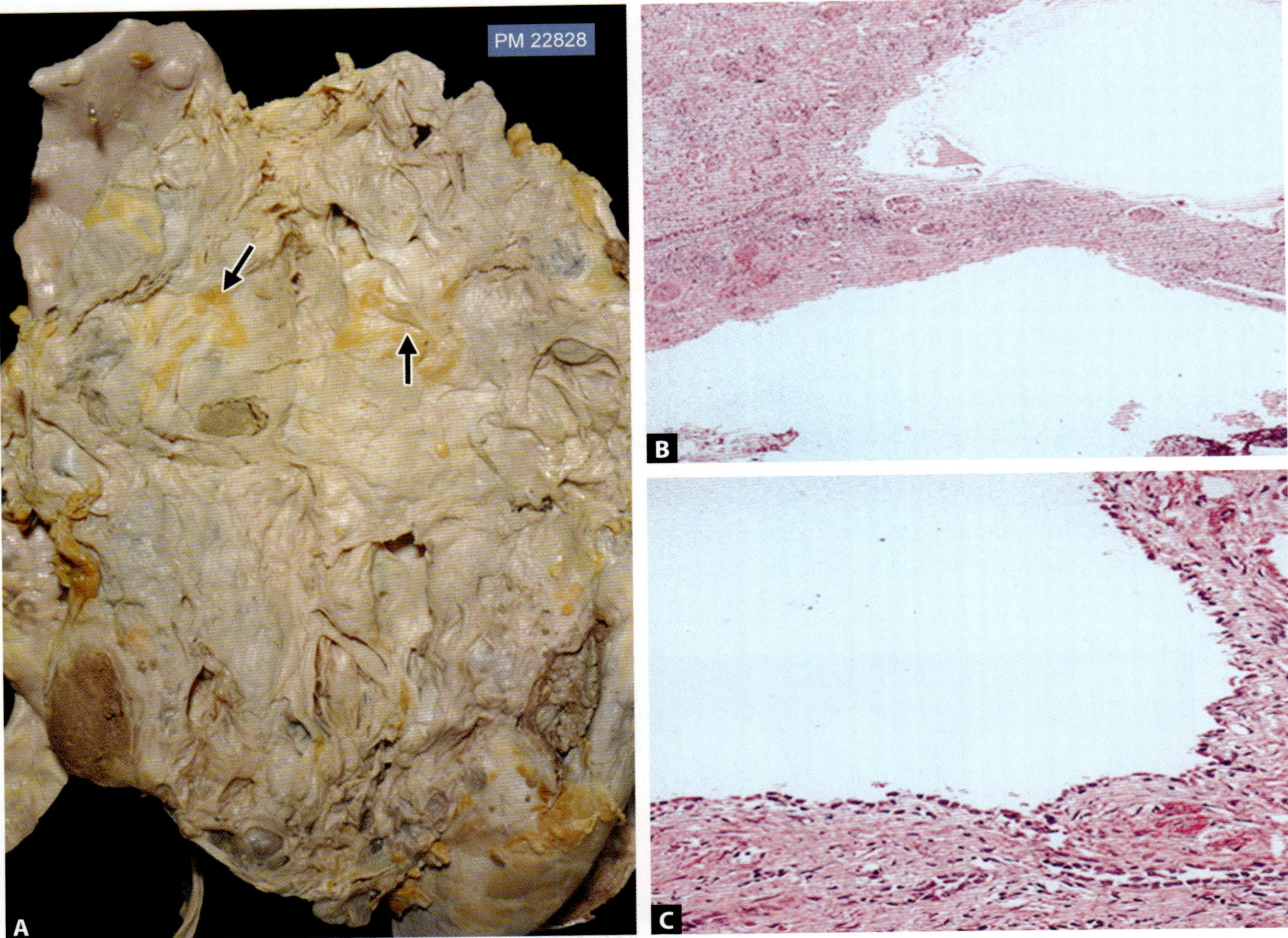

Figs 2A–C: (A) Cut section of the kidney showing multiple large cysts. Wall of few cysts shows yellowish staining with hemosiderin (arrows); (B) Photomicrographs from the kidney show multiple cysts with a flattened lining and adjacent renal parenchyma; (C) Cyst lined by cuboidal epithelium.

noted. There was left ventricular hypertrophy (wall measuring 1.7 cm) along with concentric hypertrophy (Figs 4E and F). The brain was within normal limits, weighed 1,440 g. No aneurysm was seen.

FINAL AUTOPSY DIAGNOSIS: PM 22828

47 Years Male

- Autosomal dominant polycystic kidney disease with acute on chronic tubulointerstitial nephritis, cyst infection and nephrolithiasis.
- Left ventricular hypertrophy
- Liver—changes of shock, septicemia and bile duct hamartomas
- Grade 3 atherosclerosis.

AUTOSOMAL DOMINANT POLYCYSTIC KIDNEY DISEASE

Autosomal dominant polycystic kidney disease has a clearly familial autosomal dominant mode of transmission, affects 1 in every 400–1,000 live births and puts a heavy load on the dialysis units worldwide. Patients present with flank pain, hematuria, lithiasis, cyst infection and hypertension. By the beginning of fourth decade, with progressive enlargement of the cysts (derived from the tubules), kidneys get enlarged, can be palpated and ultrasonographic diagnosis can be made. Both kidneys are affected, but earlier on, there is an asymmetric enlargement. Extrarenal manifestations include cysts in the liver (in two-thirds cases), pancreas (in 10% cases), aneurysms in the brain or extracranial locations, mitral valve prolapse and diverticuli in the colon. Hypertension occurs

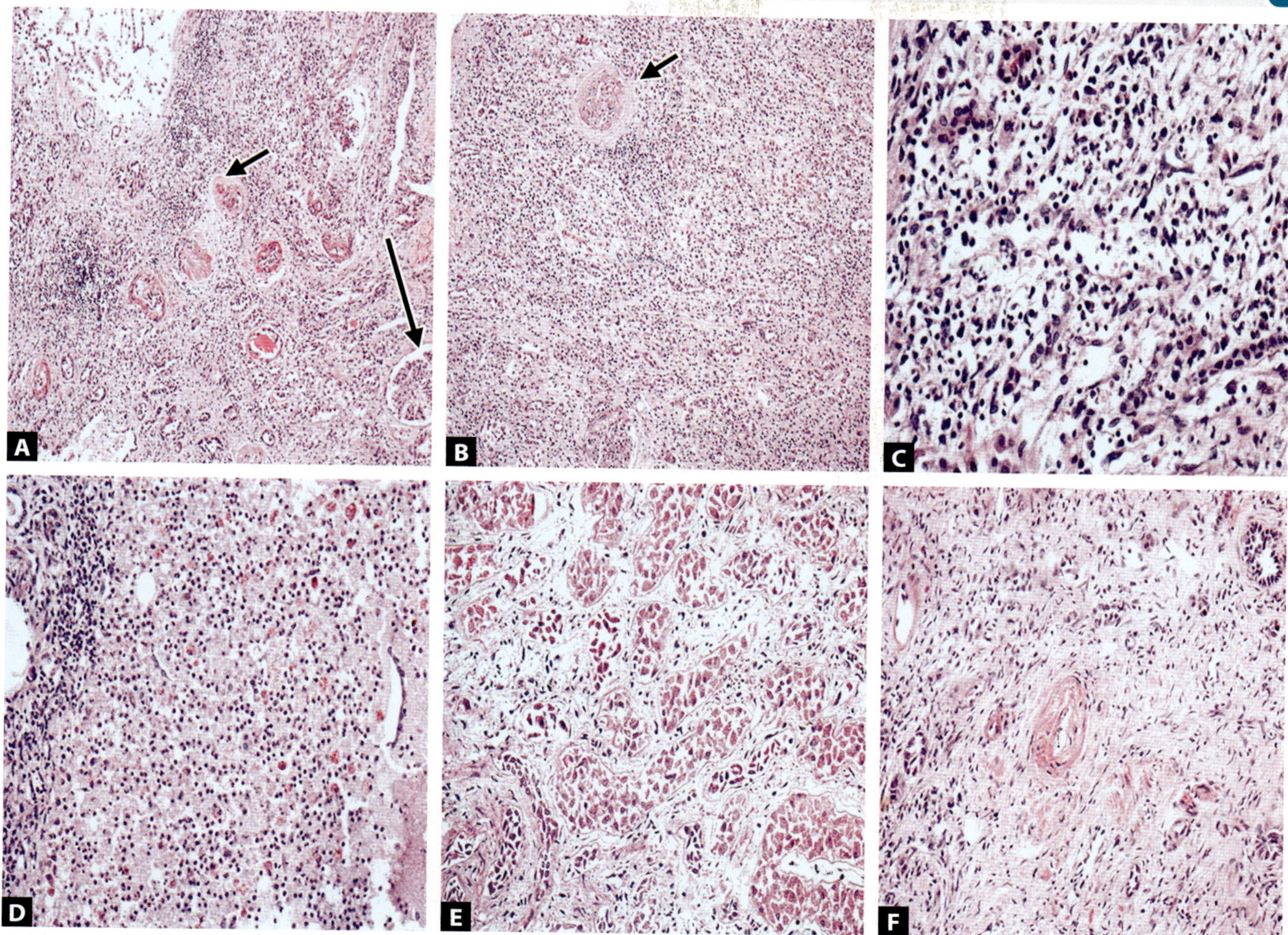

Figs 3A–F: (A and B) Renal parenchyma showing dense inflammation, tubular loss, prominent intralobular vessels, scattered normal glomeruli (long arrow), and periglomerular fibrosis (small arrow). Cysts showing dense collections of (C) Polymorphs and (D) Macrophages; (E) Tubules showing shedding of the epithelium with interstitial edema; (F) Renal parenchyma showing fibrosis, tubular loss and intralobular vessel showing medial hypertrophy.

in a half to two-thirds of the patients, much before the renal derangement starts and accelerates the disease process, leading to end-stage renal disease. Hypertension occurs due to involvement of the renin–angiotensin–aldosterone, nitric oxide and sympathetic nervous systems. Renal failure starts to set in after 40 years of age and by the age of 70 years, two-thirds of the patients land up with end-stage renal disease. Patients also have back or flank pain, gross or microscopic hematuria, renal concentrating defect and proteinuria. Renal concentrating defect occurs due to disruption of the medullary architecture by the cysts and due to intrinsic hyposensitivity of ADPKD collecting duct epithelia to arginine vasopressin. The disease is now considered as one of the primary ciliopathies.

In ADPKD, mutations are found in two genes *PKD1* (located on chromosome 16p13.3) and *PKD2* (located on chromosome 4q13-q23), both of which show a large number of different mutations and encode polycystin 1 and 2, respectively. Majority, i.e. 80–85%, patients show *PKD1* mutations and the remaining show *PKD2*. A third gene *PKD3* is under evaluation. Earlier onset of symptoms, i.e. cyst formation, hypertension and renal insufficiency occurs in patients with *PKD1* mutations. Inherited background genes and environmental factors also contribute to the disease expression. Polycystin 1, an epithelial cell membrane receptor, is needed for differentiation and division of the tubular epithelial cells. Polycystin 2 modulates intracellular levels of Ca^{2+}.

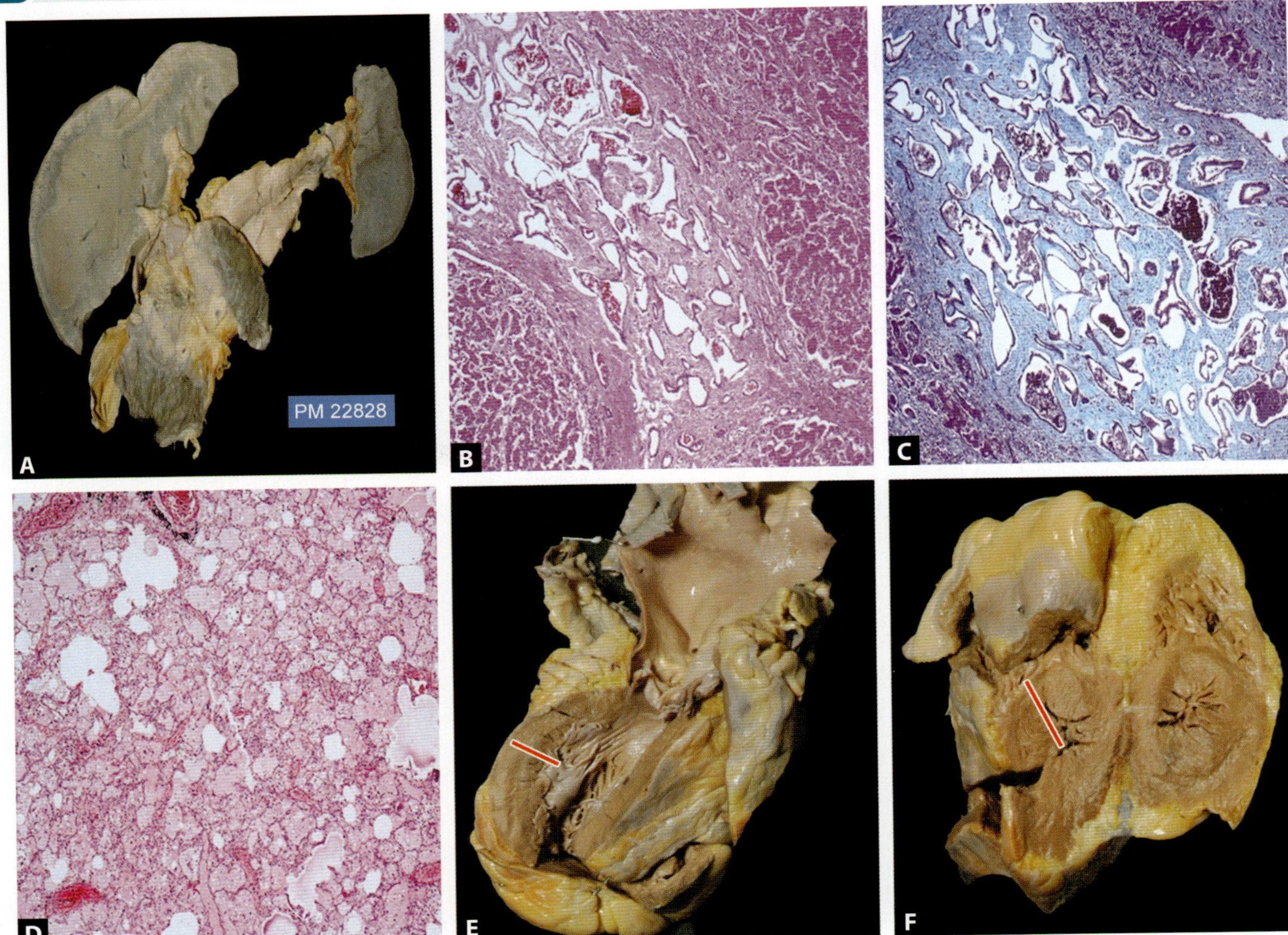

Figs 4A–F: (A) Organ complex composed of slice of liver, spleen, pancreas, C loop of the duodenum, and gall bladder. The liver and pancreas do not show any cysts. Photomicrographs of the liver show (B and C) Von Meyenburg complexes showing small clusters of dilated, angulated bile ducts embedded in a fibrous stroma, better highlighted in the Massons trichrome stain in "C"; (D) Photomicrograph of the lung showing alveoli filled with edema fluid; (E) Out flow tract of the enlarged heart showing left ventricular hypertrophy (red line); (F) Heart showing concentric hypertrophy.

On ultrasonography, the following criteria are considered for patients at high risk of developing ADPKD in the presence of family history—(1) Age ≤30 years—minimum of two cysts in one or both kidney; (2) Age 30–60 years—two cysts in each kidney; (3) Age > 60 years—four cysts in each kidney. If no cyst is identified by the age of 30 years, then occurrence of ADPKD is unlikely. In ADKPD, CT/MRI show enlarged kidneys with multiple cysts with both low and high (due to infection, hemorrhage) signal intensity. Phenotypic variability is a deterrent in establishing a diagnosis of ADPKD.

Grossly the kidneys are massively enlarged, distorted with multiple cysts which are unilocular, oval or round, ranging in size from millimeters to several centimeters, containing clear to turbid fluid which can be hemorrhagic. The pelvis and calyces cannot be appreciated. As age advances, the number and size of the cysts increases and the functional renal parenchyma goes on decreasing. Lectin staining has demonstrated that the cysts arise from all parts of the excretory nephron. Most severely affected are the collecting ducts and distal nephrons. Microscopically the cysts are lined by flat to cuboidal epithelium which can proliferate, giving rise to hyperplastic papillae or small polyps. The intervening renal parenchyma in due course of time shows inflammation and fibrosis.

A revolution in the treatment of ADPKD is the use of arginine vasopressin (AVP)–V2 receptor inhibitor in patients

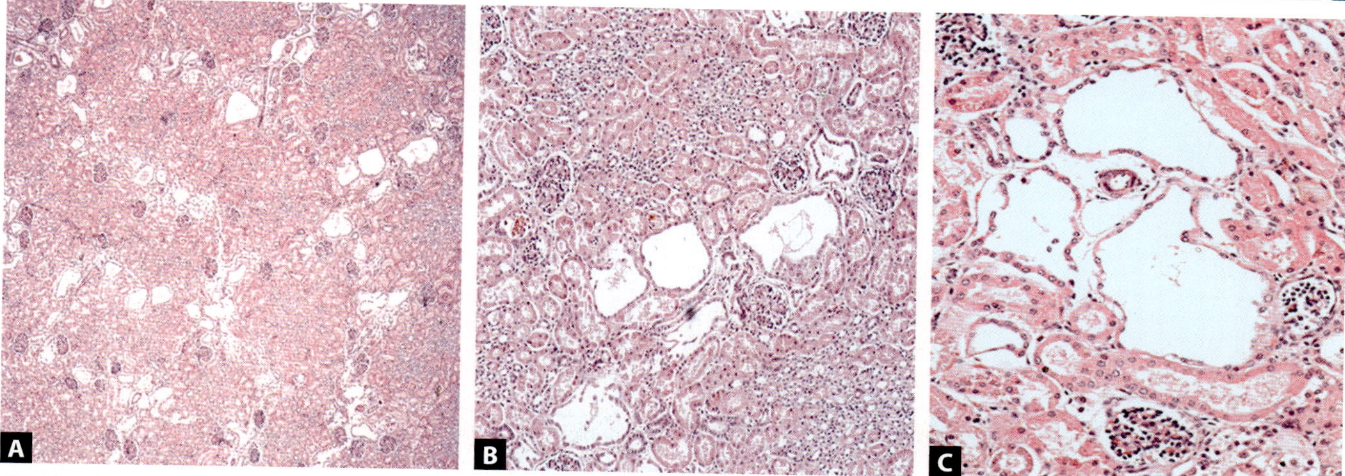

Figs 5A–C: Photomicrographs from the kidney of a baby with father having autosomal dominant polycystic kidney disease. (A–C) Show small cysts present diffusely, both in the cortex and medulla. Other components of the kidney are normal.

with subclinically detected disease. The distal nephrons and collecting ducts are sensitive to vasopressin and they are most affected in ADPKD. A constant action of AVP in mammals is to avoid dehydration. If one consumes more water, AVP levels decrease to make the urine more dilute. So the epithelial cells of the cysts are stimulated to secrete fluid and the AVP levels in ADPKD patients are high to compensate for the low concentrating capacity. Thus the AVP effect in them leads to cyst formation and starting patients on AVP receptor inhibitor will delay the cyst formation.

Children diagnosed with ADKPD before one and a half years of life are said to have "very early onset" (VEO) ADKPD. These children present with oligohydramnios, hypertension, pain abdomen, micro/gross hematuria and proteinuria. Screening children with a positive family history of ADPKD is now being done in many centers. This can detect the affected children and timely measures can be adopted to reduce the disease progression. About 33% children have documented hypertension and many of these have left ventricular hypertrophy. Thus, control of blood pressure of both hypertensive and normotensive children by using AVP-V2 receptor inhibitor, averts left ventricular hypertrophy and renal dysfunction. Figures 5A–C show photomicrographs from a 3-month-old baby who had a positive family history of ADKPD. Baby died of some other cause and the renal functions were normal. Both kidneys were normal grossly but microscopy revealed small cysts present diffusely, both in the cortex and medulla. Other components of the kidney were normal.

Resection in ADPKD (bilateral) is done when complications become very severe like recurrent infections, bleeding and severe pain or before renal transplantation. Figures 6A and B show right nephrectomy specimen in a 48-year-old male, a known case of ADKPD with positive family history. Nephrectomy was done due to recurrent severe infection and severe bleeding. The cysts however revealed hemorrhagic fluid and many contained blood clots.

COMMENTARY—INDEX CASE: PM 22828

This was a 47-year-old male who came to our institute for treatment of urethral stricture and was detected to have ADPKD with a positive family history. A few months later he was again admitted with a diagnosis of cyst infection for which he was treated. A month later he came with fever, abdominal pain, burning micturition and generalized weakness. Urine examination revealed red blood cells, pus cells and mild proteinuria. He was hypertensive since 15 years and was on treatment. There was anemia, hypoproteinemia, hypoalbuminemia, mildly raised creatinine, hyponatremia and hypokalemia; urine and blood culture grew ***E. coli*** and blood culture 2 days before his demise grew ***Klebsiella pneumoniae***. He was being treated for cyst infection, but succumbed to his illness. At autopsy there was ADPKD with tubulointerstitial nephritis, cyst infection, septicemic changes, left ventricular hypertrophy and features of shock. Surprisingly the renal functions were still well-maintained.

TAKE HOME MESSAGE

- Cyst infection is an ominous complication of ADKPD.
- A revolution in the treatment of ADPKD is the use of AVP-V2 receptor inhibitor in patients with subclinically detected disease.

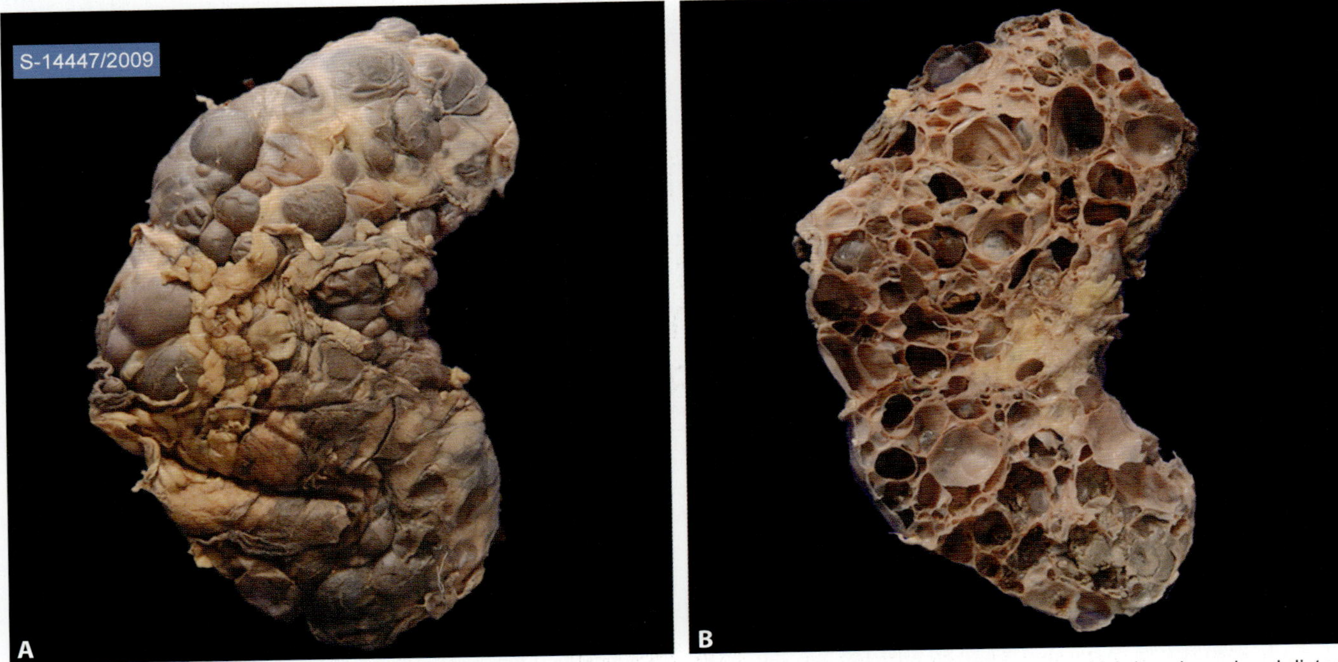

Figs 6A and B: (A) Case of autosomal dominant polycystic kidney disease—resected specimen of right kidney which is enlarged and distorted. Capsular aspect shows multiple cysts of varying sizes, most of them containing hemorrhagic fluid and some of them also containing clots; (B) Cut section of the kidney showing multiple, round to oval, well-defined cysts.

SUGGESTED READING

4. Cadnapaphornchai MA. Autosomal dominant polycystic kidney disease in children. Curr Opin Pediatr. 2015;27(2):193-200.
1. Hill GS. Cystic and dysplastic diseases of the kidney: genetic. In: Hill GS (Ed). Uropathology, Volume 1. Edinburgh, New York: Churchill Livingstone; 1989. pp. 135.
2. Jennette JC, Olson JL, Schwartz MM, Silva FG (Eds). Cystic diseases and developmental kidney defects. Hepinstall's Pathology of the Kidney, Volume 2, 6th edition. Lippincott: Williams & Wilkins; 2007. p. 1258.
3. Polubothu S, Richardson A, Kerecuk L, et al. Autosomal dominant polycystic kidney disease in children. BMJ. 2016; 353:i29.

CONTRIBUTIONS BY:

1. Dr Vikrant, Junior Resident, Department of Pathology (In taking gross photographs)
2. Dr RK Vasishta, Professor and Head, Department of Histopathology (Consultation)
3. Dr Vinay Sakhuja, Ex-Professor and Head, Department of Nephrology (Clinician In-Charge)
4. Dr SK Singh, Professor, Department of Urology (Urologist In-Charge)

Post Graduate Institute of Medical Education and Research, (PGIMER), Chandigarh, India.

CASE 89

Co-existing Glomerulocystic Kidney Disease and Renal Tubular Dysgenesis with Late Onset Oligohydramnios and Renal Failure at D2 of Life: PM 28154

Nandita Bharadwaj Kakkar

HIGHLIGHTS OF THE CASE

This baby has a co-existing renal tubular dysgenesis (RTD) which is autosomal recessive and glomerulocystic kidney (GCK) disease group 1—sporadic ? mutation. These are rare disorders and both being seen together, has not been reported in literature.

Keywords: Renal tubular dysgenesis, glomerulocystic kidney disease, co-existence, autosomal recessive.

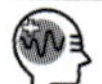

CLINICAL DETAILS

Baby had Three Admissions in PGIMER

First Admission NICU, Date of Birth: 14.03.2017, Date of Discharge: 05.04.2017, Duration of Stay: 21 Days

A primigravida, aged 25 years, was undergoing a supervised pregnancy at an outside facility. Antenatal ultrasonography done at 9/18/26 weeks of gestation was reported as normal. However, at 30 weeks gestation, she was detected to have oligohydramnios. At 34 weeks gestation, mother had bleeding per vaginum (indeterminate abruption) with no pain. Ultrasonography revealed a single live fetus with cephalic presentation, severe oligohydramnios and no congenital malformation. She was referred to PGIMER, Chandigarh. She delivered a male baby by spontaneous vaginal delivery; at 34 weeks gestation, baby weighed 1,910 g (AGA) with APGAR of 5, 8, 9. Baby required positive pressure ventilation for 30 seconds. Thereafter, baby was managed in NICU for hypoxic ischemic encephalopathy stage I and respiratory distress with nasal prong continuous positive airway pressure followed by invasive and noninvasive ventilation for a total duration of 7 days. X-ray chest was suggestive of pneumonia. Initially, he was treated with ciprofloxacin and amikacin, upgraded to meropenem on D2. Blood culture sent on D2 grew *Stenotrophomonas* and he was managed with levofloxacin as per sensitivity report. He received morphine infusion for persistent pulmonary hypertension.

Baby passed urine on D1, but developed oliguria (UOP <1 mL/Kg/hr) and azotemia on D2. Ultrasonography of kidneys/ureters/bladder (KUB) revealed atypical appearance of the kidneys with increased cortical echogenicity, size being 4.7–4.8 cm each and fetal lobulations being present. Features were suggestive of autosomal recessive polycystic kidney disease (ARPKD). He continued to have worsening azotemia, fluid retention and persistent hyponatremia.

Investigations and Course of Management

Hemoglobin: 9.2–12.8 g/dL, TLC—12,800/μL, DLC—N31, L37, M23, E7 and platelets—1,93000/μL. There was a persistent hyponatremia (Na^+: 121–130 mEq/L) along with hyperkalemia (K^+: 4.6–7.6 mEq/L). Serum urea—69–103 mg%, serum creatinine—rose from 3.4 mg% to 9.3 mg%. Liver function tests were normal. Blood gas analysis revealed metabolic acidosis.

He was managed with restricted fluid, sodium supplementation and furosemide infusion till 25.3.2017. Subsequently, urinary output improved. Hyperkalemia was treated with kayexalate. Renal biopsy was deferred. Peritoneal dialysis was considered to be nonproductive. Baby initially had encephalopathy, so was put on tube feeds. Gradually spoon feeds were introduced and hiked and breast feed was also started. The prognosis was explained to the parents and was discharged on fluid restriction, hydrochlorthiazide, kayexalate, oral bicarbonate, along with calcium and vitamin D supplements. Both parents underwent ultrasonography (KUB) which was within normal limits. No cysts were identified in any one of them and there was no history of any kidney disease in the family with special reference to the grandparents. Clinical diagnosis was Autosomal recessive polycystic kidney disease with renal failure.

Second admission: **12.04.2017 to 13.04.2017, 2 days**. Baby came for follow-up. He had pallor (Hb—6.4 g/dL) and was given blood transfusion. He continued to be acidotic.

Third Admission, Date of Admission: 29.04.2017, Date of Death: 07.05.2017, Duration of Hospital Stay: 8 Days

Baby was readmitted with complaints of loose stools, vomiting and rales since 1 day. The stools were 4–5/day, large watery, not containing any blood or mucus. There was no fever, cough, altered sensorium or any seizures. He was accepting feeds and vitals were stable. On examination there was no icterus, cyanosis, edema, rash, bleeds or any lymphadenopathy. The abdomen was soft and there was no organomegaly. Baby was lethargic, hypotonia was present and bilateral deep tendon reflexes were elicitable. There were no meningeal signs.

Investigations

Hemoglobin—9.4 g/dL, TLC—23,090/µL, DLC—N31, L52, M15, E2, platelets—52,000/µL, serum urea—163–244 mg%, serum creatinine—7.8–9.2 mg%, total proteins—4.08 gms, $Na^+/K^+/CL^-$ —128/3.5/108 mEq/L. Procalcitonin levels were 48.33 ng/mL. Despite all measures, baby succumbed to his illness on D53 of life. A partial autopsy was performed after taking consent from the parents.

AUTOPSY FINDINGS: PM 28154

A partial autopsy was performed via an abdominothoracic incision. Baby weighed 2,500 g (born at 34 weeks gestation and lived for 53 days), Anthropometric measurements-head/chest/abdominal circumference—32/29/31 cm, crown rump—2 cm, foot length—6.5 cm. There were low set ears and no other external abnormality was noted. The ***kidneys*** (Figs 1A–C) were small in size and together weighed 18 g (normal for this age—28 g) and measured 3 × 2 × 1 cm each. The reniform shape was perfectly maintained and fetal lobulations were well discernable. The capsular aspect showed innumerable small pinhead-sized cysts, present diffusely, measuring 1–2 mm. Mild dilatation of the ureters was appreciable in the lower part and the urinary bladder was normal, but mildly thickened. On cut section, a moderate pelvicalyceal system dilatation was noted on both sides (Figs 2A and B). The cysts were appreciable only in the periphery of the cortex, in the subcapsular location and also in the medullary extension of the cortex (Figs 2A and B; Fig 3). No cyst was seen in the medulla. On microscopic examination as seen on gross (Figs 4A and B), the cysts were present in the peripheral cortex and no cyst was seen in the medulla. The glomeruli (Figs 4C and D) were closely packed and exhibited a prominent glomerulocystic change which involved practically all the glomeruli. Some glomeruli showed collapsed capillary tufts covered by prominent layer of visceral epithelial cells (Figs 5A–C). The Bernstein's criteria of labeling the kidney "glomerulocystic" was fulfilled, i.e. enlarged Bowman's space i.e 2 to 3 times the normal and more than 5% cysts contained atrophic glomeruli. Periglomerular fibrosis, glomerular calcification, interstitial inflammation, fibrosis and thickening/disorganization of the muscular wall of the small arteries was noted (Figs 5D and E). The cortical tubules were reduced in number and few were lined by densely packed columnar cells. No features of dysplasia, i.e. no primitive duct was seen. Medulla appeared normal but showed some dilated tubules. The urinary bladder showed mild hypertrophy of the detrusor muscle. Immunohistochemistry (Figs 6A–D) was also done as a diagnosis of renal tubular dysgenesis (RTD) was suspected on microscopy and because there was a persistent/nonresponding hyponatremia. The tubules in between the glomeruli (supposed to be proximal convoluted tubules PCT) were negative for CD10 and positive for EMA, CK7 and E-cadherin, indicating thereby the absence of proximal convoluted tubules and meaning thereby that the tubules present in between the glomeruli were either distal convoluted tubules, loops of Henle or collecting ducts. The medullary tubules (Figs 7A–D) stained strongly for CK7, EMA and E-cadherin and were negative for CD10. These features are consistent with a diagnosis of RTD. The liver (Figs 8A and B) did not show any features of ductal plate malformation. The lungs (Figs 8C and D) together weighed 65 g and there was no hypoplasia. Microscopy revealed alveolar hemorrhage, mild bronchopulmonary dysplasia and features of persistent pulmonary hypertension (Fig 8E). Other organs including the heart were within normal limits.

FINAL AUTOPSY DIAGNOSIS: PM 28154

D53 Male, Late Onset Oligohydramnios with Oliguria and Renal Failure at D2 of Life

- Renal tubular dysgenesis co-existing with Glomerulocystic kidney disease (GCKD)—Group 1 sporadic, nonsyndromal, nonfamilial/familial.
- Pulmonary hemorrhage, mild bronchopulmonary dysplasia and persistent pulmonary hypertension.

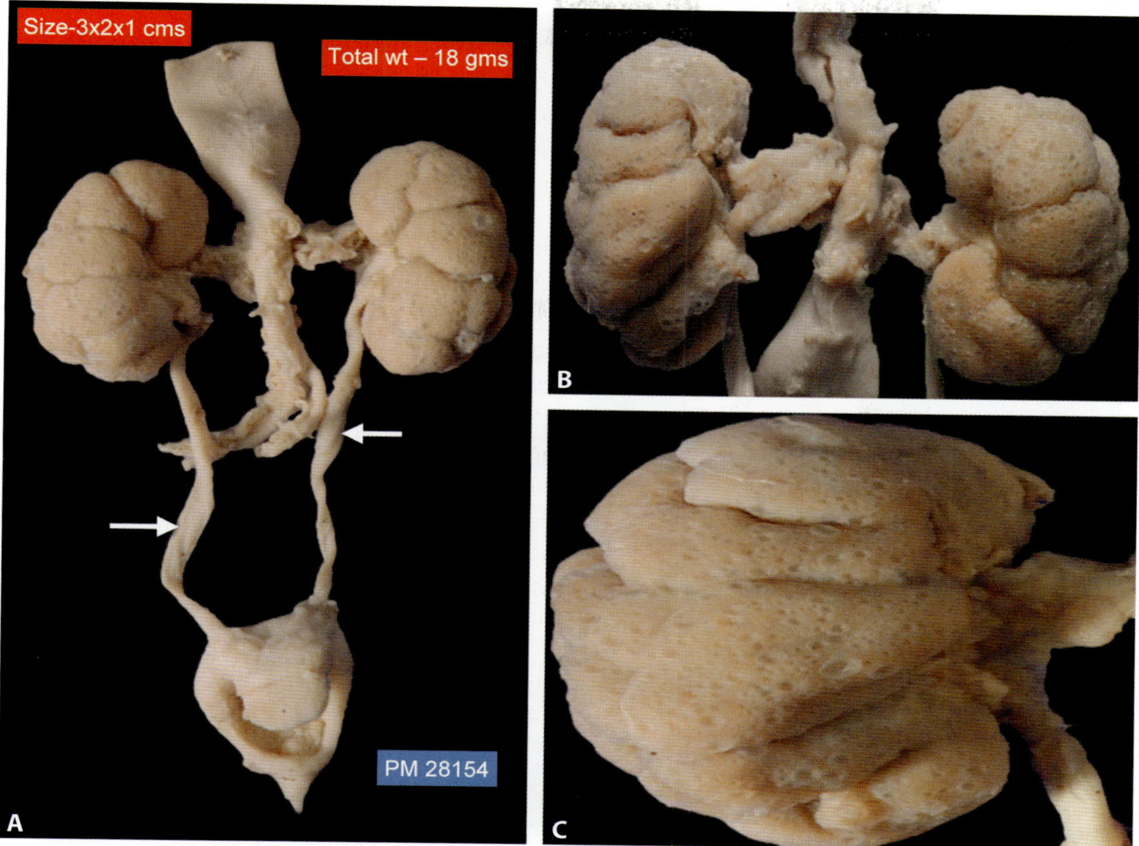

Figs 1A–C: (A and B) Kidneys are small in size, together weigh 18 g, and show maintained reniform shape/fetal lobulations. Appear sponge-like due to the tiny cysts present diffusely. The ureters show mild dilatation in the lower/mid portion (arrows). The urinary bladder is normal-sized but shows thickening; (C) Close-up view of the right kidney showing innumerable, tiny and pinhead-sized cysts on the capsular aspect present diffusely.

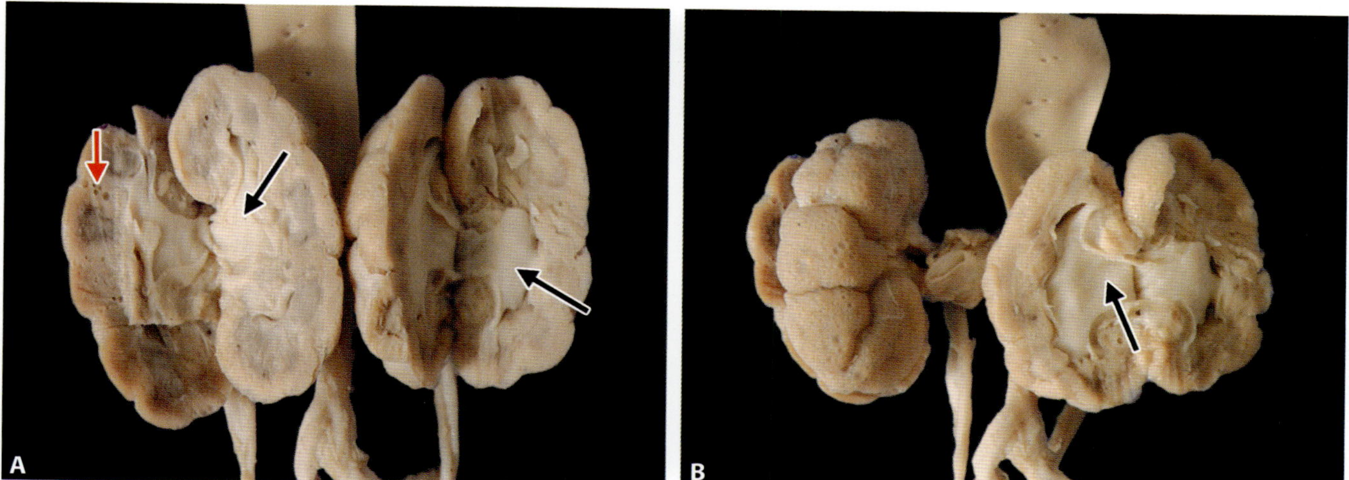

Figs 2A and B: Cut section of the kidney shows a distinct corticomedullary distinction with the medulla showing a darker hue due to congestion. The pelvicalyceal system shows moderate degree of dilatation (black arrows). Please note that the tiny cysts are seen only in the peripheral cortex in the subcapsular location and also in the medullary extension of the cortex (red arrow). No cyst seen in the medulla.

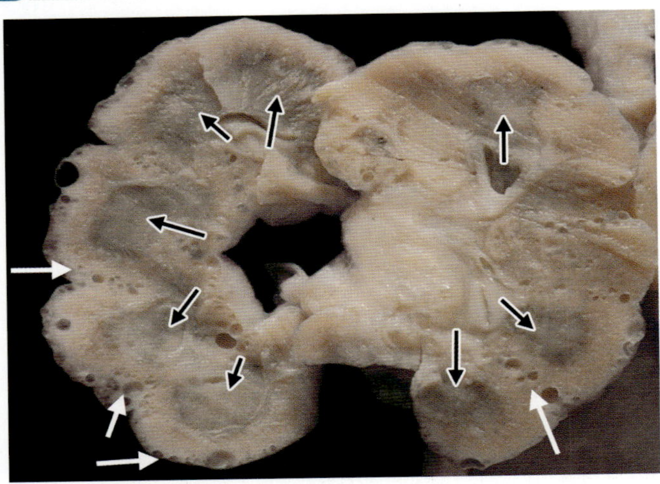

Fig 3: Cut section of the kidney shows a distinct corticomedullary distinction with the medulla showing congestion (black arrows). The tiny cysts are seen only in the peripheral cortex in the subcapsular location and also in the medullary extension of the cortex (white arrows). No cyst is seen in the medulla.

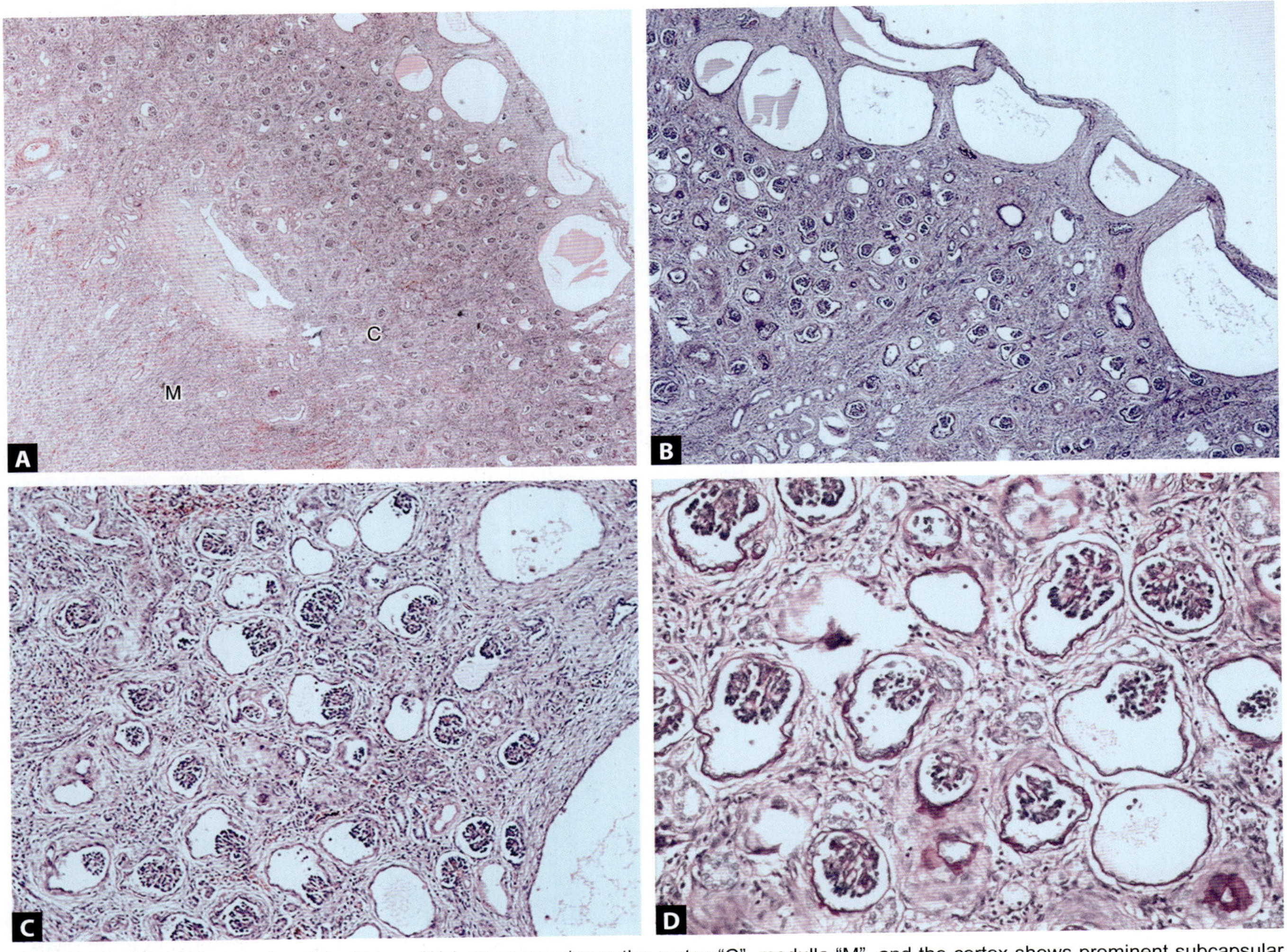

Figs 4A–D: Photomicrographs of the kidney (A) Low power shows the cortex "C", medulla "M", and the cortex shows prominent subcapsular cysts. No cyst is seen in the medulla; (B) Periodic acid–Schiff stain shows peripherally placed cortical cysts and marked approximation of the glomeruli along with prominent glomerular cysts; (C and D) Cortex showing a prominent glomerulocystic change with a paucity of cortical tubules.

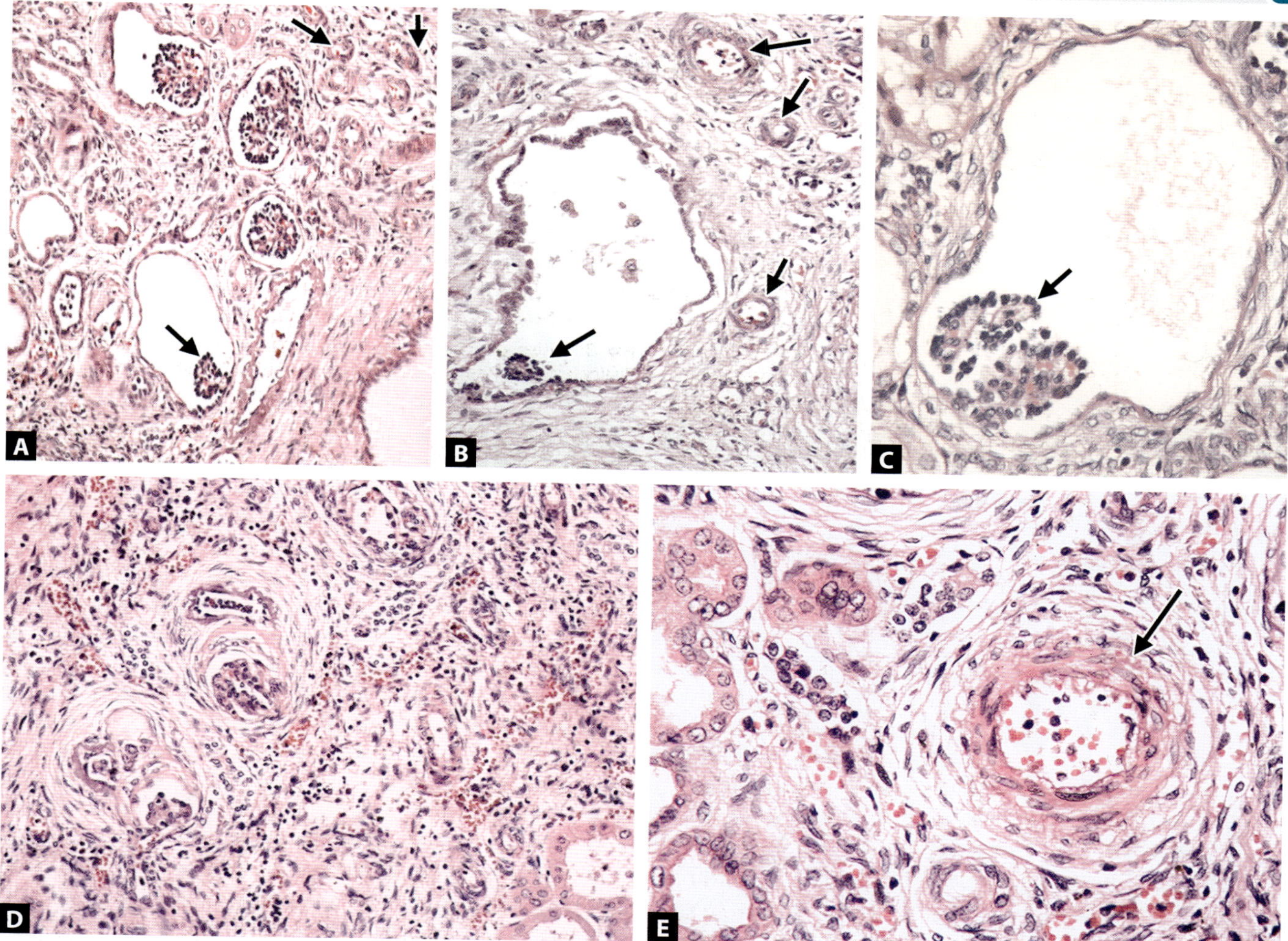

Figs 5A–E: Photomicrographs of the kidney shows (A to C) Prominent glomerulocysts with atrophic glomeruli lying within them (arrows). In addition prominent arterioles are seen in both "A" and "B" in the upper right corner (arrows); (D) Cortex shows areas with periglomerular fibrosis and interstitial inflammation; (E) Cortex shows prominent arterioles showing medial hypertrophy (arrow).

RENAL TUBULAR DYSGENESIS

Renal tubular dysgenesis is a life-threatening, autosomal recessive disorder characterized by the total absence or a poor development of proximal convoluted tubules. This entity leads to a late onset oligohydramnios and presents in the early neonatal period with oliguria, renal failure, persistent hyponatremia and respiratory distress (due to pulmonary hypoplasia). Mutations occur in the genes encoding the major components of the renin–angiotensin system (RAS) leading to either nonproduction or defective formation of angiotensin 2. Thus this is a genetically heterogeneous disorder. Ossification defects of the skull, i.e. patent cranial fontanelles are generally seen along with. RTD may be acquired (secondary RTD) in fetuses exposed during pregnancy to drugs (given to the mother) like RAS blockers and nonsteroidal anti-inflammatory drugs. It has been seen in fetuses with severe liver disease like congenital hemochromatosis, renal artery stenosis, major cardiac malformations and in the donor twin of severe twin-to-twin transfusion syndrome. All this basically leads to hypoperfusion of the kidney and absence of angiotensin 2 production/action which further leads to accumulation of renin. Ultrasonography of the kidneys, however appears normal. The diagnosis is confirmed on microscopic examination by proving the absence of proximal convoluted tubules in between the glomeruli in the cortex, by the use of immunostains. The proximal convoluted tubules show strong positivity with CD10 and are negative for EMA, CK7 and E-cadherin. The latter three immunostains however mark the distal convoluted tubules, loops of Henle and the

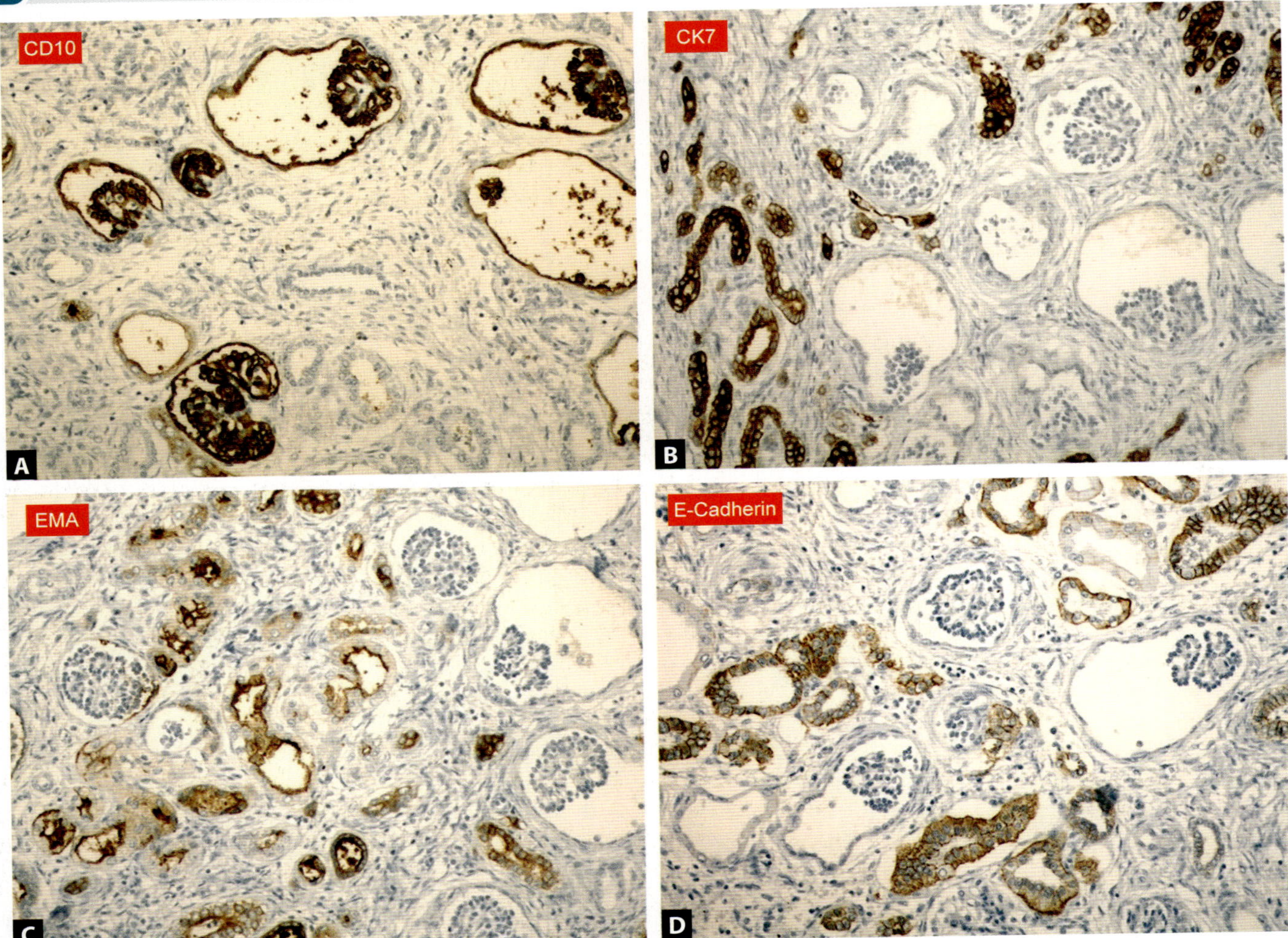

Figs 6A–D: (A) CD10 immunostain stains the glomeruli. The tubules seen in between are negative indicating that they are not proximal convoluted tubules; (B to D) CK7, EMA and E-cadherin immunostains show strong positivity in the cortical tubules indicating thereby that they are not proximal convoluted tubules, but distal tubules/loop of Henle's/collecting ducts. The glomeruli are negative for these stains.

collecting ducts. On microscopic examination, in RTD, there is an approximation of the glomeruli in the cortex due to paucity of tubules, the tubules present are lined by densely packed columnar cells and there is a prominent thickening and disorganization of the muscular wall of small arteries (from arcuate to afferent arterioles).

GLOMERULOCYSTIC KIDNEY

The term glomerulocystic kidney is an umbrella under which reside a large number of entities categorized into three major groups by Bernstein J. The ***Bernstein's criteria*** of labeling the kidney "glomerulocystic" is: (1) Bowman's space—2–3 times the normal and (2) More than 5% cysts contain atrophic glomeruli. Glomerulocystic kidney is thus a heterogeneous term.

***Group 1*:** Glomerulocystic kidney disease—true GCKD: nonsyndromal (heritable/sporadic). (1) Heritable—ADPKD in neonates or infants. (2) Dominant GCKD (non PKD/PKD type) in older individuals. (3) Familial hypoplastic autosomal dominant GCKD (HNF1beta gene mutation) associated with pyelocalyceal abnormalities. (4) Sporadic, nonsyndromal, nonfamilial/familial GCKD. The sporadic cases are due to new mutations.

***Group 2*:** Glomerular cysts as a component of other cystic diseases, i.e. diffuse cystic dysplasia, Meckel–Gruber, Ivemark syndrome (renal hepatic pancreatic dysplasia), prune belly syndrome and glutaric aciduria type 2.

***Group 3*:** Syndromal glomerulocystic kidneys seen in heritable malformation syndromes like tuberous sclerosis,

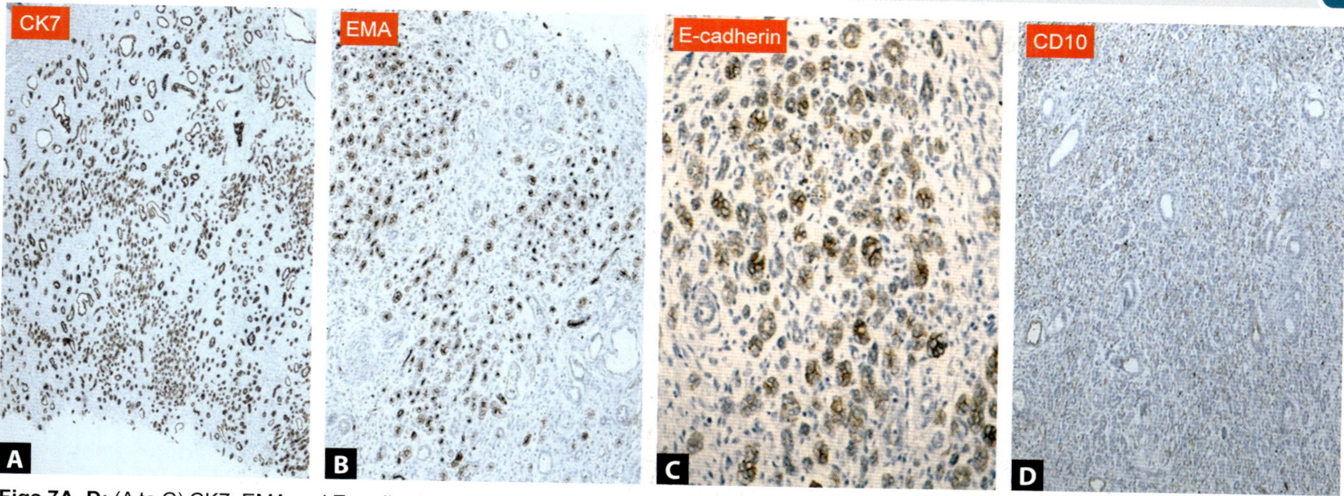

Figs 7A–D: (A to C) CK7, EMA and E-cadherin immunostains show strong positivity in the medullary tubules (as they should) indicating that they are distal tubules/loop of Henle's/collecting ducts; (D) CD10 immunostain is negative in the medullary tubules.

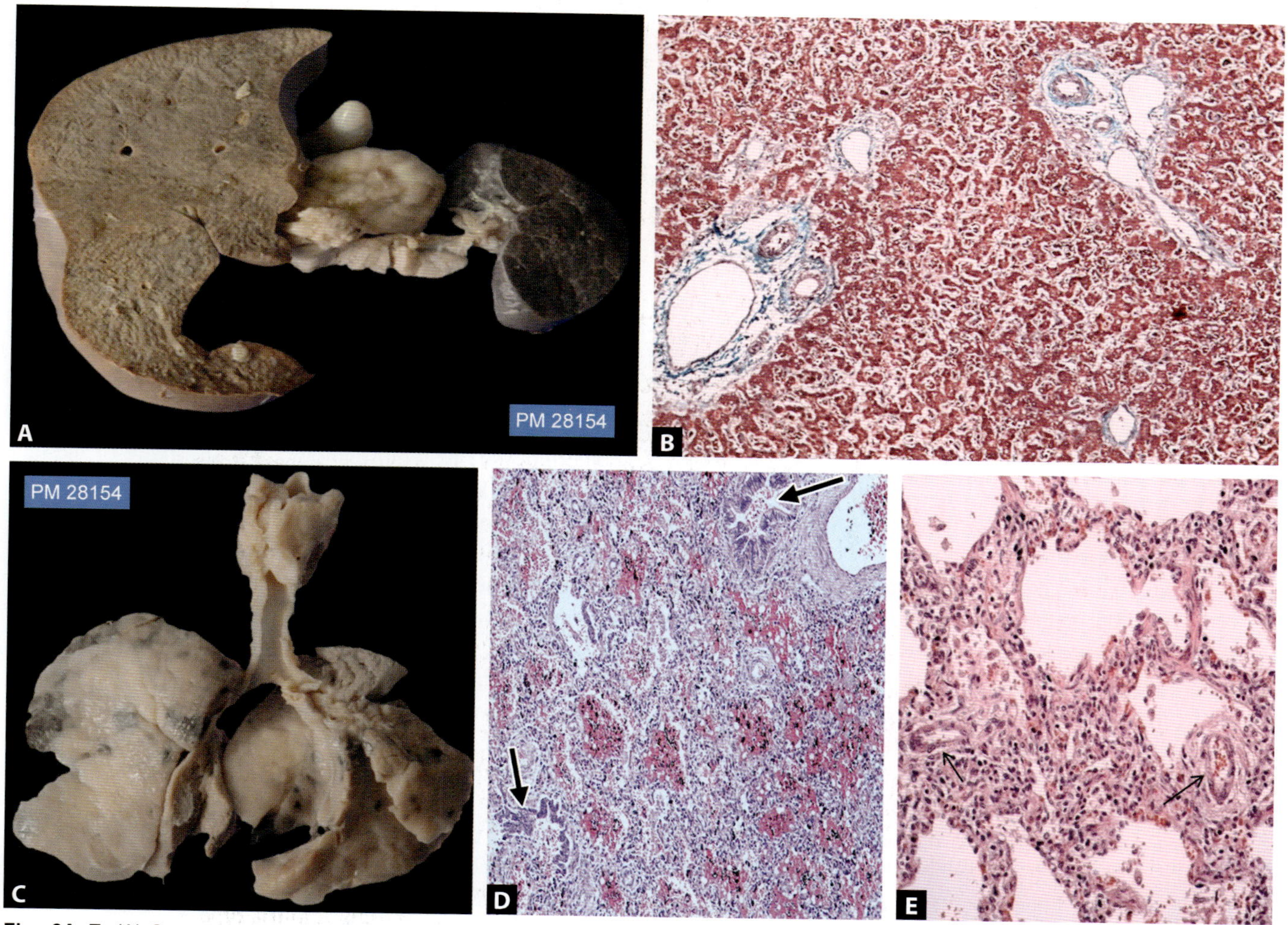

Figs 8A–E: (A) Organ complex of the liver, pancreas, 'c' loop of the duodenum, and slice of spleen; (B) Massons trichrome stain of the liver shows normal portal tracts, which do not show ductal plate malformation; (C) Both lungs show areas of hemorrhage; (D) Photomicrograph of the lung showing alveolar hemorrhage and bronchioles show mild bronchopulmonary dysplasia (arrows); (E) Lung showing prominent inter-acinar arterioles (arrows) indicating pulmonary arterial hypertension.

orofaciodigital syndrome Type 1, brachymesomelia-renal syndrome, trisomy 13, short rib-polydactyly syndromes, Jeune asphyxiating thoracic dystrophy syndrome, Zellweger cerebrohepatorenal syndrome, familial juvenile nephronophthisis, etc.

A fourth category has been added, i.e. acquired, which is associated with hemolytic uremic syndrome. Group 1 is the true GCKD. Glomerulocystic kidney associated with other cystic renal disorders and heritable syndromes, i.e. Group 2 and 3, shows specific manifestations of the basic disease along with a prominent glomerulocystic change, thus giving the kidney a label of being "glomerulocystic". This can surely be called "secondary glomerulocystic change" but not GCKD.

True Glomerulocystic Kidney Disease (GCKD)—Group 1

This is said to be the true category of glomerulocystic kidneys and is labeled as "glomerulocystic kidney disease", i.e. GCKD. Majority of these cases are seen in newborns and young children and a small number are seen in adolescents and adults. They can be both sporadic and familial (polycystic kidney disease, i.e. PKD type or non-PKD type). Some of the babies with GCKD, have positive family history, i.e. one parent has autosomal dominant polycystic kidney disease (ADPKD). They have PKD1 mutations on short arm of chromosome 16 and are thus labeled as infantile onset of polycystic kidney disease. Glomerulocystic change is said to be commonly seen in ADPKD, especially when the cysts are small. The other categories are:

- Some familial forms do not show the PKD type mutations, ? new mutations.
- Familial hypoplastic (autosomal dominant) glomerulocystic disease is rare, seen in few families, show defective pyelocalyceal anatomy detected by ultrasonography. The kidneys are small in size.
- Sporadic type of GCKD is very much like the PKD type of GCKD, but without the family history. They are said to occur because of new mutations and occur as commonly as the familial type. They may show enlarged or normal-sized kidneys and cysts are present diffusely in the cortex. The medullary pyramids may be abnormal with dilated collecting ducts, surrounding fibrosis and lesser number of vasa recta. Oligohydramnios generally occurs early. There is dilatation of the Bowman's capsule along with the attached proximal convoluted tubule which is lined by a layer of flattened epithelium and house rudimentary glomerular tufts. The kidney can be enlarged, normal-sized or small in size. Ten percent cases show a mild degree of ductal plate malformation.

There are many unanswered questions, i.e. whether sporadic GCKD with new mutations is a category of classical ADPKD or are they different ?

COMMENTARY—INDEX CASE: PM 28154

This was a male baby born by a normal vaginal delivery, at 34 weeks gestation, to a primigravida, aged 25 years who came with antepartum hemorrhage. The baby weighed 1,910 g (AGA) with an APGAR of 5, 8, 9. Antenatal ultrasonography done at 9/18/26 weeks of gestation was reported as normal. There was late onset oligohydramnios which was detected at 30 weeks gestation. Baby developed oliguria, renal failure and respiratory distress on D2 of life. Initially the ultrasonography was suggestive of a recessive polycystic kidney disease and on review a possibility of glomerulocystic disease was rendered with diffusely scattered multiple tiny cysts, concentrated along subcapsular area, poor corticomedullary differentiation and a size of 47–48 mm. There was persistent hyponatremia, hyperkalemia, metabolic acidosis, infections and a persistently rising serum creatinine or urea. Baby succumbed to his illness on D53 of life. Both parents underwent ultrasonography (KUB) which was within normal limits. There was no history of any kidney disease in the grandparents or in any other member of the family.

Autopsy revealed RTD co-existing with GCKD—Group 1 in the index case sporadic, nonsyndromal, nonfamilial/familial. The GCKD in the index case is probably nonfamilial as there is no family history, but whether this cannot be said with full certainty. The point now is—(1) Whether this baby has two different distinct disorders associated by chance or (2) Are these two entities related, i.e. does RTD show a glomerulocystic histomorphology? We are aware of the fact that GCK is a heterogeneous entity and can be seen with various syndromes or as a component of other cystic diseases. The index case showed a mild dilatation of the lower part of the ureters, the urinary bladder did show a mild hypertrophy and there was mild dilatation of the pelvicalyceal system. So was there some partial obstruction at the level of the urethra, which led to glomerulocystic change in the both the kidneys? This could be a plausible explanation. (3) Referring to Case 90-PM 28255 (18 weeks, MTP) where a classical posterior urethral valve leads to "glomerulocystic change" along with bilateral congenital hydroureteronephrosis with marked dysplasia, hypertrophied urinary bladder and dilated posterior urethra. In this case (PM 28255), the renal cysts were present diffusely, as well as peripherally in the cortical rim, with no corticomedullary distinction and with the hallmark of dysplasia, i.e. primitive ducts. The "index case" however showed corticomedullary distinction with cysts present only in the peripheral cortex, in the subcapsular location and in the medullary extensions of the cortex, just like what is seen in the true GCKD, i.e. Group 1 and no dysplasia was noted. Hence, I feel that both the theories could be plausible here, i.e. the "glomerulocystic kidney" could be due to obstruction as stated above in point number 2 or it could be the true GCKD—Group 1 sporadic, nonsyndromal, nonfamilial/familial. But the latter seems more plausible. So this baby has a co-existing RTD which is autosomal recessive and glomerulocystic kidney disease group 1—sporadic ? new mutation. So, in the next pregnancy the mother should be kept on a very good follow-up. Before 20 weeks gestation, she should be fully evaluated by ultrasonography and amniocentesis should be done for ruling out RTD, which has a 25% chance of recurrence.

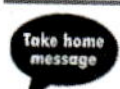

TAKE HOME MESSAGE

- Renal tubular dysgenesis is a life-threatening, autosomal recessive disorder characterized by the total absence or a poor development of proximal convoluted tubules.
- Persistent hyponatremia with early onset renal failure, paucity of cortical tubules with negative staining for CD10 and positive staining for EMA, CK7 and E-cadherin clinches the diagnosis.
- Glomerulocystic kidney is a heterogeneous entity under which there is true GCKD—nonsyndromal (heritable or sporadic) or glomerulocystic change could be seen as a component of other cystic disorders or heritable syndromes.

SUGGESTED READING

1. Bernstein J. Glomerulocystic kidney disease-nosological considerations. Pediatr Nephrol. 1993;7:464-70.
2. Bissler JJ, Siroky BJ, Yin H. Glomerulocystic kidney disease. Pediatr Nephrol. 2010;25(10):2049-50.
3. Dedeoglu IO, Fisher JE, Springate JE, et al. Spectrum of glomerulocystic kidneys: a case report and review of the literature. Pediatr Pathol Lab Med. 1996;16(6):941-9.
4. Genest R, Lage JM. Absence of normal appearing proximal tubules in the fetal and neonatal kidney: prevalence and significance. Hum Pathol. 1991;22(2):147-53.
5. Gubler MC. Renal tubular dysgenesis. Pediatr Nephrol. 2014;29(1):51-9.
6. Gupta K, Vankalakunti M, Sachdeva MUS. Glomerulocystic kidney disease and its rare associations: an autopsy report of two unrelated cases. Diagn Pathol. 2007;2:12.
7. Gusmano R, Caridi G, Marini M, et al. Glomerulocystic kidney disease in a family. Nephrol Dial Transplant. 2002; 17:813-8.
8. Lacoste M, Cai Y, Guicharnaud L, et al. Renal tubular dysgenesis, a not uncommon autosomal recessive disorder leading to oligohydramnios: role of the renin angiotensin system. J Am Soc Nepharol. 2006;17(8):2253-63.
9. Landau D, Shalev H, Shulman H, et al. Oligohydramnion, renal failure and no pulmonary hypoplasia in glomerulocystic kidney disease. Pediatr Nephrol. 2000;14:319-21.
10. Sahay M, Gowrishankar s. Glomerulocystic disease. NDT Plus. 2010;3(4):349-50.
11. Taxy JB, Filmer RB. Glomerulocystic kidney. Report of a case. Arch Pathol Lab Med. 1976;100:186-8.

CONTRIBUTIONS BY:

1. Dr Jayshree M, Additional Professor, Department of Pediatrics (Clinician In-Charge)
2. Dr Karthi N, Professor, Department of Pediatrics (Clinician In-Charge)
3. Dr Venkataseshan S, Professor, Department of Pediatrics—Neonatology Division (Clinician In-Charge)
4. Dr Arun Baranwal, Professor, Department of Pediatrics (Compilation of clinical details)
5. Mr Gurpreet Singh, Laboratory Technician, Immunohistochemistry, Department of Histopathology

Post Graduate Institute of Medical Education and Research, Chandigarh, India.

CASE 90

Glomerulocystic Kidney Associated with Posterior Urethral Valve—A Rare Association: PM 28255

Nandita Bharadwaj Kakkar

HIGHLIGHTS OF THE CASE

This is a classical case of posterior urethral valve leading to bilateral congenital hydronephrosis with marked dysplasia, bilateral hydroureters, hypertrophied urinary bladder and a dilated posterior urethra. Grossly and microscopically the kidneys fitted into the criteria of being called "glomerulocystic". Thus, this case illustrates that "glomerulocystic kidney" can be seen as a component of other renal cystic disorders or syndromes.

Keywords: Glomerulocystic kidney, bladder outlet obstruction, posterior urethral valve, dysplasia, primitive duct.

CLINICAL DETAILS

Date of Medical Termination of Pregnancy: 24.06.2017

This was a 26-year-old female, gravida 3, with two previous abortions, both were induced due to marital discord during her first marriage. She remarried, conceived for the third time and came for her routine antenatal check-up. Level 2 ultrasonography revealed single live intrauterine fetus, moderately reduced liquor, distended urinary bladder (3.9 cm), posterior urethra dilated, both ureters dilated, both kidneys measured 1.8–1.9 cm with increased echogenicity and mild cardiomegaly. A diagnosis of bladder outlet obstruction consistent with posterior urethral valve was made. Medical termination of pregnancy was done at 19 weeks gestation and the baby was sent for autopsy after taking consent from the parents.

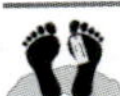

AUTOPSY FINDINGS: PM 28255

It was a male baby weighing 175 g. Crown-heal/crown-rump—17/11 cm, head/chest/abdominal circumference—14/13/15 cm and foot length—2.5 cm. The abdomen was visibly distended. On opening the abdomen, the urinary bladder was markedly distended and contained urine. Both ***kidneys*** (Fig 1A) measured 1.3 × 1 × 0.5 cm, the reniform shape was maintained and fetal lobulations were discernable. The capsular aspect (Figs 1A and C) showed tiny pinhead-sized cysts present diffusely, giving it a spongy appearance. Cut section of the kidney (Figs 1B and D) revealed dilatation of the pelvicalyceal system with a thin peripheral rim of renal tissue, showing no corticomedullary differentiation and riddled with tiny cysts, present diffusely, giving it a spongy appearance. Both ureters were dilated and the urinary bladder was enlarged, hypertrophied and contained urine (Figs 1A and B). The posterior part of the urethra (Figs 2A and B) was dilated and the obstruction, i.e. a posterior urethral valve was present beyond it. Microscopic examination of the ***kidneys*** (Figs 2C–E) revealed lobar disorganization, small cysts, predominantly confined to the peripheral cortex, but in areas they were present more diffusely in the entire rim of renal tissue. No corticomedullary distinction was identifiable. A large percentage of the cysts were glomerular (Figs 3A–F), showing dilatation of the Bowman's space 2–3 times the normal and more than 5% cysts contained atrophic glomeruli, thus fulfilling the Bernstein criteria of calling the kidney "glomerulocystic". In some cysts the atrophic glomeruli could be seen as small excrescences (Figs 3D and E). In between the glomeruli (Figs 4A and B), plenty of primitive ducts with a collar of immature mesenchyme could be seen. Foci of extramedullary hematopoiesis were seen. The would be medulla (Fig 4C) also showed metaplastic tissue, i.e. immature mesenchyme and primitive ducts. There was bilateral ureteric dilatation, urinary bladder was hypertrophied and the posterior urethra was dilated, distal to which the obstruction, i.e. the posterior urethral valve was discernable. The degree of ureteric and bladder abnormality was compatible with the renal parenchymal disarray and dysplasia. The ***lungs*** (Figs 4D and E) were normal in

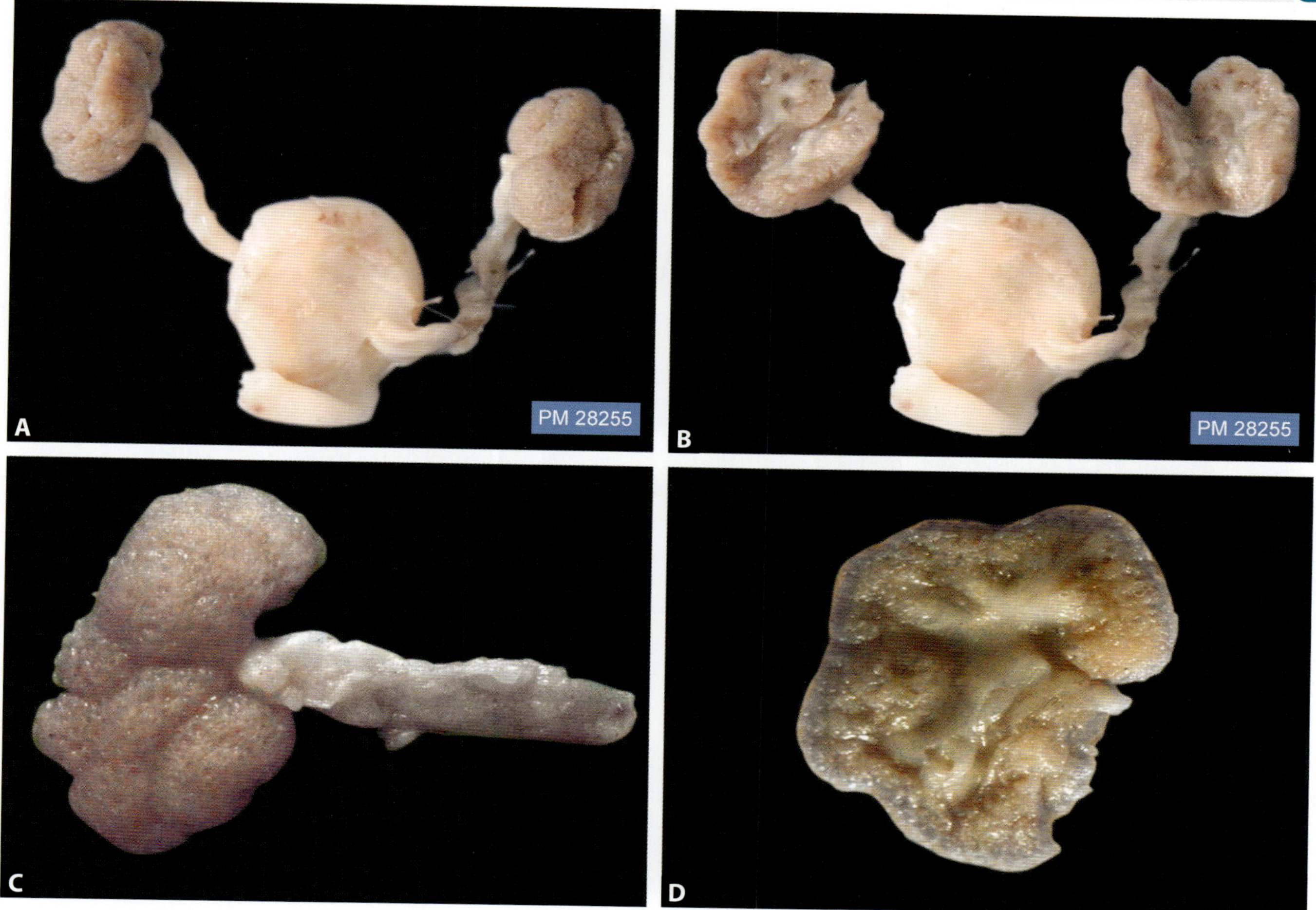

Figs 1A–D: (A) Gross picture of the kidneys showing maintained reniform shape/fetal lobulations. Tiny cysts are present diffusely on the capsular aspect giving a sponge like appearance, ureters are dilated, and the urinary bladder is hypertrophied; (B) Cut section of the kidneys showing dilated pelvicalyceal system; (C) Capsular aspect of the kidney showing tiny pinhead-sized cysts present diffusely giving it a spongy-like appearance. Note the normal fetal lobulations and maintained reniform shape. The ureter is dilated; (D) Cut section of the kidney showing dilatation of the pelvicalyceal system and a thin rim of renal tissue showing no corticomedullary distinction, but studded with tiny cysts present diffusely.

weight and there was no hypoplasia. Microscopy showed pseudoglandular stage, compatible with period of gestation. The heart was within normal limits. No cardiomegaly was noted. The liver (Figs 4F and G) was normal grossly and showed extramedullary hematopoiesis compatible with period of gestation. No ductal plate malformation was seen. Other organs including brain were within normal limits.

FINAL AUTOPSY DIAGNOSIS: PM 28255

MTP done at 19 Weeks Gestation for Bladder Outlet Obstruction

- Posterior urethral valve leading to - Congenital bilateral hydroureteronephrosis with marked dysplasia, hypertrophied urinary bladder and dilated posterior urethra.
- Glomerulocystic kidney (Group 2), secondary to Posterior urethral valve.

For glomerulocystic kidney—Refer to PM 28154 - Case 89

For posterior urethral valve—Refer to PM 18485 - Case 82

COMMENTARY—INDEX CASE: PM 28255

This is a classical case of posterior urethral valve leading to bilateral congenital hydronephrosis with dysplasia, bilateral hydroureters, hypertrophied urinary bladder and a dilated posterior urethra. Grossly the kidneys (index case) showed a maintained reniform shape, fetal lobulations were discernable, each measured 1.3 × 1 × 0.5 cm and the capsular aspect was sponge like, with tiny pinhead-sized cysts.

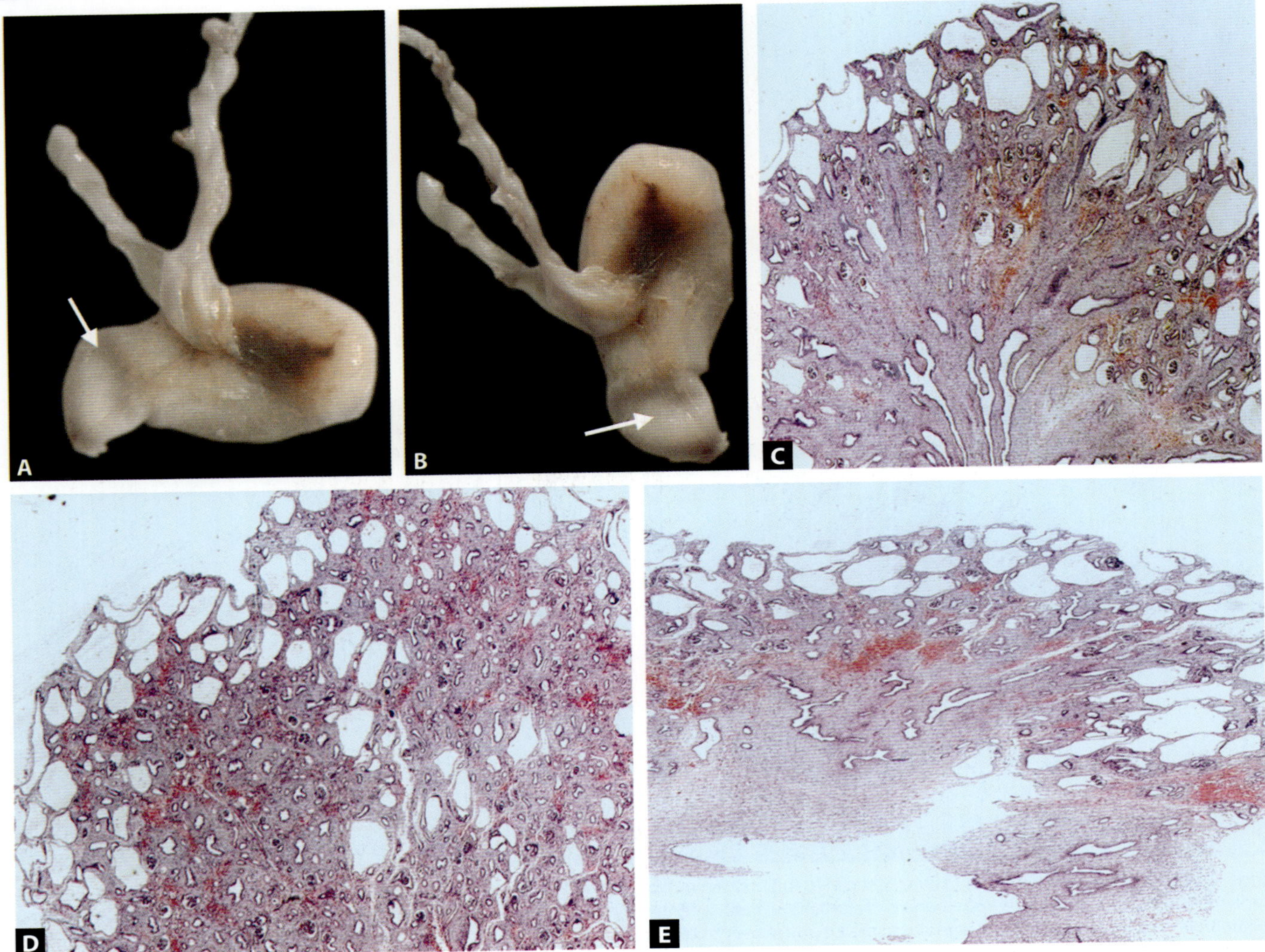

Figs 2A–E: (A and B) Gross picture of the hypertrophied urinary bladder and dilated posterior urethra (white arrows) proximal to the posterior urethral valve; (C to E) Photomicrographs of the kidney at low power showing innumerable peripherally placed cysts with the inner cortex and would be medulla showing metaplastic renal parenchyma.

Cut section of the kidneys revealed dilatation of the pelvicalyceal system with a thin peripheral rim of renal tissue showing no corticomedullary differentiation and riddled with tiny cysts, present diffusely (in the entire rim) giving it a spongy appearance. This external gross appearance of the kidneys is seen in autosomal recessive polycystic kidney disease and in true glomerulocystic kidney disease (Group 1). In autosomal recessive polycystic kidney, the cut section however shows a sunray appearance, wherein longitudinal cysts starting from the medulla end just below the capsular surface and there is no pelvicalyceal dilatation. In true glomerulocystic kidney disease, i.e. Group 1, the external appearance is the same with maintained reniform shape/fetal lobulations and the capsular aspect sponge like, with tiny pinhead-sized cysts. But the cut section generally shows a distinct corticomedullary distinction and the cysts are truly peripheral, present only in the cortex, with no cyst seen in the medulla.

On microscopic examination, the kidneys in the index case can be termed as "glomerulocystic" as a prominent glomerulocystic change was present fulfilling the Bernstein criteria of "Bowman's space—2 to 3 times the normal and more than 5% cysts contained atrophic glomeruli". A large number of cysts in the index case were glomerulocysts with a dilated Bowman's space and many cysts contained an atrophic or rudimentary glomeruli seated at one end. There was no corticomedullary distinction and the entire rim of renal tissue was riddled with cysts. This is however not seen in the true glomerulocystic kidney disease, i.e. Group 1,

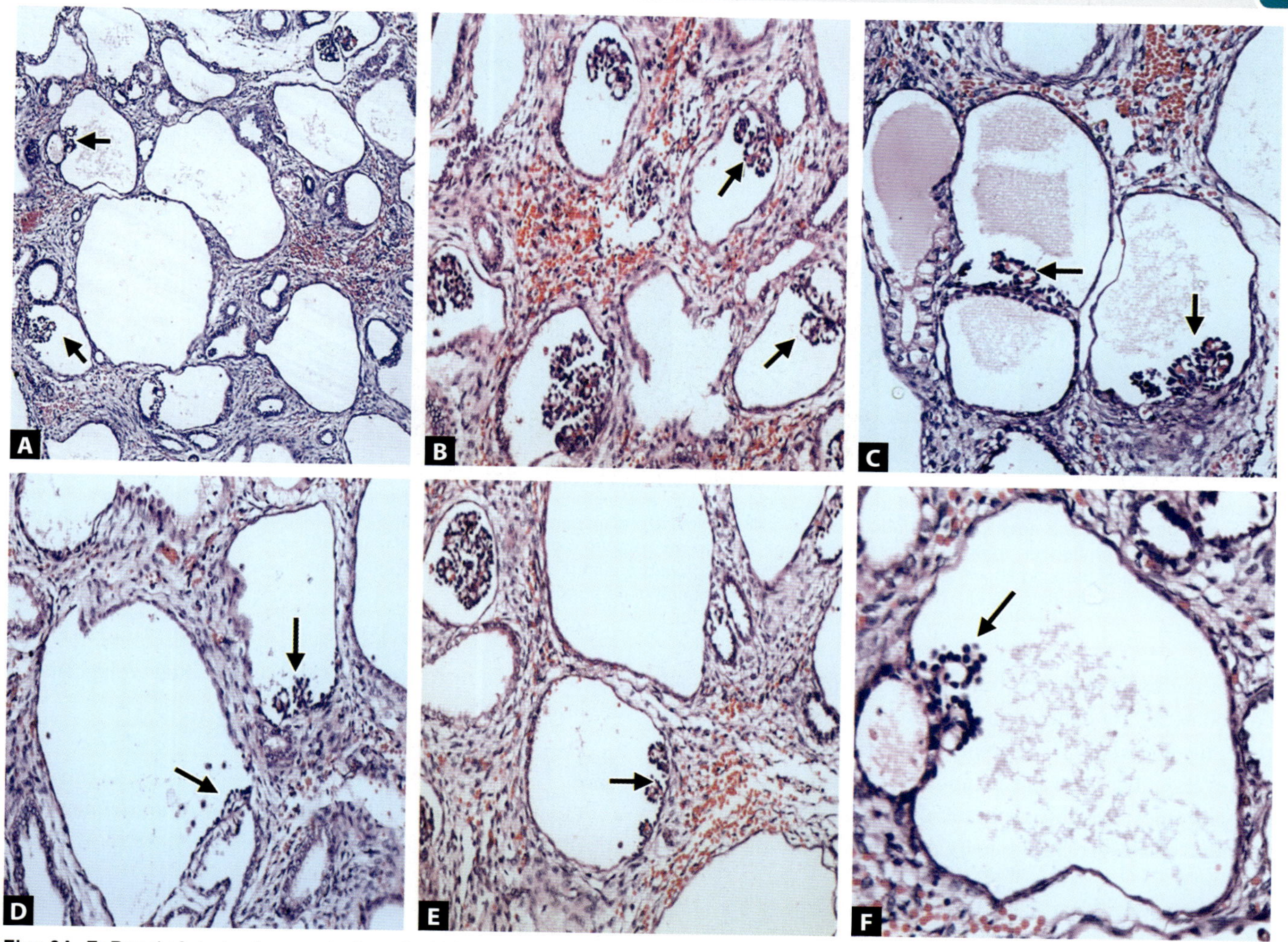

Figs 3A–F: Panel of photomicrographs from the kidney showing a prominent glomerulocystic change with markedly distended glomerular space and many cysts showing atrophic glomerular tufts (arrows).

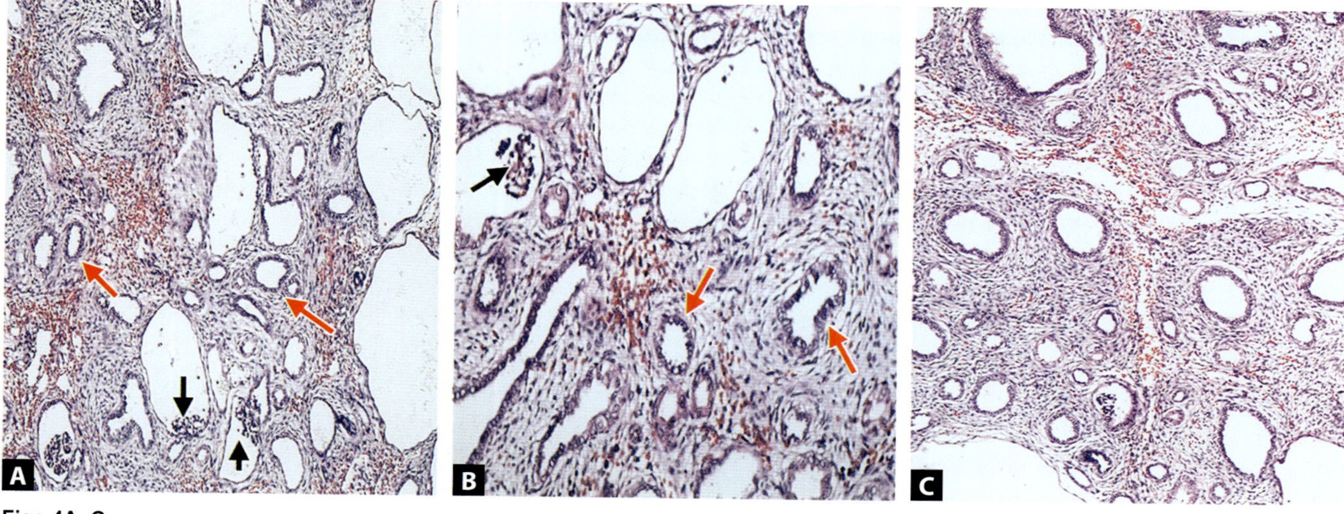

Figs 4A–C:

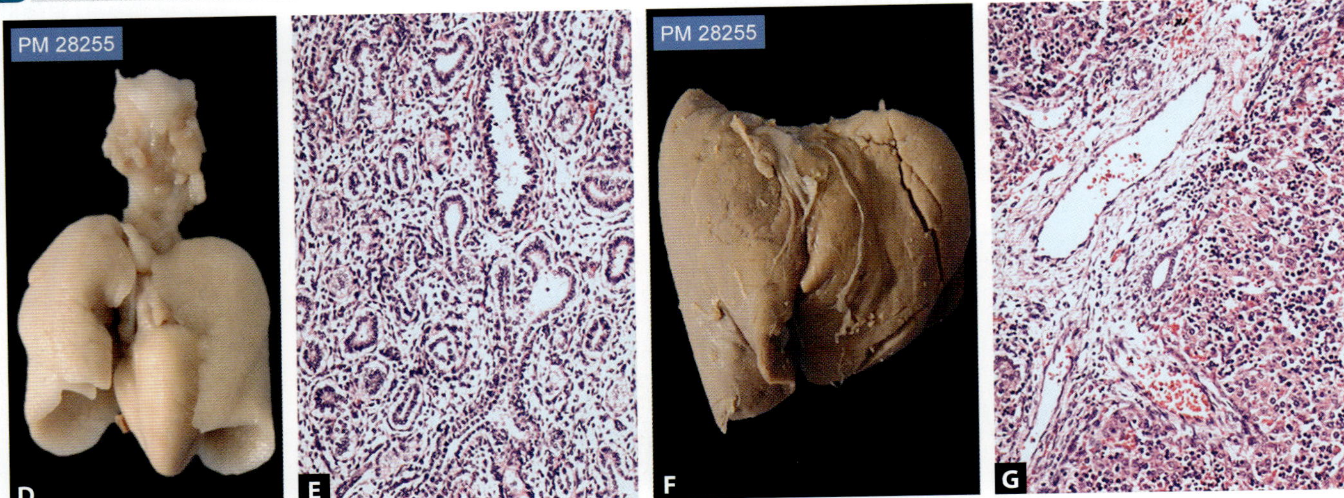

Figs 4D–G: (A and B) Photomicrograph of the kidney showing cysts, many glomerular cysts with remnant of atrophic glomeruli (black arrows). In between the cysts are seen primitive ducts with a collar of immature mesenchyme (red arrows); (C) Medullary region showing clusters of primitive ducts embedded in immature mesenchymel; (D) Organ complex comprising of both lungs and the heart which are normal; (E) Photomicrograph of the lung showing pseudoglandular stage of development; (F) Gross picture of the normal liver; (G) Liver shows prominent extramedullary hematopoiesis and a normal portal tract with no ductal plate abnormality.

where the cysts are seen only in the peripheral cortex and corticomedullary distinction is generally present, although at times the medullary development may be abnormal. Glomerular cysts can be seen as a component of other cystic diseases or syndromes, i.e. diffuse cystic dysplasia, Meckel–Gruber, Ivemark syndrome, prune belly syndrome, glutaric aciduria type 2, etc. Glomerulocystic kidney associated with posterior urethral valve has not been reported.

TAKE HOME MESSAGE

- Glomerulocystic kidney can be seen as a component of other cystic diseases or syndromes.

CONTRIBUTIONS BY:

1. Dr Vanita Suri, Professor and Head, Department of Obstetrics and Gynecology (Clinician In-Charge)
2. Dr Pranjali Vasisht, Fellow, Post-Doctoral Course, Pediatric Pathology

Post Graduate Institute of Medical Education and Research, Chandigarh, India.

Section 15F: Syndromes

CASE 91-92

Meckel–Gruber Syndrome: PM 20070, PM 26190

Nandita Bharadwaj Kakkar

CASE 91: PM 20070

HIGHLIGHTS OF THE CASE

An unbooked primigravida delivered a fresh still birth at 33 weeks gestation, wherein ultrasonography at admission revealed a brain abnormality, ? microcephaly ?? anencephaly and bilateral enlarged, echogenic kidneys, ? autosomal recessive polycystic kidney disease (ARPKD). At autopsy a diagnosis of Meckel–Gruber syndrome was made as there was anencephaly, polydactyly, bilateral multicystic dysplastic kidneys and ductal plate malformation.

Keywords: Meckel–Gruber syndrome, autosomal recessive, multicystic dysplastic kidneys, encephalocele, ductal plate malformation, polydactyly, autopsy.

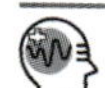

CLINICAL DETAILS

A primigravida, at 33 weeks gestation, underwent an assisted breech vaginal delivery. The baby was a fresh still birth, female with multiple congenital malformations. The pregnancy was unsupervised. There was no history of bleeding per vaginum, fever, drug intake or consanguinity. A day before being referred to our institute, there was leaking per vaginum and handling by a midwife. Ultrasonography done at admission revealed a single live fetus, breech, placenta in upper uterine segment, liquor grossly reduced, head small and skull vault appeared to be deformed, ? microcephaly ?? anencephaly, no definite evidence of spina bifida, mild scoliotic deformity of the spine present, bilateral kidneys enlarged and echogenic ? ARPKD. Soon after admission, intrauterine death occurred and baby was born by assisted breech vaginal delivery. Baby was sent for autopsy after permission from the parents.

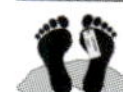

AUTOPSY FINDINGS CASE 91: PM 20070

The baby was a fresh still birth, female and weighed 1,900 g. There was anencephaly and all four limbs showed polydactyly. The abdomen was distended and congenital talipes equinovarus (CTEV) was noted. The kidneys together weighed 302 g, were symmetrically, massively, enlarged (10 × 8 × 4 cm and 9.5 × 8 × 4 cm), fetal lobulations were prominent and no cysts were seen on the surface (Fig 1A). Cut section (Fig 1B) showed small rounded cysts present diffusely and no corticomedullary distinction was appreciated. The ureters and urinary bladder were normal. Microscopic examination of the kidneys (Figs 1C–E and 2A–C) revealed small round to oval cysts, present diffusely and the intervening areas showed classical primitive ducts surrounded by a collar of immature mesenchyme, proliferating nerves, abortive glomeruli and tubules, cartilage and foci of extramedullary hematopoiesis. Overall features were those of bilateral multicystic dysplastic kidneys. The liver (Fig 2D) weighed 85 g and was firm to feel. Microscopic examination (Fig 2E) revealed expanded portal tracts containing plenty of abnormally angulated biliary channels along with porto-portal bridging fibrosis, consistent with a diagnosis of ductal plate malformation. The lungs (Fig 2F) together weighed 15 g and were hypoplastic.

FINAL AUTOPSY DIAGNOSIS CASE 91: PM 20070

Fresh Still-birth at 33 Weeks Gestation, Weighing 1900 gms

Consistent with Meckel–Gruber syndrome

- Anencephaly
- Polydactyly (all four limbs), CTEV
- Bilateral multicystic dysplastic kidneys
- Ductal plate malformation–liver
- Hypoplastic lungs.

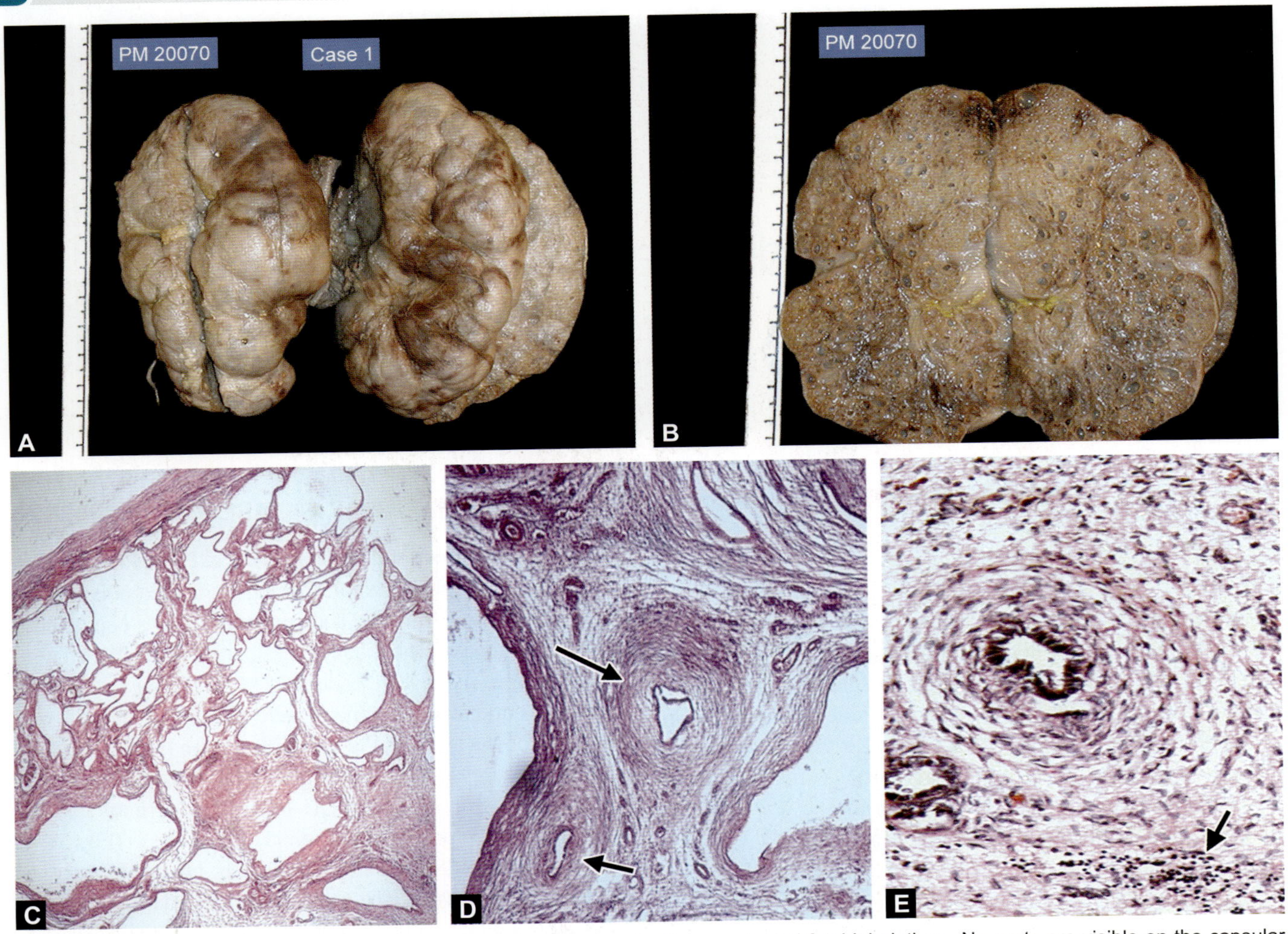

Figs 1A–E: (A) Both kidneys show bilateral symmetrical enlargement with accentuated fetal lobulations. No cysts are visible on the capsular aspect; (B) Cut section of the kidney show rounded cysts scattered diffusely. Photomicrographs of the kidney; (C) Show total parenchymal disorganization with diffusely scattered round cysts; and (D) Cysts of varying sizes with interspersed primitive ducts (arrows); (E) Classical primitive duct with a collar of immature mesenchyme and a focus of extramedullary hematopoiesis (arrow).

CASE 92: PM 26190

HIGHLIGHTS OF THE CASE

A booked primigravida underwent a medical termination of pregnancy at 16 weeks gestation in view of ultrasonographic detection of Meckel–Gruber syndrome.

CLINICAL DETAILS

A booked primigravida at 16 weeks gestation was detected on ultrasonography to have occipital encephalocele, micrognathia, bilateral enlargement of both kidneys with cysts, occupying the entire abdomen, polydactyly and flexion deformity at knees and wrists. A diagnosis of Meckel–Gruber syndrome was considered and a medical termination of pregnancy was done. Baby was sent for autopsy.

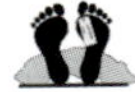

AUTOPSY FINDINGS CASE 92: PM 26190

It was female fetus weighing 64 g (16 weeks gestation). On external examination, the abdomen was distended (Fig 3A-long arrows), there was occipital encephalocele (Fig 3A-upper most arrow), micrognathia, flexion deformity at knees (Fig 3A) and wrists and polydactyly, i.e. six fingers in all four limbs (Figs 3B–E). In situ examination revealed bilateral, symmetrical, massive enlargement of both kidneys showing cysts on the capsular aspect (Figs 4A and B) and

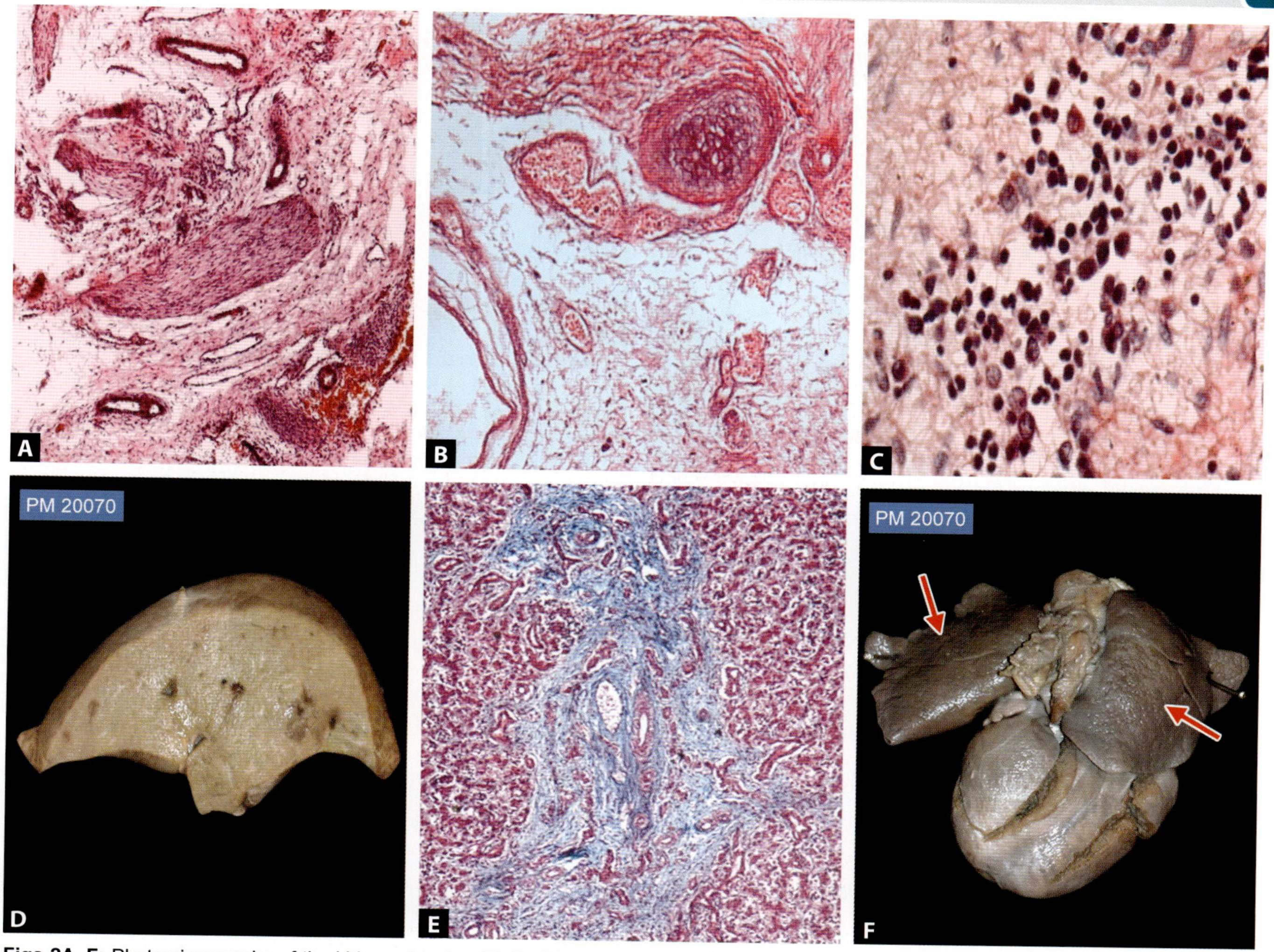

Figs 2A–F: Photomicrographs of the kidney showing (A) Proliferating nerves; (B) Metaplastic cartilage; and (C) Foci of extramedullary hematopoiesis; (D) Coronal slice of the liver which is firm to feel; (E) Photomicrograph of the liver showing expanded portal tracts with porto-portal bridging fibrosis and plenty of angulated biliary channels (Masson's trichrome stain). The sinusoids show extramedullary hematopoiesis; (F) Heart–lung complex showing bilateral lung hypoplasia (arrows).

hypoplastic lungs (Fig 4A- red arrows). Microscopy of both the kidneys revealed complete lobar disorganization and diffusely present rounded cysts with interspersed classical primitive ducts. Overall features in the kidneys were consistent with a diagnosis of bilateral multicystic dysplasia. The liver exhibited early phase of ductal plate malformation.

 FINAL AUTOPSY DIAGNOSIS: PM 26190

16 Weeks Gestation, Female Abortus, MTP, 64 gms

Consistent with Meckel–Gruber syndrome

- Anencephaly
- Polydactyly (all four limbs), CTEV
- Bilateral multicystic dysplastic kidneys
- Ductal plate malformation—liver
- Hypoplastic lungs.

MECKEL–GRUBER SYNDROME

Meckel–Gruber syndrome was first reported by Johann Friedrich Meckel way back in 1822. It was in 1934, that G B Gruber published more reports of this entity and it finally came to be known as Meckel–Gruber syndrome. Meckel-Gruber syndrome[1-3] is a lethal ciliopathy, an autosomal recessive disorder, characterized by the triad of occipital encephalocele and/or other central nervous system malformations, bilateral multicystic dysplastic kidneys and postaxial polydactyly. The fourth consistent finding seen in MKS is ductal plate malformation and instead of the triad it should be called a

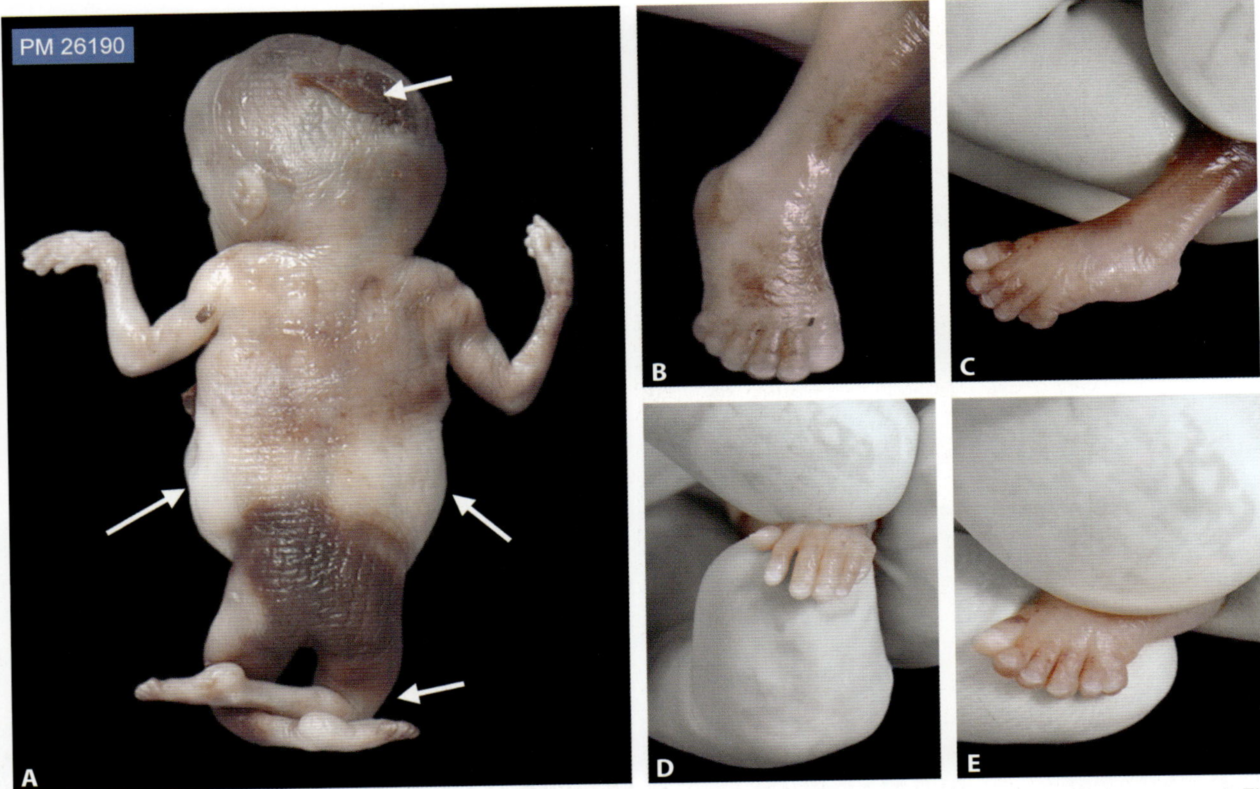

Figs 3A–E: (A) Dorsal aspect of the abortus showing abdominal distension (middle arrows) and occipital encephalocele (upper arrow). Flexion deformity of the knees is seen (lower arrow); (B and C) Polydactyly of both feet (six toes each); (D and E) Polydactyly of both hands (six fingers each).

tetrad. Being autosomal recessive, every pregnancy has a 25% chance of getting affected. Other abnormalities noted are cleft lip/palate, microphthalmia, micrognathia, webbed neck, ear anomalies, heart defects (VSD, aortic stenosis, aortic hypoplasia and aortic co-arctation), talipes, defects of the external/internal genitalia, cryptorchidism, urethral atresia and omphalocele. Other CNS abnormalities (apart from encephalocele) seen are Dandy–Walker/Arnold–Chiari malformations, cerebral/cerebellar hypoplasia, anencephaly, microcephaly, hydrocephalus, holoprosencephaly and agenesis of corpus callosum, olfactory lobes/tracts and septum pellucidum. This condition is incompatible with life and most babies are still born or die within few hours or days after birth. The live born are generally preterm babies with birth weight less than 2,500 g. Pulmonary hypoplasia is the leading cause of death. Male to female ration is equal.

This syndrome shows marked genetic heterogeneity[4] and has been mapped to 12 different loci on a number of chromosomes. These[4] are 17q21-24 (MKS1), 11q13 (MKS2), 8q21.13-q22.1 (MKS3), 12q21.31-q21.33 (MKS4), 16q12.2 (MKS5), 4p15.3 (MKS6), 3q22.1 (MKS7), 12q24.31 (MKS8), 17p11.2 (MKS9), 19q13.2 (MKS10), 16q23.1 (MKS11) and 1q32.1 (MKS12). 17q21-24 codes a part of the flagellar apparatus involved in the functioning of the cilia. The MKS3 encodes a seven-transmembrane receptor protein, meckelin. Primary cilia are organelles found on the surface of epithelial cells and help in organ development and the above mentioned proteins are involved in their correct functioning. Worldwide incidence of MKS varies from 1/13,250 to 1/140,000 live births. High incidence is seen in Finland[5] (1/9,000 live births, carrier rate 1 in 50), Belgium/Kuwait (1/3,500, carrier rate 1 in 30), Gujarati Indians[6] (1/1,300, carrier rate 1 in 18), Arab countries and Pakistan. Prevalence is higher in population with the higher consanguinity. Pregnancies with MKS show the an elevated alfa-fetoprotein level by 12 weeks gestation in amniotic fluid and after 15 weeks gestation in the maternal blood. By the 14th week of gestation, all cases of MKS on ultrasonography show occipital encephalocele, postaxial polydactyly and bilateral enlarged multicystic kidneys with unusual corticomedullary differentiation. Once the oligohydramnios sets

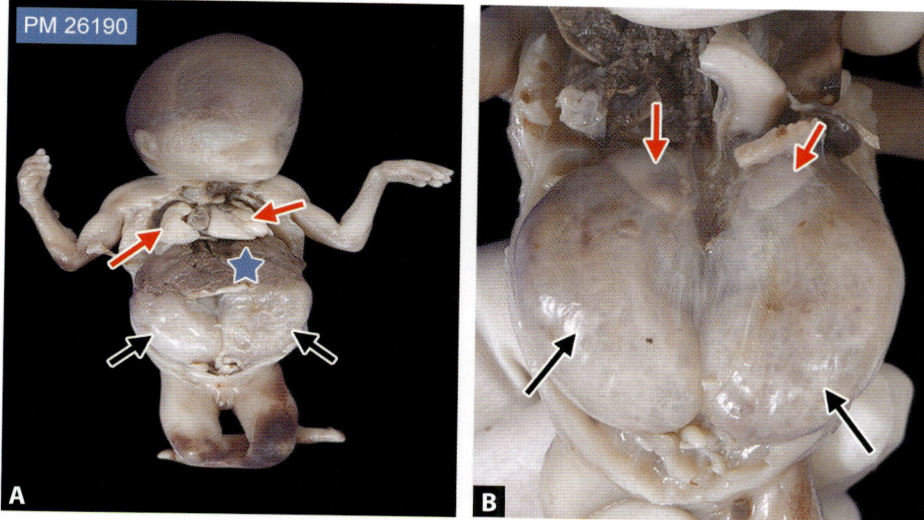

Figs 4A and B: In situ examination of the abortus showing bilateral symmetrically enlarged kidneys (black arrows) filling the entire abdominal cavity. In "A", the liver (star) is seen and both lungs are hypoplastic (red arrows). In "B", cysts are discernable below the capsule (black arrows) and adrenals (red arrows) are appreciated.

in, the detection of encephalocele and polydactyly becomes difficult. Salonen et al.[7] reported kidney and liver involvement in 100% cases, occipital encephalocele in 85% (rest had other CNS malformation) and polydactyly in 96%.

Occipital encephalocele[8] is characterized by herniation of brain components via the widened posterior fontanelle. Of the classic triad of MKS, polydactyly[9] is the most variable feature. It generally involves all four extremities. Kidneys[10] show massive bilateral symmetrical enlargement (10–20 times their normal size) with preserved fetal lobulations. Capsular aspect is smooth and does not show any cysts. Cut section shows small rounded cysts distributed all over. The ureters and urinary bladder are normal. Microscopic examination shows cysts, interspersed with primitive ducts, abortive glomeruli or tubules and other elements seen in dysplastic kidneys like foci of extramedullary hematopoiesis, proliferating nerves and metaplastic cartilage. Grossly and microscopically the main differential diagnosis is from an ARPKD. ARPKD also show a massive (10–20 times their normal size), bilateral, symmetrical enlargement of the kidneys, but the capsular aspect shows a myriad of pinhead-sized cysts, cut section shows radially arranged cysts giving a sunray appearance, microscopy shows longitudinal cysts interspersed with normal glomeruli and tubules and no dysplastic elements. Liver shows characteristic ductal plate in all cases of MKS and ARPKD. Central nervous system malformations and polydactyly are not seen in ARPKD.

COMMENTARY—INDEX CASES: PM 20070, PM 26190

They are both classical cases (33 weeks and 16 weeks gestation, respectively) of Meckel–Gruber syndrome. Both were primigravidas and their next pregnancies have a 25% of recurrence and hence proper monitoring in the subsequent pregnancy is mandatory.

TAKE HOME MESSAGE

- Meckel–Gruber syndrome is an autosomal recessive disorder.
- It is characterized by the tetrad of occipital encephalocele and/or other central nervous system malformations, bilateral multicystic dysplastic kidneys, postaxial polydactyly and ductal plate malformation.

REFERENCES

1. Barisic I, Boban L, Loane M, et al. Meckel-Gruber Syndrome: a population-based study on prevalence, prenatal diagnosis, clinical features and survival in Europe. Eur J Hum Genet. 2015;23(6):746-52.
2. Parelkar SV, Kapadnis SP, Sanghvi BV, et al. Meckel-Gruber syndrome: A rare and lethal anomaly with review of literature. J Pediatr Neurosci. 2013;8(2):154-7.
3. Wright C, Healicon R, English C, et al. Meckel syndrome: what are the minimum diagnostic criteria? J Med Genet. 1994;31(6):482-5.
4. Paavola P, Salonen R, Baumer A. Clinical and genetic heterogeneity in Meckel syndrome. Hum Genet. 1997;101(1):88-92.

5. Salonen R, Norio R. The Meckel syndrome in Finland: epidemiologic and genetic aspects. Am J Med Genet. 1984; 18(4):691-8.
6. Young ID, Rickett AB, Clerke M. High incidence of Meckel's syndrome in Gujarati Indians. J Med Genet. 1985;22: 301-4.
7. Salonen R. The Meckel syndrome: Clinicopathological findings in 67 patients. Am J Med Genet. 1984;18(4): 671-89.
8. Ahdab-Barmada M, Claassen D. A distinctive triad of malformations of the central nervous system in the Meckel-Gruber syndrome. J Neuropathol Exp Neurol. 1990;49(6):610-20.
9. Alexiev BA, Lin X, Sun CC. Meckel-Gruber syndrome: pathologic manifestations, minimal diagnostic criteria and differential diagnosis. Arch Pathol Lab Med. 2006;130(8): 1236-8.
10. Blankenberg TA, Ruebner BH, Ellis WG. Pathology of renal and hepatic anomalies in Meckel syndrome. Am J Med Gen. 1987;3:395-410.

CONTRIBUTIONS BY:

Case 91

1. Dr Sarla Malhotra, Ex-Professor and Head, Department of Obstetrics and Gynecology (Clinician In-Charge)

Case 92

1. Dr Neelam Chaudhary, Department of Obstetrics and Gynecology (Clinician In-Charge)
2, Dr Suravi Mohanty, Fellow, Post-doctoral Course Pediatric Pathology

Post Graduate Institute of Medical Education and Research, Chandigarh, India.

CASE 93-94

Prune Belly Syndrome Leading to a Markedly Distended Urinary Bladder and Hydroureteronephrosis: PM 23424, PM 25509

Nandita Bharadwaj Kakkar

CASE 93: PM 23424

HIGHLIGHTS OF THE CASE

A 23-year-old, gravida 2 mother, came for her first antenatal visit at 29 weeks gestation. Ultrasonography (USG) revealed oligohydramnios and a large (12 × 9 cm) thick-walled cystic lesion in the abdomen with mild hydronephrosis, ? pelvic cystic mass ? overdistended bladder with posterior urethral valve. Clinical possibilities were prune belly syndrome (PBS) or posterior urethral valve. Baby died at 1 hour 30 minutes of life. Autopsy was consistent with a diagnosis of PBS.

Keywords: Prune belly syndrome, congenital hydronephrosis, dysplasia, hydroureters, megacystis, cryptorchidism, Potter facies, hypoplastic lungs, autopsy.

CLINICAL DETAILS

Date of Birth: 21.11.2009, Date of Death: 21.11.2009, Lived for 1 and Half Hours.

A 23-year-old, gravida 2 mother with one live child (G1), diagnosed with Tetralogy of Fallot (G2P1001), underwent antenatal supervision of G2 in PGIMER, Chandigarh after 29 weeks gestation. The index case ***G2***, a male baby, was a preterm spontaneous normal vaginal delivery, born at 34 weeks gestation and weighed 3.2 kg at birth, i.e. was large for date. The baby was depressed at birth and the APGAR score was 1, 1, 1, 1 at 1, 5, 10, 20 minutes. The heart rate was less than 100 at 1, 5, 10 minutes, apnea was present and baby was cyanosed. The mother had a spontaneous conception and was sure of her dates. There was no history of any drug intake, or of any medical illness. She came for the first antenatal visit at 29 weeks gestation. Earliest USG was done at an outside facility at ***28 weeks*** gestation and it revealed mild hydronephrosis of both kidneys with a large abdominopelvic mass with thickened wall and multiple diverticuli ? dilated urinary bladder. ***USG at 30 + 3 weeks*** gestation at PGI showed a large thick-walled cystic lesion, 12 × 9 cm, showing multiple internal echoes, seemed to be arising from pelvic cavity, causing compression of lower vesicourethral junction, causing bilateral hydronephrosis, ? pelvic cystic mass ? overdistended bladder with posterior urethral valve. ***Fetal MRI*:** A 14 × 12 × 4 cm sized, well-defined, T2 hyperintense fetal abdominopelvic cystic lesion with small sacculations is seen. It has narrow neck inferiorly causing fetal hydroureteronephrosis. Urinary bladder is not visualized separately ? Bladder outlet obstruction due to posterior urethral valve. Antenatal pediatric surgery consultation was sought which gave a poor prognosis in view of the severe oligohydramnios. On ***external examination***, the baby had a Potter facies and other components of oligohydramnios complex, i.e. flat facies, short neck, beaked nose, low set ear, epicanthic folds, ill-formed small chest, abdominal distension with wrinkling, redundant skin over the infraumbilical abdominal wall, short legs, congenital talipes equinovarus (CTEV) and undescended testes. ***Clinical possibilities*** were: (1) Prune belly syndrome and (2) Bladder outlet obstruction due to posterior urethral valve. Baby was put on bag mask ventilation to which he did not respond. There was persistent cyanosis with saturation of 30–40%. Parents were told about the expected outcome and were not willing for further care. Compassionate care with intravenous (IV) fluid and O_2 was given and the baby expired at 1 hour 30 minutes of life.

AUTOPSY FINDINGS: PM 23424

A complete autopsy was performed. The baby weighed 3,200 g (34 weeks gestation). Anthropometric measurements—crown

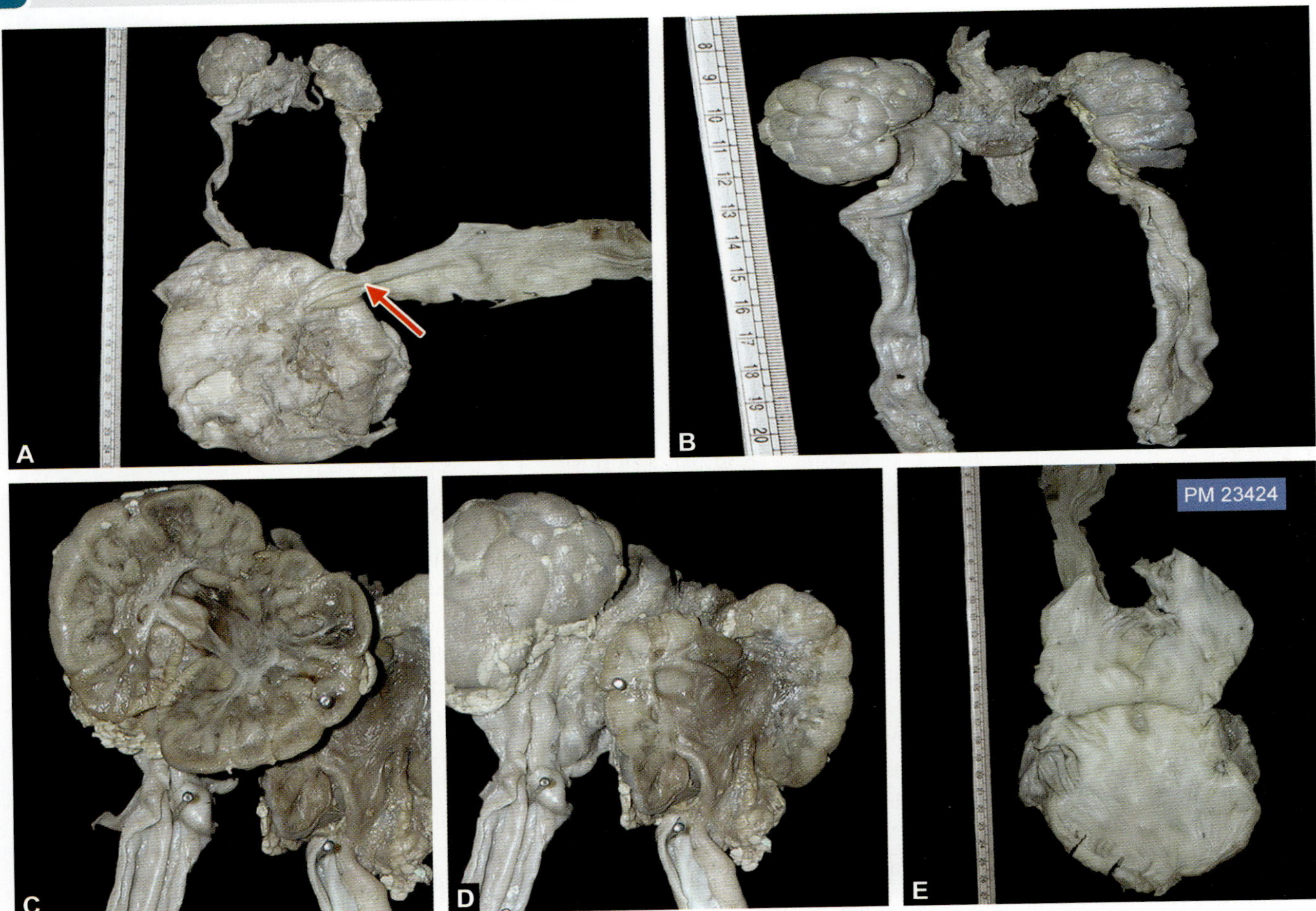

Figs 1A–E: (A) Both kidneys with dilated ureters and distended hypertrophied urinary bladder. The gut is attached blindly on the surface; (B) Enlarged kidneys with fetal lobulations and dilated tortuous ureters; (C and D) Cut section of both kidneys showing dilated pelvicalyceal system; (E) Opened up urinary bladder which is distended and has a thick wall.

heel: 43 cm, crown-rump: 29 cm, head/chest/abdominal circumference (AC): 25/26/48 cm, foot length: 5 cm. There was Potter facies with a flat face, beaked nose, bags under the eyes, epicanthic folds, low set ears and short neck. The chest was ill-formed and small. Abdominal distension along with loose wrinkled skin below the umbilicus was noted. There was bilateral CTEV. Anal opening was imperforate. The male genitalia were severely abnormal, with penile hypoplasia, urethral meatus could not be identified and a small scrotum with bilateral cryptorchidism was noted. Both kidneys (Figs 1A and B) weighed 30 g, (Normal: 17.7± 5.3), reniform shape was maintained and fetal lobulations were well seen. On cut section (Figs 1C and D), mild dilatation of the pelvicalyceal system was noted. Both the ureters were however markedly dilated (Figs 1A and B). The urinary bladder was markedly dilated with thickened wall (Figs 1A and E). The gut was blindly attached to its surface (Fig 1A- arrow). On microscopic examination, both kidneys revealed a well-preserved renal parenchyma (Figs 2A and B). No cysts were present. In the medulla, classical primitive ducts with a collar of immature mesenchyme were seen, singly as well as in clusters (Figs 2B and C-arrows). The ureters were markedly dilated and tortuous, out of proportion to the degree of renal parenchymal involvement. On microscopic examination, both the urinary bladder (Fig 2D) and the ureter (Fig 3A) showed replacement of the muscle by fibrocollagenous tissue and edema.

Overall features of bilateral congenital hydronephrosis with dysplasia, hydroureters, markedly distended/hypertrophied urinary bladder, abundant collagenous tissue seen in between the muscle fibers in the ureters/urinary bladder, wrinkled skin over the anterior abdominal wall, bilateral

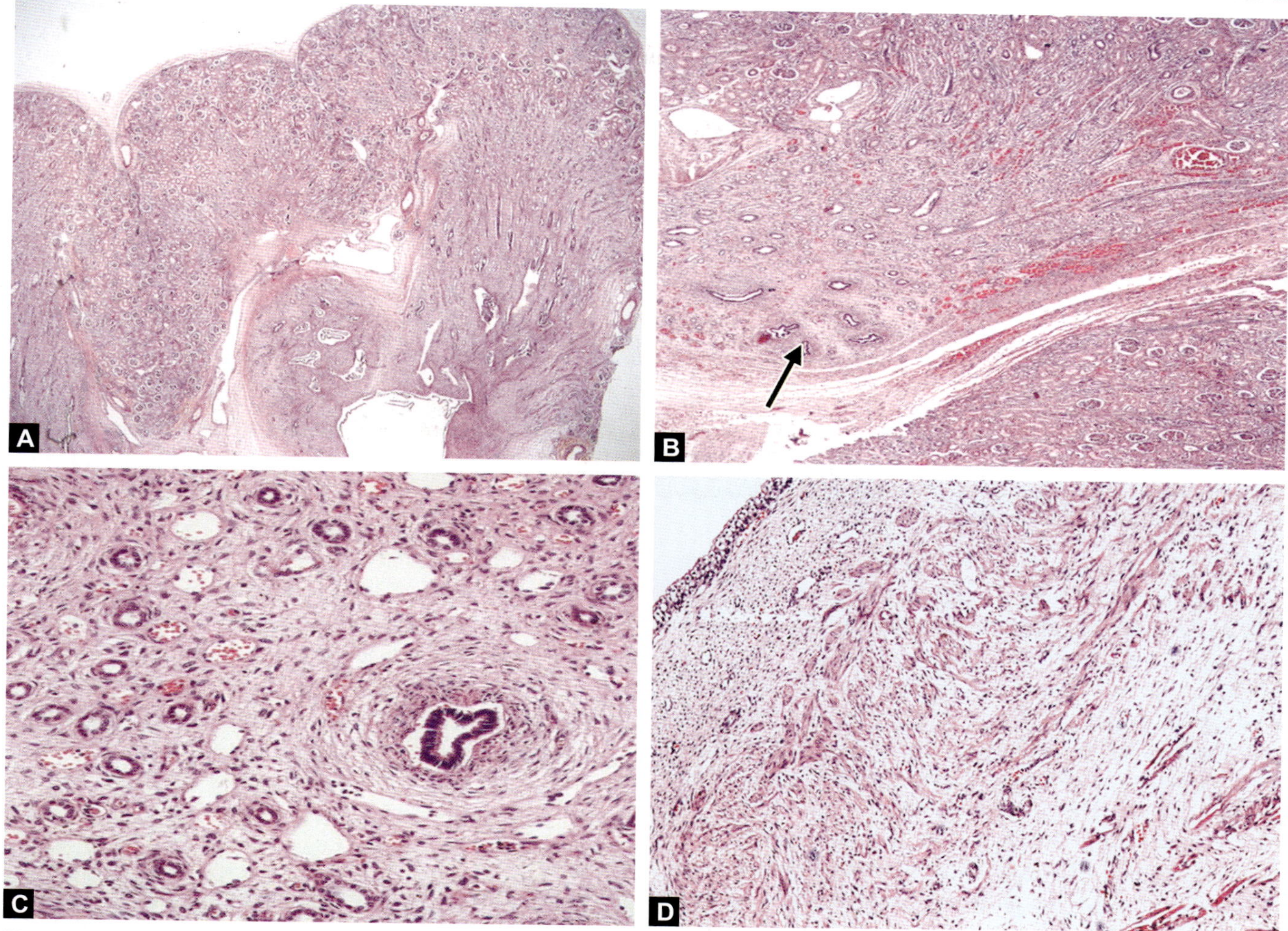

Figs 2A–D: (A and B) Photomicrograph of the kidneys showing preserved renal parenchyma. No cysts are seen. Primitive ducts seen in the medulla (arrow); (C) Primitive duct with collar of immature mesenchyme; (D) Photomicrograph of the urinary bladder showing replacement of the muscle by interweaning fibrocollagenous tissue.

cryptorchidism, hypoplastic penis without a urethral meatus, was consistent with a diagnosis of Prune belly syndrome. The lungs (Fig 3B-arrows) weighed 17 g and were hypoplastic. There was an imperforate anus and the gut was ending blindly over the urinary bladder. Other organs were within normal limits.

FINAL AUTOPSY DIAGNOSIS: PM 23424

D1 Male Baby, Lived for 1 hour 30 minutes

External appearance: Potter facies, ill-formed and small chest, abdomen distended with loose wrinkled skin, bilateral CTEV, imperforate anus, penile hypoplasia, urethral meatus not identified and small scrotum with bilateral cryptorchidism.

- Consistent with a diagnosis of (Prune Belly Syndrome (***PBS***):
    - Bilateral hydronephrosis with dysplasia, hydroureters and dilated/hypertrophied urinary bladder
    - Distended abdomen with loose wrinkled skin—"Prune belly"
    - Bilateral cryptorchidism.
- Bilateral hypoplastic lungs
- Anorectal malformation.

COMMENTARY—INDEX CASE 93: PM 23424

This is a classical case of PBS. In this case, the close differential diagnosis is posterior urethral valve. Points in favor of Pune belly syndrome are: (1) Presence of wrinkled

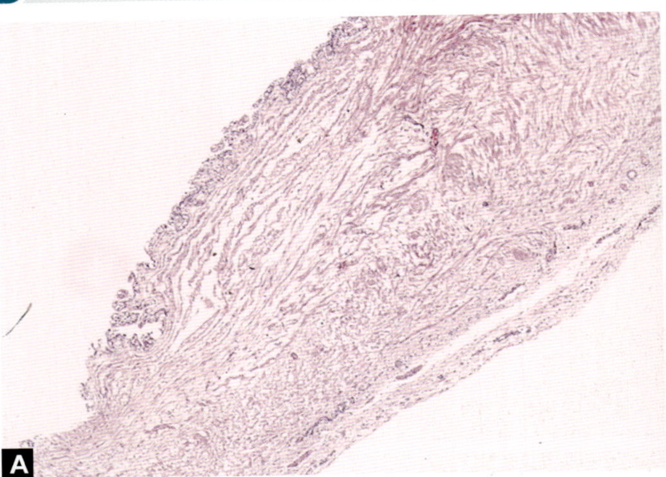

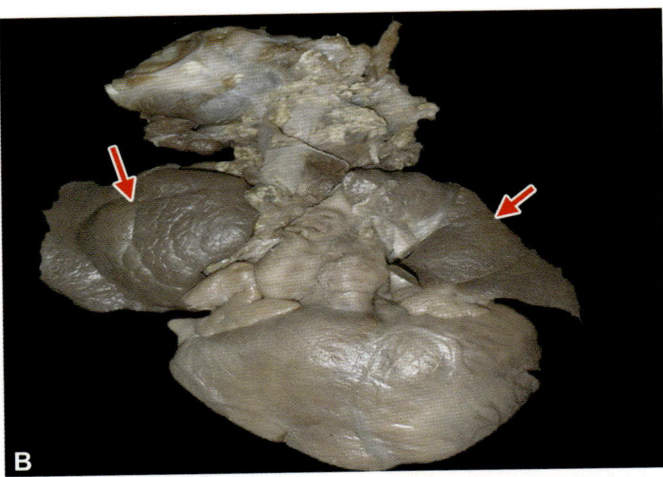

Figs 3A and B: (A) Ureter showing a thickened wall and collagenous tissue in between the muscle fibers leading to separation of the muscle fibres; (B) Heart–lung complex showing markedly hypoplastic lungs (arrows).

skin over the abdominal wall. (2) Bilateral cryptorchidism. (3) Well-preserved renal parenchyma with dysplasia seen only in the medulla. (4) Markedly distended urinary bladder showing abundant interweaning collagenous tissue. (5) Markedly dilated and tortuous ureters, out of proportion to the degree of renal parenchymal involvement. Ureters showed collagenous tissue and scanty muscle. (6) Severely abnormal male genitalia, with penile hypoplasia and unidentifiable urethral meatus. The lungs were severely hypoplastic. The normal lung weight-to-body weight ratio for term and near-term infants is 0.222 ± 0.002 and term infants is 4.4 ± 0.9. Cases in which the pulmonary hypoplasia is the direct cause of death, the lung weight is usually less than 40% of expected and is often as low as 20–30%. Histologically, the acini are small for the infant's gestational age, but alveolar and capillary development is usually consistent with the gestational age.

CASE 94: PM 25509

HIGHLIGHTS OF THE CASE

A fourth gravida with one live issue was detected with congenital malformation in her fourth pregnancy. The USG at 16 + 6 weeks revealed bilateral renal hydronephrosis, dilated ureters and a grossly distended urinary bladder, i.e. megacystis, measuring 8.5 cm in diameter. A medical termination of pregnancy (MTP) was done and the fetus was autopsied. Autopsy revealed Prune Belly Syndrome (PBS).

CLINICAL DETAILS

Medical termination of pregnancy was done on 4.7.2013, 17 + 5 week gestation.

A 28-year-old female (G4P3001), fourth gravida with one live issue and two term fetal losses was detected with congenital malformation in her fourth pregnancy. The USG at 16 + 6 weeks revealed biparietal diameter (BPD) = 15 + 3 weeks, femur length (FL) = 14 + 3 weeks, AC = 26 weeks, head circumference (HC) = 15 + 3 weeks, placentomegaly, bilateral renal hydronephrosis, dilated ureters and a grossly distended urinary bladder, measuring 8.5 cm in diameter. There was no fetal ascites or pleural effusion. A MTP was done and baby was sent for autopsy. G1 was a live born, male baby, weighed 2 kg at birth and is alive and well. G2 was a term live born male, 2.2 kg and he expired at 3 hours of life. Records however mention that the kidneys were not functioning, but there were no ultrasonographic records available. Autopsy was however not performed. G3 was a live born male, at 34 weeks gestation and weighed 1.5 kg. There was no external malformation seen, no cyanosis and the cause of death was labeled as prematurity. G4 was the index case and the pregnancy was terminated in view of the congenital malformation. It was male baby weighing 230 g, with a markedly distended abdomen.

AUTOPSY FINDINGS: PM 25509

The baby (17 + 5 weeks gestation) weighed 230 g and the abdomen was markedly distended, just like a balloon (Fig 4A). The facies were normal. The external genitalia could not be commented upon. The anthropometric measurements were—crown-heel/crown-rump length: 25/18 cm, head/chest/abdomen circumference: 12/11/18 cm, femur/foot length: 5/2 cm. The kidneys (Figs 4B and C) were mildly enlarged, measured 1 × 0.5 × 0.3 cm and showed fetal

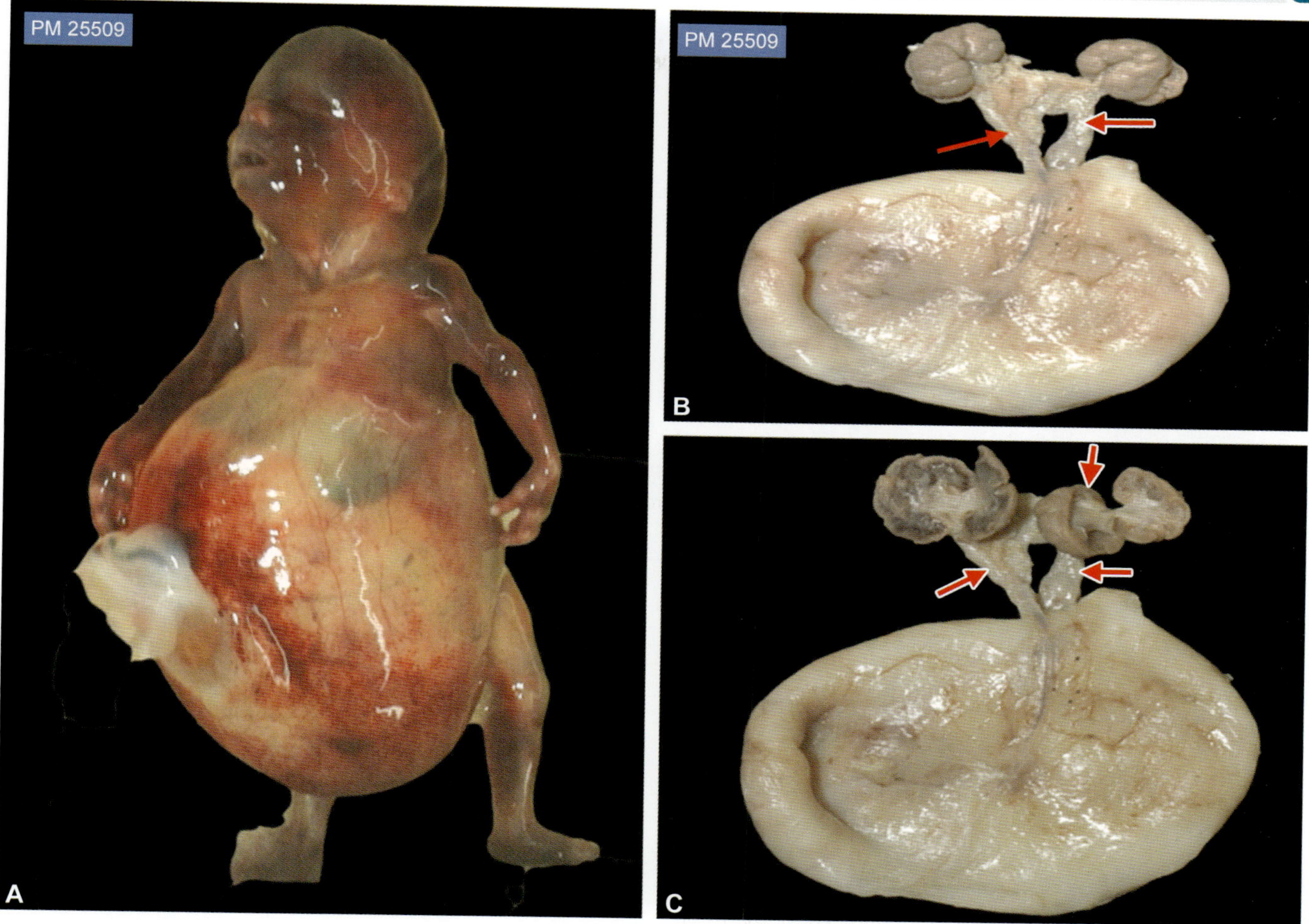

Figs 4A–C: (A) Abortus weighing 230 g and showing a markedly distended and glistening abdomen; (B) Gross photograph showing mildly enlarged kidneys with maintained fetal lobulations, dilated ureters (red arrow) and a markedly distended and glistening urinary bladder with a thick wall; (C) Cut section of both kidneys show dilatation of the pelvicalyceal system (upper arrow) and dilated ureters (red arrows).

lobulations. On cut section, the pelvicalyceal system was dilated and no cysts were appreciated. Both ureters were dilated (Figs 4B and C–arrows). The urinary bladder (Figs 4B and C) was markedly distended, contained urine, external surface was glistening, whitish in color and the wall was thick. On microscopic examination, the renal parenchyma (Figs 5A and B) was well-preserved, occasional small cyst was seen and few primitive ducts were present in the medulla (Fig 5B- arrows). There was hydronephrosis. The urinary bladder (Fig 5C) and ureter (Fig 5D) revealed extensive replacement of the detrusor muscle by fibrocollagenous tissue and edema. Marked attenuation and degeneration of the detrusor muscle fibers was noted. Both lungs were within normal limits and no hypoplasia was detected. Bilateral cryptorchidism was present.

FINAL AUTOPSY DIAGNOSIS: PM 25509

17 + 5 Weeks Gestation

- Consistent with a diagnosis of Prune Belly Syndrome (***PBS***):
  - Bilateral hydronephrosis with dysplasia, hydroureters and markedly dilated/hypertrophied urinary bladder
  - Bilateral cryptorchidism.

PRUNE BELLY SYNDROME

Prune belly syndrome is a rare congenital malformation of unknown etiology and is a triad characterized by abnormalities of the urinary tract, i.e. absence or partial obstruction of the urethra, hydroureteronephrosis with a markedly distended urinary bladder, a deficiency of abdominal musculature and bilateral cryptorchidism in males. This entity is

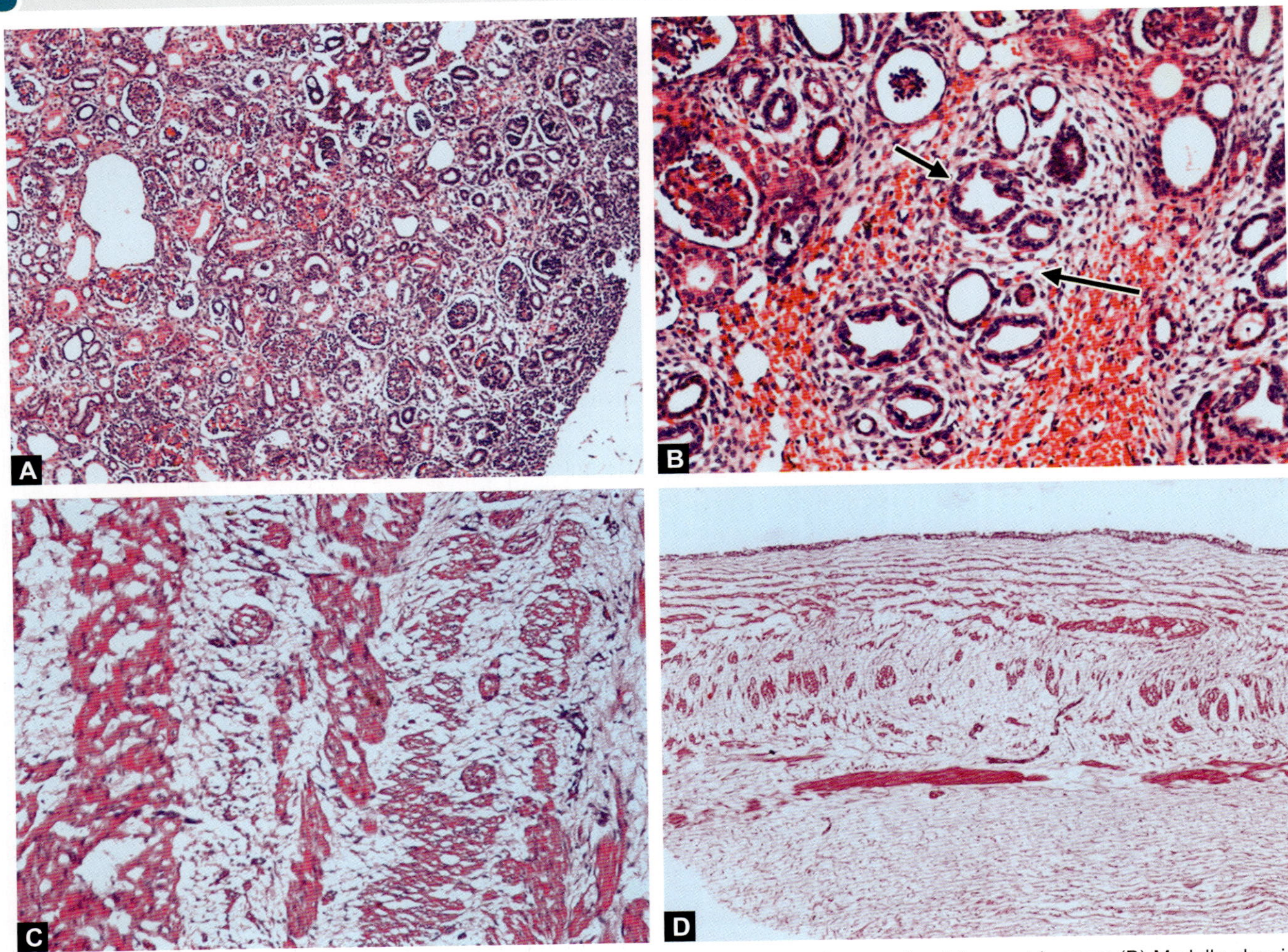

Figs 5A–D: Photomicrographs of the kidney (A) Showing preserved renal parenchyma. An occasional tiny cyst is seen; (B) Medulla showing primitive ducts (arrows); (C) Photomicrograph of the urinary bladder showing replacement of the detrusor muscle by fibrocollagenous tissue and edema; (D) Photomicrograph of the ureter showing replacement of the muscle by fibrocollagenous tissue leading to destruction of the muscle fibers.

known by a number of names like Eagle–Barrett syndrome, Obrinsky syndrome, Fröhlich syndrome and triad syndrome. It was first described by Fröhlich in 1839. Osler in 1901 coined the term "prune belly" which signifies the mass of redundant, wrinkled skin, akin to the skin of a dried prune, invariably present on the abdomen. Ninety seven percent of those affected are males, 3% are females and it affects 1 in 40,000 births. PBS is seen in twins and approximately 4% of all cases are products of twin pregnancies. It is also associated with trisomy 21 and 18 and shows an increased incidence of Tetralogy of Fallot and ventriculoseptal defects. Antenatal ultrasound shows oligo or anhydramnios, megacystis, hydronephrosis and hyperechogenic kidneys.

Pathology of Prune Belly Syndrome

The abdominal musculature forms a mass of wrinkled and redundant skin and on microscopic examination the muscle shows a reduced number of muscle fibers and those present are hypertrophied. The ***kidneys*** and ureters vary in appearance depending upon the degree of obstruction. Kidneys show normal reniform shape with fetal lobulations, well-developed cortex and mild to moderate degree of hydronephrosis. The kidneys are usually normal to small sized, but still show dilatation of the pelvicalyceal system. The renal parenchyma is well-preserved and dysplastic changes, i.e. the primitive ducts are seen in the medulla. Cysts are generally not seen. The ureters are markedly dilated and tortuous, out of proportion to the degree of renal parenchymal involvement. On microscopic examination, the muscle layer of the ureters is either very scanty or absent altogether and is replaced by collagenous tissue. This explains the degree of ureteric dilatation and tortuosity. In some cases, the ureteric musculature is defective only in the lower part.

Massive vesicoureteric reflux occurs because the amuscular ureter acts as a passive conduit between the urinary bladder and the kidney. The urinary bladder is markedly dilated, i.e. megacystis and thickened. This is due to the increased collagenous tissue and not due to hypertrophy of the muscle. The intravesical pressure is abnormally low due to the marked distension and lack of compression by the abdominal musculature. Some bladders are thin with atrophy and fibrosis. Herniation of the bladder is commonly seen in patients with PBS, as the bladder is large and redundant. Patients with urethral obstruction commonly have a patent urachus, which enables the patient to survive. Normally the urachus closes in the 12th week of gestation and if it does in cases of PBS, perinatal deaths occur. In a large number of patients, the prostate is poorly developed (with absent glands) or absent altogether. On microscopic examination, the region of the prostate is replaced by smooth muscle and fibrous connective tissue. Urethral abnormalities range from total atresia, partial obstruction to megalourethra. Patients who survive urethral atresia have a patent urachus. The penis may show dorsal chordee, megalourethra and partial or complete absence of corpora cavernosa/spongiosa. Testes in majority of the cases are cryptorchid having short spermatic vessels, marked reduction of spermatogonia and Leydig cell hyperplasia. Skeletal anomalies are common, can affect 50% of patients and include pectus excavatum, scoliosis and congenital joint dislocations including that of the hip. Abnormalities associated with oligohydramnios, i.e. limb abnormalities and hypoplastic lungs are observed. Cardiac anomalies are reported in 10% of patients. Gastrointestinal abnormalities affect 30% of patients and include malrotation, atresia, stenosis and volvulus. They may be due to a persistence of the wide mesentery seen in embryonic life, with absent fixation to the posterior abdominal wall. Other abnormalities include splenic torsion, imperforate anus, anorectal agenesis, omphalocele and gastroschisis. Prognosis depends on the status of the renal function present at birth and the methods used to conserve it. Burbige et al in their series of 50 cases found that 16 babies died—14 in perinatal period and two at 3 and 6 months of age due to urosepsis. Amongst the 34 survivors, two developed renal failure and underwent transplantation and the remaining had satisfactory renal function, many have reached adulthood and one is a professional mountaineer.

Pathogenesis of Prune Belly Syndrome

This syndrome in a large number of cases is genetically determined, has been seen in twins and in consecutive siblings with a mosaic chromosome abnormality. It was seen in two siblings and their first cousin, one of which was a female with Turner syndrome. This finding and the male predominance led the researchers to believe that this condition is probably inherited as a sex-linked recessive trait. Autosomal recessive inheritance is suggested in some cases and a homozygous mutation in the muscarinic cholinergic receptor-3 gene (*CHRM3*) on chromosome 1q43 was reported in one family. Defect of mesenchymal development during early pregnancy is also considered. Pagon et al said that it could be sequelae of abdominal distension in utero due to proximal urethral obstruction. But all said and done, PBS is an obstructive nephropathy and the obstruction is urethral. Recent theories advocate that prostatic hypoplasia leads to a conformational change in the prostatic urethra during voiding, due to which there occurs a functional and transient obstruction at the junction of the glandular and penile urethra. Obstruction can also be caused by severe angulation at the prostatic and membranous urethral junction. This could be due to a lack of striated muscle in the membranous urethra or urogenital diaphragm or an additional ring of obstructive tissue acting as a flap valve due to hypoplasia of the prostate, creating a ballooning of the prostatic urethra. Thus, there is a high incidence of megalourethra observed in cases of PBS. Broadly, in PBS, there is a mesodermal arrest, which explains the involvement of the abdominal wall, genitourinary tract and the testis. The noxious insult occurs between the 6th and 10th weeks of gestation. An insult at 3 weeks of embryogenesis explains the prostatic hypoplasia and poor glandular development. The mesodermal arrest theory is supported by the histologic findings of abundance of fibrous tissue, collagen and connective tissue with sparsely placed smooth muscle throughout the urinary tract. Thus, this indicates that a mesodermal differentiation problem occurs along with obstruction. Obstruction alone will not lead to PBS. A few cases of PBS have been found to have classical or atypical posterior urethral valve.

Differences between Prune Belly Syndrome and Posterior Urethral Valve

Both posterior urethral valve and PBS are urethral obstructions and lead to bilateral hydroureteronephrosis with a distended and hypertrophied urinary bladder. But there are differences highlighted in the Table 1.

Table 1: Differences between Prune Belly Syndrome and Posterior Urethral Valve.

	Posterior urethral valve (Cases 82, 83 and 90)	*Prune belly syndrome (Cases 93 and 94)*
Abdomen	Moderately distended. No abnormalities of the musculature of the abdomen.	Markedly distended—balloon like initially and later shows loose, wrinkled and redundant abdominal skin.
Kidneys—external appearance	Enlarged, maintain basic reniform shape, capsular surface studded with cysts of varying sizes. Kidneys may show variation in size.	Kidneys vary considerably in appearance, mostly small in size or mildly enlarged, surface does not show cysts, show normal reniform shape with fetal lobulations and do not show variation in size, i.e. are of same size.
Kidneys—cut section	Marked hydronephrosis with a rim of cortex. Show plenty of cysts, mostly confined to the peripheral cortex.	Moderate hydronephrosis and have a well-developed cortex. Cysts are generally not visible on gross examination.
Kidneys—microscopy	Renal parenchyma shows complete lobar disorganization with plenty of cysts, predominantly peripheral and prominent dysplastic changes. The degree of ureteric and bladder abnormality go hand in hand with the renal parenchymal disarray and dysplasia.	The renal parenchyma is well-preserved, there is no lobar disorganization, generally few cysts may be seen and the primitive ducts are seen in the medulla. There is disparity between markedly dilated ureters or urinary bladder and relatively preserved renal parenchyma.
Ureters	Markedly dilated and tortuous. Microscopy shows marked hypertrophy of the detrusor muscle.	Markedly dilated and less tortuous. Microscopy—muscle layer is either very scanty or absent altogether and is replaced by collagenous tissue.
Urinary bladder	Distended and markedly hypertrophied. Microscopy shows marked hypertrophy of the detrusor muscle. Intravesical fluid pressure high	Markedly distended like a balloon, i.e. megacystis and thickened. Microscopy: Increased fibrocollagenous tissue replacing the muscle fibers. Few cases show marked attenuation and degeneration of the muscle fibers. Intravesical fluid pressure low due to the lack of compression of abdominal organs by the abdominal musculature.
Prostate	Prostate well-developed	Prostate is replaced by smooth muscle and fibrous connective tissue.
Testis	Occasionally cryptorchid	Generally cryptorchid
Penis	Normal	May show dorsal chordee, megalourethra and partial or complete absence of corpora cavernosa or spongiosa.
Pathogenesis	There is presence of an obstructing membrane, occurring due to an abnormal embryological development, located in the posterior male urethra.	Defect of mesenchymal development during early pregnancy
Abdominal, ureteric and urinary bladder musculature	Normal	Abnormal and leads to the marked abdominal distension, wrinkled prune belly-like abdominal skin, low intravesical fluid pressure and this also explains the disparity between markedly dilated ureters and relatively preserved renal parenchyma.

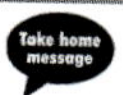

TAKE HOME MESSAGE

- Prune belly syndrome is a rare congenital malformation of unknown etiology. It is an obstructive nephropathy and the obstruction is urethral.
- This syndrome, in a large number of cases, is genetically determined.
- Broadly, in prune belly, there is a mesodermal arrest, which explains the involvement of the abdominal wall, genitourinary tract and the testis. The noxious insult occurs between the 6th and 10th weeks of gestation.
- It is a triad characterized by abnormalities of the urinary tract, i.e. hydroureteronephrosis with a markedly distended urinary bladder, wrinkled redundant skin seen over the anterior abdominal wall and bilateral cryptorchidism in males.
- Important microscopic clues to the diagnosis of prune belly syndrome: (1) Marked disparity between markedly dilated ureters/urinary bladder and relatively preserved renal parenchyma and (2) Fibrocollagenous replacement of the muscle of the ureters and urinary bladder.

SUGGESTED READING

1. Brinker MR, Palutsis RS, Sarwark JF. The orthopaedic manifestations of prune-belly (Eagle-Barrett) syndrome. J Bone Joint Surg Am. 1995;77(2):251-7.
2. Burbige KA, Amodio J, Berdon WE, et al. Prune belly syndrome: 35 years of experience. J Urol. 1987;137:86.
3. Eagle JF, Barrett GS. Congenital deficiency of abdominal musculature with associated genitourinary abnormalities: A syndrome. Report of 9 cases. Pediatrics. 1950;6(5):721-36.
4. Hill GS. Cystic and dysplastic diseases of the kidney: developmental lesions. In: Hill GS (Ed). Uropathology, Volume 1. Edinburgh, New York: Churchill Livingstone; 1989. pp. 121-6.
5. Hoagland MH, Hutchins GM. Obstructive lesions of the lower urinary tract in the prune belly syndrome. Arch Pathol Lab Med. 1987;111:154.
6. Moerman P, Fryns JP, Goddeeris P, et al. Pathogenesis of the prune-belly syndrome: a functional urethral obstruction caused by prostatic hypoplasia. Pediatrics. 1984;73:470.
7. Nunn N, Stephens FD. The triad syndrome: a composite anomaly of the abdominal wall, urinary system and testes. J Urol. 1961;86:782.
8. Obrinsky W. Agenesis of abdominal muscles with associated malformation of the genitourinary tract; a clinical syndrome. Am J Dis Child. 1949;77(3):362-73.
9. Osler W. Congenital absence of abdominal muscles, with distended and hypertrophied urinary bladder. Bull Johns Hopkins Hosp. 1901;12:331.
10. Pagon RA, Smith DW, Shepard TH. Urethral obstruction malformation complex: a cause of abdominal muscle deficiency and the "prune belly". J Pediatr. 1979;94:900.
11. Peterson DS, Fish L, Cass AA. Twins with congenital deficiency of abdominal musculature. J Urol. 1972;107:670.
12. Reinberg Y, Shapiro E, Manivel JC, et al. Prune belly syndrome in females: a triad of abdominal musculature deficiency and anomalies of the urinary and genital systems. J Pediatr. 1991;118(3):395-8.
13. Stephens FD, Gupta D. Pathogenesis of the prune belly syndrome. J Urol. 1994;152:2328-31.
14. Straub E, Spranger J. Etiology and the pathogenesis of the prune belly syndrome. Kidney Int. 1981;20:695.
15. Zugor V, Schott GE, Labanaris AP. The prune belly syndrome: urological aspects and long-term outcomes of a rare disease. Pediatr Rep. 2012;4(2):e20.

CONTRIBUTIONS BY:

Case 93

1. Dr Madhusudhan, Junior Resident, Department of Pathology (In taking gross photographs)
2. Dr Manjay Singh, Junior Resident, Department of Pediatrics (Compilation of Clinical Details)
3. Dr Kanya Mukhopadhyay, Professor, Department of Pediatrics (Clinician In-Charge)

Case 94

1. Dr Neelam Chaudhary, Department of Obstetrics and Gynecology (Clinician In-Charge)

Post Graduate Institute of Medical Education and Research, Chandigarh, India.

CASE 95

Sirenomelia with Bilateral Renal Agenesis and Multiple Other Malformations: PM 27025

Nandita Bharadwaj Kakkar

 HIGHLIGHTS OF THE CASE

Medical termination of pregnancy was done in this fetus at 18 weeks gestation due to multiple congenital malformations. Autopsy revealed sirenomelia with bilateral renal agenesis, single umbilical artery and multiple other malformations.

Keywords: Sirenomelia, renal agenesis, omphalocele, sacral agenesis, single umbilical artery, diabetes mellitus.

 CLINICAL DETAILS

Date of MTP: 10.11.2015

A gravida 3 mother, with one live child, came for her routine antenatal check-up. She was 32 years of age and was having diabetes mellitus since 5 years. Ultrasonography revealed fused lower limbs (single femur and abnormal tibia and fibula were present), abdominal wall defect and kyphoscoliosis. Medical termination of pregnancy was done at 18 weeks gestation due to major multiple congenital malformations.

 AUTOPSY FINDINGS: PM 27025

Baby was deformed and weighed 205 g. Autopsy revealed fused lower limbs, i.e. sirenomelia, low set ears, omphalocele, bilateral renal agenesis, absent ureters and urinary bladder, bilateral lung hypoplasia, markedly hypoplastic sacrum with fused pelvic bones, kyphoscoliosis, absent anus, blind ending colon, absent genitalia and a single umbilical artery. The fused lower limbs showed a single femur and abnormal tibia and fibula. The feet were deformed, partly fused with marked extension. Fingers were appreciable. The abdominal wall defect revealed herniated gastrointestinal tract and liver with a white membranous covering i.e omphalocele. Upper limbs, heart and brain were normal.

 FINAL AUTOPSY DIAGNOSIS: PM 27025

MTP done at 18 weeks in a diabetic mother.

- Sirenomelia with omphalocele, bilateral renal agenesis, lung hypoplasia, fused sacrum, anorectal malformation, absent genitalia.
- Single umbilical artery.

SIRENOMELIA

Sirenomelia is a lethal rare congenital abnormality also known as Mermaid syndrome, wherein the lower limbs show varying degrees of fusion. It is most severe form of caudal dysplasia. It occurs 1 in a 100,000 births, causes still birth, is more common in monozygotic twins and is associated with single umbilical artery and various anomalies of the urogenital tract, lower gastrointestinal tract and lumbosacral spine. The abnormalities accompanying sirenomelia appear as a spectrum. Sirenomelia shows a variety of changes, i.e. its hallmark is single lower limb with: (1) Rudimentary femur and proximal tibia/fibula. (2) Rudimentary development below the femur. (3) Two femurs and two lower long bones and no separate feet. (4) Soft tissue fusion of the lower limbs with normal long bones and everted feet. (5) Two femurs, single lower bone and single foot below. Other defects seen are—(1) Hypoplastic or abnormal sacrum, fused pelvic bones and small iliac wings. (2) Gastrointestinal tract (GI)—rectal atresia, imperforate anus, absent anus with blind ending colon, malrotation and colon ending in the cloaca. (3) Urinary tract—majority of the cases show bilateral renal agenesis and some show dysplastic kidneys. (4) Genitalia—external genitalia are absent or there may be a small phallic

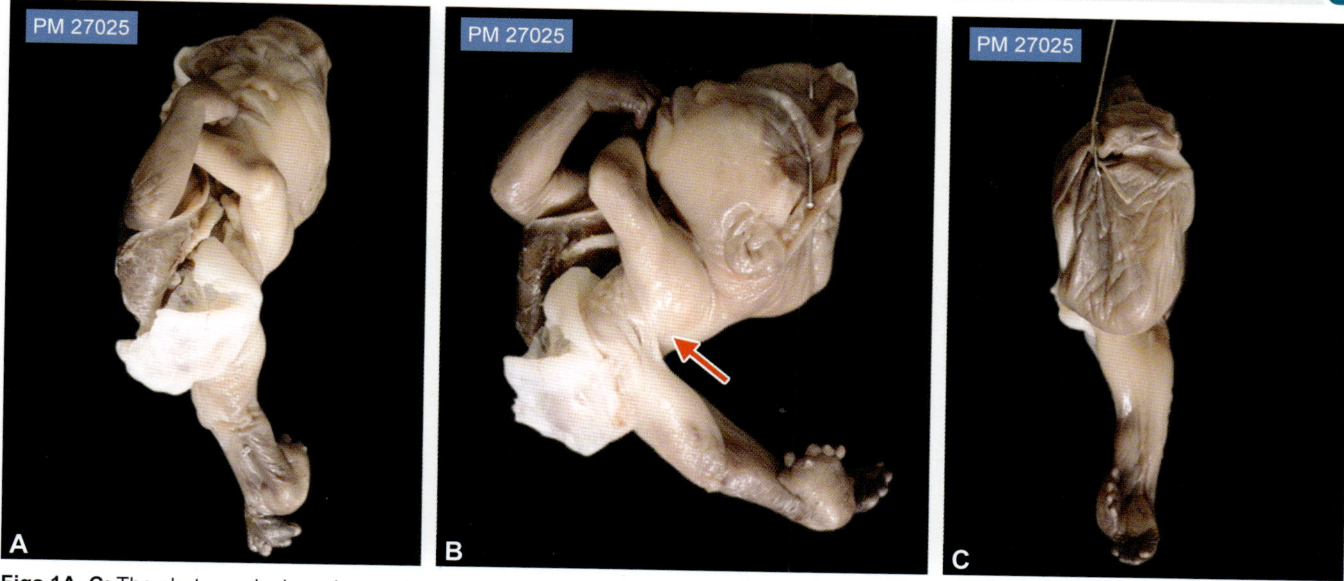

Figs 1A–C: The photographs have been taken after the autopsy. The brain has been removed. (A) Sirenomelic fetus with fused lower limbs and distorted feet. The omphalocele membrane can be seen; (B) The sacrum is markedly hypoplastic and so there is marked extension of the fused lower limb toward the back (arrow). The upper limbs are normal but contractures are seen; (C) The fused lower limb with distorted feet which are partly fused, show fingers and hyperextension.

structure. (5) Others—anencephaly, exencephaly, cervical rachischisis, cleft palate, hypoplastic lungs, exomphalos, dorsal hemivertebrae, low set ears, micrognathia and ventricular septal defect (VSD).

Differential diagnosis of sirenomelia is from caudal dysgenesis. They are considered to be two ends of the same spectrum, as they both occur due to embryonal defects in the development of the caudal region. Caudal dysgenesis does not have fused lower limbs and has a greater association with maternal diabetes than sirenomelia. However, single umbilical artery can be seen in a few cases. In caudal dysgenesis, there is a marked hypoplasia of the lower half of the body, i.e. short lower limbs, small/absent sacrum, small pelvis, vertebral anomalies of the thoracic/lumbosacral spine, short deformed lumbar spine, kyphoscoliosis, spina bifida, bilateral talipes, anorectal atresia, rectovesical fistula, imperforate anus, malrotation of the intestines, renal agenesis/ hypoplasia/dysplasia, horse shoe kidneys, absent uterus/ vagina, small phallus, absent genital opening, pulmonary hypoplasia, exomphalos, diaphragmatic hernia, esophageal atresia, VSD, truncus arteriosus, cystic hygroma, postaxial polydactyly, hydrocephalus and short neck etc. Thus, there is a marked overlap between the two entities but a fused lower limb defines sirenomelia. Infants of diabetic mothers have three to four times the incidence of congenital malformations, as compared to the general population and caudal dysgenesis and to a lesser extent sirenomelia are associated with it. Another entity that comes in the differential diagnosis is VACTERL, which has a considerable overlap with sirenomelia, the former showing more upper body segment defects and the latter showing more of lower body segment defects.

TAKE HOME MESSAGE

- Sirenomelia is a rare, lethal congenital abnormality also known as Mermaid syndrome, wherein the lower limbs show varying degrees of fusion. It is associated with multiple other malformations as the abnormalities accompanying sirenomelia appear as a spectrum.
- Differential diagnosis of Sirenomelia is from Caudal dysgenesis. They are considered to be two ends of the same spectrum and both are associated with maternal diabetes.

SUGGESTED READING

1. Duesterhoeft SM, Ernst LM, Siebert JR, et al. Five cases of caudal regression syndrome with an aberrant abdominal umbilical artery: Further support for a caudal regression-sirenomelia spectrum. Am J Med Genet A. 2007;143A:3175-84.
2. Duncan PA, Shapiro LR. Interrelationships of the hemi facial microsomia, VATER and sirenomelia phenotypes. Am J Med Genet. 1993;47:75-84.
3. Rodriguez MM. Congenital anomalies of the kidney and the urinary tract (CAKUT). Fetal and Pediatric Pathology. 2014;33:293-320.

4. Seidahmed MZ, Omer B, Abdelbasit, OB, et al. Sirenomelia and severe caudal regression syndrome. Saudi Med J. 2014; 35:36-43.

5. Thottungal AD, Charles AK, Dickinson JE, et al. Caudal dysgenesis and sirenomelia-single centre experience suggests common pathogenic basis. Am J Med Genet Part A. 2010; 152A:2578-87.

CONTRIBUTIONS BY:

1. Dr Neelam Chaudhary, Department of Obstetrics and Gynecology (Clinician In-Charge)
Post Graduate Institute of Medical Education and Research (PGIMER), Chandigarh, India.

SECTION 16

Liver Disorders Pediatric Cases

CASE 96

Coexistence of Duarte 2 Variant of Galactosemia with Niemann–Pick Disease Type B, in an Infant: PM 23108

Nandita Bharadwaj Kakkar

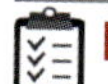

HIGHLIGHTS OF THE CASE

Coexistence of two autosomal recessive metabolic disorders is very rare. We report a novel case of classical galactosemia with Niemann–Pick disease type B. Both the disorders are inherited as autosomal recessive traits. At first instance, presence of cholestasis and reduced blood galactose-1-phosphate uridylyltransferase (GALT) activity with subsequent identification of N314D mutation in GALT gene confirmed the diagnosis of galactosemia. But persistent jaundice and splenohepatomegaly, with no improvement following the galactose free diet, led to antemortem bone aspiration biopsy, which documented large vacuolated Niemann–Pick cells. Child succumbed to his illness. The histopathology of liver showed evidence of extensive liver fibrosis confirming it to be a composite case of galactosemia and Niemann–Pick disease. Other organs also showed presence of Niemann–Pick cells.

Keywords: Galactosemia, Niemann–Pick disease, coexistence, autosomal recessive disorders, autopsy.

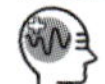

CLINICAL DETAILS

This child had two admissions in our institute.

First Admission: 26.02.2009 till 23.03.2009, Duration of Hospital Stay: 27 Days

A 5-month-old male child was admitted with history of jaundice and progressive abdominal distension since 3½ months and fever with respiratory distress in the form of rapid breathing and retractions since 4 days. The jaundice was first noted at 45 days of life and was progressive. He was passing high colored urine and clay colored stools. There was no history of lethargy, pruritis, melena or seizures. He was the second product of a nonconsanguineous marriage, was developmentally appropriate for age and was exclusively on breast feeding. On ***examination***—weight: 5.8 kg, length: 65 cm, occipitofrontal circumference: 38.5 cm, icterus +, coarse facies noted, liver: enlarged, firm in consistency (3.5 cm below right costal margin), spleen: enlarged (9 cm below left costal margin), no ascites and chest revealed bilateral crepitations.

Investigations

Hematological: Hb- 8.1 g/dL, TLC – 8300/uL, platelets- 85,000/uL, Peripheral blood film- mild anisocytosis, microcytosis, few macrocytes, elliptocytes, target cells with mild hypochromia, reticulocyte count 2%, Coagulogram- PT -24 sec (control- 12 sec), PTTK- 94 sec (control -35 sec), INR- 3.27.

Blood Biochemistry/Microbiology: Liver function tests—S bilirubin- 28 mg% with conjugated fraction of 16 mg%, serum albumin- 2.5 gm, SGOT- 546 U/L, SGPT -157 U/L (normal range: 15-45 U/L), S alkaline phosphatase - 588 U/L (Normal range: 20-250 IU/L), CRP negative, Blood/urine cultures sterile, Serology - toxoplasma, retroviral, rubella, cytomegalovirus and herpes virus - negative.

Radiology: Mebrofenin scan showed no drainage after 24 hours with impaired hepatocyte function. The ultrasonography of the abdomen showed liver with coarse echotexture, with normal portal vein and hepatic artery, no intrahepatic biliary radical dilation and gall bladder 4×1 cm. Common bile duct measured 1 cm at the porta hepatis.

Ophthalmic examination – no cataract, fundus normal.

Galactosemia work up: A reduced galactose-1-phosphate uridyl transferase (GALT) activity (36%) was observed. Galatose-1-phosphate levels were found to be 9.2 mg/100 mL packed RBC's (Normal < 1 mg/100 mL packed erythrocyte). There was presence of N314D mutation in homozygous state in exon 10 of the *GALT* gene, thus confirming the child to be galactosemic (Fig 1). Besides this, the child was also positive for 4 other genetic variations - G1105C in intron 4, G1323A and G1391A in intron 5 and a 4bp deletion in 5' untranslated region 116-119delGTCA upstream from the first methionine codon. All these variations in association with N314D are known to constitute Duarte 2 variant of galactosemia which is associated with diminished GALT activity (~40% of the normal). Patient was put on a galactose free diet and followed up.

Second Admission: Date of Admission: 11.04.2009, Date of Death: 23.04.2009, Duration of Stay: 12 Days

However, at 7 months, the baby was re-admitted with persistent jaundice, lethargy and poor feeding. On examination, he was deeply icteric with distended abdomen and an umbilical hernia. The liver and spleen were enlarged 2 and 10 cm below their respective costal margins. Hb was 7.4 g/dL, TLC: 4,600/µl, platelets: 63,000/µl and the liver function tests were markedly deranged. The INR had worsened to 4.9. Bone marrow aspiration and trephine biopsy was done, which were cellular and replete with large multivacuolated Niemann–Pick cells (Figs 2A and B). He received N-acetylcysteine with cefotaxim and supportive care, but his general condition worsened and he developed hospital acquired sepsis. Subsequently, he developed respiratory failure and refractory shock followed by cardiac arrest and succumbed to his illness.

AUTOPSY FINDINGS: PM 23108

A partial autopsy was done on this 7-month-old male infant. Externally the prosector noticed that the body of the child was deeply jaundiced. There was minimal straw-colored fluid in the peritoneal cavity. The ***liver*** weighed 155 g, as against a normal of 276 g, at this age. On cut section (Figs 2C and D), it was bile stained, firm and fibrotic. The hepatic veins, portal veins, splenic vein, superior mesenteric vein, extrahepatic biliary tract and gall bladder were within normal limits. On microscopy, there was extensive porto-portal and porto-central bridging fibrosis, with transition into cirrhosis (Fig 3A). The portal tracts (Fig 3B) showed lymphomononuclear cell infiltrate and marked periportal/periseptal cholangiolar proliferation. Canalicular cholestasis, pseudo acinar transformation, occasional giant cell transformation and focal steatosis were noted (Figs 3C and D). Few reticulin rich regenerative nodules without atypia were seen (Figs 4A and B). No periodic acid–Schiff (PAS) positive globules and no increase in hemosiderin or copper-associated proteins were noted. A diagnosis of metabolic liver

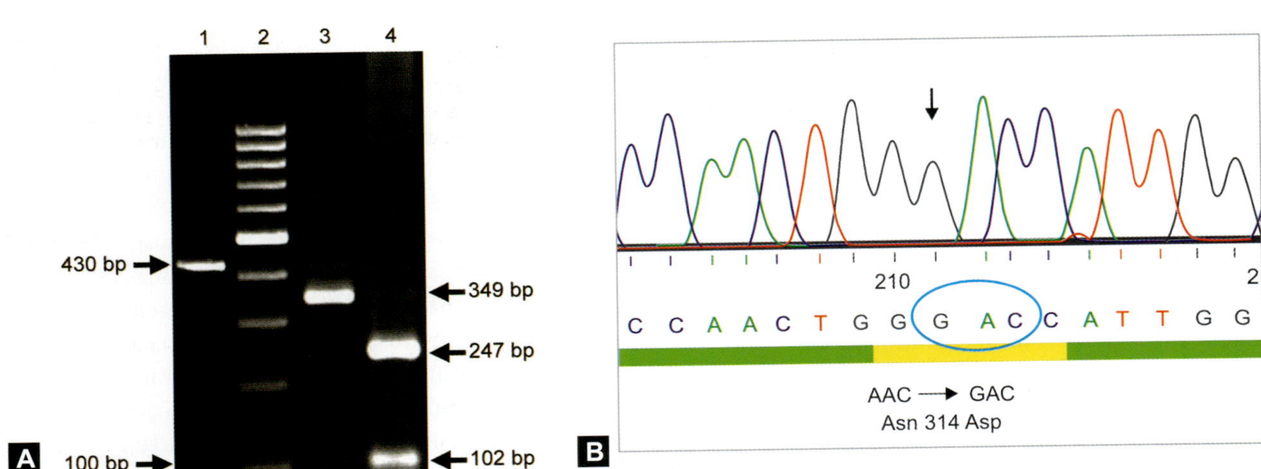

a. Detection of *N314D* mutation by Ava II restriction digestion
Lane 1: Uncut
Lane 2: 100 bp DNA Ladder
Lane 3: Wild type ({49 bp + 81 bp [not shown]})
Lane 4: Homozygous mutant [247 p + 102 bp + 81 bp (not shown)]

Figs 1A and B: (A) RFLP analysis of *N314D* mutation in exon 10 of GALT gene; (B) *GALT* gene sequence depicting substitution of A to G at nucleotide position 940 resulting in asparagine to aspartate amino acid change at codon 314.
(*Courtesy*: Dr Ramandeep singh and Dr Rajinder Prasad)

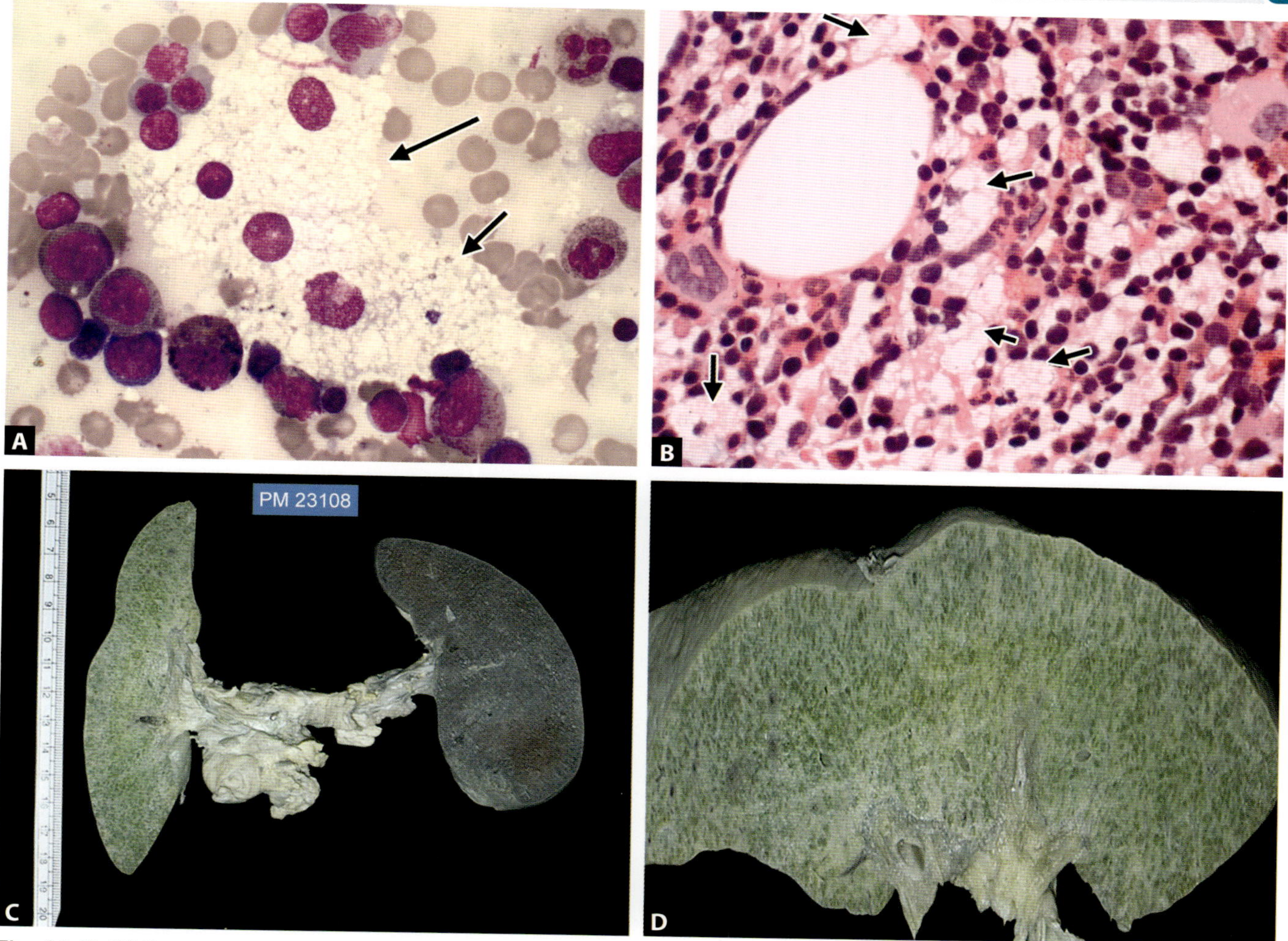

Figs 2A–D: (A) Bone marrow aspirate showing large multivacuolated Niemann–Pick cells (arrows). Giemsa stain x 1000; (B) Trephine biopsy replete with Niemann–Pick cells (arrows); (C) Organ complex comprising of a slice of the bile stained, firm and fibrotic liver, pancreas, C loop of the duodenum and the markedly enlarged spleen; (D) Coronal slice of the liver which is firm, shows extensive fibrosis and vague bile stained nodules.

disorder consistent with galactosemia with extensive fibrosis going on to cirrhosis was given. The antemortem bone marrow and at necropsy other organs like spleen, thymus, lymph nodes and bone marrow showed large foamy multivacuolated cells consistent with the morphology of Niemann–Pick cells. The liver was scrutinized diligently in this light and there were some large vacuolated Niemann–Pick cells seen amidst the fibrosis (Figs 4C and D—arrows). Oil red O stain was done on the sections from the liver and these large foamy cells showed reddish granular positivity (Fig 4E—arrow) indicating that the large vacuolated Niemann–Pick cells were camouflaged by the extensive fibrosis in the liver, due to the concomitant presence of galactosemia. The ***spleen*** (Fig 5A) showed massive enlargement and weighed 230 g, as against a normal of 25 g, at this age. No focal lesion was seen. Microscopy revealed red pulp congestion with sinusoids loaded with large foamy and multivacuolated cells (Figs 5B and C) which showed mild PAS positivity, consistent with Neimann–Pick cells. Similar large multivacuolated cells were also seen in the ***lymph nodes*** (Fig 5D), ***post mortem bone marrow*** (Figs 5E and F), ***thymus*** (Fig 6A) and in the liver amidst the fibrosis. The ganglion cells and nerve cells of the myenteric plexus (Fig 6B) of the ***gastrointestinal tract*** showed diffuse fine vacuolations indicating deposition of sphingomyelins. The ***lungs*** together weighed 160 g, were firm to feel and on microscopy revealed a diffuse alveolar damage with eosinophilic hyaline membranes (Fig 6C) lining the alveolar spaces. In addition bronchopneumonia was also seen.

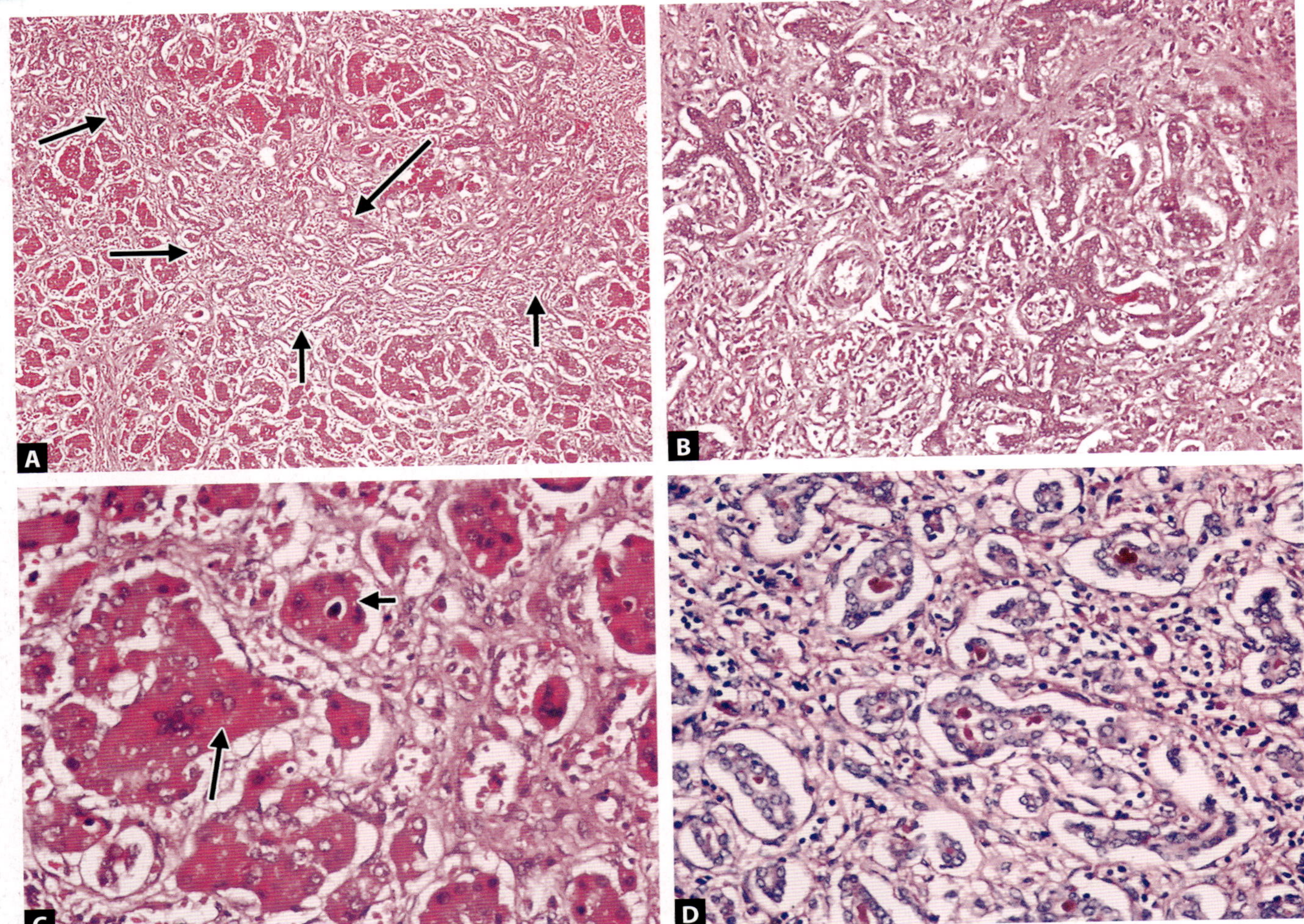

Figs 3A–D: (A) Photomicrograph from the liver showing extensive bridging fibrosis with septa showing florid periseptal cholangiolar proliferation (arrows); (B) Portal tract shows mild inflammation and marked periportal cholangiolar proliferation; (C) Liver showing giant cell (long arrow) and pseudo acinar transformation (small arrow) along with fibrosis; (D) Canalicular proliferation with cholestasis.

FINAL AUTOPSY DIAGNOSIS: PM 23108

7 Months Male

- *Galactosemia*: Duarte 2 variant with extensive fibrosis, going on to cirrhosis
- Storage disorder consistent with Niemann–Pick disease (Type B) with involvement of spleen, lymph nodes, thymus, bone marrow, liver and myenteric plexus
- Diffuse alveolar damage with bronchopneumonia.

Galactosemia—Refer to Case 97 (PM 23869).

Niemann–Pick disease—Refer to Case 96 (PM 27096)

COEXISTENCE OF DUARTE 2 VARIANT OF GALACTOSEMIA WITH NIEMANN–PICK DISEASE TYPE B

Classical galactosemia is an autosomal recessive disorder of galactose metabolism, caused by deficiency of the enzyme GALT, the gene for which is present on chromosome 9 and which manifests as infantile cholestasis with liver failure. Niemann–Pick disease is a form of lipidosis and consists of six subtypes (A–F), that are inherited as autosomal recessive traits. Niemann–Pick disease type B results from the deficiency of a lysosomal enzyme, acid sphingomyelinase encoded by sphingomyelin phosphodiesterase (*SMPD1*) gene

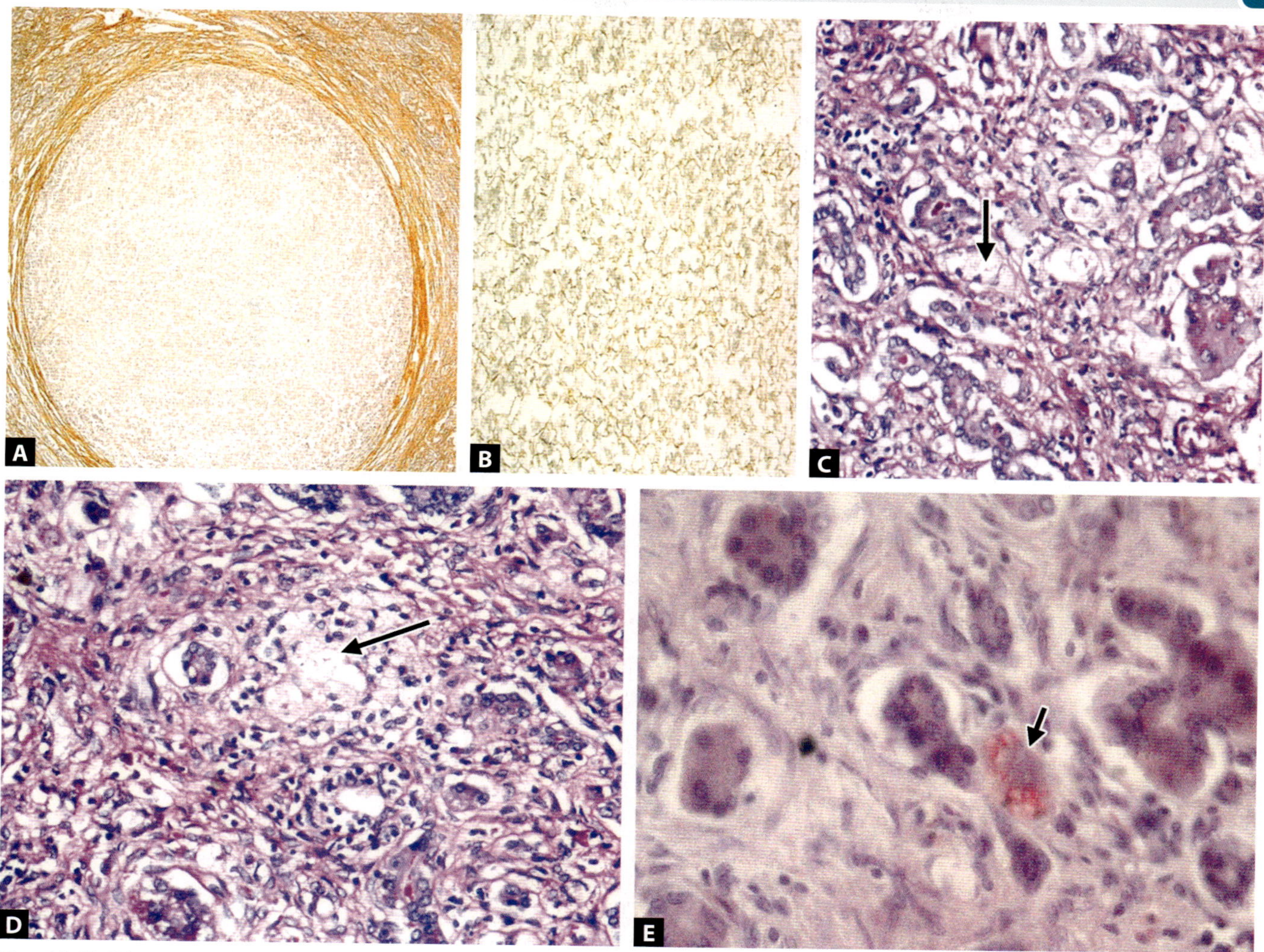

Figs 4A–E: (A) Liver showing a regenerative nodule (reticulin stain); (B) At high power, the nodule seen in the preceding picture is reticulin rich; (C and D) Liver showing large foamy, multivacuolated Niemann–Pick cells (arrows) amidst the fibrosis; (E) Oil red O stain showing positivity in the Niemann–Pick cell.

leading to the pathological accumulation of sphingomyelin and other lipids in the body. The coexistence of two autosomal recessive disorders has been very rarely documented in the literature. Since the genes for both disorders are located on different chromosomes, the most likely explanation for this atypical coexistence is the independent association of galactosemia and Niemann–Pick disease type B and is assumed to be coincidental. To the best of our knowledge, no clinical report is available on coexistence of galactosemia and Niemann–Pick disease type B.

COMMENTARY—INDEX CASE: PM 23108

The unusual co-occurrence of these two autosomal recessive disorders prompts speculation about the pathophysiological effects and treatment of both diseases in such cases. Does the presence of galactosemia worsen the course of Niemann–Pick disease or vice versa. ? There is no literature present which addresses such problems. Collaborative efforts between experts in different branches of pediatrics and genetics will be needed to find enough patients to answer such questions. However, it seems that the coexistence of these two diseases in the index case could have contributed to the severity of two disease processes, that ultimately led to the death of the child. Hepatosplenomegaly is the most prominent feature in both disorders. But massive splenomegaly in the index case was clue to storage disorder. Observed persistent jaundice throughout the course and porto-central bridging fibrosis leading to cirrhosis could be due to the

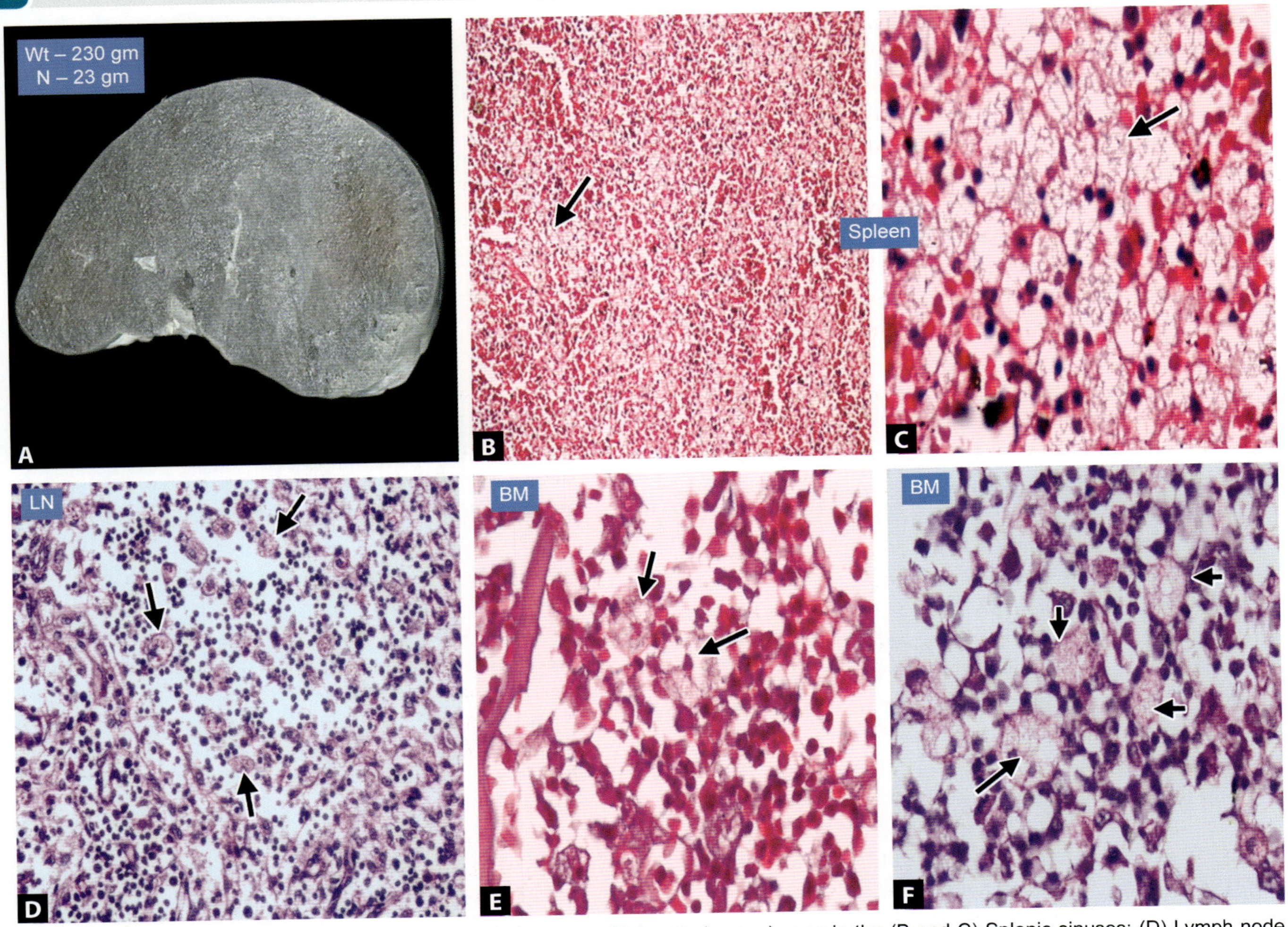

Figs 5A–F: (A) Slice of the markedly enlarged spleen. Niemann–Pick cells (arrows) seen in the (B and C) Splenic sinuses; (D) Lymph node sinuses (PAS stain); (E and F) Bone marrow.

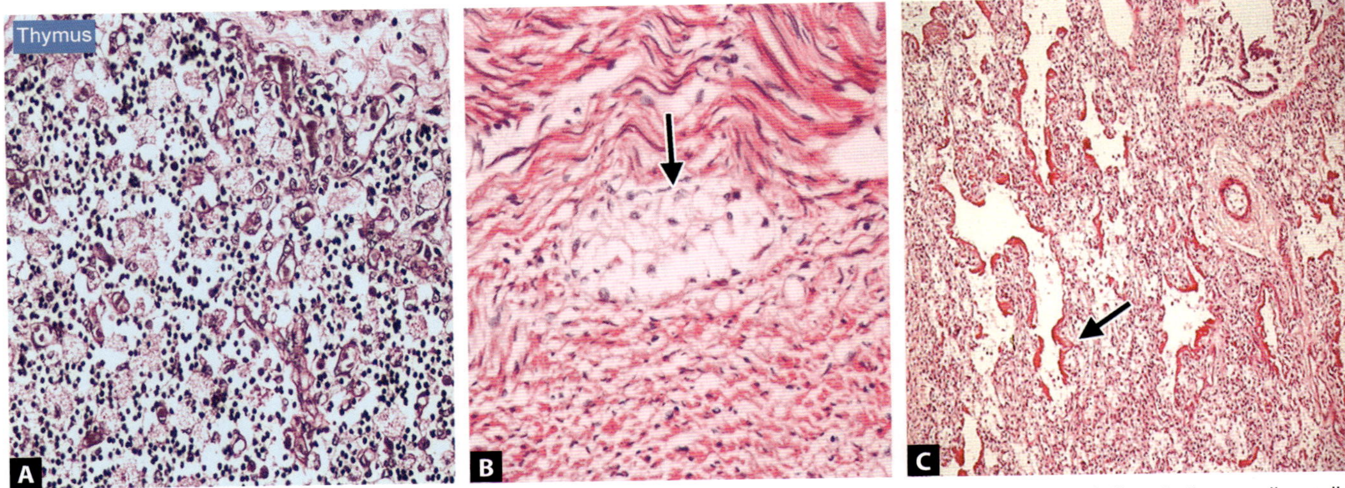

Figs 6A–C: (A) Thymus showing Niemann–Pick cells (PAS stain); (B) Myenteric plexus showing diffuse fine vacuolations in the ganglion cells (arrows); (C) Microphotograph of the lung showing hyaline membrane formation (arrow).

synergistic effect. Further, genetic analysis in the index case has revealed *N314D* mutation in exon 10 of *GALT* gene which is known to result in diminished red cell GALT enzyme activity and milder symptoms in the patients. Thereby, it is possible that presence of *N314D* mutation may have exacerbated the manifestations of Niemann–Pick disease as well as its early onset. Niemann–Pick disease is diagnosed by demonstration of foamy and multivacuolated cells in bone marrow and other organs like spleen, thymus, lymph nodes and liver. The Niemann–Pick cells were difficult to discern in the liver as they were camouflaged by the extensive fibrosis due to accompanying galactosemia.

Histopathology of the liver in the index case showed porto-portal and porto-central extensive bridging fibrosis, going on to cirrhosis, as the nodules were yet not well formed. Few regenerative nodules were however seen, which maintained the two cord pattern and reticulin stain supported this finding. Apart from that, there was periportal/periseptal cholangiolar proliferation, pseudoacinar transformation, occasional giant cells and canalicular cholestasis. Steatosis was present only focally. But our experience in autopsy cases of galactosemia says that, as the cirrhotic state is reached, the steatosis decreases and at times is not discernable.

The most important message from this case is that a wider differential diagnosis should be entertained in a patient who has an established genetic disease, but whose phenotype is highly atypical. Such features should prompt a high index of suspicion and appropriate investigations need to be done to prove or exclude a concurrent disorder, since finding yet another disease has important prognostic, management and genetic counseling implications.

TAKE HOME MESSAGE

- Coexistence of two autosomal recessive metabolic disorders is very rare, but can occur.
- Persistent jaundice and splenohepatomegaly, with no improvement following the galactose-free diet, led to antemortem bone aspiration biopsy, which documented large vacuolated Niemann–Pick cells in the index case.

SUGGESTED READING

1. Bosch AM, IJ Lodewijk, Oostheim W, et al. Identification of novel mutations in classical galactosemia. Hum Mutat. 2005;25:502.
2. Elsas LJ, Langley S, Evinger J, et al. Galactosemia: A strategy to identify new biochemical phenotypes and molecular genotypes. Am J Hum Genet. 1995;56:630-9.
3. Fretzayas A, Koukoutsakis P, Moustaki M, et al. Co-inheritance of Rotor Syndrome, G-6-PD deficiency and heterozygous thalassemia: a possible genetic interaction. J Pediatr Gastroenterol Nutr. 2001;33:211-3.
4. Motamedi MK, Khoddami M, Naseri M. Type B Niemann-Pick disease: report of a case with miliary pattern on chest X-ray. Arch Iranian Med. 2005;8:223-5.
5. Prasad R, Kaur G, Kumar S, et al. Two novel mutations (2976INSA, 4311insA) of ATP7B in a patient with Wilson's disease coexisting with glucose-6-phosphate dehydrogenase deficiency. J Gastroenterol Hepatol. 2005;20:660-2.
6. Singh R, Thapa BR, Kaur G, et al. Frequency distribution of Q188R, N314D, Duarte 1, Duarte 2 GALT variant alleles in an Indian galactosaemic population. Biochem Genet. 2012; 50:871-80.

CONTRIBUTIONS BY:

1. Dr Ramandeep Singh, PhD, Department of Biochemistry (GALT Assay - Figs 1A and B)
2. Dr Man Updesh Singh Sachdeva, Additional Professor, Department of Hematology (Figs 2A and B)
3. Dr Rajindra Prasad, Ex-Professor and Head, Department of Biochemistry (GALT Assay - Figs 1A and B)
4. Dr BR Thapa, Professor and Head, Department of Gastroenterology, Hepatology and Nutrition (Clinician In-Charge)

Post Graduate Institute of Medical Education and Research, Chandigarh, India.

CASE 97

A Classical Case of Galactosemia: PM 23869

Nandita Bharadwaj Kakkar

HIGHLIGHTS OF THE CASE

A 3-month-old male child presented with failure to thrive, diarrhea, progressive abdominal distension, weight loss, jaundice, acholic stools, conjugated hyperbilirubinemia, deranged liver function tests, coagulopathy and ascites. He was said to be doing well till 2 months of age. A clinical diagnosis of infantile cholestasis syndrome—chronic liver disease with sepsis and decompensation was made. Autopsy revealed micronodular cirrhosis with classical gross and histological features of galactosemia.

Keywords: Galactosemia, classical, micronodular cirrhosis, neonatal cholestasis syndrome, autopsy.

CLINICAL DETAILS

Date of Admission: 23.8.2010, Date of Death: 25.8.2010, Duration of Hospital Stay: 2 days

A 3-month-old male child presented with complaints of loose stools, progressive abdominal distension and weight loss since one month. He was said to be doing well till 2 months of age. There was jaundice with clay-colored stools since 5 days. The stools were loose/watery, 10–12/day and each episode lasted for 4–5 days. Stools were clay-colored for last 5 days. There was no associated vomiting. Diffuse abdominal distension was present which progressed over one month to involve the external genitalia. There was considerable weight loss (300 g over one month). There was history of mild-to-moderate, intermittent and undocumented fever for one month, which was more prominent in initial 5 days of illness. The baby was admitted at an outside facility for 15 days, where he was given antibiotics, blood transfusion and a course of chloroquine. Thereafter, he was referred to our institute. He was born to a third gravida mother with two previous issues, one male and one female, both doing well. He was born at term by normal vaginal delivery with no perinatal complications. The baby cried immediately after birth, APGAR was 7/10, birth weight was 2.5 kg and he was a product of a nonconsanguineous marriage. He was exclusively breast fed and was adequately immunized for age. On examination—weight: 3.192 kg (<5th centile), length: 53 cm (<5th centile), occipitofrontal circumference (OFC): 35 cm (< −2SD), he was irritable, emaciated with sunken eyes and prominent skin folds. Anterior fontanelle—depressed, pulse: 100/min, all pulses well palpable, respiratory rate: 28/min, afebrile, pallor +, jaundice +, dysmorphic facies noted ie pointed chin, pinched nose and long eyelashes. The liver was firm and palpable 4 cm (span 7.5 cm) below the right costal margin, spleen was not palpable and ascites was present.

Investigations and Course of Management

***Hematological*:** Hb – 5.4 g/dL, TLC 6700/uL, Coagulogram PT/PTI/PTTK – 19'/68%/38',

***Blood biochemistry/microbiology*:** Na^+- 134 mEq/L, K^+- 5.8 mEq/L, S urea 15 mg%, S creatinine 0.6 mg%, S bilirubin 13.4 mg%, conjugated fraction 7.9 mg%, AST 271 U/L, ALT 183 U/L, ALP 1847 U/L, Total proteins 5.3 gm, Alb/Glob 2.8/2.5 gm, TORCH serology – Toxoplasma, Herpes, Rubella – negative , CMV – IgM (microELISA) Positive, Blood culture negative, Ascitic tap- 80 cells (80% polyorphs), ADA 8 IU/L, Gram stain- negative.

***Radiology*:** Ultrasonography of the abdomen revealed features suggestive of hepatitis, a contracted gall bladder, ascites and bilateral renal parenchymal disease. GALT assay was not done and cataracts were not looked for.

***Course and management*:** The patient was admitted with a working diagnosis of neonatal cholestasis syndrome and started on vitamin supplements (A,D,K) along with oral rehydrating solution, zinc and probiotics for the diarrhoea. On day 3 baby developed hypothermia and became lethargic and developed cardiac arrest from which he could not be revived.

Unit's final clinical diagnosis: Infantile cholestasis syndrome-Chronic liver disease with decompensation and sepsis.

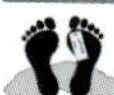

AUTOPSY FINDINGS: PM 23869

A complete autopsy was performed on this 3-month-old male child. The body weight was 3,233 g. The peritoneal cavity contained 2.2 liters of straw-colored fluid. The ***liver*** weighed 195 g, was firm and bile stained with micronodules on the capsular aspect (Fig 1A). Cut section (Fig 1B) was firm bile stained and showed micronodules. The biliary tree (Fig 1B - arrow) was dissected and found to be within normal limits. Microscopic examination revealed a complete loss of lobular architecture with formation of porto-portal and porto-central septa (bridging fibrosis), forming micronodules, well-appreciated on hematoxylin and eosin (H&E), reticulin stain and Masson's trichrome stain (Figs 1C–E). The septa showed chronic inflammation. There was marked periportal/periseptal cholangiolar proliferation (Figs 2A and B) extending into the lobule for varying distance with bile plugs and some showing infiltration by neutrophils. Immunohistochemistry with CK7 stained the neocholangioles, thus highlighting the florid periportal/periseptal cholangiolar proliferation (Fig 2C). Abundant and diffuse macrovesicular steatosis was noted (Fig 2D). Florid pseudoacinar transformation (Figs 2E and F) of the hepatic plates, also called cholestatic rosettes, wherein the hepatocytes surround a dilated canaliculus which is either empty, contains bile or some orange-colored material were noted. Cholestasis was noted in the pseudorosettes and bile ductules. Prussian blue stain revealed siderosis (2+) in the portal tracts and the hepatocytes (Fig 3A). No pericellular/intralobular fibrosis was seen, orcein stain was negative, PAS stain showed glycogen which was lost with PAS predigestion with diastase (PASD), no globules of alfa1 antitrypsin were noted and the hepatocytes did not show any nuclear irregularities or dysplasia. So, with the liver showing micronodular cirrhosis, diffuse macrovesicular steatosis, marked periportal cholangiolar proliferation, pseudoacinar transformation and cholestasis, diagnosis is consistent with metabolic liver disease, i.e. galactosemia. The ***spleen*** (Figs 3B and C) weighed 28 g and showed congestion and siderosis (confirmed by Perls stain) in the red pulp. The ***lung*** on microscopy revealed bronchopneumonia (Fig 3D) along with hemorrhages (Fig 3E). The ***adrenal gland*** showed cytomegalovirus inclusions (Fig 3F). No inclusions were seen anywhere else in the body. Other organs were within normal limits.

FINAL AUTOPSY DIAGNOSIS: PM 23869

3 Months Male with Infantile Cholestasis Syndrome

- Micronodular cirrhosis—Morphological features consistent with Galactosemia
- Ascites
- Organizing pneumonia with pulmonary hemorrhage
- Cytomegalovirus—adrenal gland.

ABOUT GALACTOSEMIA[1-4]

Galactosemia is an autosomal recessive disorder of galactose metabolism. It was first described by Von Reuss in 1908. Mammalian milk contains lactose which is split by lactase in the intestinal microvilli into glucose and galactose. Galactose is further converted into glucose and this reaction requires three steps—(1) Galactose combines with adenosine triphosphate (ATP) and in the presence of enzyme galactokinase, is converted into galactose-1-phosphate and adenosine diphosphate (ADP). (2) Galactose-1-phosphate combines with uridine diphosphate (UDP) glucose and in the presence of enzyme galactose-1-phosphate uridylyltransferase is converted to UDP galactose and glucose-1-phosphate. (3) UDP galactose in the presence of enzyme UDP galactose-4-epimerase is converted into UDP glucose. There are three types of galactosemia which occur due to mutations in *GALT*, *GALK1* and *GALE* genes on chromosome 9q13.

1. ***Galactosemia Type 1***: This is known as classic galactosemia and is the most common variant. There is a total lack of enzyme galactose 1-phosphate uridyl transferase which is involved in metabolic step 2 and encoded on the GALT gene on chromosome 9q13. Mutations in GALT gene leads to almost complete elimination of the enzyme activity, resulting in the life-threatening signs and symptoms of this disorder. It occurs in approximately 1 in 30,000 to 60,000 newborns. This entity has a very high allelic heterogeneity and more than 150 different mutations have been identified in different populations and ethnic groups in 15 countries. The most frequently cited GALT gene mutations are Q188R, N314D, S135L and K285N. N314D is further associated with two variants, Duarte 1 and Duarte 2. Missense mutations lead to extremely low to absent enzymatic activity and thus causing severe symptoms. The "Duarte" variant produces some active enzyme and hence these variants have a better prognosis. Compound heterozygotes, i.e.

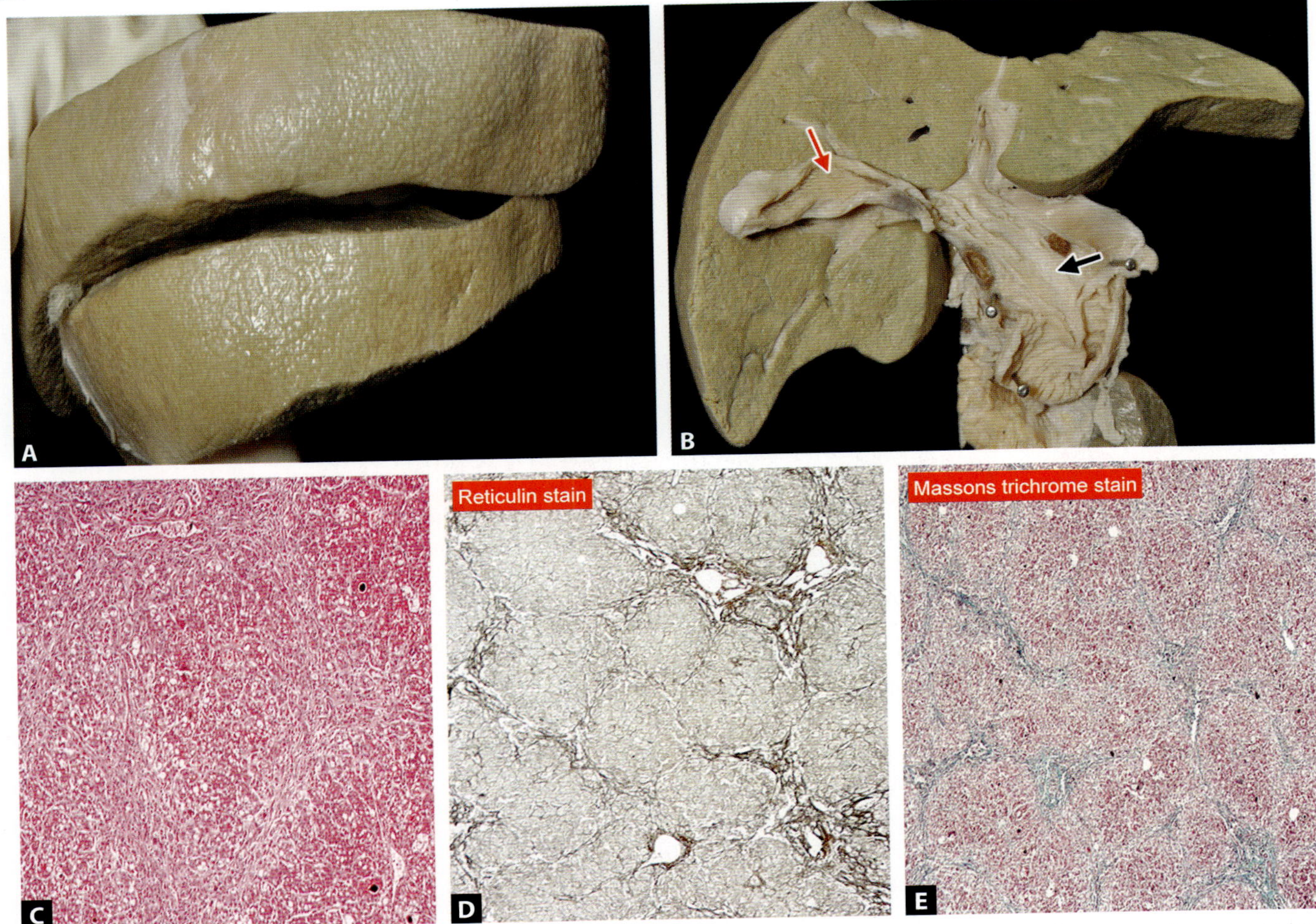

Figs 1A–E: (A) Capsular aspect of the liver showing micronodules; (B) Complex comprising of slice of liver showing micronodules, opened up biliary tract (arrow), and gall bladder (red arrow) which are normal; (C) Microphotograph of the liver at low power showing fibrous septa forming a nodule along with steatosis; (D and E) Reticulin and Masson's trichrome stain showing micronodular cirrhosis.

a classical allele with a "Duarte" allele are less severely affected. A study from our institute by Singh et al,[5] using PCR–RFLP procedure, screened 55 galactosemic infants from different regions of India for the Q188R, N314D, L218L, G1105C, G1323A, G1391A and 5'UTR-119del-GTCA changes in GALT gene. They found N314D homozygotes in 7 and N314D heterozygotes in 30 patients, i.e. in 40% cases. The second common mutation found was Q188R in three patients (one homozygous and two heterozygous), i.e. in 2.7% of cases. Of the 44 alleles carrying N314D, 43 were found to be D2 alleles and no D1 allele was detected. Thus, in the Indian population, a higher frequency of Duarte 2 allele suggests the presence of a milder form of galactosemia, which however can be managed by early diagnosis and dietary management.

2. ***Galactosemia Type 2***: This shows deficiency of enzyme galactokinase involved in reaction 1. This is a milder form of disease and occurs due to mutations on the GALK1 gene.
3. ***Galactosemia Type 3***: This shows deficiency of galactose epimerases and occurs due to mutations in the GALE gene.

As a result of the disorder in the metabolic pathway, galactose-1-phosphate accumulates in many places in the body including the liver, spleen, kidneys, heart, cerebral cortex, erythrocytes and the lens of the eye. Activation of the alternate metabolic pathways leads to the accumulation

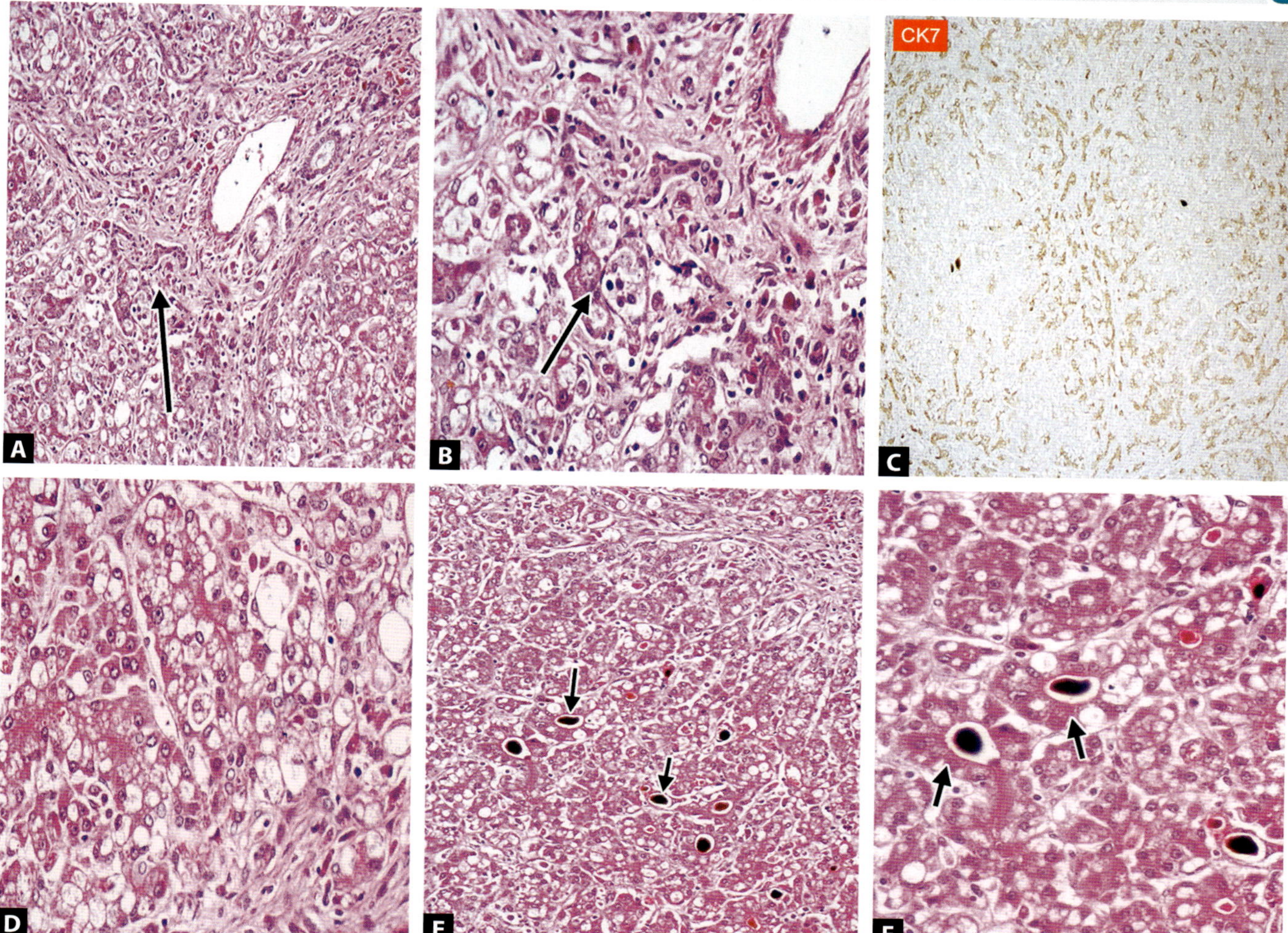

Figs 2A–F: (A and B) Liver showing periportal cholangiolar proliferation (arrows); (C) Immunohistochemistry with CK7 highlights the florid periportal cholangiolar proliferation and nodular architecture is better appreciated; (D) Hepatocytes showing diffuse macrovesicular steatosis; (E and F) Liver at low/high power showing pseudoacinar transformation with bile plugs (arrows).

in the tissues of galactitol, a polyol metabolite of galactose and galactonate, an oxidized by product of excess galactose. Thus, a shortage of any of one of the critical enzymes leads to galactose and related compounds to build up to toxic levels in the body, leading on to damage of tissues and organs, further leading on to the characteristic features of galactosemia. Heterozygous states have mild enzyme deficiency, but homozygous individuals, fully manifest the disease.

The clinical picture is variable due to the heterogeneity of mutations, but the most affected organs are the liver, eyes and brain. Children present with vomiting, diarrhea, failure to thrive right from birth, cholestatic jaundice, cataracts due to galactitol accumulation leading to water absorption, lethargy, fulminant *E. coli* sepsis, hemolytic anemia, increased intracranial pressure and cerebral edema. Severe cases may have edema, ascites and coagulopathy. Hepatomegaly occurs due to fatty change, but fibrosis sets in very fast leading to micronodular cirrhosis. CNS manifestations are nonspecific and lead to loss of neurons, gliosis and edema with predilection for the dentate nucleus of the cerebellum and olivary nuclei of the medulla. So, these babies fail to thrive from birth, vomiting/diarrhea appears within a few days, jaundice/hepatomegaly appears in the 1st week, cataracts develop in a few weeks and mental retardation is detected by 6–12 months. The only available therapy is the complete dietary restriction of galactose. This becomes difficult as fruits and vegetables also contain significant soluble galactose and there is an endogenous synthesis of galactose as well. With restriction of galactose right from birth, the liver damage and cataracts can be prevented but the neurodevelopmental

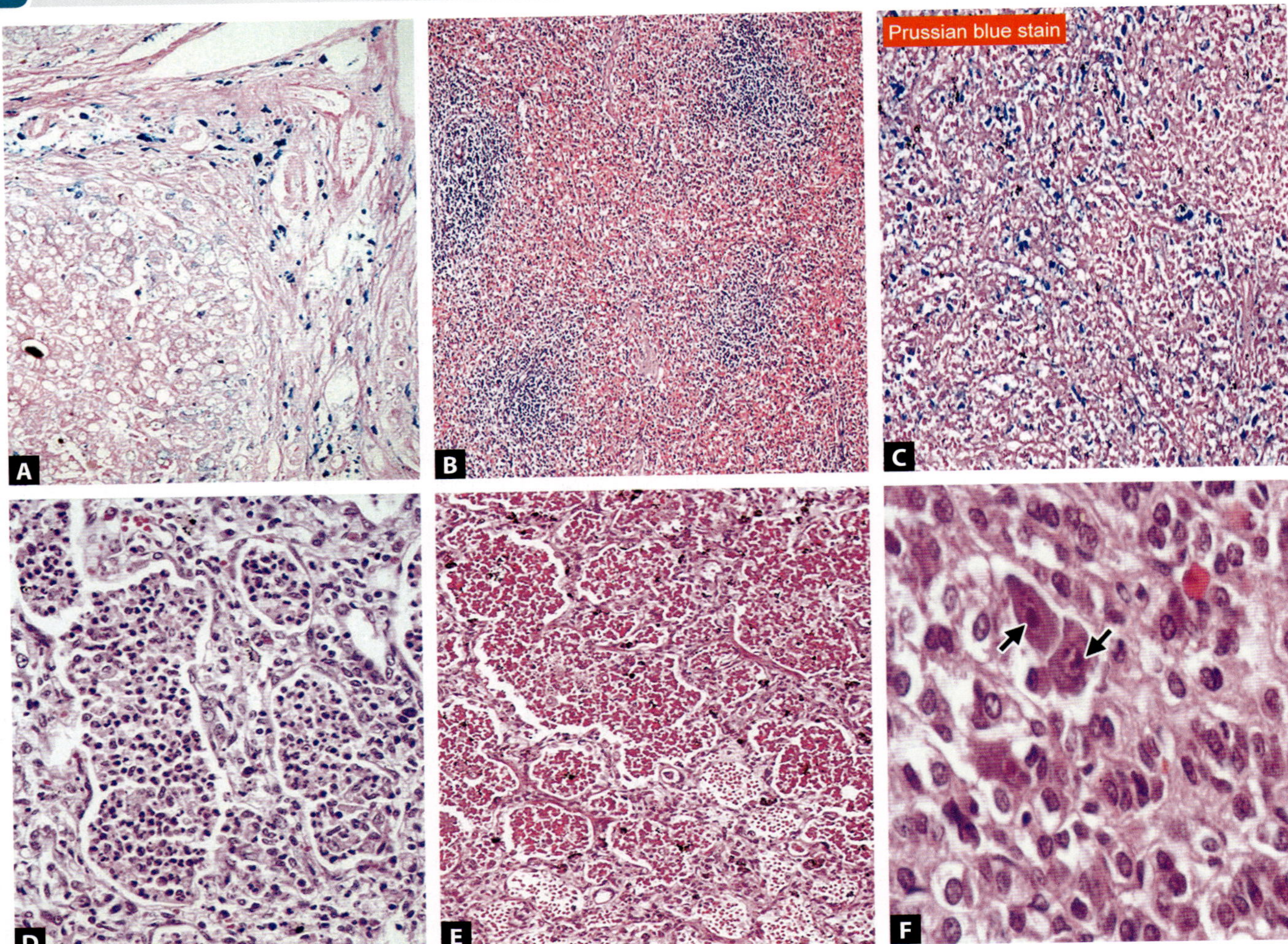

Figs 3A–F: (A) Liver section stained with Prussian blue stain showing portal and periportal siderosis (2+); (B and C) Spleen showing congestion and Perls stains highlights the siderosis (3+); (D) Microphotograph of the lung showing alveolar spaces packed with polymorphs; (E) Lung showing alveolar hemorrhage; (F) Adrenal gland showing intranuclear inclusions of CMV (arrow).

complications remain. Late complication include speech disorder, ataxia and in females a partial or complete ovarian failure. Benedict's test/chromatography are screening tests for galactosemia, wherein a non-glucose sugar is detected (with a negative glucostix test). GALT enzyme assays done in erythrocytes and biallelic mutations in the GALT gene are diagnostic tests.

Pathologic features in the liver are most distinctive and appear by 10 days of life. The liver is initially enlarged, firm and bile stained. Later on, once the fibrosis sets in, it shrinks and micronodules can be seen on the capsular aspect and on cut section. There is marked steatosis, periportal cholangiolar proliferation containing bile plugs and infiltrated by neutrophils, porto-portal/porto-central bridging fibrosis which ultimately leads to micronodular cirrhosis within 3–6 months, pseudoacinar/pseudoglandular proliferation of hepatic plates, wherein hepatocytes surround a dilated canaliculus that may be empty or contain bile, extramedullary hematopoiesis and periportal hemosiderosis. Occasional giant cell transformation and macroregenerative nodule can be seen. As the fibrosis increases, at times, the fat begins to disappear and in an occasional case of full blown cirrhosis, it is difficult to discern. Differential diagnosis includes fructosemia and tyrosinemia. Fructosemia presents with severe liver disease, when fructose is introduced in the infant's diet, at the time of weaning. Histological findings in the liver show a neonatal hepatitis-like picture with florid giant cell transformation, steatosis, fibrosis and early phases of cirrhosis rather than frank cirrhosis. Tyrosinemia is a disorder of amino acid metabolism and morphologically can mimic galactosemia. Here, liver dysfunction is precipitated by an infection, typically in the first 2 years of life. Liver in tyrosinemia is enlarged, yellow and firm with varying sized variegated (yellow, tan, green) nodules. Microscopic examination shows fatty change, cholestasis, pseudoacinar transformation, pericellular/periportal fibrosis, hemosiderosis, extramedullary hematopoiesis and varying sized large regenerative/macroregenerative nodules. These nodules may give an impression of multifocal hepatocellular carcinoma and they show more fat accumulation as compared to the adjacent liver. Periportal cholangiolar proliferation occurs, but is not striking as seen in galactosemia. Cirrhosis can be micro or macro or mixed type. Liver cell dysplasia (large and small cell type) has been noted.

COMMENTARY—INDEX CASE: PM 23869

A 3-month-old male child presented with failure to thrive, diarrhea, progressive abdominal distension, weight loss, jaundice, acholic stools, conjugated hyperbilirubinemia, deranged liver function tests, coagulopathy and ascites. He was said to be doing well till 2 months of age. A clinical diagnosis of infantile cholestasis syndrome—chronic liver disease with sepsis and decompensation was made. Autopsy revealed micronodular cirrhosis with classical gross and histological features of galactosemia.

Worth stressing points in this case are:

- The child presented at two months of age, and by three months he was frankly cirrhotic. There was ascites and coagulopathy, indicating a severe disease.
- Sepsis and pulmonary hemorrhage took away the patient.
- There was hemosiderosis in the liver and spleen and a low hemoglobin, which could be due to associated hemolytic anaemia, although the work up for it was not done.
- CMV IgM (microELISA) was positive in this case and CMV inclusions were found in the adrenal glands (a favoured site) only.

TAKE HOME MESSAGE

- Marked steatosis, periportal cholangiolar proliferation containing bile plugs and porto-portal/porto-central bridging fibrosis leading to micronodular cirrhosis within 3–6 months, pseudoacinar proliferation of hepatic plates, giant cells and extramedullary hematopoiesis are morphologic features of galactosemia.
- These patients normally present in the 1st week of life, but as seen in the index case, the child was doing well till 2 months of age.

REFERENCES

1. Elsas LJ 2nd, Lai K. The molecular biology of galactosemia. Genet Med. 1998;1(1):40-8.
2. Suzuki M, West C, Beutler E. Large-scale molecular screening for galactosemia alleles in a pan-ethnic population. Hum Genet. 2001;109(2):210-5.
3. Thompson RJ, Portmann BC, Roberts EA. Genetic and metabolic liver disease. In: Burt A, Portmann B, Ferrel L (Eds). MacSween's Pathology of the Liver, 6th edition. UK: Churchill Livingstone; 2012.
4. Maitra A. Diseases of infancy and childhood. In: Kumar V, Abbas AK, Aster JC (Eds). Robbins and Cotran Pathologic Basis of Disease, 9th edition. US: Elsevier; 2014. p. 465.
5. Singh R, Thapa BR, Kaur G, et al. Frequency distribution of Q188R, N314D, Duarte 1, Duarte 2 GALT variant alleles in an Indian galactosaemic population. Biochem Genet. 2012; 50:871-80.

CONTRIBUTIONS BY:

1. Dr Rakesh Kumar, Associate Professor, Department of Pediatrics (Compilation of Clinical Details)
2. Dr BR Thapa, Professor and Head, Department of Gastroenterology, Hepatology and Nutrition (Clinician In-Charge)

Post Graduate Institute of Medical Education and Research, Chandigarh, India.

CASE 98

Galactosemia, Double Heterozygous for N314D and Q188R Mutations, with Micronodular Cirrhosis and Absence of Steatosis: PM 25342

Nandita Bharadwaj Kakkar

HIGHLIGHTS OF THE CASE

A 5½ months old male child came with cholestatic jaundice since birth, abdominal distension with ascites, altered sensorium, hard irregular liver with hepatosplenomegaly, visible bilateral cataract, anemia, leukocytosis, thrombocytopenia, markedly deranged liver function tests, deranged coagulogram, hyponatremia, hypoglycemia and ultrasonography showing a hard echotexture of liver, increased liver size and mild intrahepatic biliary radical dilatation. A clinical diagnosis of acute on chronic liver failure—cirrhosis ? Galactosemia ? Caroli syndrome with sepsis was made. Autopsy revealed micronodular cirrhosis with morphologic features consistent with galactosemia along with diffuse nesidioblastosis. On molecular analysis, this case was double heterozygous for N314D and Q188R mutations. The odd point was that the liver revealed a marked prominence of giant cells and there was no steatosis.

Keywords: Galactosemia, double heterozygous, N314D and Q188R mutations, absence of steatosis, diffuse nesidioblastosis, giant cells prominence, autopsy.

CLINICAL DETAILS

Date of Admission: 09.04.2013, Date of Death: 13.04.2013, Duration of Hospital Stay: 4 Days

A 5½ months old male child was admitted with complaints of yellowish discoloration of body since day 4 of life, vomiting since day 8 of life, decreased urine output, poor feeding, lethargy, fever and abdominal distension since 2 days. The fever was 100°F. Vomiting was intermittent, 1–2 episodes/day, nonbilious, nonprojectile and containing ingested milk. Jaundice was persistent and proressively increased. There was history of passing clay colored stool and dark color urine at the age of 3 months. There was history of two spontaneous abortions at 8 and 12 weeks period of gestation. He was a full-term, normal vaginal delivery, baby cried immediately after birth, weighed 2.1 kg and there were no antenatal or postnatal complications. Developmental history revealed the presence of social smile, he was recognizing his mother, but there was partial neck holding. He was immunized for age and was on breast milk and cow milk (1:1 dilution). On ***examination***, there was pallor, jaundice, no fever, normal facies, respiratory rate: 52/min, no intercostal retractions, heart rate: 140/min, BP: 88/50 mm Hg, visible bilateral cataract noted, excessive hair present over forehead and pinna, no edema, cyanosis or lymphadenopathy. Anthropometry—weight: 4.7 kg (<3rd centile), occipitofrontal circumference: 37 cm (<3rd centile) and length: 58 cm (<3rd centile). Abdomen was distended, soft, overlying veins were visible but not dilated or tortuous, umbilicus was transverse, liver was palpable 4 cm below right costal margin, was firm with irregular border, spleen was firm and palpable 2 cm below left costal margin, free fluid was present and bowel sounds were noted. CNS—GCS-E1M4V1, muscle bulk normal but hypotonia noted, deep tendon reflexes elicitable and there were no cerebellar/meningeal signs. CVS and respiratory systems were within normal limits.

Investigations

Hematological: Hb 8.5 g/dL, TLC – 26,900/uL, DLC – N-55, L-36, M-7, E-2, platelets – 37000/uL, Coagulogram deranged – PT 78 secs, PT1 18%, INR 5.16 and APPT -95 sec.

Blood biochemistry/microbiology: S bilirubin 24 mg%, conjugated 15 mg%, total serum proteins 4.2 gm with albumin 1.9 gm, AST/ALT 344/269 U/L, alkaline phosphatase

336 U/l, Serum Na+ 110 mEq/L, K+-5.9 mEq/L, Ca2+/PO4-8.5/2.5 mg%, S urea 17 mg%, S creatinine 0.5 mg%, random blood sugar 44 mg%, blood culture and TORCH serology negative. Galactose-1-phosphate uridyltransferase (GALT) assay could not be done.

Radiology: Ultrasonography – liver showed heterogonous echotexture, irregular margin and mild intrahepatic biliary radical dilatation.

Units clinical diagnosis: - Acute on chronic liver failure – Cirrhosis ? Galactosemia ? Caroli's syndrome with sepsis - bacterial/fungal and bleed.

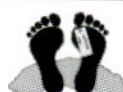

AUTOPSY FINDINGS: PM 25342

5½ Months Male Child

A partial autopsy was performed. The pleural and peritoneal cavities contained 150 mL and 300 mL of straw colored fluid, respectively. The liver (Figs 1A and B) weighed 145 g (N: 259 ± 58 g). It was shrunken and the capsular aspect showed micronodules (0.1–0.3 cm). Cut section (Fig 1B) was bile stained and showed extensive fibrosis along with micronodules. Dissection of the biliary tree revealed its patency. Microscopic examination showed diffuse effacement of the lobular architecture with formation of nodules separated by wide fibrous septa (Figs 1C and D). The septa showed bile ductular proliferation, lymphomononuclear cell infiltrate, periportal/periseptal cholangiolar proliferation (Fig 2A) highlighted by CK7 immunohistochemistry (Fig 2B) and canalicular cholestasis. The hepatocytes showed marked giant cell (Figs 2C and D) and pseudoacinar transformation (Fig 2E- arrows). There was no steatosis, pericellular fibrosis, Mallory hyaline, orcein stain did not reveal any copper-associated proteins and iron stains did not reveal any increase

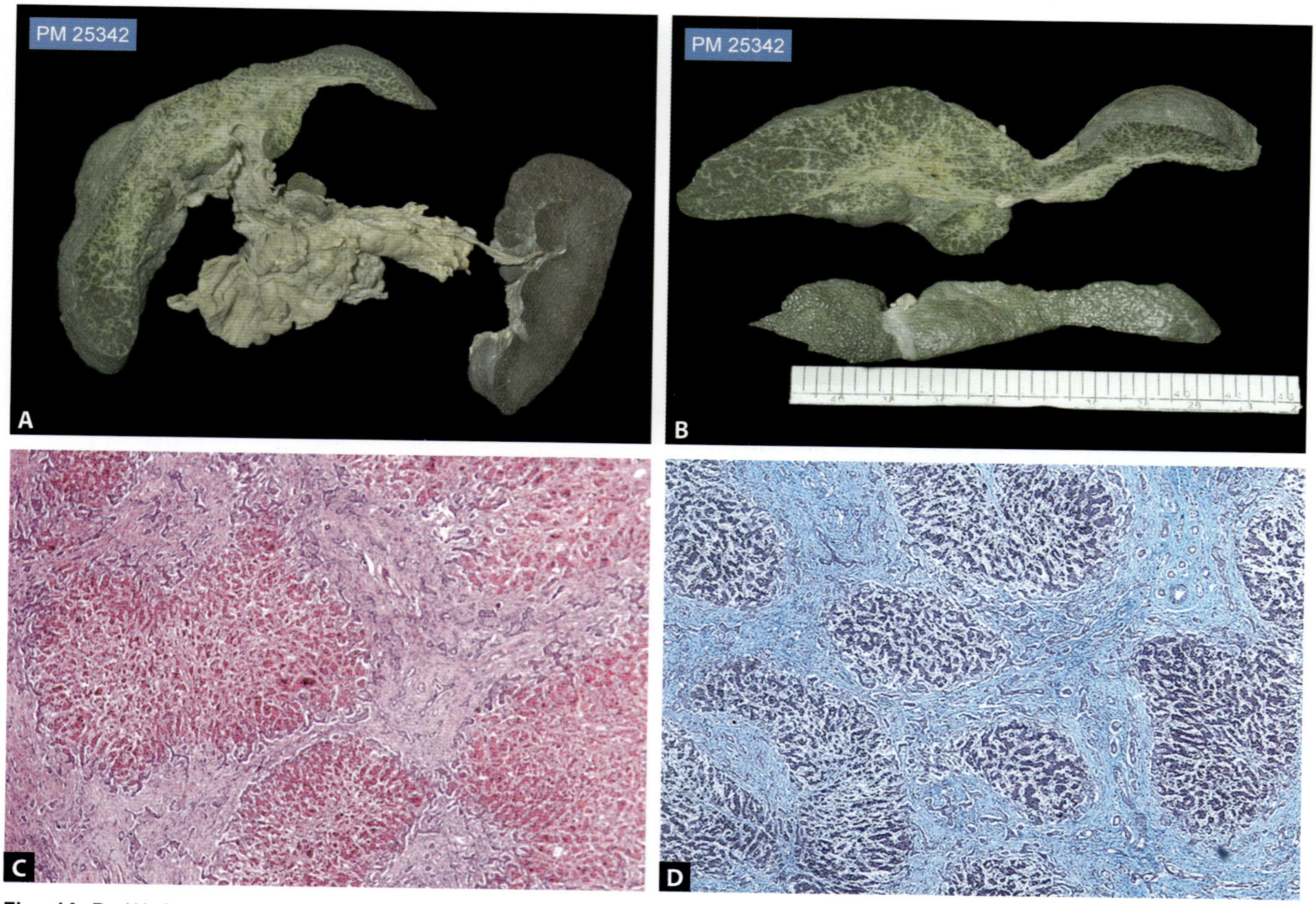

Figs 1A–D: (A) Organ complex comprising of slice of the shrunken fibrotic liver, enlarged spleen, and pancreas; (B) Coronal slice of the liver which is bile stained and shows micronodules. The capsular aspect also shows micronodules; (C) Photomicrograph of the liver showing micronodules separated by fibrous septa with bile ductular and periportal cholangiolar proliferation; (D) Masson trichrome stain highlighting the micronodules and the septa.

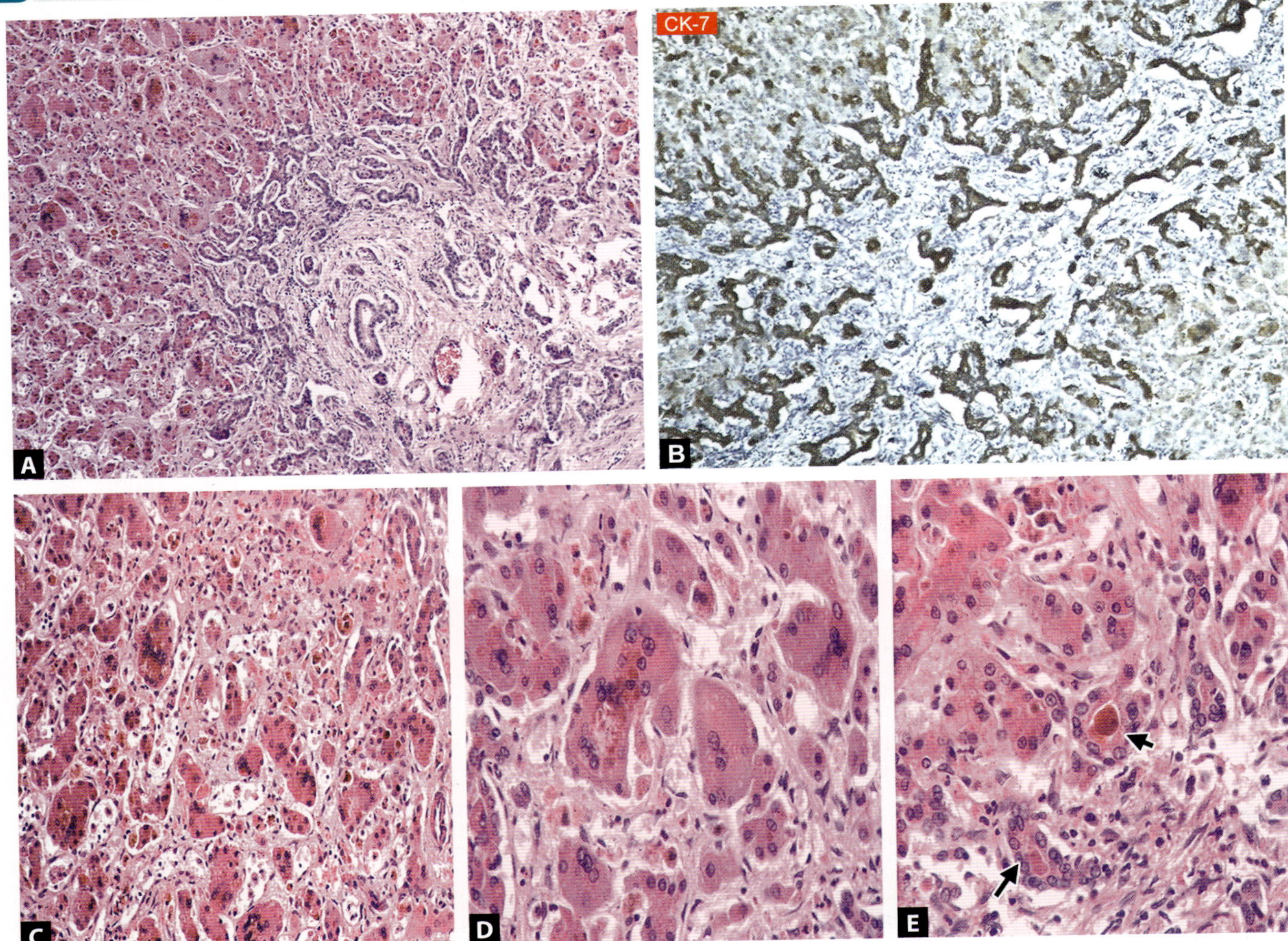

Figs 2A–E: Photomicrographs of the liver showing (A) Marked periportal cholangiolar proliferation; (B) Periportal cholangiolar proliferation highlighted by CK7 immunostain; (C and D) Extensive giant cell transformation; (E) Pseudoacinar transformation with bile plugs (arrows).

in iron. Overall features were suggestive of a metabolic liver disease, i.e. galactosemia. The complete absence of steatosis and marked giant cell transformation were the odd point, although other morphologic features in the liver were consistent with a diagnosis of galactosemia. It is seen in our experience that when frank cirrhosis sets in, the steatosis can start to disappear and may be present only focally or disappears altogether. In galactosemia, it is said that only occasional giant cell transformation is noted. But in our experience of genetically proven autopsy cases of galactosemia, marked giant cell transformation is seen. The liver tissue was sent to the Department of Biochemistry for mutational analysis of GALT gene and it was found to be double heterozygous for N314D (Figs 3A and B) and Q188R mutations (Figs 3C and D). The ***spleen*** was enlarged (54 g, N: 20 $\pm$ 7) and on microscopic examination revealed features of congestive splenomegaly. The ***pancreas*** was normal grossly, but on microscopic examination revealed diffuse nesidioblastosis, i.e. islet cell hyperplasia (Fig 4A), proven with insulin immunohistochemistry (Fig 4B). The ***lungs*** weighed 115 g, pleural dullness was noted and cut section (Fig 4C) showed consolidation and areas of hemorrhage. Microscopic examination revealed necrotizing bronchopneumonia (Fig 4D) and dilated alveolar spaces lined by hyaline membranes consistent with diffuse alveolar damage (Fig 4E). The ***kidneys*** were normal grossly and microscopic examination revealed plenty of bile casts. Other organs were within normal limits.

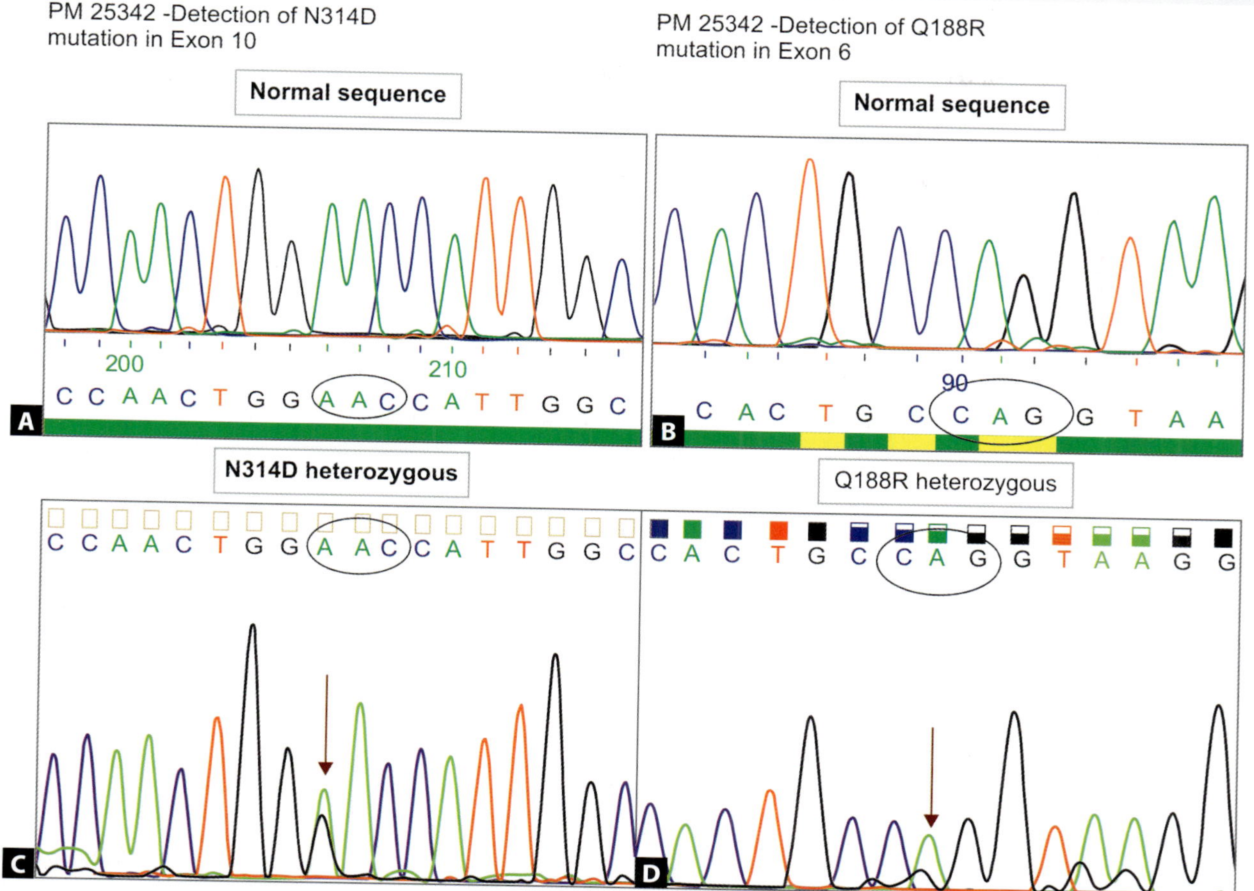

Figs 3A–D: Electropherogram of galactose-1-phosphate uridyltransferase (GALT) sequence. (A) Normal sequence—exon 10 showing wild type sequence; (B) N314D mutation—exon 10 GALT gene sequence depicting substitution of A to G at nucleotide position 940 resulting in asparagine to aspartic acid at codon 314 heterozygous state; (C) Normal sequence—wild type sequence exon 6 sequence of GALT gene; (D) Q188R mutation—exon 6 GALT gene sequence of the sample depicting substitution of A to G at nucleotide position 563 resulting in glutamine to arginine at codon 188 heterozygous state.
(*Courtesy*: Dr Rajinder Prasad)

FINAL AUTOPSY DIAGNOSIS: PM 25342

6 Months, Male Child, History of Two Previous Abortions

- Micronodular cirrhosis consistent with Galactosemia (double heterozygous for *N314D* and *Q188R* mutations)
- Portal hypertension—ascites and congestive splenomegaly
- Confluent necrotizing pneumonia with diffuse alveolar damage
- Nesidioblastosis—diffuse
- Bile cast in kidneys and pleural effusion.

Galactosemia: See case 97, PM 23869—A classical case of Galactosemia.

COMMENTARY—INDEX CASE: PM 25342

This 5½ months old male child came with cholestatic jaundice since birth, abdominal distension with ascites, altered sensorium, hard irregular liver with hepatosplenomegaly, visible bilateral cataract, anemia, leukocytosis, thrombocytopenia, markedly deranged liver function tests, deranged coagulogram, hyponatremia, hypoglycemia and ultrasonography showing enlarged liver with a hard echotexture and mild intrahepatic biliary radical dilatation. A clinical diagnosis of Acute on chronic liver failure—Cirrhosis ? Galactosemia ? Caroli's syndrome with sepsis and bleed was made.

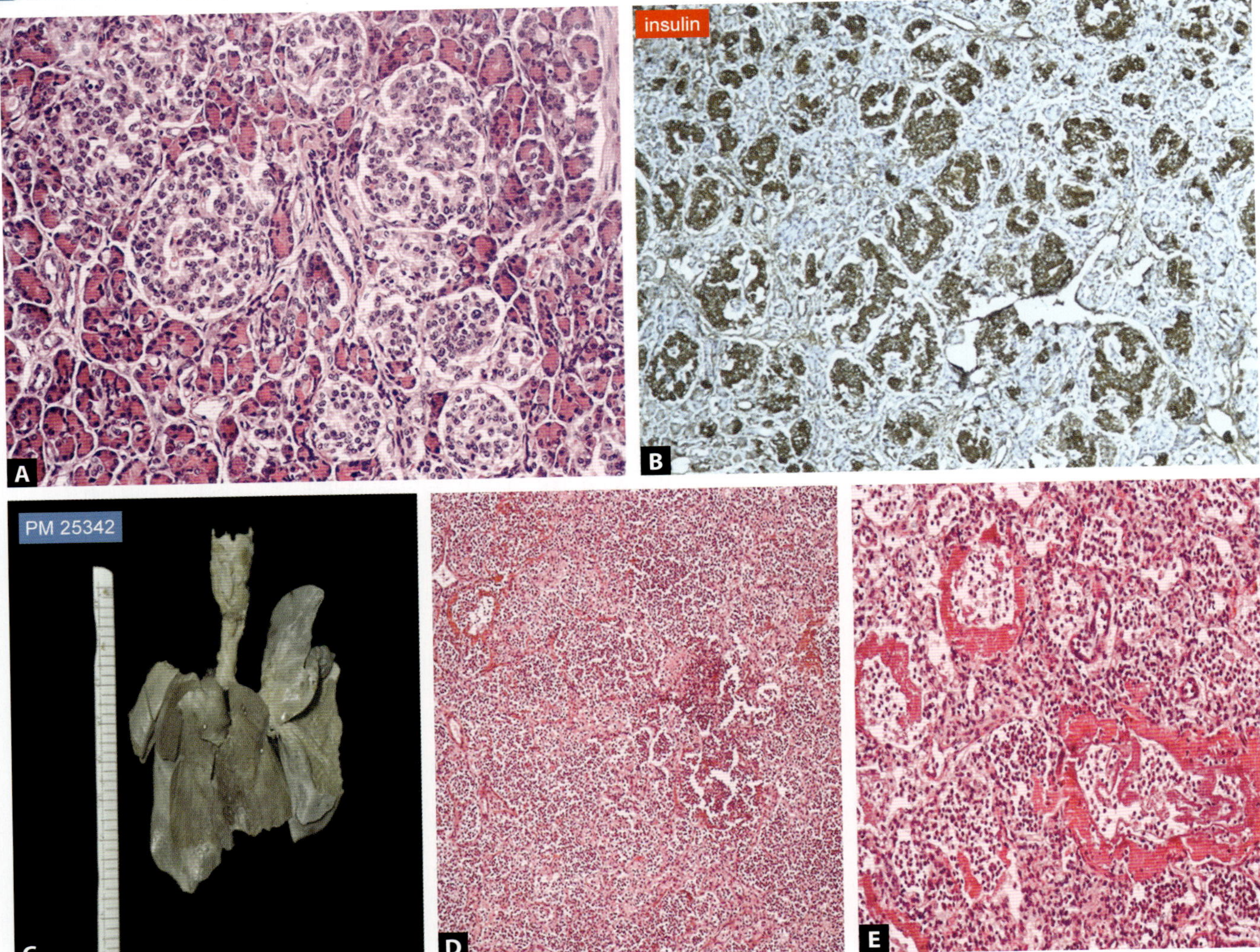

Figs 4A–E: (A) Photomicrograph of the pancreas showing diffuse islet cell hyperplasia, i.e. nesidioblastosis; (B) Insulin immunohistochemistry highlights the islet cell hyperplasia; (C) Cut section of the lung showing hemorrhages; (D) Lung showing necrotizing bronchopneumonia; (E) Dilated alveolar spaces containing neutrophils lined by hyaline membranes.

At autopsy, there was micronodular cirrhosis with morphologic features consistent with classical galactosemia along with diffuse nesidioblastosis. On molecular analysis, this case was double heterozygous for *N314D* and *Q188R* mutations. These two mutations (*N314D*> > >*Q188R*) are the most common mutations seen in galactosemic patients in our country. On histopathology there was a diagnostic problem as there was no steatosis seen in the liver and florid giant cell transformation was noted. In our experience with genetically proven cases of galactosemia, when frank cirrhosis sets in, the steatosis can start to disappear and at times is either present only focally or disappears altogether (as seen in the index case). In galactosemia, it is said that only occasional giant cell transformation is noted. But in our experience again, marked giant cell transformation has been seen in very many proven cases (e.g.—index case). So cholestatic symptoms from birth, micronodular cirrhosis, steatosis (may be absent when frank cirrhosis sets in), florid periportal cholangiolar proliferation, pseudoacinar transformation, cholestasis and giant cells (few or many) are pointers toward a diagnosis of galactosemia.

This patient had hypoglycemia and this was due to the presence of diffuse nesidioblastosis. Islet cell hyperplasia is seen in cases of tyrosinemia, but has not been documented in galactosemia. Literature says that marked giant cell transformation is seen in cases of fructosemia. Symptoms of fructosemia start to occur after weaning, but in the index case the symptoms started right from birth. Moreover, molecular diagnosis confirmed the presence of galactosemia in the index case. The terminal event was fulminant sepsis with necrotizing pneumonia and diffuse alveolar damage.

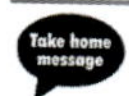

TAKE HOME MESSAGE

- Double heterozygotes manifest with severe disease as seen in the index case.
- *N314D> >Q188R* mutations are the two common mutations seen in galactosemic patients in India.
- In galactosemia, once cirrhosis sets in, steatosis can disappear or be present only focally. This can however lead to diagnostic difficulties.
- Marked giant cell transformation can be seen in galactosemia.
- With cholestatic symptoms starting from birth, galactosemia should be in the differential and GALT assay is mandatory.

SUGGESTED READING

1. Singh R, Thapa BR, Kaur G, et al. Frequency distribution of Q188R, N314D, Duarte 1, Duarte 2 GALT variant alleles in an Indian galactosaemic population. Biochem Genet. 2012; 50:871-80.

CONTRIBUTIONS BY:

1. Dr Pulkit Rastogi, Assistant Professor, Department of Histopathology.
2. Dr Vinita Garg, Junior Resident, Department of Pediatrics (Compilation of Clinical Details)
3. Dr Rajindra Prasad, Ex-Professor and Head, Department of Biochemistry (Postmortem GALT assay. Figs 3A—D)
4. Dr RK Vasishta, Professor and Head, Department of Histopathology (Consultation)
5. Dr BR Thapa, Professor and Head, Department of Gastroenterology, (Clinician In-Charge)

Post Graduate Institute of Medical Education and Research, Chandigarh, India.

CASE 99

A Case of Galactosemia, Double Heterozygous for Q188R and E308K Mutations with Early Neonatal Acute Liver Failure: PM 25552

Nandita Bharadwaj Kakkar

HIGHLIGHTS OF THE CASE

This new born female baby presented in the 1st week of life with fever, rising hyperbilirubinemia (conjugated at first and then unconjugated since day 14 of life), polymorphonuclear leukocytosis, falling hemoglobin, low platelets, raised serum glutamic oxaloacetic transaminase (SGOT)/alkaline phosphatase, coagulopathy, hypoproteinemia, hypoalbuminemia, distended abdomen, ascites, hepatosplenomegaly and bilateral congenital cataracts. She was treated on the lines of acute liver failure—galactosemia and sepsis. Autopsy revealed metabolic liver disease—consistent with galactosemia, double heterozygous for Q188R and E308K mutations with extensive pulmonary hemorrhage and 700 mL of blood tinged ascitic fluid.

Keywords: Acute liver failure, galactosemia, early presentation, coagulopathy, galactose-1-phosphate uridyl transferase (GALT) mutations, double heterozygous, *E308K* mutation, *Q188R* mutation.

CLINICAL DETAILS

Date of Birth: 05.07.13, Date of Admission: 19.07.2013, Date of Death: 27.07.2013, Duration of Hospital Stay: 8 Days

A 14-day-old female baby came with history of fever since day 2 of life which was undocumented, intermittent with no chills or diurnal variation. On day 5 of life, yellowish discoloration of body and passage of yellow colored stools was detected. Two days before admission there was melena along with loose stools. She was admitted at an outside facility, was given intravenous antibiotics and phototherapy for 4 days and was discharged on 12.07.13. After 2 days, there was rebound yellowish discoloration and she was referred to PGIMER Chandigarh. She was born to a G4P2012 mother at term through a vaginal delivery, body weight was 3.2 Kg and she cried immediately at birth, APGAR being 7, 9. She was both on breast and top feed. Mother's blood group was A+. ***Outside investigations*** revealed a TLC of 12,300/μL on day 2 and 11,520/μL on day 3 with predominant polymorphs (85–77%). Total serum bilirubin/conjugated fraction were 11.5/2.5 (day 3), 9.5/3.5 (day 4), 18.5/6.9 (day 11) and 20.7/14.7 (day 14) mg%. ***On examination***: weight = 3.2 Kg; height = 50 cm; occipitofrontal circumference = 33 cm (-2 to -3Z score); PR: 134/min; RR: 44/min; SpO2: 97%, icterus present, no pallor, edema, cyanosis or clubbing, bilateral cataract +, anterior fontanelle: 3×3 cm, bulging and pulsatile. ***Systemic examination***: abdomen distended, superficial veins dilated, liver palpable 4.5 cm below right costal margin, spans 7.7 cm, firm and nontender with regular margins; spleen palpable 2 cm below left costal margin and free fluid present. CVS: S1S2 normal, no murmur, Respiratory system: normal, CNS: E4M6V5; state to state variability present, suck and rooting: Good, Moro's complete and cry normal.

Investigations

Hematology: The hematology details are summarized in Table 1. ***Coagulogram (22/07):*** PT: 24'; PTI: 54%; aPTT: 100'; INR: 1.82; ***Ascitic fluid***: ***22/07:*** TLC: 360; DLC: predominantly polymorphs; Protein: 690 mg%; Sugar: 50 mg%; Bilirubin: 0.6 mg%; Conjugated bilirubin: 0.41 mg%. ***24/07:*** TLC: No WBC seen; Protein: 450 mg%; Sugar: 77 mg%; Bilirubin: 1.4 mg%. Culture: sterile. ***Cerebrospinal fluid (21/07)***: TLC: No WBC seen; Protein: 58 mg%; Sugar: 25 mg%; Culture: sterile. ***Blood culture and sensitivity test***: Grew yeast species.

Table 1: Hemograms.

	Hb g/dL	*TLC/µL*	*DLC(N/L/M/E)*	*Platelets/µL*
22/07/13	11.3	12,200	16/75/5/4	1,00,000
25/07/13	8.9	26,000	86/6	33,000
26/07/13	3.4	40,000	–	20,000

Table 2: Blood biochemistry.

	19/07/13	*22/07/13*	*24/07/13*	*25/07/13*
Urea (mg%)	–	22	25	27
Creatinine (mg%)	–	0.8	0.87	0.75
Ca2+ (mg%)	–	8.4	8.9	9.4
PO4 (mg)	–	4.5	5.8	4.8
TSP (gm)	–	3.5	3.87	3.94
Albumin (gm)	–	2.1	2.7	3.1
TSB (mg%)	25.5	16.8	25.54	21.99
Conjugated bilirubin (mg%)	–	10.94	14.97	14.00
SGOT (U/L)	–	130	115	74.11
SGPT (U/L)	–	NR	33.74	23.88
ALP (U/L)	–	NR	261	173

(ALP: Alkaline phosphatase; SGOT: Serum glutamic oxaloacetic transaminase; SGPT: Serum glutamate-pyruvate transaminase; TSP: Total serum proteins, TSB: Total serum bilirubin)

Blood biochemistry (Table 2): Serum electrolytes were within normal limits. ***Lipid Profile (25/07/13)***: *Cholesterol*: 61.1 mg%; Triglycerides: 308.06 mg%; HDL: 5.7 mg%; LDL: 6.02 mg%; blood sugar: 60 mg%. ***USG Abdomen 22/07***: Liver: 7 cms, echotexture normal, portal veins seen, no intrahepatic biliary radical dilatation. Spleen 6 cms. Kidneys normal in size and echotexture, Gross ascites present.

Eye Examination: Bilateral congenital cataract seen.

GALT assay could not be done.

Course in hospital: Child was treated on the lines of ***acute liver failure***. Vitamin K, Udiliv and N-acetylcysteine was given. Therapeutic ascitic tap was done twice for tense abdomen. For sepsis and secondary bacterial peritonitis, she was started on IV imipenem and vancomycin. She was initially kept nil orally, but was then started on enteral feed on day 3 of admission in the form of soya milk through orogastric tube providing 100 kcal/kg/day and protein of 2.5 g/kg/day. She was euglycemic on full feeds. For thrombocytopenia and coagulopathy, she received fresh frozen plasma and platelet concentrate. Albumin was also administered as there was hypoalbuminemia. She remained afebrile throughout the hospital stay. Preterminally, she developed acute abdominal distension with respiratory distress although her sensorium remained intact. Ascitic tap revealed frank blood. She developed refractory shock and subsequently cardiac arrest from which could not be revived. ***Units final diagnosis***: Acute liver failure (Galactosemia) with sepsis, coagulopathy and bilateral congenital cataracts.

AUTOPSY FINDINGS: PM 25552

A complete autopsy was performed. The baby was icteric, abdomen was distended and ascitic tap marks were present. The peritoneal cavity contained 700 mL of blood mixed fluid. ***Liver*** (Fig 1A) was enlarged, weighed 160 g (N: 110 g), was bile stained, firm to feel with a nutmeg appearance. There was no frank cirrhosis. Extrahepatic biliary tract was dissected out and was within normal limits. Microscopy (Figs 1B–D) revealed a distorted liver architecture with expanded portal tracts, a prominent porto-portal bridging fibrosis along with extensive portal/periportal cholangiolar/ductular proliferation. CK7 immunostain highlighted the distorted architecture by exhibiting the severe degree of cholangiolar proliferation. Reticulin stain showed reticulin rich fibers in the portal tracts and in the areas of bridging fibrosis. The Masson's trichrome stain, however weakly stained these reticulin rich fibers. The florid periportal cholangiolar proliferation (highlighted by the CK7 immunostain) was extending into the zone 2 (Figs 2A and B), sparing the perivenular hepatocytes which could be seen as forming circumscribed nodules containing fat (Fig 2C). The expanded portal tracts showed minimal lym-

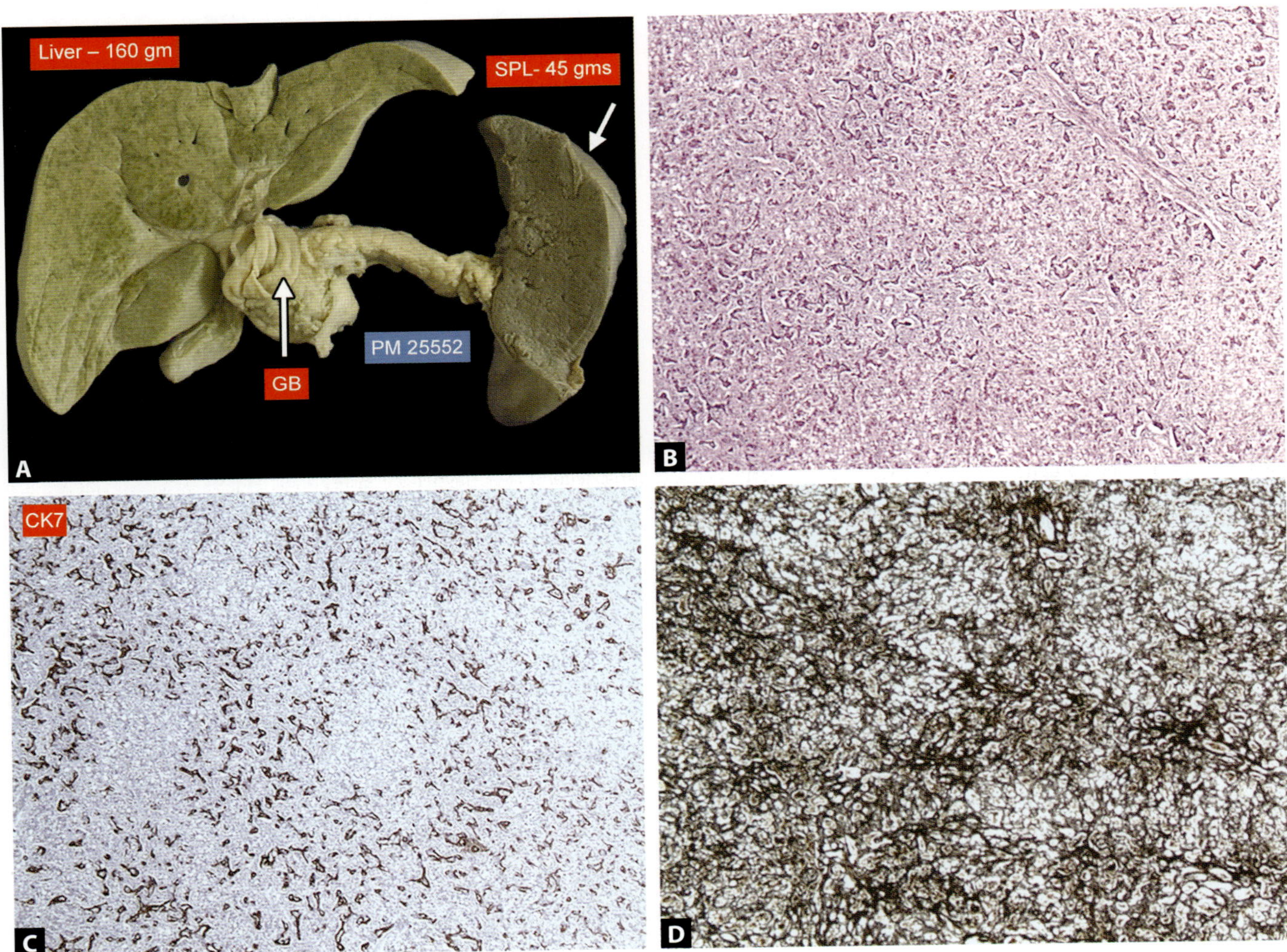

Figs 1A–D: (A) Organ complex composed of slice of the bile stained, enlarged liver showing nutmeg appearance, C loop of duodenum, pancreas, gall bladder, and slice of enlarged spleen; (B) Microphotograph of the liver at low power shows distorted liver architecture with expanded portal tracts and prominent bridging fibrosis along with extensive cholangiolar proliferation; (C) Cholangiolar proliferation better highlighted on CK7 immunostain; (D) Areas of bridging fibrosis show increased reticulin fibers.

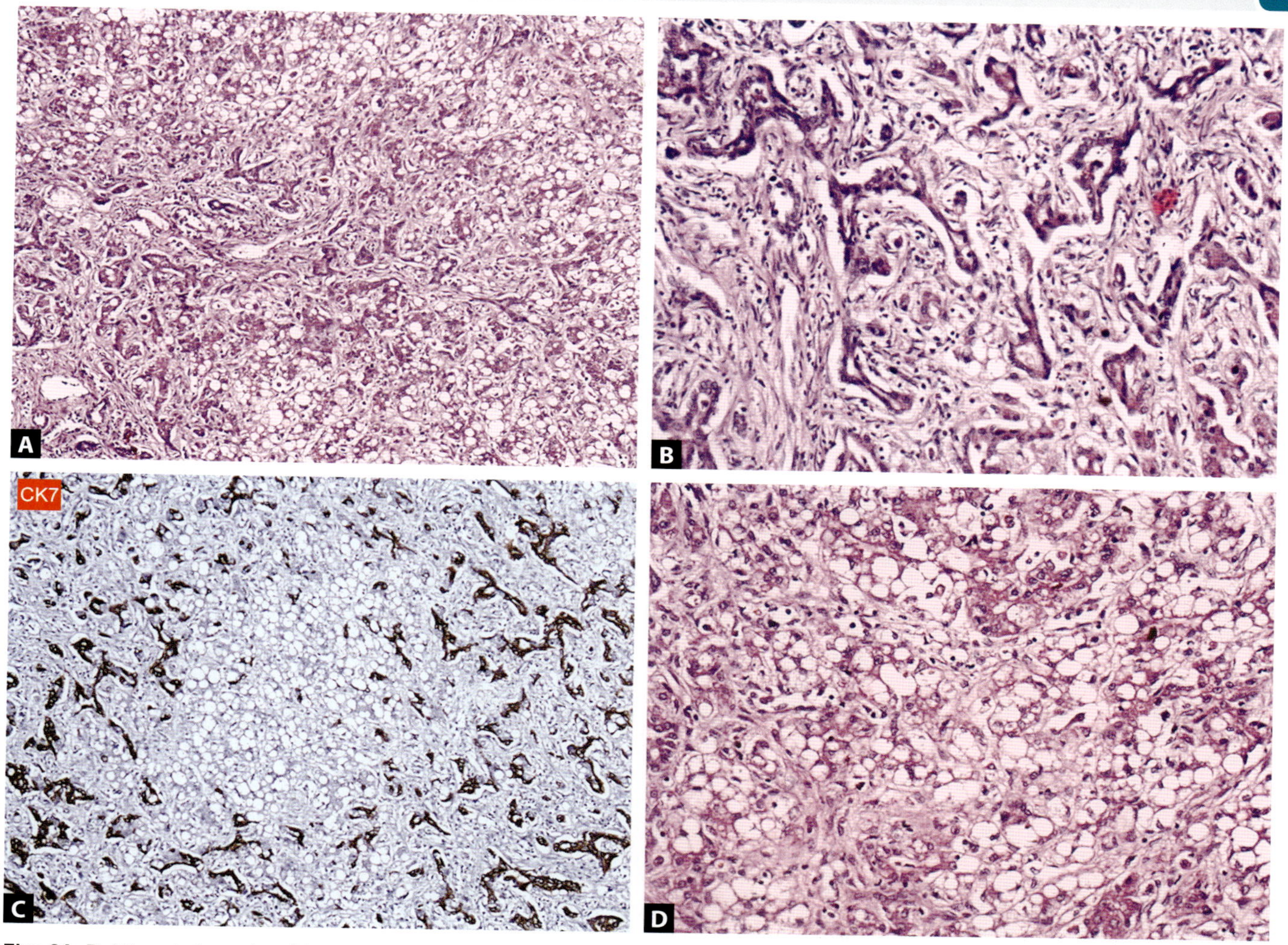

Figs 2A–D: Microphotographs of the liver. (A) Expanded portal tracts showing extensive portal/periportal cholangiolar proliferation. Adjacent hepatocytes in (A) show macrovesicular steatosis; (B) Cholangiolar proliferation at high power showing intervening fibrosis; (C) CK7 immunostain showing periportal cholangiolar proliferation and perivenular hepatocytes show diffuse macrovesicular steatosis forming a well-circumscribed nodule; (D) Diffuse macrovesicular steatosis.

phomononuclear cells (Fig 2A). The hepatocytes showed prominent macrovesicular steatosis (Figs 2A–D), pseudoacinar transformation and cholestasis (Figs 3A and B). There was no pericellular fibrosis, Mallory hyaline, iron deposition (Perls stain negative) or cola colored granules (orcein stain). The morphology was consistent a diagnosis of galactosemia with extensive fibrosis. The ***spleen*** was enlarged, weighed 45 g (N: 10 g) and on microscopy there was adequate white pulp along with congested red pulp. The ***lungs*** (Figs 3C and D) on the pleural aspect and on cut section showed areas of hemorrhage. Microscopy (Fig 3E) revealed extensive alveolar hemorrhage and early bronchopneumonia. Adrenal hemorrhage was noted. Early acute tubular necrosis was seen in the kidneys. Other organs (including the brain) were within normal limits.

Postmortem *GALT* gene mutation analysis (Fig 4) was done on the liver tissue and revealed two heterozygous mutations—*E308K* on Exon 10 and *Q188R* on Exon 6.

FINAL AUTOPSY DIAGNOSIS: PM 25552

Day 21 Female Baby

- *Metabolic liver disease*: Consistent with galactosemia with two heterozygous mutation—*E308K* on exon 10 and *Q188R* on exon 6

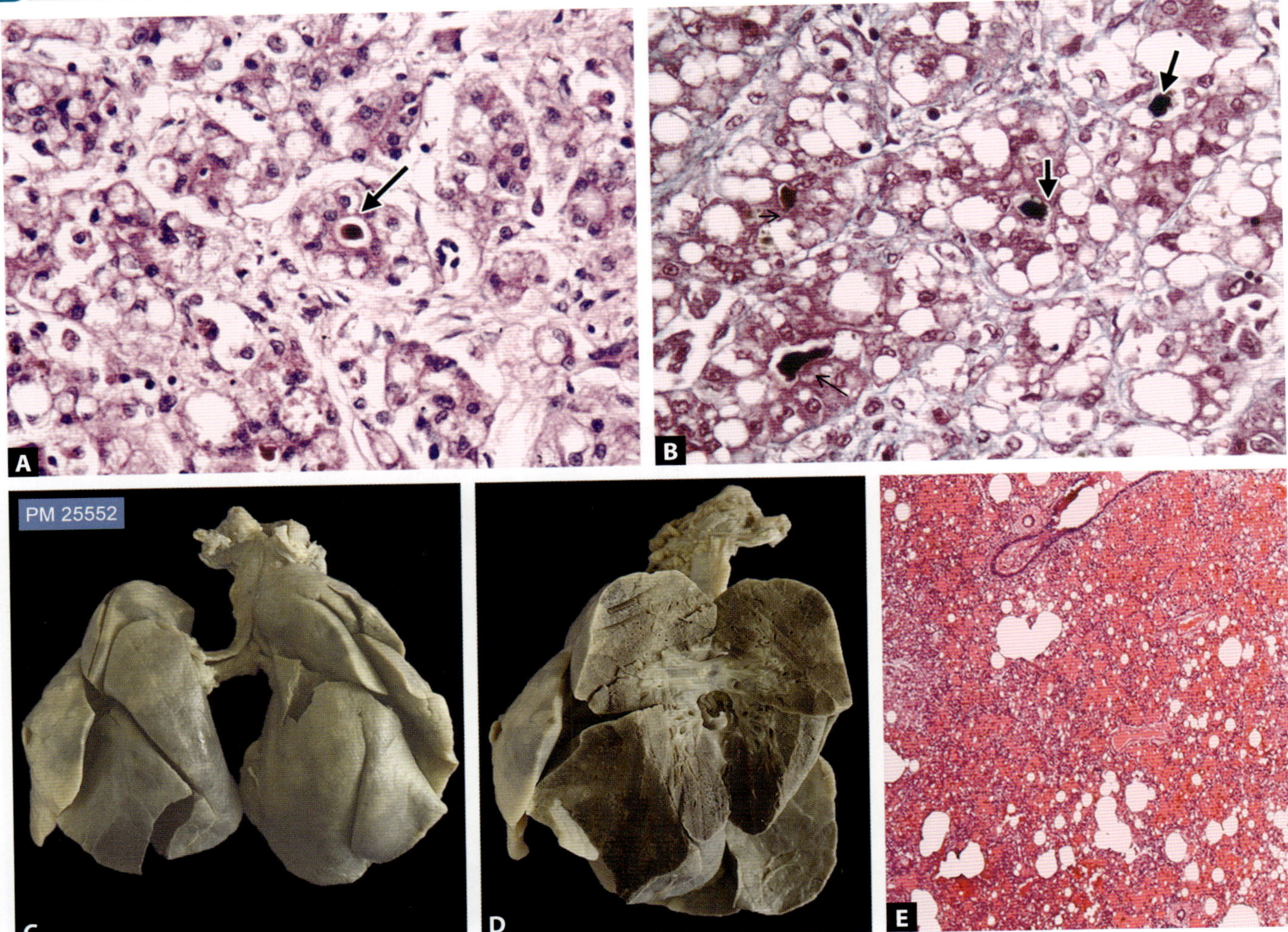

Figs 3A–E: (A and B) Liver showing pseudoacinar transformation with bile plugs (arrows); (C) Gross photograph of the lungs showing dusky discoloration of the pleura; (D) Cut section of the lungs show hemorrhage; (E) Microphotograph of the lung showing extensive alveolar hemorrhage.

- Pulmonary hemorrhage with early bronchopneumonia
- Congestive splenomegaly and ascites
- Acute tubular necrosis.

For Galactosemia—See Case 97 - PM 23869—A Classical case of Galactosemia.

COMMENTARY—INDEX CASE: PM 25552

This new born female baby presented in the first week of life with fever, rising hyperbilirubinemia (conjugated at first and then unconjugated since day 14 of life), polymorphonuclear leukocytosis, falling hemoglobin, low platelets, raised SGOT/alkaline phosphatase, coagulopathy, hypoproteinemia, hypoalbuminemia, distended abdomen, ascites, hepatosplenomegaly and bilateral congenital cataracts. She was treated on the lines of acute liver failure—galactosemia and sepsis. Autopsy revealed metabolic liver disease—consistent with galactosemia, double heterozygous for Q188R and E308K mutations with extensive pulmonary hemorrhage, early acute tubular necrosis and 700 mL of blood tinged ascitic fluid. In the west, Q188R is the most common mutation seen in galactosemic patients. In the Indian subcontinent, N314D has been found to be the most common mutation and Q188R mutation is the second most common. Although the index case was treated on lines for galactosemia, but the presence of coagulopathy and advanced disease took her away.

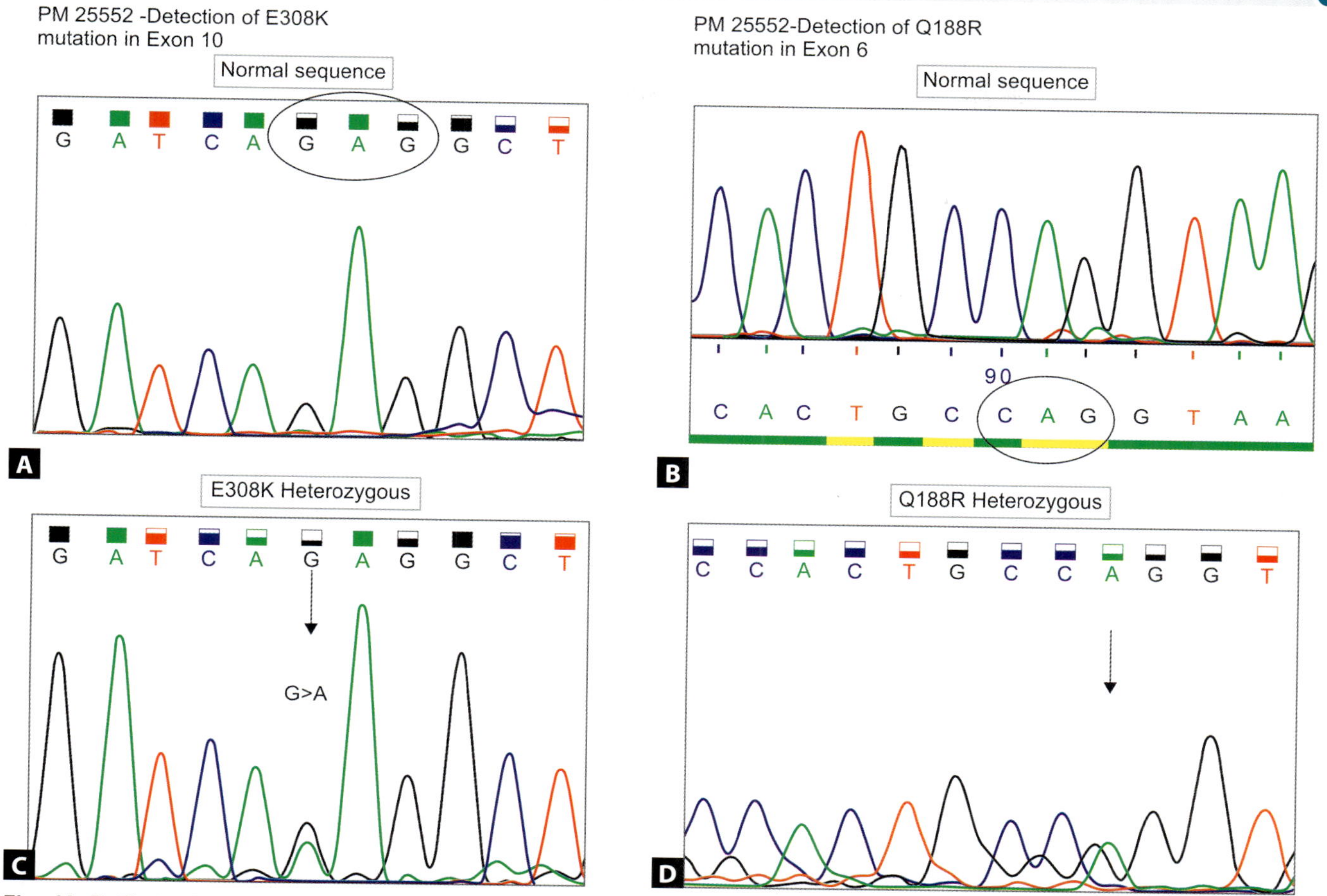

Figs 4A–D: Electropherogram of galactose-1-phosphate uridyl transferase (GALT) sequence. (A) Normal sequence—exon 10 showing wild type sequence; (B) E308K mutation—exon 10 GALT gene sequence depicting substitution of G to A at nucleotide position 922 resulting in Glutamic acid to Lysine at 308 position in heterozygous state; (C) Normal sequence—exon 6 showing wild type sequence; (D) Q188R mutation—exon 6 GALT gene sequence of the sample substitution of A to G at nucleotide position 563 resulting in glutamine to arginine at codon 188 in heterozygous state.
(*Courtesy*: Dr Rajinder Prasad)

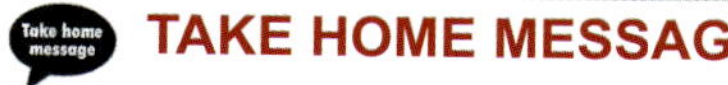

TAKE HOME MESSAGE

- Galactosemia can present in the first week of life as in the index case.
- GALT enzyme assays and biallelic mutational analysis in the GALT gene are diagnostic tests and clinch the diagnosis.

CONTRIBUTIONS BY:

1. Dr RK Vasishta, Professor and Head, Department of Histopathology (Consultation)
2. Dr Rajindra Prasad, Ex-Professor and Head, Department of Biochemistry (GALT Assay—Figs 4A–D)
3. Dr Arun Bansal, Professor, Department of Pediatrics (Compilation of Clinical Details)
4. Professor BR Thapa, Professor and Head, Department of Gastroenterology, Hepatology and Nutrition (Clinician In-Charge)

Post Graduate Institute of Medical Education and Research, Chandigarh, India.

CASE 100

Neonate with Hemolytic Disease of Newborn (Due to Rh Isoimmunization—for both Rh-D Antigen and Rh-C Antigen), Conjugated Hyperbilirubinemia, and Associated Nonsyndromic Paucity of Intrahepatic Bile Ducts: PM 27937

Nandita Bharadwaj Kakkar

HIGHLIGHTS OF THE CASE

An 11-hour-old male baby (term baby, weighing 2.4 kg at birth) presented to PGI emergency with severe jaundice (serum bilirubin: 23 mg/dL), anemia [Hb: 6 g/dL, packed cell volume (PCV): 18], encephalopathy, hepatosplenomegaly, respiratory distress and hypoglycemia in a setting of Rh isoimmunization, with direct Coombs test strongly positive for IgG. Antibodies for both Rh-D antigen and Rh-C antigen were present in the baby's sera. He underwent two double volume exchange transfusions (DVET) and was put on ventilation. Investigations revealed predominantly conjugated hyperbilirubinemia with mildly deranged liver function tests and coagulopathy. The clinical diagnosis was acute liver failure with Rh isoimmunization, ? neonatal hemochromatosis, ? glycogen storage disorder, ? galactosemia, ? tyrosinemia, ? congenital disorders of glycosylation, ? neonatal leukemia. Autopsy revealed hemolytic disease of newborn (HDN) (Rh incompatibility existed at two Rh loci, i.e. Rh-D and Rh-C) with extensive extramedullary hematopoiesis (EMH), 4 + siderosis in the liver, 1 + siderosis in the pancreas and diffuse islet cell hyperplasia along with nonsyndromic paucity of intrahepatic bile ducts (PIBD).

Keywords: Neonate, hemolytic disease of newborn, Rh isoimmunization, conjugated hyperbilirubinemia, nonsyndromic, Alagille syndrome, paucity of intrahepatic bile ducts.

CLINICAL DETAILS

Date of Admission: 21.01.2017, Date of Death: 23.01.2017, Duration of Hospital Stay: 3 Days

An Rh incompatible male neonate was referred to PGIMER at 11 hours of life with severe jaundice and serum bilirubin being 23 mg/dL at 6 hours of life along with respiratory distress. He was born at 38 + 1 week gestation to a gravida 2 mother at an outside facility, by a lower segment cesarean section, done in view of meconium-stained liquor. The baby weighed 2.4 kg, cried immediately after birth and his APGAR score documented was 8 and 9 at 1 minute and 5 minutes respectively. This was an unsupervised pregnancy and details of antenatal ultrasonography (USG) were not available. There was no history of infections or premature rupture of membranes. The mother was a known case of hypothyroidism, on thyroid supplements. The blood group of the mother was A Rh negative, father B Rh positive and baby B Rh positive. Mother did not receive anti-D in current pregnancy. She had received one dose of anti-D in the prior pregnancy, on the first postpartum day only. No anti-D was given at 28 weeks gestation. In the present pregnancy, indirect Coombs test was not done for mother. ***On examination***: Heart rate: 113/min, respiratory rate: 76/min, SaO_2: 30% going up to 79% on nasal prong oxygen, peripheral and central pulses were normal, temperature warm, capillary filling time less than 2 seconds and blood sugar was low. He was a sick looking infant with severe pallor, marked icterus and respiratory distress. The liver was palpable 6 cm and spleen 4 cm below their respective costal margins. No free fluid was noted. There was generalized hypotonia, bilateral equal sized and sluggishly reacting pupils. Cardiovascular system was within normal limits.

Investigations

Hemogram: *Pre-double volume exchange transfusion (DVET)*—Hb: 6 g/dL; PCV: 19; TLC: 118,500/uL; corrected TLC: 23,700/uL; DLC: N47, L35, M5, E3; Platelets: 33000/uL; and Reticulocyte count: 30%. Peripheral blood film showed anisopoikilocytosis, macrocytes, echinocytes, spherocytes, polychromasia, low platelets and nRBCs: 400/100 WBCs. ***Post-DVET Hemogram***—Hb: 19.7 g/dL; PCV: 51; reticulocyte count: 2.5%; TLC: 18,900/uL; DLC: N50, L35, M12, E; and Platelets: 68,000/uL. ***Coagulogram***—PT: 36 seconds (N: 12–14 seconds), INR: 2.5, aPTT: 36 seconds (N: 26–32 seconds). ***Blood group***—Baby: B Rh positive; Mother: A Rh negative; and Father: B Rh positive. ***On the baby—direct Coombs test (DCT)*** strongly positive for IgG. Baby's sera strongly positive for antibodies for both Rh-D antigen as well as Rh-C antigen. ***Blood Biochemistry***: The details of biochemistry investigations have been tabulated in Table 1. ***Post DVET***—G6PD: normal; serum ferritin: 1,995 ng/mL, CRP: 9.9 (normal <8 mg/L), blood culture: sterile. ***Radiology***: ***USG head***—within normal limits. ***USG abdomen***—liver normal echotexture, no intrahepatic biliary radical dilatation, common bile duct: 2 mm and gall bladder normally distended with anechoic contents.

Course in hospital: This 11-hour-old male baby presented to PGI emergency with severe conjugated hyperbilirubinemia and anemia in a setting of ***Rh isoimmunization***. He had respiratory failure at presentation requiring intubation and manual intermittent positive pressure respiration (IPPR) which was later shifted to pressure-synchronized intermittent-mandatory ventilation (P-SIMV) mode ventilation. He underwent DVET at 18 hours of life with O negative packed red blood cells and AB + fresh frozen plasma. Post-DVET his total serum bilirubin decreased to 17.5 mg/dL, PCV increased to 50 and intensive phototherapy was initiated. Repeat serum bilirubin at 25 hours of life increased to 20 mg/dL, so a second DVET was done at 31 hours of life. Work up revealed predominantly ***conjugated hyperbilirubinemia*** with mildly deranged liver function tests. He was noted to have prolonged puncture site bleeds and persisting encephalopathy. Possibility of primary hepatic pathology with liver failure was considered in view of deranged coagulogram, transaminitis and conjugated hyperbilirubinemia. He was further supported with two transfusions of fresh frozen plasma and three platelet transfusions, along with vitamin K, but he persisted to have bleeding. N' acetylcysteine infusion was started and intravenous immunoglobulins, 1 g/kg, were administered on day 2 in view of a clinical possibility of hemophagocytic lymphohistiocytosis. Acyclovir was also administered to cover HSV hepatitis. ***Encephalopathy*** was noted throughout hospital stay in form of decreased state to state variability, generalized hypotonia and with persistent fisting. He had transient improvement on day 2 in the form of improved tone and spontaneous activity. He also had recurrent episodes of ***hypoglycemia***, noted since admission and required maximum glucose infusion rate (GIR) of 8 mg/kg/minute, on which the blood sugar normalized. ***Respiratory failure*** required intubation at admission; IPPR for 4 hours followed by P-SIMV with minimal settings with FiO_2 of 23% for 36 hours, on which he maintained status quo. He was being considered for extubation, when he developed respiratory deterioration on day 3 of life, along with multiple episodes of endotracheal bleeds. He required high frequency oscillatory ventilation, despite which hypoxia persisted. He received intravenous antibiotics, initially cefotaxime and amikacin, later changed

Table 1: Blood Biochemistry.

Date	*Na^+/K^+*	*Urea/creatinine mg%*	*Bilirubin T/ conjugated (mg%)*	*Aspartate aminotransferase/ Alanine aminotransferase/ Alk-aline phosphatase (AST/ ALT/ALP)*	*Total proteins/ Albumin-(gm)*	*$Ca^{2+}/PO4^{3-}$*
21/01/17 Pre-double volume exchange transfusion (DVET)	130/2.7	19/0.935	23/17.3	521/100/182	2.7/1.5	8.1/4.1
21/01/17 Post DVET	138/5.3	23/0.83	15/11	203/49/207	4/2.1	9.4/11
22/01/17	138/3.6	23/1.3	16.4/11	–	–	–
23/01/17	133/3.3	24/1.2	14.9/9.4	–	–	–

to meropenem, in view of a clinical suspicion of ***early onset neonatal sepsis***. Preterminally, on day 3 of life, baby had recurrent episodes of pulmonary hemorrhage with refractory hypoxia. He soon developed shock and suffered a cardiac arrest at 72 hours of life, from which he could not be revived. ***Units final diagnosis***: Day 3 male, 2.4 kg, with acute liver failure, Rh isoimmunization, ? neonatal hemochromatosis, ? glycogen storage disorder, ? galactosaemia, ? tyrosinemia, ? congenital disorders of glycosylation ? neonatal leukemia. ***Cause of death***: Pulmonary hemorrhage secondary to disseminated intravascular coagulation (DIC) and possible sepsis.

AUTOPSY FINDINGS: PM 27937

A partial autopsy was performed on this 3-day-old male child. Baby weighed 2100 gms. The peritoneal cavity contained 20 mL of straw-colored fluid. Pleural and pericardial cavities were within normal limits. The liver (Figs 1A–C) was massively enlarged and weighed 310 g (N: 113 g). It was bile stained with a near normal texture and was not foldable on itself. No fibrosis, nodules, cirrhosis, necrosis or thrombosis was identified. The gall bladder and the extrahepatic biliary tree dissected out, were within normal limits. On microscopic examination, the architecture of the liver was maintained. There was no fibrosis at any location, i.e. portal, pericellular or any bridging fibrosis. No necrosis of hepatocytes was noted and there was no steatosis. There was, however, extensive extramedullary hematopoiesis (EMH) (Figs 1D–F) in the sinusoids and the portal tracts, composed of myeloid (MPO ++) and erythroid series of cells along with megakaryocytes. The hepatocytes and Kupffer cells were swollen

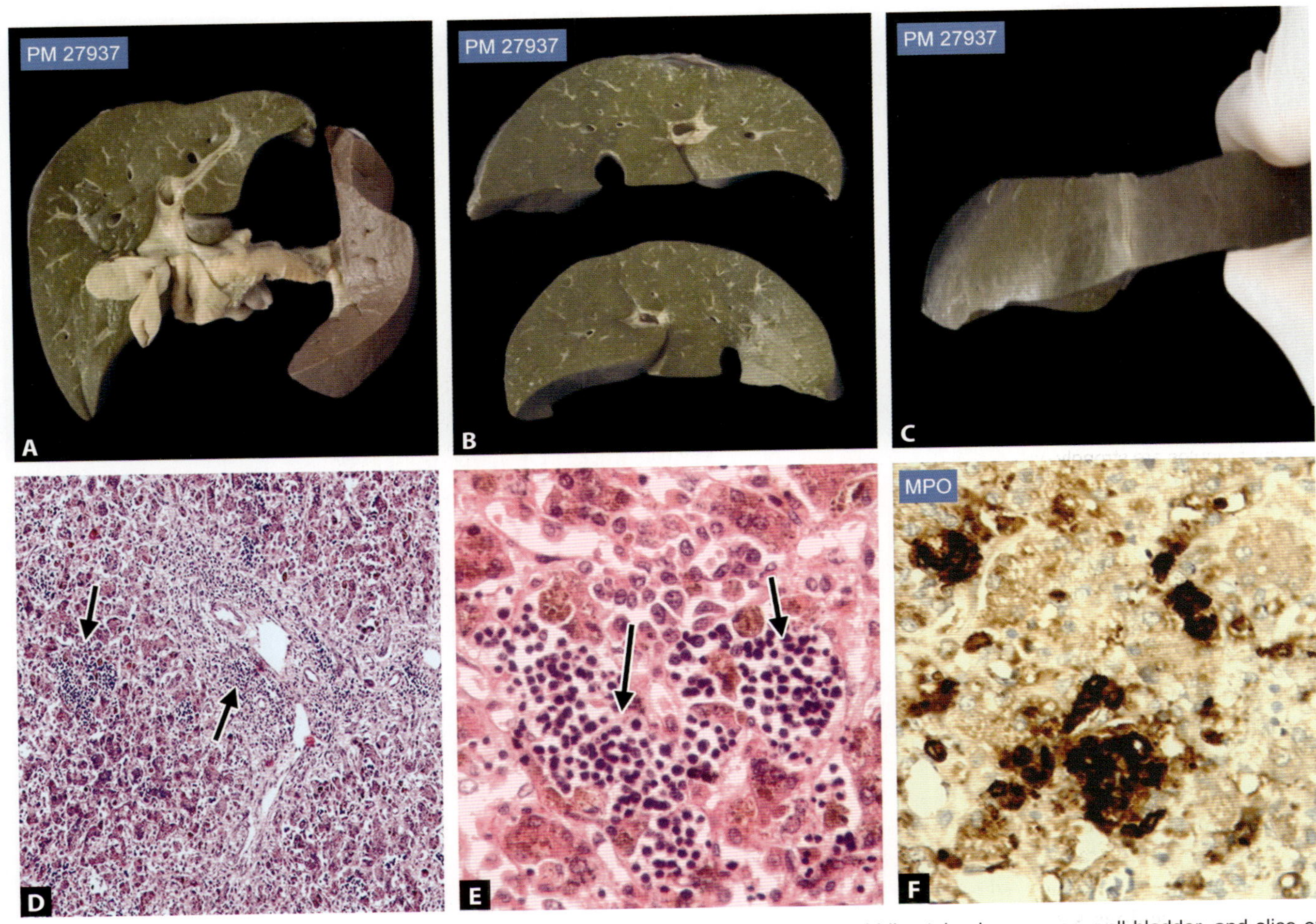

Figs 1A–F: (A) Organ complex comprising of slice of liver which is enlarged (3 times) and bile stained, pancreas, gall bladder, and slice of the enlarged spleen (six times); (B) Slices of the enlarged, bile stained liver. No fibrosis or any nodule seen; (C) Capsule of the liver shows no nodules or any wrinkling; (D and E) Microphotographs of the liver showing extensive extramedullary hematopoiesis (EMH) (arrows) in the portal tracts and in the sinusoids; (F) Myeloperoxidase immunohistochemistry shows strong positivity in the myeloid precursors in the foci of EMH in the liver.

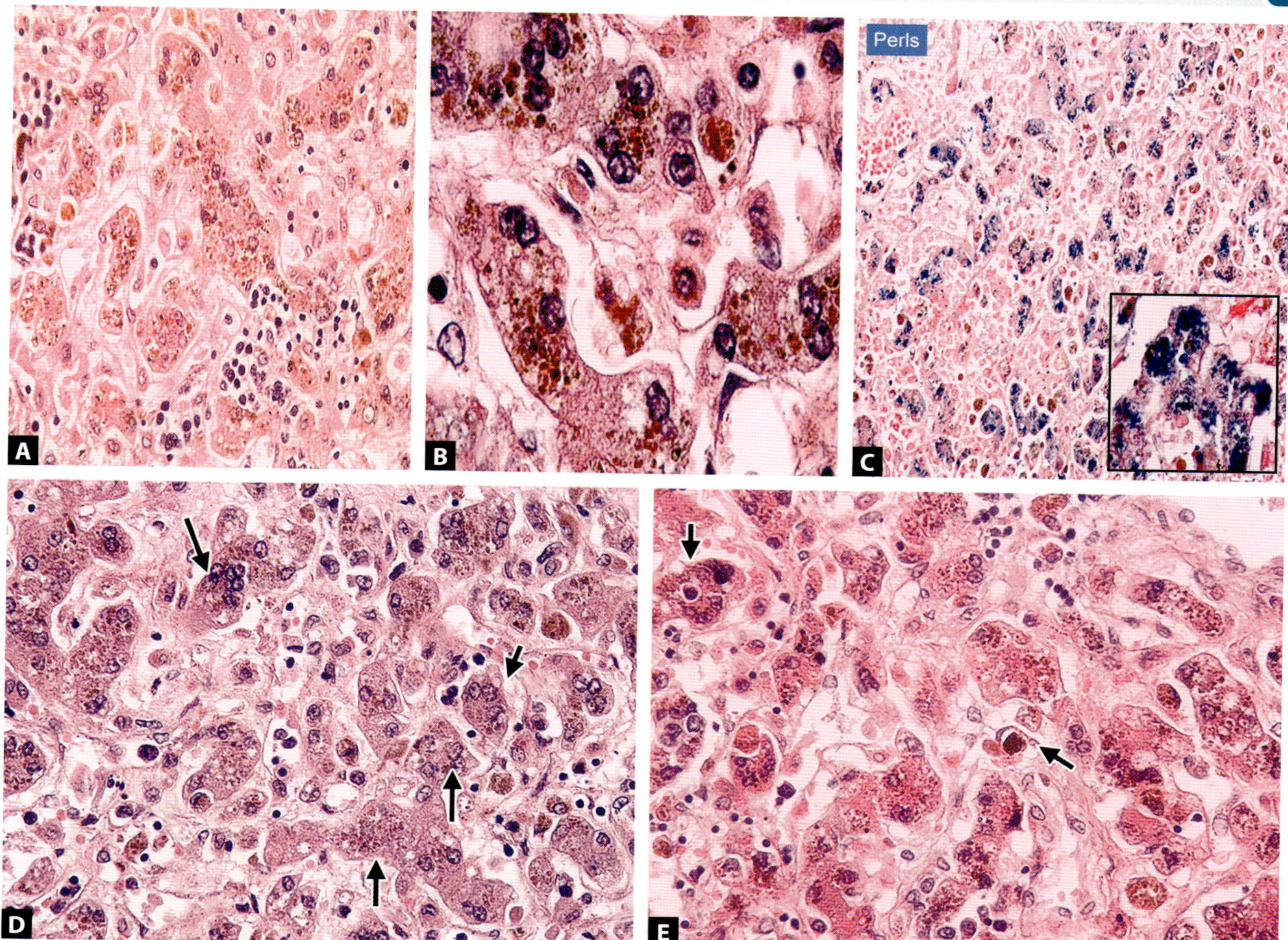

Figs 2A–E: Microphotographs of the liver showing (A and B) golden brown coarse granules in the enlarged hepatocytes and Kupffer cells; (C) The granules are strongly positive with Prussian blue stain, indicating them to be iron (4 +); (D) Hepatocytes showing giant cell transformation (arrows); (E) Hepatocytes showing acinar transformation (upper arrow) along with cholestasis both hepatocytic and canalicular (lower arrow).

and were packed with coarse golden brown-colored granules (Figs 2A and B). These granules (Fig 2C) were strongly positive (4+) for Prussian blue stain (Perls stain) for iron. Apart from this, the hepatocytes showed prominent giant cell transformation (Fig 2D), occasional acinar transformation and extensive cholestasis, which was hepatocytic, ductular and canalicular (Fig 2E). Prominent periportal cholangiolar proliferation (angulated structures) was seen which was better highlighted on CK7 immunohistochemistry (Fig 3D). Normally the portal tracts contain hepatic arteries, adjacent to which is seen a bile duct, which is small and round (Fig 3A). On a meticulous scrutiny, more than 30% of the portal tracts showed a paucity of interlobular bile ducts, i.e. the hepatic arteries were not accompanied with interlobular bile ducts (Figs 3B and C). Diagnosis—EMH with 4 + siderosis and nonsyndromic PIBD (Alagille syndrome). The ***spleen*** (Fig 4A) was massively enlarged, weighed 80 g (N: 12 g) and revealed EMH with presence of myeloid/erythroid series of cells along with megakaryocytes (Figs 4B and C). ***Pancreas*** was normal grossly and on microscopic examination (Fig 4D) revealed diffuse islet cell hyperplasia (diffuse nesidioblastosis) which was better highlighted on insulin immunohistochemistry (Fig 4E). Perls stain (Fig 4F), however, revealed 1 + positivity in the pancreatic acinar cells. The ***kidneys*** (Fig 5A) revealed extramedullary hematopoiesis in the perivascular location and in the interstitium. The ***adrenals*** (Fig 5B) showed foci of extramedullary hematopoiesis and hemorrhage. The ***lymph nodes*** (Fig 5C) were not enlarged and on microscopy showed dilatation of sinuses with evidence of erythrophagocytosis. The ***bone marrow***

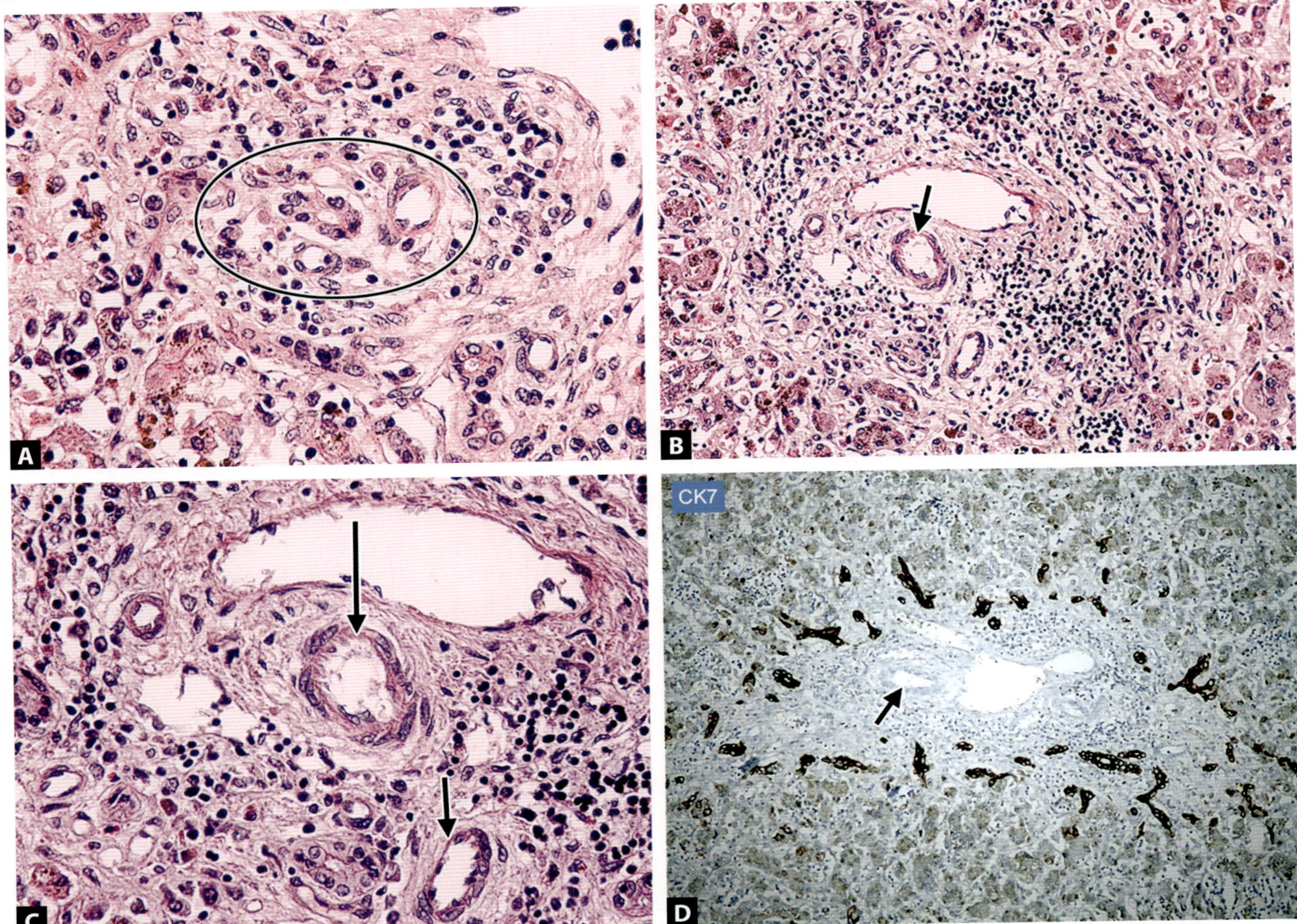

Figs 3A–D: (A) Portal tracts showing hepatic artery with a paired bile duct (circle); (B and C) Portal tract showing hepatic artery (arrows) without an accompanying bile duct, i.e. paucity; (D) CK7 immunohistochemistry showing periportal cholangiolar proliferation, hepatic artery (arrow) is seen without a bile duct.

(Figs 5D and E) showed adequate representation of all three elements with prominent erythroid hyperplasia. Perls stain was 2 +. The ***thymus*** (Fig 5F) revealed stress involution. The ***heart*** (Fig 6A) was enlarged, weighed 55 g (N: 18 g), the ductus was patent and right ventricular hypertrophy was noted. All valves were however normal. The ***lungs*** (Fig 6B) weighed 180 g and cut section showed extensive hemorrhagic consolidation. No thromboembolism was seen. On microscopic examination, there was florid pulmonary hemorrhage (Fig 6C). Intra-acinar arterioles were prominent indicating presence of persistent pulmonary hypertension. Perls stain was done and found to be negative on sections from the spleen, heart, kidneys, adrenals, lymph nodes, thymus and lungs.

FINAL AUTOPSY DIAGNOSIS: PM 27937

Day 3 Male, Term Baby (38 Weeks Gestation), 2.1 kg, good APGAR, Gravida 2 Mother, Rh Incompatibility

- *Hemolytic disease of newborn*: Rh isoimmunization (Baby's sera—direct Coombs test strongly positive for antibodies against both Rh-D antigen as well as Rh-C antigen) with:
    - Extensive extramedullary hematopoiesis in the liver, spleen, kidneys and adrenals (focal)

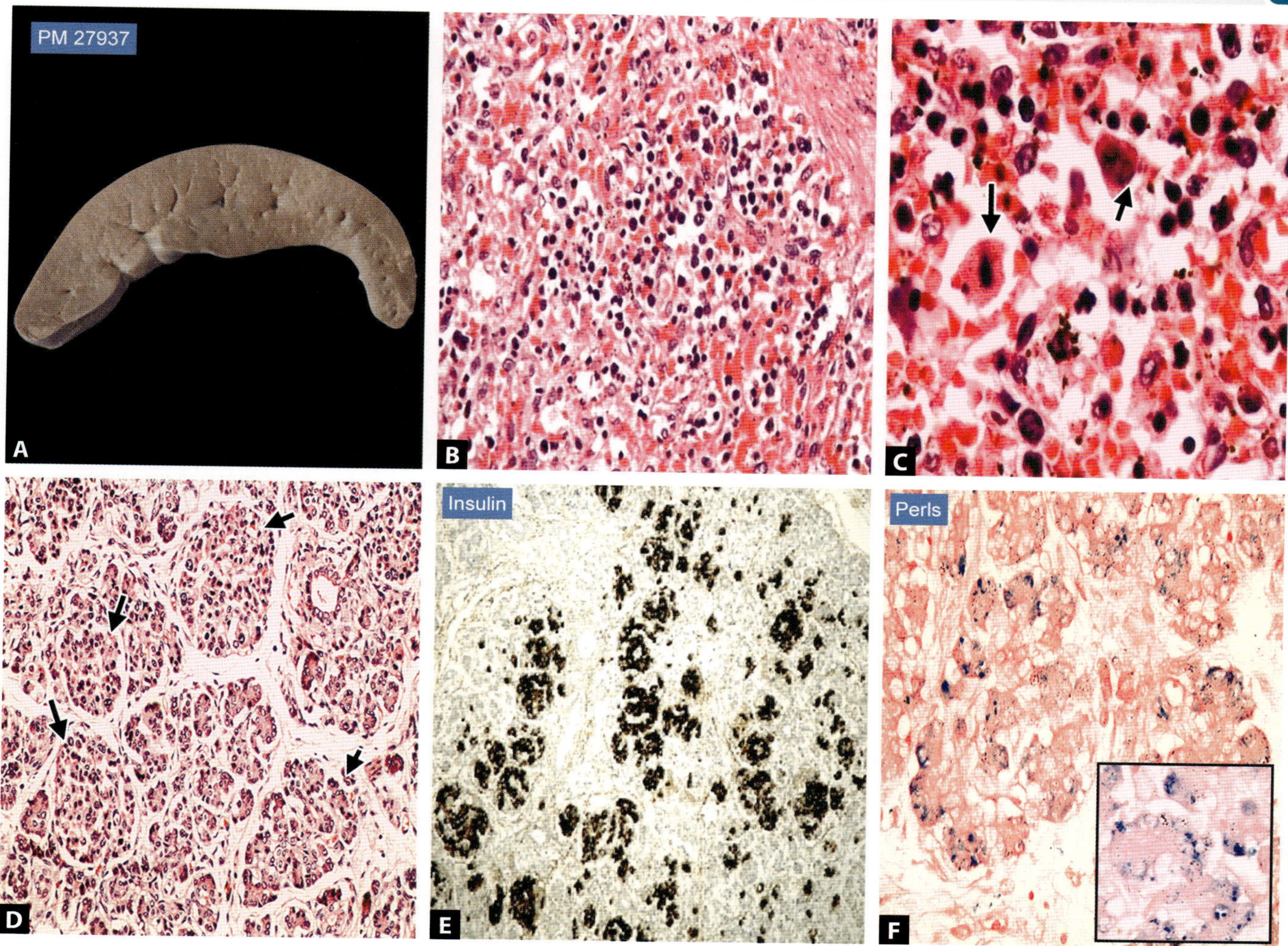

Figs 4A–F: (A) Enlarged (6 times) slice of spleen; (B) Spleen shows florid extramedullary hematopoiesis in the red pulp; (C) Splenic extramedullary hematopoiesis under oil immersion lens, showing megakaryocytes (arrows) and erythroid/myeloid series of cells. Pancreas showing; (D) Islet cell hyperplasia (arrows); (E) Insulin immunohistochemistry highlights diffuse islet cell hyperplasia; (F) Perls stain showing 1 + iron granules in the pancreatic acinar cells.

    - Siderosis—liver 4 + (hepatocytes and Kupffer cells), Pancreas 1 + (acinar cells)
    - Bone marrow—erythroid hyperplasia with increased megakaryocytes
- *Paucity of intrahepatic bile ducts*: Nonsyndromic Alagille syndrome
- Cardiomegaly with patent ductus arteriosus and right ventricular hypertrophy
- *Diffuse islet cell hyperplasia*: Diffuse nesidioblastosis
- Extensive pulmonary hemorrhage (bilateral) with persistent pulmonary hypertension
- *Erythrophagocytosis*: Lymph nodes, ? sepsis.

HEMOLYTIC DISEASE OF NEWBORN DUE TO RH ISOIMMUNIZATION

Hemolytic disease of newborn is an alloimmune disorder which begins in utero as a result of alloantibody (produced in the mother and transmitted via the placenta to the fetus) attack on the fetal red blood cells leading to their destruction. Clinically it presents as fetal anemia, unconjugated hyperbilirubinemia with peripheral blood showing plenty of nRBCs, i.e. erythroblastemia. Rh incompatibility at the D locus is associated with severe immune hemolysis in the fetus. This occurs when the mother is Rh negative and the baby is Rh

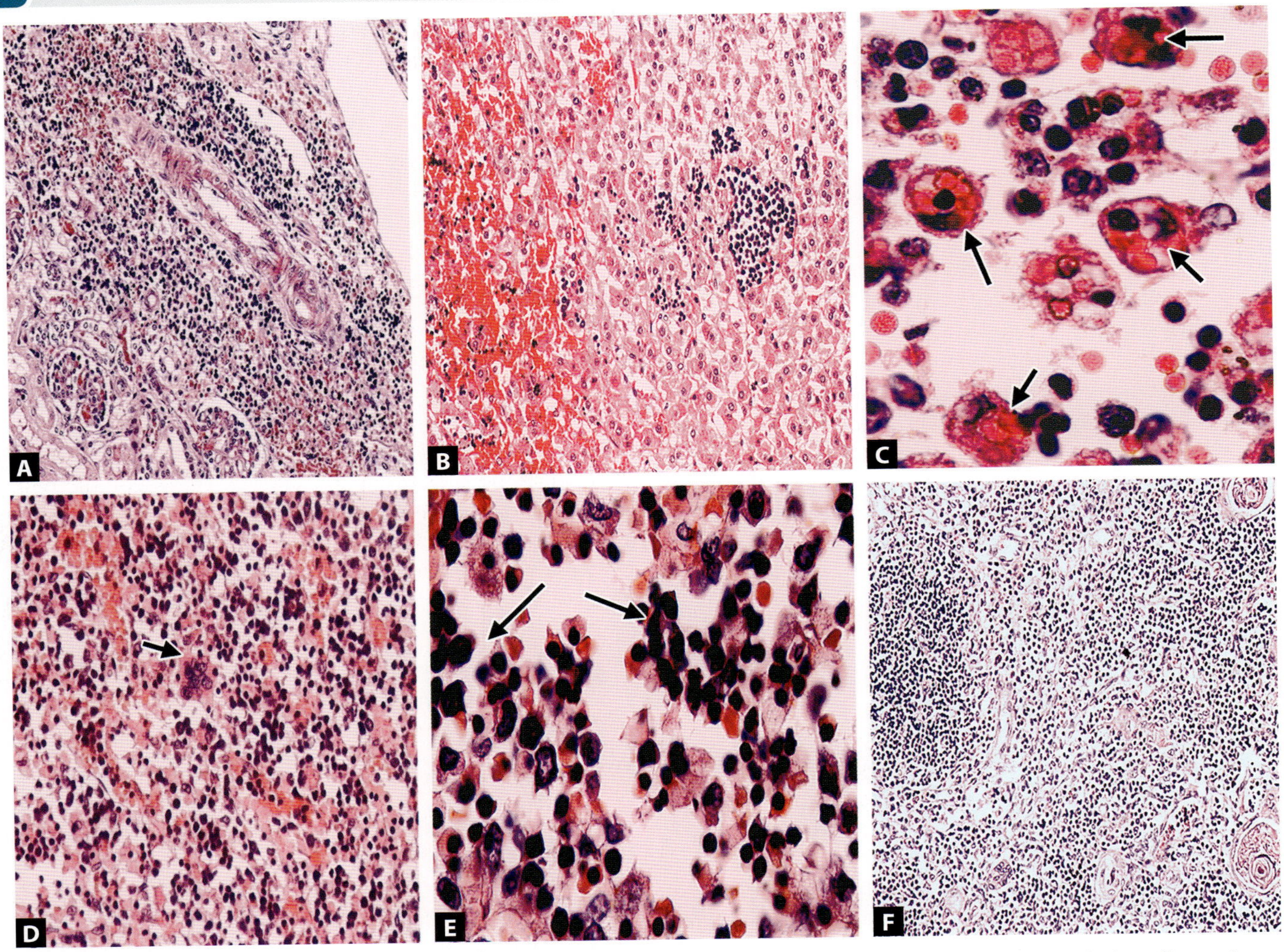

Figs 5A–F: (A) Kidneys showing extramedullary hematopoiesis; (B) Adrenal gland showing foci of extramedullary hematopoiesis and hemorrhage; (C) Lymph node shows erythrophagocytosis (arrows); (D and E) Bone marrow shows erythroid hyperplasia (arrows) and megakaryocytes; (F) Thymus shows involution.

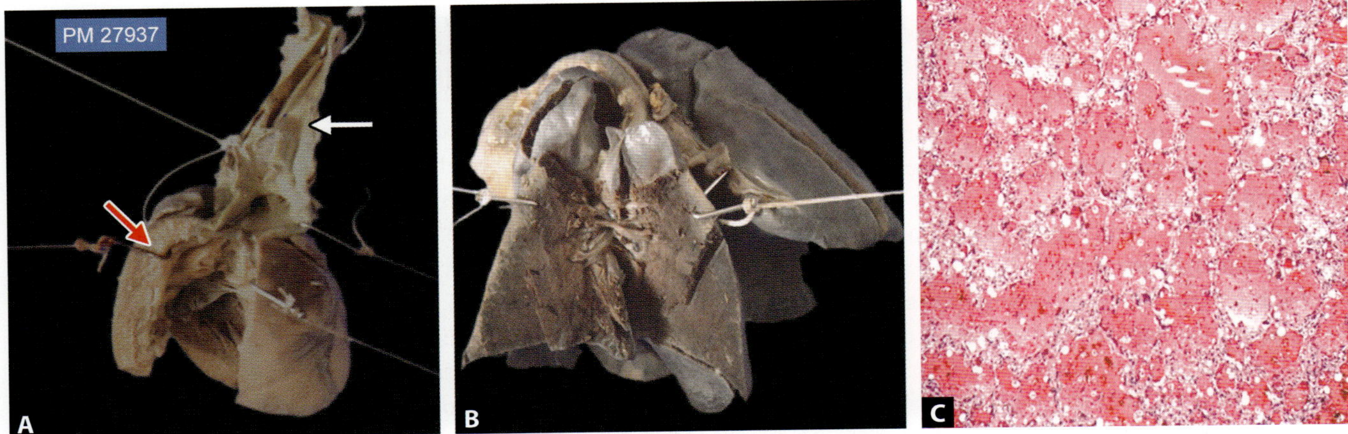

Figs 6A–C: (A) Enlarged heart showing patent ductus arteriosus (white arrow) and right ventricular hypertrophy (red arrow); (B) Lungs showing hemorrhagic consolidation; (C) Lung showing extensive alveolar hemorrhage.

positive. The Rh positive blood (0.5–1 mL of blood) of the fetus can enter the mother's circulation due to a number of reasons like trauma, placental abnormalities, amniocentesis and placental separation during first pregnancy or during an abortion. This is recognized as foreign by the mother, leading to formation of IgG antibodies which go back to the baby via the placenta and create havoc in the form of erythroblastosis fetalis. Other antigens at the Rh locus are C(R'), E(R'), c(H') and e(H') and they too can be incompatible leading to worsening of the situation as was seen in the index case. The first pregnancy is not affected unless the mother has been exposed to Rh positive blood either by blood transfusion or has had a previous abortion. Fetal cells only cross over to the mother during delivery or abortion when the placenta separates. So the mother gets immunized and produces anti-Rh antibodies which cross over in the second pregnancy.

For the prevention of Rh disease, all mothers who are Rh negative should be given an intramuscular injection of anti-Rh-D gamma globulins within 72 hours of the delivery, so that the baby's Rh + red blood cells are destroyed, before the mother's immune system recognizes them as foreign. Today, the antenatal care regimen gives an intramuscular injection of anti-Rh-D gamma globulins at 28 weeks gestation with or without a booster at 32 weeks. Maternal screening for IgG antibodies during pregnancy can be done by the indirect Coombs test. If the mother has no risk factor except for being Rh negative, anti-D titers are done at 12–16 weeks, 28–32 weeks and at 36 weeks. If there is a risk, i.e. previous abortion or previous pregnancy without monitoring or Rh + blood transfusion, then titers are determined every 4 weeks. Babies with HDN can have mild, moderate or severe disease. The most severe cases die in utero with hydrops fetalis. The neonate undergoes the following tests to make a diagnosis of HDN—direct Coombs test for the presence of immune hemolytic anemia, Hb estimation, peripheral smear for erythroblastemia and serum bilirubin levels. Antibodies against other antigens at the Rh locus, i.e. C(R'), E(R'), c(H') and e(H') should also be looked for.

Autopsy findings in HDN depend on the period of gestation. On external examination, there may be generalized edema (hydrops fetalis), more prominent on the face, icterus and effusions are noted. There is marked splenomegaly with the spleen weighing several times its normal weight. The liver is also enlarged, generally twice its weight. Both liver and spleen show EMH with myeloid/erythroid series of cells along with megakaryocytes. Large amounts of iron are present in the liver within the Kupffer cells and hepatocytes. EMH is also seen in the perivascular location in the kidneys, meninges and in the pulmonary capillaries. The lymphoid tissue of the body is hypoplastic and the thymus is small. Brain shows kernicterus.

PAUCITY OF INTRAHEPATIC BILE DUCTS (PIBD)

This is one of the rarer causes of neonatal cholestasis syndrome, wherein there is a reduction in the number of interlobular bile ducts. The pathogenesis is unknown, but points toward a failure of duct developmental or a progressive duct destruction, the latter being a more acceptable proposal. Under normal conditions, the interlobular bile duct and the hepatic arteries are paired structures, located within the portal tracts. Ideally the normal ratio of bile ducts to portal tracts is 0.9–1.8. A ratio less than 0.4 is clearly indicative of a paucity of bile ducts. This applies to neonates more than 38 weeks gestation, as below this period of gestation the ratio is normally low. Easier method of making a diagnosis is to count the number of portal tracts without a bile duct. For this, identify the arteriole in the portal tract which is easily discernable and look for a small rounded bile duct adjacent to it. Cholangiolar proliferation around the portal tracts should not be counted as interlobular bile ducts. The important differentiating factor is that the cholangioles are present in a periportal location and they are angulated. Normally 10–15% portal tracts do not have interlobular bile ducts and if the number goes beyond 30%, a paucity of bile ducts is considered. Other associated changes with paucity of bile ducts include hepatocyte swelling, giant cell transformation, acinar transformation, cholestasis (hepatocytic, canalicular or ductular), variable portal fibrosis with mild portal inflammation, variable hepatocytic necrosis and lobular inflammation. Alagille syndrome, also designated as arteriohepatic dysplasia, shows PIBD, along with facial, cardiac, ophthalmic and skeletal anomalies. This is a familial disorder, occurring 1 in 70,000 live births and said to be autosomal dominant with low penetrance and variable expressivity. Apart from the syndromic Alagille syndrome, there is a nonsyndromic Alagille syndrome where PIBD occurs without the extrahepatic manifestations. Some of the nonsyndromic cases are however associated with congenital rubella, cytomegalovirus infection, alpha1 antitrypsin deficiency, trisomy 17,18, 21 and Turner syndrome.

COMMENTARY—INDEX CASE: PM 27937

Index case was an Rh incompatible, day 1, male, neonate who came with severe jaundice (serum bilirubin: 23 mg/dL predominantly conjugated), anemia (Hb: 6 g/dL, PCV: 18), encephalopathy, respiratory distress, hepatosplenomegaly, hypoglycemia, elevated transaminases—AST >> ALT, low to normal alkaline phosphatase, lactic acidosis, coagulopathy, INR: 2.5, aPTT: normal, thrombocytopenia (DIC like picture) and hyperferritinemia. Baby was born at 38 weeks gestation to a gravida 2 mother and weighed 2.4 kg. The father's blood group was B positive and the mother's was A negative. Mother received one dose of anti-D in the prior pregnancy on the first postpartum day. In the present pregnancy, indirect Coombs test was not done and she did not receive anti-D. In the baby, however, direct Coombs test was strongly positive for IgG and antibodies for both Rh-D antigen and Rh-C antigen were present. Clinically the odd point in this case was the conjugated hyperbilirubinemia present on the first day of life. Literature search however reveals that 10–15% of children with Rh isoimmunization develop conjugated jaundice beyond 1+ week of life. Allgood et al have reported severe conjugated hyperbilirubinemia in three cases of neonatal hemolysis as early as 48 hours of life. But in the index case, there was a paucity of bile ducts, which was actually contributing to the conjugated hyperbilirubinemia. Clinically there was a strong possibility of neonatal hemochromatosis due to the presence of acute liver failure with minimally raised transaminases. This was ruled out as the liver at autopsy did not show any hepatocytic necrosis, fibrosis or any cirrhosis. There was 4 + siderosis which can be seen in hemolytic disease of newborn. Extrahepatic siderosis in the pancreas, myocardium and kidneys is seen in neonatal hemochromatosis. The hemolysis in the index case was very severe as antibodies for both Rh-D antigen as well as Rh-C antigen were present in the baby's sera, meaning thereby that incompatibility existed at two Rh loci. Thus, the severity of the problem was amplified. This could explain the siderosis seen in the pancreas. The hypoglycemia was due to the presence of diffuse islet cell hyperplasia. The baby finally succumbed to his illness due to extensive pulmonary hemorrhage.

TAKE HOME MESSAGE

- Hemolytic disease of the newborn is preventable and hence antenatal supervision is very important.
- In hemolytic disease of newborn, conjugated hyperbilirubinemia on first day of life has been occasionally seen in case reports. But in the index case it was due to an associated nonsyndromic paucity of bile ducts. Thus, it is important to look for associated primary parenchymal liver disorders under such circumstances.

SUGGESTED READING

1. Brumbaugh JE, Morgan S, Beck JC, et al. Blueberry muffin rash, hyperbilirubinemia and hypoglycemia: A case of hemolytic disease of the fetus and newborn due to anti-Kpa. J Perinatol. 2011;31:373-6.
2. Taylor SA, Whitington PF. Neonatal acute liver failure. Liver Transpl. 2016;22:677-85.
3. Whitington PF. Gestational alloimmune liver disease and neonatal hemochromatosis. Semin Liver Dis. 2012;32: 325-32.

CONTRIBUTIONS BY:

1. Dr Richa Jain, Assistant Professor, Department of Pediatrics (Hematology Oncology Division) (Compilation of Clinical Details)
2. Dr Kanya Mukhopadhyay, Professor, Department of Pediatrics (Neonatology Division) (Clinician In-Charge)
3. Dr Ashish Jain, Associate Professor, Department of Transfusion Medicine (Coombs Testing)

Post Graduate Institute of Medical Education and Research, Chandigarh, India.

CASE 101

Indian Childhood Cirrhosis: PM 24527

Nandita Bharadwaj Kakkar

HIGHLIGHTS OF THE CASE

This was a year old female child who was doing well for the first 10 months of life. Thereafter she developed fever, progressive abdominal distension, vomiting, pallor, hepatosplenomegaly, ascites, pleural effusion, anemia, deranged liver function tests and deranged coagulogram. Units final clinical diagnosis was—pneumonia with septicemia with storage disorder/chronic liver disorder; pulmonary hemorrhage/pulmonary edema. Autopsy revealed a classical case of Indian childhood cirrhosis (ICC) with portal hypertension along with acute necrotizing pneumonia, diffuse alveolar damage and extensive hemorrhage.

Keywords: Indian childhood cirrhosis, micronodular, pericellular fibrosis, cola-colored granules, orcein stain, autopsy.

CLINICAL DETAILS

Date of Admission: 20.10.2011, Date of Death: 22.10.2011, Duration of Hospital Stay: 2 days

This was a one year old girl who was admitted to PGIMER, Chandigarh on 05.10.2011, with complaints of intermittent fever (documented upto 101°F), progressive abdominal distension and occasional vomiting (nonbilious and nonprojectile) for 1½ months. She also had progressive pallor since 1 month, which was not initially associated with jaundice, edema or bleeding manifestations. There was considerable weight loss (500 g over 10 days). Patient was worked up for the possibility of hemolytic anemia and storage disorder, was given one unit packed red cell transfusion and discharged on 08.10.2011. She was readmitted again on the 20.10.2011 in Pediatric Emergency for the same complaints, with new onset cough and coryza and fever with respiratory difficulty for 7 days. She was a term baby, weighed 1,500 g at birth and born through a nonconsanguineous marriage. There was no birth asphyxia and her development milestones were appropriate for age. Her two elder siblings, both girls, were asymptomatic. There was no apparent history of contact with tuberculosis patient.

Examination**: First admission**—afebrile, pulse: 130/min, BP: normal, weight: 7 kg (<3rd centile), length: 67 cm (<3rd centile), head circumference: 42 cm (<-2SD), pallor++, a cutaneous hemangioma measuring 1 × 0.5 cm, at right mandibular area (since birth) and right eye convergent squint (since birth) were noted. No petechiae, icterus, edema, cyanosis, clubbing, facial dysmorphism or cataract was seen. Systemic examination revealed hepatomegaly (liver span 9 cm, firm, sharp margin and smooth surface), splenomegaly (8 cms below left costal margin, firm) and ejection systolic murmur heard all over precordium (best at tricuspid area). The central nervous system examination was normal. ***Second admission***—In addition, she had tachypnea, retractions with bilateral crepitations, pallor, icterus, pedal edema and hepatosplenomegaly with ascites.

Investigations and Course of Management

Hematological**:** Hb 7.9 g%, TLC - 19200, DLC – N82, L16,M2, E2, platelets 13700/uL, peripheral blood film-microcytic hypochromic, anisopoikilocytosis, few target cells and elliptocytes seen. No malarial parasite seen. Coagulogram PT-30 sec (N-14 sec), PTI – 46%, APPT – 66 sec (N-25-35 sec). Bone Marrow aspiration- Normocellular marrow spaces with adequate representation of all three hematopoietic elements. No storage cells seen. Iron stores- low. Hemoglobin electrophoresis-Normal (Hb A 95, A_2 2.4, F 2.7). HIV Serology- Non-reactive.

Blood biochemistry/microbiology: S bilirubin - 4.5 mg%, SGOT-506 U/L, SGPT-305 U/L, ALP- 181 U/L, Total proteins/ albumin- 5.5/2.0 gm, S urea- 51 mg%, S creatinine- 0.2 mg%, S. calcium -8.0 mg%, Na^+ -145 mEq/L, K^+ 4.5 mEq/L, Cl 114, Random blood sugar – 67 mg%, CRP – normal, ABG – Ph 7.1, PO2-42.8, PCO2- 49.9, HCO3- 15.1, SO2 55.6%. Ascitic fluid: 500 ml aspirated. No WBC. Sugar/ protein: 93/560 mg/dL, Gram stain and culture-normal. Blood Culture- no growth

Radiology: USG Abdomen- (20/09/11, done at an outside facility)- Liver-10.4 cm, normal echotexure. Gall bladder distended normally. Portal vein normal calibre. Spleen 9.6 cm normal echotexture and no focal lesion. At PGIMER- Hepatosplenomegaly with mild ascites;

Course and management: During the second admission she was managed as a case of pneumonia with septicaemia with a suspicion of storage disorder. Supplemental oxygen with nasal prongs, intravenous fluids and antibiotics were started. At 22 hrs of admission, patient started desaturating with pinkish frothy secretions from mouth and altered GI aspirates. Possibility of pulmonary hemmorhage/edema were considered. Endotracheal intubation was done, IPPR started and 10ml/kg FFP (Fresh frozen plasma) was given. Subsequently, she had refractory shock for which inotropic support was started. Preterminally, she had cardiac arrest but patient could not be salvaged.

Units final clinical diagnosis: Pneumonia with septicaemia with ? Storage disorder ? Chronic liver disorder. Cause of death- Pulmonary hemorrhage/pulmonary edema.

AUTOPSY FINDINGS: PM 24527

A complete autopsy was performed on this 1-year-old female child. The pleural and peritoneal cavities contained 250 mL and 500 mL of serous fluid, respectively. The liver weighed 390 g (normal for age: 300 g) was bile stained and the capsular aspect revealed tiny nodules (Fig 1A). The cut section of the liver was fibrotic and bile stained with vague nodularity (Fig 1B). The portal vein was within normal limits. On microscopic examination, the liver showed a distorted architecture with presence of micronodules separated by fibrous septa (Figs 1C and D), which were better highlighted by the Masson's trichrome stain (Figs 1E and F). The septae were infiltrated by mononuclear cell infiltrate and proliferating bile ductules (Fig 2A). A very prominent pericellular fibrosis (Figs 2B and C) was noted, with fibrosis seen around single/ groups of hepatocytes. Extensive hepatocytic damage was seen with marked feathery degeneration and abundant Mallory's hyaline (Fig 2D) present in the cytoplasm of large ballooned hepatocytes. Mallory's hyaline are the tangled skeins of intermediate filaments which appear as pink eosinophilic structures within the cytoplasm of the hepatocytes. Cholestasis (Fig 2E), both hepatocytic and canalicular, was noted. Orcein stain showed abundant cola-colored coarse granules of copper-binding proteins in the cytoplasm of the hepatocytes (Fig 2F). Prominent neutrophilic infiltrate was seen to attack the hepatocytes, stuffed with Mallory's hyaline. Perivenular fibrosis was also noted. No regenerative nodule or any steatosis was however seen. Features were those of micronodular cirrhosis consistent with the morphology of typical Indian childhood cirrhosis. The ***spleen*** weighed 100 g and on microscopic examination revealed marked congestion. ***Lungs*** together weighed 140 g and cut section showed hemorrhagic consolidation (Fig 3A). Microscopic examination (Figs 3B–D) revealed widespread alveolar hemorrhage, extensive acute necrotizing pneumonia, extensive hyaline membrane formation, a hallmark of diffuse alveolar damage and edema. The ***bone marrow*** was normal with adequate representation of all three elements with some histiocytes showing hemophagocytosis. No storage cells were seen. Other organs were within normal limits.

FINAL AUTOPSY DIAGNOSIS: PM 24527

1 Year Female Child

- Indian childhood cirrhosis—classical
- Portal hypertension—congestive splenomegaly and ascites
- Acute necrotizing pneumonia with diffuse alveolar damage and pleural effusion.

INDIAN CHILDHOOD CIRRHOSIS

Indian childhood cirrhosis is unique to the Indian subcontinent and has fascinated the scientific community for decades. It was a common killer in the 1980's, became treatable in the 1990's and is said to be rare now. ICC is very much prevalent in North India, although reports say that it has nearly disappeared. It is a form of chronic liver disease occurring in children, with age ranging between 6 months and 5 years, with the mean age of 18 months. This is a progressive liver disorder in young children associated with marked hepatic copper overload (>800 μg/g dry weight). This is due to increased dietary copper consumption in genetically susceptible individuals, resulting from the use of copper-containing utensils and cooking ware. In contrast to Wilson's disease, serum ceruloplasmin levels are normal or raised and there

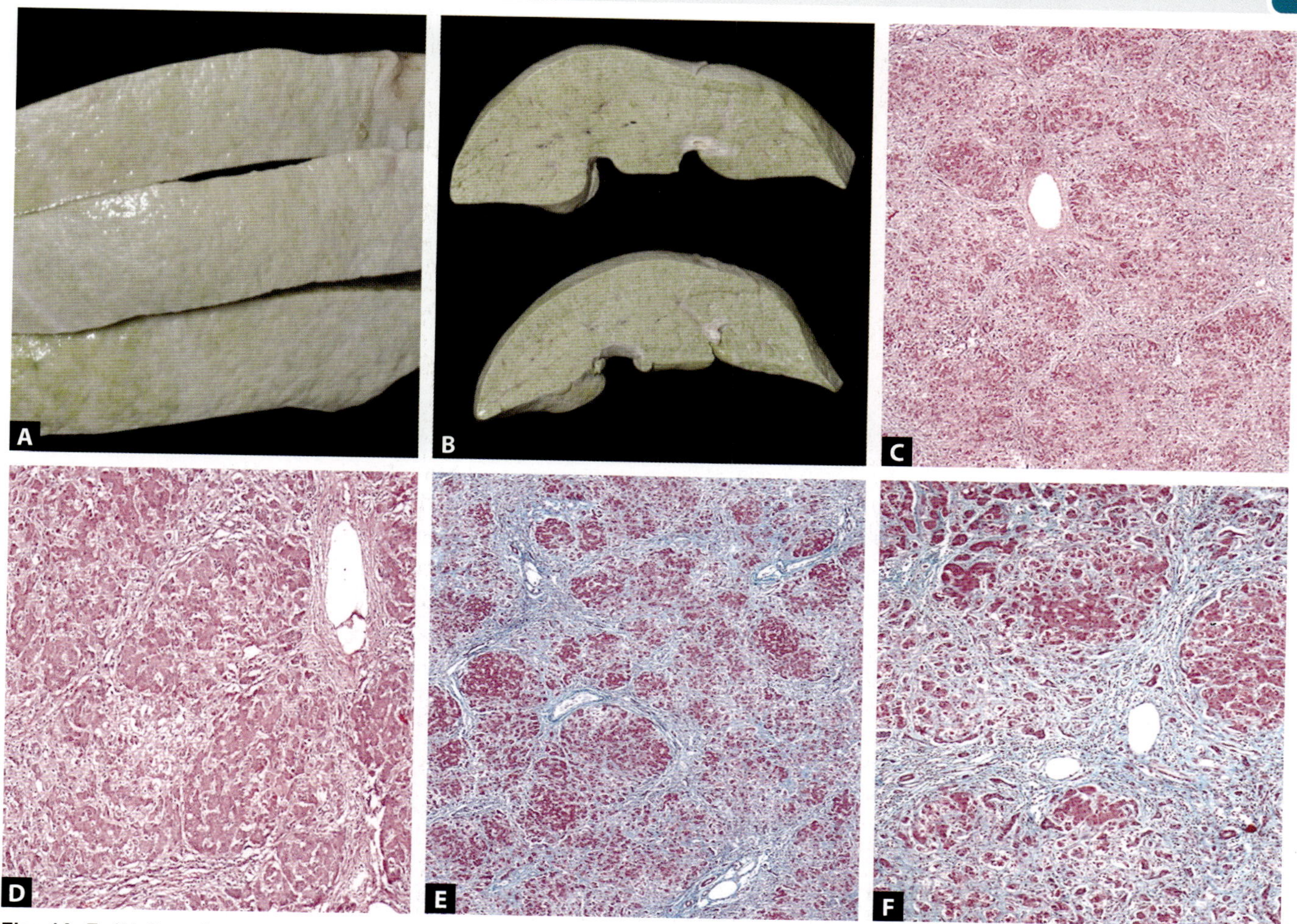

Figs 1A–F: (A) Capsular aspect of the liver showing micronodularity; (B) Coronal slices of the enlarged liver which is bile stained, firm, shows small nodules, and sharp leafy margins; (C and D) Photomicrograph of the liver showing a distorted architecture composed of micronodules cut off by fibrous septa. No steatosis is seen; (E and F) Masson's trichrome stain sharply demarcates the micronodules and the fibrous septa.

is no demonstrated linkage to the *ATP7B* gene. Males are affected more than the females and it is seen more in families with history of consanguinity. ICC is seen to affect siblings in 22% of cases. The disease is seen more in rural areas and Hindus are affected more than the Muslims and Christians.

Pathogenesis of ICC is debatable, but points toward the dietary copper toxicity. Copper in the liver is increased in ICC to more than 800 µg/g dry weight of liver, the normal being 15–55 µg/g. Hepatic copper can also be increased in the neonates (physiologic), in cases of obstructive jaundice and in chronic active hepatitis. But values more than 800 µg/g dry weight cannot be seen in the preceding conditions and it clearly distinguishes ICC from other liver disorders in the ICC age group. The only other disorder that has increased copper is Wilson's disease. Copper and brass (an alloy of 2/3rd copper and 1/3rd zinc) utensils have been extensively used in India by the traditional Hindu families. Copper is known to be cytotoxic and milk boiled in copper vessels, a very common practice in the rural India, leads to a 60 times increase in its copper levels. Studies have shown that copper binds predominantly to casein, a constituent of the milk. In the acidic environment of the stomach, casein liberates most of this bound copper, leading to its rapid absorption. Water extracts copper less avidly and storing water in copper vessels raises the copper concentration by six times only. Thus, broadly the etiology is due to the increased copper, which may be secondary to liver damage/impaired biliary copper excretion, could be the result of an inherited disorder of copper metabolism just like in Wilson's disease or may be the result of excessive copper intake. No stud-

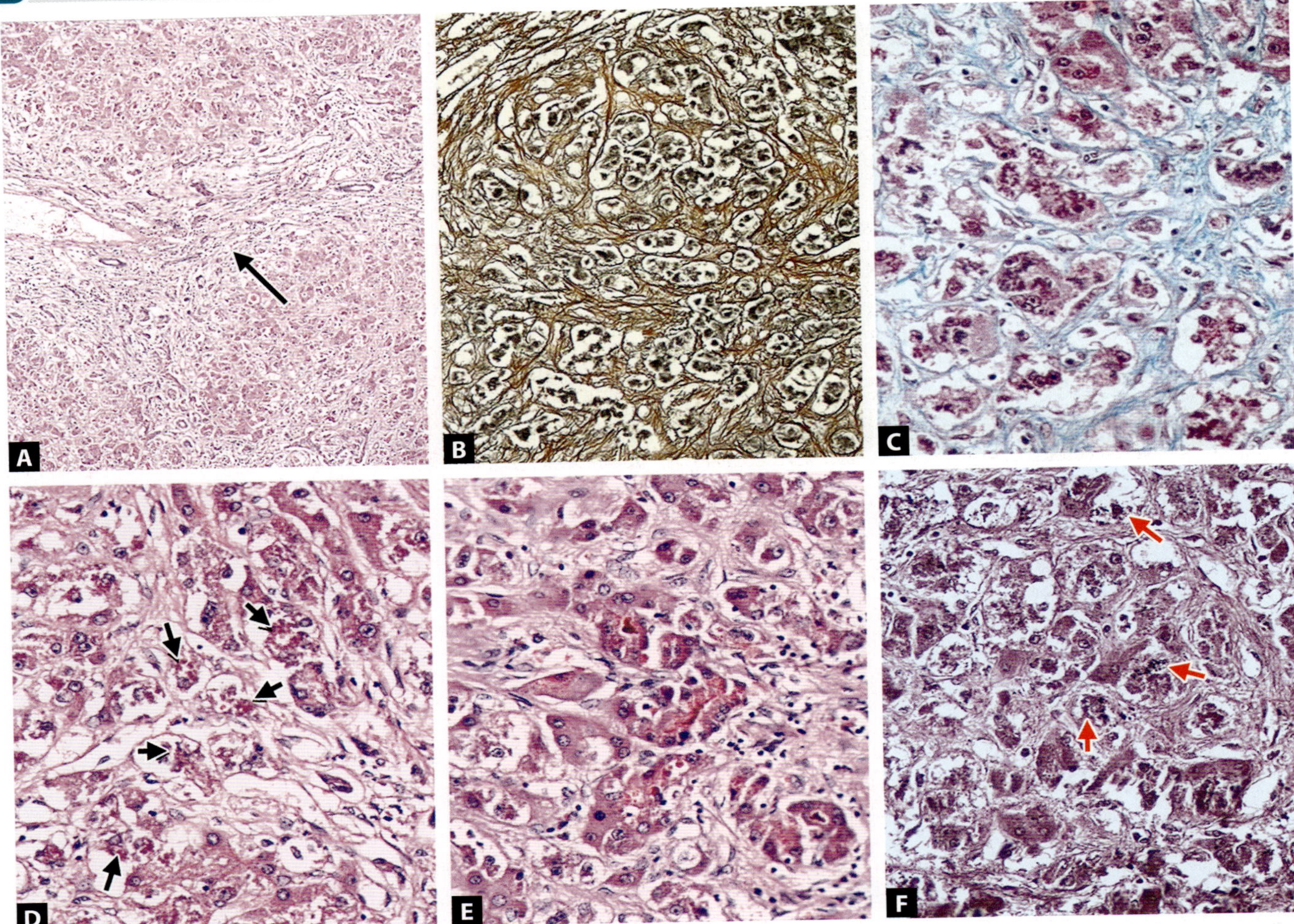

Figs 2A–F: Liver. (A) The septa showing lymphomononuclear cells and bile ductular proliferation. No steatosis is seen; (B) Reticulin stain showing prominent pericellular fibrosis; (C) Masson's (arrows) trichrome stain showing pericellular fibrosis with single or groups of hepatocytes surrounded by fibrous tissue; (D) Abundant Mallory's hyaline in the cytoplasm of the large ballooned hepatocytes; (E) Hepatocytes show pericellular fibrosis and cholestasis; (F) Orcein stain showing cola-colored coarse granules in the cytoplasm of the hepatocytes (arrows).

ies have substantiated the first two theories, but the copper ingestion theory has an epidemiological support. There are also reports where dietary copper as a source of this raised copper seemed unlikely and the most probable cause given was a defect in the metabolism of copper. Other pathogenetic mechanisms are—familial, genetic, viral, microbial, toxins and nutritional deficiencies. A combination of factors like lack of breast feeding, early introduction of animal milk in large amounts and use of copper or brass vessels for boiling or storing milk and a physiologically higher hepatic copper content in infants, all adds and sows the seed for acquiring ICC. This disease is now disappearing due to the education being given to the masses and due to the use of steel utensils. It is treatable with penicillamine and survivors have no apparent evidence of liver disease.

In the majority of cases, the disease is insidious, comprising of nonspecific complaints like excessive crying, altered appetite, irregular fever and abdominal distension. Jaundice is mostly a late manifestation, but in a few children, the disease may begin with this. The liver has a very characteristic feel, i.e. it is firm to hard with a sharp leafy margin. If not treated, ICC is fatal within a few months. The child becomes very ill with hepatosplenomegaly, ascites, jaundice, coagulopathy and edema. A unique late feature is an enlarged gall bladder which becomes palpable. This is said to be due to cholangitis and cholecystitis. Cause of death is secondary to infections, bleeding or due to hepatic coma. Liver function tests are deranged, but this cannot differentiate it from other chronic liver diseases. Histopathology remains the gold standard for diagnosis. In the National Workshop on ICC at

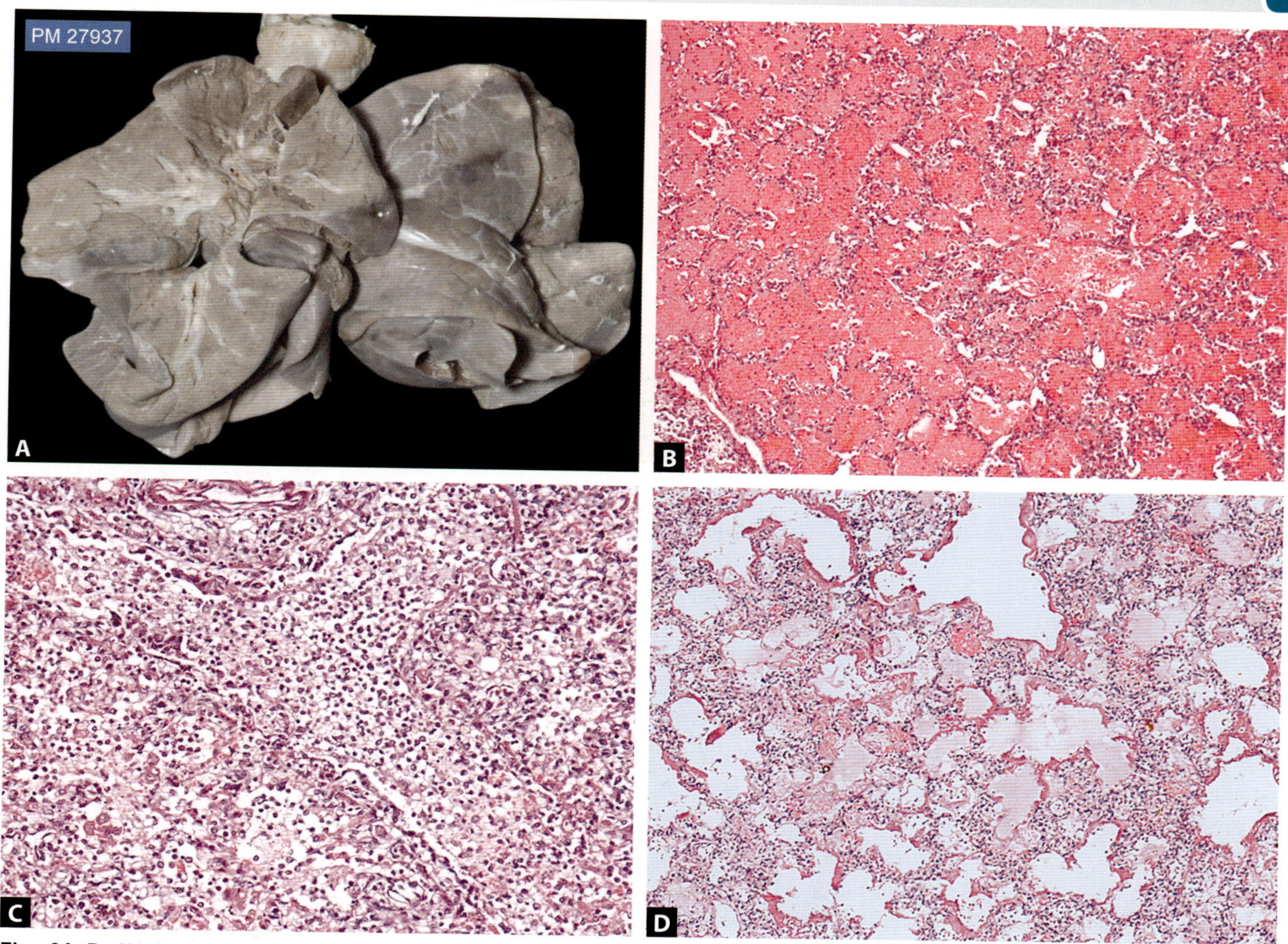

Figs 3A–D: (A) Gross photograph of the lungs which were firm and showed areas of hemorrhage. Photomicrograph of the lung showing; (B) Alveolar hemorrhage; (C) Acute bronchopneumonia; and (D) Hyaline membrane formation with edema.

Chandigarh in February 1987, criteria were laid down for the diagnosis of ICC—(1) Diffuse degeneration of hepatocytes; (2) Absence of distinct regenerative nodules; (3) Presence of abundant Mallory's hyaline; (4) Predominantly neutrophilic infiltrate; (5) Extensive pericellular fibrosis; and (6) Diffuse excess of copper-binding proteins by Orcein–rhodanine stain. The two most important features of ICC are cola-colored, coarse copper-binding proteins in the cytoplasm of the hepatocytes (Orcein stain) and the pericellular fibrosis. Diffuse hepatocytic damage is seen in 98% of cases and Mallory's hyaline is seen in one-third of the cases. Steatosis and regenerative nodules are conspicuously absent. The above features are those of classical or typical ICC. If focal steatosis or an occasional regenerative nodule is present, along with all the above features, the term atypical ICC is used.

The closest differential diagnosis is Wilson's disease (another pediatric copper storage disorder) where hepatic copper is raised to nearly the same levels as seen in ICC. Wilson's disease occurs in children more than 5 years, is an autosomal recessive condition, presentation is variable, hepatic copper is more than 800 μg/g dry weight, ceruloplasmin levels are low, histology shows nuclear glycogen and may show chronic active hepatitis like picture or cirrhosis. Orcein stain may show fine, cola-colored granules, etiology points toward deranged copper metabolism and D-penicillamine is needed life-long. ICC is seen in children in the age group of 6 months to 5 years, siblings can be affected, presentation is characteristic, hepatic copper is grossly raised (> 1000), ceruloplasmin levels are normal or high, histology shows the characteristic features described above, orcein stain demonstrates coarse cola-colored granules, etiology is due to the increased copper which could be the result of an inherited disorder of copper metabolism just like Wilson's disease or may be the result of excessive copper intake. ICC is definitely on the decline and disappearing from India, but scattered reports of ICC-like cirrhosis is appearing in the West.

COMMENTARY—INDEX CASE: PM 24527

This was a year old female child who was doing well for the first 10 months of life. Thereafter she developed fever, progressive abdominal distension, vomiting, pallor, hepatosplenomegaly, ascites, pleural effusion, anemia, deranged liver function tests and deranged coagulogram. Units final clinical diagnosis was—pneumonia with septicemia with storage disorder or chronic liver disorder; pulmonary hemorrhage/pulmonary edema. Autopsy revealed a classical case of ICC with portal hypertension along with acute necrotizing pneumonia, diffuse alveolar damage and extensive hemorrhage. Histopathology revealed a firm liver with sharp leafy margins, capsular aspect showing micronodules and the cut section firm, showing bile stained micronodules. All features of typical ICC were seen, i.e. micronodular cirrhosis, diffuse hepatocytic damage, pericellular fibrosis, neutrophilic satellitosis, Mallory's hyaline, coarse cola-colored granules on orcein staining, absence of fat/regenerative nodules and cholestasis. There was portal hypertension with congestive splenomegaly and ascites. As happens in patients of ICC, it was the pneumonia and pulmonary hemorrhage that took away the patient.

TAKE HOME MESSAGE

- Indian childhood cirrhosis is unique to the Indian subcontinent. Its incidence has declined considerably due to measures taken by the Indian Council of Medical Research, but in North India, it is still prevalent.
- It is a form of chronic liver disease associated with marked hepatic copper overload (>800 μg/g dry weight) in children, with age ranging between 6 months and 5 years, with the mean age of 18 months.
- It occurs due to increased dietary copper consumption in genetically susceptible individuals.
- Milk boiled in copper vessels, a very common practice in the rural India, leads to a 60 times increase in its copper levels and this is considered as an important cause of ICC.
- Features of typical ICC are firm, bile stained liver with sharp leafy margin along with micronodular cirrhosis, diffuse hepatocytic damage, pericellular fibrosis, neutrophilic satellitosis, Mallory's hyaline, coarse cola-colored granules on orcein staining, absence of fat or regenerative nodules and cholestasis.

Acknowledgement

This case has been published as a clinicopathological conference (CPC) in the official journal of our institute - Kakkar et al. I am still around. Journal of Postgraduate Medicine Education and Research. 2012;46(1):51-9.

SUGGESTED READING

1. Adamson M, Reiner B, Olson JL, et al. Indian childhood cirrhosis in an American child. Gastroenterology. 1992; 102(5):1771.
2. Bavdekar AR, Bhave SA, Pradhan AM, et al. Long term survival in Indian childhood cirrhosis treated with D-penicillamine. Arch Dis of Childhood. 1996;74(1):32-5.
3. Bhusnurmath SR, Walia BN, Singh S, et al. Sequential histopathologic alterations in Indian childhood cirrhosis treated with d-penicillamine. Hum Pathol. 1991;22(7):653-8.
4. Drouin E, Russo P, Tuchweber B, et al. North American Indian cirrhosis in children: a review of 30 cases. J Pediatr Gastroenterol Nutr. 2000;31(4):395-404.
5. Johncilla M, Mitchell KA. Pathology of liver in copper overload. Semin Liver Dis. 2011;31(3):239-44.
6. Pandit A, Bhave S. Present interpretation of the role of copper in Indian childhood cirrhosis. Am J Clin Nutr. 1996; 63(5):830S-5S.
7. Sriramachari S, Nayak NC. Indian childhood cirrhosis: several dilemmas resolved. Indian J Med Res. 2008;128(2):93-6.
8. Tanner MS. Role of copper in Indian childhood cirrhosis. Am J Clin Nutr. 1998;67(5 Suppl):1074S-81.
9. Yachha SK, Sharma BC, Khanduri A, et al. Current spectrum of hepatobiliary disorders in northern India. Indian Pediatr. 1997;34(10):885-90.

CONTRIBUTIONS BY:

1. Dr Mandeep Walia, Assistant Professor, Department of Pediatrics (Compilation of Clinical Details)
2. Dr S Singhi, Ex-Professor and Head, Department of Pediatrics (Clinician In-Charge)

Post Graduate Institute of Medical Education and Research, Chandigarh, India.

Abbreviations

Nandita Bharadwaj Kakkar

CPR : Cardiopulmonary resuscitation
NAD : No abnormality detected
IHBRD : Intrahepatic biliary radical dilatation
AMBU : Artificial manual breathing unit
FFP : Fresh frozen plasma
OPD : Out Patient Department
LAD : Left anterior descending artery
RCA : Right Coronary Artery
LCX : Left Circumflex Artery
VSD : Ventricular Septal Defect
ASD : Atrial Septal Defect
PAH : Pulmonary Artery Hypertension
IHC : Immunohistochemistry
CRP : C-Reactive Proteins
WNL : Within Normal Limits
H&E : Haematoxylin and eosin
RCM : Right Costal Margin
LCM : Left Costal Margin
GVHD : Graft Versus Host Disease
LVH : Left Ventriculat Hypertrophy
MCL : Mantle Cell Lymphoma
PRBC : Packed Red Blood Cells
SOL : Space Occupying Lesion
HLH : Haemophagocytic Lymphohistiocytosis
SAAG : Serum-ascites albumin gradient or gap
AFB : Acid Fast Bacilli
PDA : Patent Ductus Arteriosus
NNJ : Neonatal Jaundice
USG : Ultrasonography
RBS : Random Blood Sugar
MDR : Multi Drug Resistance
NCCT : Non Contrast Computarized Tomography
CECT : Contrast Enhenced Computarized Tomography
KUB : Kidney Urinary Bladder
ATN : Acute Tubular Necrosis
IV : Intravenous
PA : Pulmonary Artery
RV : Right Ventricle
RA : Right Atrium
LV : Left Ventricle
LA : Left Atrium
GN : Glomerulonephritis
CVA : Cardiovascular Accident
GPA : Granulomatosis with Polyangiitis
WG : Wegeners Granulomatosis
MPA : Microscopic Polyangiitis
EGPA : Eosinophilic Granulomatosis with Polyangiitis
RR : Respiratory Rate
PR : Pulse Rate
PBF : Peripheral Blood Film
SGOT : Serum Glutamic Oxaloacetic Transaminase, Also called Aspartate Aminotransferase (AST).
SGPT : Serum Glutamic Pyruvic Transaminase Also called Alanine Aminotransferase (ALT).
LFT : Liver Function Test
RFT : Renal Function Test
AFP : Alfa Feto Protein
TOF : Tetrology of Fallots
CMF : Congenital Malformation
GTCS : Generalized Tonic Clonic Seizures
MP : Malarial Parasite
Hb : Hemoglobin
TLC : Total Leucocyte Count
DLC : Differential Leucocyte Count
GI : Gastrointestinal
FNAC : Fine Needle Aspiration Cytology

PET : Positron Emission Tomography
PTI : Prothrombn Index
ANA : Antinuclear Antibodies
ANCA : Antinuclear Cytoplasmic Antibody
CCF : Congestive Cardiac Failure
HRCT : High Resolution Computarized Tomography
MPO : Myeloperoxidase
ALL : Acute Lymphoblastic Leukaemia
AML : Acute Myeloid Leukaemia
DIC : Disseminated Intravascular Coagulation
DS : Differentiation Syndrome
TMA : Thrombotic Microangiopathy

Index

Page numbers followed by *f* refer to figure and *t* refer to table.

C

D

E

F

G

I

J

K

L

N

O

R

S

U

V

W

Y

Z